Schwartz's
MANUAL OF
SURGERY

Editor-in-Chief

F. Charles Brunicardi, MD, FACS
DeBakey/Bard Professor and Chairman
Michael E. DeBakey Department of Surgery
Baylor College of Medicine
Houston, Texas

Associate Editors

Dana K. Andersen, MD, FACS
Professor and Vice-Chair
Department of Surgery
Johns Hopkins School of Medicine
Surgeon-in-Chief
Johns Hopkins Bayview Medical Center
Baltimore, Maryland

Timothy R. Billiar, MD, FACS
George Vance Foster Professor and Chairman of Surgery
Department of Surgery
University of Pittsburgh School of Medicine
Pittsburgh, Pennsylvania

David L. Dunn, MD, PhD, FACS
Vice President for Health Sciences
University at Buffalo/SUNY
Buffalo, New York

John G. Hunter, MD, FACS
Mackenzie Professor and Chairman of Surgery
Department of Surgery
Oregon Health and Science University
Portland, Oregon

Raphael E. Pollock, MD, PhD, FACS
Head, Division of Surgery
Professor and Chairman
Department of Surgical Oncology
Senator A.M. Aiken, Jr., Distinguished Chair
The University of Texas M. D. Anderson Cancer Center
Houston, Texas

Schwartz's

MANUAL OF
SURGERY

EIGHTH EDITION

Editor-in-Chief
F. Charles Brunicardi, MD, FACS

Associate Editors
Dana K. Andersen, MD, FACS
Timothy R. Billiar, MD, FACS
David L. Dunn, MD, PhD, FACS
John G. Hunter, MD, FACS
Raphael E. Pollock, MD, PhD, FACS

McGRAW-HILL
Medical Publishing Division

New York   Chicago   San Francisco   Lisbon   London   Madrid   Mexico City
Milan   New Delhi   San Juan   Seoul   Singapore   Sydney   Toronto

The McGraw·Hill Companies

Schwartz's Manual of Surgery, Eighth Edition

1234567890   DOC/DOC   09876

ISBN 0-07-144688-5

This book was set in Times Roman by TechBooks.
The editors were Marc Strauss, Christie Naglieri, and Penny Linskey.
The production supervisor was Catherine H. Saggese.
The indexer was Pamela J. Edwards.
The cover designer was Aimee Nordin.
RR Donnelley was printer and binder.

This book was printed on acid-free paper.

Library of Congress Cataloging-in-Publication Data

Schwartz's manual of surgery / editor-in-chief, F. Charles Brunicardi ; associate
    editors, Dana K. Andersen ... [et al.]. —8th ed.
        p. ; cm.
    Rev. ed. of: Principles of surgery, seventh edition, companion handbook c1999.
    Should be used in conjunction with the 8th ed. of Schwartz's principles of
surgery.
    Includes bibliographical references and index.
    ISBN 0-07-144688-5
    1. Surgery—Handbooks, manuals, etc.   I. Title: Manual of surgery.
II. Schwartz, Seymour I., 1928.   III. Brunicardi, F. Charles.   IV. Principles of
surgery, seventh edition, companion handbook.   V. Schwartz's principles of
surgery.
    [DNLM: 1. Surgical Procedures, Operative—Handbooks. WO 39 S399 2006]
    RD37.P74 2006
    617—dc22
                                                                        2005052273

INTERNATIONAL EDITION ISBN: 0-07-110518-2
Copyright © 2006, Exclusive rights by The McGraw-Hill Companies, Inc., for
manufacture and export. This book cannot be re-exported from the country to
which it is consigned by McGraw-Hill. The International Edition is not available in
North America.

NOTICE

Medicine is an ever-changing science. As new research and clinical experience broaden our knowledge, changes in treatment and drug therapy are required. The authors and the publisher of this work have checked with sources believed to be reliable in their efforts to provide information that is complete and generally in accord with the standards accepted at the time of publication. However, in view of the possibility of human error or changes in medical sciences, neither the authors nor the publisher nor any other party who has been involved in the preparation or publication of this work warrants that the information contained herein is in every respect accurate or complete, and they disclaim all responsibility for any errors or omissions or for the results obtained from use of the information contained in this work. Readers are encouraged to confirm the information contained herein with other sources. For example and in particular, readers are advised to check the product information sheet included in the package of each drug they plan to administer to be certain that the information contained in this work is accurate and that changes have not been made in the recommended dose or in the contraindications for administration. This recommendation is of particular importance in connection with new or infrequently used drugs.

Contents

vii

PART II   SPECIFIC CONSIDERATIONS

Contributors

Hardeep S. Ahluwalia, MD
Medical Dean, Housestaff
Department of Surgery
Creighton University Medical
    Center
Omaha, Nebraska
Chapter 36: Inguinal Hernias

Louis H. Alarcon, MD
Assistant Professor
Departments of Surgery and Critical
    Care Medicine
University of Pittsburgh School of
    Medicine
Pittsburgh, Pennsylvania
*Chapter 12: Physiologic Monitoring
    of the Surgical Patient*

Dana K. Andersen, MS, FACS
Professor and Vice-Chair
Department of Surgery
Johns Hopkins School of Medicine
Surgeon-in-Chief
Johns Hopkins Bayview Medical
    Center
Baltimore, Maryland
Chapter 32: Pancreas

**Peter B. Angood, MD, FACS,
    FCCM**
Professor of Surgery Anesthesia and
    Emergency Medicine
Chief, Division of Trauma and
    Critical Care
University of Massachusetts
    Medical School and
University of Massachusetts—
    Memorial Health Care System
Worcester, Massachusetts
*Chapter 11: Patient Safety, Errors,
    and Complications in Surgery*

Stanley W. Ashley, MD
Professor and Vice Chairman

Department of Surgery
Brigham and Women's
    Hospital/Harvard Medical School
Boston, Massachusetts
Chapter 27: Small Intestine

Samir S. Awad, MD
Associate Professor of Surgery
Chief, Section of Critical Care
Michael E. DeBakey Department
    of Surgery
Baylor College of Medicine
Medical Director SICU
Michael E. DeBakey Veterans
    Affairs Medical Center
Houston, Texas
*Chapter 46: ACGME Core
    Competencies*

Adrian Barbul, MD, FACS
Surgeon-in-Chief, Sinai Hospital
    of Baltimore and
Professor and Vice-Chairman,
    Department of Surgery
Johns Hopkins Medical Institutions
Baltimore, Maryland
Chapter 8: Wound Healing

**Samuel W. Beenken, MD,
    FRCS(C), FACS**
Professor of Surgery
The University of Alabama at
    Birmingham
Birmingham, Alabama
Chapter 16: The Breast

Gregory J. Beilman, MD, FACS
Associate Professor of Surgery and
    Anesthesia
University of Minnesota Medical
    School
Minneapolis, Minnesota
Chapter 5: Surgical Infections

Richard H. Bell, Jr., MD, FACS
Loyal and Edith Davis Professor and Chair
Department of Surgery
Feinberg School of Medicine
Northwestern University
Chicago, Illinois
Chapter 32: Pancreas

Robert L. Bell, MD, MA
Assistant Professor
Department of Surgery
Yale University School of Medicine
New Haven, Connecticut
Chapter 34: Abdominal Wall, Omentum, Mesentery, and Retroperitoneum

Arie Belldegrun, MD, FACS
Roy and Carol Doumani Chair in Urologic Oncology
Professor of Urology
Chief, Division of Urologic Oncology
David Geffen School of Medicine at University of California, Los Angeles
Los Angeles, California
Chapter 39: Urology

David H. Berger, MD, FACS
Associate Professor and Vice Chair
Michael E. DeBakey Department of Surgery
Baylor College of Medicine
Operative Care Line Executive
Chief, Surgical Services
Michael E. DeBakey Veterans Affairs Medical Center
Houston, Texas
Chapter 29: The Appendix
Chapter 46: ACGME Core Competencies

Alan Bienstock, MD, BS
Resident
Division of Plastic Surgery
Michael E. DeBakey Department of Surgery
Baylor College of Medicine
Houston, Texas
Chapter 43: Plastic and Reconstructive Surgery

Timothy R. Billiar, MD
George Vance Foster
Professor and Chairman
Department of Surgery
University of Pittsburgh School of Medicine
Pittsburgh, Pennsylvania
Chapter 4: Shock

Kirby I. Bland, MD, FACS
Fay Fletcher Kerner Professor and Chairman
Deputy Director, UAB Comprehensive Cancer Center
Department of Surgery
University of Alabama at Birmingham
Birmingham, Alabama
Chapter 16: The Breast

Mary L. Brandt, MD
Chief, Colorectal Clinic and Chief, Pediatric Surgery Clinic
Texas Children's Hospital, Houston, Texas
Professor of Surgery, Michael E. DeBakey Department of Surgery
Professor of Pediatrics, Baylor College of Medicine
Houston, Texas
Chapter 46: ACGME Core Competencies

F. Charles Brunicardi, MD, FACS
DeBakey/Bard Professor and Chairman
Michael E. DeBakey Department of Surgery
Baylor College of Medicine
Houston, Texas
Chapter 14: Cell, Genomics, and Molecular Surgery
Chapter 32: Pancreas
Chapter 46: ACGME Core Competencies

Kelli M. Bullard, MD, FACS
Assistant Professor of Surgery and Laboratory Medicine and Pathology
University of Minnesota

Minneapolis, Minnesota
*Chapter 28: Colon, Rectum,
and Anus*

John M. Burch, MD
Professor of Surgery
University of Colorado Health
Sciences Center
Chief of General and Vascular
Surgery
Denver Health Medical Center
Denver, Colorado
Chapter 6: Trauma

Ruth L. Bush, MD
Assistant Professor of Surgery
Division of Vascular Surgery and
Endovascular Therapy
Michael E. DeBakey Department of
Surgery
Baylor College of Medicine
Houston, Texas
Chapter 22: Arterial Disease
*Chapter 46: ACGME Core
Competencies*

Steven E. Calvano, PhD
Associate Professor
Division of Surgical Sciences
Department of Surgery
University of Medicine and
Dentistry of New Jersey—Robert
Wood Johnson Medical School
New Brunswick, New Jersey
*Chapter 1: Systemic Response to
Injury and Metabolic Support*

Rakesh K. Chandra, MD
Assistant Professor
Director, Division of Nasal and
Sinus Disorders
Residency Program Director
Department of Otolaryngology—
Head and Neck Surgery
University of Tennessee Health
Science Center
Memphis, Tennessee
*Chapter 17: Disorders of the Head
and Neck*

Changyi Chen, MD, PhD
Professor of Surgery

Division of Vascular Surgery and
Endovascular Therapy
Michael E. DeBakey Department of
Surgery
Baylor College of Medicine
Houston, Texas
Chapter 22: Arterial Disease

Orlo H. Clark, MD
Professor of Surgery
University of California, San
Francisco/Mt. Zion Medical
Center
Department of Surgery
San Francisco, California
*Chapter 37: Thyroid, Parathyroid,
and Adrenal*

Stephen B. Colvin, MD
Chief, Cardiothoracic Surgery
New York University School of
Medicine
New York, New York
*Chapter 20: Acquired Heart
Disease*

Edward E. Copeland, III, MD
Distinguished Professor of
Surgery
University of Florida College of
Medicine
Gainesville, Florida
Chapter 16: The Breast

Janice N. Cormier, MD, MPH
Assistant Professor of Surgery
Department of Surgical Oncology
The University of Texas M. D.
Anderson Cancer Center
Houston, Texas
Chapter 35: Soft Tissue Sarcomas

Joseph C. Coselli, MD
Professor and Chief
Division of Cardiothoracic
Surgery
Michael E. DeBakey Department of
Surgery
Baylor College of Medicine
Houston, Texas
*Chapter 21: Thoracic Aortic
Aneurysms and Aortic Dissection*

Steven A. Curley, MD, FACS
Professor, Department of Surgical
  Oncology
Chief, Gastrointestinal Tumor
  Surgery
The University of Texas M.D.
  Anderson Cancer Center
Houston, Texas
Chapter 30: Liver

Tom R. DeMeester, MD
The Jeffrey P. Smith Professor of
  General and Thoracic Surgery
Chairman, Department of Surgery
Keck School of Medicine,
  University of Southern California
Los Angeles, California
*Chapter 24: Esophagus and
  Diaphragmatic Hernia*

Daniel T. Dempsey, MD, FACS
Professor and Chairman of
  Surgery
Temple University School of
  Medicine
Philadelphia, Pennsylvania
Chapter 25: Stomach

Robert S. Dorian, MD
Chairman and Program Director
Department of Anesthesiology
Saint Barnabas Medical Center
Livingston, New Jersey
*Chapter 45: Anesthesia of the
  Surgical Patient*

David L. Dunn, MD, PhD
Vice President for Health Sciences
University at Buffalo/SUNY
Buffalo, New York
Chapter 5: Surgical Infections
Chapter 10: Transplantation

Xin-Hua Feng, PhD
Associate Professor of Surgery
Division of General Surgery
Michael E. DeBakey Department of
  Surgery
Baylor College of Medicine
Houston, Texas
*Chapter 14: Cell, Genomics, and
  Molecular Surgery*

Mitchell P. Fink, MD
Professor and Chairman
Department of Critical Care
  Medicine
Watson Chair in Surgery
University of Pittsburgh
Pittsburgh, Pennsylvania
*Chapter 12: Physiologic Monitoring
  of the Surgical Patient*

William E. Fisher, MD, FACS
Associate Professor of Surgery
Michael E. DeBakey Department of
  Surgery
Baylor College of Medicine
Houston, Texas
Chapter 32: Pancreas

Robert J. Fitzgibbons, Jr., MD
Harry E. Stuckenhoff Professor of
  Surgery
Department of Surgery
Creighton University School of
  Medicine
Omaha, Nebraska
Chapter 36: Inguinal Hernias

Henri R. Ford, MD
Benjamin R. Fisher Chair
Professor and Chief
Division of Pediatric Surgery
Children's Hospital of
  Pittsburgh
University of Pittsburgh School of
  Medicine
Pittsburgh, Pennsylvania
Chapter 38: Pediatric Surgery

Reginald J. Franciose, MD
Assistant Professor of Surgery
University of Colorado Health
  Sciences Center
Attending Surgeon
Denver Health Medical Center
Denver, Colorado
Chapter 6; Trauma

Aubrey C. Galloway, MD
Professor of Surgery, Cardiothoracic
  Surgery
Director, Cardiac Surgical
  Research

New York University School of
Medicine
New York, New York
*Chapter 20: Acquired Heart
Disease*

M. Sean Grady, MD, FACS
Charles Harrison Frazier Professor
and Chairman
Department of Neurosurgery
University of Pennsylvania School
of Medicine
Philadelphia, Pennsylvania
Chapter 41: Neurosurgery

Eugene A. Grossi, MD
Professor of Surgery, Cardiothoracic
Surgery
New York University School of
Medicine
New York, New York
*Chapter 20: Acquired Heart
Disease*

David J. Hackam, MD, PhD
Assistant Professor of Surgery, Cell
Biology and Physiology
University of Pittsburgh School of
Medicine
Attending Pediatric Surgeon
Co-Director, Fetal Diagnosis and
Treatment Center
Children's Hospital of Pittsburgh
Pittsburgh, Pennsylvania
Chapter 38: Pediatric Surgery

Scott L. Hansen, MD
Resident, Plastic and Reconstructive
Surgery
University of California, San
Francisco
San Francisco, California
*Chapter 15; Skin and Subcutaneous
Tissue*

Brain G. Harbrecht, MD, FACS
Associate Professor of
Surgery
Department of Surgery
University of Pittsburgh
Pittsburgh, Pennsylvania
Chapter 4: Shock

Rosemarie E. Hardin, MD
Resident
Department of Surgery
State University of New York Health
Science Medical Center
Brooklyn, New York
*Chapter 44: Surgical
Considerations in the
Elderly*

David M. Heimbach, MD, FACS
Professor of Surgery
University of Washington Burn
Center
Harborview Medical Center
Seattle, Washington
Chapter 7: Burns

James H. Holmes, MD
Burn Fellow & Acting Instructor in
Surgery
Harborview Medical Center—
University of Washington
Seattle, Washington
Chapter 7: Burns

Abhinav Humar, MD, FRCS (Can)
Associate Professor
Department of Surgery
University of Minnesota
Minneapolis, Minnesota
Chapter 10: Transplantation

John G. Hunter, MD, FACS
Mackenzie Professor and Chairman
of Surgery
Department of Surgery
Oregon Health and Science
University
Portland, Oregon
*Chapter 13: Minimally-Invasive
Surgery*
*Chapter 31: Gallbladder and
Extrahepatic Biliary
System*

**William W. Hurd, MD, FACOG,
FACS**
Nicholas J. Thompson Professor and
Chair
Department of Obstetrics and
Gynecology

Wright State University School of
    Medicine
Dayton, Ohio
Chapter 40: Gynecology

Bernard M. Jaffe, MD
Professor of Surgery
Tulane University School of
    Medicine
New Orleans, Louisiana
Chapter 29: The Appendix

Blair A. Jobe, MD
Assistant Professor
Department of Surgery
Oregon Health and Science
    University
Portland, Oregon
*Chapter 13: Minimally-Invasive
    Surgery*

Tara B. Karamlou, MD
Senior Research Fellow
Division of Cardiothoracic Surgery
Oregon Health and Science
    University
Portland, Oregon
*Chapter 19: Congenital heart
    Disease*

Hyung L. Kim, MD
Assistant Professor
Department of Urology
Department of Cellular Stress
    Biology
Roswell Park Cancer Institute
Buffalo, New York
Chapter 39: Urology

John Y. S. Kim, MD
Assistant Professor, Division of
    Plastic Surgery
Department of Surgery
Northwestern University School of
    Medicine
Chicago, Illinois
*Chapter 43: Plastic and
    Reconstructive Surgery*

Rosemary A. Kozar, MD, PhD
Associate Professor of Surgery
University of Texas-Houston

Houston, Texas
*Chapter 2: Fluid and Electrolyte
    Management of the Surgical
    Patient*

Greeta Lal, MD
Assistant Professor of Surgery
Surgical Oncology and Endocrine
    Surgery
University of Iowa Hospital and
    Clinics
Iowa City, Iowa
*Chapter 37: Thyroid, Parathyroid,
    and Adrenal*

Scott A. LeMaire, MD
Assistant Professor
Division of Cardiothoracic Surgery
Baylor College of Medicine
The Methodist DeBakey Heart
    Center
Houston, Texas
*Chapter 21: Thoracic Aortic
    Aneurysms and Aortic
    Dissection*

Edward Lin, DO, CNSP
Assistant Professor of Surgery
Division of Gastrointestinal and
    General Surgery
Surgical Metabolism Laboratory
Emory University School of
    Medicine
Atlanta, Georgia
*Chapter 1: Systemic Response to
    Injury and Metabolic Support*

Peter H. Lin, MD
Associate Professor of Surgery
Division of Vascular Surgery and
    Endovascular Therapy
Michael E. DeBakey Department of
    Surgery
Baylor College of Medicine
Houston, Texas
Chapter 22: Arterial Disease

Xia Lin, PhD
Assistant Professor of Surgery
Division of General Surgery
Michael E. DeBakey Department of
    Surgery

Baylor College of Medicine
Houston, Texas
Chapter 14: Cell, Genomics, and Molecular Surgery

Steven F. Lowry, MD, FACS
Professor and Chairman
Department of Surgery
UMDNJ - Robert Wood Johnson Medical School
New Brunswick, New Jersey
Chapter 1: Systemic Response to Injury and Metabolic Support

James D. Luketich, MD
Professor and Chief, Division of Thoracic and Foregut Surgery
University of Pittsburgh Medical Center
Pittsburgh, Pennsylvania
Chapter 18: Chest Wall, Lung, Mediastinum, and Pleura

Alan B. Lumsden, MD
Professor of Surgery
Division of Vascular Surgery and Endovascular Therapy
Michael E. DeBakey Department of Surgery
Baylor College of Medicine
Houston, Texas
Chapter 22: Arterial Disease

Michael A. Maddaus, MD, FACS
Professor and Head, Section of General Thoracic Surgery
Garamella-Lynch-Jensen Chair in Thoracic and Cardiovascular Surgery
Co-Director, Minimally Invasive Surgery Center
University of Minnesota
Minneapolis, Minnesota
Chapter 18: Chest Wall, Lung, Mediastinum, and Pleura

Stephen J. Mathes, MD
Professor of Surgery
Chief, Division of Plastic and Reconstructive Surgery

University of California, San Francisco
San Francisco, California
Chapter 15: Skin and Subcutaneous Tissue

Jeffrey B. Matthews, MD, FACS
Christian R. Holmes Professor and Chairman
Department of Surgery
University of Cincinnati
Cincinnati, Ohio
Chapter 14: Cell, Genomics, and Molecular Surgery

Rodrick McKinlay, MD
Gastrointestinal and Minimally Invasive Surgery
Rocky Mountain Associated Physicians
Salt Lake City, Utah
Chapter 33: Spleen

Funda Meric-Bernstam, MD, FACS
Assistant Professor
Department of Surgical Oncology
University of Texas M. D. Anderson Cancer Center
Houston, Texas
Chapter 9: Oncology

Gregory L. Moneta, MD
Professor and Chief Vascular Surgery
Oregon Health and Science University
Portland, Oregon
Chapter 23: Venous and Lymphatic Disease

Ernest E. Moore, MD, FACS
Professor and Vice Chairman, Department of Surgery
University of Colorado Health Sciences Center
Chief of Surgery and Trauma Services
Denver Health Medical Center
Denver, Colorado
Chapter 6: Trauma

Frederick A. Moore, MD
James H. "Red" Duke, Jr. Professor & Vice Chairman
Department of Surgery
The University of Texas Houston Medical School
Houston, Texas
Chapter 2: Fluid and Electrolyte Management of the Surgical Patient

Martina F. Mutone, MD
Clinical Assistant Professor
Indiana University/Methodist Hospital
St. Vincent Hospitals and Health Services
Indianapolis, Indiana
Chapter 40: Gynecology

Kurt Newman, MD, FACS
Executive Director and Surgeon in Chief
Joseph E. Robert, Jr. Center for Surgical Care
Children's National Medical Center
Professor of Surgery and Pediatrics
George Washington University School of Medicine
Washington, D.C.
Chapter 38: Pediatric Surgery

Liz Nguyen, MD
Surgery Resident
Baylor College of Medicine
Houston, Texas
Chapter 46: ACGME Core Competencies

Margrét Oddsdóttir, MD
Professor of Surgery
Chief of General Surgery
Landspitali–University Hospital
Hringbraut
Reykjavik, Iceland
Chapter 31: Gallbladder and the Extrahepatic Biliary System

Adrian E. Park, MD, FRCS(C), FACS
Campbell and Jeanette Plugge Professor of Surgery
Chief, Division of General Surgery, Department of Surgery, University of Maryland Medical Center
Baltimore, Maryland
Chapter 33: Spleen

Andre B. Peitzman, MD, FACS
Professor and Vice-Chairman, Department of Surgery
University of Pittsburgh Medical Center
Pittsburgh, Pennsylvania
Chapter 4: Shock

J. Martin Perez MD
Assistant Professor of Surgery
Trauma and Surgical Critical Care
University of Medicine and Dentistry of New Jersey
New Brunswick, New Jersey
Chapter 1: Systemic Response to Injury and Metabolic Support

Jeffrey H. Peters, MD, FACS
Seymour I. Schwartz Professor and Chairman
University of Rochester School of Medicine and Dentistry
Surgeon-in-Chief Strong Memorial Hospital
Department of Surgery
Rochester, New York
Chapter 24; Esophagus and Diaphragmatic Hernia

Raphael E. Pollock, MD, PhD, FACS
Head, Division of Surgery
Professor and Chairman
Department of Surgical Oncology
Senator A.M. Aiken, Jr., Distinguished Chair
The University of Texas M. D. Anderson Cancer Center
Houston, Texas
Chapter 9: Oncology
Chapter 35: Soft Tissue Sarcomas

Robert E. Rogers, MD
Emeritus Professor, Obstetrics and
    Gynecology
Indiana University School of
    Medicine
Indianapolis, Indiana
Chapter 40: Gynecology

Forrest S. Roth, MD
Fellow in Plastic Reconstructive and
    Microsurgery
Division of Plastic and
    Reconstructive Surgery
Michael E. DeBakey Department of
    Surgery
Baylor College of Medicine
Houston, Texas
*Chapter 43: Plastic and
    Reconstructive Surgery*

David A. Rothenberger, MD
Professor of Surgery
Chief, Divisions of Colon and Rectal
    Surgery and Surgical Oncology
Department of Surgery
University of Minnesota
Minneapolis, Minnesota
*Chapter 28: Colon, Rectum, and
    Anus*

Ashok K. Saluja, PhD
Professor of Surgery, Medicine, and
    Cell Biology
University of Massachusetts
    Medical School
Worcester, Massachusetts
Chapter 32: Pancreas

Paul C. Saunders, MD
Fellow
Division of Cardiothoracic Surgery
New York University School of
    Medicine
New York, New York
*Chapter 20: Acquired Heart
    Disease*

Philip R. Schauer, MD
Associate Professor of Surgery
Director of Bariatric Surgery
Chief, Minimally Invasive General
    Surgery
The University of Pittsburgh
Pittsburgh, Pennsylvania
*Chapter 26: The Surgical
    Management of Obesity*

Bruce D. Schirmer, MD, FACS
Stephen H. Watts Professor of
    Surgery
University of Virginia Health
    System
Charlottesville, Virginia
*Chapter 26: The Surgical
    Management of Obesity*

Charles F. Schwartz, MD
Assistant Professor of Surgery
Division of Cardiothoracic Surgery
New York University School of
    Medicine
New York, New York
Chapter 20: Acquired Heart Disease

Seymour I. Schwartz, MD, FACS
Distinguished Alumni Professor of
    Surgery
University of Rochester School of
    Medicine and Dentistry
Rochester, New York
*Chapter 3: Hemostasis, Surgical
    Bleeding, and Transfusion*

Neal E. Seymour, MD, FACS
Associate Professor Tufts University
    School of Medicine
Vice Chairman Department of
    Surgery
Baystate Medical Center
Springfield, Massachusetts
*Chapter 34: Abdominal Wall,
    Omentum, Mesentery, and
    Retroperitoneum*

Mark L. Shapiro, MD
Assistant Professor of Surgery
Department of Surgery
Division of Trauma and Critical Care
University of Massachusetts
    Medical School
Worcester, Massachusetts
*Chapter 11: Patient Safety, Errors,
    and Complications in Surgery*

Ram Sharony, MD
Minimally Invasive Cardiac Surgery Fellow
Division of Cardiothoracic Surgery
New York University Medical Center
New York, New York
Chapter 20: Acquired Heart Disease

Irving Shen, MD
Assistant Professor of Surgery
Division of Cardiothoracic Surgery
Oregon Health and Science University
Portland, Oregon
Chapter 19: Congenital Heart Disease

Saleh M. Shenaq, MD
Chief, Division of Plastic Surgery
Professor of Surgery
Michael E. DeBakey Department of Surgery
Baylor College of Medicine
Houston, Texas
Chapter 43: Plastic and Reconstructive Surgery

Timothy D. Sielaff, MD, PhD, FACS
Associate Professor
Department of Surgery
University of Minnesota
Minneapolis, Minnesota
Chapter 30: Liver

Michael L. Smith, MD
Resident
Department of Neurosurgery
University of Pennsylvania School of Medicine
Philadelphia, Pennsylvania
Chapter 41: Neurosurgery

Dempsey Springfield, MD
Professor and Chairman
Department of Orthopaedics
The Mount Sinai School of Medicine
New York, New York
Chapter 42: Orthopedics

Gregory P. Sutton, MD
Director, Gynecologic Oncology
St. Vincent Oncology Center
St. Vincent Hospitals and Health Services
Indianapolis, Indiana
Chapter 40: Gynecology

Ross M. Ungerleider, MD
Professor of Surgery
Chief, Division of Cardiothoracic Surgery
Oregon Health and Science University
Portland, Oregon
Chapter 19: Congenital Heart Disease

Randal S. Weber, MD, FACS
Hubert L. and Olive Stringer, Distinguished Professor and Chairman
Department of Head and Neck Surgery
University of Texas M.D. Anderson Cancer Center
Houston, Texas
Chapter 17: Disorders of the Head and Neck

Richard O. Wein, MD
Assistant Professor
Department of Otolaryngology and Communicative Sciences
University of Mississippi Medical Center
Jackson, Mississippi
Chapter 17: Disorders of the Head and Neck

Edward E. Whang, MD
Assistant Professor of Surgery
Brigham and Women's Hospital
Harvard Medical School
Boston, Massachusetts
Chapter 27: Small Intestine

David M. Young, MD, FACS
Associate Professor of Plastic Surgery
Department of Surgery

University of California, San
  Francisco
San Francisco, California
*Chapter 15: Skin and Subcutaneous
  Tissue*

Eser Yuksel, MD
Assistant Professor Plastic
  Surgery
Division of Plastic Surgery
Baylor College of Medicine
Adjunct Assistant Professor
Department of Bioengineering
Rice University
ONEP Plastic Surgery Institute,
  Istanbul
*Chapter 43: Plastic and
  Reconstructive Surgery*

Michael E. Zenilman, MD
Clarence and Mary Dennis Professor
  and Chairman
Department of Surgery
State University of New York
  Downstate Medical Center
Brooklyn, New York
*Chapter 44: Surgical
  Considerations in the Elderly*

Michael J. Zinner, MD
Moseley Professor of Surgery
Harvard Medical School
Surgeon-in-Chief and Chairman
Department of Surgery
Brigham and Women's Hospital
Boston, Massachusetts
Chapter 27: Small Intestine

Preface

This manual, crafted for easy portability and convenient reference by surgical students and house officers, is intended as a supplement to the eighth edition of *Schwartz's Principles of Surgery*. These condensed chapters, edited by their original authors, provide a concise synopsis of each chapter and are meant as a companion to the main text. I am grateful for the efforts of all whom contributed and their willingness and dedication to further the education of students of surgery.

I also express my deep appreciation to Katie Elsbury, who worked with the contributors, the publisher, and with me in every step of the production of this book.

F. Charles Brunicardi, MD, FACS
Editor-in-Chief

PART I | BASIC CONSIDERATIONS

1 | Systemic Response to Injury and Metabolic Support

J. Martin Perez, Edward Lim, Steven E. Calvano,
and Stephen F. Lowry

The inflammatory response to injury is designed to restore tissue function and eradicate invading microorganisms. Injuries of limited duration are usually followed by functional restoration with minimal intervention. By contrast, major insults to the host are associated with an overwhelming inflammatory response that, without appropriate and timely intervention, can lead to multiple-organ failure and adversely impact patient survival. Therefore, understanding how the inflammatory response is mobilized and controlled provides a functional framework on which interventions and therapeutics are formulated for the surgical patient.

This chapter addresses the hormonal, immunologic, and cellular responses to injury. Alterations of metabolism and nutrition in injury states are discussed in continuum because the utilization of fuel substrates during injury also is subject to the influences of hormonal and inflammatory mediators.

THE SYSTEMIC INFLAMMATORY RESPONSE SYNDROME

The systemic response to injury can be broadly compartmentalized into two phases: (1) a proinflammatory phase characterized by activation of cellular processes designed to restore tissue function and eradicate invading microorganisms, and (2) an antiinflammatory (*counterregulatory* phase) that is important for preventing excessive proinflammatory activities and restoring homeostasis in the individual (Table 1-1).

CENTRAL NERVOUS SYSTEM REGULATION OF INFLAMMATION

Reflex Inhibition of Inflammation

The central nervous system (CNS), via autonomic signaling, has an integral role in regulating the inflammatory response that is primarily involuntary. The autonomic system regulates heart rate, blood pressure, respiratory rate, gastrointestinal (GI) motility, and body temperature. The autonomic nervous system also regulates inflammation in a reflex manner, much like the patellar tendon reflex. The site of inflammation sends afferent signals to the hypothalamus, which in turn rapidly relays opposing antiinflammatory messages to reduce inflammatory mediator release by immunocytes.

Afferent Signals to the Brain

The CNS receives immunologic input from both the circulation and neural pathways. Areas of the CNS devoid of blood–brain barrier admit the passage of inflammatory mediators such as tumor necrosis factor (TNF)-α. Fevers, anorexia, and depression in illness are attributed to the humoral (circulatory) route of inflammatory signaling. Although the mechanism for vagal sensory input is not fully understood, it has been demonstrated that afferent stimuli

3

	Definition
	...ble source of microbial insult
	...more of following criteria
	...mperature $\geq 38°C$ or $\leq 36°C$
	...eart rate ≥ 90 beats/min
	...espiratory rate ≥ 20 breaths/min or
	...aco_2 ≤ 32 mm Hg or mechanical
	...ventilation
	White blood cell count $\geq 12,000/\mu L$ or $\leq 4000/\mu L$ or $\geq 10\%$ band forms
Sepsis	Identifiable source of infection + SIRS
Severe sepsis	Sepsis + organ dysfunction
Septic shock	Sepsis + cardiovascular collapse (requiring vasopressor support)

to the vagus nerve include cytokines (e.g., TNF-α and interleukin [IL]-1), baroreceptors, chemoreceptors, and thermoreceptors originating from the site of injury.

Cholinergic Antiinflammatory Pathways

Acetylcholine, the primary neurotransmitter of the parasympathetic system, reduces tissue macrophage activation. Furthermore, cholinergic stimulation directly reduces tissue macrophage release of the proinflammatory mediators TNF-α, IL-1, IL-18, and high mobility group protein (HMG-1), but not the antiinflammatory cytokine IL-10. The attenuated inflammatory response induced by cholinergic stimuli was further validated by the identification of acetylcholine (nicotinic) receptors on tissue macrophages.

In summary, vagal stimulation reduces heart rate, increases gut motility, dilates arterioles, and causes pupil constriction, and regulates inflammation. Unlike the humoral antiinflammatory mediators, signals discharged from the vagus nerve are targeted at the site of injury or infection. Moreover, this cholinergic signaling occurs rapidly in real time.

HORMONAL RESPONSE TO INJURY

Hormone Signaling Pathways

Hormones are chemically classified as *polypeptides* (e.g., cytokines, glucagon, and insulin), *amino acids* (e.g., epinephrine, serotonin, and histamine), or *fatty acids* (e.g., glucocorticoids, prostaglandins, and leukotrienes [LT]). Most hormone receptors generate signals by one of three major overlapping pathways: (1) *receptor kinases* such as insulin and insulin-like growth factor receptors, (2) *guanine nucleotide-binding* or *G-protein receptors* such as neurotransmitter and prostaglandin receptors, (3) *ligand-gated ion channels,* which permit ion transport when activated. Membrane receptor activation leads to amplification via secondary signaling pathways. Hormone signals are further mediated by intracellular receptors with binding affinities for both the hormone itself, and for the targeted gene sequence on the deoxyribonucleic acid (DNA). The classic example of a cytosolic hormonal receptor is the glucocorticoid (GC) receptor.

TABLE 1-2 Hormones Regulated by the Hypothalamus, Pituitary, and Autonomic System

Hypothalamic Regulation
Corticotropin-releasing hormone
Thyrotropin-releasing hormone
Growth hormone-releasing hormone
Luteinizing hormone-releasing hormone

Anterior Pituitary Regulation
Adrenocorticotropic hormone
Cortisol
Thyroid-stimulating hormone
Thyroxine
Triiodothyronine
Growth hormone
Gonadotrophins
Sex hormones
Insulin-like growth factor
Somatostatin
Prolactin
Endorphins

Posterior Pituitary Regulation
Vasopressin
Oxytocin

Autonomic System
Norepinephrine
Epinephrine
Aldosterone
Renin-angiotensin system
Insulin
Glucagon
Enkephalins

Hormones of the hypothalamic-pituitary-adrenal (HPA) axis influences the physiologic response to injury and stress (Table 1-2), but some with direct influence on the inflammatory response or immediate clinical impact will be highlighted.

Adrenocorticotropic Hormone

Adrenocorticotropic hormone (ACTH) is synthesized and released by the anterior pituitary. In healthy humans, ACTH release is regulated by circadian signals with high levels of ACTH occurring late at night until the hours immediately before sunrise. During injury, this pattern is dramatically altered. Elevations in corticotropin-releasing hormone and ACTH are typically proportional to the severity of injury. Pain, anxiety, vasopressin, angiotensin II, cholecystokinin, vasoactive intestinal polypeptide (VIP), catecholamines, and proinflammatory cytokines are all prominent mediators of ACTH release in the injured patient.

Cortisol and Glucocorticoids

Cortisol is the major glucocorticoid in humans and is essential for survival during significant physiologic stress. Following injury, the degree of cortisol elevation is dependent on the degree of systemic stress. For example, burn patients have elevated circulating cortisol levels for up to 4 weeks, whereas lesser injuries may exhibit shorter periods of cortisol elevation.

Cortisol potentiates the actions of glucagon and epinephrine that manifest as hyperglycemia. Cortisol stimulates gluconeogenesis, but induces insulin resistance in muscles and adipose tissue. In skeletal muscle, cortisol induces protein degradation and the release of lactate that serve as substrates for hepatic gluconeogenesis. During injury, cortisol potentiates the release of free fatty acids, triglycerides, and glycerol from adipose tissue providing additional energy sources.

Acute adrenal insufficiency (AAI) secondary to exogenous glucocorticoid administration can be a life-threatening complication most commonly seen in acutely ill patients. These patients present with weakness, nausea, vomiting, fever, and hypotension. Objective findings include hypoglycemia from decreased gluconeogenesis, hyponatremia, and hyperkalemia. Insufficient mineralocorticoid (aldosterone) activity also contributes to hyponatremia and hyperkalemia.

Glucocorticoids have long been employed as immunosuppressive agents. Immunologic changes associated with glucocorticoid administration include thymic involution, depressed cell-mediated immune responses reflected by decreases in T-killer and natural killer cell functions, T-lymphocyte blastogenesis, mixed lymphocyte responsiveness, graft-versus-host reactions, and delayed hypersensitivity responses. With glucocorticoid administration, monocytes lose the capacity for intracellular killing but appear to maintain normal chemotactic and phagocytic properties. For neutrophils, glucocorticoids inhibit intracellular superoxide reactivity, suppress chemotaxis, and normalize apoptosis signaling mechanisms. However, neutrophil phagocytosis function remains unchanged. Clinically, glucocorticoids has been associated with modest reductions in proinflammatory response in septic shock, surgical trauma, and coronary artery bypass surgery. However, the appropriate dosing, timing, and duration of glucocorticoid administration have not been validated.

Macrophage Inhibitory Factor

Macrophage inhibitory factor (MIF) is a glucocorticoid antagonist produced by the anterior pituitary that potentially reverses the immunosuppressive effects of glucocorticoids. MIF can be secreted systemically from the anterior pituitary and by T lymphocytes situated at the sites of inflammation. MIF is a proinflammatory mediator that potentiates gram-negative and gram-positive septic shock.

Growth Hormones and Insulin-Like Growth Factors

During periods of stress, growth hormone (GH), mediated in part by the secondary release of insulin-like growth factor-1 (IGF-1), promotes protein synthesis and enhances the mobilization of fat stores. IGF, formerly called somatomedin C, circulates predominantly in bound form and promotes amino acid incorporation, cellular proliferation, skeletal growth, and attenuates proteolysis. In the liver, IGFs are mediators of protein synthesis and glycogenesis. In adipose tissue, IGF increases glucose uptake and fat utilization. In skeletal muscles, IGF increases glucose uptake and protein synthesis. The decrease in protein synthesis and observed negative nitrogen balance following injury is attributed in part to a reduction in IGF-1 levels. GH administration has improved the clinical course of pediatric burn patients. Its use in injured adult patients remains unproven.

Catecholamines

The hypermetabolic state observed following severe injury is attributed to activation of the adrenergic system. Norepinephrine (NE) and epinephrine (EPI) are increased 3- to 4-fold in plasma immediately following injury, with elevations lasting 24–48 hours before returning toward baseline levels.

In the liver, EPI promotes glycogenolysis, gluconeogenesis, lipolysis, and ketogenesis. It also causes decreased insulin release, but increases glucagon secretion. Peripherally, EPI increases lipolysis in adipose tissues and induces insulin resistance in skeletal muscle. These collectively manifest as stress-induced hyperglycemia, not unlike the effects of cortisol on blood sugar.

Like cortisol, EPI enhances leukocyte demargination with resultant neutrophilia and lymphocytosis. However, EPI occupation of β receptors present on leukocytes ultimately decreases lymphocyte responsiveness to mitogens.

In noncardiac surgical patients with heart disease, perioperative β-receptor blockade also reduced sympathetic activation and cardiac oxygen demand with significant reductions in cardiac-related deaths.

Aldosterone

The mineralocorticoid aldosterone is synthesized, stored, and released, via ACTH stimulation, in the adrenal zona glomerulosa. The major function of aldosterone is to maintain intravascular volume by conserving sodium and eliminating potassium and hydrogen ions in the early distal convoluted tubules of the nephrons.

Patients with aldosterone deficiency develop hypotension and hyperkalemia, whereas patients with aldosterone excess develop edema, hypertension, hypokalemia, and metabolic alkalosis.

Insulin

Hormones and inflammatory mediators associated with stress response inhibit insulin release. In conjunction with peripheral insulin resistance following injury, this results in stress-induced hyperglycemia and is in keeping with the general catabolic state immediately following major injury.

In the healthy individual, insulin exerts a global anabolic effect by promoting hepatic glycogenesis and glycolysis, glucose transport into cells, adipose tissue lipogenesis, and protein synthesis. During injury, insulin release is initially suppressed followed by normal or excessive insulin production despite hyperglycemia.

Activated lymphocytes express insulin receptors, and activation enhances T-cell proliferation and cytotoxicity. Tight control of glucose levels in the critically ill has been associated with significant reductions in morbidity and mortality.

Acute Phase Proteins

The acute phase proteins are nonspecific biochemical markers produced by hepatocytes in response to tissue injury, infection, or inflammation. IL-6 is a potent inducer of acute phase proteins that can include proteinase inhibitors, coagulation and complement proteins, and transport proteins. Only C-reactive protein (CRP) has been consistently used as a marker of injury response because of its dynamic reflection of inflammation. The accuracy of CRP appears to surpass that of the erythrocyte sedimentation rate.

MEDIATORS OF INFLAMMATION

Cytokines

Cytokines are the most potent mediators of the inflammatory response. When functioning locally at the site of injury or infection, cytokines eradicate invading microorganisms and promote wound healing. Overwhelming production of proinflammatory cytokines in response to injury can cause hemodynamic instability (e.g., septic shock) or metabolic derangements (e.g., muscle wasting). If uncontrolled, the outcome of these exaggerated responses is end-organ failure and death. The production of antiinflammatory cytokines serves to oppose the actions of proinflammatory cytokines. To view cytokines merely as proinflammatory or antiinflammatory oversimplifies their functions, and overlapping bioactivity is the rule (Table 1-3).

Heat Shock Proteins

Hypoxia, trauma, heavy metals, local trauma, and hemorrhage all induce the production of intracellular heat shock proteins (HSPs). HSPs are intracellular protein modifiers and transporters that are presumed to protect cells from the deleterious effects of traumatic stress. The formation of HSPs requires gene induction by the heat shock transcription factor.

Reactive Oxygen Metabolites

Reactive oxygen metabolites are short-lived, highly reactive molecular oxygen species with an unpaired outer orbit. Tissue injury is caused by oxidation of unsaturated fatty acids within cell membranes. Activated leukocytes are potent generators of reactive oxygen metabolites. Furthermore, ischemia with reperfusion also generates reactive oxygen metabolites.

Oxygen radicals are produced by complex processes that involve anaerobic glucose oxidation coupled with the reduction of oxygen to superoxide anion. Superoxide anion is an oxygen metabolite that is further metabolized to other reactive species such as hydrogen peroxide and hydroxyl radicals. Cells are generally protected by oxygen scavengers that include glutathione and catalases.

Eicosanoids

The eicosanoid class of mediators, which encompasses prostaglandins (PGs), thromboxanes (TXs), LTs, hydroxy-icosatetraenoic acids (HETEs), and lipoxins (LXs), are oxidation derivatives of the membrane phospholipid arachidonic acid (eicosatetraenoic acid). Eicosanoids are secreted by virtually all nucleated cells except lymphocytes. Products of the cyclooxygenase pathway include all of the prostaglandins and thromboxanes. The lipoxygenase pathway generates the LT and HETE.

Eicosanoids are synthesized rapidly on stimulation by hypoxic injury, direct tissue injury, endotoxin, NE, vasopressin, angiotensin II, bradykinin, serotonin, acetylcholine, cytokines, and histamine. COX-2, a second cyclooxygenase enzyme, converts arachidonate to prostaglandin E_2 (PGE_2). PGE_2 increases

TABLE 1-3 Cytokines and Their Sources

Cytokine	Source	Comment
TNF-α	*Macrophages/monocytes* Kupffer cells Neutrophils NK cells Astrocytes Endothelial cells T lymphocytes Adrenal cortical cells Adipocytes Keratinocytes Osteoblasts Mast cells Dendritic cells	Among earliest responders following injury; half-life <20 min; activates TNF-receptor-1 and -2; induces significant shock and catabolism
IL-1	*Macrophages/monocytes* B and T lymphocytes NK cells Endothelial cells Epithelial cells Keratinocytes Fibroblasts Osteoblasts Dendritic cells Astrocytes Adrenal cortical cells Megakaryocytes Platelets Neutrophils Neuronal cells	Two forms (IL-α and IB-β); similar physiologic effects as TNF-α; induces fevers through prostaglandin activity in anterior hypothalamus; promotes β-endorphin release from pituitary; half-life <6 min
IL-2	*T lymphocytes*	Promotes lymphocyte proliferation, immunoglobulin production, gut barrier integrity; half-life <10 min; attenuated production following major blood loss leads to immunocompromise; regulates lymphocyte apoptosis
IL-3	*T lymphocytes* Macrophages Eosinophils Mast cells	
IL-4	*T lymphocytes* Mast cells Basophils Macrophages B lymphocytes Eosinophils Stromal cells	Induces B-lymphocyte production of IgG4 and IgE, mediators of allergic and anthelmintic response; downregulates TNF-α, IL-1, IL-6, IL-8
IL-5	*T lymphocytes* Eosinophils Mast cells Basophils	Promotes eosinophil proliferation and airway inflammation
IL-6	*Macrophages* B lymphocytes Neutrophils Basophils Mast cells Fibroblasts	Elicited by virtually all immunogenic cells; long half-life; circulating levels proportional to injury severity; prolongs activated neutrophil survival

(*continued*)

TABLE 1-3 *Continued*

Cytokine	Source	Comment
	Endothelial cells Astrocytes Synovial cells Adipocytes Osteoblasts Megakaryocytes Chromaffin cells Keratinocytes	
IL-8	*Macrophages/monocytes* T lymphocytes Basophils Mast cells Epithelial cells Platelets	Chemoattractant for neutrophils, basophils, eosinophils, lymphocytes
IL-10	*T lymphocytes* B lymphocytes Macrophages Basophils Mast cells Keratinocytes	Prominent anti-inflammatory cytokine; reduces mortality in animal sepsis and ARDS models
IL-12	*Macrophages/monocytes* Neutrophils Keratinocytes Dendritic cells B lymphocytes	Promotes T_H1 differentiation; synergistic activity with IL-2
IL-13	*T lymphocytes*	Promotes B-lymphocyte function; structurally similar to IL-4; inhibits nitric oxide and endothelial activation
IL-15	*Macrophages/monocytes* Epithelial cells	Anti-inflammatory effect; promotes lymphocyte activation; promotes neutrophil phagocytosis in fungal infections
IL-18	*Macrophages* Kupffer cells Keratinocytes Adrenal cortical cells Osteoblasts	Similar to IL-12 in function; elevated in sepsis, particularly gram-positive infections; high levels found in cardiac deaths
IFN-γ	*T lymphocytes* NK cells Macrophages	Mediates IL-12 and IL-18 function; half-life, days; found in wounds 5–7 days after injury; promotes ARDS
GM-CSF	*T lymphocytes* Fibroblasts Endothelial cells Stromal cells	Promotes wound healing and inflammation through activation of leukocytes
IL-21	*T lymphocytes*	Preferentially secreted by T_H2 cells; structurally similar to IL-2 and IL-15; activates NK cells, B and T lymphocytes; influences adaptive immunity
HMGB-I	*Monocytes/lymphocytes*	High mobility group box chromosomal protein; DNA transcription factor; late (downstream) mediator of inflammation (ARDS, gut barrier disruption); induces "sickness behavior"

ARDS = acute respiratory distress syndrome; GM-CSF = granulocyte-macrophage colony-stimulating factor; IFN = interferon; IgE = immunoglobulin E; IgG = immunoglobulin G; IL = interleukin; NK = natural killer; T_H1 = T helper subset cell 1; T_H2 = T helper subset cell 2; TNF = tumor necrosis factor.

fluid leakage from blood vessels, but a rising PGE_2 level over several hours eventually feeds back to COX-2 and induces the formation of the antiinflammatory lipoxin from neutrophils. Nonsteroidal antiinflammatory drugs (NSAIDs) reduce the PGE_2 levels by COX-2 acetylation and increases lipoxin production. COX-2 activity also can be inhibited by glucocorticoids.

Eicosanoids have diverse effects systemically on endocrine and immune function, neurotransmission, and vasomotor regulation Eicosanoids are implicated in acute lung injury, pancreatitis, and renal failure. LT are effective promoters of leukocyte adherence, neutrophil activation, bronchoconstriction, and vasoconstriction.

Eicosanoids are involved in the regulation of glucose, with the products of the cyclooxygenase pathway inhibiting pancreatic β-cell release of insulin, whereas products of the lipoxygenase pathway promote β-cell activity. Hepatocyte PGE_2 receptors, when activated, inhibit gluconeogenesis. PGE_2 also can inhibit hormone-stimulated lipolysis.

Fatty Acid Metabolites

Fatty acid metabolism potentially has a role in the inflammatory response. Omega-6 fatty acids, most commonly the primary lipid source in enteral nutrition formulas, also serve as precursors of inflammatory mediators, such as the eicosanoids, and are associated with injury and the stress response. Animal studies substituting omega-3 for omega-6 fatty acids have demonstrated attenuated inflammatory response in hepatic Kupffer cells as measured by TNF and IL-1 release and PGE_2 production.

Kallikrein-Kinin System

Bradykinins are potent vasodilators that are produced through kininogen degradation by the serine protease kallikrein. Kinins increase capillary permeability and tissue edema, evoke pain, inhibit gluconeogenesis, and increase bronchoconstriction. An increase in renin secondary to reduced renal perfusion promotes sodium and water retention via the renin-angiotensin system.

Increased bradykinin levels are observed following hypoxia, reperfusion, hemorrhage, sepsis, endotoxemia, and tissue injury. These elevations are proportional to the magnitude of injury and mortality. Clinically, bradykinin antagonists in septic shock studies have only demonstrated modest reversal in gram-negative sepsis, but no overall improvement in survival.

Serotonin

The neurotransmitter serotonin (5-hydroxytryptamine, 5-HT) is a tryptophan derivative that is found in chromaffin cells of the intestine and in platelets. Serotonin stimulates vasoconstriction, bronchoconstriction, and platelet aggregation. Although serotonin is clearly released at sites of injury, its role in the inflammatory response is unclear.

Histamine

Histamine is derived from histidine and stored in neurons, skin, gastric mucosa, mast cells, basophils, and platelets. There are two receptor types (H_1 and H_2) for histamine binding. H_1 receptor binding stimulates bronchoconstriction, intestinal motility, and myocardial contractility. H_2 receptor binding inhibits histamine release. Both H_1 and H_2 receptor activation induce hypotension, peripheral pooling of blood, increased capillary permeability, decreased venous return, and myocardial failure. The rise in histamine levels has been documented in hemorrhagic shock, trauma, thermal injury, endotoxemia, and sepsis.

CYTOKINE RESPONSE TO INJURY

Tumor Necrosis Factor

TNF-α is among the earliest and most potent mediators of the inflammatory host responses. TNF-α synthesis occurs in monocytes/macrophages and T cells, which are abundant in the peritoneum, splanchnic tissues, and liver (Kupffer cells). Although the half-life of TNF-α is less than 20 minutes, this is sufficient to evoke marked muscle catabolism and cachexia during stress, hemodynamic changes, and activate mediators distally in the cytokine cascade. TNF-α also promotes coagulation activation, the expression or release of adhesion molecules, prostaglandin E_2, platelet-activating factor (PAF), glucocorticoids, and eicosanoids.

Soluble TNF receptors (sTNFRs) are proteolytically cleaved extracellular domains of membrane-associated TNFRs that are elevated and readily detectable in acute inflammation. sTNFRs retain their affinity for the binding of TNF-α and therefore compete with the cellular receptors for the binding of free TNF-α. This may represent a counterregulatory response to excessive systemic TNF-α activity or serve as a carrier of bioactive TNF-α.

Interleukin-1

IL-1 (IL-1α and IL-1β) is primarily released by activated macrophages and endothelial cells. IL-1α is predominantly cell membrane–associated and exerts its influence via cellular contacts. IL-1β is more readily detectable in the circulation and is similar in its effects to TNF-α. High doses of either IL-1 or TNF-α initiate a state of hemodynamic decompensation. At low doses, they can produce the same response only if administered simultaneously. TNF-α and IL-1 appear to have synergy in the inflammatory response. IL-1 is predominantly a local mediator with a half-life of approximately 6 minutes. IL-1 induces the febrile response to injury by stimulating local prostaglandin activity in the anterior hypothalamus.

Endogenous IL-1 receptor antagonists (IL-1ra) also are released during injury and serve as an endogenous auto-regulator of IL-1 activity.

Interleukin-2

IL-2 is a primary promoter of T-lymphocyte proliferation, immunoglobulin production, and gut barrier integrity. Partly because of its circulation half-life of less than 10 minutes, IL-2 has not been readily detectable following acute injury. Attenuated IL-2 expression associated with major injuries or perioperative blood transfusions potentially contribute to the transient immunocompromised state of the surgical patient.

Interleukin-4

IL-4 is produced by activated type 2 T-helper (T_H2) lymphocytes and is particularly important in antibody-mediated immunity and in antigen presentation. IL-4 also induces class switching in differentiating B lymphocytes to produce predominantly IgG_4 and IgE, which are important immunoglobulins in allergic and anthelmintic responses. IL-4 has potent antiinflammatory properties against activated macrophages by downregulating the effects of IL-1, TNF-α, IL-6, and IL-8, and oxygen radical production. IL-4 also appears to increase macrophage susceptibility to the antiinflammatory effects of glucocorticoids.

Interleukin-6

TNF-α and IL-1 are potent inducers of IL-6 production from virtually all cells and tissues, including the gut. Circulating IL-6 levels appear to be proportional to the extent of tissue injury during an operation, more so than the duration of the surgical procedure itself. Recent evidence has demonstrated both a proinflammatory role and an antiinflammatory role for IL-6. IL-6 is an important mediator of the hepatic acute phase response during injury and convalescence, induces neutrophils activation, and paradoxically delays the disposal of activated neutrophils.

Interleukin-8

IL-8 is a chemoattractant and a potent activator of neutrophils. Expression and activity is similar to that of IL-6 after injury and has been proposed as an additional biomarker for the risk of multiple-organ failure. IL-8 does not produce the hemodynamic instability characteristic of TNF-α and IL-1.

Interleukin-10

IL-10 has emerged as a modulator of TNF-α activity. Experimental evidence has demonstrated that neutralization of IL-10 during endotoxemia increases monocyte TNF-α production and mortality, but restitution of IL-10 reduces TNF-α levels and the associated deleterious effects.

Interferon-γ

Human T-helper lymphocytes activated by bacterial antigens and interleukins readily produce IFN-γ. When released into the circulation, IFN-γ is detectable in vivo by 6 hours and may be persistently elevated for as long as 8 days. Injured tissues, such as operative wounds, also demonstrate the presence of IFN-γ production 5–7 days after injury. IFN-γ has important roles in activating circulating and tissue macrophages. Alveolar macrophage activation mediated by IFN-γ may induce acute lung inflammation after major surgery or trauma.

Granulocyte-Macrophage Colony-Stimulating Factor

Granulocyte-macrophage colony-stimulating factor (GM-CSF) delays apoptosis (programmed cell death) of macrophages and neutrophils. This growth factor is effective in promoting the maturation and recruitment of functional leukocytes necessary for normal inflammatory cytokine response, and potentially in wound healing. The delay in apoptosis may contribute to organ injury such as that found in acute respiratory distress syndrome (ARDS).

High Mobility Group Box-1

DNA transcription factor, HMGB-1, is released 24–48 hours after the onset of sepsis. The appearance of HMGB-1 is contrast to the early appearances of TNF-α, IL-1, IL-6, and IL-8. Clinically, HMGB-1 peak levels are associated with ARDS and mortality. As a late mediator of the inflammatory response, anti-HMGB-1 strategies may be utilized to modify the inflammatory response.

CELLULAR RESPONSE TO INJURY

Gene Expression and Regulation

In the inflammatory response, cytokine production involves rapid ribonucleic acid (RNA) transcription and translation or protein synthesis. These proteins can further be modified in the cytosol for specific functions. In essence, these cytosolic modifications supplement the primary regulatory mechanisms within the nucleus.

How a particular gene is activated depends on the orderly assemblage of transcription factors to specific DNA sequences immediately upstream to the target gene, known as the *promoter region*. The DNA binding sites are the *enhancer sequences,* and proteins that inhibit the initiation of transcription are *repressors*. Transcription factors become important during the inflammatory response because the ability to control the pathways leading to their activation means the ability to regulate the manner and magnitude by which a cell can respond to an injury stimulus.

Cell Signaling Pathways

Heat Shock Proteins

HSPs, also known as stress proteins, are produced by cells in response to injury or tissue ischemia. HSPs are essential for the ability of cells to overcome stress. HSPs' primary role are to attenuate the inflammatory response by reducing oxygen metabolites, promoting T_H2 cell proliferation, and inhibiting nuclear factor (NF)-κB activation.

G-Protein Receptors

Guanosine-5′-triphosphate (GTP)-binding proteins (G-proteins), with activation of an adjacent effector protein, are the largest family of signaling receptors for cells and include many of the pathways associated with the inflammatory response. The two major second messengers of the G-protein pathway are (a) formation of cyclic adenosine monophosphate (cAMP), and (b) calcium, released from the endoplasmic reticulum. An increase in cellular cAMP can activate gene transcription.

G-protein/calcium activation requires activation of the effector phospholipase C and phosphoinositols. G-protein signaling activates protein kinase C (PKC), which can in turn activate NF-κB and other transcription factors.

Ligand-Gated Ion Channels

These receptor channels, when activated by a ligand, permit rapid flux of ions across the cell membrane. Neurotransmitters function by this pathway, and an example of such a receptor is the nicotinic acetylcholine receptor.

Receptor Tyrosine Kinases

Receptor tyrosine kinases have significant intracellular tyrosine kinase domains. Examples of these receptors include insulin and various hormone growth factors (e.g., platelet-derived growth factor [PDGF], IGF-1, epidermal growth factor [EGF], and vascular endothelial growth factor [VEGF]).

Activation of protein kinase receptors is important for gene transcription and cell proliferation.

Janus Kinase/Signal Transduction and Activator of Transcription (STAT) Signaling

Janus kinase (JAK) is the receptor for many cytokines. Ligand receptor interaction leads to receptor dimerization and enzymatic activation results in propagation through the JAK domains of the receptors. JAK mediated signaling via STAT mediated transcription can activate different T-cell responses during injury and inflammation.

Suppressors of Cytokine Signaling

Suppressors of cytokine signaling (SOCS) specifically block JAK and STAT activation and regulate the signaling of certain cytokines. A deficiency of SOCS activity may render a cell hypersensitive to certain stimuli such as inflammatory cytokines and growth hormones.

Mitogen-Activated Protein Kinases

The mitogen-activated protein kinase (MAPK) pathway is a major cellular inflammatory signaling pathway with regulatory roles over cell proliferation and cell death. The three major isoforms are the JNK (c-Jun NH_2-terminal kinase), ERK (extracellular regulatory protein kinase), and p38 kinase. The JNK pathway has clear links, via TNF-α and IL-1, to the inflammatory response with a regulatory role in apoptosis. The p38 kinase is activated in response to endotoxin, viruses, interleukins, TNF-α, and transforming growth factor (TGF)-β. P38-kinase activation triggers the recruitment and activation of leukocytes. MAPK isoforms exhibit appreciable "cross-talk," which can modulate the inflammatory response.

Nuclear Factor-κB

NF-κB activates genes important for the activation of proinflammatory cytokines and acute phase proteins. NF-κB is really a complex of smaller proteins, and the p50-p65 heterodimer complex is the most widely studied. Cytosolic NF-κB is maintained by binding to the inhibitor protein I-κB. When a cell is exposed to an inflammatory stimulus (TNF-α or IL-β), a series of phosphorylation events leads to I-κB degradation. Low intracellular I-κB appears to prolong the inflammatory response and enhanced activity of NF-κB appears to delay the apoptosis of activated immune cells.

Toll-Like Receptors and CD14

Lipopolysaccharide (LPS), an endotoxin, is an important mediator of gram-negative sepsis syndrome. LPS recognition and activation of the inflammatory response by immune cells occurs primarily by the toll-like receptor-4 (TLR4) mechanism. LPS-binding proteins (LBPs) carry LPS to the CD14/TLR4 complex, which sets into motion cellular mechanisms that activate MAPK, NF-κB, and cytokine gene promoters. TLR4 is primarily the receptor for gram-negative endotoxins and TLR2 is the counterpart for gram-positive sepsis. The fact that some patient populations are more susceptible to infectious complications than others recently has been associated with specific point mutations in the TLR gene.

Tumor Necrosis Factor and CD95-Induced Apoptosis

Apoptosis is the principal mechanism by which senescent or dysfunctional cells, including macrophages and neutrophils, are systematically disposed of without activating other immunocytes or inducing an inflammatory response. The cellular environment created by systemic inflammation disrupts the normal apoptotic machinery in activated immunocytes, consequently prolonging the inflammatory response.

Several proinflammatory cytokines (e.g., TNF-α, IL-1, IL-3, IL-6, GM-CSF, granulocyte colony-stimulating factor [G-CSF], and IFN-γ) and bacterial products (e.g., endotoxin) have been shown to delay macrophage and neutrophil apoptosis in vitro, whereas IL-4 and IL-10 accelerate apoptosis in activated monocytes.

In acute inflammation, the response of the immunocyte to TNF-α is perhaps the most widely investigated. This cytokine exerts its biologic effects by binding to specific cellular receptors, tumor necrosis factor receptor (TNFR)-1 (55 kDa) and TNFR-2 (75 kDa). When TNFR-1 is exclusively activated, it precipitates circulatory shock reminiscent of severe sepsis. However, exclusive activation of TNFR-2 fails to induce any inflammatory responses or shock.

The activation of NF-κB and JNK is believed to be the major antiapoptotic, and therefore proinflammatory, factor; it is signal induced by TNFR-1 and TNFR-2. It is well known that TNF-α–induced NF-κB activation delays cell death and is associated with the activation of diverse genes that include proinflammatory mediators. Exaggerated peripheral blood monocyte NF-κB activation has been associated with higher mortality rates in patients with septic shock.

The CD95 (Fas) receptor shares much of its intracellular structure with TNFR-1. Unlike TNFR-1, the only known function of CD95 is to initiate programmed cell death. Neutrophils and macrophages express CD95, and this expression may have important implications in the cellular contribution to the inflammatory response. In fact, both clinical sepsis and experimental endotoxemia have demonstrated prolonged survival of neutrophils and diminished responsiveness to CD95 stimuli.

Cell-Mediated Inflammatory Response

Platelets

Clot formation at the site of injury releases inflammatory mediators and serves as the principal chemoattractant for neutrophils and monocytes. The migration of platelets and neutrophils through the vascular endothelium occurs within 3 hours of injury and is mediated by serotonin release, platelet-activating factor, and prostaglandin E_2. Platelets can enhance or reduce neutrophil-mediated tissue injury by modulating neutrophil adherence to the endothelium and subsequent respiratory burst. Platelets are an important source of eicosanoids and vasoactive mediators. NSAIDs irreversibly inhibit thromboxane production.

Lymphocytes and T-Cell Immunity

Injury, surgical or traumatic, is associated with acute impairment of cell-mediated immunity and macrophage function. T-helper lymphocytes are functionally divided into two subgroups, referred to as T_H1 and T_H2. In severe infections and injury, there appears to be a reduction in T_H1 (cell-mediated immunity) cytokine production, with a lymphocyte population shift toward the

T_H2 response and its associated immunosuppressive effects. In patients with major burns, a shift to a T_H2 cytokine response has been a predictor of infectious complications. However, studies in patients undergoing major surgery have demonstrated a postoperative reduction in T_H1 cytokine production that is not necessarily associated with increased T_H2 response. Nevertheless, depressed T_H1 response and systemic immunosuppression following major insults to the host may be a useful paradigm in predicting the subset of patients who are prone to infectious complications and poor outcome.

Eosinophils

Eosinophils are characteristically similar to neutrophils in that they migrate to inflamed endothelium and release cytoplasmic granules that are cytotoxic. Eosinophils preferentially migrate to sites of parasitic infection and allergen challenge. Major activators of eosinophils include IL-3, GM-CSF, IL-5, platelet-activating factor, and complement anaphylatoxins C3a and C5a.

Mast Cells

Tissue resident mast cells are important as first-responders to sites of injury. Activated mast cells produce histamine, cytokines, eicosanoids, proteases, and chemokines. The immediate results are vasodilation, recruitment of other immunocytes, and capillary leakage. TNF-α is secreted rapidly by mast cells because of the abundant stores within granules. Mast cells also can synthesize a variety of cytokines and migration-inhibitory factor (MIF).

Monocytes

In clinical sepsis, nonsurviving patients with severe sepsis have an immediate reduction in monocyte surface TNFR expression with failure to recover, whereas surviving patients have normal or near-normal receptor levels from the onset of clinically defined sepsis.

Thus, TNFR expression potentially can be used as a prognostic indicator of outcome in patients with systemic inflammation. There is also decreased CD95 expression following experimental endotoxemia in humans, which correlates with diminished CD95-mediated apoptosis. Taken together, the reduced receptor expression and delayed apoptosis may be a mechanism for prolonging the inflammatory response during injury or infection.

Neutrophils

Neutrophils mediate important functions in every form of acute inflammation, including acute lung injury, ischemia/reperfusion injury, and inflammatory bowel disease. G-CSF is the primary stimulus for neutrophil maturation. Inflammatory mediators from a site of injury induce neutrophil adherence to the vascular endothelium and promote eventual cell migration into the injured tissue. Neutrophil function is mediated by a vast array of intracellular granules that are chemotactic or cytotoxic to local tissue and invading microorganisms.

ENDOTHELIUM-MEDIATED INJURY

Neutrophil-Endothelium Interaction

Increased vascular permeability during inflammation is intended to facilitate oxygen delivery and immunocyte migration to the sites of injury. However, neutrophils migration and activation at sites of injury may contribute to the cytotoxicity of vital tissues and result in organ dysfunction. Ischemia/reperfusion (I/R) injury potentiates this response by unleashing oxygen metabolites, lysosomal enzymes that degrade tissue basal membranes, cause microvascular thrombosis, and activate myeloperoxidases. The recruitment of circulating neutrophils to endothelial surfaces is mediated by concerted actions of adhesion molecules referred to as selectins that are elaborated on cell surfaces.

Nitric Oxide

Nitric oxide (NO) is derived from endothelial surfaces in response to acetylcholine stimulation, hypoxia, endotoxin, cellular injury, or mechanical shear stress from circulating blood. NO promotes vascular smooth muscle relaxation, reduces microthrombosis, and mediates protein synthesis in hepatocytes. NO is formed from oxidation of L-arginine, a process catalyzed by nitric oxide synthase (NOS). NO is a readily diffusible substance with a half-life of a few seconds. NO spontaneously decomposes into nitrate and nitrite.

In addition to the endothelium, NO formation also occurs in neutrophils, monocytes, renal cells, Kupffer cells, and cerebellar neurons.

Prostacyclin

Although it is an arachidonate product, prostacyclin (PGI_2) is another important endothelium-derived vasodilator synthesized in response to vascular shear stress and hypoxia. PGI_2 shares similar functions with NO, inducing vasorelaxation and platelet deactivation by increasing cAMP. Clinically, it has been used to reduce pulmonary hypertension, particularly in the pediatric population.

Endothelins

Endothelins (ETs) are elaborated by vascular endothelial cells in response to injury, thrombin, transforming growth factor-β (TGF-β), IL-1, angiotensin II, vasopressin, catecholamines, and anoxia. ET is a 21-amino-acid peptide with potent vasoconstricting properties. Of the peptides in this family (e.g., ET-1, ET-2, and ET-3), endothelial cells appear to exclusively produce ET-1. ET-1 appears to be the most biologically active and the most potent known vasoconstrictor. It is estimated to be 10 times more potent than angiotensin II. The maintenance of physiologic tone in vascular smooth muscle depends on the balance between NO and ET production. Increased serum levels of ETs correlate with the severity of injury following major trauma, major surgical procedures, and in cardiogenic or septic shock.

Platelet-Activating Factor

Platelet-activating factor (PAF), an endothelial-derived product, is a natural phospholipid constituent of cell membranes, which under normal physiologic conditions is minimally expressed. During acute inflammation, PAF is released by neutrophils, platelets, mast cells, and monocytes, and is expressed at the outer leaflet of endothelial cells. PAF can further activate neutrophils and platelets and increase vascular permeability. Human sepsis is associated with a reduction in PAF-acetylhydrolase levels, which is the endogenous inactivator of PAF. Indeed, PAF-acetylhydrolase administration in patients with severe sepsis has shown some reduction in multiple organ dysfunction and mortality.

Atrial Natriuretic Peptides

Atrial natriuretic peptides (ANPs) are a family of peptides released primarily by atrial tissue, but are also synthesized by the gut, kidney, brain, adrenal glands, and endothelium. They induce vasodilation and fluid and electrolyte excretion. ANPs are potent inhibitors of aldosterone secretion and prevent reabsorption of sodium.

SURGICAL METABOLISM

The initial hours following surgical or traumatic injury are metabolically associated with a reduced total body energy expenditure and urinary nitrogen wasting. Following resuscitation and stabilization of the injured patient, a reprioritization of substrate utilization ensues to preserve vital organ function and for the repair of injured tissue. This phase of recovery also is characterized by augmented metabolic rates and oxygen consumption, enzymatic preference for readily oxidizable substrates such as glucose, and stimulation of the immune system.

Understanding the collective alterations, as a consequence of the inflammatory response, in amino acid (protein), carbohydrate, and lipid metabolism lays the foundation on which clinical metabolic and nutritional support can be implemented.

Metabolism Following Injury

Injuries or infections induce unique neuroendocrine and immunologic responses that differentiate injury metabolism from that of unstressed fasting. The magnitude of metabolic expenditure appears to be directly proportional to the severity of insult, with thermal injuries and severe infections having the highest energy demands. The increase in energy expenditure is mediated in part by sympathetic activation and catecholamine release.

Lipid Metabolism Following Injury

Lipids serve as a nonprotein and noncarbohydrate fuel sources that minimize protein catabolism in the injured patient, and lipid metabolism potentially influences the structural integrity of cell membranes and the immune response during systemic inflammation. Fat mobilization (lipolysis) occurs mainly in response to catecholamine stimulus of the hormone-sensitive triglyceride lipase. Other hormonal influences on lipolysis include adrenocorticotropic hormone, catecholamines, thyroid hormone, cortisol, glucagon, growth hormone release, reduction in insulin levels, and increased sympathetic stimulus.

Lipid absorption. Adipose tissue provides fuel for the host in the form of free fatty acids and glycerol during critical illness and injury. Oxidation of 1 g of fat yields approximately 9 kcal of energy. Although the liver is capable of synthesizing triglycerides from carbohydrates and amino acids, dietary and exogenous sources provide the major source of triglycerides. Dietary lipids are not readily absorbable in the gut, but require pancreatic lipase and phospholipase within the duodenum to hydrolyze the triglycerides into free fatty acids and monoglycerides. The free fatty acids and monoglycerides are then readily absorbed by gut enterocytes, which resynthesize triglycerides by esterification of the monoglycerides with fatty acylcoenzyme A (acyl-CoA). Long-chain triglycerides (LCTs), defined as those with 12 carbons or more, undergo esterification and enter the circulation through the lymphatic system as chylomicrons. Shorter fatty acid chains directly enter the portal circulation and are transported to the liver by albumin carriers. Hepatocytes use free fatty acids as a fuel source during stress states, but can also synthesize phospholipids or triglycerides (very-low-density lipoproteins) during fed states. Systemic tissue (e.g., muscle and the heart) can use chylomicrons and triglycerides as fuel by hydrolysis with lipoprotein lipase at the luminal surface of capillary endothelium. Trauma or sepsis suppresses lipoprotein lipase activity in both adipose tissue and muscle, presumably mediated by TNF-α.

Lipolysis and fatty acid oxidation.   Periods of energy demand are accompanied by free fatty acid mobilization from adipose stores. In adipose tissues, triglyceride lipase hydrolyzes triglycerides into free fatty acids and glycerol. Free fatty acids enter the capillary circulation and are transported by albumin to tissues requiring this fuel source (e.g., heart and skeletal muscle). Insulin inhibits lipolysis and favors triglyceride synthesis by augmenting lipoprotein lipase activity and intracellular levels of glycerol-3-phosphate. The use of glycerol for fuel depends on the availability of tissue glycerokinase, which is abundant in the liver and kidneys.

Free fatty acids absorbed by cells is conjugated with acyl-CoA within the cytoplasm and transported across membranes by the carnitine shuttle. Medium-chain triglycerides (MCTs), defined as those 6 to 12 carbons in length, bypass the carnitine shuttle and readily cross the mitochondrial membranes. This accounts in part for why MCTs are more efficiently oxidized than LCTs. Ideally, the rapid oxidation of MCTs makes them less prone to fat deposition, particularly within immune cells and the reticuloendothelial system—a common finding with lipid infusion in parenteral nutrition. However, in animal studies, exclusive use of MCTs as fuel is associated with higher metabolic demands and toxicity, as well as essential fatty acid deficiency.

Fatty acyl-CoA undergoes mitochondrial β-oxidation, which produces acetyl-CoA. Each acetyl-CoA molecule subsequently enters the tricarboxylic acid (TCA) cycle for further oxidation to yield 12 adenosine triphosphate (ATP) molecules, carbon dioxide, and water. Excess acetyl-CoA molecules serve as precursors for ketogenesis. Unlike glucose metabolism, oxidation of fatty acids requires proportionally less oxygen and produces less carbon dioxide. This is frequently quantified as the ratio of carbon dioxide produced to oxygen consumed for the reaction, and is known as the *respiratory quotient* (RQ). An RQ of 0.7 would imply greater fatty acid oxidation for fuel, whereas an RQ of 1 indicates greater carbohydrate oxidation (*overfeeding*). An RQ of 0.85 suggests the oxidation of equal amounts of fatty acids and glucose.

Ketogenesis.   Carbohydrate depletion slows acetyl-CoA entry into the TCA cycle secondary to depleted TCA intermediates and enzyme activity. Increased lipolysis and reduced systemic carbohydrate availability during starvation diverts excess acetyl-CoA toward hepatic ketogenesis. A number of extrahepatic tissues, but not the liver itself, are capable of utilizing ketones for fuel. Ketosis represents a state in which hepatic ketone production exceeds extrahepatic ketone use.

The rate of ketogenesis appears to be inversely related to the severity of injury. Major trauma, severe shock, and sepsis attenuate ketogenesis by increasing insulin levels and by rapid tissue oxidation of free fatty acids.

Carbohydrate Metabolism

Ingested and enteral carbohydrates are primarily digested in the small intestine, in which pancreatic and intestinal enzymes reduce the complex carbohydrates to dimeric units. Disaccharidases are further broken down into hexose units such as glucose and galactose, which require energy dependent transport for primary absorption.

Carbohydrate metabolism primarily refers to the utilization of glucose. The oxidation of 1 g of carbohydrate yields 4 kcal, but administered sugar solutions such as that found in intravenous fluids or parenteral nutrition provides only 3.4 kcal/g of dextrose. The primary goal for maintenance glucose administration in surgical patients serves to minimize muscle wasting. The exogenous administration of small amounts of glucose (approximately 50 g/d) facilitates fat entry into the TCA cycle and reduces ketosis. Studies providing exogenous glucose to septic and trauma patients never have been shown to fully suppress amino acid degradation for gluconeogenesis. This suggests that during periods of stress, other hormonal and proinflammatory mediators have profound influence on the rate of protein degradation and that some degree of muscle wasting is inevitable. Insulin has been shown to reverse protein catabolism during severe stress by stimulating protein synthesis in skeletal muscles and inhibits hepatocyte protein degradation.

In cells, glucose is phosphorylated to form glucose-6-phosphate (G6P). G6P can be polymerized during glycogenesis or catabolized in glycogenolysis. Glucose catabolism occurs by cleavage to pyruvate or lactate (pyruvic acid pathway) or by decarboxylation to pentoses (pentose shunt).

Excess glucose from overfeeding, as reflected by RQs greater than 1.0, can result in conditions such as glucosuria, thermogenesis, and conversion to fat (lipogenesis). Excessive glucose administration results in elevated carbon dioxide production, which may be deleterious in patients with suboptimal pulmonary function.

Injury and severe infections acutely induce a state of peripheral glucose intolerance, despite ample insulin production several-fold above baseline. This may occur in part because of reduced skeletal muscle pyruvate dehydrogenase activity following injury, which diminishes the conversion of pyruvate to acetyl-CoA and subsequent entry into the TCA cycle. The consequent accumulation of 3-carbon structures (e.g., pyruvate and lactate) is shunted to the liver as substrate for gluconeogenesis. Unlike the nonstressed subject, the hepatic gluconeogenic response to injury or sepsis cannot be suppressed by exogenous or excess glucose administration, but rather persists in the hypermetabolic, critically ill patient. Hepatic gluconeogenesis, arising primarily from alanine and glutamine catabolism, provides a ready fuel source for tissues such as those of the nervous system, wounds, and erythrocytes, which do not require insulin for glucose transport. The elevated glucose concentrations also provide a necessary energy source for leukocytes in inflamed tissues and in sites of microbial invasions. Glycogen stores within skeletal muscles can be mobilized as a ready fuel source by epinephrine activation of β-adrenergic receptors.

PROTEIN AND AMINO ACID METABOLISM

The average protein intake in healthy, young adults ranges from 80 to 120 g/d, and every 6 g of protein yields approximately 1 g of nitrogen. The degradation of 1 g of protein yields approximately 4 kcal of energy, almost the same as for carbohydrates.

Following injury the initial systemic proteolysis, mediated primarily by glucocorticoids, increases urinary nitrogen excretion to levels in excess of 30 g/day, which roughly corresponds to a loss in lean body mass of 1.5 percent per day. An injured individual who does not receive nutrition for 10 days can theoretically lose 15 percent lean body mass. Therefore amino acids cannot be considered a long-term fuel reserve, and indeed excessive protein depletion (25–30 percent of lean body weight) is not compatible with sustaining life.

Protein catabolism following injury provides substrates for gluconeogenesis and for the synthesis of acute phase proteins. Radiolabeled amino acid incorporation studies and protein analyses confirm that skeletal muscles are preferentially depleted acutely following injury, whereas visceral tissues (e.g., the liver and kidney) remain relatively preserved. The accelerated urea excretion following injury is also associated with the excretion of intracellular elements such as sulfur, phosphorus, potassium, magnesium, and creatinine. Conversely, the rapid use of elements such as potassium and magnesium during recovery from major injury may indicate a period of tissue healing.

The net changes in protein catabolism and synthesis correspond to the severity and duration of injury. The rise in urinary nitrogen and negative nitrogen balance can be detected early following injury and peak by 7 days. This state of protein catabolism may persist for as long as 3–7 weeks. The patient's prior physical status and age appear to influence the degree of proteolysis following injury or sepsis.

NUTRITION IN THE SURGICAL PATIENT

The goal of nutritional support in the surgical patient is to prevent or reverse the catabolic effects of disease or injury. Although several important biologic parameters have been used to measure the efficacy of nutrition regimens, the ultimate validation for nutritional support should be improvement in clinical outcome and restoration of function.

Estimating Energy Requirements

Nutritional assessment determines the severity of nutrient deficiencies or excess and aids in predicting nutritional requirements. Elements of nutritional assessment include weight loss, chronic illnesses, or dietary habits that influence the quantity and quality of food intake. Social habits predisposing to malnutrition and the use of medications that may influence food intake or urination should also be investigated. Physical examination seeks to assess loss of muscle and adipose tissues, organ dysfunction, and subtle changes in skin, hair, or neuromuscular function reflecting frank or impending nutritional deficiency. Anthropometric data including weight change, skinfold thickness, and arm circumference muscle area and biochemical determinations (i.e., creatinine excretion, albumin, prealbumin, total lymphocyte count, and transferrin) may be used to substantiate the patient's history and physical findings. Nutritional assessment remains an imprecise method for the detection of malnutrition and prediction of patient outcome. Appreciation for the stresses and natural history of the disease process, in combination with nutritional assessment, remains the basis for identifying patients in acute or anticipated need of nutritional support.

A fundamental goal of nutritional support is to meet the energy requirements for metabolic processes, core temperature maintenance, and tissue repair. The requirement for energy may be measured by indirect calorimetry or estimated from urinary nitrogen excretion, which is proportional to resting energy expenditure. However, the use of indirect calorimetry, particularly in the critically ill patient, is labor-intensive and often leads to overestimation of caloric requirements.

Basal energy expenditure (BEE) may also be estimated using the Harris-Benedict equations:

$$\text{BEE (men)} = 66.47 + 13.75\,(W) + 5.0\,(H) - 6.76\,(A)\,\text{kcal/d}$$
$$\text{BEE (women)} = 655.1 + 9.56\,(W) + 1.85\,(H) - 4.68\,(A)\,\text{kcal/d}$$

where W = weight in kilograms, H = height in centimeters, and A = age in years.

These equations, adjusted for the type of surgical stress, are suitable for estimating energy requirements in over 80 percent of hospitalized patients. It has been demonstrated that the provision of 30 kcal/kg per day will adequately meet energy requirements in most postsurgical patients, with low risk of overfeeding. Following trauma or sepsis, energy substrate demands are increased, necessitating greater nonprotein calories beyond calculated energy expenditure. These additional nonprotein calories provided after injury are usually 1.2 to 2.0 times greater than calculated resting energy expenditure (REE), depending on the type of injury. It is seldom appropriate to exceed this level of nonprotein energy intake during the height of the catabolic phase.

The second objective of nutritional support is to meet the substrate requirements for protein synthesis. An appropriate nonprotein calorie-to-nitrogen ratio of 150:1 (e.g., 1 g N = 6.25 g protein) should be maintained, which is the basal calorie requirement provided to prevent use of protein as an energy source. There is now greater evidence suggesting that increased protein intake, and a lower calorie-to-nitrogen ratio of 80:1 to 100:1, may benefit healing in selected hypermetabolic or critically ill patients. In the absence of severe renal or hepatic dysfunction precluding the use of standard nutritional regimens, approximately 0.25 to 0.35 g of nitrogen per kilogram of body weight should be provided daily.

Vitamins and Minerals

The requirements for vitamins and essential trace minerals usually can be easily met in the average patient with an uncomplicated postoperative course. Therefore vitamins are usually not given in the absence of preoperative deficiencies. Patients maintained on elemental diets or parenteral hyperalimentation require complete vitamin and mineral supplementation. Essential fatty acid supplementation may also be necessary, especially in patients with depletion of adipose stores.

Overfeeding

Overfeeding usually results from overestimation of caloric needs, as occurs when actual body weight is used to calculate the BEE in such patient populations as the critically ill with significant fluid overload and the obese. Indirect calorimetry can be used to quantify energy requirements, but frequently overestimates BEE by 10–15 percent in stressed patients, particularly if they are on a ventilator. In these instances, estimated dry weight should be obtained from preinjury records or family members.

Adjusted lean body weight also can be calculated. Clinically, increased oxygen consumption, increased CO_2 production, fatty liver, suppression of leukocyte function, and increased infectious risks have all been documented with overfeeding.

ENTERAL NUTRITION

Rationale for Enteral Nutrition

Enteral nutrition generally is preferred over parenteral nutrition based on reduced cost and associated risks of the intravenous route. Laboratory models have long demonstrated that luminal nutrient contact reduces intestinal mucosal atrophy when compared with parenteral or no nutritional support. Studies comparing postoperative enteral and parenteral nutrition in patients undergoing GI surgery have demonstrated reduced infection complications and acute phase protein production when fed by the enteral route. Yet, prospectively randomized studies for patients with adequate nutritional status (albumin $\geq$ 4 g/dL) undergoing GI surgery demonstrate no differences in outcome and complications when administered enteral nutrition compared to maintenance intravenous fluids alone in the initial days following surgery. At the other extreme, recent meta-analysis for critically ill patients demonstrates a 44 percent reduction in infectious complications in those receiving enteral nutritional support over those receiving parenteral nutrition. Most prospectively randomized studies for severe abdominal and thoracic trauma demonstrate significant reductions in infectious complications for patients given early enteral nutrition when compared with those who are unfed or receiving parenteral nutrition.

Recommendations for instituting early *enteral* nutrition to surgical patients with moderate malnutrition (albumin = 2.9 to 3.5 g/dL) can only be made by inferences because of a lack of data directly pertaining to this population. It is prudent to offer enteral nutrition based on measured energy expenditure of the recovering patient, or if complications arise that may alter the anticipated course of recovery (e.g., anastomotic leaks, return to surgery, sepsis, or failure to wean from the ventilator). Other clinical scenarios with substantiated benefits from enteral nutritional support include permanent neurologic impairment, oropharyngeal dysfunction, short-bowel syndrome, and bone marrow transplantation patients.

Data support the use of early enteral nutritional support following major trauma and in patients who are anticipated to have prolonged recovery after surgery. Healthy patients without malnutrition undergoing uncomplicated surgery can tolerate 10 days of partial starvation (with maintenance intravenous fluids only) before any significant protein catabolism occurs. Earlier intervention is likely indicated in patients with poorer preoperative nutritional status.

Initiation of enteral nutrition should occur immediately after adequate resuscitation, most readily determined by adequate urine output. Presence of bowel sounds and the passage of flatus or stool are not absolute requisites for initiating enteral nutrition, but feedings in the setting of gastroparesis should be administered distal to the pylorus. Enteral feeding should also be offered to patients with short-bowel syndrome or clinical malabsorption, but caloric needs, essential minerals, and vitamins should be supplemented with parenteral modalities.

Enteral Formulas

The functional status of the GI tract determines the type of enteral solutions to be used. Patients with an intact GI tract will tolerate complex enteral solutions. In patients with malabsorption such as in inflammatory bowel diseases, absorption may be improved by provision of dipeptides, tripeptides, and MCTs. However, MCTs are deficient in essential fatty acids, which necessitates supplementation with some LCT.

In general, factors that influence the choice of enteral formula include the extent of organ dysfunction (e.g., renal, pulmonary, hepatic, or GI), the nutrient needs to restore optimal function and healing, and the cost of specific products.

Immune-enhancing formulas. These formulas are fortified with special nutrients that are purported to enhance various aspects of immune or solid organ function. Such additives include glutamine, arginine, branched-chain amino acids, omega-3 fatty acids, nucleotides, and beta-carotene. Although several trials have proposed that one or more of these additives reduce surgical complications and improve outcome, these results have not been uniformly corroborated by other trials. The addition of amino acids to these formulas generally doubles the amount of protein (nitrogen) found in standard formula; however, their use can be cost-prohibitive.

High-protein formulas. High-protein formulas are available in isotonic and nonisotonic mixtures and are proposed for critically ill or trauma patients with high protein requirements. These formulas comprise nonprotein calorie-to-nitrogen ratios between 80:1 and 120:1.

Elemental formulas. These formulas contain predigested nutrients and provide proteins in the form of small peptides. Complex carbohydrates are limited, and fat content, in the form of MCTs and LCTs, is minimal. The primary advantage of such a formula is ease of absorption, but the inherent scarcity of fat, associated vitamins, and trace elements limits its long-term use as a primary source of nutrients. Because of its high osmolarity, dilution or slow infusion rates are usually necessary, particularly in critically ill patients. These formulas have been used frequently in patients with malabsorption, gut impairment, and pancreatitis, but their cost is significantly higher than that of standard formulas.

Renal-failure formulas. The primary benefits of the renal formula are the lower fluid volume and concentrations of potassium, phosphorus, and magnesium needed to meet daily calorie requirements. This formulation almost exclusively contains essential amino acids and has a high nonprotein-to-calorie ratio; however, it does not contain trace elements or vitamins.

Pulmonary-failure formulas. In these formulas, fat content is usually increased to 50 percent of the total calories, with a corresponding reduction in carbohydrate content. The goal is to reduce CO_2 production and alleviate ventilation burden for failing lungs.

Access for Enteral Nutritional Support

The available techniques and repertoire for enteral access have provided multiple options for feeding the gut. Table 1-4 summarizes the presently used methods and preferred indications.

TABLE 1-4 Options for Enteral Feeding Access

Access option	Comments
Nasogastric tube	Short-term use only; aspiration risks; nasopharyngeal trauma; frequent dislodgment
Nasoduodenal/nasojejunal	Short-term use; lower aspiration risks in jejunum; placement challenges (radiographic assistance often necessary)
Percutaneous endoscopic gastrostomy (PEG)	Endoscopy skills required; may be used for gastric decompression or bolus feeds; aspiration risks; can last 12–24 months; slightly higher complication rates with placement and site leaks
Surgical gastrostomy	Requires general anesthesia and small laparotomy; may allow placement of extended duodenal/jejunal feeding ports; laparoscopic placement possible
Fluoroscopic gastrostomy	Blind placement using needle and T-prongs to anchor to stomach; can thread smaller catheter through gastrostomy into duodenum/jejunum under fluoroscopy
PEG-jejunal tube	Jejunal placement with regular endoscope is operator dependent; jejunal tube often dislodges retrograde; two-stage procedure with PEG placement, followed by fluoroscopic conversion with jejunal feeding tube through PEG
Direct percutaneous endoscopic jejunostomy (DPEJ)	Direct endoscopic placement with enteroscope; placement challenges; greater injury risks
Surgical jejunostomy	Commonly applied during laparotomy; general anesthesia; laparoscopic placement usually requires assistant to thread catheter; laparoscopy offers direct visualization of catheter placement
Fluoroscopic jejunostomy	Difficult approach with injury risks; not commonly done

Nasoenteric tubes. Nasogastric feeding should be reserved for those with intact mental status and protective laryngeal reflexes to minimize risks of aspiration. Even in intubated patients, nasogastric feedings can often be recovered from tracheal suction. Nasojejunal feedings are associated with fewer pulmonary complications, but access past the pylorus requires greater effort to accomplish. Blind insertion of nasogastric feeding tubes is fraught with misplacement, and air instillation with auscultation is inaccurate for ascertaining proper positioning. Radiographic confirmation is usually required to verify the position of the nasogastric feeding tube.

Small bowel feeding is more reliable for delivering nutrition than nasogastric feeding. Furthermore, the risks of aspiration pneumonia can be reduced by 25 percent with small bowel feeding when compared with nasogastric feeding. The disadvantages of nasoenteric feeding tubes are clogging, kinking, inadvertent displacement or removal, and nasopharyngeal complications. If nasoenteric feeding will be required for longer than 30 days, access should be converted to a percutaneous one.

Percutaneous endoscopic gastrostomy. The most common indications for percutaneous endoscopic gastrostomy (PEG) placement include impaired swallowing mechanisms, oropharyngeal or esophageal obstruction, and major facial trauma. It is frequently utilized for debilitated patients requiring caloric supplementation, hydration, or frequent medication dosing. It is also appropriate for patients requiring passive gastric decompression. Relative contraindications for PEG placement include ascites, coagulopathy, gastric varices, gastric neoplasm, and lack of a suitable abdominal site.

If endoscopy is not available or technical obstacles preclude PEG placement, the interventional radiologist can attempt the procedure percutaneously under fluoroscopic guidance. If this is also unsuccessful, surgical gastrostomy or small-bowel tube placement can be considered.

Although PEG tubes enhance nutritional delivery, facilitate nursing care, and are superior to nasogastric tubes, serious complications can occur in approximately 3 percent of patients. These complications include wound infection, necrotizing fasciitis, peritonitis, aspiration, leaks, dislodgment, bowel perforation, enteric fistulas, bleeding, and aspiration pneumonia. For patients with significant gastroparesis or gastric outlet obstruction, feedings through PEG tubes are hazardous. In this instance, the PEG tube can be used for decompression and to allow access for converting the PEG tube to a transpyloric feeding tube.

Surgical gastrostomy and jejunostomy. In a patient undergoing complex abdominal or trauma surgery, thought should be given during surgery to the possible routes for subsequent nutritional support, because laparotomy affords direct access to the stomach or small bowel. The only absolute contraindication to feeding jejunostomy is distal intestinal obstruction. Relative contraindications include severe edema of the intestinal wall, radiation enteritis, inflammatory bowel disease, ascites, severe immunodeficiency, and bowel ischemia. Needle-catheter jejunostomies can also be done with a minimal learning curve. The biggest drawback is usually related to clogging and knotting of the 6F catheter.

Abdominal distention and cramps are common adverse effects of early enteral nutrition and usually managed by temporarily discontinuing feeds and resuming at a lower infusion rate.

Pneumatosis intestinalis and small bowel necrosis are infrequent but significant problems associated with patients receiving jejunal tube feedings. Several contributing factors have been proposed, including the hyperosmolar consistency of enteral solutions, bacterial overgrowth, fermentation, and metabolic breakdown products. The common pathophysiology is believed to be bowel distention and consequent reduction in bowel wall perfusion. Risk factors for these complications include cardiogenic and circulatory shock, vasopressor use, diabetes mellitus, and chronic obstructive pulmonary disease. Therefore, enteral feedings in the critically ill patient should be delayed until adequate resuscitation has been achieved.

PARENTERAL NUTRITION

Parenteral nutrition involves the continuous infusion of a hyperosmolar solution containing carbohydrates, proteins, fat, and other necessary nutrients through an indwelling catheter inserted into the superior vena cava. To obtain the maximum benefit, the ratio of calories to nitrogen must be adequate (at least 100 to 150 kcal/g nitrogen), and both carbohydrates and proteins must be infused simultaneously. When the sources of calories and nitrogen are given at different times, there is a significant decrease in nitrogen utilization. These nutrients can be given in quantities considerably greater than the basic caloric and nitrogen requirements. Clinical trials and meta-analysis of parenteral feeding in the perioperative period have suggested that preoperative nutritional support may benefit some surgical patients, particularly those with extensive malnutrition. Short-term use of parenteral nutrition in critically ill patients (i.e., duration <7 days) when enteral nutrition may have been instituted is associated with higher rates of infectious complications. Following severe injury, parenteral nutrition is associated with higher rates of infectious risks when compared with enteral feeding. However, parenteral feeding still has fewer infectious complications compared with no feeding at all.

Rationale for Parenteral Nutrition

The principal indications for parenteral nutrition are found in seriously ill patients suffering from malnutrition, sepsis, or surgical or accidental trauma, when use of the GI tract for feedings is not possible. In some instances, intravenous nutrition may be used to supplement inadequate oral intake. The safe and successful use of parenteral nutrition requires proper selection of patients with specific nutritional needs, experience with the technique, and an awareness of the associated complications. As with enteral nutrition, the fundamental goals are to provide sufficient calories and nitrogen substrate to promote tissue repair and to maintain the integrity or growth of lean tissue mass. Listed below are situations in which parenteral nutrition has been used in an effort to achieve these goals:

1. Newborn infants with catastrophic GI anomalies, such as tracheoesophageal fistula, gastroschisis, omphalocele, or massive intestinal atresia.
2. Infants who fail to thrive because of GI insufficiency associated with short-bowel syndrome, malabsorption, enzyme deficiency, meconium ileus, or idiopathic diarrhea.
3. Adult patients with short-bowel syndrome secondary to massive small bowel resection (<100 cm without colon or ileocecal valve, or <50 cm with intact ileocecal valve and colon).
4. Enteroenteric, enterocolic, enterovesical, or high-output enterocutaneous fistulas (>500 mL/d).
5. Surgical patients with prolonged paralytic ileus following major operations (>7–10 days), multiple injuries, blunt or open abdominal trauma, or patients with reflex ileus complicating various medical diseases.
6. Patients with normal bowel length but with malabsorption secondary to sprue, hypoproteinemia, enzyme or pancreatic insufficiency, regional enteritis, or ulcerative colitis.
7. Adult patients with functional GI disorders such as esophageal dyskinesia following cerebrovascular accident, idiopathic diarrhea, psychogenic vomiting, or anorexia nervosa.
8. Patients with granulomatous colitis, ulcerative colitis, and tuberculous enteritis, in which major portions of the absorptive mucosa are diseased.
9. Patients with malignancy, with or without cachexia, in whom malnutrition might jeopardize successful delivery of a therapeutic option.

10. Failed attempts to provide adequate calories by enteral tube feedings or high residuals.
11. Critically ill patients who are hypermetabolic for more than 5 days or when enteral nutrition is not feasible.

Conditions *contraindicating* hyperalimentation include the following:

1. Lack of a specific goal for patient management, or in cases in which instead of extending a meaningful life, inevitable dying is delayed.
2. Periods of hemodynamic instability or severe metabolic derangement (e.g., severe hyperglycemia, azotemia, encephalopathy, hyperosmolality, and fluid-electrolyte disturbances) requiring control or correction before attempting hypertonic intravenous feeding.
3. Feasible GI tract feeding; in the vast majority of instances, this is the best route by which to provide nutrition.
4. Patients with good nutritional status.
5. Infants with less than 8 cm of small bowel, because virtually all have been unable to adapt sufficiently despite prolonged periods of parenteral nutrition.

Total Parenteral Nutrition

Total parenteral nutrition (TPN), also referred to as central parenteral nutrition, requires access to a large-diameter vein to deliver the entire nutritional requirements of the individual. Dextrose content is high (15–25 percent) and all other macro- and micronutrients are deliverable by this route.

Peripheral Parenteral Nutrition

The lower osmolarity of the solution used for peripheral parenteral nutrition (PPN), secondary to reduced dextrose (5–10 percent) and protein (3 percent) levels, allows for its administration via peripheral veins. Some nutrients cannot be supplemented because of inability to concentrate them in small volumes. Therefore PPN is not appropriate for repleting patients with severe malnutrition. It can be considered if central routes are not available or if supplemental nutritional support is required. Typically, PPN is used for short periods (< 2 weeks).

Intravenous Access Methods

Temporary or short-term access can be achieved with a 16-gauge, percutaneous catheter inserted into a subclavian or internal jugular vein and threaded into the superior vena cava. More permanent access, with the intention of providing long-term or home parenteral nutrition, can be achieved by placement of a catheter with a subcutaneous port for access, by tunneling a catheter with a substantial subcutaneous length, or threading a long catheter through the basilic or cephalic vein into the superior vena cava.

COMPLICATIONS OF PARENTERAL NUTRITION

Technical Complications

One of the more common and serious complications associated with long-term parenteral feeding is sepsis secondary to contamination of the central venous catheter. Complications related to catheter insertion such as pneumothorax, hemothorax, subclavian artery injury, thoracic duct injury, cardiac arrhythmia, air embolism, catheter embolism, and cardiac perforation with tamponade have also been described. Contamination of solutions should be considered, but is rare when proper pharmacy protocols have been followed. This problem occurs more frequently in patients with systemic sepsis, and in many cases is because of hematogenous seeding of the catheter with bacteria. It is prudent to delay reinserting the catheter by 12–24 hours, especially if bacteremia is present.

Metabolic Complications

Hyperglycemia may develop with normal rates of infusion in patients with impaired glucose tolerance or in any patient if the hypertonic solutions are administered too rapidly. This is a particularly common complication in latent diabetics and in patients subjected to severe surgical stress or trauma. Treatment of the condition consists of volume replacement with correction of electrolyte abnormalities and the administration of insulin. This complication can be avoided with careful attention to daily fluid balance and frequent monitoring of blood sugar levels and serum electrolytes.

Increasing experience has emphasized the importance of not overfeeding the parenterally nourished patient. This is particularly true of the depleted patient in whom excess calorie infusion may result in carbon dioxide retention and respiratory insufficiency. Additionally, excess feeding also has been related to the development of hepatic steatosis or marked glycogen deposition in selected patients. Cholestasis and formation of gallstones are common in patients receiving long-term parenteral nutrition. Mild but transient abnormalities of serum transaminase, alkaline phosphatase, and bilirubin may occur in many parenterally nourished patients. Failure of the liver enzymes to plateau or return to normal over 7–14 days should suggest another etiology.

Intestinal Atrophy

Lack of intestinal stimulation is associated with intestinal mucosal atrophy, diminished villous height, bacterial overgrowth, reduced lymphoid tissue size, reduced IgA production, and impaired gut immunity. The full clinical implications of these changes are not well realized, although bacterial translocation has been demonstrated in animal models. The most efficacious method to prevent these changes is to provide nutrients enterally. In patients requiring total parenteral nutrition, it may be feasible to infuse small amounts of trophic feedings via the GI tract.

Special Formulations

Glutamine and Arginine

Glutamine is the most abundant amino acid in the human body, comprising nearly two-thirds of the free intracellular amino acid pool. Of this, 75 percent is found within the skeletal muscles. In healthy individuals, glutamine is considered a nonessential amino acid because it is synthesized within the skeletal muscles and the lungs. Glutamine is a necessary substrate for nucleotide synthesis in most dividing cells, and hence provides a major fuel source for enterocytes. It also serves as an important fuel source for immunocytes such as lymphocytes and macrophages, and a precursor for glutathione, a major intracellular antioxidant. During stress states such as sepsis, or in tumor-bearing hosts, peripheral glutamine stores are rapidly depleted and the amino acid is preferentially shunted as a fuel source toward the visceral organs and tumors, respectively. These situations create, at least experimentally, a glutamine-depleted environment, with consequences including enterocyte and immunocyte starvation.

Arginine, also a nonessential amino acid in healthy subjects, first attracted attention for its immunoenhancing properties, wound-healing benefits, and improved survival in animal models of sepsis and injury. As with glutamine, the benefits of experimental arginine supplementation during stress states are diverse. Clinical studies in which arginine was administered enterally have demonstrated net nitrogen retention and protein synthesis compared to isonitrogenous diets in critically ill and injured patients and following surgery for certain malignancies. Some of these studies also are associated with in vitro evidence of enhanced immunocyte function. The clinical utility of arginine in improving overall patient outcome remains an area of investigation.

Omega-3 Fatty Acids

The provision of omega-3 polyunsaturated fatty acids (canola oil or fish oil) displaces omega-6 fatty acids in cell membranes, which theoretically reduce the proinflammatory response from prostaglandin production.

Nucleotides

RNA supplementation in solutions is purported, at least experimentally, to increase cell proliferation, provide building blocks for DNA synthesis, and improve T-helper cell function.

Suggested Readings

Henneke P, Golenbock DT: Innate immune recognition of lipopolysaccharide by endothelial cells. *Crit Care Med* 30:S207, 2002.

Lin E, Calvano SE, Lowry SF: Inflammatory cytokines and cell response in surgery. *Surgery* 127:117, 2000.

Lin E, Lowry SF: Human response to endotoxin. *Sepsis* 2:255, 1999.

Marshall JC, Vincent J-L, Fink MP, et al: Measures, markers, and mediators: Toward a staging system for clinical sepsis. A report of the Fifth Toronto Sepsis Roundtable, Toronto, Ontario, Canada, October 25–26, 2000. *Crit Care Med* 31:1560, 2003.

Vincent J-L, Sun Q, Dubois M-J: Clinical trials of immunomodulatory therapies in severe sepsis and septic shock. *Clin Infect Dis* 34:1084, 2002.

Wilmore DW: From Cuthbertson to fast-track surgery: 70 years of progress in reducing stress in surgical patients. *Ann Surg* 236:643, 2002.

Cerra FB, Benitez MR, Blackburn GL, et al: Applied nutrition in ICU patients: A consensus statement of the American College of Chest Physicians. *Chest* 111:769, 1997.

Guirao X: Impact of the inflammatory reaction on intermediary metabolism and nutrition status. *Nutrition* 18:949, 2002.

Heslin MJ, Brennan MF: Advances in perioperative nutrition: Cancer. *World J Surg* 24:1477, 2000.

Zhou Y-P, Jiang Z-M, Sun Y-H, et al: The effect of supplemental enteral glutamine on plasma levels, gut function, and outcome in severe burns: A randomized, double-blind, controlled clinical trial. *J Parenter Enteral Nutr* 27:241, 2003.

2 | Fluid and Electrolyte Management of the Surgical Patient

Rosemary A. Kozar and Frederick A. Moore

Fluid and electrolyte management are paramount to the care of the surgical patient. Changes in both fluid volume and electrolyte composition occur preoperatively, intraoperatively, and postoperatively, and in response to trauma and sepsis.

BODY FLUIDS

Total Body Water

Water constitutes approximately 50–60 percent of total body weight. The relationship between total body weight and total body water (TBW) is primarily a reflection of body fat. As a result, young, lean males have a higher proportion of body weight as water than older adult or obese individuals. The highest percentage of TBW is found in newborns, with approximately 80 percent of their total body weight composed of water. This decreases to about 65 percent by 1 year of age and thereafter remains fairly constant.

Fluid Compartments

TBW is divided into two functional fluid compartments, the extracellular and intracellular. The extracellular fluid compartment comprises about one third of the TBW and the intracellular compartment the remaining two thirds. The extracellular water comprises 20 percent of the total body weight and is divided between plasma (5 percent of body weight) and interstitial fluid (15 percent of body weight).

Composition of Fluid Compartments

The extracellular fluid compartment is balanced between the principal cation—sodium and the principal anions—chloride and bicarbonate. The intracellular fluid compartment is composed primarily of the cations, potassium and magnesium, and of the anions, phosphate and proteins. Proteins add to the osmolality of the plasma and contribute to the balance of forces that determine fluid balance across the capillary endothelium. Water is distributed evenly throughout all fluid compartments of the body. Sodium, however, is confined to the extracellular fluid compartment, and because of its osmotic and electrical properties, it remains associated with water. Therefore, sodium-containing fluids are distributed throughout the extracellular fluid and add to the volume of both the intravascular and interstitial spaces.

Osmotic Pressure

The movement of water across a cell membrane depends primarily on osmosis. The principal determinants of osmolality are the concentrations of sodium,

32

glucose, and urea (blood urea nitrogen [BUN]): serum osmolality = 2 sodium + glucose/18 + BUN/2.8.

The osmolality of the intracellular and extracellular fluids is maintained between 290 and 310 mOsm in each compartment. Because cell membranes are permeable to water, any change in osmotic pressure in one compartment is accompanied by a redistribution of water until the effective osmotic pressure between compartments is equal.

CLASSIFICATION OF BODY FLUID CHANGES

Normal Exchange of Fluid and Electrolytes

Daily water losses for the average adult include about 1 L in urine, 250 mL in stool, and 600 mL as insensible losses. Insensible losses occur through both the skin (75 percent) and lungs (25 percent) and by definition is pure water. Insensible losses can be increased by fever, hypermetabolism, and hyperventilation. To clear the products of metabolism, the kidneys must excrete a minimum of 500–800 mL of urine per day, regardless of the amount of oral intake.

Disturbances in Fluid Balance

Extracellular volume deficit is the most common fluid disorder in surgical patients and can be either acute or chronic. Acute volume deficit is associated with cardiovascular and central nervous system (CNS) signs, although chronic deficits display tissue signs, such as a decrease in skin turgor and sunken eyes, in addition to cardiovascular and CNS signs (Table 2-1). Sodium concentration does not necessarily reflect volume status, and therefore may be high, normal, or low when a volume deficit is present. The most common etiology of volume deficit in surgical patients is a loss of gastrointestinal (GI) fluids from nasogastric suction, vomiting, diarrhea, or fistula. Additionally, sequestration secondary to soft-tissue injuries, burns, and intraabdominal processes such as peritonitis, obstruction, or prolonged surgery also can lead to volume deficits.

Extracellular volume excess may be iatrogenic or secondary to renal dysfunction, congestive heart failure, or cirrhosis. Both plasma and interstitial volumes are increased.

TABLE 2-1 Signs and Symptoms of Volume Disturbances

System	Volume deficit	Volume excess
Generalized	Weight loss Decreased skin turgor	Weight gain Peripheral edema
Cardiac	Tachycardia Orthostasis/hypotension Collapsed neck veins	Increased cardiac output Increased central venous pressure Distended neck veins Murmur
Renal	Oliguria Azotemia	
Gastrointestinal	Ileus	Bowel edema
Pulmonary		Pulmonary edema

Concentration Changes

Hyponatremia

A low serum sodium level occurs when there is an excess of extracellular water relative to sodium. Extracellular volume can be high, normal, or low. For most cases of hyponatremia, sodium concentration is decreased as a consequence of either sodium depletion or dilution. Dilutional hyponatremia frequently results from excess extracellular water and therefore is associated with a high extracellular volume status. Postoperative patients are particularly prone to increased secretion of antidiuretic hormone, which increases reabsorption of free water from the kidneys with subsequent volume expansion and hyponatremia. Physical signs of volume overload are usually absent and laboratory evaluation reveals hemodilution. Depletional causes of hyponatremia result from either a decreased intake or increased loss of sodium-containing fluids. Etiologies include decreased sodium intake, GI losses, or renal losses. Depletional hyponatremia often is accompanied by extracellular volume deficit.

Hyponatremia also can be seen with an excess of solute relative to free water, such as with untreated hyperglycemia or mannitol administration. When evaluating hyponatremia in the presence of hyperglycemia, the corrected sodium concentration should be calculated: for every 100-mg/dL increment in plasma glucose above normal the plasma sodium should decrease by 1.6 mEq/L. Lastly, extreme elevations in plasma lipids and proteins can cause pseudohyponatremia, because there is no true decrease in extracellular sodium relative to water.

Signs and symptoms of hyponatremia (Table 2-2) are dependent on the degree of hyponatremia and the rapidity with which it occurred. Clinical manifestations are primarily CNS in etiology and are related to cellular water intoxication and associated increases in intracranial pressure.

TABLE 2-2 Clinical Manifestations of Abnormalities in Serum Sodium

Body system	Hyponatremia
Central nervous system	Headache, confusion, hyper- or hypoactive deep tendon reflexes, seizures, coma, increased intracranial pressure
Musculoskeletal	Weakness, fatigue, muscle cramps/twitching
Gastrointestinal	Anorexia, nausea, vomiting, watery diarrhea
Cardiovascular	Hypertension and bradycardia if significant increases in intracranial pressure
Tissue	Lacrimation, salivation
Renal	Oliguria

Body system	Hypernatremia
Central nervous system	Restlessness, lethargy, ataxia, irritability, tonic spasms, delirium, seizures, coma
Musculoskeletal	Weakness
Cardiovascular	Tachycardia, hypotension, syncope
Tissue	Dry sticky mucous membranes, red swollen tongue, decreased saliva and tears
Renal	Oliguria
Metabolic	Fever

Hypernatremia

Hypernatremia results from either a loss of free water or a gain of sodium in excess of water. Like hyponatremia, it can be associated with an increased, normal, or decreased extracellular volume.

Hypervolemic hypernatremia usually is caused either by iatrogenic administration of sodium-containing fluids or mineralocorticoid excess as seen in hyperaldosteronism, Cushing's syndrome, and congenital adrenal hyperplasia. Urine sodium is typically greater than 20 mEq/L and urine osmolarity is greater than 300 mOsm/L. Normovolemic hypernatremia can be associated with renal (diabetes insipidus, diuretics, renal disease) or nonrenal (GI or skin) causes of water loss.

Lastly, hypovolemic hypernatremia can be because of either renal or nonrenal water loss. Renal causes include diabetes insipidus, osmotic diuretics, adrenal failure, and renal tubular diseases. The urine sodium concentration is less than 20 mEq/L and urine osmolarity is less than 300 to 400 mOsm/L. Nonrenal water loss can occur secondary to GI fluid losses or skin fluid losses such as fever or tracheotomies. Additionally, thyrotoxicosis can cause water loss as can the use of hypertonic glucose solutions for peritoneal dialysis. With nonrenal water loss, the urine sodium concentration is less than 15 mEq/L and the urine osmolarity is greater than 400 mOsm/L.

Symptoms of hypernatremia are rare until the serum sodium concentration exceeds 160 mEq/L. As symptoms are related to hyperosmolarity, CNS effects predominate (Table 2-2).

Composition Changes: Etiology and Diagnosis

Potassium Abnormalities

Although only 2 percent of the total body potassium is located within the extracellular compartment, this small amount is critical to cardiac and neuromuscular function.

Hyperkalemia. Hyperkalemia is caused by an excessive potassium intake, increased release of potassium from cells, or impaired excretion by the kidneys. Increased intake can be either from oral or intravenous supplementation, and from blood transfusions. Cell breakdown can release potassium in association with hemolysis, rhabdomyolysis, crush injuries, and GI hemorrhage. Acidosis can raise serum potassium levels by causing a shift of potassium ions to the extracellular compartment. Because aldosterone plays an important role in stimulating potassium secretion from the collecting ducts, any drug (like spironolactone and angiotensin-converting enzyme [ACE] inhibitors) that interferes with aldosterone activity inhibits potassium secretion. Impaired potassium excretion also occurs with renal insufficiency and renal failure.

Symptoms of hyperkalemia are primarily GI, neuromuscular, and cardiovascular. GI symptoms include nausea, vomiting, intestinal colic, and diarrhea; neuromuscular symptoms range from weakness to ascending paralysis to respiratory failure. Electrocardiogram (ECG) changes that may be seen with hyperkalemia include: peaked T waves, flattened P wave, prolonged PR interval (first-degree block), widened QRS complex, sine wave formation, and ventricular fibrillation.

Hypokalemia. Hypokalemia may be caused by inadequate intake, excessive renal excretion (hyperaldosteronism, medications such as diuretics that increase potassium excretion, or drugs such as penicillin that promote renal tubular loss of potassium), loss in GI secretions (direct loss of potassium in stool or renal potassium loss from vomiting or high nasogastric output), or intracellular shifts (as seen with metabolic alkalosis or insulin therapy). In cases in which potassium deficiency is because of magnesium depletion, potassium repletion is difficult unless hypomagnesemia is first corrected.

The symptoms of hypokalemia include ileus, constipation, weakness, fatigue, diminished tendon reflexes, paralysis, and cardiac arrest (pulseless electrical activity or asystole). ECG changes suggestive of hypokalemia include: U waves, T-wave flattening, ST-segment changes, and arrhythmias.

Magnesium Abnormalities

Hypermagnesemia. Hypermagnesemia is rare but can be seen with impaired renal function and excess intake in the form of total parenteral nutrition or magnesium-containing laxatives and antacids. Symptoms may be GI (nausea and vomiting), neuromuscular (weakness, lethargy, and decreased reflexes), or cardiovascular (hypotension and arrest). ECG changes are similar to those seen with hyperkalemia.

Hypomagnesemia. Hypomagnesemia results from poor intake (starvation, alcoholism, prolonged use of intravenous fluids, and total parenteral nutrition), increased renal excretion (alcohol, most diuretics, and amphotericin B), GI losses (diarrhea), malabsorption, acute pancreatitis, diabetic ketoacidosis, and primary aldosteronism.

Magnesium depletion is characterized by neuromuscular and CNS hyperactivity, and symptoms are similar to those of calcium deficiency, including hyperactive reflexes, muscle tremors, and tetany with a positive Chvostek's sign. Severe deficiencies can lead to delirium and seizures. ECG changes include: prolonged QT and PR intervals, ST-segment depression, flattening or inversion of P waves, Torsades de pointes, and arrhythmias. Hypomagnesemia can produce hypocalcemia and lead to persistent hypokalemia. When hypokalemia or hypocalcemia coexist with hypomagnesemia, magnesium should be aggressively replaced to assist in restoring potassium or calcium homeostasis.

Calcium Abnormalities

Although only approximately 50 percent of serum calcium is found in the ionized form, it is the ionized fraction that is responsible for neuromuscular stability. Total serum calcium is affected by albumin concentration, so that total serum calcium should be adjusted down by 0.8 mg/dL for every 1 g/dL decrease in albumin. Unlike changes in albumin, changes in pH will affect the ionized calcium concentration. Acidosis decreases protein binding, thereby increasing the ionized fraction of calcium.

Hypercalcemia. Primary hyperparathyroidism malignancy (associated bony metastasis or because of secretion of parathyroid hormone–related protein) accounts for most cases of symptomatic hypercalcemia. Symptoms of hypercalcemia include neurologic (depression, confusion, stupor, or coma), musculoskeletal (weakness and back and extremity pain), renal (polyuria and polydipsia as kidneys lose their ability to concentrate), and GI (anorexia, nausea, vomiting, constipation, abdominal pain, and weight loss). Cardiac symptoms include hypertension, cardiac arrhythmias, and a worsening of digitalis toxicity. ECG changes of hypercalcemia include shortened QT interval, prolonged PR and QRS intervals, increased QRS voltage T-wave flattening and widening, and AV block.

Hypocalcemia. Etiologies of hypocalcemia include pancreatitis, massive soft tissue infections such as necrotizing fasciitis, renal failure, pancreatic and small-bowel fistulas, hypoparathyroidism, toxic shock syndrome, abnormalities in magnesium, and tumor lysis syndrome. Additionally, transient hypocalcemia commonly occurs following removal of a parathyroid adenoma as atrophy of the remaining glands and avid bone uptake of calcium occurs. Hungry bone syndrome can develop postoperatively in secondary or tertiary hyperparathyroidism as bone is being rapidly remineralized, requiring high-dose calcium supplementation. Additionally, malignancies associated with increased osteoclastic activity such as breast and prostate cancer can lead to hypocalcemia from increased bone formation. Calcium precipitation with organic anions is also a cause of hypocalcemia, such as that seen with hyperphosphatemia (tumor lysis syndrome or rhabdomyolysis), pancreatitis (chelation with free fatty acids), or massive blood transfusion (citrate).

Asymptomatic hypocalcemia may occur with hypoproteinemia (normal ionized calcium), but symptoms can develop with alkalosis (decreased ionized calcium). Symptoms are neuromuscular and cardiac in origin, including paresthesias, muscle cramps, carpopedal spasm, stridor, tetany, and seizures. Patients will demonstrate hyperreflexia and positive Chvostek's and Trousseau's sign. Decreased cardiac contractility and heart failure also can accompany hypocalcemia, as do the following ECG changes: prolonged QT interval, T-wave inversion, heart block, and ventricular fibrillation.

Phosphorus Abnormalities

Hyperphosphatemia. Hyperphosphatemia can be because of decreased urinary excretion or increased intake or production of phosphorus. Most cases of hyperphosphatemia are seen in patients with impaired renal function. Hypoparathyroidism or hyperthyroidism also can decrease urinary excretion of phosphorus and thus lead to hyperphosphatemia. Increased release of endogenous phosphorus can be seen in association with cell destruction, such as with rhabdomyolysis, tumor lysis syndrome, hemolysis, sepsis, severe hypothermia, or malignant hyperthermia. Excessive phosphate administration (phosphorus-containing laxatives) also may lead to elevated phosphate levels. Most cases of hyperphosphatemia are asymptomatic, but significant hyperphosphatemia can lead to metastatic soft tissue calcium-phosphorus complexes.

Hypophosphatemia. Decreased intake can lead to hypophosphatemia and occurs with malnutrition or decreased GI absorption. Most cases are because of an intracellular shift of phosphorus as occurs in association with respiratory alkalosis, insulin therapy, refeeding syndrome, and hungry bone syndrome. Symptoms are related to adverse effects on the oxygen availability of tissue and to a decrease in high-energy phosphates and can be manifested as cardiac dysfunction or muscle weakness.

Acid-Base Balance

Compensation for acid-base derangements is either respiratory or metabolic. Changes in ventilation in response to metabolic abnormalities are mediated by

TABLE 2-3 Predicted Changes in Acid-Base Disorders

Disorder	Predicted change
Metabolic	
Metabolic acidosis	$Pco_2 = 1.5 \times HCO_3^- + 8$
Metabolic alkalosis	$Pco_2 = 0.7 \times HCO_3^- + 21$
Respiratory	
Acute respiratory acidosis	$\Delta pH = (Pco_2 - 40) \times 0.008$
Chronic respiratory acidosis	$\Delta pH = (Pco_2 - 40) \times 0.003$
Acute respiratory alkalosis	$\Delta pH = (40 - Pco_2) \times 0.008$
Chronic respiratory alkalosis	$\Delta pH = (40 - Pco_2) \times 0.017$

hydrogen-sensitive chemoreceptors. Acidosis stimulates the chemoreceptors to increase ventilation whereas alkalosis decreases their activity and thus decreases ventilation. The kidneys provide compensation for respiratory abnormalities by either increasing or decreasing bicarbonate reabsorption for respiratory acidosis or alkalosis, respectively. Unlike the prompt change in ventilation that occurs with metabolic abnormalities, the compensatory response in the kidneys to respiratory abnormalities is delayed. Table 2-3 lists the predicted compensatory changes in response to metabolic or respiratory derangements. If the expected change in pH is exceeded, then a mixed acid-base abnormality may be present.

Metabolic Derangements

Metabolic acidosis. In evaluating a patient with metabolic acidosis, first measure the anion gap (AG), which is an index of unmeasured anions: AG = [Na] − [Cl + HCO$_3$]. The normal AG is less than 12 mmol/L.

Metabolic acidosis with an increased AG occurs from either exogenous acid ingestion (ethylene glycol, salicylate, or methanol) or endogenous acid production of β-hydroxybutyrate and acetoacetate in ketoacidosis, lactate in lactic acidosis, or organic acids in renal insufficiency. One of the most common causes of severe metabolic acidosis in surgical patients is lactic acidosis. With shock, lactate is produced as a by-product of inadequate tissue perfusion. The treatment is to restore perfusion with volume resuscitation rather than to attempt to correct the abnormality with exogenous bicarbonate. The administration of bicarbonate for the treatment of metabolic acidosis is controversial and the overzealous administration of bicarbonate can lead to metabolic alkalosis, which shifts the oxyhemoglobin dissociation curve to the left, interfering with oxygen unloading at the tissue level. An additional disadvantage is that sodium bicarbonate can actually exacerbate intracellular acidosis. There are commercially available buffers that do not increase CO_2 production and avoid intracellular acidosis, including Carbicarb and tromethamine. Carbicarb is an equimolar mixture of sodium bicarbonate and sodium carbonate that combines with hydrogen ions, producing bicarbonate rather than CO_2. This buffer, however, is not yet available for use in humans. An alternative buffer is tris-hydroxymethyl aminomethane (THAM). THAM is excreted by the kidneys and therefore should be used with caution in patients with renal insufficiency. Side effects include hyperkalemia and hypoglycemia.

Metabolic acidosis with a normal anion gap results from either acid administration (HCl or NH_4^+) or a loss of bicarbonate from GI sources such as diarrhea, fistulas, ureterosigmoidostomy, or from renal loss. The bicarbonate loss is accompanied by a gain of chloride, thus the AG remains unchanged.

Metabolic alkalosis. Surgical patients with pyloric obstruction (seen in infants with pyloric stenosis or adults with duodenal ulcer disease) can develop hypochloremic, hypokalemic, or metabolic alkalosis. Unlike vomiting associated with an open pylorus, vomiting with an obstructed pylorus results only in the loss of gastric fluid, which is high in chloride and hydrogen, and thus a hypochloremic alkalosis. Initially the urinary bicarbonate level is high to compensate for the alkalosis. Hydrogen ion reabsorption also ensues with an accompanied potassium ion excretion. Additionally, in response to the volume deficit, aldosterone-mediated sodium reabsorption is accompanied by potassium excretion. The resulting hypokalemia leads to the excretion of hydrogen ions in the face of alkalosis, a paradoxic aciduria. Treatment includes replacement of the volume deficit with isotonic saline and potassium once adequate urine output is ensured.

Respiratory Derangements

Respiratory acidosis. This condition is associated with the retention of CO_2 secondary to decreased alveolar ventilation. As compensation is primarily renal, it is a delayed response. Treatment is directed at the underlying cause and at measures to ensure adequate ventilation.

Respiratory alkalosis. Most cases of respiratory alkalosis are acute in nature and secondary to alveolar hyperventilation. Etiologies include pain or anxiety, neurologic disorders (meningitis, trauma), drugs (such as salicylates), fever or gram-negative bacteremia, thyrotoxicosis, or hypoxemia. Acute hypocapnia can cause an uptake of potassium and phosphate into cells and increased binding of calcium to albumin, leading to symptomatic hypokalemia, hypophosphatemia, and hypocalcemia, with subsequent arrhythmias, paresthesias, muscle cramps, and seizures. Treatment should be directed at the underlying cause, but also may require direct treatment of the hyperventilation.

FLUID AND ELECTROLYTE THERAPY

Parenteral Solutions

The type of fluid administered depends on the patient's volume status and the type of concentration or compositional abnormality present. Both lactated Ringer's solution and normal saline are considered isotonic and are useful in replacing GI losses and extracellular volume deficits. Lactated Ringer's solution is slightly hypotonic in that it contains 130 mEq of sodium, which is balanced by 109 mEq of chloride and 28 mEq of lactate. Lactate is more stable than bicarbonate and is converted into bicarbonate in the liver following infusion. Sodium chloride is mildly hypertonic, containing 154 mEq of sodium that is balanced by 154 mEq of chloride, which may lead to a hyperchloremic metabolic acidosis. It is an ideal solution, however, for correcting volume deficits associated with hyponatremia, hypochloremia, and metabolic alkalosis.

The less concentrated sodium solutions, such as 0.45 percent sodium chloride, are useful to replace ongoing GI losses and for maintenance fluid therapy in the postoperative period. The addition of 5 percent dextrose (50 g of dextrose per liter) supplies 200 kcal/L, and it always is added to solutions containing less than 0.45 percent sodium chloride to maintain osmolality and thus prevent lysis of red blood cells (RBCs) that may occur with rapid infusion of hypotonic fluids.

Alternative Resuscitative Fluids

A number of alternative solutions for volume expansion and resuscitation are now available. Hypertonic saline solutions (3.5 percent and 5 percent) are used for correction of severe sodium deficits whereas a 7.5 percent solution has been used as a treatment modality in patients with closed-head injuries and as a potential resuscitative fluid. Renewed interest in this solution has occurred with recent evidence of its antiinflammatory and immunomodulatory properties.

Colloids have long been debated as effective volume expanders compared to isotonic crystalloids. Because of their molecular weight, they are confined to the intravascular space and their infusion results in more efficient plasma volume expansion. However, under conditions of severe hemorrhagic shock, capillary membrane permeability increases, permitting colloids to enter the interstitial space, which can worsen edema and impair tissue oxygenation. There are four major types of colloids available: albumin, dextrans, hetastarch, and gelatins, which are described by their molecular weight and size. Colloid solutions with smaller size particles and lower molecular weights exert a greater oncotic effect, but are retained within the circulation for a shorter period of time than larger and higher molecular weight colloids.

Albumin (molecular weight 70,000) is prepared from pooled human plasma and is available as either a 5 or 25 percent solution. Because it is a derivative of blood, it can be associated with allergic reactions. Albumin has been shown to induce renal failure and impair pulmonary function when used for resuscitation of hemorrhagic shock.

Dextrans are glucose polymers produced by bacteria grown on sucrose media and are available as either 40,000 (dextran 40) or 70,000 (dextran 70) molecular-weight solutions. They lead to initial volume expansion because of their osmotic effect, but are associated with alterations in blood viscosity. Thus dextrans are used primarily to lower blood viscosity rather than as volume expanders. Dextrans have, however, been used in association with hypertonic saline to help maintain intravascular volume.

Hydroxyethyl starch solutions are another group of alternative plasma expanders. Hetastarch is the only hydroxyethyl starch approved for use in the United States. It has a limited role in massive resuscitation because of its associated coagulopathy and hyperchloremic acidosis. Hextend is a modified, balanced, high-molecular-weight hydroxyethyl starch also available in the United States that is suspended in a lactate-buffered solution, rather than in saline. Unlike Hetastarch, no adverse effects on coagulation with Hextend other than the known effects of hemodilution have been demonstrated. Hextend has not been tested in massive resuscitation, and not all clinical studies show consistent results.

Gelatins are the fourth group of colloids and are produced from bovine collagen. The two major types are urea-linked gelatin and succinylated gelatin (modified fluid gelatin, Gelofusine). Gelofusine has been used abroad with mixed results and is currently not approved for use in the United States.

Correction of Life-Threatening Electrolyte Abnormalities

Sodium

Hypernatremia. Treatment of hypernatremia entails treatment of the associated water deficit. In hypovolemic patients, volume should be restored with normal saline. Once adequate volume status has been achieved, the water deficit is replaced using a hypotonic fluid. To estimate the water deficit required to correct hypernatremia use the following formula:

$$\text{Water deficit (L)} = \frac{\text{serum sodium} - 140}{140} \times \text{TBW}$$

Estimate TBW as 50 percent of lean body mass in men and 40 percent in women.

The rate of fluid administered should be titrated to achieve a decrease in serum sodium of no more than 1 mEq/h and 12 mEq/L for treatment of acute hypernatremia. Even slower correction should be undertaken with chronic hypernatremia (0.7 mEq/L/h), as overly rapid correction can lead to cerebral edema and herniation. The type of fluid depends on the severity and ease of correction. Caution also should be exercised when using 5 percent dextrose in water to avoid overly rapid correction.

Hyponatremia. In patients with normal renal function, symptomatic hyponatremia does not occur until the serum sodium level is greater than or equal to 120 mEq/L. If neurologic symptoms are present, 3 percent normal saline should be used to increase the sodium by no more than 1 mEq/L/h until the serum sodium level reaches 130 mEq/L or neurologic symptoms are improved. Correction of asymptomatic hyponatremia should increase the sodium level by no more than 0.5 mEq/L to a maximum increase of 12 mEq/L per day, and even slower in chronic hyponatremia. The rapid correction of hyponatremia can lead to pontine myelinolysis, with seizures, weakness/paresis, akinetic movements, and unresponsiveness, and may result in permanent brain damage and death.

Potassium

Hyperkalemia. The goal is to reduce total body potassium, shift potassium from extracellular to intracellular, and to protect cells from the effects of increased potassium. All patients should have exogenous sources of potassium discontinued. Potassium can be removed from the body with a cation-exchange resin, such as Kayexalate, which binds potassium in exchange for sodium. Measures should also include shifting potassium intracellularly with glucose and bicarbonate. Glucose alone will cause a rise in insulin secretion, but in the acutely ill this response may be blunted and therefore both glucose and insulin are recommended. Circulatory overload and hypernatremia may result from the administration of Kayexalate and bicarbonate. When ECG changes are present, calcium chloride or calcium gluconate (5–10 mL of 10 percent solution) should also be administered to counteract the myocardial effects of hyperkalemia. It should be used cautiously in patients on digitalis as digitalis toxicity may occur. Dialysis should be considered when conservative measures fail.

Hypokalemia. Oral repletion is adequate for mild and asymptomatic hypokalemia. If intravenous repletion is required, usually no more than 10–20 mEq/L/h is advisable in an unmonitored setting. This can be increased to 40 mEq/L/h when accompanied by ECG monitoring, and even higher if cardiac arrest is imminent from a malignant arrhythmia. Caution should be exercised when oliguria or impaired renal function is coexistent.

Magnesium

Hypermagnesemia. Treatment consists of measures to withhold exogenous sources of magnesium, correct volume deficit and acidosis if present. To manage symptoms, calcium chloride (5–10 mL) will antagonize the cardiovascular effects. If elevated levels or symptoms persist, dialysis is indicated.

Hypomagnesemia. Correction can be oral or intravenous. For severe deficits (<1.0 mEq/L) or symptoms, administer 1–2 g of magnesium sulfate intravenously over 15 min or over 2 min if secondary to torsades de pointes (irregular ventricular arrhythmia). Simultaneous calcium gluconate will counteract the adverse side effects of a rapidly rising magnesium level and correct hypocalcemia, which is frequently associated with hypomagnesemia.

Calcium

Hypercalcemia. Treatment is required for symptomatic hypercalcemia which usually occurs when the serum level exceeds 12 mg/dL. The initial treatment is aimed at repleting the associated volume deficit and then inducing a brisk diuresis with normal saline.

Hypocalcemia. Symptomatic hypocalcemia should be treated with intravenous 10 percent calcium gluconate until serum levels are 7–9 mg/dL. Associated deficits in magnesium, potassium, and pH also must be corrected. Hypocalcemia will be refractory to treatment if hypomagnesemia is not first corrected.

Phosphorus

Hyperphosphatemia. Either phosphate binders (sucralfate or aluminum-containing antacids) or calcium acetate tablets (if hypocalcemia is present) can be used as treatment modalities. Dialysis is reserved for patients with renal failure.

Hypophosphatemia. Both oral and intravenous supplementation are available.

Preoperative Fluid Therapy

Maintenance fluids can be calculated using the following formula:

For the first 0 to 10 kg	Give 100 mL/kg per day
For the next 10 to 20 kg	Give an additional 50 mL/kg per day
For weight > 20 kg	Give 20 mL/kg per day

Preoperative volume deficits also should be considered in patients presenting with obvious GI loss and in patients with poor oral intake. Less obvious are third-space losses that occur with GI obstruction, peritoneal or bowel inflammation, ascites, crush injuries, burns, and severe soft-tissue infections.

Once a volume deficit is diagnosed, prompt fluid replacement should be instituted, usually with an isotonic crystalloid. If symptomatic electrolyte abnormalities accompany volume deficit, the abnormality should be corrected to the extent that the acute symptom is relieved prior to surgical intervention.

Intraoperative Fluid Therapy

With the induction of anesthesia, compensatory mechanisms are lost and hypotension will develop if volume deficits are not appropriately corrected prior to surgery. In addition to measured blood loss, open abdominal surgeries are associated with continued third-space losses. Large soft tissue wounds, complex fractures, and burns also must be considered.

Postoperative Fluid Therapy

Therapy should be based on the patient's current estimated volume status and projected ongoing fluid losses. Both preexisting deficits and third space losses should be included along with the maintenance fluids. Initial fluids should be isotonic and then can be changed to 0.45 percent saline with added dextrose after the initial 24–48 hr. If normal renal function and adequate urine output are present, potassium may be added to the intravenous fluids.

Special Considerations in the Postoperative Patient

Volume excess is a common disorder in the postoperative period. The earliest sign of volume overload is weight gain. The average postoperative patient who is not receiving nutritional support should lose approximately one-quarter to one-half pound per day. Peripheral edema may not necessarily be associated with volume overload, as overexpansion of total extracellular fluid may exist in association with a deficit in the circulating plasma volume.

Volume deficits also can be encountered in surgical patients if preoperative losses were not completely corrected, intraoperative losses were underestimated, or postoperative losses were greater than appreciated. In most cases of volume deficit, replacement with an isotonic fluid will be sufficient.

ELECTROLYTE ABNORMALITIES IN SPECIFIC SURGICAL PATIENTS

Neurologic Patients

Syndrome of Inappropriate Secretion of Antidiuretic Hormone

Syndrome of inappropriate secretion of antidiuretic hormone (SIADH) can occur following head injury or surgery to the CNS, but it also is seen with drugs (such as morphine, nonsteroidals, and oxytocin) and in a number of pulmonary (pneumonia, abscess, and tuberculosis) and endocrine disease states (hypothyroidism and glucocorticoid deficiency), and malignancies (most notably small-cell cancer of the lung, but also pancreatic carcinoma, thymoma, and Hodgkin' disease). It should be considered in patients who are euvolemic and hyponatremic with elevated urine sodium (> 20 mEq/L) and urine osmolality. Antidiuretic hormone (ADH) stimulation is considered inappropriate in that it is not caused by osmotic or volume-related conditions. Correction of the underlying problem should be attempted. In most cases, restriction of free water will correct the problem. The goal is to achieve net water balance, but to avoid volume depletion that compromises renal function. Furosemide also can be used to induce free water loss.

Diabetes Insipidus

Diabetes insipidus (DI) is a disorder of antidiuretic hormone stimulation and is manifested by dilute urine in the face of hypernatremia. Central DI results from a defect in antidiuretic hormone secretion, and nephrogenic DI from a defect in end-organ responsiveness to ADH. Central DI is frequently seen in association with pituitary surgery or injury (closed-head injury or anoxic encephalopathy).

Nephrogenic DI occurs in association with hypokalemia, radiocontrast dye, and drugs such as aminoglycosides and amphotericin. In patients tolerating oral intake, volume status is usually normal as thirst stimulates increased intake. Volume depletion can occur in patients incapable of oral intake. The diagnosis can be confirmed by documenting an increase in urine osmolality in response to a period of water deprivation. If mild, free water replacement is all that is needed. In more severe cases, vasopressin (5 units subcutaneously) can be added.

Cerebral Salt Wasting

Cerebral salt wasting is a diagnosis of exclusion that occurs in patients with a cerebral lesion and renal wasting of sodium and chloride with no other identifiable cause. Natriuresis in a patient with a contracted extracellular volume should prompt the diagnosis. Hyponatremia occurs as a secondary event, differentiating it from SIADH.

Malnourished Patients: Refeeding Syndrome

This is a potentially lethal condition that can occur with rapid and excessive feeding of patients with severe underlying malnutrition because of starvation, alcoholism, delayed enteral or parenteral support, anorexia nervosa, or massive weight loss in obese patients. With refeeding, a shift in metabolism from fat to carbohydrate stimulates insulin release, resulting in the cellular uptake of phosphate, magnesium, potassium, and calcium. Because of blunted basal insulin secretion, severe hyperglycemia may also arise. Symptoms include cardiac arrhythmias, confusion, respiratory failure, and even death. To prevent refeeding syndrome, caloric repletion should be instituted slowly.

Acute Renal Failure Patients

There are a number of fluid and electrolyte abnormalities specific to patients with acute renal failure. Oliguric renal failure requires close monitoring of serum potassium. Treatment should be instituted early and may need to include dialysis. Hyponatremia is common in established renal failure and derives from the breakdown of proteins, carbohydrates, and fats, and administered free water. Dialysis is required for severe hyponatremia. Hypocalcemia, hypermagnesemia, and hyperphosphatemia also are associated with acute renal failure. Metabolic acidosis is commonly seen with renal failure, as the kidneys lose their ability to clear acid by-products. Bicarbonate may be used but dialysis is frequently required.

Cancer Patients

Hypocalcemia can be seen following removal of a thyroid or parathyroid tumor or following a central neck dissection by damage to the parathyroid glands. Hungry bone syndrome produces hypocalcemia following parathyroid surgery for secondary or tertiary hyperparathyroidism when calcium is rapidly taken up by bones. Prostate and breast cancer can result in increased osteoblastic activity that increases bone formation thereby decreasing serum calcium. Hypomagnesemia is a side effect of ifosfamide and cisplatin therapy. Hypophosphatemia can be seen with hyperparathyroidism as phosphorus reabsorption is decreased, although oncogenic osteomalacia increases urinary excretion of phosphorus. Acute hypophosphatemia can occur as rapidly proliferating malignant cells take up phosphorus in acute leukemia or from hungry bone syndrome following parathyroidectomy. Tumor lysis syndrome or bisphosphonates can also cause hyperphosphatemia.

Malignancy is the most common etiology of hypercalcemia. Bone destruction from bony metastasis is seen with breast or renal cell cancer, but also can occur with multiple myeloma. With Hodgkin and non-Hodgkin lymphoma, hypercalcemia results from increased calcitriol formation, which in turn increases absorption of calcium from both the GI tract and bone. Humoral hypercalcemia of malignancy is a common cause of hypercalcemia in cancer patients. As parathyroid-related protein is secreted, it binds to parathyroid receptors, stimulating calcium resorption from bone and decreasing renal excretion of calcium. The treatment of hypercalcemia of malignancy should begin with saline volume expansion and then a loop diuretic. A variety of drugs also are available. Bisphosphonates (etidronate and pamidronate) inhibit bone resorption and osteoclastic activity. They act slowly (within 48 hr) but last for up to 15 days. Calcitonin also is effective by inhibiting bone resorption and increasing renal excretion of calcium. It acts quickly (2–4 hr), but its use is limited by the development of tachyphylaxis. Corticosteroids may decrease tachyphylaxis and can be used alone to treat hypercalcemia. Gallium nitrates are potent inhibitors of bone resorption. They display a long duration of action but can cause nephrotoxicity. Mithramycin blocks osteoclastic activity but can be associated with liver, renal, and hematologic abnormalities, and therefore its use is limited to the treatment of Paget disease of the bone. For patients in whom hypercalcemia is severe and refractory, or who are unable to tolerate volume expansion (because of pulmonary edema or congestive heart failure), dialysis is an option.

Suggested Readings

Bushinsky DA, Monk RD: Calcium. *Lancet* 352:306, 1998.

European Resuscitation Council: Part 8. Advanced challenges in resuscitation. Section 1: Life-threatening electrolyte abnormalities. *Resuscitation* 46:253, 2000.

Gluck SL: Acid-base. *Lancet* 352:474, 1998.

Jonge E, Levi M: Effects of different plasma substitutes on blood coagulation: A comparative review. *Crit Care Med* 291:1261, 2001.

Kapoor M, Chan G: Fluid and electrolyte abnormalities. *Crit Care Clin* 17:571, 2001.

Lucas CE: The water of life: A century of confusion. *J Am Coll Surg* 192:86, 2001.

Miller M: Syndromes of excess antidiuretic hormone release. *Crit Care Clin* 17:11, 2001.

Moore FA, McKinley BA, Moore EE: The next generation in shock resuscitation. *Lancet* 363:1988, 2004.

Rotstein OD: Novel strategies for immunomodulation after trauma: Revisiting hypertonic saline as a resuscitative strategy for hemorrhagic shock. *J Trauma* 49:580, 2000.

Singh S, Bohn D, Carlotti APCP: Cerebral salt wasting: Truths, fallacies, theories, and challenges. *Crit Care Med* 30:2575, 2002.

3 | Hemostasis, Surgical Bleeding, and Transfusion

Seymour I. Schwartz

BIOLOGY OF HEMOSTASIS

Hemostasis is a complex process that prevents or terminates blood loss from the intravascular space, provides a fibrin network for tissue repair, and ultimately, removes the fibrin when it is no longer needed. Four major physiologic events participate in this process.

Vascular Constriction

This is the initial response to injury, even at the capillary level. Vasoconstriction begins prior to platelet adherence as a reflex response to various stimuli. It is subsequently linked to platelet plug and fibrin formation. The vasoconstrictors thromboxane A_2 (TXA_2) and serotonin are released during platelet aggregation. Local physical factors, including the extent and orientation of injury to the blood vessel, also may influence the degree of bleeding.

Platelet Function

Platelets normally number 150,000–400,000/mm^3, with an average life span of 10 days. They contribute to hemostasis by two processes. *Primary hemostasis* is a reversible process that is not affected by heparin administration. Platelets adhere to the subendothelial collagen of disrupted vascular tissue. This process requires von Willebrand factor (vWF), a protein congenitally absent in von Willebrand disease. The platelets expand and initiate a release reaction, recruiting additional platelets. The resulting aggregate forms a plug, sealing the disrupted vessel. ADP, TXA_2, and serotonin are the prominent mediators in this process. Opposing these mediators are prostacyclin, endothelium-derived relaxing factor (EDRF), and prostaglandin E_2 (PGE_2), which are vasodilators and inhibit aggregation. The second process by which platelets act, which is irreversible, involves *fibrinogen-dependent degranulation*. Platelet factor 3 is released, acting at several points in the coagulation cascade. Platelet-derived mediators also influence the subsequent fibrinolytic process.

Coagulation

Coagulation refers to a cascade of zymogen activation that ultimately results in the cleavage of fibrinogen to insoluble fibrin that stabilizes the platelet plug. The *intrinsic* pathway is initiated by exposure of coagulation factors to subendothelial collagen at the site of vascular damage. The *extrinsic* pathway is activated by tissue factors (glycoproteins). The two pathways converge at activated factor X (Xa), which, in turn, cleaves prothrombin to thrombin. All the coagulation factors except thromboplastin, factor VIII, and Ca^{2+} are synthesized in the liver. Factors II, VII, IX, and X are dependent on vitamin K.

Fibrinolysis

The patency of blood vessels is maintained by lysis of fibrin deposits and by antithrombin III (which neutralizes several of the proteases in the complement cascade). Fibrinolysis depends on plasmin, which is derived from the precursor plasma protein plasminogen. Plasmin lyses fibrin, the fragments of which interfere with platelet aggregation.

TESTS OF HEMOSTASIS AND BLOOD COAGULATION

The most valuable part of this assessment is a careful history and physical examination. Specific questions should be asked to determine if there was a prior history of transfusion, untoward bleeding during a major surgical procedure, any bleeding after a minor operation, any spontaneous bleeding, or any family history of bleeding difficulties.

The history should include a list of medications and underlying medical disorders (e.g., malignancy, liver or kidney disease) that may affect normal hemostasis. Laboratory studies also provide important clues of hemostatic ability.

Platelet count. Spontaneous bleeding rarely occurs with a platelet count of greater than $50,000/mm^3$. Platelet counts in this range are usually adequate to provide hemostasis following trauma or surgical procedures if other hemostatic factors are normal.

Bleeding time. This assesses the interaction between platelets and a damaged blood vessel and the formation of a platelet plug. Deficiencies in platelet number, platelet function, or some coagulation factors will yield a prolonged bleeding time.

Prothrombin time (PT). This test measures the extrinsic pathway of blood coagulation. Thromboplastin, a procoagulant, is added with calcium to an aliquot of citrated plasma, and the clotting time is determined. The test will detect deficiencies in factors II, V, VII, and X or fibrinogen.

Partial thromboplastin time (PTT). A screen of the intrinsic clotting pathway, the PPT will determine abnormalities in factors VIII, IX, XI, and XII. This test has a high sensitivity; only extremely mild deficiencies in factor VIII or IX will be missed. The PTT, used in conjunction with the PT, can help place a clotting defect in the first or second stage of the clotting process.

Thrombin time (TT). This screen detects abnormalities in fibrinogen and will detect circulating anticoagulants and inhibitors of anticoagulation.

Tests of fibrinolysis. Fibrin degradation products (FDPs) can be measured immunologically. Falsely positive results (> 10 mg/mL) may be seen in liver disease, kidney disease, thromboembolic disorders, and pregnancy.

EVALUATION OF THE SURGICAL PATIENT AS A HEMOSTATIC RISK

Preoperative Evaluation of Hemostasis

Rapaport has suggested four levels of concern (given the patient's history and the proposed operation) that should dictate the extent of preoperative testing.

Level I: The history is negative, and the procedure is relatively minor (e.g., breast biopsy or hernia repair). No screening tests are recommended.

Level II: The history is negative and a major operation is planned, but significant bleeding is not expected. A platelet count, blood smear, and PTT are recommended to detect thrombocytopenia, circulating anticoagulant, or intravascular coagulation.

Level III: The history is suggestive of defective hemostasis, and the patient is to undergo a procedure in which hemostasis may be impaired, such as operations using pump oxygenation or cell savers. This level also applies to situations where minimal postoperative bleeding could be detrimental, such as intracranial operations. A platelet count and bleeding time should be done to assess platelet function. A PT and PTT should be used to evaluate coagulation, and the fibrin clot should be checked to screen for abnormal fibrinolysis.

Level IV: These patients have a known hemostatic defect or a highly suggestive history. The same tests suggested for level III should be checked, and a hematologist should be consulted. In case of an emergency, assessment of platelet aggregation and a TT are indicated to detect dysfibrinogenemia or a circulating anticoagulant.

Patients with liver disease, obstructive jaundice, kidney failure, or malignancy should have the platelet count, PT, and PTT checked preoperatively.

CONGENITAL DEFECTS IN HEMOSTASIS

Classical Hemophilia (Factor VIII Deficiency)

Classical hemophilia (hemophilia A) is a sex-linked recessive disorder in which there is a failure to synthesize normal factor VIII. The incidence is approximately 1 in 10,000 to 1 in 15,000 persons. Spontaneous mutations account for almost 20 percent of cases. Clinical expression of the disease is highly variable.

The severity of the clinical manifestations is related to the degree of factor deficiency. Spontaneous bleeding and severe complications are the rule when virtually no factor VIII activity can be detected. Concentrations of approximately 5 percent of normal may produce no spontaneous bleeding, yet there may be severe bleeding with trauma or surgical therapy.

Significant bleeding is usually first noted when the subject is a toddler. At that time the child may be subject to bleeding into joints, epistaxis, and hematuria. Intracranial bleeding, associated with trauma in half the cases, accounts for 25 percent of deaths. Hemarthrosis is the most characteristic orthopedic problem. Retroperitoneal bleeding or intramural intestinal hematoma also may occur, causing nausea, vomiting, or crampy abdominal pain. Upper gastrointestinal examination may demonstrate uniform thickening of mucosal folds ("picket fence" or "stack of coins" appearance).

Treatment. The plasma concentration of factor VIII necessary to provide hemostatic integrity is normally quite small (as little as 2–3 percent). Once serious bleeding begins, however, much higher levels (30 percent) of activity are required to achieve hemostasis. The half-life of factor VIII is 8–12 h; after an initial transfusion, its half-life is approximately 4 h. One unit of factor VIII is considered to be the amount present in 1 mL normal plasma. Cryoprecipitate concentrates of factor VIII contain 9.6 units/mL. The amount of activity suggested to be repleted varies according to the severity of the lesion. To calculate the amount of factor VIII needed: 1 unit/kg of body weight will yield approximately a 2 percent rise in activity. Half this amount is subsequently administered every 4–6 h to maintain a safe level.

Wet-frozen cryoprecipitate is preferred for replacement in patients with mild hemophilia, since it provides the lowest risk of viral hepatitis. Factor VIII concentrates are preferred in severe disease. In mild hemophilia A and mild von Willebrand disease, dDAVP, a synthetic derivative of vasopressin, has been used to produce a dose-dependent increase in all factor VIII activities and release plasminogen activator. Following major surgical treatment of a hemophiliac, transfusion replacement of factor VIII should be continued for at least 10 days. Even relatively minor procedures should be supplemented with factor VIII to achieve levels above 25–30 percent.

Christmas Disease (Factor IX Deficiency)

Factor IX deficiency is clinically indistinguishable from factor VIII deficiency. It is also inherited as an X-linked recessive disease with variable expression. The clinically severe form of the disease has a level of less than 1 percent of normal activity. Half the patients belong to this group.

Treatment. All patients require substitution therapy when major or minor surgery is performed. Current therapy involves the administration of factor IX concentrate. The initial half-life is shorter than that of factor VIII; its steady-state half-life is much longer (18–40 h). A number of factor IX concentrates are available. Konyne contains 10–60 units/mL of factor IX but has been associated with thromboembolic complications. Newer preparations have had additional clotting factors removed, and the incidence of thromboembolic events is lower. During severe hemorrhage, treatment should be directed to achieving levels of 20–50 percent of normal for the first 3–5 days and then maintaining a plasma level of 20 percent for approximately 10 days. Plasma activity should be monitored during the course of therapy. The development of antibodies occurs in about 10 percent of patients.

von Willebrand Disease

von Willebrand disease occurs in approximately 1 in 1000 individuals. The clinically severe form of the disease occurs much less frequently. This disorder is usually transmitted as an autosomal dominant trait, but recessive inheritance may occur. The disease is characterized by abnormal vWF and a decrease in the level of factor VIII:C (procoagulant) activity, which corrects the clotting abnormality in hemophilia A. Characteristically, patients with this disease have a prolonged bleeding time, but this is less consistent than the factor VIII:C reduction. A given patient may have an abnormal bleeding time on one occasion and a normal bleeding time an another. Ristocetin fails to cause platelet aggregation in about 70 percent of patients with this disease.

Clinical manifestations. Clinical manifestations are usually minimal until trauma or surgery makes them apparent. Spontaneous bleeding is often limited to the skin or mucous membranes. Epistaxis and menorrhagia are relatively common. Serious bleeding following minor surgery is not uncommon.

Treatment. Treatment is directed at correcting the bleeding time and factor VIII R:vWF (the von Willebrand factor). Only cryoprecipitate is effective (10–40 units/kg q12h). Replacement therapy should start 1 day before surgery, and the duration of therapy should be the same as that described for classic hemophilia.

ACQUIRED HEMOSTATIC DEFECTS

Platelet Abnormalities

Thrombocytopenia, the most common abnormality of hemostasis in the surgical patient, may be due to massive blood loss, medications, or a variety of disease processes. Heparin-induced thrombocytopenia is notable for being reported in 0.6 percent of patients receiving heparin and is thought to be immune mediated. The lowest platelet counts occur after 4–15 days of initial therapy and after 2–9 days in patients receiving subsequent courses.

Abnormalities in platelet number also may be accompanied by abnormalities in function. Uremia affects bleeding time and platelet aggregation. Defects in platelet aggregation and secretion occur in patients with thrombocytopenia, polycythemia, or myelofibrosis.

Treatment. A count greater than $50,000/mm^3$ requires no specific therapy. Thrombocytopenia due to acute alcoholism, drug effect, or viral infection generally will correct within 1–3 weeks. Severe thrombocytopenia may be due to vitamin B_{12} or folate deficiency. This condition is usually responsive to the appropriate nutrient therapy. In patients with idiopathic thrombocytopenia or lupus erythematosus, a platelet count of less than $50,000/mm^3$ may respond to steroid therapy or plasmapheresis. Splenectomy alone should not be performed to correct thrombocytopenia associated with splenomegaly due to portal hypertension.

Prophylactic platelet administration in not routinely required following massive blood transfusions. One unit of platelets contains approximately 5.5×10^5 platelets and would be expected to increase the circulating platelet count by $10,000/mn^3$ in a 70-kg man. In patients refractory to standard platelet transfusion, the use of human leukocyte antigen (HLA)–compatible platelets has proved effective.

Acquired Hypofibrinogenemia-Defibrination Syndrome (Fibrinogen Deficiency)

This is rarely an isolated defect because deficiencies in factors II, VI, and VIII and platelets usually accompany this state. Most patients with acquired hypofibrinogenemia suffer from disseminated intravascular coagulation (DIC). DIC is caused by the introduction of thromboplastic material into the circulation. This syndrome has been seen with a retained dead fetus, separation of the placenta, and amniotic fluid embolism. Defibrination has been observed in association with extracorporeal circulation, disseminated carcinoma, lymphoma, and a variety of infections (including both gram-negative and gram-positive sepsis).

It is difficult to distinguish DIC from secondary fibrinolysis because both show prolongation in the TT, PTT, and PT. The combination of a low platelet count, a positive plasma protamine test, reduced fibrinogen, and increased FDPs (taken in the context of the patient's underlying disease) is highly suggestive of the syndrome.

The prime consideration in treatment is relieving the underlying medical problem. The use of intravenous fluids is indicated to maintain volume. If there is active bleeding, hemostatic factors should be replaced with fresh frozen plasma, cryoprecipitate, and platelet concentrates as needed. Most studies show that heparin is not indicated in acute forms of DIC but is indicated for purpura fulminans or venous thromboembolism. Fibrinolytic inhibitors may be used to block the accumulation of FDPs. They should not be used without prior effective antithrombotic treatment with heparin.

Fibrinolysis

The acquired hypofibrinogenemic state in the surgical patient also may be due to pathologic fibrinolysis. This can be seen in patients with metastatic prostatic carcinoma, shock, sepsis, hypoxia, neoplasia, cirrhosis, and portal hypertension. A reduction in fibrinogen and factors V and VIII is seen, since they all are substrates for the enzyme plasmin. Thrombocytopenia is not an accompaniment of the purely fibrinolytic state. Treatment of the underlying disorder (if identified) is warranted. ϵ-Aminocaproic acid (EACA), an inhibitor of fibrinolysis, also may be useful.

Myeloproliferative Diseases

Thrombocytopenia can be treated by standard therapy for the underlying disease. Ideally, the hematocrit should be kept below 48 percent and the platelet count less than $400,000/mm^3$. In a study with polycythemic patients undergoing major surgical procedures, 46 percent had complications perioperatively, including a 16 percent mortality (in 80 percent of whom the disease was not under control). Hemorrhage is the most common complication in this group, followed by thrombosis and infection. Preoperative use of antiplatelet agents (e.g., aspirin, dipyridamole) and anticoagulants has been suggested in these patients.

LIVER DISEASE

Advanced liver disease may result in decreased synthesis of the coagulation factors II, V, VII, X, and XIII. Also, there may be increased fibrinolysis due to the failure of the liver to clear plasminogen activators.

ANTICOAGULATION AND BLEEDING

Spontaneous bleeding may be a complication of anticoagulant therapy, with an incidence proportional to the degree of anticoagulation. Surgical therapy may be necessary in patients receiving anticoagulant therapy. The risk of thrombotic complications is increased when anticoagulant therapy is suddenly discontinued and may be due to a "rebound phenomenon." When the clotting time is less than 25 min in the heparinized patient or when the PT is less than 1.5 times control, reversal of anticoagulant therapy may not be necessary. If an emergent surgical procedure is necessary, anticoagulation can be reversed. Heparin can be reversed with protamine sulfate (1 mg protamine per 1000 units heparin). Bleeding is infrequently related to hypoprothrombinemia if the prothrombin concentration is greater than 15 percent. Warfarin can be discontinued several days before surgery. If emergency surgery is required, parenteral vitamin K_1 can be used. Reversal may take up to 6 h, so fresh frozen plasma may be needed.

LOCAL HEMOSTASIS

The goal of local hemostasis is to prevent the flow of blood from incised or transected blood vessels. The techniques may be classified as mechanical, thermal, or chemical.

Mechanical

The oldest mechanical device to effect closure of a bleeding point or to prevent blood from entering an area of disruption is digital pressure. The finger has the advantage of being the least traumatic means of hemostasis. Diffuse bleeding from multiple transected vessels may be controlled by mechanical techniques, including direct pressure over the bleeding area, pressure at a distance, or generalized pressure. Direct pressure is preferable and is not attended by the danger of tissue necrosis associated with a tourniquet. Gravitational suits have been used to create generalized pressure.

The hemostat represents a temporary mechanical device to stem bleeding. Ligature replaces a hemostat as a permanent method of hemostasis of a single vessel.

Thermal

Cautery effects hemostasis by denaturation of proteins, which results in coagulation of large areas of tissue. Cooling also has been applied to control bleeding and acts by increasing the local intravascular hematocrit and decreasing the blood flow by vasoconstriction. Cryogenic surgery uses temperatures between -20 ($-4°F$) and $-180°C$ ($-292°F$).

Chemical

Some chemicals act as vasoconstrictors, others are procoagulants, and others have hygroscopic properties that aid in plugging disrupted blood vessels. Epinephrine is a vasoconstrictor, but because of its considerable absorption and systemic effects, it is generally used only on areas of mucosal oozing. Local hemostatic materials include gelatin foam, cellulose, and micronized collagen.

TRANSFUSION

Approximately 14 percent of all inpatient operations include blood transfusions. Blood provides transportation of oxygen to meet the body's metabolic demands and removes carbon dioxide.

Replacement Therapy

Banked whole blood is stored at $4°C$ ($39.2°F$) and has a storage life of up to 35 days. Up to 70 percent of transfused erythrocytes remain in the circulation 24 h after transfusion; 60 days after transfusion, approximately 50 percent of the cells will survive. Banked blood is rarely indicated.

Banked blood is a poor source of platelets. Factors II, VII, IX, and XI are stable in banked blood. Factor VIII rapidly deteriorates during storage. During the storage of whole blood, red cell metabolism and plasma protein degradation result in chemical changes in the plasma, including increases in lactate, potassium, and ammonia and a decrease in pH.

Typing and cross-matching. Serologic compatibility is routinely established for donor and recipient A, B, O, and Rh groups. As a rule, Rh-negative recipients should be transfused only with Rh-negative blood. In the patient receiving repeated transfusions, serum drawn less than 48 h before cross-matching should be used. Emergency transfusion can be performed with group O blood. If it is known that the prospective recipient is group AB, group A blood is preferable.

Fresh whole blood. This term refers to blood given within 24 h of its collection.

Packed red cells and frozen red cells. Packed cells have approximately 70 percent of the volume of whole blood. Use of frozen cells markedly reduces the risk of infusing antigens to which the patients have previously been sensitized. The red cell viability is improved, and the ATP and 2,3-diphosphoglycerate (2,3-DPG) concentrations are maintained.

Platelet concentrates. Platelet transfusions should be used for thrombocytopenia due to massive blood loss replaced with stored blood, thrombocytopenia due to inadequate production, and qualitative platelet disorders. Isoantibodies are demonstrated in about 5 percent of patients after 1–10 transfusions, 20 percent after 10–20 transfusions, and 80 percent after more than 100 transfusions. HLA-compatible platelets minimize this problem.

Fresh frozen plasma and volume expanders. Factors V and VIII require plasma to be fresh or freshly frozen to maintain activity. The risk of hepatitis is the same as that of whole blood or packed red cells. In emergency situations, lactated Ringer solution can be administered in amounts two to three times the estimated blood loss. Dextran or lactated Ringer solution with albumin can be used for rapid plasma expansion.

Concentrates. Antihemophilic concentrates are prepared from plasma with a potency of 20–30 times that of fresh frozen plasma. The simplest factor VIII concentrate is plasma cryoprecipitate. Albumin also may be used as a concentrate (25 g has the osmotic equivalent of 500 mL), with the advantage of being hepatitis-free.

INDICATIONS FOR REPLACEMENTS OF BLOOD OR ITS ELEMENTS

Volume replacement. The most common indication for blood transfusion in the surgical patient is the restoration of circulating blood volume. The hematocrit can be used to estimate blood loss, but up to 72 h is required to establish a new equilibrium after a significant blood loss.

In the normal person, reflex mechanisms allow the body to accommodate up to moderate-size blood losses. Significant hypotension develops only after about a 40 percent loss of blood volume.

Loss of blood during operation may be estimated by weighing the sponges (representing about 70 percent of the true loss). For patients who have normal preoperative blood values, Table 3-1 shows replacement recommendations.

Improvement in oxygen-carrying capacity. Transfusion should be performed only if treatment of the underlying anemia does not provide adequate blood counts for the patient's clinical condition. In general, raising hemoglobin levels above 7–8 g/dL provides little additional benefit. A whole blood substitute, Fluosol-DA, provides oxygen-carrying capacity in the absence of blood products.

TABLE 3-1 Blood Replacement Recommendations

Percentage of total blood volume loss	Replacement
20	Crystalloid solutions
20–50	Crystalloids and red cell concentrates (RBCs)
Above 50	Crystalloids, RBCs, and albumin or plasma
Continued bleeding above 50	Crystalloids, RBCs, fresh frozen plasma, and albumin or plasma

Replacement of clotting factors. Supplemental platelets or clotting factors may be required in the treatment of certain hemorrhagic conditions. Fresh frozen plasma is used in the treatment of a coagulopathy in patients with liver disease, but its efficacy is very low. The rigid use of PT and PTT to anticipate the effect of fresh frozen plasma is not justified. If fibrinogen is required, a plasma level greater than 100 mg/dL should be maintained.

Massive transfusion. This term refers to a single transfusion of greater than 2500 or 5000 mL over a 24-h period. A number of problems may accompany the use of massive transfusion, including thrombocytopenia, impaired platelet function, deficiency in factors V, VIII, and XI, and the increased acid load of stored blood products.

With large transfusions, a heater may be used to warm the blood, since hypothermia may result in decreased cardiac output and an acidosis.

Complications (Table 3-2)

Hemolytic reactions from blood group incompatibilities are usually manifest by a sensation of warmth and pain along the site of transfusion, flushing in the face, pain in the lumbar region, and constricting pain in the chest. The patient additionally may experience chills, fever, and respiratory distress. In anesthetized patients, two signs of reaction are abnormal bleeding and continued hypotension in the face of adequate replacement. The morbidity and mortality of hemolytic reactions are high and include oliguria, hemoglobinuria, hypotension, jaundice, nausea, and vomiting. The transfusion should be stopped immediately if a transfusion reaction is suspected. Samples of the recipient and donor blood should be sent for comparison with pretransfusion samples. Renal function should be monitored following a suspected transfusion reaction. Renal toxicity is affected by the rate of urinary excretion and the pH. Alkalinization of the urine prevents precipitation of hemoglobin.

TABLE 3-2 Complications of Transfusion

Complication	Risk per unit blood product
Infectious	
Hepatitis C	1:3300
Human immunodeficiency virus	1:40,000–1:225,000
Human T-lymphocyte virus (I and II)	1:50,000
Hepatitis B	1:200,000
Immunologic	
Fever, chills, urticaria	1:50–1:100
Hemolytic reaction	1:1000
Fatal hemolytic reaction	1:100,000

Febrile and allergic reactions. These occur in approximately 1 percent of transfusions. They appear as urticaria and fever occurring within 60–90 min of the start of the transfusion. Occasionally, the allergic reaction is severe enough to cause anaphylactic shock. Treatment consists of antihistamines, epinephrine, and steroids, depending on the severity of the reaction.

Transmission of disease. Posttransfusion viral hepatitis is the most common fatal complication of blood transfusion. Other viral illnesses may be transmitted (e.g., cytomegalovirus, human immunodeficiency virus, etc.), as well as several bacterial species.

Additional, less frequent complications include

Embolism: Intravenous volumes of less than 200 mL are generally well tolerated by normal adults.
Volume overload: The patient's risk is related to underlying cardiac reserve.
Bacterial sepsis: Gram-negative organisms and *Pseudomonas* predominate.
Thrombophlebitis: More commonly seen with prolonged infusions.

Suggested Readings

Schwartz SI: Hemostasis, Surgical Bleeding, and Transfusion, chap. 3 in *Principles of Surgery,* 7th ed.

4 | Shock

Andrew B. Peitzman, Brian G. Harbrecht, and Timothy R. Billiar

Shock may be defined as inadequate delivery of oxygen and nutrients to maintain normal tissue and cellular function. The resultant cellular injury is initially reversible; if the hypoperfusion is severe enough and prolonged, the cellular injury becomes irreversible. The clinical manifestations of shock are the result of stimulation of the sympathetic and neuroendocrine stress responses, inadequate oxygen delivery, and end-organ dysfunction. Inadequate oxygen delivery is presumed to be the pathologic defect in shock. The management of the patient in shock is empiric; securing the airway and restoration of vascular volume and tissue perfusion often occur prior to definitive diagnosis.

The failure of physiologic systems to buffer the organism against external forces results in organ and cellular dysfunction, what is clinically recognized as shock.

Six types of shock have been described: hypovolemic, septic (vasodilatory), neurogenic, cardiogenic, obstructive, and traumatic shock. Hypovolemic shock, the most common type, results from loss of circulating blood volume. This may result from loss of whole blood (hemorrhagic shock), plasma, interstitial fluid (bowel obstruction), or a combination. Vasogenic shock results from decreased resistance within capacitance vessels, usually seen in sepsis. Neurogenic shock is a form of vasogenic shock in which spinal cord injury or spinal anesthesia causes vasodilatation because of acute loss of sympathetic vascular tone. Cardiogenic shock results from failure of the heart as a pump, as in arrhythmias or acute heart failure. Obstructive shock, caused by pulmonary embolism or tension pneumothorax, results in depressed cardiac output, which results from mechanical impediment to circulation rather than a primary cardiac failure. In traumatic shock, the soft-tissue injury and long-bone fractures that occur in association with blood loss yield an upregulation of proinflammatory mediators that is more complex than simple hemorrhagic shock. The clinical dilemma faced in a patient with shock is that the etiology may not be immediately apparent. Inadequate treatment results in ongoing hypoperfusion and activation of inflammatory mediators. Thus, treatment of the patient in shock is initially empiric, although the underlying etiology of the shock state is investigated.

Core principles in the early management of the critically ill or injured patient include: (1) definitive control of the airway, (2) prompt control of active hemorrhage (generally in the operating room, as delay in control of ongoing bleeding increases mortality), (3) volume resuscitation with red blood cells and crystalloid solution while operative control of bleeding is achieved (operating room resuscitation), (4) unrecognized or inadequately corrected hypoperfusion increases morbidity and mortality, and (5) care that excessive fluid resuscitation is monitored as it may exacerbate bleeding. Thus, both inadequate and uncontrolled volume resuscitation are harmful.

PATHOPHYSIOLOGY

Shock is defined as tissue hypoperfusion that is insufficient to maintain normal aerobic metabolism. The initial insult, whether hemorrhage, injury, or infection, initiates both a neuroendocrine and inflammatory mediator response. The magnitude of the physiologic response is proportional to both the degree and the duration of the shock. Although the quantitative nature of the physiologic response in shock will vary with the etiology of shock, the qualitative nature of the response to shock is similar, with common pathways in all types of shock. Persistent hypoperfusion will result in hemodynamic derangements, end-organ dysfunction, cell death, and death of the patient if treated late or inadequately. Hemorrhagic shock most often is seen clinically; bleeding and resuscitation produce a "whole body" ischemia-reperfusion injury. The physiologic responses to hypovolemia are directed at preservation of perfusion to the heart and brain. To this end, vasoconstriction occurs, fluid excretion is curtailed, and fluid is shifted into the intravascular space. The major mechanisms achieving this response are: (1) prompt increase in cardiac contractility and peripheral vascular tone via the autonomic nervous system, (2) hormonal response to preserve salt and intravascular volume, and (3) changes in the local microcirculation to regulate regional blood flow. With substantial physiologic compensatory mechanisms for small volume blood loss, predominantly through the neuroendocrine response, hemodynamics may be maintained. This represents the compensated phase of shock. With continued hypoperfusion often not apparent clinically, cell death and tissue injury are ongoing and the decompensation phase of shock evolves. At this point in treatment, the cellular dysfunction can be reversed with appropriate volume resuscitation. If volume loss continues or volume resuscitation is insufficient, a vicious physiologic cycle will develop. With persistent hypoperfusion with low cardiac output, regional tissue hypoperfusion and progressive tissue and microcirculatory changes induce cardiovascular decompensation. This progression to the irreversible phase of shock often is insidious and recognized only in retrospect. Sufficient tissue injury and cell death have occurred to this point that continued volume resuscitation fails to reverse the process. Ultimately, even massive quantities of fluid resuscitation and vasopressors fail to maintain adequate blood pressure. As discussed later in this chapter, this vasodilatory response probably represents the common late phase of all forms of shock, regardless of etiology.

NEUROENDOCRINE RESPONSE

The goal of the neuroendocrine response to hemorrhage is to maintain perfusion to the heart and the brain, even at the expense of other organ systems. Peripheral vasoconstriction occurs and fluid excretion is inhibited. The mechanisms include autonomic control of peripheral vascular tone and cardiac contractility, hormonal response to stress and volume depletion, and local microcirculatory mechanisms that are organ specific and regulate regional blood flow. The initial stimulus is loss of circulating blood volume in hemorrhagic shock. The magnitude of the neuroendocrine response is based on both the volume of blood lost and the rate at which it is lost.

Afferent Signals

Afferent impulses transmitted from the periphery are processed within the central nervous system (CNS) and activate the reflexive effector responses or efferent impulses. These effector responses are designed to expand plasma volume, maintain peripheral perfusion and tissue oxygen delivery, and restore homeostasis. Stimuli that can produce the neuroendocrine response include hypocolemia, pain, hypoxemia, hypercarbia, acidosis, infection, changes in temperature, emotional arousal, or hypoglycemia. The sensation of pain from injured tissue is transmitted via the spinothalamic tracts, resulting in activation of the hypothalamic-pituitary-adrenal axis, and activation of the autonomic nervous system (ANS) to induce direct sympathetic stimulation of the adrenal medulla to release catecholamines.

Baroreceptors in the atria of the heart become activated with low-volume hemorrhage or mild reductions in right atrial pressure. Receptors in the aortic arch and carotid bodies respond to alterations in pressure or stretch of the arterial wall, responding to larger reductions in intravascular volume or pressure. These receptors normally inhibit induction of the ANS. When activated, these baroreceptors diminish their output, thus disinhibiting the effect of the ANS. The autonomic nervous system then increases its output, principally via sympathetic activation at the vasomotor centers of the brain stem, producing centrally mediated constriction of peripheral vessels.

Chemoreceptors in the aorta and carotid bodies are sensitive to changes in oxygen tension, H^+ ion concentration, and CO_2 levels. Stimulation of the chemoreceptors results in vasodilatation of the coronary arteries, slowing of the heart rate, and vasoconstriction of the splanchnic and skeletal circulation.

Efferent Signals

Cardiovascular Response

Hemorrhage results in diminished venous return to the heart and decreased cardiac output. This is compensated by increased cardiac heart rate and contractility, and venous and arterial vasoconstriction. Stimulation of sympathetic fibers innervating the heart leads to activation of β_1-adrenergic receptors that increase heart rate and contractility in this attempt to increase cardiac output. Increased myocardial oxygen consumption occurs as a result of the increased workload; thus, myocardial oxygen supply must be maintained or myocardial dysfunction will develop.

Direct sympathetic stimulation of the peripheral circulation via the activation of α_1-adrenergic receptors on arterioles induces vasoconstriction and causes a compensatory increase in systemic vascular resistance and blood pressure. Selective perfusion to tissues occurs because of regional variations in arteriolar resistance, with blood shunted away from less essential organ beds such as the intestine, kidney, and skin. In contrast, the brain and heart have autoregulatory mechanisms that attempt to preserve their blood flow despite a global decrease in cardiac output. Direct sympathetic stimulation also induces constriction of venous vessels, decreasing the capacitance of the circulatory system and accelerating blood return to the central circulation.

Increased sympathetic output induces catecholamine release from the adrenal medulla. Catecholamine levels peak within 24–48 hours of injury, and then return to baseline. The majority of the circulating epinephrine is produced by the adrenal medulla, whereas norepinephrine is derived from synapses of the sympathetic nervous system. Catecholamine effects on peripheral tissues include stimulation of hepatic glycogenolysis and gluconeogenesis to increase circulating glucose availability to peripheral tissues, an increase in skeletal muscle glycogenolysis, suppression of insulin release, and increased glucagon release.

Hormonal Response

The stress response includes activation of the autonomic nervous system as discussed above, and activation of the hypothalamic-pituitary-adrenal axis. Shock stimulates the hypothalamus to release corticotropin-releasing hormone, that results in the release of adrenocorticotropic hormone (ACTH) by the pituitary. ACTH subsequently stimulates the adrenal cortex to release cortisol. Cortisol acts synergistically with epinephrine and glucagon to induce a catabolic state. Cortisol stimulates gluconeogenesis and insulin resistance, resulting in hyperglycemia and muscle cell protein breakdown and lipolysis to provide substrates for hepatic gluconeogenesis. Cortisol causes retention of sodium and water by the nephrons of the kidney. In the setting of severe hypovolemia, ACTH secretion occurs independently of cortisol negative feedback inhibition.

The renin-angiotensin system is activated in shock. Decreased renal artery perfusion, β-adrenergic stimulation, and increased renal tubular sodium concentration cause the release of renin from the juxtaglomerular cells. Renin catalyzes the conversion of angiotensinogen (produced by the liver) to angiotensin I, which is then converted to angiotensin II by angiotensin-converting enzyme (ACE) produced in the lung. Although angiotensin I has no significant functional activity, angiotensin II is a potent vasoconstrictor of both splanchnic and peripheral vascular beds, and also stimulates the secretion of aldosterone, ACTH, and antidiuretic hormone (ADH). Aldosterone, a mineralocorticoid, acts on the nephron to promote reabsorption of sodium, and as a consequence, water. Potassium and hydrogen ions are lost in the urine in exchange for sodium.

The pituitary also releases vasopressin or ADH in response to hypovolemia, changes in circulating blood volume sensed by baroreceptors and left atrial stretch receptors, and increased plasma osmolality detected by hypothalamic osmoreceptors. Epinephrine, angiotensin II, pain, and hyperglycemia increase production of ADH. ADH acts on the distal tubule and collecting duct of the nephron to increase water permeability, decrease water and sodium losses, and preserve intravascular volume. Also known as arginine vasopressin, ADH acts as a potent mesenteric vasoconstrictor, shunting circulating blood away from the splanchnic organs during hypovolemia. Vasopressin also increases hepatic gluconeogenesis and increases hepatic glycolysis.

Circulatory Homeostasis

Preload

At rest, the majority of the blood volume is within the venous system. Venous return to the heart generates ventricular end-diastolic wall tension, a major determinant of cardiac output. With decreased arteriolar inflow, there is active contraction of the venous smooth muscle and passive elastic recoil in the thin-walled systemic veins. This increases venous return to the heart, thus maintaining ventricular filling.

Ventricular Contraction

The Frank-Starling curve describes the force of ventricular contraction as a function of its preload. This relationship is based on force of contraction being determined by initial muscle length. Intrinsic cardiac disease will shift the

Frank-Starling curve and alter mechanical performance of the heart. Additionally, cardiac dysfunction has been demonstrated experimentally in burns and in hemorrhagic, traumatic, and septic shock.

Afterload

Afterload is the force that resists myocardial work during contraction. Arterial pressure is the major component of afterload influencing the ejection fraction. This vascular resistance is determined by precapillary smooth muscle sphincters. Blood viscosity will also increase vascular resistance. As afterload increases in the normal heart, stroke volume can be maintained by increases in preload. In shock, with decreased circulating volume and therefore diminished preload, this compensatory mechanism to sustain cardiac output is impeded.

Cellular Effects

As oxygen tension within cells decreases, there is a decrease in oxidative phosphorylation and the generation of adenosine triphosphate (ATP) slows or stops. When oxygen delivery is impaired so severely that mitochondrial respiration cannot be sustained, the state is called "dysoxia." As oxidative phosphorylation slows, the cells shift to anaerobic glycolysis that allows for the production of ATP from the breakdown of cellular glycogen. Under aerobic conditions, pyruvate, the end-product of glycolysis, is fed into the Krebs cycle for further oxidative metabolism. Under hypoxic conditions, the mitochondrial pathways of oxidative catabolism are impaired, and pyruvate is instead converted into lactate. The accumulation of lactic acid and inorganic phosphates is accompanied by a reduction in pH, resulting in intracellular metabolic acidosis.

Decreased intracellular pH (intracellular acidosis) can alter the activity of cellular enzymes, lead to changes in cellular gene expression, impair cellular metabolic pathways, and impede cell membrane ion exchange. Acidosis also leads to changes in cellular calcium (Ca2+) metabolism and Ca2+-mediated cellular signaling, which alone can interfere with the activity of specific enzymes and cell function. These changes in the normal cell function may progress to cellular injury or cell death.

As cellular ATP is depleted under hypoxic conditions, the activity of the membrane Na+, K+-ATPase slows, and thus the maintenance of cellular membrane potential and cell volume is impaired. Na+ accumulates intracellularly, whereas K$^+$ leaks into the extracellular space. The net gain of intracellular sodium is accompanied by a gain in intracellular water and the development of cellular swelling. This influx is associated with a reduction in extracellular fluid volume. The changes in cellular membrane potential impair a number of cellular physiologic processes that are dependent on the membrane potential, such as myocyte contractility, cell signaling, and the regulation of intracellular Ca2+ concentrations. Once intracellular organelles such as lysosomes or cell membranes rupture, the cell will undergo death by necrosis.

Apoptosis has been detected in trauma patients with ischemia-reperfusion injury, in which both lymphocyte and intestinal epithelial cell apoptosis occur in the first 3 hours of injury. The intestinal mucosal cell apoptosis may compromise bowel integrity and lead to translocation of bacteria and endotoxins into the portal circulation during shock. Lymphocyte apoptosis also has been hypothesized to contribute to the immune suppression that is observed in trauma patients.

Tissue hypoperfusion and cellular hypoxia result not only in intracellular acidosis, but also in systemic metabolic acidosis as metabolic by-products of anaerobic glycolysis exit the cells. The systemic changes in acid/base status may lag behind changes at the tissue level. In the setting of acidosis, the oxyhemoglobin dissociation curve is shifted toward the right. The decreased affinity of hemoglobin in erythrocytes for oxygen results in increased O_2 release and increased tissue extraction of oxygen. Additionally, hypoxia stimulates the production of erythrocyte 2, 3-diphosphoglycerate (2, 3-DPG), further contributing to the right shift of the oxyhemoglobin dissociation curve, promoting O_2 availability to the tissues during shock.

In addition to induction of changes in cellular metabolic pathways, shock also induces changes in cellular gene expression. The DNA binding activity of a number of nuclear transcription factors is altered by hypoxia and the production of oxygen radicals or nitrogen radicals that are produced at the cellular level by shock. Expression of other gene products such as heat-shock proteins, vascular endothelial growth factor (VEGF), inducible nitric oxide synthase (iNOS), and cytokines also is clearly increased by shock. Many of these shock-induced gene products, such as cytokines, have the ability themselves to subsequently alter gene expression in specific target cells and tissues. The involvement of multiple pathways emphasizes the complex, integrated, and overlapping nature of the response to shock.

Microcirculation

Shock induces profound changes in tissue microcirculation that are thought to contribute to organ function, organ dysfunction, and the systemic consequences of severe shock. These changes have been studied most extensively in models of sepsis and hemorrhage. After hemorrhage, larger arterioles vasoconstrict, most likely because of sympathetic stimulation, whereas smaller, distal arterioles dilate, presumably because of local mechanisms. Furthermore, flow at the capillary level is heterogeneous, with endothelial cell swelling and the aggregation of leukocytes producing diminished capillary perfusion in some vessels both during shock and following resuscitation. In sepsis, similar changes in microcirculatory function can also be demonstrated. Regional differences in blood flow can be demonstrated after proinflammatory stimuli, and the microcirculation in many organs is heterogeneous; blood flow is heterogenous between and within organ systems. In hemorrhagic shock, correction of hemodynamic parameters and oxygen delivery and consumption generally restores tissue oxygenation. In contrast, regional tissue dysoxia often persists in sepsis, despite restoration of oxygen delivery and consumption variables. Whether this defect in oxygen extraction is the result of regional hypoxia or a defect in the pathways of mitochondrial respirations is not resolved. Shunting of oxygen from the microcirculation has been proposed as a possible etiology of the regional dysoxia seen in sepsis, despite adequate oxygen delivery.

The decreases in capillary perfusion and blood flow result in diminished capillary hydrostatic pressure. The changes in hydrostatic pressure promote an influx of fluid from the extravascular or extracellular space into the capillaries to increase circulating volume. However, these changes are associated with further loss of intracellular fluid volume because of increased cellular swelling. Resuscitation with volumes of fluid sufficient to restore the extracellular fluid deficit are associated with improved outcome after shock.

Capillary occlusion from endothelial cell swelling and neutrophil sludging and adherence may prevent restoration of capillary flow after adequate resuscitation, and is termed no-reflow. The nonperfused capillary beds further compound the ischemic injury. Neutrophil sludging in the capillaries with adherence to endothelial cells results in release of proinflammatory mediators by these cells. Neutrophil depletion in animals subjected to hemorrhagic shock produces fewer capillaries with no-reflow and lower mortality.

IMMUNE AND INFLAMMATORY RESPONSE

Alterations in the activity of the innate host immune system can be responsible for both the development of shock (distributive or septic shock following severe infection), and the pathophysiologic sequelae of shock such as the proinflammatory changes seen following hemorrhage or multisystem trauma. When these predominantly paracrine mediators gain access to the systemic circulation, they can induce a variety of metabolic changes that are collectively referred to as the host inflammatory response. Understanding of the intricate, redundant, and interrelated pathways that comprise the inflammatory response to shock continues to expand. Despite limited understanding of how many therapeutic interventions impact the host response to illness, inappropriate or excessive inflammation appears to be an essential event in the development of acute respiratory distress syndrome (ARDS), multiple organ dysfunction syndrome (MODS), and posttraumatic immunosuppression that can prolong recovery.

The immune response to shock encompasses the elaboration of mediators with both proinflammatory and antiinflammatory properties. Furthermore, new mediators, new relationships between mediators, and new functions of known mediators are continually being identified. As new pathways are uncovered, understanding of the immune response to injury and the potential for therapeutic intervention by manipulating the immune response following shock will expand. What seems clear at present, however, is that the innate immune response can help restore homeostasis, or if it is excessive, promote cellular and organ dysfunction.

Multiple mediators have been implicated in the host immune response to shock. It is likely that some of the most important mediators have yet to be discovered, and the roles of many known mediators have not been defined. A comprehensive description of all of the mediators and their complex interactions is beyond the scope of this chapter (see Chapter 1 for a comprehensive review of the inflammatory mediators).

CELLULAR HYPOPERFUSION

Hypoperfused cells and tissues experience what has been termed oxygen debt. The oxygen debt is the deficit in tissue oxygenation over time that occurs during shock. When oxygen delivery is limited, oxygen consumption can be inadequate to match the metabolic needs of cellular respiration, creating a deficit in oxygen requirements at the cellular level. The measurement of oxygen deficit uses calculation of the difference between the estimated oxygen demand and the actual value obtained for oxygen consumption. Under normal circumstances, cells can "repay" the oxygen debt during reperfusion. The magnitude of the oxygen debt correlates with the severity and duration of hypoperfusion. Surrogate values for measuring oxygen debt include base deficit and lactate levels.

FORMS OF SHOCK

Hemorrhagic or Hypovolemic Shock

The most common cause of shock in the surgical or trauma patient is loss of circulating volume from hemorrhage. Acute blood loss results in reflexive decreased baroreceptor stimulation from stretch receptors in the large arteries, resulting in decreased inhibition of vasoconstrictor centers in the brain stem, increased chemoreceptor stimulation of vasomotor centers, and diminished output from atrial stretch receptors. These changes increase vasoconstriction and peripheral arterial resistance. Hypovolemia also induces sympathetic stimulation, leading to epinephrine and norepinephrine release, activation of the renin-angiotensin cascade, and increased vasopressin release. Peripheral vasoconstriction is prominent, although lack of sympathetic effects on cerebral and coronary vessels and local autoregulation promote maintenance of cardiac and CNS blood flow.

Diagnosis

Treatment of shock is initially empiric. The airway must be secured and volume infusion for restoration of blood pressure initiated while the search for the cause of the hypotension is pursued. Shock in a trauma patient and postoperative patient should be presumed to be because of hemorrhage until proven otherwise. The clinical signs of shock may be evident with an agitated patient, including cool clammy extremities, tachycardia, weak or absent peripheral pulses, and hypotension. Such apparent clinical shock results from at least 25–30 percent loss of the blood volume. However, substantial volumes of blood may be lost before the classic clinical manifestations of shock are evident. Thus when a patient is significantly tachycardiac or hypotensive, this represents both significant blood loss and physiologic decompensation. The clinical and physiologic response to hemorrhage has been classified according to the magnitude of volume loss. Loss of up to 15 percent of the circulating volume (700–750 mL for a 70-kg patient) may produce little in terms of obvious symptoms, although loss of up to 30 percent of the circulating volume (1.5 L) may result in mild tachycardia, tachypnea, and anxiety. Hypotension, marked tachycardia [pulse > 110–120 beats per minute (bpm)], and confusion may not be evident until more than 30 percent of the blood volume has been lost; loss of 40 percent of circulating volume (2 L) is immediately life-threatening, and generally requires operative control of bleeding. Young healthy patients with vigorous compensatory mechanisms may tolerate larger volumes of blood loss while manifesting fewer clinical signs despite the presence of significant peripheral hypoperfusion. These patients may maintain a near-normal blood pressure until a precipitous cardiovascular collapse occurs. Older adult patients may be taking medications that either promote bleeding (e.g., warfarin or aspirin), or mask the compensatory responses to bleeding (e.g., β blockers). Additionally, atherosclerotic vascular disease, diminishing cardiac compliance with age, inability to elevate heart rate or cardiac contractility in response to hemorrhage, and overall decline in physiologic reserve decrease the older adult patient's ability to tolerate hemorrhage.

In management of trauma patients, understanding the patterns of injury of the patient in shock will help direct the evaluation and management. Identifying the sources of blood loss in patients with penetrating wounds is relatively simple because potential bleeding sources will be located along the known or suspected path of the wounding object. Patients with penetrating injuries who are in shock usually require operative intervention. Patients who suffer multisystem injuries from blunt trauma have multiple sources of potential hemorrhage. Blood loss sufficient to cause shock is generally of a large volume, and there are a limited number of sites that can harbor sufficient extravascular blood volume to induce hypotension (e.g., external, intrathoracic, intraabdominal, retroperitoneal, and long bone fractures). In the nontrauma patient, the gastrointestinal tract must always be considered as a site for blood loss. Substantial blood loss externally may be suspected from prehospital medical reports documenting a substantial blood loss at the scene of an accident, history of massive blood loss from wounds, visible brisk bleeding, or presence of a large hematoma adjacent to an open wound. Injuries to major arteries or veins with associated open wounds may cause massive blood loss rapidly. Direct pressure must be applied and sustained to minimize ongoing blood loss. Persistent bleeding from uncontrolled smaller vessels can, over time, precipitate shock if inadequately treated.

When major blood loss is not immediately visible, internal (intracavitary) blood loss should be suspected. Each pleural cavity can hold 2–3 L of blood and can therefore be a site of significant blood loss. Diagnostic and therapeutic tube thoracostomy may be indicated in unstable patients based on clinical findings and clinical suspicion. In a more stable patient, a chest radiograph may be obtained to look for evidence of hemothorax. Major retroperitoneal hemorrhage typically occurs in association with pelvic fractures, which is confirmed by pelvic radiography in the resuscitation bay. Intraperitoneal hemorrhage is probably the most common source of blood loss inducing shock. The physical exam for detection of substantial blood loss or injury is insensitive and unreliable; large volumes of intraperitoneal blood may be present before physical exam findings are apparent. Findings with intraabdominal hemorrhage include abdominal distension, abdominal tenderness, or visible abdominal wounds. Hemodynamic abnormalities generally stimulate a search for blood loss prior to the appearance of obvious abdominal findings. Adjunctive tests are essential in the diagnosis of intraperitoneal bleeding; intraperitoneal blood may be rapidly identified by diagnostic ultrasound or diagnostic peritoneal lavage.

Treatment

Control of ongoing hemorrhage is an essential component of the resuscitation of the patient in shock. As mentioned above, treatment of hemorrhagic shock is instituted concurrently with diagnostic evaluation to identify a source. Patients who fail to respond to initial resuscitative efforts should be assumed to have ongoing active hemorrhage from large vessels and require prompt operative intervention. The appropriate priorities in these patients are to (1) secure the airway, (2) control the source of blood loss, and (3) intravenous volume resuscitation. Identifying the body cavity harboring active hemorrhage will help focus operative efforts; however, because time is of the essence, rapid treatment is essential and diagnostic laparotomy or thoracotomy may be indicated. The actively bleeding patient cannot be resuscitated until control of ongoing hemorrhage is achieved.

Patients who respond to initial resuscitative efforts, but then deteriorate hemodynamically, frequently have injuries that require operative intervention. The magnitude and duration of their response will dictate whether diagnostic maneuvers can be performed to identify the site of bleeding. However, hemodynamic deterioration generally denotes ongoing bleeding for which some form of intervention (such as an operation or interventional radiology) is required. Patients who have lost significant intravascular volume, but hemorrhage is controlled or abated, will often respond to resuscitative efforts if the depth and duration of shock have been limited.

A subset of patients exists who fail to respond to resuscitative efforts despite adequate control of ongoing hemorrhage. These patients have ongoing fluid requirements despite adequate control of hemorrhage, have persistent hypotension despite restoration of intravascular volume necessitating vasopressor support, and may exhibit a futile cycle of uncorrectable hypothermia, hypoperfusion, acidosis, and coagulopathy that cannot be interrupted despite maximum therapy. These patients have deteriorated to decompensated or irreversible shock with peripheral vasodilation and resistance to vasopressor infusion. Mortality is inevitable once the patient manifests shock in its terminal stages.

Cardiogenic Shock

Cardiogenic shock is defined clinically as circulatory pump failure leading to diminished forward flow and subsequent tissue hypoxia, in the setting of adequate intravascular volume. Hemodynamic criteria include sustained hypotension (i.e., SBP <90 mmHg for at least 30 min), reduced cardiac index (<2.2 L/min per square meter), and elevated pulmonary artery wedge pressure (>15 mmHg). Mortality rates for cardiogenic shock are 50 to 80 percent. Acute, extensive myocardial infarction (MI) is the most common cause of cardiogenic shock; a smaller infarction in a patient with existing left ventricular dysfunction may also precipitate shock. Cardiogenic shock complicates 5–10 percent of acute MIs. Conversely, cardiogenic shock is the most common cause of death in patients hospitalized with acute MI. Although shock may develop early after myocardial infarction, it is typically not found on admission. Seventy-five percent of patients who have cardiogenic shock complicating acute MIs develop signs of cardiogenic shock within 24 h after onset of infarction (average 7 h). Recognition of the patient with occult hypoperfusion is critical to prevent progression to obvious cardiogenic shock with its high mortality rate; early initiation of therapy to maintain blood pressure and cardiac output is vital. Rapid assessment, adequate resuscitation, and reversal of the myocardial ischemia are essential in optimizing outcome in patients with acute MI. Prevention of infarct extension is a critical component. Large segments of nonfunctional but viable myocardium contribute to the development of cardiogenic shock after MI. In the setting of acute MI, expeditious restoration of coronary perfusion is mandatory to minimize mortality; the extent of myocardial salvage decreases exponentially with increased time to restoration of coronary blood flow. Inadequate cardiac function can be a direct result of cardiac injury, including profound myocardial contusion, blunt cardiac valvular injury, or direct myocardial damage (Table 4-1). The pathophysiology of cardiogenic shock involves a vicious cycle of myocardial ischemia which causes myocardial dysfunction, which results in more myocardial ischemia. When sufficient mass of the left ventricular wall is necrotic or ischemic and fails to pump, the stroke volume decreases. Decreased compliance results from myocardial ischemia, and compensatory increases in left ventricular filling pressures progressively occur.

TABLE 4-1 Causes of Cardiogenic Shock

Acute myocardial infarction
Pump failure
Mechanical complications
Acute mitral regurgitation from papillary muscle rupture
Ventricular septal defect
Free-wall rupture
Pericardial tamponade
Right ventricular infarction

Other causes of cardiogenic shock
End-stage cardiomyopathy
Myocarditis
Severe myocardial contusion
Prolonged cardiopulmonary bypass
Septic shock with severe myocardial depression
Left ventricular outflow obstruction
Aortic stenosis
Hypertrophic obstructive cardiomyopathy
Obstruction to left ventricular filling
Mitral stenosis
Left atrial myxoma
Acute mitral regurgitation
Acute aortic insufficiency

Source: Hollenberg SM, Kavinsky CJ, Parillo JE. Cardiogenic Shock. Ann Int. Med 131:47, 1999.

Diagnosis

Rapid identification of the patient with pump failure and institution of corrective action are essential in preventing the ongoing spiral of decreased cardiac output from injury causing increased myocardial oxygen needs that cannot be met, leading to progressive and unremitting cardiac dysfunction. In evaluation of possible cardiogenic shock, other causes of hypotension must be excluded, including hemorrhage, sepsis, pulmonary embolism, and aortic dissection.

Confirmation of a cardiac source for the shock requires electrocardiogram and urgent echocardiography. Other useful diagnostic tests include chest radiograph, arterial blood gases, electrolytes, complete blood count, and cardiac enzymes. Invasive cardiac monitoring, which is generally not necessary, can be useful to exclude right ventricular infarction, hypovolemia, and possible mechanical complications.

Making the diagnosis of cardiogenic shock involves the identification of cardiac dysfunction or acute heart failure in a susceptible patient. Because patients with blunt cardiac injury typically have multisystem injury, hemorrhagic shock from intraabdominal bleeding, intrathoracic bleeding, and bleeding from fractures must be excluded. Relatively few patients with blunt cardiac injury will develop cardiac pump dysfunction. Those who do generally exhibit cardiogenic shock early in their evaluation. Therefore, establishing the diagnosis of blunt cardiac injury is secondary to excluding other etiologies for shock and establishing that cardiac dysfunction is present. Invasive hemodynamic monitoring with a pulmonary artery catheter may uncover evidence of diminished cardiac output and elevated pulmonary artery pressure.

Treatment

After ensuring that an adequate airway is present and ventilation is sufficient, attention should be focused on support of the circulation. Intubation and mechanical ventilation are often required, if only to decrease work of breathing and facilitate sedation of the patient. Rapidly excluding hypovolemia and establishing the presence of cardiac dysfunction is essential. Treatment of cardiac dysfunction includes maintenance of adequate oxygenation to ensure adequate myocardial oxygen delivery and judicious fluid administration to avoid fluid overload and development of cardiogenic pulmonary edema. Electrolyte abnormalities, commonly hypokalemia and hypomagnesemia, should be corrected. Pain is treated with intravenous morphine sulfate or fentanyl. Significant dysrhythmias and heart block must be treated with antiarrhythmic drugs, pacing, or cardioversion if necessary.

When profound cardiac dysfunction exists, inotropic support may be indicated to improve cardiac contractility and cardiac output. Dobutamine primarily stimulates cardiac $\beta 1$ receptors to increase cardiac output, but may also vasodilate peripheral vascular beds, lower total peripheral resistance, and lower systemic blood pressure through effects on β_2 receptors. Ensuring adequate preload and intravascular volume is therefore essential prior to instituting therapy with dobutamine. Dopamine stimulates α receptors (vasoconstriction), β_1 receptors (cardiac stimulation), and β_2 receptors (vasodilation), with its effects on β receptors predominating at lower doses. Dopamine may be preferable to dobutamine in treatment of cardiac dysfunction in hypotensive patients. Tachycardia and increased peripheral resistance from dopamine infusion may worsen myocardial ischemia. Titration of both dopamine and dobutamine infusions may be required in some patients.

Epinephrine stimulates α and β receptors and may increase cardiac contractility and heart rate; however, it also may have intense peripheral vasoconstrictor effects that impair further cardiac performance. Catecholamine infusions must be carefully controlled to maximize coronary perfusion, although minimizing myocardial oxygen demand. Balancing the beneficial effects of impaired cardiac performance with the potential side effects of excessive reflex tachycardia and peripheral vasoconstriction requires serial assessment of tissue perfusion using indices such as capillary refill, character of peripheral pulses, adequacy of urine output, or improvement in laboratory parameters of resuscitation such as pH, base deficit, and lactate. Invasive monitoring is generally necessary in these unstable patients. The phosphodiesterase inhibitors amrinone and milrinone may be required on occasion in patients with resistant cardiogenic shock. These agents have long half-lives and induce thrombocytopenia and hypotension, and use is reserved for patients unresponsive to other treatment.

Patients whose cardiac dysfunction is refractory to cardiotonics may require mechanical circulatory support with an intraaortic balloon pump (IABP). Intraaortic balloon pumping increases cardiac output and improves coronary blood flow by reduction of systolic afterload and augmentation of diastolic perfusion pressure. Unlike vasopressor agents, these beneficial effects occur without an increase in myocardial oxygen demand. IABP can be inserted at the bedside in the ICU via the femoral artery through either a cutdown or using the percutaneous approach. Aggressive circulatory support of patients with cardiac dysfunction from intrinsic cardiac disease has led to more widespread application of these devices and more familiarity with their operation by both physicians and critical care nurses.

Preservation of existing myocardium and preservation of cardiac function are priorities of therapy for patients who have suffered an acute myocardial infarction. Ensuring adequate oxygenation and oxygen delivery, maintaining adequate preload with judicious volume restoration, minimizing sympathetic discharge through adequate relief of pain, and correcting electrolyte imbalances are all straightforward nonspecific maneuvers that may improve existing cardiac function or prevent future cardiac complications. Anticoagulation and aspirin are given for acute myocardial infarction. Although thrombolytic therapy reduces mortality in patients with acute myocardial infarction, its role in cardiogenic shock is less clear. Patients in cardiac failure from an acute MI may benefit from pharmacologic or mechanical circulatory support in a manner similar to that of patients with cardiac failure related to blunt cardiac injury. Additional pharmacologic tools may include the use of β blockers to control heart rate and myocardial oxygen consumption, nitrates to promote coronary blood flow through vasodilatation, and ACE inhibitors to reduce ACE-mediated vasoconstrictive effects that increase myocardial workload and myocardial oxygen consumption.

Current guidelines of the American Heart Association (AHA) recommend percutaneous transluminal coronary angiography (PTCA) for patients with cardiogenic shock, ST elevation, left bundle-branch block, and age younger than 75 years. Early definition of coronary anatomy and revascularization is the pivotal step in treatment of patients with cardiogenic shock from acute MI. When feasible, PTCA (generally with stent placement) is the treatment of choice. Coronary artery bypass grafting (CABG) seems to be more appropriate for patients with multiple vessel disease or left main coronary artery disease.

Vasodilatory Shock (Septic Shock)

In vasodilatory shock, hypotension results from failure of the vascular smooth muscle to constrict appropriately. Vasodilatory shock is characterized by both peripheral vasodilatation with resultant hypotension, and resistance to treatment with vasopressors. Despite the hypotension, plasma catecholamine levels are elevated and the renin-angiotensin system is activated in vasodilatory shock. The most frequently encountered form of vasodilatory shock is septic shock. Other causes of vasodilatory shock include hypoxic lactic acidosis, carbon monoxide poisoning, decompensated and irreversible hemorrhagic shock, terminal cardiogenic shock, and postcardiotomy shock (Table 4-2). Thus, vasodilatory shock seems to represent the final common pathway for profound and prolonged shock of any etiology.

Septic shock is a by-product of the body's response to invasive or severe localized infection, typically from bacterial or fungal pathogens. In the attempt to eradicate the pathogens, the immune and other cell types (e.g., endothelial cells) elaborate soluble mediators that enhance macrophage and neutrophil killing effector mechanisms, increase procoagulant activity and fibroblast activity to localize the invaders, and increase microvascular blood flow to enhance delivery of killing forces to the area of invasion. When this response is overly exuberant or becomes systemic rather than localized, manifestations of sepsis may be evident. These findings include enhanced

TABLE 4-2 Causes of Vasodilatory Shock

Sepsis
Prolonged and severe hypotension
Hemorrhagic shock
Cardiogenic shock
Cardiopulmonary bypass
Inadequate tissue oxygenation
Hypoxic lactic acidosis
Carbon monoxide poisoning

Source: Modified from Landry DW, Oliver JA: Mechanisms of disease: The pathogenesis of vasodilatory shock. NEJM 345;588, 2001.

cardiac output, peripheral vasodilation, fever, leukocytosis, hyperglycemia, and tachycardia. In septic shock, the vasodilatory effects are due in part to the upregulation of the inducible isoform of nitric oxide synthase (iNOS or NOS 2) in the vessel wall. iNOS produces large quantities of nitric oxide for sustained periods of time. This potent vasodilator suppresses vascular tone and renders the vasculature resistant to the effects of vasoconstricting agents.

Diagnosis

Attempts to standardize terminology have led to the establishment of criteria for the diagnosis of sepsis in the hospitalized adult. These criteria include manifestations of the host response to infection, in addition to identification of an offending organism. The terms sepsis, severe sepsis, and septic shock are used to quantify the magnitude of the systemic inflammatory reaction. Patients with sepsis have evidence of an infection, and systemic signs of inflammation (e.g., fever, leukocytosis, and tachycardia). Hypoperfusion with signs of organ dysfunction is termed severe sepsis. Septic shock requires the presence of the above, associated with more significant evidence of tissue hypoperfusion and systemic hypotension. Beyond the hypotension, maldistribution of blood flow and shunting in the microcirculation further compromise delivery of nutrients to the tissue beds.

Recognizing septic shock begins with defining the patient at risk. The clinical manifestations of septic shock will usually become evident and prompt the initiation of treatment before bacteriologic confirmation of an organism or the source of an organism is identified. In addition to fever, tachycardia, and tachypnea, signs of hypoperfusion such as confusion, malaise, oliguria, or hypotension may be present. These should prompt an aggressive search for infection including a thorough physical exam, inspection of all wounds, evaluation of intravascular catheters or other foreign bodies, obtaining appropriate cultures, and adjunctive imaging studies as needed.

Treatment

Evaluation of the patient in septic shock begins with an assessment of the adequacy of their airway and ventilation. Severely obtunded patients and patients whose work of breathing is excessive require intubation and ventilation to prevent respiratory collapse. Because vasodilation and decrease in total peripheral resistance may produce hypotension, fluid resuscitation and restoration of circulatory volume with balanced salt solutions is essential. Empiric antibiotics must be chosen carefully based on the most likely pathogens (gram-negative rods, gram-positive cocci, and anaerobes), because the portal of entry of the offending organism and its identity may not be evident until culture data return or imaging studies are completed. Knowledge of the bacteriologic profile of infections in an individual unit can be obtained from most hospital infection control departments and will suggest potential responsible organisms. Antibiotics should be tailored to cover the responsible organisms once culture data are available, and if appropriate, the spectrum of coverage narrowed. Long-term empiric broad-spectrum antibiotic use should be minimized to reduce the development of resistant organisms, and to avoid the potential complications of fungal overgrowth and antibiotic-associated colitis from overgrowth of *Clostridium difficile*. Intravenous antibiotics will be insufficient to adequately treat the infectious episode in the settings of infected fluid collections, infected foreign bodies, and devitalized tissue. These situations may require multiple operations to ensure proper wound hygiene and healing.

The majority of septic patients have hyperdynamic physiology with supranormal cardiac output and low systemic vascular resistance. On occasion, septic patients may have low cardiac output despite volume resuscitation and even vasopressor support. Mortality in this group is high. Despite the increasing incidence of septic shock over the past several decades, the overall mortality rates have changed little. Recent evidences indicate the benefit of immediate goal-directed resuscitation in improving outcomes in sepsis.

After first-line therapy of the septic patient with antibiotics, intravenous fluids, and intubation if necessary, vasopressors may be necessary to treat patients with septic shock. Catecholamines are the vasopressors used most often. Occasionally, patients with septic shock will develop arterial resistance to catecholamines. Arginine vasopressin, a potent vasoconstrictor, is often efficacious in this setting. A recent study also reported significant positive impact of tight glucose management on outcome in critically ill patients. Mortality in patients receiving intensive insulin treatment is significantly lower and most notable in the patients requiring longer than 5 days in the intensive care unit (ICU).

Recent studies have reported benefit from intravenous infusion of recombinant human activated protein C for severe sepsis. Activated protein C is an endogenous protein that promotes fibrinolysis and inhibits thrombosis and inflammation. Treatment with activated protein C has been shown to reduce 28-day mortality rate from 31–25 percent; a reduction in relative risk of death of 19.4 percent.

The observation that severe sepsis is often associated with adrenal insufficiency or glucocorticoid receptor resistance has generated renewed interest in therapy for septic shock with corticosteroids. Seven-day treatment with low doses of hydrocortisone and fludrocortisone significantly and safely lowers the risk of death in patients with septic shock and relative adrenal insufficiency. Adrenal insufficiency is established in critically ill patients using a corticotropia stimulator test.

Neurogenic Shock

Neurogenic shock refers to diminished tissue perfusion as a result of loss of vasomotor tone to peripheral arterial beds. Loss of vasoconstrictor impulses results in increased vascular capacitance, decreased venous return, and decreased cardiac output. Neurogenic shock is usually secondary to spinal cord injuries from vertebral body fractures of the cervical or high thoracic region that disrupt sympathetic regulation of peripheral vascular tone. Rarely, a spinal cord injury without bony fracture, such as an epidural hematoma impinging on the spinal cord, can produce neurogenic shock. Sympathetic input to the heart, which normally increases heart rate and cardiac contractility, and input to the adrenal medulla, which increases catecholamine release, may also be disrupted, preventing the typical reflex tachycardia that occurs with hypovolemia. Acute spinal cord injury results in activation of multiple secondary injury mechanisms: (1) vascular compromise to the spinal cord with loss of autoregulation, vasospasm, and thrombosis, (2) loss of cellular membrane integrity and impaired energy metabolism, and (3) neurotransmitter accumulation and release of free radicals. Importantly, hypotension contributes to the worsening of acute spinal cord injury as the result of further reduction in blood flow to the spinal cord. Management of acute spinal cord injury with attention to blood pressure control, oxygenation, and hemodynamics, essentially optimizing perfusion of an already ischemic spinal cord, seems to result in improved neurologic outcome. Patients with hypotension from spinal cord injury are best monitored in an intensive care unit, and carefully followed for evidence of cardiac or respiratory dysfunction.

Diagnosis

Acute spinal cord injury may result in bradycardia, hypotension, cardiac dysrhythmias, reduced cardiac output, and decreased peripheral vascular resistance. The severity of the spinal cord injury seems to correlate with the magnitude of cardiovascular dysfunction. Patients with complete motor injuries are over five times more likely to require vasopressors for neurogenic shock, as compared to those with incomplete lesions. The classic description of neurogenic shock consists of decreased blood pressure associated with bradycardia (absence of reflexive tachycardia because of disrupted sympathetic discharge), warm extremities (loss of peripheral vasoconstriction), motor and sensory deficits indicative of a spinal cord injury, and radiographic evidence of a vertebral column fracture. Patients with multisystem trauma that includes spinal cord injuries often have head injuries that may make identification of motor and sensory deficits difficult in the initial evaluation. Furthermore, associated injuries may occur that result in hypovolemia, further complicating the clinical presentation. In the multiply injured patient, other causes of hypotension including hemorrhage, tension pneumothorax, and cardiogenic shock must be sought and excluded.

Treatment

After the airway is secured and ventilation is adequate, fluid resuscitation and restoration of intravascular volume will often improve perfusion in neurogenic shock. Most patients with neurogenic shock will respond to restoration of intravascular volume alone, with satisfactory improvement in perfusion and resolution of hypotension. Administration of vasoconstrictors will improve peripheral vascular tone, decrease vascular capacitance, and increase venous return, but should only be considered once hypovolemia is excluded as the cause of the hypotension, and the diagnosis of neurogenic shock established. If the patient's blood pressure has not responded to what is felt to be adequate volume resuscitation, dopamine may be used first. A pure α agonist, such as phenylephrine may be used primarily or in patients unresponsive to dopamine.

Specific treatment for the hypotension is often of brief duration, as the need to administer vasoconstrictors typically lasts 24–48 hours. On the other hand, life-threatening cardiac dysrhythmias and hypotension may occur up to 14 days after spinal cord injury.

Obstructive Shock

Commonly, mechanical obstruction of venous return in trauma patients is because of the presence of tension pneumothorax. Cardiac tamponade occurs when sufficient fluid has accumulated in the pericardial sac to obstruct blood flow to the ventricles. The hemodynamic abnormalities in pericardial tamponade are because of elevation of intracardiac pressures with limitation of ventricular filling in diastole with resultant decrease in cardiac output. Acutely, the pericardium does not distend; thus small volumes of blood may produce cardiac tamponade. If the effusion accumulates slowly (e.g., in the setting of uremia, heart failure, or malignant effusion), the quantity of fluid producing cardiac tamponade may reach 2000 mL. The major determinant of the degree of hypotension is the pericardial pressure. With either cardiac tamponade or tension pneumothorax, reduced filling of the right side of the heart from either increased intrapleural pressure secondary to air accumulation (tension pneumothorax), or increased intrapericardial pressure precluding atrial filling secondary to blood accumulation (cardiac tamponade) results in decreased cardiac output associated with increased central venous pressure.

Diagnosis and Treatment

The diagnosis of tension pneumothorax should be made on clinical examination. The classic findings include respiratory distress (in an awake patient), hypotension, diminished breath sounds over one hemithorax, hyperresonance to percussion, jugular venous distention, and shift of mediastinal structures to the unaffected side with tracheal deviation. In most instances, empiric treatment with pleural decompression is indicated rather than delaying to wait for radiographic confirmation. When a chest tube cannot be immediately inserted, such as in the prehospital setting, the pleural space can be decompressed with a large caliber needle. Immediate return of air should be encountered with rapid resolution of hypotension. Unfortunately, not all of the clinical manifestations of tension pneumothorax may be evident on physical exam. Practically, three findings are sufficient to make the diagnosis of tension pneumothorax: respiratory distress or hypotension, decreased lung sounds, and hypertympany to percussion. Chest x-ray findings that may be visualized include deviation of mediastinal structures, depression of the hemidiaphragm, and hypo-opacification with absent lung markings. As discussed above, definitive treatment of a tension pneumothorax is immediate tube thoracostomy. The chest tube should be inserted rapidly, but carefully, and should be large enough to evacuate any blood that may be present in the pleural space. Our preference is via the fourth intercostal space (nipple level) at the anterior axillary line.

Cardiac tamponade results from the accumulation of blood within the pericardial sac, usually from penetrating trauma or chronic medical conditions such as heart failure or uremia. Although precordial wounds are most likely to injure the heart and produce tamponade, any projectile or wounding agent that passes in proximity to the mediastinum can potentially produce tamponade. Blunt cardiac rupture, a rare event in trauma victims who survive long enough to reach the hospital, can produce refractory shock and tamponade in the multiply injured patient. The manifestations of cardiac tamponade may be catastrophic such as total circulatory collapse and cardiac arrest, or they may be more subtle. A high index of suspicion is warranted to make a rapid diagnosis. Patients who present with circulatory arrest from cardiac tamponade require emergency pericardial decompression, usually through a left thoracotomy (see Chapter 6 for indications for this maneuver). Cardiac tamponade may also be associated with dyspnea, orthopnea, cough, peripheral edema, chest pain, tachycardia, muffled heart tones, jugular venous distention, and elevated central venous pressure. The triad of Beck consists of hypotension, muffled heart tones, and neck vein distention. Unfortunately, absence of these clinical findings may not be sufficient to exclude cardiac injury and cardiac tamponade. Muffled heart tones may be difficult to appreciate in a busy trauma center and jugular venous distention and central venous pressure may be diminished by coexistent bleeding. Therefore, patients at risk for cardiac tamponade whose hemodynamic status permits additional diagnostic tests frequently require additional diagnostic maneuvers to confirm cardiac injury or tamponade.

Invasive hemodynamic monitoring may support the diagnosis of cardiac tamponade if elevated central venous pressure, pulsus paradoxus (i.e., decreased systemic arterial pressure with inspiration), or elevated right atrial and right ventricular pressure by pulmonary artery catheter are present. These hemodynamic profiles suffer from lack of specificity, the duration of time required to obtain them in critically injured patients, and their inability to exclude cardiac injury in the absence of tamponade. Chest radiographs may provide information on the possible trajectory of a projectile, but rarely are diagnostic because the acutely filled pericardium distends poorly. Echocardiography has become the preferred test for the diagnosis of cardiac tamponade. Good results in detecting pericardial fluid have been reported, but the yield in detecting pericardial fluid depends on the skill and experience of the ultrasonographer, body habitus of the patient, and absence of wounds that preclude visualization of the pericardium. Pericardiocentesis to diagnose pericardial blood and potentially relieve tamponade may be used. Performing pericardiocentesis under ultrasound guidance has made the procedure safer and more reliable. An indwelling catheter may be placed for several days in patients with chronic pericardial effusions. Needle pericardiocentesis may not evacuate clotted blood and has the potential to produce cardiac injury, making it a poor alternative in busy trauma centers.

Diagnostic pericardial window represents the most direct method to determine the presence of blood within the pericardium. The procedure is best performed in the operating room under general anesthesia. It can be performed through either the subxiphoid or transdiaphragmatic approach. Adequate equipment and personnel to rapidly decompress the pericardium, explore the injury, and repair the heart should be present. Once the pericardium is opened and tamponade relieved, hemodynamics usually improve dramatically and formal pericardial exploration can ensue. Exposure of the heart can be achieved by extending the incision to a median sternotomy, performing a left anterior thoracotomy, or performing bilateral anterior thoracotomies ("clamshell").

Traumatic Shock

The systemic response after trauma, combining the effects of soft-tissue injury, long-bone fractures, and blood loss, is clearly a different physiologic insult than simple hemorrhagic shock. Multiple organ failure, including ARDS, develops relatively often in the blunt trauma patient, but rarely after pure hemorrhagic shock (such as a gastrointestinal bleed). The hypoperfusion deficit in traumatic shock is magnified by the proinflammatory activation that occurs following the induction of shock. In addition to ischemia or ischemia-reperfusion, accumulating evidence demonstrates that even simple hemorrhage induces proinflammatory activation that results in many of the cellular changes typically ascribed only to septic shock. Treatment of traumatic shock is focused on correction of the individual elements to diminish the cascade of proinflammatory activation, and includes prompt control of hemorrhage, adequate volume resuscitation to correct oxygen debt, débridement of nonviable tissue, stabilization of bony injuries, and appropriate treatment of soft tissue injuries.

ENDPOINTS IN RESUSCITATION

Shock is defined as inadequate perfusion to maintain normal organ function. With prolonged anaerobic metabolism, tissue acidosis and oxygen debt accumulate. Thus the goal in the treatment of shock is restoration of adequate organ perfusion and tissue oxygenation. Resuscitation is complete when oxygen debt is repaid, tissue acidosis is corrected, and aerobic metabolism restored. Clinical confirmation of this endpoint remains a challenge.

Resuscitation of the patient in shock requires simultaneous evaluation and treatment; the etiology of the shock often is not initially apparent. Hemorrhagic shock, septic shock, and traumatic shock are the most common types of shock encountered on surgical services. To optimize outcome in bleeding patients, early control of the hemorrhage and adequate volume resuscitation, including both red blood cells and crystalloid solutions, are necessary. Expedient operative resuscitation is mandatory to limit the magnitude of activation of multiple mediator systems and to abort the microcirculatory changes, which may evolve insidiously into the cascade that ends in irreversible hemorrhagic shock. Attempts to stabilize an actively bleeding patient anywhere but in the operating room are inappropriate. Any intervention that delays the patient's arrival in the operating room for control of hemorrhage increases mortality thus the important concept of operating room resuscitation of the critically injured patient.

Endpoints in resuscitation can be divided into systemic or global parameters, tissue-specific parameters, and cellular parameters. Global endpoints include vital signs, cardiac output, pulmonary artery wedge pressure, oxygen delivery and consumption, lactate, and base deficit (Table 4-3).

Assessment of Endpoints in Resuscitation

Oxygen Transport

Attaining supranormal oxygen transport variables has been proposed as a means to correct oxygen debt. However, evidence is insufficient to support the routine use of a strategy to maximize oxygen delivery in a group of unselected patients.

Inability to repay oxygen debt is a predictor of mortality and organ failure; the probability of death has been directly correlated to the calculated oxygen debt in hemorrhagic shock. Direct measurement of the oxygen debt in the resuscitation of patients is difficult. The easily obtainable parameters of

TABLE 4-3 Endpoints in Resuscitation

Systemic/global
Lactate
Base deficit
Cardiac output
Oxygen delivery and consumption

Tissue-specific
Gastric tonometry
Tissue pH, oxygen, carbon dioxide levels
Near infrared spectroscopy

Cellular
Membrane potential
Adenosine triphosphate (ATP)

arterial blood pressure, heart rate, urine output, central venous pressure, and pulmonary artery occlusion pressure are poor indicators of the adequacy of tissue perfusion. Therefore, surrogate parameters have been sought to estimate the oxygen debt; serum lactate and base deficit have been shown to correlate with oxygen debt.

Lactate

Lactate is generated by conversion of pyruvate to lactate by lactate dehydrogenase in the setting of insufficient oxygen. Lactate is released into the circulation and is predominantly taken up and metabolized by the liver and kidneys. The liver accounts for approximately 50 percent and the kidney for about 30 percent of whole body lactate uptake. Elevated serum lactate is an indirect measure of the oxygen debt, and therefore an approximation of the magnitude and duration of the severity of shock. The admission lactate level, highest lactate level, and time interval to normalize the serum lactate are important prognostic indicators for survival. In contrast, individual variability of lactate may be too great to permit accurate prediction of outcome in any individual case. Base deficit and volume of blood transfusion required in the first 24 hours of resuscitation may be better predictors of mortality than the plasma lactate alone.

Base Deficit

Base deficit is the amount of base in millimoles that is required to titrate 1 L of whole blood to a pH of 7.40 with the sample fully saturated with O_2 at $37°C$ ($80.6°F$) and a $PaCO_2$ of 40 mmHg. It is usually measured by arterial blood gas analysis in clinical practice as it is readily and quickly available. The mortality of trauma patients can be stratified according to the magnitude of base deficit measured in the first 24 hours after admission. In a retrospective study of over 3000 trauma admissions, patients with a base deficit worse than 15 mmol/L had a mortality of 70 percent. Base deficit can be stratified into mild (3–5), moderate (6–14) and severe (≥ 15) categories, with a trend toward higher mortality with worsening base deficit in patients with trauma. Both the magnitude of the perfusion deficit as indicated by the base deficit and the time required to correct it are major factors determining outcome in shock.

Indeed, when elevated base deficit persists (or lactic acidosis) in the trauma patient, ongoing bleeding is often the etiology. Trauma patients admitted with a base deficit greater than 15 mmol/L required twice the volume of fluid infusion and 6 times more blood transfusion in the first 24 hours, as compared to patients with mild acidosis. Transfusion requirements increased as base deficit worsened and ICU and hospital lengths of stay increased. Mortality increased as base deficit worsened; the frequency of organ failure increased with greater base deficit. The probability of trauma patients developing ARDS has been reported to correlate with severity of admission base deficit and lowest base deficit within the first 24 hours postinjury. Persistently high base deficit is associated with abnormal oxygen utilization and higher mortality. Monitoring base deficit in the resuscitation of trauma patients assists in assessment of oxygen transport and efficacy of resuscitation.

Factors that may compromise the utility of the base deficit in estimating oxygen debt are the administration of bicarbonate, hypothermia, hypocapnia (overventilation), heparin, ethanol, and ketoacidosis. However, the base deficit remains one of the most widely used estimates of oxygen debt for its clinical relevance, accuracy, and availability.

Controversies about Fluids Used for Resuscitation

No differences in overall mortality, length of stay, or incidence of pulmonary edema have been noted in comparison of crystalloid to colloids in fluid resuscitation of critically ill patients. Subgroup analysis suggested a significant survival advantage in trauma patients in favor of crystalloid resuscitation. A systematic review of 30 randomized trials of human albumin administration in 1419 critically ill patients similarly noted an increased risk of mortality with the use of albumin infusion in treatment of hypovolemia, burns, and hypoalbuminemia. Additionally, albumin is several times more expensive than crystalloid solutions. The expense of the infusion of albumin-containing solution cannot be justified.

Several papers have suggested improved outcome with the use of hypertonic saline in the treatment of hemorrhagic shock. The clinical trials have shown marginal benefit with the infusion of hypertonic saline (7.5 percent sodium chloride). The benefit of hypertonic saline solutions may be immunomodulatory, in addition to shifting of fluids from intracellular compartments.

Use of Blood in Transfusion

Volume resuscitation in the trauma patient requires restoration of intravascular volume and repletion of sufficient oxygen-carrying capacity with red blood cell transfusion. Delay of transfusion of red blood cells in the actively bleeding trauma patients increases mortality.

Hypotensive Resuscitation

Reasonable conclusions controlled hypotension in the setting of uncontrolled hemorrhage include: any delay in surgery for control of hemorrhage increases mortality; with uncontrolled hemorrhage attempting to achieve normal blood pressure may increase mortality, particularly with penetrating injuries and short transport times; a goal of systolic blood pressure of 80–90 mmHg may be adequate in the patient with penetrating injury; and profound hemodilution should be avoided by early transfusion of red blood cells. For the patient with blunt injury, in which the major cause of death is a closed head injury, the increase in mortality with hypotension in the setting of brain injury must be avoided. In this setting, a systolic blood pressure of 110 mmHg would seem to be more appropriate.

Suggested Readings

Chambers NK, Buchman TG: Shock at the Millennium. Walter B. Cannon and Alfred Blalock. Shock 13:497, 2000.

Wiggers CJ: Experimental hemorrhagic shock, in Physiology of Shock. New York: Commonwealth, 1950, p. 121.

Bickell WH, Wall MJ, Pepe PE, et al: Immediate versus delayed resuscitation for hypotensive patients with penetrating torso injuries. N Engl J Med 331:1105, 1994.

Peitzman AB, Billiar TR, Harbrecht BG, et al: Hemorrhagic shock. Curr Prob Surg 32:925, 1995.

Landry DW, Oliver JA: Mechanisms of disease: The pathogenesis of vasodilatory shock. N Engl J Med 345:588, 2001.

Fink MP: Intestinal epithelial hyperpermeability: Update on the pathogenesis of gut mucosal barrier dysfunction in critical illness. Curr Opin Crit Care 9:143, 2003.

Rivers E, Nguyen B, Harstad S, et al: Early goal-directed therapy in the treatment of severe sepsis and septic shock. N Engl J Med 345:1368, 2001.

Rutherford EJ, Morris JA Jr., Reed GW, et al: Base deficit stratifies mortality and determines therapy. J Trauma 33:417, 1992.

Mann DV, Robinson MK, Rounds ID, et al: Superiority of blood over saline resuscitation from hemorrhagic shock. Ann Surg 226:653, 1997.

5 | Surgical Infections

Gregory J. Beilman and David L. Dunn

Although treatment of infection has been an integral part of the surgeon's practice since the dawn of time, the body of knowledge that led to the present field of surgical infectious disease was derived from the evolution of germ theory and antisepsis. Application of the latter to clinical practice, concurrent with the development of anesthesia, was pivotal in allowing surgeons to perform complex procedures that were previously associated with high rates of morbidity and mortality because of postoperative infections. Until recently the occurrence of infection related to the surgical wound was the rule rather than the exception. The development of modalities to effectively prevent and treat infection has occurred only within the last several decades.

The first intraabdominal operation to treat infection via "source control" (i.e., surgical intervention to eliminate the source of infection) was appendectomy. McBurney's classic report on early operative intervention for appendicitis was presented before the New York Surgical Society in 1889. Sir Alexander Fleming in 1928 noted a zone of inhibition around a mold colony (*Penicillium notatum*) that serendipitously grew on a plate of Staphylococcus, and he named the active substance penicillin. This first effective antibacterial agent subsequently led to the development of hundreds of potent antimicrobials, set the stage for their use as prophylaxis against postoperative infection, and became a critical component of the armamentarium to treat aggressive, lethal surgical infections.

Concurrent with the development of numerous antimicrobial agents were advances in the field of clinical microbiology. Many new microbes were identified, including numerous anaerobes; the autochthonous microflora of the skin, gastrointestinal tract, and other parts of the body that the surgeon encountered in the process of an operation were characterized in great detail. Subsequently, the initial clinical observations of surgeons such as Frank Meleney, William Altemeier, and others provided the observation that aerobes and anaerobes could synergize to cause serious soft tissue and severe intraabdominal infection.

The discovery of the first cytokines began to allow insight into the organism's response to infection, and led to an explosion in our understanding of the host inflammatory response. Expanding knowledge of the multiple pathways activated during the response to invasion by infectious organisms has permitted the design of new therapies targeted at modifying the inflammatory response to infection. Preventing and treating this process of multiple-organ failure during infection is one of the major challenges of modern critical care and surgical infectious disease.

PATHOGENESIS OF INFECTION

Host Defenses

The mammalian host possesses several layers of endogenous defense mechanisms that serve to prevent microbial invasion, limit proliferation of microbes within the host, and contain or eradicate invading microbes. They include site-specific defenses that function at the tissue level, and components that freely circulate throughout the body in both blood and lymph. Systemic host defenses

78

are recruited to a site of infection, a process that begins immediately on introduction of microbes into a sterile area of the body. Perturbation of one or more components of these defenses (e.g., via immunosuppressants, chronic illness, and burns) may have substantial negative impact on resistance to infection.

Entry of microbes into the mammalian host is precluded by the presence of a number of barriers that possess either an epithelial (integument) or mucosal (respiratory, gut, and urogenital) surface. However, barrier function is not solely limited to physical characteristics: host barrier cells may secrete substances that limit microbial proliferation or prevent invasion. Also, resident or commensal microbes (endogenous or autochthonous host microflora) adherent to the physical surface and to each other may preclude invasion, particularly of virulent organisms (colonization resistance).

The most extensive physical barrier is the integument or skin. In addition to the physical barrier posed by the epithelial surface, the skin harbors its own resident microflora that may block the attachment and invasion of noncommensal microbes. Microbes also are held in check by chemicals that sebaceous glands secrete and by the constant shedding of epithelial cells. Diseases of the skin (e.g., eczema and dermatitis) are associated with overgrowth of skin commensal organisms, and barrier breaches invariably lead to the introduction of these microbes.

The respiratory tract possesses several host defense mechanisms that facilitate the maintenance of sterility in the distal bronchi and alveoli under normal circumstances. In the upper respiratory tract, respiratory mucus traps larger particles including microbes. Smaller particles arriving in the lower respiratory tract are cleared via phagocytosis by pulmonary alveolar macrophages. Any process that diminishes these host defenses can lead to development of bronchitis or pneumonia.

The urogenital, biliary, pancreatic ductal, and distal respiratory tracts do not possess resident microflora in healthy individuals, although microbes may be present if these barriers are affected by disease or if microorganisms are introduced from an external source. In contrast, significant numbers of microbes are encountered in many portions of the gastrointestinal tract, with vast numbers being found within the oropharynx and distal colorectum, although the specific organisms differ. Organisms ingested into the stomach from the oropharynx are routinely killed in the highly acidic, low-motility environment of the stomach during the initial phases of digestion. Thus, small numbers of microbes populate the gastric mucosa (approximately 10^2–10^3 colony-forming units [CFU]/mL); this population expands in the presence of drugs or disease states that diminish gastric acidity. Microbes that are not destroyed within the stomach enter the small intestine, in which a certain amount of microbial proliferation takes place, such that approximately 10^5–10^8 CFU/mL are present in the terminal ileum.

The relatively low-oxygen, static environment of the colon is accompanied by the exponential growth of microbes that comprise the most extensive host endogenous microflora. Anaerobic microbes outnumber aerobic species approximately 100:1 in the distal colorectum, and approximately 10^{11}–10^{12} CFU/g are present in feces. Large numbers of facultative and strict anaerobes (*Bacteroides fragilis* and other species) and several orders of magnitude fewer aerobic microbes (*Escherichia coli* and other Enterobacteriaceae species, *Enterococcus faecalis* and *E. faecium*, *Candida albicans* and other Candida species) are present.

Once microbes enter a sterile body compartment (e.g., pleural or peritoneal cavity) or tissue, host defenses act to limit and/or eliminate pathogens. Initially, several primitive and relatively nonspecific host defenses act to contain the nidus of infection. Within the peritoneal cavity, unique host defenses exist, including a diaphragmatic pumping mechanism whereby small particles within peritoneal fluid are expunged from the abdominal cavity via specialized structures on the undersurface of the diaphragm. Concurrently, containment by the omentum, the so-called "gatekeeper" of the abdomen and intestinal ileus, serves to wall off infection, albeit with the likely result of abscess formation.

Microbes also immediately encounter host defense mechanisms that reside within the tissues of the body. These include resident macrophages and complement (C) proteins and immunoglobulins (Ig, antibodies). Resident macrophages secrete a wide array of substances in response to the above-mentioned processes, which appear to regulate the cellular components of the host defense response. Macrophage cytokine synthesis is upregulated and includes secretion of tumor necrosis factor-alpha (TNF-α), interleukins (IL)-1, 6, and 8; and interferon-γ (INF-γ) within the tissue milieu, and, depending on the magnitude of the host defense response, the systemic circulation. Concurrently, a counterregulatory response is initiated consisting of binding proteins (TNF-BP), cytokine receptor antagonists (IL-1ra), and antiinflammatory cytokines (IL-4 and IL-10).

The interaction of microbes with these first-line host defenses leads to microbial opsonization (C1q, C3bi, and IgFc), phagocytosis, and extracellular (C5b6-9 membrane attack complex) and intracellular microbial destruction (phagocytic vacuoles). The classical and alternate complement pathways are activated both via direct contact with and via IgM and IgG binding to microbes (IgM > IgG), leading to the release of a number of different complement protein fragments (C3a, C4a, C5a) that are biologically active, acting to markedly enhance vascular permeability. Bacterial cell wall components and a variety of enzymes that are expelled from leukocyte phagocytic vacuoles during microbial phagocytosis and killing act in this capacity as well.

Simultaneously, the release of substances chemotactic to polymorphonuclear leukocytes (PMNs) in the bloodstream takes place. These consist of C5a, microbial cell wall peptides containing N-formyl-methionine, and macrophage cytokines such as IL-8. This process of host defense recruitment leads to further influx of inflammatory fluid and PMNs into the area of incipient infection, a process that begins within several minutes and may peak within hours or days. The magnitude of the response is related to several factors: (1) the initial number of microbes, (2) the rate of microbial proliferation in relation to containment and killing by host defenses, (3) microbial virulence, and (4) the potency of host defenses. In regard to the latter, drugs or disease states that diminish any or multiple components of host defenses are associated with higher rates and potentially more grave infections.

Definitions

Several possible outcomes can occur subsequent to microbial invasion and the interaction of microbes with resident and recruited host defenses: (1) eradication; (2) containment, often leading to the presence of purulence—the hallmark of chronic infection (e.g., a furuncle in the skin and soft tissue or abscess within the parenchyma of an organ or potential space); (3) locoregional infection (cellulitis, lymphangitis, and aggressive soft tissue infection) with or without distant spread of infection (metastatic abscess); or (4) systemic infection (bacteremia or fungemia). The latter represents the failure of resident and recruited host defenses at the local level, and is associated with significant morbidity and mortality in the clinical setting. Additionally, it is not uncommon that disease progression occurs such that serious locoregional infection is associated with concurrent systemic infection. A chronic abscess also may intermittently drain and/or be associated with bacteremia.

Infection is defined by identification of microorganisms in host tissue or the blood stream, plus an inflammatory response to their presence. At the site of infection the classic findings of rubor, calor, and dolor in areas such as the skin or subcutaneous tissue are common. Most infections in normal individuals with intact host defenses are associated with these local manifestations, plus systemic manifestations such as elevated temperature, elevated white blood cell (WBC) count, tachycardia, or tachypnea. The systemic manifestations noted above comprise the systemic inflammatory response syndrome (SIRS). SIRS can be caused by a variety of disease processes, including pancreatitis, polytrauma, malignancy, and transfusion reaction, and infection. SIRS caused by infection is termed sepsis, and is mediated by the production of a cascade of proinflammatory mediators produced in response to exposure to microbial products. These products include lipopolysaccharide (endotoxin, LPS) derived from gram-negative organisms and many others. Patients have developed sepsis if they have met clinical criteria for SIRS and have evidence of a local or systemic source of infection. Severe sepsis is characterized as sepsis (defined above) combined with the presence of new-onset organ failure. Severe sepsis is the most common cause of death in noncoronary critical care units, with more than 200,000 deaths occurring annually in the United States. With respect to clinical criteria, a patient with sepsis and the need for ventilatory support, with oliguria unresponsive to aggressive fluid resuscitation, or with hypotension requiring vasopressors should be considered to have developed severe sepsis. Septic shock is a state of acute circulatory failure identified by the presence of persistent arterial hypotension (systolic blood pressure < 90 mmHg) despite adequate fluid resuscitation, without other identifiable causes. Septic shock is the most severe manifestation of infection, occurring in approximately 40 percent of patients with severe sepsis; it has an attendant mortality rate of 60–80 percent.

MICROBIOLOGY OF INFECTIOUS AGENTS

Bacteria

Table 5-1 lists common pathogens of surgical interest. Bacteria are responsible for the majority of surgical infections. Specific species are identified using Gram stain and growth characteristics on specific media. The Gram stain allows rapid classification of bacteria by color: gram-positive bacteria stain blue and gram-negative bacteria stain red. Bacteria are classified based on a number of additional characteristics including morphology [cocci and bacilli], the pattern of division (e.g., single organisms, groups of organisms in pairs [diplococci], clusters [staphylococci], and chains [streptococci]), and the presence and location of spores.

Gram-positive bacteria that frequently cause infections in surgical patients include aerobic skin and enteric organisms. Aerobic skin commensals are the most frequent cause of surgical site infections (SSIs); enterococci can cause nosocomial infections (urinary tract infections [UTIs] and bacteremia)

TABLE 5-1 Common Pathogens in Surgical Patients

Gram-positive aerobic cocci

Staphylococcus aureus
Staphylococcus epidermidis
Streptococcus pyogenes
Streptococcus pneumoniae
Enterococcus faecium, E. faecalis

Gram-negative aerobic bacilli

Escherichia coli
Haemophilus influenzae
Klebsiella pneumoniae
Proteus mirabilis
Enterobacter cloacae, E. aerogenes
Serratia marcescens
Acinetobacter calcoaceticus
Citrobacter freundii
Pseudomonas aeruginosa
Xanthomonas maltophilia

Anaerobes

Gram-positive
  Clostridium perfringens, C. tetani, C. septicum
  Clostridium difficile
  Peptostreptococcus spp.
Gram-negative
  Bacteroides fragilis
  Fusobacterium spp.

Other bacteria

Mycobacterium avium-intracellulare
Mycobacterium tuberculosis
Nocardia asteroides
Legionella pneumophila
Listeria monocytogenes

Fungi

Aspergillus fumigatus, A. niger, A. terreus, A. flavus
Blastomyces dermatitidis
Candida albicans
Candida glabrata, C. paropsilosis, C. krusei
Coccidiodes immitis
Cryptococcus neoformans
Histoplasma capsulatum
Mucor/Rhizopus

Viruses

Cytomegalovirus
Epstein-Barr virus
Hepatitis B, C viruses
Herpes simplex virus
Human immunodeficiency virus
Varicella zoster virus

in immunocompromised or chronically ill patients, but are of relatively low virulence in healthy individuals.

There are many gram-negative bacterial species capable of causing infection in surgical patients. Most gram-negative organisms of interest to the surgeon belong to the family Enterobacteriaceae. Other gram-negative bacilli of note include Pseudomonas species, including *Pseudomonas aeruginosa* and *P. fluorescens* and Xanthomonas species.

Anaerobic organisms are unable to grow or divide poorly in air because of the absence of the enzyme catalase. Common anaerobes in the gastrointestinal (GI) tract include *Bacteroides fragilis*, which typically contribute to mixed infections.

Infection because of *Mycobacterium tuberculosis* was once one of the most common causes of death in Europe, causing one in four deaths in the seventeenth and eighteenth centuries. This organism and other related organisms (*M. avium-intracellulare* and *M. leprae*) are known as acid-fast bacilli and are typically slow-growing. Deoxyribonucleic acid (DNA)-based analysis is increasingly providing a means for preliminary, rapid detection.

Fungi

Fungi are typically identified by use of special stains (e.g., potassium hydroxide [KOH], India ink, methenamine silver, or Giemsa). Identification is assisted by observation of branching and septation in stained specimens or in culture. Fungi of relevance to surgeons include those that cause nosocomial infections in surgical patients as part of polymicrobial infections or fungemia (e.g., Candida albicans and related species), rare causes of aggressive soft tissue infections (e.g., Mucor, Rhizopus, and Absidia species), and so-called opportunistic pathogens that cause infection in the immunocompromised host (e.g., Aspergillus species, *Blastomyces dermatitidis*, *Coccidioides immitis*, and *Cryptococcus neoformans*).

Viruses

Because of their small size and necessity for growth within cells, viruses are difficult to culture, requiring a longer time than is typically optimal for clinical decision making. Recent advances in technology have allowed for the identification of viral DNA or ribonucleic acid (RNA) using methods such as polymerase chain reaction. Most viral infections in surgical patients occur in the immunocompromised host, particularly those receiving immunosuppression to prevent rejection of a solid organ allograft. Relevant viruses include adenoviruses, cytomegalovirus, Epstein-Barr virus, herpes simplex virus, and varicella-zoster virus. Surgeons must be aware of the manifestations of hepatitis B and C virus, and human immunodeficiency virus infections, including their capacity to be transmitted to health care workers (described below).

PREVENTION AND TREATMENT OF SURGICAL INFECTIONS

General Principles

Maneuvers to diminish the presence of exogenous (surgeon and operating room environment) and endogenous (patient) microbes are termed prophylaxis, and consist of the use of mechanical, chemical, and antimicrobial modalities, or a combination of these methods.

The host resident microflora of the skin (patient and surgeon) and other barrier surfaces represent a potential source of microbes that can invade the body during trauma, thermal injury, or elective or emergent surgical intervention. A number of maneuvers are typically utilized to prevent spread of these organisms to the operative area, including preoperative scrub by operating room personnel, preoperative skin preparation (with clipping, not shaving), and intraoperative aseptic technique. Additional maneuvers are prudent when undertaking bowel surgery. Preparation of areas of the body such as the distal colorectum requires that body waste in the form of bacteria-laden feces be removed to the greatest extent possible. Current practice includes a clear liquid diet, a cathartic preparation (e.g., polyethylene glycol or buffered-saline laxative), and adequate oral hydration for 12–24 hours prior to colonic resection to flush the contents of the colon.

Although these modalities result in a significant reduction of microbial inoculum, they are not capable of sterilizing the hands of the surgeon or the skin or epithelial surfaces of the patient. This suggests the use of prophylactic antimicrobial agents, especially in patients undergoing procedures associated with the ingress of significant numbers of microbes (e.g., colonic resection) or in whom the consequences of infection carry increased risk (e.g., prosthetic vascular graft infection).

Source Control

The primary precept of surgical infectious disease therapy consists of drainage of all purulent material, debridement of all infected, devitalized tissue, and debris, and/or removal of foreign bodies at the site of infection, plus remediation of the underlying cause of infection. Other treatment modalities such as antimicrobial agents, although critical, are of secondary importance to effective surgery regarding treatment of surgical infections and overall outcome. Rarely, if ever, can an aggressive surgical infection be cured only by the administration of antibiotics, and never in the face of inadequate source control. Finally, it has been well-demonstrated that delay in operative intervention, whether because of misdiagnosis or the need for additional diagnostic studies, is associated with increased morbidity and mortality.

Appropriate Use of Antimicrobial Agents

Table 5-2 shows a classification of antimicrobial agents, mechanisms of action, and spectrum of activity. Prophylaxis consists of the administration of appropriate antimicrobial agent(s) prior to initiation of surgical procedures to reduce the number of microbes that enter the operative site. Timing of prophylaxis for surgery is critical: patients should receive a dose of agent within 30 minutes prior to creating the incision. Agents are selected according to their activity against microbes likely to be present at the surgical site. For the majority of infections not involving the GI tract or biliary/pancreatic tract a dose of first generation cephalosporin is appropriate (e.g., cephazolin). For cases involving the GI/biliary/pancreatic tracts, any one of a number of agents may be utilized (e.g., cefotetan, ampicillin-sulbactam, ertapenem, many others). Use of these prophylactic measures constitutes the current standard of care in North America. By definition, prophylaxis is limited to the time prior to and during the operative procedure; in the vast majority of cases only a single dose of antibiotic is required. However, patients who undergo prolonged procedures in which the duration of the operation exceeds the serum drug

TABLE 5-2 Antimicrobial Agents

Antibiotic class, generic name	Trade name	Mechanism of action	Organism								
			S. pyogenes	MSSA	MRSA	S. epidermidis	Enterococcus	VRE	E. coli	P. aeruginosa	Anaerobes
Penicillins		Cell wall synthesis inhibitors (bind penicillin-binding protein)									
Penicillin G			1	0	0	0	+/−	0	0	0	1
Nafcillin	Nallpen, Unipen		1	1	0	+/−	0	0	0	0	0
Piperacillin	Pipracil		1	0	0	0	+/−	0	1	1	+/−
Penicillin/beta lactamase inhibitor combinations		Cell wall synthesis inhibitors/beta lactamase inhibitors									
Ampicillin-sulbactam	Unasyn		1	1	0	+/−	1	+/−	1	0	1
Ticarcillin-clavulanate	Timentin		1	1	0	+/−	+/−	0	1	1	1
Piperacillin-tazobactam	Zosyn		1	1	0	1	+/−	0	1	1	1
First-generation cephalosporins		Cell wall synthesis inhibitors (bind penicillin-binding protein)									
Cephazolin, cephalexin	Ancef, Keflex		1	1	0	+/−	0	0	1	0	0
Second-generation cephalosporins		Cell wall synthesis inhibitors (bind penicillin-binding protein)									
Cefoxitin	Mefoxin		1	1	0	+/−	0	0	1	0	1
Cefotetan	Cefotan		1	1	0	+/−	0	0	1	0	1−

(continued)

85

TABLE 5-2 *Continued*

Antibiotic class, generic name	Trade name	Mechanism of action	S. pyogenes	MSSA	MRSA	S. epidermidis	Enterococcus	VRE	E. coli	P. aeruginosa	Anaerobes
Cefuroxime	Ceftin	Cell wall synthesis inhibitors (bind penicillin-binding protein)	1	1	0	+/–	0	0	1	0	0
Third- and fourth-generation cephalosporins											
Ceftriaxone	Rocefin		1	1	0	+/–	0	0	1	0	0
Ceftazidime	Fortaz		1	+/–	0	+/–	0	0	1	1	0
Cefepime	Maxipime		1	1	0	+/–	0	0	1	1	0
Cefotaxime	Cefotaxime		1	1	0	+/–	0	0	1	+/–	0
Carbapenems		Cell wall synthesis inhibitors (bind									
Imipenem-cilastatin	Primaxin	penicillin-binding protein)	1	1	0	1	+/–	0	1	1	1
Meropenem	Merrem		1	1	0	1	0	0	1	1	1
Ertapenem	Invanz		1	1	0	1	0	0	1	+/–	1
Aztreonam	Azactam	Cell wall synthesis inhibitor (bind penicillin-binding protein)	0	0	0	0	0	0	1	1	0
Aminoglycosides		Alteration of cell membrane, binding and inhibition of 30S ribosomal unit									
Gentamicin			0	1	0	+/–	1	0	1	1	0
Tobramycin, amikacin			0	1	0	+/–	0	0	1	1	0

Fluoroquinolones

Generic	Trade	Mechanism of action									
Ciprofloxacin	Cipro	Inhibit topoisomerase II and IV (DNA synthesis inhibition)	+/−	1	0	1	0	0	0	1	0
Gatifloxacin	Tequin		1	1	+/−	1	+/−	0	1	+/−	+/−
Levofloxacin	Levaquin		1	1	0	1	0	0	1	+/−	0
Glycopeptides		Cell wall synthesis inhibition									
Vancomycin	Vancocin	(peptidoglycan synthesis inhibition)	1	1	1	1	1	0	0	0	0
Quinupristin-Dalfopristin	Synercid	Inhibits 2 sites on 50S ribosome (protein synthesis inhibition)	1	1	1	1	1	1	1	0	+/−
Linezolid	Zyvox	Inhibits 50S ribosomal activity (protein synthesis inhibition)	1	1	1	1	1	1	0	0	+/−
Daptomycin	Cubicin	Binds bacterial membrane, results in depolarization, lysis	1	1	1	1	1	1	0	0	0
Rifampin		Inhibits DNA-dependent RNA polymerase	1	1	1	1	+/−	0	0	0	0
Clindamycin	Cleocin	Inhibits 50S ribosomal activity (protein synthesis inhibition)	1	1	0	0	0	0	0	0	1
Metronidazole	Flagyl	Production of toxic intermediates (free radical production)	0	0	0	0	0	0	0	0	1

(continued)

TABLE 5-2 *Continued*

Antibiotic class, generic name	Trade name	Mechanism of action	S. pyogenes	MSSA	MRSA	S. epidermidis	Enterococcus	VRE	E. coli	P. aeruginosa	Anaerobes
							Organism				
Macrolides		Inhibit 50S ribosomal activity (protein synthesis inhibition)									
Erythromycin			1	+/–	0	+/–	0	0	0	0	0
Azithromycin	Zithromax		1	1	0	0	0	0	0	0	0
Clarithromycin	Biaxin		1	1	0	0	0	0	0	0	0
Trimethoprim-sulfamethoxazole	Bactrim, Septra	Inhibits sequential steps of folate metabolism	+/–	1	0	+/–	0	0	1	0	0
Tetracyclines		Bind 30S ribosomal unit (protein synthesis inhibition)									
Minocycline	Minocin		1	1	0	0	0	0	0	0	+/–
Doxycycline	Vibromycin		1	+/–	0	0	0	0	1	0	+/–

E. coli = *Escherichia coli*; MRSA = methicillin-resistant *Staphylococcus aureus*; MSSA = methicillin-sensitive *Staphylococcus aureus*; P. aeruginosa = *Pseudomonas aeruginosa*; S. epidermidis = *Staphylococcus epidermidis*; S. pyogenes = *Streptococcus pyogenes*; VRE = vancomycin-resistant enterococcus.

1 = Reliable activity; +/– = variable activity; 0 = no activity.

The sensitivities presented are generalizations. The clinician should confirm sensitivity patterns at the locale where the patient is being treated since these patterns may vary widely depending on location.

88

half-life should receive an additional dose or doses of the antimicrobial agent. There is no evidence that administration of postoperative doses of an antimicrobial agent provides additional benefit.

Empiric therapy comprises the use of an antimicrobial agent or agents when the risk of a surgical infection is high, based on the underlying disease process (e.g., ruptured appendicitis), or when significant contamination during surgery has occurred (e.g., inadequate bowel preparation or considerable spillage of colon contents). Prophylaxis merges into empiric therapy in situations in which the risk of infection increases markedly because of intraoperative findings. Empiric therapy also often is employed in critically ill patients in whom a potential site of infection has been identified and severe sepsis or septic shock occurs. Invariably, empiric therapy should be limited to a short course of drug (3–5 days), and should be curtailed as soon as possible based on microbiologic data (i.e., absence of positive cultures) coupled with improvements in the clinical course of the patient.

Similarly, empiric therapy merges into therapy of established infection in some patients as well. However, among surgical patients, the manner in which therapy is employed, particularly in relation to the use of microbiologic data (culture and antibiotic sensitivity patterns), differs depending on whether the infection is monomicrobial or polymicrobial. Monomicrobial infections frequently are nosocomial infections occurring in postoperative patients, such as UTIs, pneumonia, or catheter-related infection. In polymicrobial infections, culture results are less helpful because it is invariably difficult to identify all microbes that comprise the initial polymicrobial inoculum. For this reason, the antibiotic regimen should not be modified solely on the basis of culture information, as it is less important than the clinical course of the patient. In clinical trials of antimicrobial therapy for appendicitis including antimicrobials with activity against appropriate gram-negative and anaerobic organisms, most failures could not be attributed to antibiotic selection, but rather were because of the inability to achieve effective source control.

Duration of antibiotic administration should be decided at the time the drug regimen is prescribed. As noted above, prophylaxis is limited to a single dose administered immediately prior to creating the incision. Empiric therapy should be limited to 3–5 days or less, and should be curtailed if the presence of a local site or systemic infection is not revealed.

In the later phases of postoperative antibiotic treatment of serious intraabdominal infection, the absence of an elevated WBC count, lack of band forms of PMNs on peripheral smear, and lack of fever ($<38.2°C$ [100.5°F]) provide close to complete assurance that infection has been eradicated. Under these circumstances, antibiotics can be discontinued with impunity.

Allergy to antimicrobial agents must be considered prior to prescribing them. Penicillin allergy is quite common, the reported incidence ranging from 0.7–10 percent. Although avoiding the use of any beta-lactam drug is appropriate in patients who manifest significant allergic reactions to penicillins, the incidence of cross-reactivity appears highest for carbapenems, much lower for cephalosporins (approximately 5–7 percent), and extremely small or nonexistent for monobactams. Severe allergic manifestations to a specific class of agents, such as anaphylaxis, generally preclude the use of any agents in that class, except under circumstances in which use of a certain drug represents a lifesaving measure.

INFECTIONS OF SIGNIFICANCE IN SURGICAL PATIENTS

Surgical Site Infections

SSIs are infections of the tissues, organs, or spaces exposed by surgeons during performance of an invasive procedure. SSIs are associated with considerable morbidity and occasional lethality, and substantial health care costs and patient inconvenience and dissatisfaction. The development of SSIs is related to three factors: (1) the degree of microbial contamination of the wound during surgery, (2) the duration of the procedure, and (3) host factors such as diabetes, malnutrition, obesity, immune suppression, and a number of other underlying disease states (Table 5-3). By definition, an incisional SSI has occurred if a surgical wound drains purulent material or if the surgeon judges it to be infected and opens it.

Surgical wounds are classified based on the presumed magnitude of the bacterial load at the time of surgery (Table 5-4). Clean wounds (class I) include those in which no infection is present; only skin microflora potentially contaminate the wound, and no hollow viscus that contains microbes is entered. Class ID wounds are similar except that a prosthetic device (e.g., mesh or valve) is inserted. Clean/contaminated wounds (class II) include those in which a hollow viscus such as the respiratory, alimentary, or genitourinary tracts with indigenous bacterial flora is opened under controlled circumstances without significant spillage of contents. Contaminated wounds (class III) include open

TABLE 5-3. Risk Factors for Development of Surgical Site Infections

Patient factors
Older age
Immunosuppression
Obesity
Diabetes mellitus
Chronic inflammatory process
Malnutrition
Peripheral vascular disease
Anemia
Radiation
Chronic skin disease
Carrier state (e.g., chronic *Staphylococcus* carriage)
Recent operation

Local factors
Poor skin preparation
Contamination of instruments
Inadequate antibiotic prophylaxis
Prolonged procedure
Local tissue necrosis
Hypoxia, hypothermia

Microbial factors
Prolonged hospitalization (leading to nosocomial organisms)
Toxin secretion
Resistance to clearance (e.g., capsule formation)

TABLE 5-4. Wound Class, Representative Procedures, and Expected Infection Rates

Wound class	Examples of cases	Expected infection rates
Clean (class I)	Hernia repair, breast biopsy	1.0–5.4 percent
Clean/contaminated (class II)	Cholecystectomy, elective GI surgery	2.1–9.5 percent
Contaminated (class III)	Penetrating abdominal trauma, large tissue injury, enterotomy during bowel obstruction	3.4–13.2 percent
Dirty (class IV)	Perforated diverticulitis, necrotizing soft tissue infections	3.1–12.8 percent

accidental wounds encountered early after injury, those with extensive introduction of bacteria into a normally sterile area of the body because of major breaks in sterile technique (e.g., open cardiac massage), gross spillage of viscus contents such as from the intestine, or incision through inflamed, albeit nonpurulent, tissue. Dirty wounds (class IV) include traumatic wounds in which a significant delay in treatment has occurred and in which necrotic tissue is present, those created in the presence of overt infection as evidenced by the presence of purulent material, and those created to access a perforated viscus accompanied by a high degree of contamination.

The National Nosocomial Infection Surveillance (NNIS) risk index is commonly used to classify infection risk as well, and assesses three factors: (1) American Society of Anesthesiologists (ASA) Physical Status score greater than 2, (2) class III/IV wound, and (3) duration of operation greater than the 75th percentile for that particular procedure, to refine the risk of infection beyond that achieved by use of wound classification alone. Intriguingly, the risk of SSIs for class I wounds varies from approximately 1–2 percent for patients with low NNIS scores, to approximately 15 percent for patients with high NNIS scores (e.g., long operations and/or high ASA scores), and it seems clear that additional refinements are required.

Surgical management of the wound is also a critical determinant of the propensity to develop an SSI. In healthy individuals, class I and II wounds may be closed primarily, although skin closure of class III and IV wounds is associated with high rates of incisional SSIs (approximately 25–50 percent). The superficial aspects of these latter types of wounds should be packed open and allowed to heal by secondary intention, although selective use of delayed primary closure has been associated with a reduction in incisional SSI rates.

Effective therapy for incisional SSIs consists solely of incision and drainage without the addition of antibiotics. Antibiotic therapy is reserved for patients in whom evidence of severe cellulitis is present, or who manifest signs of concurrent sepsis. Although culture results are of epidemiologic interest, they rarely serve to direct therapy because antibiotics are not routinely withheld until results are known.

Intraabdominal Infections

Microbial contamination of the peritoneal cavity is termed peritonitis or intraabdominal infection, and is classified according to etiology. Primary microbial peritonitis occurs when microbes invade the normally sterile confines of the peritoneal cavity via hematogenous dissemination from a distant source of infection or direct inoculation. This process is more common among patients who retain large amounts of ascites, and in those being treated for renal failure via peritoneal dialysis. These infections invariably are monomicrobial and rarely require surgical intervention. Treatment consists of administration of an antibiotic to which the organism is sensitive. Removal of indwelling devices (e.g., peritoneal dialysis catheter or peritoneovenous shunt) may be required for effective therapy of recurrent infections.

Secondary microbial peritonitis occurs subsequent to contamination of the peritoneal cavity because of perforation or severe inflammation and infection of an intraabdominal organ. Examples include appendicitis, perforation of any portion of the GI tract, or diverticulitis. As noted previously, effective therapy requires source control to resect the diseased organ; débridement of necrotic, infected tissue and debris; and administration of antimicrobial agents directed against aerobes and anaerobes. A combination of agents or single agents with a broad spectrum of activity can be used for this purpose; conversion of a parenteral to an oral regimen when the patient's ileus resolves provides results similar to those achieved with intravenous antibiotics. Effective source control and antibiotic therapy is associated with low failure rates and a mortality rate of approximately 5–6 percent; inability to control the source of infection leads to mortality greater than 40 percent. The response rate to effective source control and use of appropriate antibiotics has remained approximately 70–90 percent over the past several decades.

Patients in whom standard therapy fails develop an intraabdominal abscess, leakage from a gastrointestinal anastomosis leading to postoperative peritonitis, or tertiary (persistent) peritonitis. The latter is a poorly understood entity that is more common in immunosuppressed patients in whom peritoneal host defenses do not effectively clear or sequester the initial secondary microbial peritoneal infection. Microbes such as *E. faecalis* and *E. faecium*, *S. epidermidis*, *C. albicans*, and *P. aeruginosa* can be identified, typically in combination, and may be selected based on their lack of responsiveness to the initial antibiotic regimen, coupled with diminished activity of host defenses. Unfortunately, even with effective antimicrobial agent therapy, this disease process is associated with mortality rates in excess of 50 percent.

Formerly, the presence of an intraabdominal abscess mandated surgical reexploration and drainage. Today, the vast majority of such abscesses can be effectively diagnosed via abdominal computed tomographic (CT) imaging techniques and drained percutaneously. Surgical intervention is reserved for those individuals who harbor multiple abscesses, those with abscesses in proximity to vital structures such that percutaneous drainage would be hazardous, and those in whom an ongoing source of contamination (e.g., enteric leak) is identified. The necessity of antimicrobial agent therapy and precise guidelines that dictate duration of catheter drainage have not been established. A short course (3–7 days) of antibiotics that possess aerobic and anaerobic activity seems reasonable, and most practitioners leave the drainage catheter in situ until it is clear that cavity collapse has occurred, output is less than 10–20 mL/day, no evidence of an ongoing source of contamination is present, and the patient's clinical condition has improved.

Infections of the Skin and Soft Tissue

These infections can be classified according to whether or not surgical intervention is required. For example, superficial skin and skin structure infections such as cellulitis, erysipelas, and lymphangitis invariably are effectively treated with antibiotics alone, although a search for a local source of infection should be undertaken. Generally, drugs that possess activity against the gram-positive skin microflora that are causative are selected. Furuncles or boils may drain spontaneously or require surgical incision and drainage. Antibiotics are prescribed if significant cellulitis is present or if cellulitis does not rapidly resolve after surgical drainage. The astute clinician should be aware of the emerging incidence of community acquired methicillin-resistant Staphylococcus aureus in the setting of unresolving cellulitis after simple drainage, and consider culture of these wounds.

Aggressive soft tissue infections are rare, difficult to diagnose, and require immediate surgical intervention plus administration of antimicrobial agents. Failure to do so results in an extremely high mortality rate (approximately 80–100 percent), and even with rapid recognition and intervention, current mortality rates remain approximately 30–50 percent. These infections are classified based on the soft tissue layer(s) of involvement (e.g., skin and superficial soft tissue, deep soft tissue, and muscle) and the pathogen(s) that cause them.

Patients at risk for these types of infections include those who are older adult, immunosuppressed, or diabetic; those who suffer from peripheral vascular disease; or those with a combination of these factors. Additionally, over the last decade, aggressive necrotizing soft tissue infections among healthy individuals because of streptococci have been described. The diagnosis of necrotizing soft tissue infection is most commonly clinical. Not surprisingly, patients often develop sepsis syndrome or septic shock without an obvious cause. Affected areas include the extremities, perineum, trunk, and torso. Careful examination should be undertaken for an entry site from which grayish, turbid semipurulent material ("dishwater pus") can be expressed, and for the presence of skin changes (bronze hue or brawny induration), blebs, or crepitus. The patient often develops pain at the site of infection that appears to be out of proportion to any of the physical manifestations. Any of these findings mandates immediate surgical intervention, which should consist of exposure and direct visualization of potentially infected tissue (including deep soft tissue, fascia, and underlying muscle) and radical resection of affected areas. Radiologic studies should be undertaken only in patients in whom the diagnosis is not seriously considered, as they delay surgical intervention and frequently provide confusing information. Antimicrobial agents directed against gram-positive and gram-negative aerobes and anaerobes (e.g., vancomycin plus a carbapenem), and high-dose aqueous penicillin G (16,000 to 20,000 units/day) should be administered. Approximately 60–70 percent of such infections are polymicrobial, the remainder being caused by a single organism such as *P. aeruginosa*, *Clostridium perfringens*, or *Streptococcus pyogenes*. Most patients should be returned to the operating room on a scheduled basis for evaluation and further debridement, if necessary. Antibiotic therapy can be refined based on culture and sensitivity results, particularly in the case of monomicrobial soft tissue infections.

Postoperative Nosocomial Infections

Surgical patients are prone to develop a wide variety of nosocomial infections during the postoperative period, which include SSIs, UTIs, pneumonia, and bacteremic episodes. SSIs are discussed above, and the latter types of nosocomial infections are related to prolonged use of indwelling tubes and catheters for the purpose of urinary drainage, ventilation, and venous and arterial access, respectively.

The presence of a postoperative UTI should be considered based on urinalysis demonstrating WBCs or bacteria, a positive test for leukocyte esterase, or a combination of these elements. The diagnosis is established after greater than 104 CFU/mL of microbes are identified by culture techniques in symptomatic patients, or greater than 105 CFU/mL in asymptomatic individuals. Treatment with a single antibiotic that achieves high levels in the urine is appropriate. Postoperative surgical patients should have indwelling urinary catheters removed as quickly as possible, typically within 1–2 days, as long as they are mobile.

Prolonged mechanical ventilation is associated with an increased incidence of pneumonia, and is frequently because of pathogens common in the nosocomial environment. Frequently these organisms are highly resistant to many different agents. The diagnosis is established based on clinical criteria of purulent sputum, fever, elevated WBC, and roentgenographic evidence of one or more areas of pulmonary consolidation. Consideration should be given to performing bronchoalveolar lavage to obtain samples to assess by Gram stain and to performing a culture to assess for the presence of microbes. Surgical patients should be weaned from mechanical ventilation as soon as feasible to reduce the incidence of this complication.

Infection associated with indwelling intravascular catheters has become a common problem among hospitalized patients. Because of the complexity of many surgical procedures, these devices are increasingly used for physiologic monitoring, vascular access, drug delivery, and parenteral nutrition. Among the several million catheters inserted each year in the United States, approximately 25 percent will become colonized, and approximately 5 percent will be associated with bacteremia. Many patients who develop intravascular catheter infections are asymptomatic, often exhibiting an elevation in the WBC count. Blood cultures obtained from a peripheral site and drawn through the catheter that reveal the presence of the same organism increase the index of suspicion for the presence of a catheter infection. Obvious purulence at the exit site of the skin tunnel, severe sepsis syndrome because of any type of organism when other potential causes have been excluded, or bacteremia because of gram-negative aerobes or fungi should lead to catheter removal.

Sepsis

A number of studies have demonstrated the importance of empiric antimicrobial agent therapy in patients who develop severe sepsis concurrent with fluid resuscitation, metabolic support, and control of any site-specific source of infection. Use of institutional and unit-specific sensitivity patterns and knowledge of likely pathogens are critical in selecting an appropriate agent. Retrospective reviews demonstrate that appropriate initial therapy is associated with a two- to threefold reduction in mortality.

A number of new therapies for treatment of patients with severe sepsis have recently been demonstrated to be of significant benefit in patients with severe sepsis or septic shock. Drotrecogin alpha (activated), also known as Xigris, is a recombinant form of human-activated protein C. The use of this agent in a series of patients with sepsis syndrome has been associated with a 6 percent overall reduction in mortality (31–25 percent, $p = 0.005$). Evaluation of the surgical cohorts of several grouped trials suggests that the benefits of this agent are confined to those patients with at least two organ failures (e.g., elevated lactate plus respiratory failure). The use of this agent should be considered in patients with severe infection who have completed their source control procedure, and who develop severe sepsis with at least two organs failing. Current recommendations are a dose of 24 μg/kg per h given for 96 h. The infusion should be interrupted for procedures or surgery, or for significant life-threatening bleeding.

A number of investigators have revisited the issue of corticosteroids for the treatment of septic shock. A number of randomized, controlled trials have demonstrated the benefit of replacement doses of corticosteroids in patients with severe shock states. In patients who develop septic shock, these authors currently initiate low-dose hydrocortisone (100 mg/8 h) after performing a corticotropin stimulation test (baseline cortisol level, corticotropin 250 mcg intravenously, cortisol level 1 h later). Adrenal insufficiency is identified if the baseline cortisol level is less than 34 mcg/dL, or if an increase of less than 9 mcg/dL occurs after corticotropin stimulation. Low-dose steroid therapy should be discontinued in patients with normal adrenal function.

Blood-Borne Pathogens

Although alarming to contemplate, the risk of human immunodeficiency virus (HIV) transmission from patient to surgeon is low. By December 31, 2001, there had been six cases of surgeons with HIV seroconversion from a possible occupational exposure, from a total of 470,000 HIV cases to that date reported to the Centers for Disease Control and Prevention (CDC). The risks for acquiring HIV infection are related to the prevalence of HIV infection in the population being cared for, the probability of transmission from a percutaneous injury suffered while caring for an infected patient, the number of such injuries sustained, and the use of postexposure prophylaxis. Annual calculated risks for acquiring HIV infection in Glasgow, Scotland, ranged from one in 200,000 for general surgeons not utilizing postexposure prophylaxis to as low as one in 10,000,000 with use of routine postexposure prophylaxis after significant exposures. Postexposure prophylaxis begun early for HIV significantly decreases the risk of seroconversion for health care workers with occupational exposure to HIV.

Transmission of HIV (and other infections spread by blood and body fluid) from patient to health care worker can be minimized by observation of universal precautions, which include the following: (1) routine use of barriers (such as gloves and/or goggles) when anticipating contact with blood or body fluids, (2) washing of hands and other skin surfaces immediately after contact with blood or body fluids, and (3) careful handling and disposal of sharp instruments during and after use.

Hepatitis B virus (HBV) is a DNA virus that only affects humans. Primary infection with HBV generally is self-limited (approximately 6 percent of those infected are older than 5 years of age), but can progress to a chronic carrier state. Death from chronic liver disease or hepatocellular cancer occurs in roughly 30 percent of chronically infected persons. Surgeons and other health care workers are at high risk for this blood-borne infection and should receive the HBV vaccine. In the postexposure setting, hepatitis B immune globulin (HBIG) confers approximately 75 percent protection from HBV infection.

Hepatitis C virus (HCV), previously known as non-A, non-B hepatitis, is a RNA flavivirus first identified specifically in the late 1980s. This virus is confined to humans and chimpanzees. A chronic carrier state develops in 75–80 percent of patients with the infection, with chronic liver disease occurring in three fourths of patients developing chronic infection. The number of new infections per year has declined since the 1980s because of the incorporation of testing of the blood supply for this virus. Fortunately, HCV virus is not transmitted efficiently through occupational exposures to blood, with the seroconversion rate after accidental needlestick reported to be approximately 2 percent.

Suggested Readings

Rutkow E: Appendicitis: The quintessential American surgical disease. Arch Surg 133:1024, 1998.

Dunn DL, Simmons RL: The role of anaerobic bacteria in intra-abdominal infections. Rev Infect Dis 6:S139, 1984.

Angus DC, Linde-Zwirble WT, Lidicer J, et al: Epidemiology of severe sepsis in the United States. Crit Care Med 29:1303, 2001.

Rozycki GS, Tremblay L, Feliciano DV, et al: Three hundred consecutive emergent celiotomies in general surgery patients: Influence of advanced diagnostic imaging techniques and procedures on diagnosis. Ann Surg 235:681, 2002.

Solomkin JS, Meakins JL Jr., Allo MD, et al: Antibiotic trials in intra-abdominal infections. A critical evaluation of study design and outcome reporting. Ann Surg 200:29, 1984.

Barie PS: Modern surgical antibiotic prophylaxis and therapy—less is more. Surg Infect 1:23, 2000.

Martone WJ, Nichols RL: Recognition, prevention, surveillance, and management of surgical site infections. Clin Infect Dis 33:S67, 2001.

Solomkin JS, Mazuski JE, Baron EJ, et al: Infectious Diseases Society of America. Guidelines for the selection of anti-infective agents for complicated intra-abdominal infections. Clin Infect Dis 37:997, 2003.

Malangoni MA: Necrotizing soft tissue infections: Are we making any progress? Surg Infect 2:145, 2001.

Hoffken G, Niederman MS: Nosocomial pneumonia: The importance of a de-escalating strategy for antibiotic treatment of pneumonia in the ICU. Chest 122:2183, 2002.

Centers for Disease Control and Prevention: Updated US Public Health Service guidelines for the management of occupational exposures to HBV, HCV, and HIV and recommendations for post-exposure prophylaxis. MMWR 50:23, 2001.

6 | Trauma

Jon M. Burch, Reginald J. Franciose,
and Ernest E. Moore

INITIAL EVALUATION AND RESUSCITATION OF THE INJURED PATIENT

Airway Management

Insuring an adequate airway is the first priority because efforts to restore cardiovascular integrity will be futile unless the oxygen content of the blood is adequate. Simultaneously, all blunt trauma patients require cervical spine immobilization until injury is ruled out. This can be accomplished with a hard (Philadelphia) collar or sand bags on both sides of the head taped to the back board.

Patients who are conscious and have a normal voice, in general, do not require further evaluation or early attention to their airway. Patients who have an abnormal voice or altered mental status require further airway evaluation. Direct laryngoscopic inspection will often reveal blood, vomit, or soft tissue swelling as sources of airway obstruction. Suctioning may afford immediate relief in many patients. Altered mental status is the most common indication for intubation because of the patient's inability to protect their airway. Options for airway access include nasotracheal, orotracheal, or surgical. Nasotracheal intubation can only be accomplished in patients who are breathing spontaneously and is contraindicated in the apneic patient. Nasotracheal intubation is primarily employed by paramedics in the field.

Orotracheal intubation can be performed in patients with potential cervical spine injuries provided that manual in-line cervical immobilization is maintained. The advantages of orotracheal intubation are the direct visualization of the vocal cords, the ability to use larger diameter endotracheal tubes, and applicability to apneic patients. The disadvantage is that conscious patients usually require neuromuscular blockade or deep sedation. Those who attempt rapid sequence induction must be thoroughly familiar with the details and contraindications of the procedure (see Chapter 45). Patients in whom attempts at intubation have failed or are precluded because of extensive facial injuries require a surgical airway. Cricothyroidotomy is preferred over tracheostomy in most emergent situations.

Breathing

All injured patients should receive supplemental oxygen therapy and be monitored by pulse oximetry. The following conditions may constitute an immediate threat to life because of inadequate ventilation: (1) tension pneumothorax, (2) open pneumothorax, or (3) flail chest/pulmonary contusion. The diagnosis of tension pneumothorax is implied by the finding of respiratory distress in combination with any of the following physical signs: tracheal deviation away from the affected side, decreased breath sounds on the affected side, distended neck veins or systemic hypotension, or subcutaneous emphysema on the affected side. Immediate tube thoracostomy is indicated without awaiting chest radiograph confirmation.

An open pneumothorax or sucking chest wound occurs with full-thickness loss of the chest wall permitting a free communication between the pleural space and the atmosphere. Definitive treatment requires wound closure and tube thoracostomy.

Flail chest occurs when four or more ribs are fractured in at least two locations. Paradoxical movement of this free floating segment of chest wall may occasionally be sufficient to compromise ventilation. However, it is of greater physiologic importance that patients with flail chest frequently have an underlying pulmonary contusion. Respiratory failure in these patients may not be immediate and frequent reevaluation is warranted. The initial chest radiograph usually underestimates the degree of pulmonary contusion.

Circulation

A first approximation of the patient's cardiovascular status is obtained by palpating peripheral pulses. In general, a systolic blood pressure of 60 mm Hg is required for the carotid pulse to be palpable, 70 mm Hg for the femoral pulse and 80 mm Hg for the radial pulse.

External control of hemorrhage should be obtained before restoring circulating volume. Manual compression and splints will frequently control extremity hemorrhage. Blind clamping should be avoided because of the risk to adjacent structures, particularly nerves. Digital control of hemorrhage for penetrating injuries of the head, neck, thoracic outlet, groin, and extremities is key. A gloved finger should be placed through the wound directly on the bleeding vessel applying only enough pressure to control active bleeding. The surgeon performing this maneuver must then walk with the patient to the operating room for definitive treatment. Scalp lacerations through the galea aponeurotica tend to bleed profusely; and can be controlled with Rainey clips or a large nylon continuous stitch.

Intravenous access for fluid resuscitation is begun with two peripheral catheters, 16 gauge or larger in an adult. Blood should be drawn simultaneously and sent for typing and hematocrit. Venous lines for volume resuscitation should be short with a large diameter. Saphenous vein cut downs at the ankle or percutaneous femoral vein catheter introducers are preferred. Secondary central venous introducers should be placed in the OR in the event vena caval crossclamping is performed. If two attempts at percutaneous peripheral access are unsuccessful, in hypovolemic children younger than 6 years of age, interosseous cannulation should be performed in the proximal tibia or distal femur if the tibia is fractured.

Initial Fluid Resuscitation

Initial fluid resuscitation is a 1 L intravenous bolus of normal saline, Ringer lactate, or other isotonic crystalloid in an adult or 20 mL/kg Ringer lactate in a child. This is repeated one time in an adult and twice in a child prior to administering red blood cells. Classic signs and symptoms of shock are tachycardia, hypotension, tachypnea, mental status changes, diaphoresis and pallor. None of these signs or symptoms taken alone can predict the patient's organ perfusion status. When viewed as a constellation, they can help to evaluate the patient's response to treatment.

There are several caveats that must be kept in mind. Individuals in good physical condition, particularly trained athletes with a low resting pulse rate, may manifest only a relative tachycardia. Patients on β-blocking medications

TABLE 6-1 Signs and Symptoms for Different Classes of Shock

	Class I	Class II	Class III	Class IV
Blood loss (mL)	Up to 750	750–1500	1500–2000	>2000
Blood loss (%BV)	Up to 15%	15–30%	30–40%	>40%
Pulse rate	<100	>100	>120	>140
Blood pressure	Normal	Normal	Decreased	Decreased
Pulse pressure (mm Hg)	Normal or increased	Decreased	Decreased	Decreased
Respiratory rate	14–20	20–30	30–40	>35
Urine output (mL/h)	>30	20–30	5–15	Negligible
CNS/mental status	Slightly anxious	Mildly anxious	Anxious and confused	Confused and lethargic

BV = blood volume; CNS = central nervous system.

may not be able to increase their heart rate in response to stress. In children relative bradycardia can occur with severe blood loss and is an ominous sign. On the other hand, hypoxia, pain, apprehension, and stimulant drugs (cocaine, amphetamines) will produce a tachycardia. In healthy patients blood volume must decrease by 30–40 percent before hypotension occurs (Table 6-1). Younger patients with good sympathetic tone can maintain systemic blood pressure with severe intravascular deficits.

Acute changes in mental status can be caused by hypoxia, hypercarbia, hypovolemia or may be an early sign of increasing intracranial pressure (ICP). A deterioration in mental status may be subtle and may not progress in a predictable fashion. Previously cooperative patients may become anxious and combative as they become hypoxic; whereas, a patient agitated from drugs or alcohol may become somnolent if hypovolemic shock develops. Urine output is a sensitive indicator of organ perfusion. Adequate urine output is .5 mL/kg/h in an adult, 1 mL/kg/h in a child, and 2 mL/kg/h in an infant younger than 1 year of age.

Based on the initial response to fluid resuscitation, hypovolemic injured patients will separate themselves into three broad categories: responders, transient responders, and nonresponders.

Persistent Hypotension (Nonresponders)

The spectrum of disease in this category ranges from nonsurvivable multisystem injury to problems as simple as a tension pneumothorax. An evaluation of the patient's neck veins and central venous pressure (CVP) is an important early maneuver. CVP determines right ventricular preload; and in otherwise healthy trauma patients, its measurement yields objective information regarding the patient's overall volume status. A hypotensive patient with a CVP less than 5 cm H_2O is hypovolemic and is likely to have ongoing hemorrhage. A hypotensive patient with a CVP greater than 15 cm H_2O is likely to be in cardiogenic shock.

In trauma patients the differential diagnosis of cardiogenic shock is a short list: 1) tension pneumothorax, 2) pericardial tamponade, 3) myocardial contusion or infarction, and 4) air embolism. Tension pneumothorax is the most frequent cause of cardiac failure. Traumatic pericardial tamponade most often is associated with penetrating injury to the heart. As blood leaks out of the injured heart, it accumulates in the pericardial sac. When the pressure exceeds that of the right atrium, right ventricular preload is reduced. With acute tamponade as little as 100 mL of blood within the pericardial sac can produce life-threatening hemodynamic compromise. The usual presentation is a patient with a penetrating injury in proximity to the heart who is hypotensive and has distended neck veins or an elevated CVP. Ultrasonography (US) in the emergency department using a subxiphoid or parasternal view is extremely helpful. Once the diagnosis of cardiac tamponade is established, pericardiocentesis should be performed. Evacuation of as little as 15–25 mL of blood may dramatically improve the patient's hemodynamic profile. While pericardiocentesis is being performed, preparation should be made for emergent transport to the OR. If pericardiocentesis is unsuccessful and the patient remains severely hypotensive (SBP <70 mm Hg) emergency department thoracotomy should be performed. This is best accomplished using a left anterolateral thoracotomy, longitudinal pericardiotomy anterior to the phrenic nerve, followed by evacuation of the pericardial sac and temporary control of the cardiac injury. The patient is then transported to the OR for definitive repair.

Myocardial contusion from direct myocardial impact occurs in approximately one third of patients sustaining significant blunt chest trauma. The diagnostic criteria for myocardial contusion include specific electrocardiograph abnormalities, but serial cardiac enzyme determinations lack sensitivity, and are not predictive of complications. Life-threatening complications of ventricular arrhythmias and cardiac pump failure occur in less than 5 percent and less than 1 percent of patients, respectively.

Air embolism is a frequently overlooked lethal complication of pulmonary injury. It occurs when air from an injured bronchus enters an adjacent injured pulmonary vein and returns to the left heart. Air accumulation in the left ventricle impedes diastolic filling; and during systole, it is pumped into the coronary arteries disrupting coronary perfusion. The typical scenario is a patient with a penetrating chest injury who appears hemodynamically stable but suddenly arrests after being intubated and placed on positive pressure ventilation. The patient should be placed in the Trendelenburg position to trap the air in the apex of the left ventricle. Emergency thoracotomy is followed by cross clamping the pulmonary hilum on the side of the injury to prevent further introduction of air. Air is aspirated from the apex of the left ventricle with an 18-gauge needle and 50-mL syringe. Vigorous open cardiac massage is used to force the air bubbles through the coronary arteries. The highest point of the aortic root is also aspirated to prevent air from entering the coronaries or embolizing to the brain. The patient should be kept in Trendelenburg and the hilum clamped until the pulmonary venous injury is controlled.

Persistent hypotension with flat neck veins because of uncontrolled hemorrhage is associated with a high mortality. A rapid search for the source or sources of hemorrhage including abdominal ultrasound, anteroposterior chest and pelvic radiographs, which usually will indicate the regions of the body responsible for the blood loss. Type O red blood cells (O negative for women of childbearing age) or type-specific red blood cells should be administered and the patient taken directly to the OR for exploration. For patients with a sustained systolic blood pressure of less than 70 mm Hg despite blood administration, emergency department thoracotomy should be considered. The clearest indication for this procedure is penetrating chest trauma. The goal of emergency department thoracotomy for thoracic injuries is control of hemorrhage; for abdominal injuries the goal is to sustain central circulation and limit abdominal blood loss by clamping the descending thoracic aorta.

Transient Responders

Hypotensive patients who transiently respond to fluid administration usually have some degree of active hemorrhage. Those with penetrating injuries should be taken to the OR for exploration. Those with multiple blunt injuries constitute a diagnostic dilemma. It is during these diagnostic evaluations where the greatest hazard exists because monitoring is compromised, and the environment is suboptimal to deal with acute problems.

SECONDARY SURVEY

Once the conditions which constitute an immediate threat to life have been addressed or excluded, the patient is examined in a systematic fashion, literally head to toe, to identify all occult injuries. Special attention should be given to the patient's back, axillae, and perineum because injuries in these areas are easily overlooked. All patients should undergo digital rectal examination and a Foley catheter should be inserted to decompress the bladder, obtain a urine specimen, and monitor urine output. Stable patients at risk for urethral injury should undergo urethrography before catheterization. A nasogastric tube should be inserted to decrease the risk of gastric aspiration and to allow inspection of the contents for blood suggestive of occult gastroduodenal injury.

For patients with severe blunt trauma, anterior/posterior chest and pelvic radiographs should be obtained as soon as possible. For patients with truncal gunshot wounds, posterior/anterior and lateral radiographs of the chest and abdomen are warranted. It also is helpful to mark the entrance and exit sites with metallic clips.

Mechanisms and Patterns of Injury

Evaluation and decision making are far more difficult in blunt than in penetrating trauma. In general, more energy is transferred over a wider area during blunt trauma than from a gunshot wound (GSW) or stab wound (SW). Injuries involving high energy transfer include auto-pedestrian accidents, motor vehicle accidents in which the car's change of speed exceeds 20 mph or in which the patient has been ejected, motorcycle accidents, and falls from heights greater than 20 feet. The greatest risk factors from the field associated with life-threatening injures are death of another occupant in the vehicle and an extrication time greater than 20 min.

Patients who have sustained high energy transfer trauma have certain patterns of injury related to the mechanism. When unrestrained drivers suffer frontal impacts, their heads strike the windshield, their chests and upper abdomens hit the steering column, and their legs or knees contact the dashboard. The resultant injuries frequently include facial fractures, cervical spine fractures, laceration of the thoracic aorta, myocardial contusion, injury to the spleen and liver, and fractures of the pelvis and lower extremities.

Penetrating injuries are classified according to the wounding agent (i.e., SWs, GSWs, or shotgun wounds [SGW]). Experience in urban trauma centers indicate that high velocity GSWs (bullet speed greater than 2000 ft/s) are infrequent in the civilian setting. Close-range (<7 meters) SGWs are tantamount to high velocity wounds because the entire energy of the load is delivered to a small area. Long-range SGWs result in a diffuse pellet pattern in which pellets are dispersed and of comparatively low energy.

Regional Assessment and Special Diagnostic Tests

Head

The Glasgow Coma Scale (GSC) should be determined for all injured patients (Table 6-2). It is calculated by adding the scores of the best motor response, best verbal response, and eye opening. Scores range from 3 (the lowest) to 15 (normal). Scores of 13–15 indicate mild head injury; 9–12, moderate injury; and less than 9, a severe injury. The GSC is useful for both triage and prognosis.

Examination of the head should focus on potentially treatable neurologic injuries. Of great importance are the presence of lateralizing findings, e.g., a unilateral dilated pupil unreactive to light, asymmetric movement of the extremities either spontaneously or in response to noxious stimuli, or a unilateral Babinski sign suggests a treatable intracranial mass lesion or major structural damage.

Epidural hematomas occur when blood accumulates between the skull and dura and are caused by disruption of the middle meningeal artery or other small arteries in that potential space from a skull fracture. Subdural hematomas occur between the dura and cortex and are caused by venous disruption or laceration of the parenchyma of the brain.

Because of the underlying brain injury, prognosis is much worse with subdural hematomas. Intraparenchymal hematomas and contusions can occur anywhere within the brain. Diffuse hemorrhage into the subarachnoid space may cause vasospasm and reduce cerebral blood flow. Diffuse axonal injury (DAI) results from high speed deceleration injury and represents direct axonal damage. On computed tomography (CT) a blurring of the gray/white matter interface may be seen along with multiple small punctate hemorrhages. Early evidence of DAI on CT scan is associated with a poor outcome. Magnetic

TABLE 6-2 Glasgow Coma Scale[a]

		Adults	Infants/children
Eye opening	4	Spontaneous	Spontaneous
	3	To voice	To voice
	2	To pain	To pain
	1	None	None
Verbal	5	Oriented	Alert, normal vocalization
	4	Confused	Cries but consolable
	3	Inappropriate words	Persistently irritable
	2	Incomprehensible words	Restless, agitated, moaning
	1	None	None
Motor response	6	Obeys commands	Spontaneous, purposeful
	5	Localizes pain	Localizes pain
	4	Withdraws	Withdraws
	3	Abnormal flexion	Abnormal flexion
	2	Abnormal extension	Abnormal extension
	1	None	None

[a]Score is calculated by adding the scores of the best motor response, best verbal response, and eye opening. Scores range from 3 (the lowest) to 15 (normal).

resonance imaging (MRI) often can identify DAI with greater precision than CT.

Significant penetrating injuries usually are produced by bullets from hand guns. While the diagnosis usually is obvious, in some instances, wounds in the auditory canal, mouth and nose can be elusive.

Neck

In evaluating the neck of blunt trauma victims, all patients should be assumed to have cervical spine injuries until proven otherwise. The presence of posterior midline pain or tenderness should provoke a thorough radiologic evaluation. The three view cervical spine series: lateral with visualization of C7-T1, anterior/posterior, and transoral odontoid views will detect most significant fractures. CT will identify almost all fractures but miss some subluxations. MRI is presently considered the most definitive test.

Spinal cord injuries can be complete or partial. Complete injuries have loss of motor function and sensation two or more levels below the bony injury. Patients with high spinal cord disruption are at risk for spinal shock because of physiologic disruption of sympathetic fibers. Central cord syndrome usually occurs in older persons who suffer hyperextension injuries. Motor function and pain and temperature sensation are preserved in the lower extremities but diminished in the upper extremities. Anterior cord syndrome is characterized by diminished motor function and pain and temperature sensation below the level of the injury. Position, vibratory sensation, and crude touch are maintained. Brown-Sequard syndrome is usually the result of a penetrating injury in which the right or left half of the spinal cord is transected. This rare lesion is characterized by the ipsilateral loss of motor function, proprioception, and vibratory sensation, whereas pain and temperature sensation are lost on the contralateral side.

Selective management of penetrating neck wounds are based on the neck divided into three zones. Zone one is between the clavicles and cricoid cartilage, zone two is between the cricoid cartilage and the angle of the mandible, and zone three is above the angle of mandible. Hemodynamically stable patients with zone one injuries should undergo angiography of the great vessels, soluble contrast esophagram followed by barium esophagram, esophagoscopy, and bronchoscopy. An alternate is CT scanning to determine which of these studies is needed.

Unstable patients with zone two injuries or those with evidence of airway compromise, an expanding hematoma, or significant external hemorrhage should be explored promptly. Stable patients without the above findings are observed for 12 h. Patients with right-to-left transcervical GSWs, however, may warrant diagnostic evaluation depending on the trajectory.

Patients with zone three penetrating injuries require carotid and vertebral angiography if there is evidence of arterial bleeding because 1) exposure of the distal internal carotid and vertebral arteries is difficult, 2) the internal carotid artery may have to be ligated, a maneuver associated with a high risk of stroke and 3) active hemorrhage from the external carotid and vertebral arteries can be controlled by selective embolization.

Chest

Most chest injuries are evaluated by physical examination and chest radiographs. Patients with large air leaks following tube thoracostomy and those who are difficult to ventilate should undergo fiberoptic bronchoscopy to search for bronchial tears or foreign bodies.

Perhaps the most feared occult injury in trauma is a tear of the descending thoracic aorta. Widening of the mediastinum on AP chest radiograph suggests this injury. The widening is caused by the formation of a hematoma around the injured aorta, which is temporarily contained by the mediastinal pleura. However, it is well established that this injury can occur with an entirely normal chest radiograph, although the incidence is approximately 5 percent. Because of this and the dire consequences of missing the diagnosis, dynamic CT scanning is frequently performed based on mechanism of injury. Aortic tears usually occur just distal to the left subclavian artery where the aorta is tethered by the ligamentum arteriosum. In 2–5 percent of cases the tear occurs in the ascending aorta, transverse arch or at the diaphragm.

Penetrating thoracic trauma is evaluated by physical examination, plain posteroanterior (PA) and lateral chest radiographs with metallic markings of entrance and exit wounds and CVP measurement. Based on the estimated trajectory of the missile or blade, bronchoscopy may be indicated to evaluate the trachea. Patients at risk for esophageal injury should undergo esophagoscopy and then a soluble contrast esophagram looking for extravasation of contrast. If no extravasation is seen, a barium esophagram should be performed for greater detail. Failure to identify esophageal injuries leads to fulminant mediastinitis, which often is fatal.

Abdomen

The abdomen is a diagnostic black box. Physical examination of the abdomen is unreliable, however, the presence of abdominal rigidity or gross abdominal distention in a patient with truncal trauma is an indication for prompt surgical exploration. Drugs, alcohol, head, and spinal cord injuries frequently complicate physical examination. It may also be impractical in patients who require general anesthesia for the treatment of other injuries.

The diagnostic approach to penetrating and blunt abdominal trauma differ substantially. Anterior truncal GSWs between the fourth intercostal space and the pubic symphysis whose trajectory by radiograph or entrance/exit wound suggests peritoneal penetration should undergo laparotomy. GSWs to the back or flank are more difficult to evaluate because of the greater thickness of tissue between the skin and the abdominal organs, SWs that penetrate the peritoneal cavity are less likely to injure intraabdominal organs. Anterior and lateral stab wounds to the trunk should be explored under local anesthesia in the emergency department to determine whether the peritoneum has been violated. Injuries that do not penetrate the peritoneal cavity do not require further evaluation. For SWs to the abdomen, diagnostic peritoneal lavage (DPL) sensitivity for detecting intraabdominal injury exceeds 95 percent. The results of DPL are considered to be grossly positive if more than 10 mL of free blood can be aspirated. If less than 10 mL is withdrawn, a liter of normal saline is instilled and the effluent is sent to the laboratory for red blood cell count, amylase alkaline phosphatase, and bilirubin levels. A red blood cell count greater than $100,000/\mu L$ is considered positive. The detection of bile or of vegetable or fecal material, or the observation of effluent draining through a chest tube, a nasogastric tube, or a Foley catheter also constitutes a positive result.

SWs to the lower chest present a unique diagnostic opportunity. After the administration of adequate local anesthesia and extension of the wound as necessary, a finger is placed into the thoracic cavity to palpate the diaphragm.

Confirmation of diaphragm penetration is an indication for laparotomy. For similar cases when a hole is not palpable but risk of a diaphragmatic injury exists, a DPL should be performed. A red cell count in the effluent of greater than 10,000 is considered positive when evaluating for a diaphragmatic injury. For red cell counts between 1,000 and 10,000, thoracoscopy should be considered.

Blunt abdominal trauma is currently evaluated by US in most major trauma centers with CT in selected cases to refine the diagnosis. Although this method is exquisitely sensitive for detecting intraperitoneal fluid collections larger than 250 mL, it is relatively poor for staging solid organ injuries. DPL is still appropriate for patients whose condition cannot be explained by US.

CT remains an important diagnostic tool because of its specificity for hepatic, splenic, and renal injuries. CT is indicated primarily for hemodynamically stable patients who are candidates for nonoperative therapy. The role of laparoscopy remains to be clarified, but it may expand with the availability of a smaller laparoscope that can be inserted under local anesthesia.

Pelvis

Blunt injury to the pelvis can produce complex fractures. Plain radiographs may reveal gross abnormalities, but CT scans are often necessary to assess the pelvis for stability. Sharp spicules of bone can lacerate the rectum or vagina and bladder. Gross blood on urinalysis may not always occur, and a cystogram should be performed if more than a few red cells are seen. Urethral injuries are suspected by the findings of blood at the meatus, scrotal, or perineal hematomas, and a high reading prostate on rectal exam.

Urethrograms should be done in stable patients prior to placing the Foley catheter to avoid false passage stricture. Major vascular injuries are uncommon in blunt pelvic trauma; however, disruption of the iliofemoral system may occur. Angiography is indicated if thrombosis of the arterial system is suspected. Surgeons should be aware that life threatening hemorrhage can be associated with pelvic fractures. The source may be the lower lumbar arteries and veins or branches of the internal iliac arteries and veins. These injuries are frequently not amenable to surgical repair and usually occur with disruption of the posterior elements of the pelvis. Evaluation of penetrating injuries of the pelvis is similar to blunt injuries in stable patients.

Extremities

Injury of the extremities from any cause requires plain radiographs to evaluate fractures. Ligamentous injuries, particularly those of the knee and shoulder when related to sports activities, can be imaged with MRI. In general, vascular diagnosis is limited to the arterial system unless there is uncontrolled external venous hemorrhage or venous injuries are uncovered during operative exploration. Physical diagnosis will localize arterial injuries in many instances. In general, hard signs constitute indications for operative exploration.

Controversy in vascular trauma is the management of patients with soft signs of injury, particularly in those with injuries in proximity to major vessels. One approach has been to measure systolic pressures using the Doppler and compare the injured side with the uninjured side. If the pressures are within 10 percent of each other a significant injury is excluded and no further evaluation is performed. If the difference is greater than 10 percent, an arteriogram is indicated. Others argue that there are occult injuries, such as pseudoaneurysms or injuries of the profunda femoris or peroneal arteries, which may not be sampled with this technique. If hemorrhage occurs from these injuries, compartment syndrome and limb loss may occur.

TREATMENT

General Considerations

There has been a remarkable change in operative approach over the past 20 years. In general, faster techniques are employed, and shorter more frequent operations have become common. For example, at the authors' institution, virtually all suture lines are created with a continuous single layer. There is no evidence that this method is less secure than interrupted multilayer techniques, and it is clearly faster. Drains, once considered mandatory for many parenchymal injuries and some anastomoses, have virtually disappeared. Fluid collections which accumulate in a delayed fashion are now effectively managed by interventional radiologists. Injuries once thought to mandate resection, such as splenic injuries, are now managed with suture repair or even nonoperatively. The treatment of most colonic injuries is primary repair.

The management of patients with multiple injuries requires the early establishment of therapeutic priorities. While the concept of life over limb and limb over cosmesis seems obvious, decision making can be subtle.

Closed head injuries are common with both abdominal and thoracic trauma. A patient hits a tree while skiing. Evaluation reveals an epidural hematoma with an 8-mm midline shift and hypotension with free intraperitoneal fluid. Fortunately, a craniotomy and laparotomy can and should be done simultaneously. In fact, craniotomy for trauma can be performed concurrent with almost any procedure.

Another dilemma is a serious fracture, e.g., an open comminuted femoral fracture, in a patient who has just undergone a major thoracoabdominal procedure. Patients in this condition do not tolerate additional blood or thermal energy loss well and are at risk for sudden death. Consequently, the open femoral fracture will have to be deferred until the patient's metabolic situation improves despite increasing the risk of osteomyelitis and even limb loss.

Transfusion Practices and the Blood Bank

Fresh whole blood, arguably the optimal replacement material for shed blood, is no longer available. Therefore, whole blood must be recreated from its component parts: packed red blood cells (pRBCs), fresh frozen plasma (FFP), and platelet packs. Most trauma patients receive between one and five units of pRBCs and no other components. However, major trauma centers and their associated blood banks have the capability of transfusing tremendous quantities of blood components. It is not unusual to see 100 component units transfused during one procedure and have the patient survive. Red cell transfusion rates (a seldom used figure) of 20–40 units of packed red cells per hour are not uncommon in severely injured patients.

The causal relationship of core hypothermia, metabolic acidosis and postinjury coagulopathy has been observed in a number of studies. The pathophysiology is multifactorial and includes inhibition of temperature dependent enzyme activated coagulation cascades, platelet dysfunction, endothelial abnormalities, and a poorly understood fibrinolytic activity.

Primary hemostasis relies on platelet adherence and aggregation to injured endothelium resulting in the formation of the platelet plug. A platelet count of 50,000/mm^3 is considered adequate for tissue hemostasis if they are normal. However, platelet dysfunction is a well documented complication of massive transfusion which is clearly aggravated by associated hypothermia. Consequently, the recommended target is greater than 100,000 cells per mm^3 for platelet transfusion.

Blood typing, and to a lesser extent, crossmatching is essential to avoid life-threatening intravascular hemolytic transfusion reactions. A complete type and crossmatch requires from 20–45 min. Therefore, trauma patients requiring emergency transfusions are given type O, type-specific, or biologically compatible red blood cells. As a crosscheck for ABO compatibility, one of the many steps of the crossmatch (e.g., a saline crossmatch) often is performed. The administrative and laboratory time required is approximately 5 min, and the risk of intravascular hemolysis is about 0.05 percent. The risk increases to 1.0 percent with a history of previous transfusions or pregnancy and up to 3.0 percent with both.

Prophylactic Measures

Injured patients undergoing an operation should receive presumptive antibiotics. Presently, the authors use second generation cephalosporins for laparotomies and first generation cephalosporins for all other operations. Additional doses should be administered during the procedure based on blood loss and the half-life of the antibiotic. The role of postoperative antibiotics in trauma patients remains to be defined, but the trend has been to reduce the duration. Tetanus prophylaxis is administered to all patients according to published guidelines.

Deep venous thrombosis and other venous complications occur more often in injured patients than generally believed. This is particularly true for patients with major fractures of the pelvis and lower extremities, those with coma or spinal cord injury and probably in those with injury of the large veins in the abdomen and lower extremities. The authors employ pulsatile compression stockings in all injured patients and selectively place inferior vena caval filters in addition for those at very high risk. The role of inferior vena caval filters has expanded in removable devices. Low-molecular-weight heparins (LMWHs) have been shown effective in patients with orthopedic injuries, but its utility in patients with other injuries remains to be elucidated.

Principles and Techniques of Vascular Repair

A knowledge of vascular surgical techniques is essential for surgeons caring for injured patients. Life- or limb-threatening injuries occur everywhere in the body; bullets, knives, fractures, and shearing forces do not discriminate between visceral and vascular structures. General surgery requires precision in the scale of millimeters; vascular surgery requires precision on the scale of tenths of millimeters. Visual magnification is necessary for many repairs. A complete set of instruments specifically designed for vascular surgery should always be available. These sets must contain the clamps, tissue forceps, scissors, and needle holders necessary to control and repair vessels ranging from the thoracic aorta to the tibial arteries using sutures ranging from 3-0 to 7-0.

The initial control of vascular injuries should be accomplished digitally by applying just enough pressure directly on the bleeding site to stop the hemorrhage. Some bleeding vessels may need to be gently pinched between the thumb and index finger. These maneuvers, along with suction, usually create a dry enough field to safely permit the dissection necessary to define the injury. In general sharp dissection with fine scissors is preferable to blunt dissection because the latter may aggravate the injury. Once a sufficient length of vessel is available a vascular thumb forceps is used to grasp the vessel. If the vessel is not transected, forceps can be placed directly across the injury. This will minimize or eliminate bleeding while the dissection necessary for clamping is completed. If the vessel is transected (or nearly so) digital control is maintained on one side while the other is occluded with a thumb forceps. The vessel is then sharply mobilized to allow an appropriate vascular clamp to be applied. When definitive control of all injuries is achieved, heparinized saline (50 units/mL) is injected into the proximal and distal ends of the injured vessel to prevent thrombosis. The exposed intima and media at the site of the injury is highly thrombogenic and small clots often form. These clots should be carefully removed to prevent thrombosis or embolism when the clamps are removed. Because of the frequency with which embolism occurs, routine balloon catheter exploration of the distal vessel has been recommended. Ragged edges of the injury site should be judiciously débrided using sharp dissection.

Injuries of the large veins such as the vena cavae, innominate, and iliac veins pose a special problem for hemostasis. Numerous large tributaries make adequate hemostasis difficult to achieve, and their thin walls render them susceptible to further or additional iatrogenic injury. When such an injury is encountered, tamponade with a folded laparotomy pad held directly over the bleeding site usually will establish hemostasis sufficient to prevent exsanguination. If hemostasis is not adequate to expose the vessel proximal and distal to the injury, sponge sticks can be strategically placed on either side of the injury and carefully adjusted to improve hemostasis. This maneuver requires both skill and discipline to maintain a dry field. On occasion the operative field will be sufficient to delineate and repair the injury. However, it is often difficult or impossible for the assistant or assistants to maintain complete control of hemorrhage with sponge sticks. In this situation, the vessel can be exposed on either side of the sponge stick and a vascular clamp applied. The clamp can then be sequentially advanced toward the injury until hemostasis is complete.

Some arteries and most veins can be ligated without significant sequelae. Arteries for which repair should always be attempted include the carotid, innominate, brachial, superior mesenteric, proper hepatic, renal, iliac, femoral, popliteal, and the aorta. In the forearm and lower leg at least one of the two palpable vessels should be salvaged. The list of veins for which repair should be attempted is short: the superior vena cava, the inferior vena cava proximal to the renal veins and the portal vein. There are notable vessels not listed for which repair is not necessary (e.g., the subclavian artery and the superior mesenteric vein). The surgeon must keep in mind that there are few absolutes when discussing the treatment of vascular injuries. The portal vein can be ligated successfully provided adequate fluid is administered to compensate for the dramatic but transient edema which occurs in the bowel. If the alternative to ligation in exsanguination, the correct decision is obvious. On the other hand, ligation of some vessels such as the popliteal vein and left or right branch of the portal vein may result in morbidity for the patient which is not life threatening. Therefore, the authors' attempt to repair all arteries larger than 3 mm and all veins larger than 10-mm diameter depending on the patient's physiologic condition.

Within the last decade, some arterial injuries have been treated by observation without subsequent complications. These include small pseudoaneurysms, intimal dissections, small intimal flaps, and A-V fistulas in the extremities, and occlusions of small (<2 mm) arteries. Follow-up angiography is obtained within 2–4 weeks to ensure that healing has occurred.

Lateral suture is appropriate for small arterial injuries with little or no loss of tissue. End to end anastomosis is used if the vessel is transected or nearly so. The severed ends of the vessel are mobilized and small branches are ligated and divided as necessary to obtain the desired length. Arterial defects of 1–2 cm usually can be bridged. The surgeon should not be reluctant to divide small branches to obtain additional length because most injured patients have normal vasculature and the preservation of potential collateral flow is not as important as in atherosclerotic surgery. To avoid postoperative stenosis, particularly in smaller arteries, some techniques such as beveling or spatulation should be used so that the completed anastomosis is slightly larger in diameter than the native artery.

Interposition grafts are employed when end to end anastomosis cannot be accomplished without tension and despite mobilization. For vessels less than 6 mm in diameter, autogenous saphenous vein from the groin should be used because polytetrafluoroethylene (PTFE) grafts less than 6 mm in diameter have a prohibitive rate of thrombosis. In practice, injuries of the brachial, popliteal and internal carotid arteries require the saphenous vein for interposition grafting. When the saphenous vein is harvested for treating an arterial injury in the lower extremity, it should be taken from the contralateral extremity. Because the status of the ipsilateral venous system is unknown, the saphenous on that side may become an important tributary. Larger arteries must be bridged by artificial grafts. Some authorities have advocated the use of free internal iliac arterial grafts because of the greater thickness and strength of its wall compared to the saphenous vein. The authors believe that this vessel in unnecessarily tedious to remove and has no advantage over the saphenous vein.

Transposition procedures can be used when an artery has a bifurcation of which one vessel can safely be ligated. Injuries of the proximal internal carotid can be treated by mobilizing the adjacent external carotid, dividing it distal to the internal injury and performing an end to end anastomosis between it and the distal internal carotid. The proximal stump of the internal carotid is oversewn in such a way as to avoid a blind pocket where a clot may form. Injuries of the ipsilateral external and contralateral common iliac arteries can be handled in a similar fashion provided flow is maintained in at least one internal iliac artery. Arterial injuries often are grossly contaminated from enteric or external sources. Many surgeons are naturally reluctant to place artificial grafts in situ in this circumstance. The situation arises most often with aortic or iliac arterial injuries when the colon is also injured. For the aorta there are few options. Ligation of the aorta with unilateral or bilateral axillofemoral bypass can be performed. However, these are lengthy procedures, which are prone to thrombosis and infection. Furthermore, most patients who require an aortic graft will not tolerate the time required to perform an axillofemoral bypass. Therefore, even in the presence of fecal contamination, it has been common practice to use PTFE or Dacron in situ for aortic injuries. Every effort is made to remove and control contamination following the control of hemorrhage, but before the graft is brought into the operative field. This includes copious irrigation of the abdominal cavity and changing of drapes, gowns, gloves and instruments. Following placement of the graft, it is covered with peritoneum or omentum prior to definitive treatment of the enteric injuries.

Suture selection for arterial injuries is based on the diameter of the vessel being repaired. The use of progressively finer suture for smaller diameter vessels encourages the inclusion of less tissue with more closely placed sutures which is necessary for success. When performing anastomoses where the vessels are tethered (e.g., the thoracic and abdominal aorta), these authors employ the parachute technique to ensure precision placement of the posterior suture line. If this technique is used, traction on both ends of the suture must be maintained, or leakage from the posterior aspect of the suture line is probable. A single temporary suture 180 degrees from the posterior row often is used to maintain alignment.

Venous injuries are inherently more difficult to repair successfully because of their propensity to thrombose. Small injuries without loss of tissue can be treated with lateral suture. More complex repairs often fail. It should be noted that thrombosis does not occur acutely but rather gradually over 1–2 weeks. Advantage can be taken of this fact because adequate collateral circulation, sufficient to avoid acute venous hypertensive complications, usually develops within several days. Therefore, it is reasonable to use PTFE for venous interposition grafting and accept a gradual but eventual thrombosis while buying time for collateral circulation to develop. On the other hand, chronic venous hypertensive complications in the lower extremities often can be avoided with any level of ligation by: 1) elastic bandages carefully applied in the OR at the end of the procedure and 2) continuous elevation of the lower extremities to 30 degrees. These measures should be maintained for 1 week. The patient is then ambulated. If no edema occurs with the bandages removed, elevation is no longer necessary. It is a reasonable precaution to have the patient wear compressive stockings up to the knee for a few months afterward.

There are several circumstances where a more aggressive approach should be considered. Ligation of the superior vena cava has been associated with sudden blindness because of compression of the optic nerve from venous hypertension. Ligation of suprarenal vena cava is believed to be associated with acute renal failure from venous hypertension. Chronic venous insufficiency of the lower extremities may be caused by ligation of the infrarenal vena cava or any in-line vein below that level, particularly the popliteal vein. Interposition grafting can be considered in these situations but the choice of material is problematic. One option is to use artificial material because it is rapidly available in hemodynamically correct sizes. The drawback is that thrombosis is inevitable when placed below the renal veins. Artificial grafts have performed satisfactorily in cases of suprarenal vena caval and superior vena caval replacement. The jugular vein can be used to replace similar sized vessels (e.g., the portal or femoral). The saphenous vein is too small to replace any important vein. Panel grafts and spiral grafts constructed around a mandrel (chest tube) using saphenous vein occasionally have been performed. These procedures are extremely tedious and have no apparent advantage over ligation in most instances.

The technology employed by interventional radiologists is advancing at an incredible pace. They have the ability to cannulate virtually any artery in the body and either dilate it, place an intraluminal filter, stent or graft in it or occlude it. At present their services are most valuable for treating arterial or venous injuries which are surgically inaccessible such as stent placement in the internal carotid artery near or in the base of the skull, controlling hemorrhage in hepatic injuries or pelvic fractures.

Staged Operations, Abdominal Compartment Syndrome and Nonoperative Management

The most common causes of death for trauma patients are head injury, exsanguination from cardiovascular injuries, and sepsis with multiple-organ failure. Another cause of death has become apparent as the capability of delivering massive quantities of red blood cells and other components developed. Surgeons are now able to continue to operate on the most severely injured patients until a constellation of metabolic derangements develop. These are characterized by the triad of an obvious coagulopathy, profound hypothermia, and metabolic acidosis. Hypothermia from evaporative and conductive heat loss and diminished heat production occurs despite warming blankets and blood warmers. The metabolic acidosis of shock is exacerbated by aortic clamping, vasopressors, massive transfusions, and impaired myocardial performance. Coagulopathy is caused by dilution, hypothermia and acidosis. Each of these factors reinforces the others resulting in a critically ill patient who is at high risk for a fatal arrhythmia. This downward spiral has been referred to as the bloody vicious cycle.

Heat loss appears to be the central event because neither of the other components can be corrected until core temperature returns toward normal. Laboratory and mathematical heat exchange models have demonstrated that evaporative heat loss from an open abdomen is by far the greatest source. A concomitant open thoracic cavity greatly accelerates the rate of the patient's deterioration and can cause the syndrome by itself. This is the rationale for the immediate abdominal closure and the reason it has been successful.

Staged operations are indicated when a coagulopathy develops and core temperature drops below 34°C (93.2°F). A refractory acidosis almost always exists. Several unorthodox techniques can be used to expedite wound closure. Bleeding raw surfaces, often of the liver, are packed with laparotomy pads. Small enteric injuries are closed with staples, and large ones are stapled on both sides with stapling devices and the damaged segment removed. Clamps may be left on unrepaired vascular injuries, or the vessels are ligated. Injuries of the pancreas and kidneys are not treated if they are not bleeding. No drains are placed, and the abdomen is closed with sharp towel clips placed 2 cm apart which include only the skin. Towel clips are used because they do not cause bleeding as needles do and they can be applied very rapidly, usually in 60–90 s. The closure of just the skin allows for the abdominal or thoracic cavities to accommodate a greater volume without increased pressure. The clips are covered with a towel, and a plastic adhesive sheet is placed over the towel to prevent excessive fluid from draining onto the patient's bedding. Cold wet drapes are removed, and the patient is covered from head to toe with layers of warm blankets. It should be noted that many of these unorthodox treatments, including the creation of closed loop bowel obstructions and unrepaired renal injuries are not compatible with survival. However, reoperation is planned within 2–24 h, and the treatments are tolerated well within that time frame. Furthermore, the goal is to complete the procedure as soon as possible or the patient will certainly die. If the surgeon believes that the patient's metabolic problems can be corrected in a short time (2 h or less), the patient may remain in the OR while additional blood products are administered and rewarming measures are instituted. Patients who are in very poor condition and will require several h for metabolic corrections should be transferred to the surgical intensive care unit (SICU). If the patient's condition improves as evidenced by normalization of coagulation studies, the correction of acid/base balance, and a core temperature of at least 36°C (96.8°F) he should be returned to the OR for removal of packs and definitive treatment of his injuries.

There are several complications associated with this treatment. Failure to identify noncoagulopathic hemorrhage can lead to exsanguination. Most patients with coagulopathic hemorrhage will have a gradual decrease in the need for pRBCs, FFP, and platelets and an improvement in coagulation studies count as temperature rises. Patients with vascular hemorrhage will not, and they must be returned to the OR for reexploration.

A second complication is referred to as the abdominal or thoracic compartment syndrome. These entities are caused by an acute increase in intracavitary pressure. In the abdomen the compliance of the abdominal wall and the diaphragm permit the accumulation of many liters of fluid before intraabdominal pressure (IAP) increases. There are primarily two sources for this fluid, blood and edema. Blood accumulates because of the coagulopathy or missed vascular injury described above. The cause of edema is multifactorial. Ischemia and reperfusion cause capillary leakage; loss of oncotic pressure occurs; and in the case of the small bowel which is often eviscerated, prolongation and narrowing of veins and lymphatics caused by traction impairs venous and lymphatic drainage. The resulting edema may be dramatic. Similar phenomena occur in the chest. As fluid continues to accumulate, the compliant limit of the abdominal cavity is eventually exceeded; and IAP increases. When IAP exceeds 15 mmHg, serious physiologic changes begin to occur. The lungs are compressed by the upward displacement of the diaphragm. This causes a decrease in functional residual capacity, increased airway pressure and, ultimately, hypoxia. Cardiac output decreases because of diminished venous return to the heart and increased afterload. Blood flow to every intraabdominal organ is reduced because of increased venous resistance. As IAP exceeds 25–30 mmHg, life-threatening hypoxia and anuric renal failure occur. Cardiac output is further reduced but can be returned toward normal with volume expansion and inotropic support. However, the only method for treating hypoxia and renal failure is to decompress the abdominal cavity by opening the incision. This results in an immediate diuresis and a resolution of hypoxia. Failure to decompress the abdominal cavity will eventually cause lethal hypoxia and/or organ failure. There have been a few reports of sudden hypotension when the abdomen is opened. However, volume loading to enhance cardiac output has largely eliminated this problem. IAP is measured using the Foley catheter. Because the bladder is a passive reservoir at low volumes (50–100 mL), it imparts no intrinsic pressure but can transmit IAP. Fifty mL of saline are injected into the aspiration port of the urinary drainage tube with an occlusive clamp placed across the tube just distal to the port. The saline is used to create a standing column of fluid between the bladder and port, which can transmit IAP to a recording device. The needle in the port is connected to a CVP manometer using a three way stopcock. The manometer is filled with saline and opened to the drainage tube. IAP is read at the meniscus with manometer zeroed at the pubic symphysis. Bladder pressures measured in this fashion are both reliable and consistent. Pressures less than 15 mmHg do not require decompression.

In the chest similar phenomena occur. Edema of the heart and lungs develops and the heart may also dilate. Blood accumulation is rarely a problem because of the use of chest tubes. However, the diagnosis usually is apparent in the OR because the heart tolerates compression poorly. Attempts to close the chest in this setting are associated with profound hypotension, and it becomes obvious that an alternative method of closure is necessary. At present the most popular material used to accommodate the addition of volume in the chest or abdomen is a 3-L plastic urologic irrigation bag, which has been cut open and sterilized. The bag is sewn to the skin or fascia using no. 2 nylon suture with a simple running technique. As many as four bags may need to be sewn together to cover a large defect. Closed suction drains are placed beneath the plastic to remove blood and serous fluid which inevitably accumulate. The entire closure is covered with a iodinated plastic adhesive sheet to simplify nursing care. Patients whose renal function has not been impaired will have a diuresis. Exogenous fluids are held to a minimum to facilitate the resolution of edema. Definitive wound closure can usually be performed in 48–72 h.

Patients who develop sepsis and multiple-organ failure (MOF) are problematic and do not resolve their edema until sepsis and MOF resolve. This may require several weeks. The bags have been left in place up to 3 weeks with the patient surviving. However, the authors make every effort to at least close the skin over the viscera to decrease protein and heat loss and to inhibit infection. If these attempts are unsuccessful and the abdomen remains open with granulating tissue exposed, lateral traction forces of the abdominal wall will eventually cause an enteric fistula. The risk of developing a fistula increases rapidly after 2 weeks with an open abdomen. These problems are extremely difficult to treat. Several approaches have been used to avoid this catastrophic complication including polyglycolic acid or polypropylene mesh sewn to the fascia, split thickness skin grafts placed directly on the bowel, musculocutaneous flaps, and traction devices. Of these options skin grafts appear to have the greatest success although the abdominal wall hernia will eventually require reconstruction.

Nonoperative treatment for blunt injuries of the liver, spleen, and kidneys is now the rule rather than the exception. Up to 90 percent of children and 50 percent of adults are treated in this manner. As interventional radiology continues to advance, these numbers will certainly increase. The primary requirement for this therapy is hemodynamic stability. The extent of the patient's injuries should be delineated by CT. Recurrent hemorrhage from the liver and kidneys has been infrequent, but delayed hemorrhage or rupture of the spleen is an important consideration in the decision to pursue nonoperative management. The patient should be monitored in the intensive care unit for at least the first 24 h. Because CT will miss some enteric injuries, frequent abdominal examination should be performed. Usually the fall in hematocrit will stabilize within 24 h. If the hematocrit continues to fall, angiography with embolization of bleeding sites should be considered particularly for hepatic and renal injuries. CT usually is repeated at least once during the hospitalization to assess major hepatic or splenic lesions requiring transfusion. Gradually increasing activity is permitted following discharge. Patients involved in contact or high impact sports such as football should have complete healing of the injury documented radiographically before resuming participation. This can take several months.

Complications of nonoperative treatment include continuing hemorrhage, delayed hemorrhage, necrosis of liver, spleen or kidney from embolization, abscess, biloma, and urinoma. Hemorrhage may be treated by interventional radiology although open operative control is often necessary. Most infectious complications can be treated by percutaneous drainage. Bilomas are usually resorbed.

HEAD

Injuries of the Brain

General principles of the management of cerebral injuries have changed in recent years. Attention is now focused on maintaining or enhancing cerebral perfusion rather than merely lowering ICP. For example, it has been found that hyperventilation to a $PaCO_2$ less than 30 mmHg to induce cerebral vasoconstriction actually exacerbates cerebral ischemia despite decreasing ICP. These secondary iatrogenic cerebral injuries cause more harm than previously appreciated. Other treatments or conditions which must be avoided include decreased cardiac output because of the excessive use of osmotic diuretics, sedatives or barbiturates, and hypoxia. Nevertheless, the measurement of ICP is still important and is efficiently accomplished with a ventriculostomy tube. The tube also permits the withdrawal of cerebrospinal fluid which is the safest method for lowering ICP. Although an ICP of 10 mmHg is believed to be the upper limit of normal, therapy is not usually initiated until the ICP reaches 20 mmHg. Cerebral perfusion pressure (CPP) is an important measurement which is used to monitor therapy. CPP is equal to the mean arterial pressure (MAP) minus the ICP, and 60 mmHg is the lowest acceptable pressure. This figure can be adjusted by either lowering ICP or raising MAP. In practice, both are manipulated. Paralysis, sedation, osmotic diuresis, and barbiturate coma are all still used with coma being the last resort. The goal of fluid therapy is to achieve a euvolemic state, and arbitrary fluid restriction is avoided. Whether boosting MAP with pressors or inotropes in patients with an elevated ICP resistant to treatment improves outcome is unclear, although recent data suggests it does. Moderate hypothermia may also be helpful by decreasing metabolic requirement.

Indications for operative intervention for space occupying hematomas are based on the amount of midline shift, the location of the clot, and the patient's ICP. Greater than 5 mm of shift is usually considered an indication for evacuation. However this is not an absolute rule. Smaller hematomas causing less shift in treacherous locations, such as the posterior fossa, may require drainage because of the threat of brainstem compression or herniation. Removal of small hematomas may also improve ICP and CPP in patients with an elevated ICP, which is refractory to medical therapy. The treatment of DAI includes the control of cerebral edema and general supportive care. These authors frequently employ percutaneous tracheostomy for airway control and percutaneous endoscopic gastrostomy for enteral access in head injured patients whose recovery is unlikely or prolonged. Prognosis is related to GSC. Serious head injuries, GSC 3–8, have a poor prognosis, and an institutional existence is almost a certainty. Mild brain injury, GSC 13–15, have a good prognosis; independent living is probable. However, neuropsychiatric testing often reveals significant abnormalities.

General surgeons in small or rural communities without emergency neurosurgical coverage may be required to perform a burr hole in one life-saving circumstance. This occurs in a patient with an epidural hematoma. As blood from a torn vessel, usually the middle meningeal artery, accumulates, the temporal lobe if forced medially, which compresses the third cranial nerve and eventually the brainstem. This sequence of events results in the typical clinical course: 1) initial loss of consciousness, 2) awakening and a lucid interval, 3) recurrent loss of consciousness with a unilaterally fixed, dilated pupil, and 4) cardiac arrest. Because these patients do not usually have a serious underlying cortical injury, chance for a complete recovery often is possible. The burr hole should be made on the same side as the dilated pupil. The goal of the procedure is not to control the hemorrhage but to decompress the intracranial space. Because a craniotomy is required for the control of hemorrhage, the patient's head should be loosely wrapped with a thick layer of gauze to absorb the bleeding, and he should be transferred to a facility with emergency neurosurgical capability for a craniotomy.

NECK

Blunt Injury

Cervical Spine

Blunt trauma may involve the cervical spine, spinal cord, larynx, carotid, and vertebral arteries, and the jugular veins. Treatment of injuries to the cervical spine is based on the level of injury, the stability of the spine, the presence of subluxation, the extent of angulation, and the extent of neurologic deficit. In general, cautious axial traction in line with the mastoid process is used to reduce subluxations. A halo-vest combination can accomplish this and also provide rigid external fixation for definitive treatment when left in place for 3–6 months. Today this device is the treatment of choice for many cervical spine injuries. Surgical fusion usually is reserved for those with neurologic deficit, those who demonstrate angulation greater than 11 degrees on flexion and extension radiographs, or those who remain unstable after external fixation.

Spinal Cord

Injuries of spinal cord, particularly complete injuries, remain essentially untreatable. Approximately 3 percent of patients who present with flaccid quadriplegia actually have concussive injuries, and these patients represent the very few who seem to have miraculous recoveries. A recent prospective randomized study comparing methylprednisolone with placebo demonstrated a significant improvement in outcome (usually one or two spinal levels) for those who received the corticosteroid within 8 h of injury. The standard dosage is 30 mg/kg given as an intravenous bolus followed by a 5.4 mg/kg infusion administered over the next 23 h. Patients with spinal cord injuries are also at high risk for deep venous thrombosis and pulmonary embolus. Prophylactic anticoagulation is essential.

Larynx

The larynx may be fractured by a direct blow which can result in airway compromise. A hoarse voice is highly suggestive. A cricothyroidotomy, or tracheostomy if time permits, should be done to protect the airway in cases of severe fracture. The larynx is anatomically repaired with fine wires and sutures. If direct repair of internal laryngeal structures is necessary, the thyroid cartilage is split longitudinally in the midline and opened like a book. This is referred to as a laryngeal fissure.

Carotid and Vertebral Arteries

Blunt injury to the carotid or vertebral arteries may cause dissection, thrombosis, or pseudoaneurysm. More than half the patients have a delayed diagnosis. Facial contact resulting in hypertension and rotation appears to be the mechanism. To reduce delayed recognition, the authors employ angiography in patients at risk to identify these injuries before neurologic symptoms develop. The injuries frequently occur at or extend into the base of the skull and are usually not surgically accessible. Currently accepted treatment for thrombosis and dissection is anticoagulation with heparin followed by Coumadin for 3 months. Pseudoaneurysms also occur near the base of the skull. If they are small, they can be followed with repeat angiography. If enlargement occurs consideration should be given to the placement of a stent across the aneurysm by an interventional radiologist. Another possibility is to approach the intracranial portion of the carotid by removing the overlying bone and performing a direct repair. This method has only recently been described and has been performed in a limited number of patients.

Thrombosis of the internal jugular veins caused by blunt trauma can occur unilaterally or bilaterally. These injuries are usually discovered incidentally and are generally asymptomatic. Bilateral thrombosis can aggravate cerebral edema in patients with serious head injuries. Stent placement should be considered in such patients if their ICP remains elevated. Laryngeal edema resulting in airway compromise can also occur.

Penetrating Injuries

Penetrating injuries in zones two or three that require operative intervention are explored using an incision along the anterior border of the sternocleidomastoid muscle. If bilateral exploration is necessary, the inferior end of the incision can be extended to the opposite side. Midline wounds or significant bilateral injuries can be exposed via a large collar incision at the appropriate level. Alternatively, bilateral anterior sternocleidomastoid incisions can be employed.

Carotid and Vertebral Arteries

Exposure of the distal carotid artery in zone three is difficult. The first step is to divide the ansa cervicalis and mobilize the hypoglossal nerve. Next, the portion of the posterior belly of the digastric muscle which overlies the internal carotid is resected. The glossopharyngeal and vagus nerves are mobilized and retracted as necessary. If accessible, the styloid process and attached muscles are removed. At this point anterior displacement of the mandible may be helpful, and various methods for accomplishing this have been devised. Some authorities have advocated division and elevation of the vertical ramus. However, two remaining structures still prevent exposure of the internal carotid to the base of the skull: the parotid gland and facial nerve. Excessive anterior traction on the mandible or parotid may damage the facial nerve, particularly the mandibular branch. Unless the surgeon is willing to resect the parotid and divide the facial nerve, division of the ramus is seldom helpful.

All penetrating carotid injuries should be repaired if possible. Inaccessible carotid injuries near the base of the skull can be treated by interventional radiologists with a stent if the anatomy of the injury is favorable. Otherwise the artery will need to be thrombosed or ligated. If ligation is necessary the patient should be anticoagulated with heparin followed by Coumadin for 3 months. This treatment may prevent a stroke by inhibiting the generation of thrombi from the surface of the clot at the circle of Willis while the endothelium heals. Without anticoagulation the risk of stoke with ligation has been approximately 20–30 percent, and most strokes occur a few days after ligation. Tangential wounds of the internal jugular vein should be repaired by lateral venorrhaphy, but extensive wounds are efficiently addressed by ligation.

Vertebral artery injuries usually result from penetrating trauma although thrombosis and pseudoaneurysms can occur from blunt injury. The diagnosis is made by angiography or when significant hemorrhage is noted posterior to the carotid sheath during neck exploration. Exposure of the vertebral artery above C6 where it enters its bony canal is complicated by the overlying anterior elements of the canal and the tough fascia covering the artery between the elements. The artery is approached through an anterior neck incision by retracting the contents of carotid sheath laterally. The muscular attachments to the elements are removed. Care must be taken to avoid injury to the cervical spinal nerves which are located directly behind and lateral to the bony canal. Some authorities have recommended using a high speed burr to remove the anterior element of the canal thereby avoiding the venous plexus between the elements. The authors have not found this to be a problem and have often carefully excised the fascia between the elements and lifted the artery out of its canal with a tissue forceps. The treatment for vertebral artery injuries is ligation both proximal and distal to the injury. There is rarely, if ever, an indication for repair. Neurologic complications are uncommon. Exposure of the vertebral artery above C2 is extremely difficult. Rather than using a direct operative approach these authors expose the vessel below C5, outside the bony canal, clamp the artery proximally, and insert a no. 3 balloon tipped catheter. The catheter is advanced to the level of the injury or distal to it, and the balloon is inflated with saline until back bleeding stops. The tube to the catheter is crimped over on itself and secured in this position with several heavy silk sutures. The catheter is trimmed so that it can be left in the wound under the skin. The proximal end of the artery is ligated. One week later the catheter is removed under local anesthesia. Rebleeding has not occurred in these authors' experience. The same approach can be used for the distal internal carotid. An alternative approach is to have the interventional radiologist place coils to induce thrombosis proximal and distal to the injury if the lesion is diagnosed by angiography. Injuries of the proximal vertebral can be exposed by a median sternotomy with a neck extension.

Trachea and Esophagus

Injuries of the trachea are repaired with a running 3-0 absorbable monofilament suture. Tracheostomy is not required in most patients. Esophageal injuries are repaired in a similar fashion. If an esophageal wound is large, or if tissue is missing, a sternocleidomastoid muscle pedicle flap is warranted, and a closed suction drain is a reasonable precaution. The drain should be near but not in contact with the esophageal or any other suture line. It can be removed in 7–10 days if the suture line remains secure. Care must be taken when exploring the trachea and esophagus to avoid iatrogenic injury to the recurrent laryngeal nerve.

Penetrating injuries of the neck often create wounds in adjacent hollow structures, e.g., the trachea and esophagus or carotid artery and esophagus. If, following repair, theses adjacent suture lines are in contact, the stage is set for devastating postoperative fistulous complications. To avoid these complications, viable tissue should routinely be interposed between adjacent suture lines. Viable strips of the sternocleidomastoid muscle or strap muscles are useful for this purpose.

Thoracic Outlet

Great Vessels

While most injuries of the great vessels of the thoracic outlet (zone one) are caused by penetrating trauma, the innominate and subclavian arteries are occasionally injured from blunt trauma. As mentioned previously angiography is desirable for planning the incision. If this is not possible because of hemodynamic instability, a reasonable approach can be inferred from the chest radiograph and the location of the wounds. If the patient has a left hemothorax, a left third or fourth interspace anterolateral thoracotomy should be performed because the proximal left subclavian artery may be injured. Hemorrhage can be controlled digitally until the vascular injury is delineated. Additional incisions or extensions are often required. A third or fourth interspace right anterolateral thoracotomy may be used for thoracic outlet injury presenting with hemodynamic instability and a right hemothorax. A median sternotomy with a right clavicular extension can also be used. Unstable patients with injuries near the sternal notch may have a large mediastinal hematoma or have lost blood directly to the outside. These patients should be explored via a median sternotomy.

If angiography has identified an arterial injury, a more direct approach can be employed. A median sternotomy is used for exposure of the innominate, proximal right carotid and subclavian, and the proximal left carotid arteries. The proximal left subclavian artery presents a unique challenge. Because it arises from the aortic arch far posteriorly, it is not readily approached via median sternotomy. A posterolateral thoracotomy provides excellent exposure but severely limits access to other structures and is not recommended. The best option is to create a full thickness flap of the upper chest wall. This is accomplished with a third or fourth interspace anterolateral thoracotomy for proximal control, a supraclavicular incision with a resection of the medial third of the clavicle, and a median sternotomy which links the two horizontal incisions. The ribs can be cut laterally for additional exposure, which allows the flap to be folded laterally with little effort. This incision has been referred to as a book or trap door thoracotomy for obvious reasons. The mid-portion of the subclavian artery is accessible by removing the proximal third of either clavicle, with the skin incision made directly over the clavicle. Muscular attachments are stripped away, and the clavicle is divided with a Gigli saw. The medial remnant of the clavicle is forcefully elevated. The periosteum is dissected from the posterior aspect of the bone until the sternoclavicular joint is reached. The capsular attachments are cut with a heavy scissors or knife and the bone is discarded. The periosteum and underlying fascia is very tough and must be sharply incised along the direction of the vessel. The subclavian vein is mobilized and the artery is directly underneath. The anterior scalene is divided for injuries just proximal to the thyrocervical trunk; the relatively small phrenic nerve should be identified on its anterior aspect and spared. Iatrogenic injury to cords of the brachial plexus can occur.

The great vessels are rather fragile and are easily torn during dissection or crushed with a clamp. For this reason some advocate oversewing proximal injuries of the artery on the side of the aortic arch and sewing a graft onto a new location on the arch. The graft is then sewn to the artery without tension. Technical details of the repair are similar to those described in the Principles and Techniques of Vascular Repair section.

Trachea and Esophagus

The trachea and esophagus are difficult to approach at the thoracic outlet. The combination of a neck incision and a high anterolateral thoracotomy may be used. Alternatively, these structures can be approached via a median sternotomy provided the left innominate vein and artery are divided. Temporary division of the innominate artery is tolerated well in otherwise healthy people, but the vessel should be repaired following treatment of the tracheal or esophageal injury. The vein does not need to be repaired. As in the neck, adjacent suture lines should be separated by viable tissue. A portion of the sternocleidomastoid can be rotated down for this purpose.

Chest

The most common life-threatening complications from both blunt and penetrating thoracic injury are hemothorax, pneumothorax, or a combination of both. Approximately 85 percent of these patients can be treated definitively with a chest tube. Because of the viscosity of blood at various stages of coagulation, a 36F or larger chest tube should be used. If one tube fails to completely evacuate the hemothorax (a "caked hemothorax"), a second tube should be placed. If the second chest tube does not remove the blood, a thoracotomy should be performed because of the risk of life-threatening hemorrhage. Common sources of blood loss include intercostal vessels, internal thoracic artery, pulmonary parenchyma, and the heart. Less common sources are the great vessels, aortic arch, azygous vein, superior vena cava, and inferior vena cava. Blood may also enter the chest from an abdominal injury through a perforation or tear in the diaphragm. Table 6-3 lists indications for operative treatment of penetrating thoracic injuries.

The indications for thoracotomy in blunt trauma are based on specific preoperative diagnoses. These include pericardial tamponade, tear of the descending thoracic aorta, rupture of a mainstem bronchus, and rupture of the esophagus. Thoracotomy for hemothorax in the absence of the above diagnoses is rarely indicated. A shattered chest wall that produces a hemothorax is better treated by the interventional radiologist with embolization.

TABLE 6-3 Indications for Operative Treatment of Penetrating Thoracic Injuries

Caked hemothorax
Large air leak with inadequate ventilation or persistent collapse of the lung
Drainage of more than 1500 mL of blood when chest tube is first inserted
Continuous hemorrhage of more than 200 mL/h for ≥ 3 consecutive h
Esophageal perforation
Pericardial tamponade

Thoracic Incisions

The selection of incisions is important and depends on the organs being treated. For exploratory thoracotomy for hemorrhage, the patient is supine and an anterolateral thoracotomy is performed. Depending on findings, the incision can be extended across the sternum or even further for a bilateral anterolateral thoracotomy. The fifth interspace usually is preferred unless the surgeon has a precise knowledge of which organs are injured and that exposure would be enhanced by selecting a different interspace. The heart, lungs, aortic arch, great vessels, and esophagus are accessible with these incisions.

The heart can also be approached via a median sternotomy. Because little else can be done in the chest through this incision, it is usually reserved for stab wounds of the anterior chest in patients who present with pericardial tamponade. Posterolateral thoracotomies are rarely used because ventilation is impaired in the dependent lung, and the incision cannot be extended. There are two specific exceptions. Injuries of the posterior aspect of the trachea or mainstem bronchi near the carina are inaccessible from the left or from the front. The only possible approach is through the right chest using a posterolateral thoracotomy. A tear of the descending thoracic aorta can only be repaired through a left posterolateral thoracotomy. Because the authors use left heart bypass for these procedures, the patient's hips and legs are rotated toward the supine position to gain access to the left groin for femoral artery cannulation. It is also helpful for optimal exposure to resect the fourth rib and enter the chest through its bed.

Heart

Most cardiac injuries are the result of penetrating trauma, and any part of the heart is susceptible. Control of hemorrhage while the heart is being repaired is crucial and several techniques can be used. The atria can be clamped with a Satinsky vascular clamp. Digital control and suturing beneath the finger is possible anywhere in the heart although the technique requires skill and a long, curved cardiovascular needle. The reality of blood borne viral infections raises the question if this method should ever be used today. If the hole is small, a peanut sponge clamped in the tip of a hemostat can be placed into the wound or the blood loss may be accepted while sutures are being placed. For larger holes a 16F Foley catheter with a 30-mL balloon can be inflated with 10 mL of saline. Gentle traction on the catheter will control hemorrhage from any cardiac wound because wounds too large for balloon tamponade are incompatible with survival. Suture placement with the balloon inflated is problematic. Usually the ends of the wound are closed progressively toward the middle until the amount of blood loss is acceptable with the balloon removed. The use of skin staples for the temporary control of hemorrhage has become popular particularly when emergency department thoracotomy has been performed. It has the advantages of reducing the risk of needle stick injury to the surgeon or assistant and does not mandate the attention required by a balloon catheter. In most instances, however, hemostasis is neither perfect nor definitive. Inflow occlusion of the heart, by clamping the superior and inferior vena cavae can be performed for short periods, and this may be essential for the treatment of extensive or multiple wounds and for those that are difficult to expose.

Trauma surgeons accept the fact that interior structures of the heart may be damaged, which impair cardiac output. However, immediate repair of valvular damage or acute septal defects is rarely necessary and requires total cardiopulmonary bypass, which has a high mortality in this situation. Most patients who survive to make it to the hospital do well with only external repair. Following recovery, the heart can be thoroughly evaluated; and if necessary secondary repair can be performed under more controlled conditions. Coronary artery injuries also pose difficult problems. Ligation leads to acute infarction distal to the tie; but again, reconstruction requires bypass. The right coronary artery can probably be ligated anywhere but the resultant arrhythmias may be extremely resistant to treatment. The left anterior descending and circumflex cannot be ligated proximally without causing a large infarct. Such injuries are extremely rare and usually produce death in the field.

Blunt cardiac injury can present in several ways. A sharp blow to the pericardium can provoke ventricular fibrillation. This is referred to as a commotio cordis and is inevitably fatal unless it is recognized immediately and resuscitation implemented. The heart can also be contused. Most of these patients present with new arrhythmias, e.g., a bundle branch block or premature ventricular contractions. Cardiac enzymes have not been helpful in making the diagnosis. Finally, the heart can rupture. The right atrium and right ventricle are most susceptible but survival is possible provided the diagnosis is suspected.

Lungs, Trachea and Bronchi

Pulmonary injuries requiring operative intervention usually result from penetrating injury. Formerly the entrance and exit wounds were oversewn to control hemorrhage. This set the stage for air embolism, which occasionally caused sudden death in the OR, or in the immediate postoperative period. A recent development, pulmonary tractotomy, has been employed to reduce this problem and the need for pulmonary resection. Linear stapling devices are inserted directly into the injury tract and are positioned to cause the least degree of devascularization. Two staple lines are created and the lung is divided between. This allows direct access to the bleeding vessels and leaking bronchi. No effort is made to close the defect. Lobectomy or pneumonectomy is rarely necessary. Lobectomy is only indicated for a completely devascularized or destroyed lobe. Parenchymal injuries severe enough to require pneumonectomy are rarely survivable, and major pulmonary hilar injuries necessitating pneumonectomy are usually lethal in the field.

Injuries of the trachea are managed in the same fashion described above. Because exposure can be difficult, provisions should be made to deflate the lung on the operative side by using a double lumen endotracheal tube (a double-lumen tube is seldom needed for cardiac or pulmonary injury). Repair of mainstem bronchial injuries and tracheal injuries near the carina may result in a complete loss of ventilation when the overlying pleura is opened even if a double lumen tube is used. Gases from the ventilator will preferentially escape from the injury and neither lung will be ventilated. Digital occlusion of the injury can control air loss if the injury is small. Larger injuries are an imminent threat to life. To avoid this catastrophe, a 6–7-mm cuffed endotracheal tube should be on the operative field and a second ventilator available. If ventilation is inadequate, the surgeon can insert and inflate the endotracheal tube into the main bronchus on the opposite side through the injury to permit ventilation of one lung while the injury is repaired. Eventually the tube will have to be removed to close the defect but the remaining hole can be controlled digitally. Alternatively, it may be possible for the anesthesiologist to cannulate the opposite bronchus although little time is available.

Esophagus

The majority of esophageal injuries are caused by penetrating trauma through blunt disruption. Because of their proximity, combined tracheoesophageal injuries do occur. Many authors recommend the interposition of viable muscle between the repairs to prevent tracheoesophageal fistula.

Descending Thoracic Aorta

Conceptually, two techniques have been advocated. The simpler technique, often referred to as "clamp and sew," is accomplished with the application of vascular clamps proximal and distal to the injury and repairing or replacing the damaged portion of the aorta. This method results in transient hypoperfusion of the spinal cord distal to the clamps and all abdominal organs. Large doses of vasodilators are also required to reduce afterload and avoid acute left heart failure. If the clamping time is short, less than 30 min, paraplegia has been uncommon. Longer clamping times have been associated with paraplegia in approximately 10 percent of patients. Unfortunately, clamping times of less than 30 min have been difficult to achieve for many tears requiring complex repair. The second method has been to employ left heart bypass. With this method a volume of oxygenated blood is siphoned from the left heart and pumped into the distal aorta. Flow rates of 2–3 L appear to provide adequate protection by maintaining a distal perfusion pressure greater than 65 mmHg. These authors prefer this method. The left superior pulmonary vein is cannulated to remove blood from the heart rather than the left atrium because the vein is tougher and less prone to tear. The left femoral artery is cannulated to return the blood to the distal aorta. A centrifugal pump is employed because it is not as thrombogenic as a roller pump and, strictly speaking, heparinization is not required. This can be a significant benefit in a patient with multiple injuries, particularly in those with intracranial hemorrhage. However, occasional small cerebral infarcts have occurred, and 5,000–10,000 units of heparin is usually administered unless contraindicated by associated injuries.

Once bypass is initiated, the proximal vascular clamp is applied between the left common carotid and left subclavian; and the distal clamp is placed distal to the injury. The left subclavian is clamped separately. The hematoma is entered, and the injury evaluated. In most patients a short gelatin sealed Dacron graft is placed, usually 18–22 mm in diameter. Primary repair without a graft is possible in some patients. A 3-0 polypropylene suture is used for the anastomoses or suture lines. Air and clot are flushed from the aorta between two clamps and the subclavian artery prior to tying the final suture. Following completion of the repair, the clamps are removed; and the patient is weaned from the pump. The cannulae are removed, and the vessels are repaired. A recent meta-analysis comparing clamp-and-sew with left heart bypass revealed a significantly lower incidence of paraplegia when the pump is used.

Injuries of the transverse arch do occur from blunt trauma. The proximal clamp can usually be placed between the innominate and left carotid arteries without cerebral infarction. The proximal clamp, however, cannot be placed proximal to the innominate artery. A possible approach to injuries in which the clamps completely exclude the cerebral circulation is with profound hypothermia and circulatory arrest (see Chapter 21).

Small intimal flaps of the thoracic aorta without hematomas can be treated nonoperatively. Intraluminal mediastinal stents may also provide a solution but their role remains to be defined. Penetrating injuries of the thoracic aorta are rare and do not afford enough time to set up the pump. Therefore, there is no choice but to use the clamp-and-sew technique. Partially occluding clamps should be used if possible.

Abdomen

Emergent Abdominal Exploration

All abdominal explorations in adults are performed using a long midline incision because of its versatility. For children younger than 6 years, a transverse incision may be advantageous. If the patient has been in shock or is currently unstable, no attempt should be made to control bleeding from the abdominal wall until major sources of hemorrhage have been identified and controlled. The incision should be made with a scalpel rather than with an electrosurgical unit because it is faster. Liquid and clotted blood are rapidly evacuated with multiple laparotomy pads and suction. Additional pads are then placed in each quadrant to localize hemorrhage and the aorta is palpated to estimate blood pressure.

If exsanguinating hemorrhage is encountered on opening the abdomen, it is usually caused by injury to the liver, aorta, inferior vena cava or iliac vessels. If the liver is the source, the hepatic pedicle should be immediately clamped (a Pringle maneuver) and the liver compressed posteriorly by tightly packing several laparotomy pads between the hepatic injury and the underside of the right anterior chest wall. This combination of maneuvers will temporarily control the hemorrhage from virtually all survivable hepatic injuries.

If exsanguinating hemorrhage is originating near the midline in the retroperitoneum, direct manual pressure is applied with a laparotomy pad, and the aorta is exposed at the diaphragmatic hiatus and clamped. The same approach is used in the pelvis except that the infrarenal aorta can be clamped, which is both easier and safer because splanchnic and renal ischemia are avoided. Injuries of the iliac vessels pose a unique problem for emergency vascular control. Because there are so many large vessels in proximity, multiple vascular injuries are common. Furthermore, venous injuries are not controlled with aortic clamping. A helpful maneuver in these instances is pelvic vascular isolation. For stable patients with large midline hematomas, clamping the aorta proximal to the hematoma is also a wise precaution. Many surgeons take a few moments, once overt hemorrhage has been controlled, to identify obvious sources of enteric contamination and minimize further spillage. This can be accomplished with a running suture or with Babcock clamps.

Any organ can be injured by either blunt or penetrating trauma, however, certain organs are injured more often depending on the mechanism. In blunt trauma, organs which cannot yield to impact by elastic deformation are most likely to be injured. The solid organs, liver, spleen, and kidneys, are representative of this group. For penetrating trauma organs with the largest surface area when viewed from the front are most prone to injury (i.e., the small bowel, liver, and colon). Because bullets and knives usually follow straight lines, adjacent structures are commonly injured (e.g., the pancreas and duodenum).

All abdominal organs are systematically examined by visualization, palpation, or both. Missed injuries are a serious problem with often fatal results. In penetrating trauma missed injuries can occur if wound tracks are not followed their entire distance. A second common reason is failure to explore retroperitoneal structures such as the ascending and descending colons, the second and third portion of the duodenum and ureters. Furthermore, injuries of the aorta or vena cava may be temporarily tamponaded by overlying structures. If the retroperitoneum is opened and the injury overlooked, delayed massive hemorrhage may occur following abdominal closure. Blunt abdominal injuries are usually obvious; but injuries of the pancreas, duodenum, bladder, and even the aorta can be overlooked.

Vascular Injuries

Injury to the major arteries and veins in the abdomen are a technical challenge to the surgeon and are often fatal. All vessels are susceptible to injury with penetrating trauma. While vascular injuries in blunt trauma are far less common all vessels also can be injured. Several vessels are notoriously difficult to expose. These include the retrohepatic vena cava, suprarenal aorta, the celiac axis, the proximal superior mesenteric artery, the junction of the superior mesenteric, splenic and portal veins, and the bifurcation of the vena cava. The suprarenal aorta, celiac axis, proximal superior mesenteric and left renal arteries can all be exposed by left medial visceral rotation. Division of the left crus of the diaphragm will permit access to the aorta above the celiac axis. The maneuver is much more difficult and time consuming than it first appears. In contrast mobilization of the right colon and a Kocher maneuver will expose the entire vena cava except the retrohepatic portion, and it is technically simple. This is referred to as a right medial visceral rotation.

The junction of the superior mesenteric, splenic, and portal veins can be exposed by dividing the neck of the pancreas. This provides excellent exposure of this difficult area. Management of the transected pancreas will be discussed below.

The bifurcation of the vena cava is obscured by the right common iliac artery. This vessel should be divided to expose extensive vena caval injuries of this area. The artery must be repaired after the venous injury is treated.

Liver

The lower costal margins impair visualization and a direct approach to the liver. The right lobe can be mobilized by dividing the right triangular and coronary ligaments. The right lobe can then be rotated medially into the surgical field. Mobilization of the left lobe is accomplished in the same fashion. On occasion it may be necessary to extend the midline abdominal incision into the chest. This is best accomplished with a median sternotomy.

The Pringle maneuver is one of the most useful techniques for evaluating the extent of hepatic injuries. The Pringle maneuver will differentiate between hemorrhage from the hepatic artery and portal vein, which ceases when the clamp is applied, and that from the hepatic veins and retrohepatic vena cava, which will not.

Techniques for the temporary control of hemorrhage from the liver are necessary when dealing with an extensive injury to provide the anesthesiologist with sufficient time to restore circulating blood volume before proceeding.

The temporary hemostatic techniques, which have proven most useful are manual hepatic compression, the Pringle maneuver and perihepatic packing. Manual compression of a bleeding hepatic injury may be a lifesaving maneuver. The addition of laparotomy pads on the surface of the liver distributes digital forces and lessens the chance of aggravating the injury. Manual compression is best suited for immediate attempts to prevent exsanguination and for periodic control during a complex procedure.

Perihepatic packing also is capable of controlling hemorrhage from most hepatic injuries, and it has the advantage of freeing the surgeon's hands. The right costal margin is elevated, and the pads are strategically placed over and around the bleeding site. Additional pads should be placed between the liver, diaphragm, and anterior chest wall until the bleeding has been controlled. Fortunately, hemorrhage from the left lobe can usually be controlled by mobilizing the lobe and compressing it between the surgeon's hands.

The Pringle maneuver often is used as an adjunct to packing for the temporary control of the arterial hemorrhage. Properly applied, a Pringle maneuver will eliminate all hepatopetal flow. The length of time that a Pringle maneuver can remain in place without causing irreversible ischemic damage to the liver is unknown. Several authors have documented a Pringle maneuver applied for over 1 h without appreciable hepatic damage.

Special techniques have been developed for controlling hemorrhage from juxtahepatic venous injuries. These formidable procedures include hepatic vascular isolation with clamps, the atriocaval shunt, and the Moore-Pilcher balloon. Hepatic vascular isolation with clamps is accomplished by the application of a Pringle maneuver, clamping the aorta at the diaphragm and clamping of the suprarenal and suprahepatic vena cavae.

The atriocaval shunt was designed to achieve hepatic vascular isolation while permitting venous blood to enter the heart from below the diaphragm. After a few early successes, enthusiasm for the shunt declined as mortality rates with its use ranged from 50–80 percent. A variation of the original atriocaval shunt has been the substitution of 9-mm endotracheal tube for the usual large chest tube. While this change may seem trivial, surrounding the suprarenal vena cava for a snare tourniquet is extremely difficult because exsanguinating hemorrhage must be controlled by posterior compression of the liver which severely restricts access to that segment of the vena cava.

An alternative to the atriocaval shunt is the Moore-Pilcher balloon. This device is inserted through the femoral vein and advanced into the retrohepatic vena cava. The catheter itself is hollow, and placed holes below the balloon permit blood to flow into the right atrium from the inferior vena cava.

Numerous methods for the definitive control of hepatic hemorrhage have been developed. Minor lacerations may be controlled with manual compression applied directly to the injury site. For similar injuries which do not respond to compression, topical hemostatic techniques have been successful. Small bleeding vessels may be controlled with electrocautery. Microcrystalline collagen can be used. The powder is placed on a clean 4x4 sponge and applied directly to the oozing surface. Topical thrombin can also be applied to minor bleeding injuries by saturating either a gelatin foam sponge or a microcrystalline collagen pad and applying it to the bleeding site.

Fibrin glue appears to be an effective topical agent. Fibrin glue is made by mixing concentrated human fibrinogen (cryoprecipitate) with bovine thrombin and calcium. Commercially available products are also available with a variety of delivery systems.

Suturing of the hepatic parenchyma remains an effective hemostatic technique. Although this treatment has been maligned as a cause of hepatic necrosis, hepatic sutures often are used for persistently bleeding lacerations less than 3 cm in depth. It is also an appropriate alternative for deeper lacerations if the patient will not tolerate further hemorrhage. The preferred suture is 2-0 or 0 chromic attached to a large, curved, blunt needle. Venous hemorrhage because of penetrating wounds which traverse the central portion of the liver can be managed by suturing the entrance and exit wounds with horizontal mattress sutures.

Hepatotomy with selective ligation of bleeding vessels in an important technique usually reserved for transhepatic penetrating wounds. Hepatotomy is performed using the finger fracture technique. The dissection continues until the bleeding vessels are identified and controlled. An alternative to suturing the entrance and exit wounds of a transhepatic injury or extensive hepatotomy is the use of an intrahepatic balloon. These authors' method is to tie a large Penrose drain to a hollow catheter and ligate the opposite end of the drain. The balloon is then inserted into the bleeding wound and inflated with soluble contrast media. If the control of the hemorrhage is successful, a stopcock or clamp is used to occlude the catheter and maintain the inflation. The catheter is left in the abdomen and removed at a subsequent operation 24–48 h later.

Hepatic arterial ligation may be appropriate for patients with recalcitrant arterial hemorrhage from deep within the liver. Its primary role is in transhepatic injuries when application of the Pringle maneuver results in the cessation of arterial hemorrhage. While ligation of the right or left hepatic artery is well-tolerated in humans, ligation of the proper hepatic artery (distal to the origin of the gastroduodenal artery) is not necessarily associated with survival. An uncommon but perplexing hepatic injury is the subcapsular hematoma. This lesion occurs when the parenchyma of the liver is disrupted by blunt trauma, but the Glisson capsule remains intact. Subcapsular hematomas discovered during an exploratory laparotomy which involve less than 50 percent if the surface of the liver and are not expanding or ruptured, should be left alone. Hematomas that are expanding during an operation may require exploration. These lesions often are caused by uncontrolled arterial hemorrhage, and packing alone may not be successful. An alternative strategy would be to pack the liver to control venous hemorrhage, close the abdomen, and transport the patient to the angiographic suite for hepatic arteriography and embolization of the bleeding vessel. Ruptured hematomas require exploration and selective ligation, with or without packing.

Resectional débridement is indicated for the removal of peripheral portions of nonviable hepatic parenchyma. The mass of tissue removed should rarely exceed 25 percent of the liver. It should be reserved for patients who are in good metabolic condition and who will tolerate additional blood loss. An alternative for patients with extensive unilobar injuries is anatomic hepatic resection. However, the mortality rate for trauma patients exceeds 50 percent in most series. A reasonable indication for anatomic lobectomy occurs in patients whose hemorrhage has been controlled by perihepatic packing and/or arterial ligation but whose left or right lobe is nonviable. Because the mass of the remaining necrotic liver is large and the risk of subsequent infection is high, it should be removed as soon as the patient's condition permits.

Omentum has been used to fill large defects in the liver. Rationale for the use of the omentum to fill defects is that it provides an excellent source for macrophages, and that it fills a potential dead space with viable tissue. The omentum can also provide a little additional support for parenchymal sutures and often is strong enough to prevent them from cutting through the Glisson capsule. Closed suction drains should be used if bile is seen oozing from the liver and in most patients with deep central injuries.

Complications following significant hepatic trauma include hemorrhage, infection, and various fistulas. Postoperative hemorrhage can be expected in a considerable percentage of patients treated with perihepatic packing. In most instances where postoperative hemorrhage is suspected, the patient is best served by returning him to the OR. Arteriography with embolization may be considered in selected patients.

Infections within and around the liver occur in about 3 percent of patients. Perihepatic infections develop more often in victims of penetrating trauma than blunt trauma. Persistent elevation of temperature and white blood cell count after the third or fourth postoperative day should prompt a search for intraabdominal infection. Many perihepatic infections can be treated with CT-guided drainage. Infected hematomas and infected necrotic liver require open operative intervention.

Bilomas are loculated collections of bile which may or may not be infected. If infected, the biloma is essentially an abscess and should be treated as such. If sterile, it will eventually be reabsorbed. Biliary ascites is caused by disruption of a major bile duct. Reoperation with the establishment of appropriate drainage is the prudent course.

Biliary fistulas occur in approximately 3 percent of patients with hepatic injuries. They are usually of little consequence and most will close without specific treatment.

Because hemorrhage from hepatic injuries often is treated without identifying and controlling each individual bleeding vessel, arterial pseudoaneurysms may develop. They may rupture into a bile duct resulting in hemobilia, which is characterized by intermittent episodes of right upper quadrant pain, upper gastrointestinal hemorrhage, and jaundice. If the aneurysm ruptures into a portal vein, portal venous hypertension with bleeding esophageal varices may occur. Each of these complications is best managed with hepatic arteriography and embolization.

Gall Bladder and Extrahepatic Bile Ducts

Injuries of the gallbladder are treated by lateral suture or cholecystectomy, whichever is easier. If lateral suture is performed, absorbable suture should be used. Injuries of the extrahepatic bile ducts are a challenge. If ducts are of normal size and texture (i.e., small in diameter and thin walled). These factors usually preclude primary repairs except for the smallest lacerations. Some injuries can be treated by the insertion of a T-tube through the wound or by lateral suture using 4-0 to 6-0 monofilament absorbable suture. Virtually all transections and any injury associated with significant tissue loss will require a Roux-en-y choledochojejunostomy. Injuries of the hepatic ducts are almost impossible to satisfactorily repair under emergency circumstances. One approach is to intubate the duct for external drainage and attempt a repair when the patient recovers. Alternatively, the duct can be ligated if the opposite lobe is normal and uninjured. For patients who are critically ill, the common duct also can be treated by intubation with external drainage.

Spleen

Splenic injuries are treated nonoperatively, by splenic repair, partial splenectomy, or resection depending on the extent of the injury and the condition of the patient. Enthusiasm for splenic salvage has been driven by the evolving trend toward nonoperative management of solid organ injuries and the rare but often fatal complication of overwhelming postsplenectomy infection (OPSI). These infections are caused by encapsulated bacteria and are very resistant to treatment. OPSI occurs most often in young children and immunocompromised adults.

To safely remove or repair the spleen it should be mobilized to the extent that it can be brought to the surface of the abdominal wall. This requires division of the attachments between the spleen and splenic flexure of the colon. Next, an incision is made in the peritoneum and endoabdominal fascia beginning at the inferior pole, a centimeter or two away from the spleen, and continuing posteriorly and superiorly until the esophagus is encountered. It often is helpful to rotate the operating table 20 degrees to the patient's right so that the weight of abdominal viscera aids in their own retraction. A plane can then be established between the spleen and pancreas and Gerota fascia, which can be extended to the aorta.

Hilar injuries or a pulverized splenic parenchyma usually are treated by splenectomy. Splenectomy also is indicated for lesser splenic injuries in patients with multiple abdominal injuries who have developed a coagulopathy; and it usually is necessary in patients with failed splenic salvage attempts. Partial splenectomy can be used in patients in whom only a portion of the spleen has been destroyed, usually the superior or inferior half. When placing horizontal mattress sutures across a raw edge, gentle compression of the parenchyma by an assistant will facilitate hemostasis. Drains are never used after completion of the repair or resection. If splenectomy is performed, pneumococcal vaccine is routinely given.

Diaphragm

In blunt trauma the diaphragm is injured on the left in 75 percent of cases, presumably because the liver diffuses some of the energy on the right side. For both blunt and penetrating trauma the diagnosis is suggested by an abnormality of the diaphragmatic shadow on chest radiograph. The typical injury from blunt trauma is a large tear in the central tendon. Regardless of etiology, acute injuries are repaired through an abdominal incision. The laceration is closed with a 0- monofilament permanent suture using a simple running technique.

Duodenum

Duodenal hematomas are caused by a direct blow to the abdomen, and they occur more often in children than adults. The diagnosis is suspected by the onset of vomiting following blunt abdominal trauma; barium examination of the duodenum reveals either the coiled spring sign or obstruction. Most duodenal hematomas in children can be managed nonoperatively. Resolution of the obstruction occurs in the majority of patients in 7–14 days. If surgical intervention becomes necessary, evacuation of the hematoma is associated with equal success but fewer complications than bypass procedures. A new approach is laparoscopic evacuation if the obstruction persists more than 7 days.

Duodenal perforations can be caused by both blunt and penetrating trauma. Blunt injuries are difficult to diagnose because the contents of the duodenum have a neutral pH, few bacteria and often are contained by the retroperitoneum. Mortality may exceed 30 percent if the lesion is not identified and treated within 24 h. The perforations are not reliably identified by initial oral contrast CT examinations; and, therefore, these authors often obtain contrast radiographs with soluble contrast followed with barium if necessary. Most perforations of the duodenum can be treated by primary repair. Occasionally, penetrating injuries will damage only the pancreatic aspect of the second or third portion. Because the duodenum cannot be adequately mobilized to repair the injury directly, the wound should be extended laterally or the duodenum divided so that the pancreatic aspect can be sutured from the inside.

Challenges arise when there is a substantial loss of duodenal tissue. Extensive injuries of the first portion of the duodenum can be repaired by débridement and anastomosis. In contrast, the second portion is tethered to the head of the pancreas by its blood supply and the ducts of Wirsung and Santorini so that the length of duodenum that can be mobilized from the pancreas is limited to approximately a centimeter and will do little to alleviate tension on a suture line. As a result, suture repair of the second portion when tissue is lost often results in an unacceptably narrow lumen, and end-to-end anastomosis is virtually impossible; therefore, more sophisticated repairs are required. For extensive injuries proximal to the accessory papilla, débridement, and end-to-end anastomosis is appropriate. For lesions between the accessory papilla and the papilla of Vater, a vascularized jejunal graft, either a patch or tubular interposition graft, may be required. A Roux-en-y duodenojejunostomy is also appropriate. Duodenal injuries with tissue loss distal to the papilla of Vater and proximal to the superior mesenteric vessels are best treated by Roux-ex-Y duodenojejunostomy. Duodenum and proximal jejunum are drained into the jejunum.

Injuries to the third and fourth portions of the duodenum with tissue loss pose other problems. Owing to the notoriously short mesentery of the third and fourth portions of the duodenum, mobilization is limited because of the risk of ischemia. It is the preference of these authors to resect the third and fourth portions and perform a duodenojejunostomy on the right side of the superior mesenteric vessels.

An important adjunct for complex duodenal repairs is the pyloric exclusion technique. By occluding the pylorus and performing a gastrojejunostomy, the gastrointestinal steam can be diverted away from the duodenal repair. If a fistula does develop, it is functionally an end fistula, which is easier to manage and more likely to close than a lateral fistula. To perform a pyloric exclusion, a gastrostomy is first made on the greater curvature as close to the pylorus as possible. The pylorus is then grasped with a Babcock clamp via the gastrostomy and oversewn with a 0 polypropylene suture. A gastrojejunostomy restores gastrointestinal continuity. Experience has shown that the absorbable sutures do not last long enough to be effective, and even heavy polypropylene will give way in 3–4 weeks in most patients. A linear staple line across the outside the pylorus provides the most permanent pyloric closure.

Pancreas

Blunt pancreatic transection at the neck of the pancreas can occur with a direct blow to the abdomen. As an isolated injury it is more difficult to detect than blunt duodenal rupture; however, a missed pancreatic injury is more benign. Because the main pancreatic duct is transected, the patient will develop a pseudocyst or pancreatic ascites, but there is little inflammation because the pancreatic enzymes remain inactivated. The diagnosis can occasionally be made with CT using fine cuts through the pancreas.

Optimal management of pancreatic trauma is determined by the location of the injury and whether or not the main pancreatic duct is injured. Pancreatic injuries in which the pancreatic duct is not injured may be treated by drainage or left alone. In contrast, pancreatic injuries associated with a ductal injury always require treatment. Direct exploration of perforations or lacerations will confirm the diagnosis of a ductal injury in most instances. This leaves a small but significant percentage of patients whom the diagnosis is in doubt, and more invasive investigations may be required. One recommendation has been to perform operative pancreatography. This procedure requires direct access to the duct either by way of a duodenotomy or following resection of the tail of the pancreas.

An expeditious alternative to pancreatography is to pass a 1.5–2.0-mm coronary artery dilator into the main duct via the papilla and observe the pancreatic wound. If the dilator is seen in the wound, a ductal injury is confirmed.

A third method for identifying pancreatic ductal injuries is the use of endoscopic retrograde pancreatography (ERP). This technique may be difficult to perform in an anesthetized patient in the OR, but the surgeon can assist by manipulating the duodenum or occluding the distal portion to facilitate air insufflation. ERP is very helpful in the delayed diagnosis of a ductal injury or in those patients who are too sick to explore adequately during the initial operation.

Rather than accepting the risks of pancreatography or aggressive local exploration, a final option for identifying ductal injuries in the head of the pancreas is to do nothing other than drain the pancreas. If pancreatic fistula or pseudocyst develops, the diagnosis is confirmed. Fortunately, the majority of pancreatic fistulas will close spontaneously with only supportive care.

There are two options for treating injuries of the neck, body, and tail when the main duct is transected. Distal pancreatectomy with or without splenectomy is the preferred approach. The spleen can be preserved by dissecting the pancreas from the splenic vein.

For injuries to the head of the pancreas that involve the main pancreatic duct but not the intrapancreatic bile duct, distal pancreatectomy alone rarely is indicated because the risk of pancreatic insufficiency is significant if more than 85–90 percent of the gland is resected. A more limited resection from the site of the injury to the neck of the pancreas, with preservation of the pancreaticoduodenal vessels and common duct, will allow for closure of the injured proximal pancreatic duct. Pancreatic function can then be preserved by a Roux-en-y pancreatojejunostomy with the distal pancreas.

In contrast to injuries of the pancreatic duct, the diagnosis of injuries to the intrapancreatic common bile duct is simple. The first method is to squeeze the gallbladder and observe the pancreatic wound. If bile is seen leaking from the pancreatic wound, the presence of an injury is established. Operative cholangiography is diagnostic in questionable cases. If a patient with an intrapancreatic bile duct injury is critically ill, external drainage can be used until the patient is fit for definitive treatment. For most injuries division of the common bile duct superior to the first portion of the duodenum, ligation of the distal common duct, and reconstruction with a Roux-en-y choledochojejunostomy is recommended.

While many authorities advocate routine drainage of all pancreatic injuries, these authors do not drain contusions, lacerations in which the probability of a major ductal injury is small or pancreatic anastomoses. We do drain pancreatic injuries when there is a possible major ductal injury although we cannot identify it. If a drain is desirable, closed suction devices are associated with fewer infectious complications than sump or Penrose drains. Nutritional support is important and electrolyte replacement may be necessary.

Pancreaticoduodenal Injuries

Because the pancreas and duodenum are in physical contact, combined pancreaticoduodenal injuries are not uncommon. These lesions are dangerous because of the risk of duodenal suture line dehiscence and the development of a lateral duodenal fistula. The simplest treatment is to repair the duodenal injury and drain the pancreatic injury. This method is appropriate for combined injuries without major duodenal tissue loss and without pancreatic or biliary ductal injuries. With more extensive injuries, consideration should be given to providing additional protection by adding a pyloric exclusion.

While most pancreatic and duodenal injuries can be treated with relatively simple procedures, a few will require a pancreatoduodenectomy. Examples of such injuries include transection of both the intrapancreatic bile duct and the main pancreatic duct in the head of the pancreas, avulsion of the papilla of Vater from the duodenum, and destruction of the entire second portion of the duodenum.

Colon

There are two conceptually different methods for treating colonic injuries: primary repair and colostomy. Primary repairs include lateral suture of perforations and resection of the damaged colon with reconstruction by ileocolostomy or colocolostomy. The advantage of primary repairs is that definitive treatment is carried out at the initial operation. The disadvantage is that leakage may occur. Several different styles of colostomies have been used to manage colonic injuries. In some instances the injured colon can be exteriorized like a loop colostomy. The injured area can be resected and an end colostomy or ileostomy performed, and the distal colon can be brought to the abdominal wall as a mucous fistula or oversewn and left in the abdominal cavity. The advantage of colostomy is avoiding a suture line in the abdomen. The disadvantage is that a second operation is required to close the colostomy. Often overlooked disadvantages are the complications associated with the creation of a colostomy, some of which may be fatal.

Numerous large retrospective and several prospective studies have now clearly demonstrated that primary repair is safe and effective in the majority of patients with penetrating injuries. Colostomy is still appropriate in a few patients but the current dilemma is how to select them. The authors' approach is to repair all injuries regardless of the extent and location and reserve colostomy for patients with protracted shock who are also candidates for damage control. The theory used to support this approach is that systemic factors are more important than local factors in determining whether a suture line will heal. When a colostomy is required, performing a loop colostomy proximal to a distal repair should be avoided because a proximal colostomy does not protect a distal suture line. All suture lines and anastomoses are performed with the running single layer technique.

Complications related to the colonic injury and its treatment may include intraabdominal abscess, fecal fistula, wound infection, and stomal complications. Intraabdominal abscess occurs in approximately 10 percent of patients and most are managed with percutaneous drainage. Fistulas occur in 1–3 percent of patients and usually present as an abscess or wound infection, which after drainage, is followed by continuous fecal output. Most colonic fistulas will heal spontaneously. Wound infection can be effectively avoided by leaving the skin and subcutaneous tissue open and relying on healing by secondary intention or delayed primary closure.

Stomal complications include necrosis, stenosis, obstruction and prolapse. Taken together they occur in approximately 5 percent of patients, and most require reoperation. Necrosis is a particularly serious complication which must be recognized and treated promptly. Failure to do so can result in life-threatening septic complications including necrotizing fasciitis.

Rectum

Rectal injuries differ from colonic injuries in two important ways, mechanisms of injury and accessibility. The rectum is often injured by GSW, rarely by SW, and frequently by acts of auto-eroticism and high pressure injuries caused by air guns or water under high pressure as used in golf course irrigation systems. The second difference is limited access to the rectum because of the surrounding bony pelvis.

The diagnosis is suggested by the course of projectiles, the presence of blood on digital examination of the rectum and history. Patients in whom a rectal injury is suspected should undergo proctoscopy. Hematomas, contusions, lacerations and gross blood may be seen. If the diagnosis is still in question, radiograph examinations with soluble contrast enemas are indicated. At times, it may be difficult to determine whether an injury is present. These authors believe that these patients should be treated as if they do have an injury.

The portion of the rectum proximal to the peritoneal reflection is referred to as the intraperitoneal segment and that distal to the reflection as the extraperitoneal segment. Injuries of the intraperitoneal portion (including its posterior aspect) are treated as previously outlined in the section on colonic injuries. Access to extraperitoneal injuries is so restricted, that indirect treatment usually is required. While colostomies proximal to a suture line are avoided in patients with colonic injuries, there is often no option in patients with extraperitoneal injuries; and sigmoid colostomies are appropriate for most patients. Properly constructed loop colostomies are preferred because they are quick and easy to fashion, and they provide total fecal diversion. Essential elements include: 1) adequate mobilization of the sigmoid colon so the loop will rest on the abdominal wall without tension, 2) maintenance of the spur of the colostomy above the level of the skin, 3) longitudinal incision in the tenia coli, and 4) immediate maturation in the OR using 3-0 braided absorbable suture.

If a perforation is inadvertently uncovered during dissection, it should be repaired as described above. Otherwise, it is not necessary to explore the extraperitoneal rectum to repair a perforation. If the injury is extensive the rectum should be divided at the level of injury, the distal rectum oversewn, and an end colostomy created. In rare instances where the anal sphincters have been destroyed, and abdominoperineal resection may be necessary.

Extraperitoneal injuries of the rectum should be drained via a retroanal incision. The drains, either Penrose or closed-suction, should be placed close to the perforation and should be left in until they fall out spontaneously or drainage diminishes. Irrigation of the distal rectum is advocated by some authorities. It may be of benefit in a patient whose rectum is loaded with feces. If it is done, the irrigation solution should be isotonic and the anus should be mechanically dilated to avoid forcing feces out of a perforation. If the patient has a concomitant bladder injury and adjacent suture lines are created, a flap of viable omentum should be placed between.

Complications are similar in frequency and nature to colonic injuries. Pelvic osteomyelitis may also occur. Bone biopsy should be performed to secure the diagnosis and bacteriology. Culture specific intravenous antibiotics should be administered for 2–3 months. Débridement may be necessary.

Stomach and Small Intestine

Gastric injuries can occasionally be missed if a wound is located within the mesentery of the lesser curvature or high in the posterior fundus. The stomach should be clamped at the pylorus and inflated with air or methylene blue colored saline if there is any question. Patients with injuries which damage both nerves of Latarjet or both vagi should have a drainage procedure (see Chapter 25). If the distal antrum or pylorus are severely damaged it can be reconstructed with a Billroth I or II procedure. Although the authors emphasize the single layer running suture line, a running two-layer suture line is preferred for the stomach because of its rich blood supply.

With the almost universal use of CT for the diagnosis of blunt abdominal injury, injury to the small intestine can be missed. Wounds of the mesenteric border also can be missed if the exploration is not comprehensive. Most injuries are treated with a lateral single layer running suture. Multiple penetrating injuries often occur close together. Judicious resections with end to end anastomosis may be appropriate.

Kidneys

There are two unique aspects to the diagnosis and treatment of renal injuries. First, virtually all injuries can be diagnosed by CT. Second, the fact that there are two identical organs makes the sacrifice of one a viable therapeutic option. Nearly 95 percent of all blunt renal injuries are treated nonoperatively. The diagnosis is suspected by the finding of microscopic or gross hematuria, and confirmed by CT. Most cases of urinary extravasation and hematuria will resolve in a few days with bed rest. Persistent gross hematuria can be treated by embolization. Persistent urinomas can be drained percutaneously. Operative treatment occasionally is necessary for similar lesions that do not respond to these less-invasive measures.

If a perinephric hematoma is encountered during laparotomy from blunt trauma, exploration is indicated if it is expanding or pulsatile. Very large hematomas should be explored because of the risk of a major vascular injury. If emergent vascular control is necessary, a large curved vascular clamp can easily be placed across the hilum from below with the clamp parallel to the vena cava and aorta.

Hemostatic and reconstructive techniques used to treat blunt renal injuries are similar to those used to treat the liver and spleen, although two additional concepts are employed: 1) the collecting system should be closed separately, and 2) the renal capsule preserved to close over the repair of the collecting system. Permanent sutures should be avoided because of the risk of calculus formation. If nephrectomy is being considered and the status of the opposite kidney is unknown, it should be palpated. The presence of a palpably normal opposite kidney is assurance that the patient will not be rendered anephric by a unilateral nephrectomy. Unilateral renal agenesis occurs in one in 1000 patients.

The renal arteries and veins are uniquely susceptible to traction injury caused by blunt trauma. This causes thrombus formation resulting in high-grade stenosis or thrombosis. These injuries can be detected by CT. If the patient does not have more urgent injuries and treatment and repair can be accomplished within 1–3 h of admission, it should be attempted. If repair is not possible within this time frame, leaving the kidney in situ does not necessarily lead to hypertension or abscess formation. Isolated renal vein injuries can occur from blunt trauma. The vein may either be torn or avulsed from the vena cava. In either case a large hematoma develops that often leads to an operation and nephrectomy.

All penetrating wounds to kidneys are explored. Bleeding perforations and lacerations are treated using the same hemostatic techniques as described above. Renal vascular injuries are common following penetrating trauma. Injuries involving the collecting system should be closed separately if they are large. Small perforations which penetrate the collecting system can be controlled by suture of the capsule and parenchyma. Perforations of the renal pelvis should be meticulously repaired with fine sutures, and drains should be employed selectively.

Ureters

Injuries of the ureters from external trauma are rare. They occur in a few patients with pelvic fractures and are uncommon in penetrating trauma. The diagnosis in blunt trauma may be made by CT or retrograde uterography. More often the injury is not identified until a complication (e.g., a urinoma) becomes apparent. In penetrating trauma ureteral injuries are discovered during the exploration of the retroperitoneum. If an injury is suspected but not identified, methylene blue or indigo carminate are administered intravenously. Staining of the tissue by the dye may facilitate identification of the injury. Most injuries can be repaired primarily using the same technique described above for small arteries. The suture these authors use is 5-0 absorbable monofilament. When the ureter is mobilized, the dissection should be at least a centimeter away from the ureter to avoid injury to its delicate vascular plexus. The kidney can also be mobilized to gain length. Injuries of the distal ureter can be treated by reimplantation. The psoas hitch and Boari flap may be helpful in selected distal ureteral injuries. If the patient is critically ill and being considered for a staged laparotomy, or if the surgeon is uncomfortable with ureteral repair, the ureter can be ligated on both sides of the injury and a nephrostomy performed.

Bladder

Bladder injuries are diagnosed by cystography, CT, or during laparotomy. A postvoid view enhance the accuracy of cystography. Blunt ruptures of the intraperitoneal portion are closed with a running single layer closure using 3-0 absorbable monofilament suture. Blunt extraperitoneal rupture is treated with a Foley catheter; direct operative repair is not necessary. The Foley can be removed in 10–14 days. Penetrating bladder injuries are treated in the same fashion although injuries near the trigone should be repaired through an incision in the dome to avoid injury to the intravesicular ureter.

Urethra

Blunt disruption of the posterior urethra is managed by bridging the defect with a Foley catheter. This requires passing catheters through the urethral meatus and through an incision in the bladder. Strictures are not uncommon but can be managed electively. Penetrating injuries are treated by direct repair.

Pelvis

Pelvic fractures can cause exsanguinating retroperitoneal hemorrhage without associated major vascular injury; branches of the internal iliac vessels and the lower lumbar arteries often are responsible. Hemorrhage also comes from small veins and from the cancellous portion of the fractured bones. Most pelvic fractures which cause life-threatening hemorrhage involve disruption of the posterior elements (i.e., the sacroiliac joints and associated ligaments) and often are biomechanically unstable.

A hemodynamically unstable patient may be bleeding from sources other than the pelvis, for example, the spleen. However, large retroperitoneal hematomas also can cause a hemoperitoneum particularly if overlying peritoneum ruptures. Determining the source of hemorrhage is a dilemma. These authors have employed US to aid in this decision. If US is unequivocally positive, the blood is assumed to be coming from an injury unrelated to the pelvic fracture; and a laparotomy is performed. If the US is negative, attention is directed toward treating the pelvic fracture. Clearly, the decision to operate or not may be wrong; and the plan may need to be altered accordingly.

Several methods have been employed to control hemorrhage associated with pelvic fractures. These include immediate external fixation, angiography with embolization, pelvic volume reduction and pelvic packing. No single technique is effective for treating all fractures and there is little agreement among specialists regarding which should be used. Anterior external fixation will decrease pelvic volume, tamponade bleeding and prevent secondary hemorrhage. Many orthopedic surgeons remain unconvinced of the efficacy of external fixation for grossly unstable posterior fractures. Tightly wrapping the pelvis with a sheet and taping the knees together reduces pelvic volume and is employed in the trauma center of these authors. Angiography with embolization is very effective for controlling arterial hemorrhage, but arterial hemorrhage occurs in only 10–20 percent of patients. Pelvic packing may control venous hemorrhage.

Because of the options available and differences of opinion regarding treatment, these authors have found it desirable to reach agreements with the other specialists involved including orthopedic surgeons, interventional radiologists, the blood bank, and anesthesiologists. These agreements avoid the time lost to unnecessary debate.

Another clinical challenge is the open pelvic fracture. In many instances the wounds are located in the perineum and the risk of pelvic sepsis and osteomyelitis is high. To reduce the risk of infection, a sigmoid colostomy is recommended. The pelvic wound is manually débrided and the wound is then left to heal by secondary intention.

Extremities

Most injuries of the extremities are within the domain of the orthopedic and plastic surgeons except for isolated vascular injuries that have been discussed above. There are two extremity injuries, however, which need to be emphasized: 1) vascular injuries associated with fractures and 2) compartment syndromes.

Vascular Injuries with Fractures

Vascular injuries associated with fractures are rare but serious, and amputation rates of more than 50 percent have been noted. These injuries can be caused by both blunt and penetrating trauma. Particular fractures and dislocations are more likely to be associated with vascular injury than others. In the upper extremity, a fractured clavicle or first rib may lacerate the distal subclavian artery. The axillary artery may be injured in patients with dislocations of the shoulder or proximal humeral fractures. Supracondylar fractures of the distal humerus and dislocations of the elbow are associated with brachial arterial injuries. In all the above fractures and dislocations, vascular injuries are uncommon.

In the lower extremity, the orthopedic injury most commonly associated with vascular injury is dislocation of the knee, where the popliteal artery and/or vein may be injured in as many as 30 percent of patients. The popliteal vessels may also be injured in patients with supracondylar fractures of the femur or tibial plateau fractures.

Three different mechanisms can produce paralysis and numbness in an injured extremity: ischemia, nerve injury and compartment syndrome. As a result, failure to accurately perform and document the neuromuscular function of the injured extremity can and will lead to missed injuries and improper treatment.

A rational approach would be to consider all the above options based on the condition of the patient's extremity. If the extremity is clearly viable and there is no hemorrhage from the vascular injury, the fracture should be treated first. If the limb is at risk from ischemia, prompt revascularization is required. When little or no fracture manipulation is anticipated, definitive vascular repair is performed first. If extensive manipulation is required in a ischemic extremity, temporary shunts can be placed followed by vascular repair after the fracture has been treated.

Combined orthopedic and vascular injuries frequently occur in open fractures, and the use of external fixation devices for these injuries has become common. Unfortunately, these devices may significantly hinder vascular repair because of their location and bulk. Preoperative planning should avoid this technical problem.

Because of the severity of combined orthopedic and vascular injuries, the need for immediate amputation may arise. When the primary nerve is transected in addition to a fracture and arterial injury, such as the popliteal nerve, popliteal artery and distal femur, primary amputation should be strongly considered. This difficult clinical decision is best reached through a collaborative effort.

Compartment Syndrome

Compartment syndromes can occur anywhere in the extremities. As in the abdomen, the pathophysiology is an acute increase in pressure in a closed space, which impairs blood flow to the structures within. The etiologies of extremity compartment syndromes include arterial hemorrhage into a compartment, venous ligation or thrombosis, crush injuries, infections, crotalid envenomation, and ischemia/reperfusion. In conscious patients, pain is the prominent symptom. Active or passive motion of involved muscles increases the pain. Progression to paralysis can occur. The most prone site is in the anterior compartment of the leg; a well described early sign is paresthesia or numbness between the first and second toes caused by pressure on the deep peroneal nerve.

In comatose or obtunded patients, the diagnosis is more difficult to secure. A compatible history, firmness of the compartment to palpation and diminished mobility of the joint are suggestive. The absence of a pulse distal to the affected compartment, a frozen joint, and myoglobinuria are late signs and suggest a poor prognosis. As in the abdomen, compartment pressure can be measured. The small handheld Stryker device is a convenient tool for this purpose. Pressures greater than 45 mm Hg usually require operative intervention. Patients with pressures between 30 and 45 mm Hg should be watched closely.

Treatment for compartment syndrome is fasciotomy. Note that the soleus must be detached from the tibia to decompress the deep flexor compartment.

Prognosis is related to the severity, duration, and etiology of the compartment syndrome. Those who develop compartment syndrome from crush injuries, crotalid envenomation, and particularly ischemia/reperfusion have a poor prognosis. Fasciotomy should still be attempted although infection and amputation are a frequent outcome.

7 | Burns

James H. Holmes and David M. Heimbach

Thermal burns and related injuries are a major cause of death and disability in the United States and worldwide. The interactive multidisciplinary team has proven to be the least expensive and most efficient method of treating major burn injury, of which the initial acute care is only a small part of the total treatment. Burn patients often require years of supervised rehabilitation, reconstruction, and psychosocial support.

EPIDEMIOLOGY

In the United States, approximately 1.1 million individuals annually are burned seriously enough to seek health care; approximately 45,000 of these require hospitalization, and approximately 4500 die. More than 90 percent of burns are preventable, with nearly one-half being smoking-related or because of substance abuse.

The annual number of burn deaths in the United States has decreased from approximately 15,000 in 1970 to around 4500 at present. Over the same period, the burn size associated with a 50 percent mortality rate has increased from 30 percent of the total body surface area (TBSA) to greater than 80 percent TBSA in otherwise healthy young adults. The duration of hospital stay has been cut in half. Almost 95 percent of the patients admitted to burn centers in the United States now survive, and over one-half of them return to preburn levels of physical and social functioning within 12–24 months following injury. The quality of burn care is no longer measured only by survival, but also by long-term function and appearance.

As with other forms of trauma, burns frequently affect children and young adults. In children less than 8 years of age, the most common burns are scalds, usually from the spilling of hot liquids. In older children and adults, the most common burns are flame-related, usually the result of house fires, the ill-advised use of flammable liquids as accelerants, or are smoking- or alcohol-related. Chemicals or hot liquids, followed by electricity, and then molten or hot metals most often cause work-related burns. The hospital expenses and the societal costs related to time away from work or school are staggering.

Etiology

Cutaneous burns are caused by the application of heat, cold, or caustic chemicals to the skin. When heat is applied to the skin, the depth of injury is proportional to the temperature applied, duration of contact, and thickness of the skin.

Scald Burns

Scalds, usually from hot water, are the most common cause of burns in civilian practice. Water at 60°C (140°F) creates a deep partial-thickness or full-thickness burn in 3 seconds. At 69°C (156°F), the same burn occurs in 1 second. As a reference point, freshly brewed coffee generally is about 82°C

(180°F). Exposed areas of skin tend to be burned less deeply than clothed areas, as the clothing retains the heat and keeps the hot liquid in contact with the skin for a longer period of time. Immersion scalds are always deep, severe burns. Deliberate scalds, many times immersion injuries, are responsible for about 5 percent of the pediatric admissions to burn centers. The physician should note any discrepancy between the history provided by the caregiver and the distribution or probable cause of a burn. Any suspicious burn requires in-patient admission and must be reported promptly to the appropriate authorities. Scald burns from grease or hot oil are usually deep partial-thickness or full-thickness burns, as the oil or grease may be in the range of 200°C (400°F). Tar and asphalt burns are a special kind of scald. The tar should be removed by application of a petroleum-based ointment or a nontoxic solvent (e.g., Medisol or sunflower oil) under a dressing. The dressing should be removed and the ointment or solvent reapplied frequently until the tar has dissolved. Only then can the extent of the injury and the depth of the burn be estimated accurately.

Flame Burns

Flame burns are the second most common mechanism of thermal injury. Although the incidence of injuries caused by house fires has decreased with the use of smoke detectors, smoking-related fires, improper use of flammable liquids, motor vehicle collisions, and ignition of clothing by stoves or space heaters are responsible for most flame burns. Patients whose bedding or clothes have been on fire rarely escape without some full-thickness burns.

Flash Burns

Flash burns are next in frequency. Explosions of natural gas, propane, butane, petroleum distillates, alcohols, and other combustible liquids, and electrical arcs cause intense heat for a brief time period. Clothing, unless it ignites, is protective. Flash burns generally have a distribution over all exposed skin, with the deepest areas facing the source of ignition. Flash burns are typically superficial or partial-thickness, their depth depending on the amount and kind of fuel that explodes. However, electrical arc burns and those from gasoline are often full-thickness and require grafting.

Contact Burns

Contact burns result from contact with hot metals, plastic, glass, or hot coals. They are usually limited in extent, but are invariably deep. The exhaust pipes of motorcycles cause a classic burn of the medial lower leg that although small, usually requires excision and grafting. Contact burns are often fourth-degree burns, especially those in unconscious or postictal patients, and those caused by molten materials.

Burn Prevention

More than 90 percent of all burns are preventable, and ongoing prevention and education efforts seem to be the most effective means to impact burn incidence. Individual burn centers, the American Burn Association (ABA), and the International Society for Burn Injury (ISBI) have produced numerous public service announcements regarding hot water, carburetor flashes, grilling-related burns, scalds, and other kinds of burn injury.

HOSPITAL ADMISSION AND BURN CENTER REFERRAL

The severity of symptoms from smoke inhalation and the magnitude of associated burns dictate the need for hospital admission and specialized care. Any patient who has a symptomatic inhalation injury or more than trivial burns should be admitted to a hospital. As a rule of thumb, if the burns cover more than 5 to 10 percent total body surface area (TBSA), the patient should be referred to a designated burn center. In the absence of burns, admission depends on the severity of respiratory symptoms, presence of premorbid medical problems, and the social circumstances of the patient.

Burn Center Referral Criteria

The ABA has identified the following injuries as those requiring referral to a burn center after initial assessment and stabilization at an emergency department:

1. Partial-thickness and full-thickness burns totaling greater than 10 percent TBSA in patients younger than 10 or older than 50 years of age.
2. Partial-thickness and full-thickness burns totaling greater than 20 percent TBSA in other age groups.
3. Partial-thickness and full-thickness burns involving the face, hands, feet, genitalia, perineum, or major joints.
4. Full-thickness burns greater than 5 percent TBSA in any age group.
5. Electrical burns, including lightning injury.
6. Chemical burns.
7. Inhalation injury.
8. Burn injury in patients with preexisting medical disorders that could complicate management, prolong the recovery period, or affect mortality.
9. Any burn with concomitant trauma (e.g., fractures) in which the burn injury poses the greatest risk of morbidity or mortality. If the trauma poses the greater immediate risk, the patient may be treated initially in a trauma center until stable, before being transferred to a burn center. The physician's decisions should be made with the regional medical control plan and triage protocols in mind.
10. Burn injury in children admitted to a hospital without qualified personnel or equipment for pediatric care.
11. Burn injury in patients requiring special social, emotional, and/or long-term rehabilitative support, including cases involving suspected child abuse.

EMERGENCY CARE

Care at the Scene

Airway

Once flames are extinguished, initial attention must be directed to the airway. Any patient rescued from a burning building or exposed to a smoky fire should be placed on 100 percent oxygen via a nonrebreather mask if there is any suspicion of smoke inhalation. If the patient is unconscious or in respiratory distress, endotracheal intubation should be performed by appropriately trained personnel.

Other Injuries and Transport

Once an airway is secured, the patient is assessed for other injuries. Emergency medical personnel should place an intravenous line and begin fluid administration with lactated Ringer (LR) solution at a rate of approximately 1 L/h in the case of an adult with a severe burn; otherwise, a maintenance rate is appropriate assuming no concomitant, nonthermal trauma. For transport, the patient should be kept warm and wrapped in a clean sheet or blanket. Sterility is not required. Before or during transport, constricting clothing and jewelry should be removed from burned parts, because local swelling begins almost immediately.

Cold Application

Small burns, particularly scalds, may be treated with immediate application of cool water. It has been mathematically demonstrated that cooling cannot reduce skin temperature enough to prevent further tissue damage, but there is evidence in animals that cooling delays edema formation. Iced water should never be used, even on the smallest of burns.

Emergency Room Care

The primary rule for the emergency physician is to ignore the burn. As with any form of trauma, the airway, breathing, and circulation protocol (ABC) must be strictly followed. Although a burn is a dramatic injury, a careful search for other life-threatening injuries is the first priority. Only after making an overall assessment of the patient's condition should attention be directed to the burn.

Emergency Assessment of Inhalation Injury

The patient's history is an integral part of assessing the extent of their injuries. Inhalation injury should be suspected in anyone with a flame burn, and assumed until proven otherwise in anyone burned in an enclosed space. Careful inspection of the mouth and pharynx should be done early, and endotracheal intubation performed as needed. Hoarseness and expiratory wheezes are signs of potentially serious airway edema or inhalation injury. Copious mucus production and carbonaceous sputum (i.e., expectorated sputum and not just black flecks in the saliva) are also positive signs, but their absence does not rule out inhalation injury. Carboxyhemoglobin levels should be obtained, and elevated levels or any symptoms of carbon monoxide (CO) poisoning are presumptive evidence of associated inhalation injury. A decreased P-to-F ratio, the ratio of arterial oxygen pressure (Pao_2) to the percentage of inspired oxygen (Fio_2), is one of the earliest indicators of smoke inhalation. A ratio of less than 250 is an indication for endotracheal intubation rather than for increasing the Fio_2.

Fluid Resuscitation in the Emergency Room

As burns approach 20 percent TBSA, local proinflammatory cytokines enter the circulation and result in a systemic inflammatory response. The microvascular leak, permitting loss of fluid and protein from the intravascular compartment into the extravascular compartment, becomes generalized. Resuscitation begins by starting intravenous LR solution at a rate tailored to the extent of the burn using the Parkland/Baxter formula (Table 7-1), as both over- and under-resuscitation are deleterious. Burn patients requiring intravenous resuscitation

TABLE 7-1 Formulas for Estimating Adult Burn Patient Resuscitation Fluid Needs

	Electrolyte	Colloid	D_5W
Colloid formulas			
Evans	Normal saline 1.0 mL/kg/% burn	1.0 mL/kg/% burn	2000 mL
Brooke	Lactated Ringer solution 1.5 mL/kg/% burn	0.5 mL/kg	2000 mL
Slater	Lactated Ringer solution 2 L/24 h	Fresh frozen plasma 75 mL/kg/24 h	
Crystalloid formulas			
Parkland	Lactated Ringer solution	4 mL/kg/% burn	
Modified Brooke	Lactated Ringer solution	2 mL/kg/% burn	
Hypertonic saline formulas			
Hypertonic saline solution (Monafo)—Volume to maintain urine output at 30 mL/h;fluid contains 25 mEq Na/L			
Modified hypertonic (Warden)—Lactated Ringer solution + 50 mEq NaHCO$_3$ (180 mEq Na/L) to maintain urine output at 30–50 mL/h; lactated Ringer solution to maintain urine output at 30–50 mL/h beginning 8 h postburn			
Dextran formula (Demling)—Dextran 40 in saline: 2 mL/kg/h for 8 h; lactated Ringer solution: volume to maintain output at 30 mL/h; fresh frozen plasma: 0.5 mL/kg/h for 18 h beginning 8 h postburn			

Source: Reproduced with permission from Warden GD: Burn shock resuscitation. *World J Surg* 16:16, 1992.

should have a Foley catheter placed and urine output monitored hourly, the goal being 30 mL/h in adults and 1.0 mL/kg per h in young children.

Patients with burns covering less than 50 percent TBSA usually can begin resuscitation via two large-bore peripheral intravenous lines. Upper extremities are preferable, even if the intravenous line must pass through burned skin or eschar. Patients with burns greater than 50 percent TBSA, or those who have associated medical problems, are at the extremes of age, or have concomitant inhalation injuries should have additional central venous access established with invasive hemodynamic monitoring.

Tetanus Prophylaxis

Burns are tetanus-prone wounds. The need for tetanus prophylaxis is determined by the patient's current immunization status.

Gastric Decompression

Many burn centers begin enteral feeding on admission. If patient transport is via air ambulance or is going to take more than a few hours, the safest course is usually to decompress the stomach with a nasogastric tube.

Pain Control

During the initial phase of burn care, medications should be given intravenously, as subcutaneous and intramuscular injections are variably absorbed. Pain control is best managed with intravenous doses of an opiate until analgesia is adequate without inducing hypotension.

Psychosocial Care

Psychosocial care should begin immediately. The patient and family must be comforted and given a realistic assessment regarding the prognosis of the burns. If the patient is a child, and if the circumstances of the burn are suspicious, physicians in all states are required by law to report any suspected case of child abuse to local authorities.

Care of the Burn Wound

After all other assessments have been completed, attention should be directed to the burn itself. If the patient is to be transferred within 24 h of injury, the wounds can be minimally dressed in gauze. However, the size of the burn should always be calculated to establish the proper level of fluid resuscitation, and pulses distal to circumferential deep burns should be monitored.

Escharotomy

Thoracic escharotomy. The adequacy of oxygenation and ventilation must be monitored continuously throughout the resuscitation period. Ventilation may be compromised by chest wall inelasticity related to a deep circumferential burn of the thorax. Pressures required for ventilation increase and arterial PCO_2 rises. When required, escharotomies are performed bilaterally in the anterior axillary lines. If there is significant extension of the burn onto the adjacent abdominal wall, the escharotomy incisions should be extended to this area by a transverse incision along the costal margins.

Escharotomy of the extremities. Edema formation in the tissues under the tight, unyielding eschar of a circumferential burn on an extremity may produce significant vascular compromise that, if left unrecognized and untreated, will lead to permanent, serious neuromuscular and vascular deficits. All jewelry must be removed from the extremities to avoid distal ischemia. Skin color, sensation, capillary refill, and peripheral pulses must be assessed hourly in any extremity with a circumferential burn. The occurrence of any of the following signs or symptoms may indicate poor perfusion of a distal extremity warranting escharotomy: cyanosis, deep tissue pain, progressive paresthesia, progressive decrease or absence of pulses, or the sensation of cold extremities. An ultrasonic flowmeter (Doppler) is a reliable means for assessing arterial blood flow, the need for an escharotomy, and also can be used to assess adequacy of circulation after an escharotomy.

When necessary, escharotomies may be done as bedside procedures with a sterile field and scalpel or electrocautery. Local anesthesia is unnecessary as full-thickness eschar is insensate; however, intravenous opiates or anxiolytics should be used. The incision, which must avoid major neurovascular and musculotendinous structures, should be placed along the mid-medial or mid-lateral aspect of the extremity. To permit adequate separation of the cut edges for decompression, the incision should be carried down through the eschar, which includes devitalized dermis, to the subcutaneous fat. The incision should extend the length of the constricting full-thickness burn and across involved joints. When a single escharotomy incision does not result in restoring adequate distal perfusion, a second escharotomy incision on the contralateral aspect of the extremity should be performed. Digital escharotomy is controversial in its efficacy and rarely required.

BURN SEVERITY

The severity of any burn injury is related to the size and depth of the burn, and to the part of the body that has been burned. Burns are the only truly quantifiable form of trauma. The single most important factor in predicting burn-related mortality, need for specialized care, and the type and likelihood of complications is the overall size of the burn as a proportion of the patient's TBSA. Treatment plans, including initial resuscitation and subsequent nutritional requirements, are directly related to the size of burn.

Burn Size

A general idea of the burn size can be made by using the rule of nines. Each upper extremity accounts for 9 percent of the TBSA, each lower extremity accounts for 18 percent, the anterior and posterior trunk each account for 18 percent, the head and neck account for 9 percent, and the perineum accounts for 1 percent. Although the rule of nines is reasonably accurate for adults, a number of more precise charts have been developed that are particularly helpful in assessing pediatric burns. For smaller burns, an accurate assessment of size can be made by using the patient's palmar hand surface, including the digits, which amounts to approximately 1 percent of TBSA.

Burn Depth

Along with burn size and patient age, the depth of the burn is a primary determinant of mortality. Burn depth is also the primary determinant of the patient's long-term appearance and functional outcome.

Burns not extending all the way through the dermis leave behind epithelium-lined skin appendages, including sweat glands and hair follicles with attached sebaceous glands. When dead dermal tissue is removed, epithelial cells swarm from the surface of each appendage to meet swarming cells from neighboring appendages, forming a new, fragile epidermis on top of a thinned and scarred dermal bed. Skin appendages vary in depth, and the deeper the burn, the fewer the appendages that contribute to healing, and the longer the burn takes to heal. The longer the burn takes to heal, the less dermis remains, the greater the inflammatory response, and the more severe the scarring.

With aggressive surgical treatment, an accurate estimation of burn depth is crucial. Burns that heal within 3 weeks usually do so without hypertrophic scarring or functional impairment, although long-term pigmentary changes are common. Burns that take longer than 3 weeks to heal often produce unsightly hypertrophic scars, frequently lead to functional impairment, and provide only a thin, fragile epithelial covering for many weeks or months. State-of-the-art burn care involves early excision and grafting of all burns that will not heal within 3 weeks. The challenge is to determine which burns will heal within 3 weeks, and are thus better treated by nonoperative wound care.

Burn depth is dependent on the temperature of the burn source, the thickness of the skin, the duration of contact, and the heat-dissipating capability of the skin. Burns are classified according to increasing depth as epidermal (first-degree), superficial and deep partial-thickness (second-degree), full-thickness (third-degree), and fourth-degree. Many burns have a mixture of clinical characteristics, making precise classification difficult.

Shallow Burns

Epidermal burns (first-degree). As implied, these burns involve only the epidermis. They do not blister, but become erythematous because of dermal vasodilation, and are quite painful. Over 2–3 days the erythema and pain subside. By about the fourth day, the injured epithelium desquamates in the phenomenon of peeling, which is well known after sunburn.

Superficial partial-thickness (second-degree). Superficial partial-thickness burns include the upper layers of dermis, and characteristically form blisters with fluid collection at the interface of the epidermis and dermis. When blisters are removed, the wound is pink and wet. The wound is hypersensitive, and the burns blanch with pressure. If infection is prevented, superficial partial-thickness burns heal spontaneously in less than 3 weeks, and do so without functional impairment. They rarely cause hypertrophic scarring, but in pigmented individuals the healed burn may never completely match the color of the surrounding normal skin.

Deep Burns

Deep partial-thickness (second-degree). Deep partial-thickness burns extend into the reticular layers of the dermis. They also blister, but the wound surface is usually a mottled pink-and-white color immediately after the injury because of the varying blood supply to the dermis (white areas have little to no blood flow and pink areas have some blood flow). The patient complains of discomfort rather than pain. When pressure is applied to the burn, capillary refill occurs slowly or may be absent. The wound often is less sensitive to pinprick than the surrounding normal skin. If not excised and grafted, and if infection is prevented, these burns will heal in 3–9 weeks, but invariably do so with considerable scar formation. Unless active physical therapy is continued throughout the healing process, joint function can be impaired, and hypertrophic scarring is common.

Full-thickness (third-degree). Full-thickness burns involve all layers of the dermis and can heal only by wound contracture, epithelialization from the wound margin, or skin grafting. They appear white, cherry red, or black, and may or may not have deep blisters. Full-thickness burns are described as being leathery, firm, and depressed when compared with adjoining normal skin, and they are insensate. The difference in depth between a deep partial-thickness burn and a full-thickness burn may be less than 1 mm. The clinical appearance of full-thickness burns can resemble that of deep partial-thickness burns. They may be mottled in appearance, rarely blanch on pressure, and may have a dry, white appearance. In some cases, the burn is translucent, with clotted vessels visible in the depths. Some full-thickness burns, particularly immersion scalds, have a red appearance and initially may be confused with superficial partial-thickness burns. However, they can be distinguished because they do not blanch with pressure. Full-thickness burns develop a classic burn eschar, a structurally intact but dead and denatured dermis that if left in situ over days and weeks, separates from the underlying viable tissue.

Fourth-degree. Fourth-degree burns involve not only all layers of the skin, but also subcutaneous fat and deeper structures. These burns almost always have a charred appearance, and frequently only the cause of the burn gives a clue to the amount of underlying tissue destruction. Electrical burns, contact burns, some immersion burns, and burns sustained by patients who are unconscious at the time of burning may all be fourth-degree.

Assessment of Burn Depth

The standard technique for determining burn depth has been clinical observation of the wound. A burn is a dynamic process for the first few days; a burn appearing shallow on day 1 may appear considerably deeper by day 3. Furthermore, the kind of topical wound care used can dramatically change the appearance of the burn. Evaluation by an experienced surgeon regarding whether a partial-thickness burn will heal in 3 weeks is about 70 percent accurate. Other techniques to quantify burn depth involve (1) the ability to detect dead cells or denatured collagen (e.g., biopsy, ultrasound, and vital dyes), (2) assessment of changes in blood flow (e.g., fluorometry, laser Doppler, and thermography), (3) analysis of the color of the wound (e.g., light reflectance methods), and (4) evaluation of physical changes, such as edema (e.g., nuclear magnetic resonance imaging). Nonetheless, the most common modality of burn depth estimation used in state-of-the-art burn care today is still clinical observation.

THE PHYSIOLOGIC RESPONSE TO BURN INJURY

Burn patients with or without inhalation injury commonly manifest an inflammatory process involving the entire organism; the term systemic inflammatory response syndrome (SIRS) summarizes that condition. SIRS with infection (i.e., sepsis syndrome) is a major factor determining morbidity and mortality in thermally injured patients. Pathologic alterations of the metabolic, cardiovascular, gastrointestinal, and coagulation systems occur, with resulting hypermetabolism; increased cellular, endothelial, and epithelial permeability; classic hemodynamic alterations; and often extensive microthrombosis. The cardiovascular manifestations of SIRS largely disappear within 24–72 hours, but the patient remains in a hypermetabolic state until wound coverage is achieved.

Burn Shock

Burn shock is a complex process of circulatory and microcirculatory dysfunction that is not easily or fully repaired by fluid resuscitation. Tissue trauma and hypovolemic shock result in the formation and release of local and systemic mediators, which produce an increase in vascular permeability and microvascular hydrostatic pressure. Most mediators act to increase permeability by altering venular endothelial integrity. The early phase of burn edema, lasting from minutes to an hour, is attributed to mediators such as histamine, products of platelet activation, eicosanoids, and proteolytic products of the coagulation, fibrinolytic, and kinin cascades. Vasoactive amines may also act by increasing microvascular blood flow or vascular pressures, accentuating the burn edema.

In addition to the loss of microvascular integrity, thermal injury also causes changes at the cellular level. The reduction in cardiac output after burn injury is a result of cellular shock, hypovolemic shock, and increased systemic vascular resistance (SVR) because of sympathetic stimulation from the release of multiple mediators. The cardiac myocyte shock state is a result of impaired calcium homeostasis and subsequent intracellular signaling dysregulation.

Metabolic Response to Burn Injury

Hypermetabolism

Resting energy expenditure (REE) after burn injury can be as much as 100 percent above predictions based on standard calculations for size, age, sex, and weight. Some debate persists regarding the genesis of this phenomenon, but increased heat loss from the burn wound and increased beta-adrenergic stimulation are probably primary factors. On average, the REE is approximately 1.3 times the predicted basal metabolic rate (BMR) obtained using the Harris-Benedict equation.

Glucose metabolism is elevated in almost all critically ill patients, including those with burn injuries. Gluconeogenesis and glycogenolysis are increased in burn patients, as are plasma insulin levels. The basal rate of glucose production is elevated despite this hyperinsulinemic state. Hyperglycemia complicates the acute management of many significant burns and may be related to increased mortality and decreased graft take. Further, hyperglycemia may exacerbate muscle catabolism in burn patients although not influencing REE. Exogenous insulin administration to achieve euglycemia has been shown to decrease donor site healing time and decrease length of stay, although ameliorating skeletal muscle catabolism.

Lipolysis occurs at a rate in excess of the requirements for fatty acids as an energy source because of alterations in substrate cycling. In burn patients, the majority of released fatty acids are not oxidized, but rather re-esterified into triglycerides, resulting in fat accumulation in the liver. The acute and long-term consequences of this hepatic steatosis are unclear. β blockade using propranolol appears promising as a means to manipulate peripheral lipolysis and potentially prevent hepatic steatosis.

Proteolysis is increased in burn patients. Following utilization, protein is excreted primarily in the urine as urea. This results in an increased efflux of amino acids from the skeletal muscle pool, including the gluconeogenic amino acids alanine and glutamine (Gln). Protein intake greater than 1 g/kg per day has been recommended for all thermally injured patients, and for burn patients with normal renal function, the recommended protein intake is 2 g/kg per day. Beneficial effects of Gln supplementation, or its metabolic precursors, have been demonstrated in burn patients. The precise mechanisms by which direct and indirect Gln supplementation improves outcome remain unclear. The anabolic steroid oxandrolone also has been shown to improve donor-site healing time, diminish weight loss, and blunt protein catabolism during the acute phase of burn wound healing.

Neuroendocrine Response

Catecholamines are massively elevated following burn injury, and appear to be the major endocrine mediators of the hypermetabolic response in thermally injured patients. Pharmacologic beta-blockade using propranolol diminishes the intensity of postburn hypermetabolism. Conversely, growth hormone (GH) levels are attenuated following thermal injury. Although early studies of exogenous GH as an anticatabolic agent were promising in the pediatric population, ultimately its use has been supplanted by less expensive, safer, and equally effective pharmacotherapies such as propranolol and oxandrolone.

Immunologic Response to Burn Injury

The immune status of the burn patient has a profound impact on outcome in terms of survival and major morbidity. Many mediators are released from both injured and uninjured tissues at the wound site where they exert local and systemic effects. The timetable of induction/suppression and physiologic sequela are similar in patients suffering thermal and nonthermal trauma.

FLUID MANAGEMENT

Proper fluid management is critical to survival following major thermal injury. An aggressive approach to fluid therapy has led to reduced mortality rates in the first 48 hours postburn; nonetheless, approximately 50 percent of the deaths still occur within the first 10 days after burn injury, owing to multiple-organ failure syndrome (MOFS) and overwhelming sepsis. One of the principal causes, particularly of MOFS, is inadequate fluid resuscitation and maintenance. Fluid management following successful resuscitation from burn shock is equally as important.

Burn Resuscitation

The primary goal of fluid resuscitation is to ensure end-organ perfusion by replacing fluid that is sequestered as a result of the thermal injury. Support of the burned patient in this manner is principally aimed at the first 24–48 hours after injury, when the rate of development of hypovolemia is maximal. A critical concept to understand is that massive fluid shifts occur even although total body water initially remains unchanged. What actually changes is the volume of each fluid compartment, with intracellular and interstitial volumes increasing at the expense of intravascular volume.

Multiple resuscitation formulas, employing various solutions at different volumes and rates, have evolved over time (see Table 7-1). However, neither consensus statements nor evidence-based guidelines have emerged demonstrating the superiority of one formula over another. Nonetheless, accepted recommendations continue to be that resuscitation should proceed in a manner sufficient to maintain end-organ perfusion and abrogate electrolyte disturbances, although being flexible and amenable to individual patient differences, regardless of the composition, volume, or infusion rate of the solution employed.

Special Considerations in Burn Shock Resuscitation

Pediatric fluid resuscitation.   The burned child represents a special challenge, as resuscitation must be much more precise than that for an adult with a similar burn. Children weighing less than 20 kg have limited glucose reserves; as such, they require the addition of dextrose-based maintenance fluids to their calculated resuscitation volumes, or profound hypoglycemia will ensue. Further, children require relatively more fluid for burn shock resuscitation than adults, with fluid requirements for children averaging approximately 6 mL/kg/ % TBSA. This is most likely reflective of the near twofold increase in urine output (1.0–1.5 mL/kg body weight per h) required to ensure adequate end-organ perfusion in children. Finally, children commonly require formal resuscitation for relatively small burns of 10–20 percent TBSA.

Inhalation injury.   Inhalation injury undoubtedly increases the fluid requirements for successful resuscitation following thermal injury, with volumes of approximately 1.5 times compared to patients without inhalation injury. Inhalation injury accompanying thermal trauma increases the magnitude of the total body injury via disproportionate increases in systemic inflammation.

Invasive hemodynamic monitoring. The use of pulmonary artery catheters (PACs), with or without goal-directed therapy, has not typically been part of burn shock resuscitation. Nonetheless, certain patients may benefit from invasive hemodynamic monitoring to try and precisely direct their resuscitation. It is generally accepted that patients with known significant premorbid cardiac or pulmonary disease, associated inhalation injury, or concomitant nonthermal trauma, and older adults might require PAC monitoring during burn resuscitation. Goal-directed, hemodynamic resuscitation in burn patients has met with mixed results. It is likely that attainment of hemodynamic goals merely represents sufficient physiologic reserve to survive the injury, and not specific salutary effects of the therapy. In fact, hemodynamic resuscitation of burn shock is universally associated with substantially increased fluid volumes and predisposes to complications of overresuscitation.

Overresuscitation. Failure to institute appropriate early fluid resuscitation following thermal injury is associated with substantially worse outcomes. With modern burn care, this has become the rare exception, and in fact, many burn patients may actually be overresuscitated. Specific complications have emerged that appear to only be attributable to excessive resuscitation, namely abdominal compartment syndrome (ACS). ACS is preventable and iatrogenic in the vast majority of patients, owing to injudicious resuscitation. Early and appropriate resuscitation following major thermal injury is of paramount importance to ensure a good outcome; however, overresuscitation may produce complications that nullify the gains.

Choice of Fluids and Rate of Administration

Most patients can be resuscitated with crystalloid, specifically LR solution. Normal saline should be avoided, as the volumes required for resuscitation invariably lead to a complicating hyperchloremic metabolic acidosis. In patients with massive burns, young children, and burns complicated by severe inhalation injury, a combination of crystalloid and colloid can be used to achieve the desired goal of end-organ perfusion while minimizing edema.

Resuscitation formulas (see Table 7-1) should only be considered general guidelines for burn shock resuscitation. Ultimately, the volume and rate of infused fluid should maintain a urine output of 30 mL/h in adults (approximately 0.5 mL/kg per h), with lower limits acceptable in the face of known renal insufficiency, and 1.0 to 1.5 mL/kg per h in children. Resuscitation is considered successful when there is no further accumulation of edema, usually between 18 and 24 h postburn, and the volume of infused fluid required to maintain adequate urine output approximates the patient's maintenance fluid volume, which is normal maintenance volume plus evaporative water loss.

Fluid Replacement Following Burn Shock Resuscitation

Colloid replacement should be used sparingly, in the form of albumin, and only after 24 hours postburn. The total daily maintenance fluid requirement in the adult patient is calculated by the following formula, where m^2 is square meters of TBSA:

$$\text{Total maintenance fluid} = (1500\,\text{mL/m}^2) + \text{evaporative water loss} \\ \times\,[(25 + \%\text{TBSA burn} \times m^2 \times 24]$$

A general guideline is that a patient will require approximately 1.5 times their normal maintenance fluids.

After initial resuscitation, urine output alone is an unreliable guide to sufficient hydration. Adult patients with major thermal injuries require a urine output of approximately 1000 to 1500 mL/24 h; children require approximately 3 to 4 mL/kg per h averaged over 24 h.

INHALATION INJURY

Of some 45,000 fire victims admitted to hospitals each year, approximately 30 percent sustain an inhalation injury. CO poisoning, thermal injury, and smoke inhalation are three distinct aspects of clinical inhalation injury. Although the symptoms and treatment of each vary, the distinct injuries may coexist and require concomitant treatment.

Carbon Monoxide Poisoning

The majority of house fire deaths can be attributed to CO poisoning. CO is a colorless, odorless, and tasteless gas with an affinity for hemoglobin (Hb) approximately 200 times that of oxygen. CO reversibly binds to Hb to form carboxyhemoglobin (COHb), which interferes with oxygen delivery to the tissues. The half-life (T1/2) of COHb when breathing room air is approximately 4 h. On 100 percent oxygen, the T1/2 is reduced to 45–60 minutes. In a hyperbaric oxygen chamber at 2 atm, it is approximately 30 minutes, and at 3 atm it is about 15–20 minutes.

Levels of COHb are easily measured, but the degree of impairment may not directly correlate with blood levels. A COHb less than 10 percent typically does not cause symptoms. At approximately 20 percent, healthy persons complain of headache, nausea, vomiting, and loss of manual dexterity. At approximately 30 percent, patients become weak, confused, and lethargic. At 40–60 percent, the patient lapses into a coma, and levels greater than 60 percent are usually fatal.

Diagnosis and Treatment

Patients burned in an enclosed space or having any signs or symptoms of neurologic impairment should be placed on 100 percent oxygen via a nonrebreather face mask while waiting for measurement of COHb levels. The use of pulse oximetry (Spo_2) to assess arterial oxygenation in the CO-poisoned patient is contraindicated, as the COHb results in erroneously elevated Spo_2 measurements. If intubation is required, then hyperventilation with 100 percent oxygen should be instituted. The use of hyperbaric oxygen (HBO) therapy remains controversial. HBO therapy in burn patients with CO poisoning is of unknown therapeutic value or efficacy, and should only be used when: (1) the COHb is greater than 25 percent, (2) a neurologic deficit exists, (3) no formal burn resuscitation is required (typically TBSA <10–15 percent), (4) pulmonary function is stable with an intact airway, and (5) interfacility transfer does not compromise burn care.

Thermal Airway Injury

The term "pulmonary burn" is a misnomer. True thermal damage to the lower respiratory tract and pulmonary parenchyma is extremely rare, unless live steam or exploding gases are inhaled.

Thermal injury to the respiratory tract is usually immediate and manifests as mucosal and submucosal erythema, edema, hemorrhage, and ulceration. It is usually limited to the upper airway (above the vocal cords) and proximal trachea for two reasons: (1) the oropharynx and nasopharynx provide an effective mechanism for heat exchange; and (2) sudden exposure to hot air typically triggers reflex closure of the vocal cords.

Patients with the greatest risk of upper airway obstruction from thermal airway injury are those injured in an explosion, with burns of the face and upper thorax, or those who have been unconscious in a fire. The presence of significant intraoral and pharyngeal injury is a clear indication for immediate endotracheal intubation.

Smoke Inhalation

Hundreds of toxic products are released during combustion (flaming) or pyrolysis (smoldering), depending on the type of fuel burned, the oxygen content of the environment, and the actual temperature of burning. Some 280 toxic substances have been identified in wood smoke alone. Petrochemical science has produced a wealth of plastic materials used in homes and automobiles, that when burned, produce nearly all of these substances, and many other products not yet characterized. Prominent by-products of incomplete combustion are oxides and hydrogenated moieties of sulfur and nitrogen, and numerous aldehydes.

After inhalation, highly soluble acidic and basic compounds rapidly dissolve in the water lining the mucosa of the respiratory tract, causing direct epithelial injury, manifested as epithelial edema, submucosal hemorrhage, and necrosis. Epithelial injury can occur at all levels of the respiratory tract, from oropharynx to alveolus. Although the chemical mechanisms of injury may be different among toxic products, the overall end-organ response is relatively homogeneous. There is an immediate loss of bronchial epithelial cilia and decreased alveolar surfactant levels. Atelectasis results, compounded by small-airway edema, and is only slowly reversed by normal ventilation. This regional hypoventilation results in worsening atelectasis, intrapulmonary shunt, and subsequent hypoxemia. Wheezing and air hunger are common early manifestations of inhalation injury.

Much of the pulmonary response appears to be related more to the severity of an associated cutaneous burn than to the degree of smoke inhalation. Without associated cutaneous thermal injury, the mortality from isolated inhalation injury is quite low. Symptomatic treatment usually leads to complete resolution of symptoms in a few days. However, in the presence of burns, inhalation injury approximately doubles the mortality rate from burns of any size.

Diagnosis

Anyone with a flame burn sustained in an enclosed space should be assumed to have an inhalation injury until proven otherwise. In obtaining a history, emphasis should be placed on findings specific to the smoke exposure and to the type of therapy instituted prior to hospitalization. The duration of exposure correlates with the severity of lung injury.

A thorough examination should be performed and include evaluation of the face and oropharyngeal airway for hoarseness, stridor, edema, or soot impaction suggesting injury; chest auscultation for wheezing or rhonchi suggesting injury to distal airways; level of consciousness associated with decreased hypoxemia, CO poisoning, or cyanide poisoning; and testing for the presence of neurologic deficits associated with CO. Copious mucus production and carbonaceous expectorated sputum are hard signs of inhalation injury, but their absence does not rule out injury. An elevated COHb or any symptoms of CO poisoning are presumptive evidence of associated smoke inhalation. Anyone suspected of smoke inhalation should have an arterial blood gas drawn. One of the earliest indicators of injury is a decreased P-to-F ratio.

The early need for bronchoscopic evaluation and diagnosis remains controversial. Aside from documenting the presence of edema, tracheal erythema, and/or carbon deposits, fiberoptic bronchoscopy (FOB) does not materially influence the treatment of smoke inhalation. It is operator-dependent, not risk-free, and yield with FOB appears to be strongly dependent on clinical suspicion of inhalation injury. Given these limitations, it is recommended that a history, physical examination, and laboratory studies be used to make the diagnosis of inhalation injury, and the use of FOB be reserved for exceptional cases requiring therapeutic FOB (e.g., expansion of lobar collapse or removal of obstructing intrabronchial secretions or casts).

Treatment

Upper airway. No standard treatment has evolved to ensure survival after smoke inhalation. In the presence of increasing oropharyngeal and laryngeal edema, rapid endotracheal intubation is indicated. A tracheostomy is never an emergency procedure and should not be used as the initial step in airway management. The incidence of postextubation stridor in burn victims is as high as 47 percent. The treatment of postextubation stridor includes the administration of nebulized racemic epinephrine and helium-oxygen (heliox) mixtures. Steroids are never indicated.

Lower airway and alveoli. Tracheobronchitis, commonly seen with inhalation injury, produces wheezing, coughing, and retained secretions. The ventilation-perfusion mismatch present in these patients can result in mild to moderate hypoxemia, varying with the degree of premorbid lung disease; therefore supplemental oxygen should be administered routinely. Although a trial of bronchodilators is indicated in patients with premorbid bronchospastic disease, the overall efficacy is questionable.

The usual presenting sign of distal airway injury is hypoxemia. Upper airway patency absolutely must be assured, and airway resistance minimized. Overall treatment for smoke inhalation is supportive, with the goal being maintenance of adequate oxygenation and ventilation until the lungs heal. The need for mechanical ventilation is determined by refractory hypoxemia. The precise mode of initial mechanical ventilation appears less important than ensuring a lung protective strategy.

Elective tracheostomy in burn patients remains controversial. Nonetheless, if the upper airway is in danger of imminent obstruction and endotracheal intubation attempts are unsuccessful, emergent cricothyroidotomy is indicated, with conversion to a formal tracheostomy soon thereafter. For patients requiring prolonged endotracheal intubation, tracheostomy should be performed at the discretion of the managing burn surgeon. There is no outcome benefit to early tracheostomy in burn patients.

Prophylactic antibiotics are not indicated with inhalation injury, which is a chemical pneumonitis. Subsequent burn wound management and treatment of eventual bacterial pneumonia may be made more difficult with the early use of antibiotics, as it rapidly leads to the selection of resistant organisms. Likewise, steroids are contraindicated with inhalation injury.

WOUND MANAGEMENT

Early Excision and Grafting

For deeper burns (i.e., deep partial-thickness and full-thickness burns), rather than waiting for spontaneous separation, the eschar is surgically removed and the wound closed via grafting techniques and/or immediate flap procedures tailored to the individual patient. This aggressive surgical approach to burn wound management is known as early excision and grafting (E&G). The optimal timing of early E&G has yet to be definitively determined; however, E&G within 3–7 days, and certainly by 10 days, following injury appears prudent. Early E&G has reduced burn mortality more than any other intervention. Early wound closure also reduces hospital stay, duration of illness, septic complications, and the need for major reconstruction, although decreasing hospital costs.

Current Status of Wound Care

Solid clinical and experimental evidence support the following conclusions:

1. Small (i.e., <20 percent) full-thickness burns and burns of indeterminate depth, if treated by an experienced surgeon, can be safely excised and grafted with a decrease in hospital stay, costs, and time away from work or school.
2. Early E&G dramatically decreases the number of painful débridements required.
3. Patients with burns of 20–40 percent TBSA will have fewer infectious wound complications if treated with early E&G.
4. In animal models, the immunosuppression and hypermetabolism associated with burns can be ameliorated by early burn wound removal.

Clinical impressions, without hard data supporting them, include the following:

1. Scarring is less severe in wounds closed early, leading to better appearance and fewer reconstructive procedures. There is no good measure of "acceptable" cosmetic appearance, and comparative studies await a consistent scale to measure results.
2. Mortality from wound infection is lower in patients with major burns after early excision. Because wounds exceeding donor skin availability cannot be closed completely until donor sites can be reharvested, definitive proof will come only when a durable permanent covering (i.e., skin substitute) can be applied in a timely fashion.

3. Mortality from other complications of major burns may be lower with early E&G. Ameliorating the stress, hypermetabolism, and overall bacterial load of the patients enables them to resist other complications. The only data to support this conclusion come from animal studies.

Technical Considerations

Excision of greater than 10 percent of TBSA should be done in a highly structured environment, preferably a dedicated burn center. Blood loss can be massive, and graft loss can be catastrophic. Smaller burns in important areas (e.g., hands, face, and feet) also require considerable experience. Excisional procedures should be performed as early as possible after the patient is stabilized, usually within a week of injury. Any burn projected to take longer than 3 weeks to heal is a candidate for E&G within the first postburn week.

Excision can be performed to include the burn and subcutaneous fat to the level of the investing fascia (fascial excision), or by tangentially removing thin slices of burned tissue until a viable bed remains (tangential excision). Fascial excision assures a viable bed for grafting, but takes longer, sacrifices potentially viable tissue, and leaves a permanent cosmetic defect. Tangential excision can create massive blood loss and risks grafting on a bed of uncertain viability, but sacrifices minimal living tissue, and leads to a superior cosmetic result. Fascial excisions are typically reserved for deeper burns; however, they can be useful in other selected patients.

If careful attention is given to sound principles of plastic surgery, the risk that there will be a need for subsequent reconstruction can be decreased. Split-thickness skin graft (STSG) junctures should be avoided over joints, and grafts should be placed transversely when possible. Adjacent pieces of STSG should be approximated carefully with a small amount of overlap. Thick STSGs (e.g., >0.015 inch) typically yield a better appearance than do thin grafts (e.g., >0.010 inch). With larger burns (>20 percent TBSA), STSGs are meshed to allow greater wound coverage per graft. However, if at all possible, cosmetically important areas should be grafted with a single sheet of STSG.

Donor Sites

As aggressive programs of early E&G developed, care and healing of donor sites became a priority. Donor sites are quite painful as they are a superficial partial-thickness injury, and appropriate dressings diminish donor site pain. Reports indicate that there is no optimal donor site dressing; however, moist wound healing is superior to dry wound healing.

Healed donor sites are still not free of complications. In addition to hypertrophic scarring and pigmentation changes, blistering for several weeks may trouble patients. Blisters are self-limiting and treated with bandages or ointments until they re-epithelialize. Donor site infections occur in approximately 5 percent of patients and can be devastating, with conversion of a partial-thickness to a full-thickness wound requiring a STSG for closure. Infection is treated aggressively with systemic and topical antibiotics.

Skin Substitutes

The ideal skin substitute must be permanent, affordable, resist hypertrophic scarring, provide normal pigmentation, and grow with developing children; however, it has yet to be developed.

Dermal Substitutes

The development of dermal substitutes has added greatly to the capabilities of the burn surgeon, especially when faced with a large burn and limited donor sites. They readily facilitate complete excision of the entire burn with wound closure. Depending on the product, grafting with STSG may be immediate or delayed until the dermal substitute has engrafted. Currently three dermal substitutes are available in the United States: INTEGRA, AlloDerm, and Dermagraft. These products are fundamentally similar in that they allow for the creation of a "neo-dermis" populated by the patient's own mesenchymal cells on which a thin STSG is placed. The use of thinner STSG allows for earlier re-cropping of donor sites, quicker closure of the complete burn, and less donor site scarring. Successful use of any one of the available dermal substitutes is technique-dependent and associated with a learning curve.

Cultured Skin

Apligraf is a Food and Drug Administration (FDA)-approved biologic dressing composed of cultured neonatal keratinocytes and fibroblasts. This allograft bioengineered product has been approved for use in chronic nonhealing ulcers, but has not yet been widely marketed for the burn patient.

Epicel is currently the only FDA-approved cultured epithelial autograft (CEA) product available. These grafts are created from a full-thickness biopsy of the patient's own skin and require 3 weeks to grow. They are quite expensive at approximately \$14,500 for 750 cm^2.

NUTRITIONAL SUPPORT

The nutritional effects of the hypermetabolic response to thermal injury are manifested as exaggerated energy expenditure and massive nitrogen loss. Nutritional support is aimed at provision of calories to match energy expenditure, although providing enough nitrogen to replace or support body protein stores.

Caloric Requirements

The magnitude of increase in the metabolic rate following thermal injury is directly proportional to the TBSA of the burn. The total energy expenditure may be elevated anywhere from 15–100 percent above basal needs. Mathematical formulas exist for the calculation of daily caloric requirements in burn patients. The formula most widely used is Long's modification of the Harris-Benedict equation (Table 7-2). Periodic determination of resting energy expenditure (REE) via indirect calorimetry may be used to allow more accurate adjustments of caloric provision. Total urine nitrogen (TUN) excretion is easy to measure, and accurately reflects the degree of catabolism. The TUN should be monitored regularly, with the goal being a persistently positive nitrogen balance. Various visceral proteins are commonly measured, typically as part of a "nutrition panel," to assess ongoing nutritional status.

TABLE 7-2 Long Modification of the Harris-Benedict Equation

Men
  BMR = (66.47 ± 13.75 weight ± 5.0 height = 6.76 age)
    × (activity factor) × (injury factor)

Women
  BMR = (655.10 ± 9.56 weight + 1.85 height = 4.68 age)
    × (activity factor) × (injury factor)

Activity factor
  Confined to bed: 1.2
  Out of bed: 1.3

Injury factor
  Minor operation: 1.20
  Skeletal trauma: 1.35
  Major sepsis: 1.60
  Severe thermal burn: 1.5

BMR = basal metabolic rate.

Carbohydrates

Carbohydrates, in the form of glucose, appear to be the best source of non-protein calories in the thermally injured patient. Provision of glucose to obligate tissues occurs at the expense of lean body mass (i.e., skeletal muscle) if adequate nutrition is not provided. The wound uses glucose by anaerobic glycolytic pathways, producing large amounts of lactate as an end product. In the liver, lactate is extracted and used for gluconeogenesis via the Cori cycle. Concomitantly, alanine, Gln, and other amino acids contribute to the increased gluconeogenesis. Increased ureagenesis, with urea derived from body protein stores, parallels the rise in hepatic glucose production. The hyperglycemia observed in burn patients is a consequence of accelerated glucose flux, not decreased peripheral utilization.

Because glucose that is obtained via gluconeogenic pathways ultimately derives from protein stores, depletion of body protein during burn hypermetabolism leads to energy deficits, malfunctioning of glucose-dependent energetic processes, and skeletal muscle wasting. High-carbohydrate enteral nutrition formulations appear to blunt this catabolism, resulting in skeletal muscle sparing. Optimal glucose oxidation during burn hypermetabolism occurs at intakes of approximately 5 mg/kg per min.

Protein

Combining glucose and protein-containing nutrients improves nitrogen balance and allows more calories to be used for the restoration of nitrogen balance than would be possible if either nutrient were used alone. Protein administration promotes synthesis of visceral and muscle protein, without appreciably affecting the rate of catabolism. Exogenous glucose retards catabolism, but exerts little effect on protein synthesis. Both mechanisms improve nitrogen balance, and sufficient glucose (approximately 7 g/kg per day) and protein (approximately 2 g/kg per day) should be components of the nutritional regimen for the severely burned catabolic patient.

The importance of Gln as a metabolic fuel source has been recognized, and it is considered a conditionally essential amino acid. During critical illness, circulating concentrations of Gln fall. Gln supplementation has been associated with improved outcomes following thermal injury.

Fat

The role of fat as a source of nonprotein calories is dependent on the extent of injury and associated hypermetabolism. Following significant thermal injury, there are alterations in substrate cycling and fatty acid oxidation that favor re-esterification and hepatic deposition of triglycerides. Fat appears to be a poor caloric source overall, and especially for the maintenance of nitrogen equilibrium and lean body mass, in burn-induced hypermetabolism. Patients with only moderate elevations in metabolic rate can use lipid calories efficiently, but these patients rarely require nutritional support.

Even more important than their energy inefficiency, fats appear to affect outcome following thermal injury. Patients fed low-fat enteral diets had fewer infectious complications, improved wound healing, shorter lengths of stay, and apparently reduced mortality compared to controls fed standard, relatively high-fat, enteral diets.

Vitamins and Minerals

Vitamin requirements in critically ill, hypermetabolic burn patients remain poorly defined. The fat-soluble vitamins (A, D, E, and K) are extensively stored in fat depots and are only slowly depleted during prolonged feeding of vitamin-free solutions. The water-soluble vitamins (B complex and C) are not stored in appreciable amounts, and are rapidly depleted. All vitamins should be supplemented. The dosage guidelines of the National Advisory Group/American Medical Association (NAG/AMA) are reasonable for burn patients unless symptoms of deficiency occur, with the exception of vitamin C. Vitamin C has an essential role in wound repair, and it is prudent to supplement the NAG/AMA recommended dose with approximately 1000 mg of vitamin C daily. Of note, all commercially available enteral feeding formulations meet NAG/AMA recommendations for vitamins and minerals.

Minerals and trace elements are essential because of their role in metabolic processes. Frequent determinations of serum levels are the best guides to electrolyte replacement. Less is known about trace element requirements after thermal injury. Zinc deficiency has been documented in burn patients; thus, empiric zinc supplementation is warranted following major burns.

Route of Administration

The route of nutritional support is important because it directly influences outcome. Total enteral nutrition (TEN) is the overwhelmingly favored mode of alimentation in the severely burned. Total parenteral nutrition (TPN) is used only when complete enteral failure is encountered, as TPN is associated with increased mortality.

In severely burned patients, gastroparesis may limit intragastric nutritional support, particularly in the early postburn period. However, immediate intragastric feeding appears to limit gastroparesis and is unquestionably safe. Even in the face of intragastric feeding intolerance, TEN should not be abandoned. Postpyloric feeding tends to work well in the burn patient with gastroparesis. Prokinetics should be used as needed.

Composition of Enteral Nutrition

In burn patients, a high-protein, high-carbohydrate, low-fat diet with fiber is optimal. As noted earlier, appropriate supplements to include Gln, vitamins, minerals, and trace elements are indicated, and add to the benefits of TEN. Immune-enhancing diets (e.g., IMPACT) offer no clear advantage over standard high-protein formulas in the burn population. Monitoring of TEN to assess tolerance and effectiveness is as important as the selection of the formula or timing of initiation. Careful nutrition and metabolic assessment can help ensure optimal support with minimal complications. Although superior to TPN, TEN still has associated complications, and any evidence of feeding intolerance should be actively investigated.

INFECTION

Infectious mortality following thermal injury has significantly declined over the past 2 decades, with the greatest reduction attributed to early E&G. However, following successful resuscitation, most acute morbidity and virtually all mortality in severely burned patients are still related to infection. Nonetheless, prophylactic systemic antibiotics are not part of modern burn care, as they do not reduce septic complications and only lead to increased bacterial resistance.

Risk Factors for Infection

The extent of burn injury as determined by TBSA is one of the major determinants of overall outcome, and the incidence of infection correlates with burn severity. Children appear to be more susceptible to systemic infection than adults for any given size burn. However, burns involving less than 20 percent TBSA in otherwise healthy individuals are rarely associated with life-threatening infection. The presence of an inhalation injury strongly correlates with infection, particularly pneumonia. Premorbid diabetes significantly increases infection rates following thermal injury, especially when coupled with poor glycemic control. Age is not an independent risk factor for infection following thermal injury.

Clinical Manifestations and Diagnosis

Hyperthermia, tachycardia, increased ventilation, and high cardiac output are part of the normal response to major burns in otherwise healthy patients.

The most important observations are related to the temporal association of physiologic events. Abrupt onset of hyperglycemia, fall in blood pressure, and decrease in urinary output should suggest the possibility that the patient is becoming unstable. If these findings are associated with development of hypothermia, feeding intolerance, and/or a falling platelet count, the patient is probably developing sepsis. Even with firm clinical evidence of sepsis, a definitive microbiologic diagnosis of infection can sometimes be difficult to obtain.

Specific Infections

Wound Infection

All burn wounds become colonized by 72 hours after injury with the patient's own flora or with endemic organisms from the treatment facility. Bacteria colonize the surface of the wound and may penetrate the avascular eschar. This colonization is invariable and without clinical significance; hence, routine early wound cultures are not efficacious and only increase costs. Bacterial proliferation may occur beneath the eschar at the viable-nonviable tissue interface, leading to eschar separation if early E&G is not practiced. In a few patients, microorganisms may breach this barrier and invade the deeper underlying viable tissue, producing wound sepsis.

The essential pathologic feature of burn wound sepsis is invasion of organisms into viable tissue, which is diagnosed via biopsy and quantitative tissue culture demonstrating greater than 105 organisms per g of tissue. Any organisms capable of invading tissue can produce burn wound sepsis. The likelihood of sepsis increases in proportion to the size of the wound. Superficial wound swab cultures should never be used to evaluate potential invasive burn wound infection. Once the diagnosis of burn wound sepsis is confirmed, appropriate parenteral antibiotics should be administered and the wound promptly excised.

Before the introduction of effective topical antimicrobial agents, up to 60 percent of the deaths in burn centers were caused by burn wound sepsis. The three agents with proven broad-spectrum antimicrobial activity when applied to the burn wound are silver sulfadiazine (SSD), mafenide acetate, and silver nitrate (Table 7-3). SSD is the most common agent used in burn centers and has antifungal properties in addition to good bacterial coverage. However, SSD does not penetrate eschar. Only mafenide acetate is able to penetrate eschar, and it is the only agent capable of suppressing dense subeschar bacterial proliferation. The main disadvantage of mafenide acetate is its carbonic anhydrase inhibition, which may produce a hyperchloremic metabolic acidosis. However, this is typically of little clinical consequence. Silver nitrate must be used before bacteria have penetrated the wound. Its disadvantages are the associated electrolyte imbalances and methemoglobinemia. Since the introduction of effective topical therapy, fungal burn wound infections, primarily involving highly invasive Phycomycetes and Aspergillus organisms, have increased.

A newly emerging variant of burn wound infection, the "melting graft-wound syndrome," was recently reported and involves progressive epithelial loss (melting) from a previously well-taken graft, healed burn wound, or healed donor site. These infections have potentially devastating consequences. As such, appropriate systemic antibiotics, topical antibiotics, and aggressive wound care are mandatory for effective treatment. Reexcision and grafting rarely are required for salvage.

Pneumonia

One result of the prolonged and improved survival of severely burned patients is that the respiratory tract has become the most common source of infection. It is generally agreed that inhalation injury increases the risk of developing pneumonia.

The diagnosis of pneumonia is confirmed by the presence of characteristic infiltrates on chest radiographs and positive cultures. The most efficacious and sensitive method of obtaining tracheobronchial specimens for microbiologic analysis remains controversial. Regardless of specimen collection methodology, colonization of the upper airway in patients requiring mechanical ventilation should not be confused with a respiratory tract infection.

Single-agent therapy is generally appropriate and efficacious regardless of the pathogen, including Pseudomonas aeruginosa. Pneumonia still carries a significant mortality rate of approximately 25 percent in mechanically ventilated burn patients. Prophylactic antibiotics should not be used, as they only select for resistant organisms and do not reduce the incidence of pneumonia. Likewise, early tracheostomy does not lower pneumonia rates in either children or adults suffering major thermal injury. Consistent infection control

TABLE 7-3 Topical Antimicrobial Agents for Burn Wound Care

Silver nitrate	Mafenide acetate	Silver sulfadiazine
Active component		
0.5 percent in aqueous solution	11.1 percent in water-miscible base	1.0 percent in water-miscible base
Spectrum of antimicrobial activity		
Gram-negative—good Gram-positive—good Yeast—good	Gram-negative—good Gram-positive—good Yeast—poor	Gram-negative—variable Gram-positive—good Yeast—good
Method of wound care		
Occlusive dressings	Exposure	Exposure or single-layer dressings
Advantages		
Painless No hypersensitivity reaction No gram-negative resistance Dressings reduce evaporative heat loss Greater effectiveness against yeasts	Penetrates eschar Wound appearance readily monitored Joint motion unrestricted No gram-negative resistance	Painless Wound appearance readily monitored when exposure method used Easily applied Joint motion unrestricted when exposure method used Greater effectiveness against yeast
Disadvantages		
Deficits of sodium, potassium, calcium, and chloride No eschar penetration	Painful on partial-thickness burns Susceptibility to acidosis as a result of carbonic anhydrase inhibition	Neutropenia and thrombocytopenia Hypersensitivity—infrequent Limited eschar penetration
Limitation of joint motion by dressings Methemoglobinemia—rare Argyria—rare Staining of environment and equipment	Hypersensitivity reactions in 7% of patients	

practices and timely extubation seem to be the only effective means to lower the incidence of pneumonia.

Vascular Catheter-Related Infections

The incidence of peripheral suppurative thrombophlebitis following thermal injury is miniscule in the modern era, as saphenous venous cutdowns have been abandoned and standard line care is routine. The true incidence of central line sepsis in burn patients is unknown. Nonetheless, routine central venous catheter changes without evidence of infection are probably unwarranted and only increase complication rates; there are no conclusive data in the burn literature to support routine catheter changes. Contrary to popular belief, the specific central line site does not appear to influence infection rates in the burn patient. However, the distance from the burn wound does appear to correlate inversely with infection, and every effort should be made to place intravenous lines as far from the burn as possible.

ELECTRICAL INJURY AND BURNS

Electrical injuries are particularly dangerous, as they can be instantaneously fatal and also put rescuers in significant danger. Injury severity depends on the amperage of the current, the pathway of current through the victim's body, and the duration of contact with the source. Electrical current sources are typically classified as either low- or high-voltage, with 1000 volts (V) being the dividing line, and distinct injuries are associated with each type. Over 95 percent of all electrical injuries and electrical burns are caused by low-voltage commercial alternating current in the range of 0–220 V. An electrical burn potentially has three different components: (1) the true electrical injury from current flow, (2) an arc or flash flame injury produced by current arcing at a temperature of approximately 4000°C (7232°F) from its source to ground, and (3) a flame injury from the ignition of clothing or surroundings.

Acute Management and Multisystem Involvement

Electrical burns are thermal injuries from very intense heat and from electrical disruption of cell membranes. As electrical current meets tissue, it is converted to heat in direct proportion to the amperage of the current and the resistance of the tissues through which it passes. The smaller the size of the body part through which the electricity passes, the more intense the heat and the less the heat is dissipated into surrounding tissue. Fingers, hands, forearms, feet, and lower legs are frequently totally destroyed by high-voltage injuries. Areas of larger volume, like the trunk, usually dissipate enough current to prevent extensive damage to viscera unless the contact point(s) are on the abdomen or chest. Although cutaneous manifestations of electrical burns may appear limited, burned skin should not be considered the only injury, as massive underlying tissue destruction may be present. Resuscitation needs are usually far in excess of what would be expected on the basis of the cutaneous burn size, and associated flame and/or flash burns often compound the problem.

Myoglobinuria frequently accompanies electrical burns, but the clinical significance appears to be minimal, as modern burn resuscitation protocols alone appear to be sufficient treatment for myoglobinuria. Cardiac damage may be present, most commonly with conduction system derangements. Even with high-voltage injuries, a normal cardiac rhythm on admission generally means that subsequent dysrhythmia is unlikely.

The nervous system is exquisitely sensitive to electricity. The most devastating injury with frequent brain damage occurs when current passes through the head, but spinal cord damage is possible whenever current has passed from one side of the body to the other. Delayed transverse myelitis can occur days or weeks after injury. Anterior spinal artery syndrome from vascular dysregulation can also precipitate spinal cord dysfunction. Damage to peripheral nerves is common and may cause permanent functional impairment. Persistent neurologic symptoms may lead to chronic pain syndromes, and posttraumatic stress disorders are apparently more common after electrical burns than thermal burns.

Cataracts are a well-recognized sequela of high-voltage electrical burns. They occur in 5–7 percent of patients, frequently are bilateral, occur even in the absence of contact points on the head, and typically manifest within 1–2 years of injury.

Wound Management

There are two unique situations in which immediate surgical treatment is indicated for patients with electrical burns. Rarely, massive deep tissue necrosis will lead to acidosis or myoglobinuria that will not resolve with standard resuscitation techniques; major débridement and/or amputation may be necessary as an emergency procedure. More commonly, injured deep tissues undergo significant swelling, increasing the risk of compartment syndrome, and potentially leading to further tissue loss. Escharotomies and fasciotomies should be performed at compartment pressures of 30 mmHg or more, or with clinical indications of compartment syndrome. Any progression of median or ulnar nerve deficit in a hand that has been electrically burned is an indication for immediate median and ulnar nerve release at the wrist. If immediate decompression or débridement is not required, definitive surgical procedures can be done in the usual time frame, between days 3 and 5.

CHEMICAL BURNS

Strong acids or alkalis cause most chemical burns. They typically are associated with industrial accidents, assaults, or the improper use of harsh household solvents and cleaners. In contrast to thermal injury, chemical burns cause progressive damage and injury until the chemicals are inactivated by reaction with tissues or diluted by therapeutic irrigation. Acid burns typically are more self-limiting than alkali burns. Acids tend to "tan" the skin, creating an impermeable barrier of coagulation necrosis debris along the leading edge of the chemical burn that limits further penetration. Alkalis combine with cutaneous lipids to create a soap, and are thus able to continue dissolving the skin until they are neutralized.

Initial Care

All involved clothing should be removed, and unlike thermal injury, the burns should be irrigated with copious amounts of tepid water. Irrigating for at least 15 minutes under a running stream of tepid water may limit the overall severity of the burn; however, care should be taken to avoid hypothermia. Neutralizing agents or antidotes are contraindicated, except with hydrofluoric acid burns. Delay deepens the chemical burn, and neutralizing agents may even produce thermal burns, as they frequently generate substantial heat on neutralization of the offending agent. Powdered chemicals should be brushed off skin and clothing.

Wound Management

A full-thickness chemical burn may appear deceptively superficial. Chemical burns should be considered deep partial-thickness or full-thickness until proven otherwise. As such, they are best treated by early E&G after full demarcation of injury.

Some chemicals, such as phenol, cause severe systemic effects, although hydrofluoric acid may cause death from hypocalcemia even after moderate exposure. Hydrofluoric acid burns are unique chemical burns in that they should be acutely treated with an antidote, calcium. Calcium gluconate should be administered intraarterially and topically, and all electrolyte abnormalities aggressively corrected.

PAIN CONTROL

All burn injuries are painful, whether the injury is simply sunburn or an extensive partial-thickness or full-thickness burn covering a large portion of the body. Attempts to manage pain in the thermally injured are frequently frustrating because of the unpredictable physiologic and psychologic reactions to the burn.

Total elimination of pain in burn patients is not possible, short of general anesthesia. The burn patient may experience acute pain from dressing changes, operative procedures, and rehabilitation therapy exercises. Patients may also have chronic background pain associated with the wound maturation process. There is a wide degree of intra- and interindividual variation with respect to the experience of burn-related pain. Pain management involves both pharmacologic and nonpharmacologic modalities.

CHRONIC PROBLEMS

Hypertrophic Scar Formation

The etiology and pathophysiology of hypertrophic scars are still incompletely understood. Burn scar hypertrophy classically develops in deeper partial-thickness and full-thickness injuries that are allowed to heal by primary intention. Hypertrophy of excised and grafted burn wounds occurs less frequently, and is partly dependent on the time from injury to excision, the site of the wound, and the patient's race or ethnicity. Delayed excision is more likely to result in hypertrophic scarring, and pigmented individuals are at an increased risk. Donor sites also can become hypertrophic, and this propensity appears to be related to graft thickness, donor site infection, and patient characteristics.

Hypertrophic scarring should be distinguished from a keloid. Both exhibit excessive collagen formation; however, a keloid grows beyond the original dimensions of the injury, although a hypertrophic scar is confined to its original anatomic boundaries. Hypertrophic scars frequently flatten with time and pressure, whereas keloids do not.

Numerous treatments have been postulated for hypertrophic scarring; however, few have proven to be efficacious. Pressure applied directly to a hypertrophic scar via various vehicles has been the most widely used treatment modality. Elasticized, custom-fitted, compression garments and silicone dressings are the most widely used and accepted pressure therapies. The most successful approach to residual hypertrophic burn scars is initial pressure therapy until the wound matures, followed by subsequent excision and grafting if necessary. Intralesional injection of corticosteroids may reduce the bulk of the hypertrophic scar mass, and may be used in combination with other treatment modalities.

Marjolin's Ulcer

Chronic ulceration of old burn scars was noted by Marjolin to predispose to malignant degeneration. Squamous cell carcinoma is most common, although basal cell carcinomas occasionally occur, and rare tumors such as malignant fibrous histiocytoma, sarcoma, and melanoma have been reported. These lesions typically appear decades after the original injury in wounds that healed primarily, but acute cases arising within a year of injury have been reported. They also can arise in grafted areas and appear to have an even longer time to occurrence when they do. The precise incidence of burn scar carcinoma is unknown.

Heterotopic Ossification

Heterotopic ossification (HO) is a rare complication of thermal injury, but is associated with significant morbidity. It most commonly occurs in patients with major full-thickness burns and typically is found adjacent to an involved joint 1–3 months after injury. The upper extremity is most commonly affected. Limitation of physical activity usually precedes radiographic evidence of calcification, which is located in the muscle and surrounding soft tissue of the joint. The precise etiology of HO is not known; however, restricted activity promotes mobilization of body calcium stores and may lead to deposition of calcium in the soft tissues.

Suggested Readings

Herndon DN, Spies M: Modern burn care. Semin Pediatr Surg 10:28, 2001.

Liao CC, Rossignol AM: Landmarks in burn prevention. Burns 26:422, 2000.

Arturson G: Forty years in burns research—the postburn inflammatory response. Burns 26:599, 2002.

Hansbrough JF: Enteral nutritional support in burn patients. Gastrointest Endosc Clin North Am 8:645, 1998.

Yu YM, Tompkins RG, Ryan CM, et al: The metabolic basis of the increase in energy expenditure in severely burned patients. J Parenter Enteral Nutr 23:160, 1999.

Murphy KD, Lee JO, Herndon DN: Current pharmacotherapy for the treatment of severe burns. Expert Opin Pharmacother 4:369, 2003.

Yowler CJ, Fratianne RB: Current status of burn resuscitation. Clin Plast Surg 27:1, 2000.

Baxter C: Fluid volume and electrolyte changes in the early post-burn period. Clin Plast Surg 1:693, 1974.

Holmes JH, Honari S, Gibran N: Excision and grafting of the large burn wound. Prob Gen Surg 20:47, 2003.

Gottschlich MM, Jenkins ME, Mayes T, et al: The 2002 Clinical Research Award. An evaluation of the safety of early vs. delayed enteral support and effects on clinical, nutritional, and endocrine outcomes after severe burns. J Burn Care Rehabil 23:401, 2002.

8 | Wound Healing

Adrian Barbul

PHASES OF WOUND HEALING

The wound healing process follows a predictable pattern that can be divided into overlapping phases defined by the cellular populations and biochemical activities: (1) hemostasis and inflammation, (2) proliferation, and (3) maturation and remodeling. This sequence of events is fluid and overlapping. All wounds need to progress through this series of cellular and biochemical events that characterizes the phases of healing to successfully re-establish tissue integrity.

Hemostasis and Inflammation

Hemostasis precedes and initiates inflammation with the ensuing release of chemotactic factors from the wound site. Wounding disrupts tissue integrity, leading to division of blood vessels and direct exposure of extracellular matrix to platelets. Exposure of subendothelial collagen to platelets results in platelet aggregation, degranulation, and activation of the coagulation cascade resulting in a fibrin clot. Platelet α granules release a number of wound-active substances such as platelet-derived growth factor (PDGF), transforming growth factor-β (TGF-β), platelet-activating factor (PAF), fibronectin, and serotonin. In addition to achieving hemostasis, the fibrin clot serves as scaffolding for the migration into the wound of inflammatory cells such as polymorphonuclear leukocytes (PMNs, neutrophils) and monocytes.

Cellular infiltration after injury follows a characteristic, predetermined sequence. PMNs are the first infiltrating cells to enter the wound site, peaking at 24–48 h. Increased vascular permeability, local prostaglandin release, and the presence of chemotactic substances such as complement factors, interleukin-1 (IL-1), tumor necrosis factor-α (TNF-α), TNF-β, platelet factor 4, or bacterial products all stimulate neutrophil migration.

The second population of inflammatory cells that invades the wound consists of macrophages. Derived from circulating monocytes, macrophages achieve significant numbers in the wound by 48–96 h postinjury and remain present until wound healing is complete.

Macrophages, like neutrophils, participate in wound débridement via phagocytosis and contribute to microbial stasis via oxygen radical and nitric oxide synthesis. The macrophage's most pivotal function is activation and recruitment of other cells via mediators such as cytokines and growth factors. By releasing such mediators as TGF-β, vascular endothelial growth factor (VEGF), insulin-like growth factor (IGF), epithelial growth factor (EGF), and lactate, macrophages regulate cell proliferation, matrix synthesis, and angiogenesis. Macrophages also play a significant role in regulating angiogenesis and matrix deposition and remodeling.

T lymphocytes comprise another population of inflammatory/immune cells that routinely invades the wound. Less numerous than macrophages, T-lymphocyte numbers peak at about 1 week postinjury and bridge the transition from the inflammatory to the proliferative phase of healing. The lymphocytes' role in wound healing is not yet fully defined.

165

Proliferation

The proliferative phase roughly spans days 4 through 12. During this phase, tissue continuity is re-established. Fibroblasts and endothelial cells are the last cell populations to infiltrate the healing wound, and the strongest chemotactic factor for fibroblasts is PDGF. On entering the wound environment, recruited fibroblasts first need to proliferate, and then become activated, to carry out their primary function of matrix synthesis and remodeling. This activation is mediated mainly by the cytokines and growth factors released from wound macrophages.

Endothelial cells also proliferate extensively during this phase of healing. These cells participate in the formation of new capillaries (angiogenesis). Endothelial cells migrate from intact venules close to the wound. Their migration, replication, and new capillary tubule formation are under the influence of such cytokines and growth factors as TNF-a, TGF-β, and VEGF.

Matrix Synthesis

Biochemistry of Collagen

Collagen is the most abundant protein in the body. Type I collagen is the major component of extracellular matrix in skin. Type III, which also normally is present in skin, becomes more prominent and important during the repair process.

Biochemically, each chain of collagen is composed of a glycine residue in every third position. The second position in the triplet is made up of proline or lysine during the translation process. The polypeptide chain that is translated from mRNA is called protocollagen. Release of protocollagen into the endoplasmic reticulum results in the hydroxylation of proline to hydroxyproline and of lysine to hydroxylysine by specific hydroxylases. Prolyl hydroxylase requires oxygen and iron as cofactors, α-ketoglutarate as co-substrate, and ascorbic acid (vitamin C) as an electron donor. In the endoplasmic reticulum, the protocollagen chain assumes an α-helical configuration after it is glycosylated by the linking of galactose and glucose at specific hydroxylysine residues. Three α-helical chains entwine to form a right-handed superhelical structure called procollagen. Although initially joined by weak, ionic bonds, the procollagen molecule becomes much stronger by the covalent cross-linking of lysine residues.

Extracellularly, the procollagen strands undergo further polymerization and cross-linking. The resulting collagen monomer is further polymerized and cross-linked by the formation of intra and intermolecular covalent bonds.

Proteoglycan Synthesis

Glycosaminoglycans comprise a large portion of the "ground substance" that makes up granulation tissue. Rarely found free, they couple with proteins to form proteoglycans. The polysaccharide chain is made up of repeating disaccharide units composed of glucuronic or iduronic acid and a hexosamine, which is usually sulfated. The disaccharide composition of proteoglycans varies from about 10 units in the case of heparan sulfate to as much as 2000 units in the case of hyaluronic acid.

The major glycosaminoglycans present in wounds are dermatan and chondroitin sulfate. Fibroblasts synthesize these compounds, increasing their concentration greatly during the first 3 weeks of healing. The interaction between collagen and proteoglycans is being actively studied. As scar collagen is deposited, the proteoglycans are incorporated into the collagen scaffolding. However, with scar maturation and collagen remodeling, the content of proteoglycans gradually diminishes.

Maturation and Remodeling

The maturation and remodeling of the scar begins during the fibroplastic phase, and is characterized by a reorganization of previously synthesized collagen. Collagen is broken down by matrix metalloproteinases (MMPs). The net wound collagen content is the result of a balance between collagenolysis and collagen synthesis. There is a net shift toward collagen synthesis and eventually the re-establishment of extracellular matrix composed of a relatively acellular collagen-rich scar.

Wound strength and mechanical integrity in the fresh wound are determined by both the quantity and quality of the newly deposited collagen. The deposition of matrix at the wound site follows a characteristic pattern: fibronectin and collagen type III constitute the early matrix scaffolding; glycosaminoglycans and proteoglycans represent the next significant matrix components; and collagen type I is the final matrix. By several weeks postinjury the amount of collagen in the wound reaches a plateau, but the tensile strength continues to increase for several more months. Fibril formation and fibril cross-linking result in decreased collagen solubility, increased strength, and increased resistance to enzymatic degradation of the collagen matrix. Scar remodeling continues for many (6–12) months postinjury, gradually resulting in a mature, avascular, and acellular scar. The mechanical strength of the scar never achieves that of the uninjured tissue.

Epithelialization

Although tissue integrity and strength are being re-established, the external barrier must also be restored. This process, beginning within 1 day of the injury, is characterized primarily by proliferation and migration of epithelial cells adjacent to the wound. Marginal basal cells at the edge of the wound lose their firm attachment to the underlying dermis, enlarge, and begin to migrate across the surface of the provisional matrix. Fixed basal cells in a zone near the cut edge undergo a series of rapid mitotic divisions, and these cells appear to migrate by moving over one another in a leapfrog fashion until the defect is covered. Once the defect is bridged, the migrating epithelial cells lose their flattened appearance, become more columnar in shape, and increase their mitotic activity. Layering of the epithelium is re-established, and the surface layer eventually keratinizes.

Re-epithelialization is complete in less than 48 h in the case of approximated incised wounds, but may take substantially longer in the case of larger wounds, in which there is a significant epidermal/dermal defect. If only the epithelium and superficial dermis are damaged, such as occurs in split-thickness skin graft (STSG) donor sites or in superficial second-degree burns, then repair consists primarily of re-epithelialization with minimal or no fibroplasia and granulation tissue formation. The stimuli for re-epithelialization remain incompletely defined; however, it appears that the process is mediated by a combination of a loss of contact inhibition; exposure to constituents of the extracellular matrix, particularly fibronectin; and cytokines produced by immune mononuclear cells. In particular EGF, TGF-β, basic fibroblast growth factor (bFGF), PDGF, and IGF-1 have been shown to promote epithelialization.

Wound Contraction

All wounds undergo some degree of contraction. For wounds that do not have surgically approximated edges, the area of the wound will be decreased by this action (healing by secondary intention). The myofibroblast has been postulated as being the major cell responsible for contraction, and it differs from the normal fibroblast in that it possesses a cytoskeletal structure. Typically this cell contains α-smooth muscle actin in thick bundles called stress fibers, giving myofibroblasts contractile capability. The α-smooth muscle actin is undetectable until day 6, and then is increasingly expressed for the next 15 days of wound healing. After 4 weeks this expression fades and the cells are believed to undergo apoptosis. Of note, undifferentiated fibroblasts may also contribute to wound contraction.

CLASSIFICATION OF WOUNDS

Wounds are classified as either acute or chronic. Acute wounds heal in a predictable manner and time frame. The process occurs with few, if any, complications, and the end result is a well-healed wound. Surgical wounds can heal in several ways. An incised wound that is clean and sutured closed is said to heal by primary intention. Often, because of bacterial contamination or tissue loss, a wound will be left open to heal by granulation tissue formation and contraction; this constitutes healing by secondary intention. Delayed primary closure, or healing by tertiary intention, represents a combination of the first two, consisting of the placement of sutures, allowing the wound to stay open for a few days, and the subsequent closure of the sutures.

Normal healing is affected by both systemic and local factors (Table 8-1). The clinician must be familiar with these factors and should attempt to counteract their deleterious effects. Complications occurring in wounds with higher risk can lead to failure of healing or the development of chronic, nonhealing wounds.

TABLE 8-1 Factors Affecting Wound Healing

Systemic
Age
Nutrition
Trauma
Metabolic diseases
Immunosuppression
Connective tissue disorders
Smoking

Local
Mechanical injury
Infection
Edema
Ischemia/necrotic tissue
Topical agents
Ionizing radiation
Low oxygen tension
Foreign bodies

Factors Affecting Wound Healing

Advanced Age

Most surgeons believe that aging produces intrinsic physiologic changes that result in delayed or impaired wound healing. Clinical experience demonstrating a decrease in wound closure rates and tensile strength with increasing age tends to support this belief.

Hypoxia, Anemia, and Hypoperfusion

Low oxygen tension has a deleterious effect on all aspects of wound healing. Fibroplasia, although stimulated initially by the hypoxic wound environment, is significantly impaired by local hypoxia. Optimal collagen synthesis requires oxygen as a cofactor, particularly for the hydroxylation steps. Increasing subcutaneous oxygen tension levels and oxygen delivery by avoiding hypovolemia or increasing the fraction of inspired oxygen (Fio_2) of inspired air for brief periods during and immediately following surgery results in enhanced collagen deposition and in decreased rates of wound infection after elective surgery.

Mild to moderate normovolemic anemia does not appear to adversely affect wound oxygen tension and collagen synthesis, unless the hematocrit falls below 15 percent.

Steroids and Chemotherapeutic Drugs

Large doses or chronic usage of glucocorticoids reduce collagen synthesis and wound strength. The major effect of steroids is to inhibit the inflammatory phase of wound healing and the release of lysosomal enzymes. The stronger the antiinflammatory effect of the steroid compound used, the greater the inhibitory effect on wound healing. Steroids used after the first 3–4 days postinjury do not affect wound healing as severely as when they are used in the immediate postoperative period. Therefore, if possible, their use should be delayed or, alternatively, forms with lesser antiinflammatory effects should be administered.

In addition to their effect on collagen synthesis, steroids also inhibit epithelialization and contraction and contribute to increased rates of wound infection, regardless of the time of administration. Steroid-delayed healing of cutaneous wounds can be stimulated to epithelialize by topical application of vitamin A. Collagen synthesis of steroid-treated wounds also can be stimulated by vitamin A.

All chemotherapeutic antimetabolite drugs adversely affect wound healing by inhibiting early cell proliferation and wound deoxyribonucleic acid (DNA) and protein synthesis.

Metabolic Disorders

Diabetes mellitus is the best known of the metabolic disorders contributing to increased rates of wound infection and impaired healing. Uncontrolled diabetes results in reduced inflammation, angiogenesis, and collagen synthesis. Additionally, the large and small vessel disease that is the hallmark of advanced diabetes contributes to local hypoxemia. Defects in granulocyte function, capillary ingrowth, and fibroblast proliferation all have been described in diabetes. In wound studies on experimental diabetic animals, insulin restores collagen synthesis and granulation tissue formation to normal levels if given during the early phases of healing. In clean, noninfected, and well-perfused experimental wounds in human diabetic volunteers, type I diabetes mellitus was noted to decrease wound collagen accumulation in the wound, independent of the degree of glycemic control. Type II diabetic patients showed no effect on collagen accretion when compared to healthy, age-matched controls. It remains unclear whether decreased collagen synthesis or an increased breakdown because of an abnormally high proteolytic wound environment is responsible.

Careful preoperative correction of blood sugar levels improves the outcome of wounds in diabetic patients. Increasing the inspired oxygen tension, judicious use of antibiotics, and correction of other coexisting metabolic abnormalities all can result in improved wound healing.

Uremia also has been associated with disordered wound healing. Experimentally, uremic animals demonstrate decreased wound collagen synthesis and breaking strength. The contribution of uremia alone to this impairment, rather than that of associated malnutrition, is difficult to assess. The clinical use of dialysis to correct the metabolic abnormalities and nutritional restoration should impact greatly on the wound outcome of such patients.

Nutrition

The clinician must pay close attention to the nutritional status of patients with wounds, because wound failure or wound infections may be no more than a reflection of poor nutrition. Although the full interaction of nutrition and wound healing is still not fully understood, efforts are being made to develop wound-specific nutritional interventions and the pharmacologic use of individual nutrients as modulators of wound outcomes.

Clinically, it is extremely rare to encounter pure energy or protein malnutrition, and the vast majority of patients exhibit combined protein-energy malnutrition. Such patients have diminished hydroxyproline accumulation (an index of collagen deposition) into subcutaneously implanted polytetrafluoroethylene tubes when compared to normally nourished patients. Furthermore, malnutrition correlates clinically with enhanced rates of wound complications and increased wound failure following diverse surgical procedures. This reflects impaired healing response and reduced cell-mediated immunity, phagocytosis, and intracellular killing of bacteria by macrophages and neutrophils during protein-calorie malnutrition.

The possible role of single amino acids in enhanced wound healing has been studied for the last several decades. Arginine appears most active in terms of enhancing wound fibroplasia. Indeed, arginine supplementation in both rats and humans has been shown to increase wound collagen deposition. Conversely, arginine deficiency in rats results in decreased wound-breaking strength and wound-collagen accumulation.

The vitamins most closely involved with wound healing are vitamin C and vitamin A. Vitamin C deficiency leads to a defect in wound healing, particularly via a failure in collagen synthesis and cross-linking. Biochemically, vitamin C is required for the conversion of proline and lysine to hydroxyproline and hydroxylysine. Vitamin C deficiency also has been associated with an increased incidence of wound infection, and if wound infection does occur, it tends to be more severe. These effects are believed to be because of an associated impairment in neutrophil function, decreased complement activity, and decreased walling-off of bacteria secondary to insufficient collagen deposition. The recommended dietary allowance is 60 mg daily. In severely injured or extensively burned patients this requirement may increase to as high as 2 g daily. There is no evidence that excess vitamin C is toxic; however, there is no evidence that supertherapeutic doses of vitamin C are of any benefit.

Vitamin A deficiency impairs wound healing, although supplemental vitamin A benefits wound healing in nondeficient humans and animals. Vitamin A increases the inflammatory response in wound healing, probably by increasing the lability of lysosomal membranes. There is an increased influx of macrophages, with an increase in their activation and increased collagen synthesis. Vitamin A directly increases collagen production and epidermal growth factor receptors when it is added in vitro to cultured fibroblasts. As mentioned before, supplemental vitamin A can reverse the inhibitory effects of corticosteroids on wound healing. Vitamin A also can restore wound healing that has been impaired by diabetes, tumor formation, cyclophosphamide, and radiation. Serious injury or stress leads to increased vitamin A requirements. In the severely injured patient, supplemental doses of vitamin A have been recommended. Doses ranging from 25,000 to 100,000 international units per day have been advocated. Vitamin A can reach toxic doses if taken in excess.

The connections between specific minerals and trace elements and deficits in wound healing are complex. Frequently, deficiencies are multiple and include macronutrient deficiencies.

Zinc is the most well-known element in wound healing and has been used empirically in dermatologic conditions for centuries. It is essential for wound healing in animals and humans. There are over 150 known enzymes for which zinc is either an integral part or an essential cofactor, and many of these enzymes are critical to wound healing. With zinc deficiency there is decreased fibroblast proliferation, decreased collagen synthesis, impaired overall wound strength, and delayed epithelialization. These defects are reversed by zinc supplementation. To date, no study has shown improved wound healing with zinc supplementation in patients who are not zinc deficient.

Infections

Wound infections continue to represent a major medical problem, both in terms of how they affect the outcome of surgical procedures, and for their impact on the length of hospital stay and medical costs. Exhaustive studies have been undertaken to examine the appropriate prophylactic treatment of operative wounds. Bacterial contaminants normally present on skin are prevented from entry into deep tissues by intact epithelium. Surgery breaches the intact epithelium, allowing bacteria access to these tissues and the blood stream. Antibiotic prophylaxis is most effective when adequate concentrations of antibiotic are present in the tissues at the time of incision. Addition of antibiotics after operative contamination has occurred is clearly ineffective in preventing postoperative wound infections.

Studies that compare operations performed with and without antibiotic prophylaxis demonstrate that class II, III, and IV procedures (see below) treated with appropriate prophylactic antibiotics have only one-third the wound infection rate of previously reported untreated series. More recently, repeat dosing of antibiotics has been shown to be essential in decreasing postoperative wound infections in operations with durations exceeding the biochemical half-life (T1/2) of the antibiotic, or in which there is large-volume blood loss and fluid replacement. In lengthy cases, those in which prosthetic implants are used, or when unexpected contamination is encountered, additional doses of antibiotic may be administered for 24 h postoperatively.

Selection of antibiotics for use in prophylaxis should be tailored to the type of surgery to be performed, operative contaminants that might be encountered during the procedure, and the profile of resistant organisms present at the institution where the surgery is performed.

The incidence of wound infection is about 5–10 percent nationwide and has not changed during the last few decades. Quantitatively, it has been shown that if the wound is contaminated with >105 microorganisms, the risk of wound infection is markedly increased, but this threshold may be much lower in the presence of foreign materials. The source of pathogens for the infection is usually the endogenous flora of the patient's skin, mucous membranes, or from hollow organs. The most common organisms responsible for wound infections in order of frequency are Staphylococcus species, coagulase-negative Streptococcus, enterococci, and *Escherichia coli*. The incidence of wound infection bears a direct relationship to the degree of contamination that occurs during the operation from the disease process itself (clean—class I, clean contaminated—class II, contaminated—class III, and dirty—class IV). Many factors contribute to the development of postoperative wound infections. Most surgical wound infections become apparent within 7–10 days postoperatively.

The mere presence of bacteria in an open wound, either acute or chronic, does not constitute an infection, because large numbers of bacteria can be present in the normal situation. Secondly, the bacteria grown may not be representative of the bacteria causing the actual wound infection. Contamination is the presence of bacteria without multiplication, colonization is multiplication without host response, and infection is the presence of host response in reaction to deposition and multiplication of bacteria. The presence of a host response helps to differentiate between infection and colonization as seen in chronic wounds. The host response that helps in diagnosing wound infection comprises cellulitis, abnormal discharge, delayed healing, change in pain, abnormal granulation tissue, bridging, and abnormal color and odor.

Chronic Wounds

Chronic wounds are defined as wounds that have failed to proceed through the orderly process that produces satisfactory anatomic and functional integrity or that have proceeded through the repair process without producing an adequate anatomic and functional result. The majority of wounds that have not healed in 3 months are considered chronic. Skin ulcers, which usually occur in traumatized or vascularly compromised soft tissue, also are considered chronic in nature, and proportionately are the major component of chronic wounds. In addition to the factors discussed above that can delay wound healing, factors such as repeated trauma, poor perfusion or oxygenation, and/or excessive inflammation may also play a role in the etiology of chronic wounds.

Unresponsiveness to normal regulatory signals also has been implicated as a predictive factor of chronic wounds. This may come about as a failure of normal growth factor synthesis, and thus an increased breakdown of growth factors within a wound environment that is markedly proteolytic because of overexpression of protease activity or a failure of the normal antiprotease inhibitor mechanisms. Fibroblasts from chronic wounds also have been found to have decreased proliferative potential, perhaps because of senescence or decreased expression of growth factor receptors. Chronic wounds occur because of various etiologic factors, and several of the most common are discussed below.

Malignant transformation of chronic ulcers can occur in any long-standing wound (Marjolin ulcer). Any wound that does not heal for a prolonged period of time is prone to malignant transformation. In patients with suspected malignant transformations, biopsy of the wound edges must be performed to rule out malignancy. Cancers arising de novo in chronic wounds include both squamous and basal cell carcinomas.

Ischemic Arterial Ulcers

These wounds occur because of a lack of blood supply and are painful at presentation. They are usually located on the most distal portions of the extremities and are associated with other symptoms of peripheral vascular disease, such as intermittent claudication, rest pain, night pain, and color changes. On examination, there may be diminished or absent pulses with decreased ankle-brachial index and poor formation of granulation tissue. Other signs of peripheral ischemia, such as dryness of skin, hair loss, scaling, and pallor can be present. The wound itself is usually shallow with smooth margins and a pale base. The management of these wounds includes revascularization and wound care. After establishing adequate blood supply, most wounds progress to heal satisfactorily.

Venous Stasis Ulcers

Although there is unanimous agreement that venous ulcers are because of venous stasis and back pressure, there is less consensus regarding what are the exact pathophysiologic pathways that lead to ulceration and impaired healing. On the microvascular level, there is alteration and distention of the dermal capillaries with leakage of fibrinogen into the tissues; polymerization of fibrinogen into fibrin cuffs leads to perivascular cuffing that can impede oxygen exchange, thus contributing to ulceration. These same fibrin cuffs and the leakage of macromolecules such as fibrinogen and α_2-macroglobulin trap growth factors and impede wound healing. Another hypothesis suggests that neutrophils adhere to the capillary endothelium and cause plugging with diminished dermal blood flow. Venous hypertension and capillary damage lead to extravasation of hemoglobin. The products of this breakdown are irritating and cause pruritus and skin damage. The resulting brownish pigmentation of skin combined with the loss of subcutaneous fat produces characteristic changes called lipodermatosclerosis. Regardless of the pathophysiologic mechanisms, the clinically characteristic picture is that of an ulcer that fails to re-epithelialize despite the presence of adequate granulation tissue.

Venous stasis occurs because of the incompetence of either the superficial or deep venous systems. Chronic venous ulcers are usually because of the incompetence of the deep venous system and are commonly painless. Stasis ulcers tend to occur at the sites of incompetent perforators, the most common being above the medial malleolus, over the Cockett perforator. On examination, the typical location combined with a history of venous incompetence and other skin changes is diagnostic. The wound is usually shallow with irregular margins and pigmented surrounding skin.

The cornerstone of treatment of venous ulcers is compression therapy. The most commonly used method is the rigid, zinc oxide–impregnated, nonelastic bandage. Most venous ulcers can be healed with perseverance and by addressing the venous hypertension. Unfortunately, recurrences are frequent.

Diabetic Wounds

Ten to 15 percent of diabetic patients run the risk of developing ulcers. There are approximately 50,000–60,000 amputations performed in diabetic patients each year in the United States. The major contributors to the formation of diabetic ulcers include neuropathy, foot deformity, and ischemia. The neuropathy is both sensory and motor. The loss of sensory function allows unrecognized injury to occur from ill-fitting shoes, foreign bodies, or other trauma. The motor neuropathy (Charcot foot) leads to collapse or dislocation of the interphalangeal or metatarsophalangeal joints, causing pressure on areas with little protection. There is also severe micro- and macrovascular circulatory impairment.

Once ulceration occurs, the chances of healing are poor. The management of diabetic wounds involves local and systemic measures. Achievement of adequate blood sugar levels is very important. Most diabetic wounds are infected, and eradication of the infectious source is paramount to the success of healing. Treatment should address the possible presence of osteomyelitis, and should employ antibiotics that achieve adequate levels both in soft tissue and bone. Wide débridement of all necrotic or infected tissue is another cornerstone of treatment. Off-loading of the ulcerated area by using specialized orthotic shoes or casts allows for ambulation while protecting the fragile wound environment. Topical application of PDGF and granulocyte-macrophage colony-stimulating factor has met with limited but significant success in achieving closure. The application of engineered skin allograft substitutes, although expensive, has also shown some success.

Decubitus or Pressure Ulcers

The incidence of pressure ulcers ranges from 2.7–9 percent in the acute care setting, in comparison to 2.4–23 percent in long-term care facilities. The expense of pressure sore management in the United States is approximately $1.3 billion annually, with an average cost of $50,000–$60,000 per ulcer. A pressure ulcer is a localized area of tissue necrosis that develops when a soft tissue is compressed between a bony prominence and an external surface. Excessive pressure causes capillary collapse and impedes the delivery of nutrients to body tissues. Pressure ulcer formation is accelerated in the presence of friction, shear forces, and moisture. Other contributory factors in the pathogenesis of pressure ulcers include immobility, altered activity levels, altered mental status, chronic conditions, and altered nutritional status. The four stages of pressure ulcer formation are as follows: stage I, nonblanchable erythema of intact skin; stage II, partial-thickness skin loss involving epidermis or dermis or both; stage III, full-thickness skin loss, but not through the fascia; and stage IV, full-thickness skin loss with extensive involvement of muscle and bone.

The treatment of established pressure ulcers is most successful when carried out in a multidisciplinary manner by involving wound care teams consisting of physicians, nurses, dietitians, physical therapists, and nutritionists. Care of the ulcer itself comprises débridement of all necrotic tissue, maintenance of a favorable moist wound environment that will facilitate healing, relief of pressure, and addressing host issues such as nutritional, metabolic, and circulatory status. Débridement is most efficiently carried out surgically, but enzymatic proteolytic preparations and hydrotherapy also are used. The wound bed should be kept moist by employing dressings that absorb secretions but do not desiccate the wound. Operative repair, usually involving flap rotation, has been found to be useful in obtaining long-term closure only in highly motivated patients.

EXCESS HEALING

Excess Dermal Scarring

Hypertrophic scars (HTSs) and keloids represent an overabundance of fibroplasia in the dermal healing process. HTSs rise above the skin level but stay within the confines of the original wound and often regress over time. Keloids rise above the skin level as well, but extend beyond the border of the original wound and rarely regress spontaneously. Both HTSs and keloids occur after trauma to the skin and may be tender, pruritic, and cause a burning sensation. Keloids are fifteen times more common in darker-pigmented ethnicities, with individuals of African, Spanish, and Asian ethnicities being especially susceptible. Men and women are equally affected. Genetically, the predilection to keloid formation appears to be autosomal dominant with incomplete penetration and variable expression.

A HTS usually develops within 4 weeks after trauma. The risk of a HTS increases if epithelialization takes longer than 21 days, independent of site, age, and race. Rarely elevated more than 4 mm above the skin level, HTSs stay within the boundaries of the wound. They usually occur across areas of tension and flexor surfaces, which tend to be at right angles to joints or skin creases. The lesions are initially erythematous and raised, and over time may evolve into pale, flatter scars.

Keloids can result from surgery, burns, skin inflammation, acne, chickenpox, zoster, folliculitis, lacerations, abrasions, tattoos, vaccinations, injections, insect bites, ear piercing, or may arise spontaneously. Keloids tend to occur 3 months to years after the initial insult, and even minor injuries can result in large lesions. They vary in size from a few millimeters to large, pedunculated lesions with a soft to rubbery or hard consistency. Although they project above surrounding skin, they rarely extend into underlying subcutaneous tissues. Certain body sites have a higher incidence of keloid formation, including the skin of the earlobe and the deltoid, presternal, and upper back regions. They rarely occur on eyelids, genitalia, palms, soles, or across joints. Keloids rarely involute spontaneously, although surgical intervention can lead to recurrence, often with a worse result.

Histologically, both HTSs and keloids demonstrate increased thickness of the epidermis with an absence of rete ridges. There is an abundance of collagen and glycoprotein deposition. Normal skin has distinct collagen bundles, mostly parallel to the epithelial surface, with random connections between bundles by fine fibrillar strands of collagen. In HTSs, the collagen bundles are flatter, more random, and the fibers are in a wavy pattern. In keloids, the collagen bundles are virtually nonexistent, and the fibers are connected haphazardly in loose sheets with a random orientation to the epithelium. The collagen fibers are larger and thicker and myofibroblasts are generally absent.

Keloidal fibroblasts have normal proliferation parameters, but synthesize collagen at a rate 20 times greater than that observed in normal dermal fibroblasts, and 3 times higher than fibroblasts derived from HTSs. Abnormal amounts of extracellular matrix such as fibronectin, elastin, and proteoglycans also are produced. The synthesis of fibronectin, which promotes clot generation, granulation tissue formation, and re-epithelialization, decreases during the normal healing process; however, production continues at high levels for months to years in HTSs and keloids. This perturbed synthetic activity is mediated by altered growth factor expression. TGF-β expression is higher in HTSs, and both HTS- and keloid-derived fibroblasts respond to lower concentrations of TGF-β than do normal dermal fibroblasts. HTSs also express increased levels of insulin-like growth factor-1, which reduces collagenase messenger ribonucleoprotein acid (mRNA) activity and increases mRNA for types I and II procollagen.

Unfortunately, the underlying mechanisms that cause HTSs and keloids are not known.

Treatment goals include restoration of function to the area, relief of symptoms, and prevention of recurrence. Many patients seek intervention because of cosmetic concerns. Because the underlying mechanisms causing keloids and HTSs remain unknown, many different modalities of treatment have been used without consistent success.

Excision alone of keloids is subject to a high recurrence rate, ranging from 45–100 percent. There are fewer recurrences when surgical excision is combined with other modalities such as intralesional corticosteroid injection, topical application of silicone sheets, or the use of radiation or pressure. Surgery is recommended for debulking large lesions or as second-line therapy when other modalities have failed. Silicone application is relatively painless and should be maintained for 24 h a day for about 3 months to prevent rebound hypertrophy. It may be secured with tape or worn beneath a pressure garment. The mechanism of action is not understood, but increased hydration of the skin, which decreases capillary activity, inflammation, hyperemia, and collagen deposition, may be involved. Silicone is more effective than other occlusive dressings and is an especially good treatment for children and others who cannot tolerate the pain involved in other modalities.

Intralesional corticosteroid injections decrease fibroblast proliferation, collagen and glycosaminoglycan synthesis, the inflammatory process, and TGF-β levels. When used alone, however, there is a variable rate of response and recurrence, therefore steroids are recommended as first-line treatment for keloids and second-line treatment for HTSs if topical therapies have failed. Intralesional injections are more effective on younger scars. They may soften, flatten, and give symptomatic relief to keloids, but they cannot make the lesions disappear nor can they narrow wide HTSs. Success is enhanced when used in combination with surgical excision. Serial injections every 2–3 weeks are required. Complications include skin atrophy, hypopigmentation, telangiectasias, necrosis, and ulceration.

Although radiation destroys fibroblasts, it has variable, unreliable results and produces poor results with 10–100 percent recurrence when used alone. It is more effective when combined with surgical excision. The timing, duration, and dosage for radiation therapy remain controversial, but doses ranging from 1500–2000 rads appear effective. Given the risks of hyperpigmentation, pruritus, erythema, paresthesias, pain, and possible secondary malignancies, radiation should be reserved for adults with scars resistant to other modalities.

Pressure aids collagen maturation, flattens scars, and improves thinning and pliability. It reduces the number of cells in a given area, possibly by creating ischemia, which decreases tissue metabolism and increases collagenase activity. External compression is used to treat HTSs, especially after burns. Therapy must begin early, and a pressure between 24 and 30 mmHg must be achieved to exceed capillary pressure, yet preserve peripheral blood circulation. Garments should be worn for 23–24 h a day for up to 1 or more years to avoid rebound hypertrophy. Scars older than 6–12 months respond poorly.

Topical retinoids also have been used as treatment for both HTSs and keloids, with reported responses of 50–100 percent. Intralesional injections of INF-γ, a cytokine released by T lymphocytes, reduce collagen types I, II, and III by decreasing mRNA and possibly by reducing levels of TGF-β. This treatment is experimental, and complications are frequent and dose-dependent. Intralesional injections of chemotherapeutic agents such as 5-fluorouracil have been used both alone and in combination with steroids. The use of bleomycin has been reported to achieve some success in older scars resistant to steroids.

Peritoneal Scarring

Peritoneal adhesions are fibrous bands of tissues formed between organs that are normally separated and/or between organs and the internal body wall. Most intraabdominal adhesions are a result of peritoneal injury, either by a prior surgical procedure or because of intraabdominal infection. Postmortem examinations demonstrate adhesions in 67 percent of patients with prior surgical procedures and in 28 percent with a history of intraabdominal infection. Intraabdominal adhesions are the most common cause (65–75 percent) of small bowel obstruction, especially in the ileum. Operations in the lower abdomen have a higher chance of producing small bowel obstruction. Following rectal surgery, left colectomy, or total colectomy, there is an 11 percent chance of developing small bowel obstruction within 1 year, and this rate increases to 30 percent by 10 years. Adhesions also are a leading cause of secondary infertility in women and can cause substantial abdominal and pelvic pain. Adhesions account for 2 percent of all surgical admissions and 3 percent of all laparotomies in general surgery.

Adhesions form when the peritoneal surface is damaged because of surgery, thermal or ischemic injury, inflammation, or foreign body reaction. The injury disrupts the protective mesothelial cell layer lining the peritoneal cavity and the underlying connective tissue. The injury elicits an inflammatory response consisting of hyperemia, fluid exudation, release and activation of white blood cells and platelets in the peritoneal cavity, activation of inflammatory cytokines, and the onset of the coagulation and complement cascades. Fibrin deposition occurs between the damaged but opposed serosal surfaces. These filmy adhesions are often transient and degraded by proteases of the fibrinolytic system, with restoration of the normal peritoneal surface. If insufficient fibrinolytic activity is present, permanent fibrous adhesions will form by collagen deposition within 1 week of the injury.

There are two major strategies for adhesion prevention or reduction. Surgical trauma is minimized within the peritoneum by careful tissue handling, avoiding desiccation and ischemia, and spare use of cautery, laser, and retractors. Fewer adhesions form with laparoscopic surgical techniques because of reduced tissue trauma. The second major advance in adhesion prevention has been the introduction of barrier membranes and gels, which separate and create barriers between damaged surfaces, allowing for adhesion-free healing. Modified oxidized regenerated cellulose and hyaluronic acid membranes or solutions have been shown to reduce adhesions in gynecologic patients, and are being investigated for their ability to prevent adhesion formation in general surgical patients.

TREATMENT OF WOUNDS

Local Care

Management of acute wounds begins with obtaining a careful history of the events surrounding the injury. The history is followed by a meticulous examination of the wound. Examination should assess the depth and configuration of the wound, the extent of nonviable tissue, and the presence of foreign bodies and other contaminants. Examination of the wound may require irrigation and débridement of the edges of the wound, and is facilitated by use of local anesthesia. Antibiotic administration and tetanus prophylaxis may be needed, and planning the type and timing of wound repair should take place.

After completion of the history, examination, and administration of tetanus prophylaxis, the wound should be meticulously anesthetized. Lidocaine (0.5–1 percent) or bupivacaine (0.25–0.5 percent) combined with a 1:100,000 to 1:200,000 dilution of epinephrine provides satisfactory anesthesia and hemostasis. Epinephrine should not be used in wounds of the fingers, toes, ears, nose, or penis, because of the risk of tissue necrosis secondary to terminal arteriole vasospasm in these structures.

Irrigation to visualize all areas of the wound and remove foreign material is best accomplished with normal saline (without additives). High-pressure wound irrigation is more effective in achieving complete débridement of foreign material and nonviable tissue. Iodine, povidone-iodine, hydrogen peroxide, and organically based antibacterial preparations have all been shown to impair wound healing because of injury to wound neutrophils and macrophages, and thus should not be used directly on the wound bed. All hematomas present within wounds should be carefully evacuated and any remaining bleeding sources controlled with ligature or cautery. If the injury has resulted in the formation of a marginally viable flap of skin or tissue, these should be resected or revascularized prior to further wound repair and closure.

Having ensured hemostasis and adequate débridement of nonviable tissues and removal of any remaining foreign bodies, irregular, macerated, or beveled wound edges should be débrided to provide a fresh edge for reapproximation. Great care must be taken to realign wound edges properly—this is particularly important for wounds that cross the vermilion border, eyebrow, or hairline.

In general, the smallest suture required to hold the various layers of the wound in approximation should be selected to minimize suture-related inflammation. Nonabsorbable or slowly absorbing monofilament sutures are most suitable for approximating deep fascial layers, particularly in the abdominal wall. Subcutaneous tissues should be closed with braided absorbable sutures, with care to avoid placement of sutures in fat.

In areas of significant tissue loss, rotation of adjacent musculocutaneous flaps may be required to provide sufficient tissue mass for closure. These flaps may be based on intrinsic blood supply, or may be moved from distant sites as free flaps and anastomosed into the local vascular bed. In areas with significant superficial tissue loss, STSG may be required and will speed formation of an intact epithelial barrier to fluid loss and infection. It is essential to ensure hemostasis of the underlying tissue bed prior to placement of STSGs, as the presence of a hematoma below the graft will prevent the graft from taking. In acute, contaminated wounds with skin loss, use of porcine xenografts or cadaveric allografts is prudent until the danger of infection passes.

After closing deep tissues and replacing significant tissue deficits, skin edges should be reapproximated for cosmesis and to aid in rapid wound healing. Skin edges may be quickly reapproximated with surgical staples or nonabsorbable monofilament sutures. Care must be taken to remove these from the wound prior to epithelialization of the skin tracts in which sutures or staples penetrate the dermal layer. Failure to remove the sutures or staples prior to 7–10 days (or 3–5 days for the face) after repair will result in a cosmetically inferior wound. Where wound cosmesis is important, the above problems may be avoided by placement of buried dermal sutures using absorbable braided sutures. This method of wound closure allows for a precise reapproximation of wound edges, and may be enhanced by application of wound closure tapes to the surface of the wound. Intradermal absorbable sutures do not require removal. Use of skin tapes alone is only recommended for closure of the smallest superficial wounds.

Recently, octyl-cyanoacrylate tissue glues have shown promise for the management of simple, linear wounds with viable skin edges. These new glues are less prone to brittleness and have superior burst-strength characteristics. Studies have shown them to be suitable for use in contaminated situations without significant risk of infection. When used in the above types of wounds, these glues appear to provide superb cosmetic results and result in significantly less trauma than sutured repair, particularly when used in pediatric patients.

Antibiotics

Antibiotic treatment of acute wounds must be based on organisms suspected to be found within the infected wound and the patient's overall immune status. When a single specific organism is suspected, treatment may be commenced using a single antibiotic. Conversely, when multiple organisms are suspected, as with enteric contamination or when a patient's immune function is impaired by diabetes, chronic disease, or medication, treatment should commence with a broad-spectrum antibiotic or several agents in combination. Lastly, the location of the wound and the quality of tissue perfusion to that region will significantly impact wound performance after injury. Antibiotics also can be delivered topically as part of irrigations or dressings, although the efficacy of this practice is questionable.

Dressings

The main purpose of wound dressings is to provide the ideal environment for wound healing. Covering a wound with a dressing mimics the barrier role of epithelium and prevents further damage. Additionally, application of compression provides hemostasis and limits edema. Occlusion of a wound with dressing material can control the level of hydration and oxygen tension within the wound thus limiting tissue desiccation. It also may allow the transfer of gases and water vapor from the wound surface to the atmosphere. Because it may enhance bacterial growth, occlusion is contraindicated in infected and highly exudative wounds.

Absorbent Dressings

Accumulation of wound fluid can lead to maceration and bacterial overgrowth. Ideally, the dressing should absorb without getting soaked through. The dressing must be designed to match the exudative properties of the wound and may include cotton, wool, and sponge.

Nonadherent Dressings

Nonadherent dressings are impregnated with paraffin, petroleum jelly, or water-soluble jelly for use as nonadherent coverage. A secondary dressing must be placed on top to seal the edges and prevent desiccation and infection.

Occlusive and Semiocclusive Dressings

Occlusive and semiocclusive dressings should only be used for clean, minimally exudative wounds. These film dressings are waterproof and impervious to microbes, but permeable to water vapor and oxygen.

Hydrocolloid and Hydrogel Dressings

Hydrocolloids and hydrogels form complex structures with water which aids in atraumatic removal of the dressing. Absorption of exudates by the hydrocolloid dressing leaves a yellowish-brown gelatinous mass after dressing removal that can be washed off. Hydrogel has high water content. Hydrogels allow a high rate of evaporation without compromising wound hydration.

Alginates

Alginates are derived from brown algae and contain long chains of polysaccharides containing mannuronic and glucuronic acid. Processed as the calcium form, alginates turn into soluble sodium alginate through ion exchange in the presence of wound exudates. The polymers gel, swell, and absorb a great deal of fluid. Alginates are used in open surgical wounds with medium exudation, and on full-thickness chronic wounds.

Medicated Dressings

Medicated dressings have long been used as a drug-delivery system. Agents delivered in the dressings include benzoyl peroxide, zinc oxide, neomycin, and bacitracin-zinc. These agents have been shown to increase epithelialization by 28 percent.

The type of dressing to be used depends on the amount of wound drainage. A nondraining wound can be covered with semiocclusive dressing. Drainage of less than 1–2 mL/day may require a semiocclusive or absorbent nonadherent dressing. Moderately draining wounds (3–5 mL/day) can be dressed with a nonadherent primary layer plus an absorbent secondary layer plus an occlusive dressing to protect normal tissue. Heavily draining wounds (>5 mL/day) require a similar dressing as moderately draining wounds, but with the addition of a highly absorbent secondary layer.

Mechanical Devices

The VAC (vacuum-assisted closure) system assists in wound closure by applying localized negative pressure to the surface and margins of the wound. This negative pressure therapy is applied to a special foam dressing cut to the dimensions of the wound and positioned in the wound cavity or over a flap or graft. The continuous negative pressure is very effective in removing exudates from the wound. This form of therapy has been found to be effective for chronic open wounds (diabetic ulcers and stages 3 and 4 pressure ulcers), acute and traumatic wounds, flaps and grafts, and subacute wounds (i.e., dehisced incisions).

Skin Replacements

All wounds require coverage to prevent evaporative losses and infection and to provide an environment that promotes healing. Both acute and chronic wounds may demand use of skin replacement, and several options are available.

Conventional Skin Grafts

Split- or partial-thickness grafts consist of the epidermis plus part of the dermis, although full-thickness grafts retain the entire dermis. Autologous grafts are transplants from one site on the body to another; allogeneic grafts (allografts, homografts) are transplants from a living nonidentical donor or cadaver to the host; and xenogeneic grafts (heterografts) are taken from another species (e.g., porcine). Split-thickness grafts require less blood supply to restore skin function. The dermal component of full-thickness grafts lends mechanical strength and resists wound contraction better, resulting in improved cosmesis. Allogeneic and xenogeneic grafts are subject to rejection, and may contain pathogens.

The use of skin grafts or bioengineered skin substitutes and other innovative treatments cannot be effective unless the wound bed is adequately prepared.

Skin Substitutes

Skin substitutes promote healing, either by stimulating host cytokine generation or by providing cells that may also produce growth factors locally. Their disadvantages include limited survival, high cost, and the need for multiple applications.

Composite substitutes provide both the dermal and epidermal components essential for permanent skin replacement. The acellular (e.g., native collagen or synthetic material) component acts as a scaffold, promotes cell migration and growth, and activates tissue regeneration and remodeling. The cellular elements re-establish lost tissue and associated function, synthesize extracellular matrix components, produce essential mediators such as cytokines and growth factors, and promote proliferation and migration.

Cultured epithelial autografts (CEAs) represent expanded autologous or homologous keratinocytes. CEAs are expanded from a biopsy of the patient's own skin, will not be rejected, and can stimulate re-epithelialization and the growth of underlying connective tissue. Keratinocytes harvested from a biopsy roughly the size of a postage stamp are cultured with fibroblasts and growth factors and grown into sheets that can cover large areas and give the appearance of normal skin. Until the epithelial sheets are sufficiently expanded, the wound must be covered with an occlusive dressing or a temporary allograft or xenograft.

Viable fibroblasts can be grown on bioabsorbable or nonbioabsorbable meshes to yield living dermal tissue that can act as a scaffold for epidermal growth. Fibroblasts stimulated by growth factors can produce type I collagen and glycosaminoglycans which adhere to the wound surface to permit epithelial cell migration, and adhesive ligands (e.g., the matrix protein fibronectin), which promote cell adhesion. This approach has the virtue of being less time-consuming and expensive than culturing keratinocyte sheets.

Growth Factor Therapy

It is believed that nonhealing wounds result from insufficient or inadequate growth factors in the wound environment. Although there is a large body of work demonstrating the effects of growth factors in animals, translation of these data into clinical practice has met with limited success.

At present, only platelet-derived growth factor BB (PDGF-BB) is currently approved by the Food and Drug Administration (FDA) for treatment of diabetic foot ulcers. Application of recombinant human PDGF-BB in a gel suspension to these wounds increases the incidence of total healing and decreases healing time.

Suggested Readings

Witte MB, Barbul A: General principles of wound healing. Surg Clin NA 77:509–528, 1997.

Singer AJ, Clark RAF: Cutaneous wound repair. N Engl J Med 341:738–746, 1999.

Williams JZ, Barbul A: Nutrition and Wound Healing. Surgical Clinics of North America 83:571–596, 2003.

Cross KJ, Mustoe TA: Growth factors in wound healing. Surgical Clinics of North America 83:531–545, 2003.

Rahban SR, Garner WL: Fibroproliferative scars. Clin Plastic Surg 30:77–89, 2003.

Werner S, Grose R: regulation of wound healing by growth factors and cytokines. Physiol Rev 83:835–870, 2002.

9 | Oncology

Funda Meric-Bernstam and Raphael E. Pollock

As the population ages, oncology is becoming a larger portion of surgical practice. Modern cancer therapy is multidisciplinary, involving the coordinated care of surgeons, medical oncologists, radiation oncologists, reconstructive surgeons, pathologists, radiologists, and primary care physicians. Primary (or definitive) therapy refers to en bloc resection of tumor with adequate margins of normal tissues and in some cases regional lymph nodes. Adjuvant therapy refers to radiation therapy and systemic therapies, including chemotherapy, immunotherapy, hormonal therapy, and increasingly, biologic therapy. The primary goal of surgical and radiation therapy is local and regional control. On the other hand, the primary goal of systemic therapies is systemic control by treating distant foci of subclinical disease to prevent recurrence. Surgeons must be familiar with adjuvant therapies to coordinate multidisciplinary care. Knowledge of cancer epidemiology, etiology, staging and natural history is also required to determine the optimal surgical therapy.

EPIDEMIOLOGY

Basic Principles of Cancer Epidemiology

The term incidence refers to the number of new cases occurring; incidence usually is expressed as the number of new cases per 100,000 persons per year. Mortality refers to the number of deaths occurring and is expressed as the number of deaths per 100,000 persons per year. Incidence and mortality data are usually available through cancer registries.

The incidence of cancer is variable by geography. This is due in part to genetic differences and in part to differences in environmental and dietary exposures. Epidemiologic studies that monitor trends in cancer incidence and mortality have tremendously enhanced our understanding of the etiology of cancer.

The two types of epidemiologic studies that are conducted most often to investigate the etiology of cancer and the effect of prevention modalities are cohort studies and case-control studies. Cohort studies follow a group of people who initially do not have a disease over time and measure the rate of development of a disease. In cohort studies, a group that is exposed to a certain environmental factor or intervention usually is compared to a group that has not been exposed (e.g., smokers vs. nonsmokers). Case-control studies compare a group of patients affected with a disease to a group of individuals without the disease for a given exposure. The results are expressed in terms of an odds ratio, or relative risk. A relative risk less than 1 indicates a protective effect, although a relative risk greater than 1 indicates an increased risk of developing the disease with exposure.

Cancer Incidence and Mortality in the United States

In the year 2003, an estimated 1,334,100 new cases of invasive cancer will be diagnosed in the United States. Furthermore, an estimated 556,500 people will die from cancer in the United States in the same year. The most common

183

causes of cancer death in men are cancers of the lung and bronchus, prostate, and colon and rectum; in women, the most common cancers are of the lung and bronchus, breast, and colon and rectum.

Trends in Cancer Incidence and Mortality

Cancer deaths accounted for 23 percent of all deaths in the United States in 2000, second only to deaths from heart disease, which accounted for 29.6 percent of total deaths. As the life expectancy of the human population increases because of reductions in other causes of death such as infections and cardiovascular disease, cancer is becoming the leading cause of death. Cancer is already the leading cause of death among women aged 40–79 and among men aged 60–79.

Cancer incidence increased by 0.3 percent per year in females during the period from 1987 to 1999, but it stabilized in males between 1995 and 1999. Interestingly, prostate cancer rates increased dramatically between 1988 and 1992, and declined between 1992 and 1995. These trends are thought to reflect the extensive use of prostate-specific antigen (PSA) screening, leading to the earlier diagnosis of prostate cancers.

From 1992 to 1999, for all cancer types combined, cancer death rates decreased by 1.5 percent per year in males and by 0.6 percent per year in females. In fact, the 5-year survival rates from 1974 to 1998 reveal improvement in relative survival rates for cancers in almost all sites. How much of this improvement reflects actual improvement of cancer therapy and how much simply reflects earlier diagnosis of tumors with stage-for-stage outcome remaining unchanged, is not yet known.

Global Statistics on Cancer Incidence and Mortality

It has been estimated that there were a total of 10.1 million new cancer cases around the world in 2000, a number 22 percent higher than estimates for 1990. The most common cancers in terms of new cases were lung cancer (1.2 million), breast cancer (1.05 million), colon-rectum (945,000), stomach (876,000), and liver (564,000) in 2000. The most common causes of death because of cancer in 2000 were cancers of the lung (1.1 million), stomach (647,000), and liver cancer (549,000).

Stomach Cancer

The incidence of stomach cancer varies significantly among different regions of the world. The age-adjusted incidence is highest in Japan. The difference in risk by country is presumed to be because of differences in dietary factors and in the incidence of infection with *Helicobacter pylori*, which is known to play a major role in gastric cancer development. Fortunately, a steady decline is being observed in the incidence and mortality rates of gastric cancer. This may be related to improvements in preservation and storage of foods.

Breast Cancer

The incidence of breast cancer is high in all of the most highly developed regions except Japan, including the United States and Canada, Australia, and Northern and Western Europe. The highest breast cancer incidence is in the United States and the lowest is in China. Although breast cancer has been linked to cancer susceptibility genes, mutations in these genes account for only 5–10 percent of breast tumors, suggesting that the wide geographic variations in breast cancer incidence are not because of geographic variations in the prevalence of these genes. Most of the differences, therefore, are attributed to differences in reproductive factors, diet, and other environmental differences. Indeed, breast cancer risk increases significantly in females who have migrated from Asia to America. Overall, the incidence of breast cancer is rising in most countries.

Colon and rectal cancer. The incidence of colon and rectal cancer is higher in developed countries than developing countries. The incidence rates are highest in Australia/New Zealand, North America, and Northern and Western Europe. These geographic differences are thought to reflect environmental exposures and are presumed to be mainly dietary differences.

Liver cancer. Eighty percent of liver cancers occur in developing countries. The incidence of liver cancer is especially high in China and other countries in Eastern Asia. Worldwide, the major risk factors for liver cancer are infection with hepatitis viruses and consumption of foods contaminated with aflatoxin. Hepatitis B immunization in children has recently been shown to reduce the incidence of hepatitis infection in China, Korea, and West Africa. Whether this will translate into a reduction in the incidence in liver cancer in these regions will soon be determined.

Prostate cancer. The incidence of prostate cancer is dramatically higher in North America than in China, Japan, and the rest of Asia, and even in Northern and Western Europe. A considerable part of the international differences in prostate cancer incidence is thought to reflect differences in diagnostic practices. As previously mentioned, the introduction of PSA screening has led to a significant increase in the diagnosis of prostate cancer in the United States.

Esophageal cancer. Geographic variations in the incidence of esophageal cancer are also striking. The highest incidence of this cancer is in Southern Africa and China. These geographic differences are attributed to nutritional deficiencies and exposures to exogenous carcinogens. Esophageal cancer in North America and Europe is attributed to tobacco and alcohol use.

The mortality rates of different cancers also vary significantly among countries. This is attributable not only to variations in incidence but also to variations in survival after a cancer diagnosis. Survival rates are influenced not only by treatment patterns but also by variations in cancer screening practices, which affect the stage of cancer at diagnosis. For example, the 5-year survival rate of stomach cancer is much higher in Japan, where the cancer incidence is high enough to warrant mass screening and is presumed to lead to earlier diagnosis. In the case of prostate cancer, the mortality rates diverge much less than the incidence rates among countries. Survival rates for prostate cancer are much higher in North America than in developing countries (88 vs. 41 percent). It is possible that the extensive screening practices in the United States allow discovery of cancers at an earlier, more curable stage; however, it is also possible that this screening leads to discovery of more latent, less biologically aggressive cancers, which may not have caused death even if they had not been identified.

CANCER BIOLOGY

Cell Proliferation and Transformation

In normal cells, cell growth and proliferation are under strict control. In cancer cells, cells become unresponsive to normal growth controls, leading to uncontrolled growth and proliferation. Abnormally proliferating, transformed cells outgrow normal cells in the culture dish (i.e., in vitro) and commonly display several abnormal characteristics. These include loss of contact inhibition (i.e., cells continue to proliferate after a confluent monolayer is formed); an altered appearance and poor adherence to other cells or the substratum; loss of anchorage-dependence for growth; immortalization; and gain of tumorigenicity (i.e., the ability to give rise to tumors when injected into an appropriate host).

Cancer Initiation

Tumorigenesis is proposed to have three steps: initiation, promotion, and progression. Initiating events may lead a single cell to acquire a distinct growth advantage, such as gain of function of genes known as oncogenes, or loss of function of genes known as tumor suppressor genes. Subsequent events can lead to accumulations of additional deleterious mutations in the clone.

Cancer is a disease of clonal progression as tumors arise from a single cell and accumulate mutations that confer on the tumor an increasingly aggressive behavior. Most tumors are thought to go through a progression from benign lesions to in situ tumors to invasive cancers (e.g., atypical ductal hyperplasia to ductal carcinoma in situ to invasive ductal carcinoma of the breast). Fearon and Vogelstein proposed the model for colorectal tumorigenesis. Colorectal tumors arise from the mutational activation of oncogenes coupled with mutational inactivation of tumor suppressor genes, the latter being the predominant change. Mutations in at least four or five genes are required for formation of a malignant tumor, although fewer changes suffice for a benign tumor. Although genetic mutations often occur in a preferred sequence, a tumor's biologic properties are determined by the total accumulation of its genetic changes.

Gene expression is a multistep process that starts from transcription of a gene into messenger ribonucleic acid (mRNA) and then translation of this sequence into the functional protein. There are several controls at each level. In addition to alterations at the genome level, alterations at the transcription level (e.g., methylation of the DNA leading to transcriptional silencing), or at the mRNA processing, mRNA stability, mRNA translation, or protein stability levels, can alter critical proteins and thus contribute to tumorigenesis.

Cell-Cycle Dysregulation in Cancer

The proliferative advantage of tumor cells is a direct result of their ability to bypass quiescence. Mutations or alterations in the expression of cell-cycle proteins, growth factors, growth factor receptors, intracellular signal transduction proteins, and nuclear transcription factors all can lead to disturbance of the basic regulatory mechanisms that control the cell cycle, allowing unregulated cell growth and proliferation.

The cell cycle is divided into four phases. During the synthetic or S phase, the cell generates a single copy of its genetic material, although in the mitotic or M phase, the cellular components are partitioned between the two identical daughter cells. The G1 and G2 phases represent gap phases during which the cells prepare themselves for completion of the S and M phases, respectively.

When cells cease proliferation, they exit the cell cycle and enter the quiescent state referred to as G0.

Cell-cycle progression is regulated by a series of checkpoints that prevent cells from entering a new phase without completing the previous phase. The central regulators are serine-threonine kinases referred to as the cyclin-dependent kinases (CDKs). CDK4 and CDK6 are thought to be involved in the early G1 phase, whereas CDK2 is required to complete G1 and initiate S phase. CDK4 and CDK6 form active complexes with the D-type cyclins, cyclins D1, D2, and D3. CDK2 is activated by the cyclins E1 and E2, during the G1/S transition and by cyclins A1 and A2, during the S phase.

The principal downstream target of the activated complex of cyclin D and CDK4 or CDK6 is the retinoblastoma protein (Rb). In its hypophosphorylated form, Rb suppresses cellular growth by binding the E2F family of transcription factors. Furthermore, Rb binding to the promoter as a complex with E2F can actively repress transcription through chromatin remodeling, by recruiting proteins such as histone diacetylases and SWI/SNF complexes. Following cyclin/CDK-mediated phosphorylation, Rb releases E2F transcription factors that then activate downstream transcriptional targets involved in S phase, such as DNA polymerase alpha, cyclin A, cyclin E, and CDK1.

Regulators of CDKs can affect cell-cycle progression. CDKs are phosphorylated and activated by CDK-activating kinase. CDK inhibitors (CKIs) comprise two classes, the INK4 family and the WAF/Kip family. The INK4 family has four members: INK4A (p16), INK4B (p15), INK4C (p18), and INK4D (p19). The INK4 proteins bind CDK4 and CDK6 and prevent their association with D-type cyclins and cyclin D activation. The WAF/Kip family members include WAF1 (p21), KIP1 (p27), and KIP2 (p57). These CKIs bind and inactivate cyclin/CDK2 complexes.

Molecular alterations of human tumors have demonstrated that cell-cycle regulators are frequently mutated. Other alterations include overexpression of cyclins D1 and E, and CDK4 and CDK6, and loss of CKIs INK4A, INK4B, and KIP1.

Oncogenes

Normal cellular genes that contribute to cancer when abnormal are called oncogenes. The normal counterpart of such a gene is referred to as a protooncogene. Oncogenes are usually designated by three-letter abbreviations, such as myc or ras. Oncogenes are further designated by the prefix of "v-" for virus or "c-" for cell or chromosome, corresponding to the origin of the oncogene when it was first detected. Protooncogenes can be activated (have increased activity) or overexpressed (expressed at increased protein levels) by translocation (e.g., abl), promoter insertion (e.g., c-myc), mutations (e.g., ras), or amplification (e.g., HER2/ neu). More than 100 oncogenes have been identified.

Oncogenes may be growth factors (e.g., platelet-derived growth factor), growth factor receptors (e.g., HER2/neu), intracellular signal transduction molecules (e.g., ras), nuclear transcription factors (e.g., c-myc), or other molecules involved in the regulation of cell growth and proliferation. Growth factors are proteins that are produced and secreted by cells locally and that stimulate cell proliferation by binding specific cell-surface receptors on the same cells (autocrine stimulation) or on neighboring cells (paracrine stimulation). Persistent overexpression of growth factors can lead to uncontrolled autostimulation and neoplastic transformation. Alternatively, growth factor receptors can be aberrantly activated (turned on) through mutations, or over-expressed (continually presenting cells with growth-stimulatory signals, even in the absence of growth factors), leading cells to respond as if growth factor levels are altered. The growth-stimulating effect of growth factors and other mitogens is mediated through postreceptor signal transduction molecules. These molecules mediate the passage of growth signals from the outside to the inside of the cell and then to the cell nucleus, initiating the cell cycle and deoxyribonucleic acid (DNA) transcription. Aberrant activation or expression of cell-signaling molecules, cell-cycle molecules, or transcription factors may play an important role in neoplastic transformation.

Alterations in Apoptosis in Cancer Cells

Apoptosis (programmed cell death) is a genetically regulated program to dispose of cells. Cancer cells must avoid apoptosis if tumors are to arise. The growth of a tumor mass is dependent not only on an increase of proliferation of tumor cells but also on a decrease in their apoptotic rate. Apoptosis is distinguished from necrosis because it leads to several characteristic changes. In early apoptosis, the changes in membrane composition lead to extracellular exposure of phosphatidylserine residues, which avidly bind annexin, a characteristic used to discriminate apoptotic cells in laboratory studies. Late in apoptosis there are characteristic changes in nuclear morphology, such as chromatin condensation, nuclear fragmentation, and DNA laddering, and membrane blebbing. Apoptotic cells are then engulfed and degraded by phagocytic cells. The effectors of apoptosis are a family of proteases called caspases (cysteine-dependent and aspartate-directed proteases). The initiator caspases (e.g., 8, 9, and 10), which are upstream, cleave the downstream executioner caspases (e.g., 3, 6, and 7) that carry out the destructive functions of apoptosis.

Two principal molecular pathways signal apoptosis by cleaving the initiator caspases with the potential for cross-talk: the mitochondrial pathway and the death receptor pathway. In the mitochondrial pathway, sometimes referred to as the intrinsic pathway, death results from the release of cytochrome c from the mitochondria. Cytochrome c, procaspase-9, and apoptotic protease-activating factor-1 (Apaf-1) form an enzyme complex, referred to as the apoptosome, which activates the effector caspases. In addition to these proteins, the mitochondria contain other proapoptotic proteins such as SMAC/DIABLO. The mitochondrial pathway can be stimulated by many factors, including DNA damage, reactive oxygen species, or withdrawal of survival factors. The mitochondrial membrane permeability determines whether the apoptotic pathway will proceed. The Bcl-2 family of regulatory proteins includes proapoptotic proteins (e.g., Bax, Bad, and Bak) and antiapoptotic proteins (e.g., Bcl-2 and Bcl-xL); the activity of the Bcl-2 proteins is centered on the mitochondria, in which they regulate membrane permeability.

The second principal apoptotic pathway is the death receptor pathway, sometimes referred to as the extrinsic pathway. Cell-surface death receptors include Fas/APO1/CD95, tumor necrosis factor receptor 1 (TNFR1), and KILLER/DR5, which bind their ligands FasL, TNF, and TRAIL, respectively. When the receptors are bound by their ligands, they form a death-inducing signaling complex (DISC). At the DISC, procaspase-8 and procaspase-10 are cleaved, yielding active initiator caspases. The death receptor pathway may be regulated at the cell surface by the expression of "decoy" receptors for Fas and TRAIL.

The decoy receptors are closely related to the death receptors but lack a functional death domain, therefore they bind death ligands, but do not transmit a death signal. Another regulatory group is the FADD-like interleukin-1 protease-inhibitory proteins (FLIPs). FLIPs have homology to caspase-8; they bind to the DISC and inhibit the activation of caspase-8. Finally, inhibitors of apoptosis proteins (IAPs) block caspase-3 activation and have the ability to regulate both the death receptor and the mitochondrial pathway. The IAP family includes XIAP, cIAP1, cIAP2, NAIP, ML-IAP, ILP2, livin, apollon, and survivin. NF-κB also induces cellular resistance to apoptosis by transcriptionally activating cIAP1 and cIAP2, and other specific antiapoptotic proteins such as A20 and Mn-SOD.

In human cancers, aberrations in the apoptotic program include increased expression of Fas and TRAIL decoy receptors; increased expression of antiapoptotic Bcl-2; increased expression of IAP-related protein survivin; increased expression of c-FLIP; mutations or downregulation of proapoptotic Bax, caspase-8, APAF1, XAF1, and death receptors CD95, TRAIL-R1, and TRAIL-R2; alterations of the p53 pathway; overexpression of growth factors and growth factor receptors; and activation of the PI3-K/Akt survival pathway.

Cancer Invasion

A feature of malignant cells is their ability to invade the surrounding normal tissue. Tumors in which the malignant cells appear to lie exclusively above the basement membrane are referred to as in situ cancer, although tumors in which the malignant cells are demonstrated to breach the basement membrane, penetrating into surrounding stroma, are termed invasive cancer. The ability to invade involves changes in adhesion, initiation of motility, and proteolysis of the extracellular matrix (ECM).

Cell-to-cell adhesion in normal cells involves interactions between cell-surface proteins. Calcium adhesion molecules of the cadherin family (E-cadherin, P-cadherin, and N-cadherin) are thought to enhance the cells' ability to bind to one another and suppress invasion. Migration occurs when cancer cells penetrate and attach to the basal matrix of the tissue being invaded; this allows the cancer cell to pull itself forward within the tissue. Attachment to glycoproteins of the ECM such as fibronectin, laminin, and collagen is mediated by tumor cell integrin receptors. Integrins are a family of glycoproteins that form heterodimeric receptors for ECM molecules. In addition to regulating cell adhesion to the ECM, integrins relay molecular signals regarding the cellular environment that influence shape, survival, proliferation, gene transcription, and migration.

Serine, cysteine, and aspartic proteinases and matrix metalloproteinases (MMPs) have all been implicated in cancer invasion. Urokinase plasminogen activators (uPA) and tissue plasminogen activators (tPA) are serine proteases that convert plasminogen into plasmin. Plasmin, in return, can degrade several ECM components. Plasmin also may activate several MMPs. Plasminogen activator inhibitors (PAI-1 and PAI-2) are produced in tissues and counteract the activity of plasminogen activators.

MMPs are upregulated in almost every type of cancer. Some of the MMPs are expressed by cancer cells, although others are expressed by the tumor stromal cells. Experimental models have demonstrated that MMPs promote cancer progression by increasing cancer cell growth, migration, invasion, angiogenesis, and metastasis. The activity of MMPs is regulated by their endogenous inhibitors, including α_2-macroglobulin, membrane-bound inhibitors RECK (reversion-inducing cysteine-rich protein with kazal domains), and tissue inhibitors of MMPs (TIMP-1, -2, -3, and -4). Thus regulation of MMPs occurs at three levels: alterations of gene expression, activation of latent zymogens, and inhibition by endogenous inhibitors. Alterations of all three levels of control have been associated with tumor progression.

Angiogenesis

Angiogenesis is the establishment of new blood vessels from a preexisting vascular bed. This neovascularization is essential for tumor growth and metastasis. Tumors develop an angiogenic phenotype as a result of accumulated genetic alterations and in response to local selection pressures such as hypoxia. Many of the common oncogenes and tumor suppressor genes have been shown to play a role in inducing angiogenesis, including ras, myc, HER2/ neu, and mutations in p53.

Angiogenesis is mediated by factors produced by various cells including tumor cells, endothelial cells, stromal cells, and inflammatory cells. Several factors have been shown to be proangiogenic or antiangiogenic. Of the angiogenic stimulators, the best studied are the vascular endothelial growth factors (VEGF). The VEGF family consists of six growth factors (VEGF-A, VEGF-B, VEGF-C, VEGF-D, VEGF-E, and placental growth factor) and three receptors (VEGFR1 or Flt-1, VEGFR2 or KDR/FLK-1, and VEGFR3 or FLT4). Neuropilin 1 and 2 also may act as receptors for VEGF. VEGF is induced by hypoxia and by different growth factors and cytokines, including EGF, PDGF, TNF-α, TGF-β, and interleukin 1β (IL-1β). VEGF has various functions including increasing vascular permeability, inducing endothelial cell proliferation and tube formation, and inducing endothelial cell synthesis of proteolytic enzymes such as uPA, PAI-1, UPAR, and MMP-1. Furthermore, VEGF may mediate blood flow by its effects on the vasodilator nitric oxide and act as an endothelial survival factor, thus protecting the integrity of the vasculature. The proliferation of new lymphatic vessels, lymphangiogenesis, is also thought to be controlled by the VEGF family. Signaling in lymphatic cells is thought to be modulated by VEGFR3. Experimental studies with VEGF-C and VEGF-D have shown that they can induce tumor lymphangiogenesis and direct metastasis via the lymphatic vessels and lymph nodes.

PDGFs A, B, C, and D also play important roles in angiogenesis. PDGFs can not only enhance endothelial cell proliferation directly but also upregulate VEGF expression in vascular smooth muscle cells, promoting endothelial cell survival via a paracrine effect. The angiopoietins, angiopoietin 1 (Ang-1) and angiopoietin 2 (Ang-2), in return, are thought to regulate blood vessel maturation. Ang-1 and Ang-2 both bind endothelial cell receptor Tie-2, but only the binding of Ang-1 activates signal transduction; thus Ang-2 is an Ang-1 antagonist. Ang-1, via the Tie-2 receptor, induces remodeling and stabilization of blood vessels. Upregulation of Ang-2 by hypoxic induction of VEGF inhibits Ang-1–induced Tie-2 signaling, resulting in destabilization of vessels and making endothelial cells responsive to angiogenic signals, thus promoting angiogenesis in the presence of VEGF. Therefore the balance between these factors determines the angiogenetic capacity of a tumor. Tumor angiogenesis is regulated by several factors in a coordinated fashion. In addition to upregulation of proangiogenic molecules, angiogenesis also can be encouraged by suppression of naturally occurring inhibitors. Such inhibitors of angiogenesis include thrombospondin 1 and angiostatin.

Angiogenesis is a prerequisite not only for primary tumor growth but also for metastasis. Angiogenesis in the primary tumor, as determined by microvessel density, has been demonstrated to be an independent predictor of distant metastatic disease and survival in several cancers. Expression of angiogenic factors such as VEGFs has had prognostic value in many studies. These findings further emphasize the importance of angiogenesis in cancer biology.

Metastasis

Metastases arise from the spread of cancer cells from the primary site and the formation of new tumors in distant sites. The metastatic process consists of a series of steps that need to be successfully completed. First, the primary cancer must develop access to the circulation through either the blood circulatory system or the lymphatic system. After the cancer cells are shed into the circulation, they must survive. Next, the circulating cells lodge in a new organ and extravasate into the new tissue. Next, the cells need to initiate growth in the new tissue and eventually establish vascularization to sustain the new tumor. Overall, metastasis is an inefficient process, although the initial steps of hematogenous metastasis (the arrest of tumor cells in the organ and extravasation) are believed to be performed efficiently.

Metastases can sometimes arise several years after the treatment of primary tumors. This phenomenon is referred to as dormancy, and it remains one of the biggest challenges in cancer biology. Persistence of solitary cancer cells in a secondary site such as the liver or bone marrow is one possible contributor to dormancy. Another explanation of dormancy is that cells remain viable in a quiescent state and then get reactivated by a physiologically perturbing event. An alternate explanation is that cells establish preangiogenic metastases in which they continue to proliferate but that the proliferative rate is balanced by the apoptotic rate. Therefore, when these small metastases acquire the ability to be vascularized, substantial tumor growth can be achieved at the metastatic site, leading to clinical detection.

Several types of tumors metastasize in an organ-specific pattern. One explanation for this is mechanical and is based on the different circulatory drainage patterns of the tumors. The other explanation for preferential metastasis is what is referred to as the "seed and soil" theory, the dependence of the seed (the cancer cell) on the soil (the secondary organ). According to this theory, once cells have reached a secondary organ, their growth efficiency in that organ is based on the compatibility of the cancer cell's biology with its new microenvironment. The ability of cancer cells to grow in a specific site likely depends on features inherent to the cancer cell, features inherent to the organ, and the interplay between the cancer cell and its microenvironment.

Many of the oncogenes discovered to date, such as HER2/neu, ras, and myc, are thought to potentiate not only malignant transformation but also one or more of the steps required in the metastatic process. Metastasis also may involve the loss of metastasis suppressor genes. Laboratory work involving cancer cell lines that have been selected to have a higher metastatic potential have led to the realization that these more highly metastatic cells have a different gene expression profile than their less metastatic parental counterparts. This in turn has led to the currently held belief that the ability of a primary tumor to metastasize may be predictable by analysis of its gene expression profile.

Indeed, several studies have recently focused on identifying a gene expression profile or a "molecular signature" that is associated with metastasis. It has been shown that such a gene expression profile can be used to predict the probability of remaining free of distant metastasis. Notably, this hypothesis differs from the multistep tumorigenesis theory in that the ability to metastasize is considered an inherent quality of the tumor from the beginning. It is assumed that metastasis develops not from a few rare cells in the primary tumor that develop the ability to metastasize but that all cells in tumors with such molecular signatures develop the ability to metastasize. The reality probably lies in between in that some early genetic changes detectable in the entire tumor can give tumors an advantage in the metastatic process, although additional genetic changes can give a clone of cells additional advantages, thus allowing them to succeed in metastasis.

CANCER ETIOLOGY

Cancer Genetics

One widely held opinion is that cancer is a genetic disease that arises from an accumulation of mutations that leads to the selection of cells with increasingly aggressive behavior. These mutations may lead either to a gain of function by oncogenes or to a loss of function by tumor suppressor genes. Most of our information on human cancer genes has been gained from hereditary cancers. In the case of hereditary cancers, the individual carries a particular germline mutation in every cell. In the past decade, more than 30 genes for autosomal dominant hereditary cancers have been identified (Table 9-1). A few of these hereditary cancer genes are oncogenes, but most are tumor suppressor genes. Although hereditary cancer syndromes are rare, somatic mutations that occur in sporadic cancer have been found to disrupt the cellular pathways altered in hereditary cancer syndromes, suggesting that these pathways are critical to normal cell growth, cell cycle, and proliferation.

The following criteria may suggest the presence of a hereditary cancer:

1. Tumor development at a much younger age than usual
2. Presence of bilateral disease
3. Presence of multiple primary malignancies
4. Presentation of a cancer in the less affected sex (e.g., male breast cancer)
5. Clustering of the same cancer type in relatives
6. Cancer associated with other conditions such as mental retardation or pathognomonic skin lesions

It is crucial that all surgeons taking care of cancer patients be aware of hereditary cancer syndromes, because a patient's genetic background has significant implications for patient counseling, planning of surgical therapy, and cancer screening and prevention. Some of the more commonly encountered hereditary cancer syndromes are discussed here.

rb1 Gene and Hereditary Retinoblastoma

The rb1 gene was the first tumor suppressor to be cloned. Retinoblastoma has long been known to occur in hereditary and nonhereditary forms. In approximately 40 percent of cases of retinoblastoma in the United States, the individual has a predisposition conferred by a germline mutation. Dr. Alfred Knudson hypothesized that hereditary retinoblastoma involves two mutations, one of which is germline, although the other, nonhereditary retinoblastoma,

TABLE 9-1 Genes Associated with Hereditary Cancer

Genes	Location	Syndrome	Cancer sites and associated traits
APC	17q21	Familial adenomatous polyposis (FAP)	Colorectal adenomas and carcinomas, duodenal and gastric tumors, desmoids, medulloblastomas, osteomas
BMPR1A	10q21-q22	Juvenile polyposis coli	Juvenile polyps of the gastrointestinal tract, gastrointestinal and colorectal malignancy
BRCA1	17q21	Breast/ovarian syndrome	Breast cancer, ovarian cancer, colon cancer, prostate cancer
BRCA2	13q12.3	Breast/ovarian syndrome	Breast cancer, ovarian cancer, colon cancer, prostate cancer, cancer of the gallbladder and bile duct, pancreatic cancer, gastric cancer, melanoma
p16; CDK4	9p21; 12q14	Familial melanoma	Melanoma, pancreatic cancer, dysplastic nevi, atypical moles
CDH1	16q22	Hereditary diffuse gastric cancer	Gastric cancer
hCHK2	22q12.1	Li-Fraumeni and hereditary breast cancer	Breast cancer, soft-tissue sarcoma, brain tumors
hMLH1; hMSH2; hMSH6; hPMS1; hPMS2	3p21; 2p22-21; 2p16; 2q31-33; 7p22	Hereditary nonpolyposis colorectal cancer	Colorectal cancer, endometrial cancer, transitional cell carcinoma of the ureter and renal pelvis, and carcinomas of the stomach, small bowel, ovary, and pancreas
MEN1	11q13	Multiple endocrine neoplasia type 1	Pancreatic islet cell cancer, parathyroid hyperplasia, pituitary adenomas
MET	7q31	Hereditary papillary renal cell carcinoma	Renal cancer
NF1	17q11	Neurofibromatosis type 1	Neurofibroma, neurofibrosarcoma, acute myelogenous leukemia, brain tumors
NF2	22q12	Neurofibromatosis type 2	Acoustic neuromas, meningiomas, gliomas, ependymomas

(continued)

TABLE 9-1 *Continued*

Genes	Location	Syndrome	Cancer sites and associated traits
PTC	9q22.3	Nevoid basal cell carcinoma	Basal cell carcinoma
PTEN	10q23.3	Cowden disease	Breast cancer, thyroid cancer, endometrial cancer
rb	13q14	Retinoblastoma	Retinoblastoma, sarcomas, melanoma, and malignant neoplasms of brain and meninges
RET	10q11.2	Multiple endocrine neoplasia type 2	Medullary thyroid cancer, pheochromocytoma, parathyroid hyperplasia
SDHB; SDHC; SDHD	1p363.1-p35; 1q21; 11q23	Hereditary paraganglioma and pheochromocytoma	Paraganglioma, pheochromocytoma
SMAD4/DPC4	18q21.1	Juvenile polyposis coli	Juvenile polyps of the gastrointestinal tract, gastrointestinal and colorectal malignancy
STK11	19p13.3	Peutz–Jeghers syndrome	Gastrointestinal tract carcinoma, breast carcinoma, testicular cancer, pancreatic cancer, benign pigmentation of the skin and mucosa
p53	17p13	Li-Fraumeni syndrome	Breast cancer, soft–tissue sarcoma, osteosarcoma, brain tumors, adrenocortical carcinoma, Wilms tumor, phyllodes tumor of the breast, pancreatic cancer, leukemia, neuroblastoma
TSC1; TSC2	9q34;16p13	Tuberous sclerosis	Multiple hamartomas, renal cell carcinoma, astrocytoma
VHL	3p25	von Hippel-Lindau disease	Renal cell carcinoma, hemangioblastomas of retina and central nervous system, pheochromocytoma
WT	11p13	Wilms' tumor	Wilms' tumor, aniridia, genitourinary abnormalities, mental retardation

Source: Modified from Marsh D, Zori R. Genetic insights into familial cancers—update and recent discoveries. Cancer Lett 181(2):125–164, 2002.

is because of two somatic mutations. Thus both hereditary and nonhereditary forms of retinoblastoma involve the same number of mutations, a hypothesis known as Knudson's "two-hit" hypothesis. A "hit" may be a point mutation, a chromosomal deletion referred to as allelic loss, or a loss of heterozygosity (LOH), or silencing of an existing gene.

The rb1 gene product, the Rb protein, is a regulator of transcription that controls the cell cycle, differentiation, and apoptosis in normal development. Besides hereditary retinoblastoma, Rb protein is commonly inactivated directly by mutation in many sporadic tumors. Moreover, other molecules in the Rb pathway, such as p16, CDK4, and CDK6, have been identified in a number of sporadic tumors, suggesting that the Rb pathway is critical in malignant transformation.

p53 and Li-Fraumeni Syndrome

Li-Fraumeni syndrome (LFS) was first defined on the basis of observations of clustering of malignancies, including early onset breast cancer, soft-tissue sarcomas, brain tumors, adrenocortical tumors, and leukemia. Criteria for classic LFS in an individual (the proband) include: (1) a bone or soft-tissue sarcoma when younger than 45 years, (2) a first-degree relative with cancer before age 45 years, and (3) another first- or second-degree relative with either a sarcoma diagnosed at any age or any cancer diagnosed before age 45 years. Approximately 70 percent of LFS families have been shown to have germline mutations in the tumor suppressor p53 gene. Breast carcinoma, soft-tissue sarcoma, osteosarcoma, brain tumors, adrenocortical carcinoma, Wilms tumor, and phyllodes tumor of the breast are strongly associated; pancreatic cancer is moderately associated; and leukemia and neuroblastoma are weakly associated with germline p53 mutations. Mutations of p53 have not been detected in approximately 30 percent of LFS families, and it is hypothesized that genetic alterations in other proteins interacting with p53 function may play a role in these families.

p53 is the most commonly mutated known gene in human cancer. The p53 protein regulates cell-cycle progression and apoptotic cell death as part of stress response pathways following ionizing or ultraviolet (UV) irradiation, chemotherapy, acidosis, growth factor deprivation, or hypoxia.

BRCA1, BRCA2, and Hereditary Breast-Ovarian Cancer Syndrome

It is estimated that 5–10 percent of breast cancers are hereditary. Of women with early onset breast cancer (aged 40 years or younger), nearly 10 percent have a germline mutation in BRCA1 or BRCA2. Mutation carriers are more prevalent among women who have a first- or second-degree relative with premenopausal breast cancer or ovarian cancer at any age. The likelihood of a BRCA mutation is higher in patients who belong to a population in which founder mutations may be prevalent, such as in the Ashkenazi Jewish population. The cumulative risks for a female BRCA1 mutation carrier of developing breast cancer and ovarian cancer by age 70 have been estimated to be 87 and 44 percent, respectively. The cumulative risks of breast cancer and ovarian cancer by age 70 in BRCA2 families were estimated to be 84 and 27 percent, respectively. Besides breast and ovarian cancer, BRCA1 and BRCA2 may be associated with increased risks for several other cancers. BRCA1 confers a 4-fold increased risk for colon cancer and 3-fold increased risk for prostate cancer. BRCA2 confers a 5-fold increased risk for prostate cancer, 7-fold in men younger than 65 years. Furthermore, BRCA2 confers a 5-fold increased risk for gallbladder and bile duct cancers, 4-fold increased risk for pancreatic cancer, and 3-fold increased risk for gastric cancer and malignant melanoma.

BRCA1 was the first breast cancer susceptibility gene identified; BRCA2, was reported shortly afterward. BRCA1 and BRCA2 encode for large nuclear proteins, which have been implicated in processes fundamental to all cells, including DNA repair and recombination, checkpoint control of the cell cycle, and transcription.

APC Gene and Familial Adenomatous Polyposis

Patients affected with familial adenomatous polyposis (FAP) characteristically develop hundreds to thousand of polyps in the colon and rectum. The polyps usually appear in adolescence and, if left untreated, progress to colorectal cancer. FAP is associated with benign extracolonic manifestations that may be useful in identifying new cases, including congenital hypertrophy of the retinal pigment epithelium, epidermoid cysts, and osteomas. In addition to colorectal cancer, patients with FAP are at risk for upper intestinal neoplasms (gastric and duodenal polyps, duodenal and periampullary cancer), hepatobiliary tumors (hepatoblastoma, pancreatic cancer, and cholangiocarcinoma), thyroid carcinomas, desmoid tumors, and medulloblastomas.

The adenomatous polyposis coli (APC) tumor suppressor gene product is widely expressed in many tissues and plays an important role in cell-cell interactions, cell adhesion, regulation of β catenin, and maintenance of cytoskeletal microtubules. Alterations in APC lead to dysregulation of several physiologic processes that govern colonic epithelial cell homeostasis, including cell-cycle progression, migration, differentiation, and apoptosis. Mutations in the APC gene have been identified in FAP and in 80 percent of sporadic colorectal cancers. Furthermore, APC mutations are the earliest known genetic alterations in colorectal cancer progression, emphasizing its importance in cancer initiation.

Mismatch Repair Genes and Hereditary Nonpolyposis Colorectal Cancer

Hereditary nonpolyposis colorectal cancer (HNPCC), also referred to as Lynch syndrome, is an autosomal dominant hereditary cancer syndrome that predisposes to a wide spectrum of cancers, including colorectal cancer without polyposis. Some have proposed that HNPCC consists of at least two syndromes: Lynch syndrome I, which entails hereditary predisposition for colorectal cancer with early age of onset (approximately age 44 years) and an excess of synchronous and metachronous colonic cancers; and Lynch syndrome II, featuring a similar colonic phenotype accompanied by a high risk for carcinoma of the endometrium, transitional cell carcinoma of the ureter and renal pelvis, and carcinomas of the stomach, small bowel, ovary, and pancreas. The diagnostic criteria for HNPCC are referred to as the Amsterdam criteria, or the "3-2-1-0 rule." These criteria are met when three or more family members have histologically verified, HNPCC-associated cancers (one of whom is a first-degree relative of the other two), two or more generations are involved, at least one individual was diagnosed before age 50 years, and no individuals have FAP.

During DNA replication, DNA polymerases may introduce single nucleotide mismatches or small insertion or deletion loops. These errors are corrected through a process referred to as mismatch repair. When mismatch repair genes are inactivated, DNA mutations in other genes that are critical to cell growth and proliferation accumulate rapidly. In HNPCC, germline mutations have been identified in several genes that play a key role in DNA nucleotide mismatch repair: hMLH1 (human mutL homologue 1), hMSH2 (human mutS homologue 2), hMSH6, and hPMS1 and hPMS2 (human postmeiotic segretation 1 and 2), of which hMLH1 and hMSH2 are the most common. The hallmark of HNPCC is microsatellite instability, which occurs on the basis of unrepaired mismatches and small insertion or deletion loops. Microsatellite instability can be tested by comparing the DNA of a patient's tumor with DNA from adjacent normal epithelium, amplifying the DNA with polymerase chain reaction (PCR) using a standard set of markers, comparing the amplified genomic DNA sequences, and classifying the degree of microsatellite instability as high, low, or stable. Such microsatellite instability testing may help select patients who are more likely to have germline mutations.

PTEN and Cowden Disease

Somatic deletions or mutations in the tumor suppressor gene PTEN (phosphatase and tensin homologue deleted on chromosome 10) have been observed in a number of glioma, breast, prostate, and renal carcinoma cell lines and several primary tumor specimens. PTEN was identified as the susceptibility gene for the autosomal dominant syndrome Cowden disease (CD) or multiple hamartoma syndrome. Trichilemmomas, benign tumors of the hair follicle infundibulum, and mucocutaneous papillomatosis are pathognomonic of CD. Other common features include thyroid adenomas and multinodular goiters, breast fibroadenomas, and hamartomatous gastrointestinal polyps. The diagnosis of CD is made when an individual or family has a combination of pathognomonic major and/or minor criteria proposed by the International Cowden Consortium. CD is associated with an increased risk of breast and thyroid cancers. Breast cancer develops in 25–50 percent of affected women, and thyroid cancer develops in 3–10 percent of all affected individuals.

PTEN encodes a tyrosine phosphatase which negatively controls the PI3K signaling pathway for the regulation of cell growth and survival by dephosphorylating phosphoinositol 3,4,5-triphosphate; thus mutation of PTEN leads to constitutive activation of the PI3K/AKT signaling pathway.

RET Protooncogene and Multiple Endocrine Neoplasia Type 2

The RET gene encodes for a receptor tyrosine kinase that plays a role in proliferation, migration, and differentiation of cells derived from the neural crest. Gain-of-function mutations in the RET gene are associated with medullary thyroid carcinoma in isolation or multiple endocrine neoplasia type 2 (MEN2) syndromes. MEN2A is associated with medullary thyroid carcinoma and pheochromocytoma (in 50 percent) or parathyroid adenoma (in 20 percent), although MEN2B is associated with medullary thyroid carcinoma, marfanoid habitus, mucosal neuromas, and ganglioneuromatosis. RET mutations lead to uncontrolled growth of the thyroid c cells, and in familial medullary cancer, c-cell hyperplasia progresses to bilateral, multicentric medullary thyroid cancer. Mutations in the RET gene have also been identified in 40–60 percent of sporadic medullary thyroid cancers.

Genetic Modifiers of Risk

Individuals carrying identical germline mutations vary in regard to cancer penetrance (whether cancer will develop or not) and cancer phenotype (the tissues involved). It is thought that this variability may be because of environmental influences or, if genetic, to genetic modifiers of risk. Similarly, genetic modifiers of risk also can play a role in determining whether an individual will develop cancer after exposure to carcinogens.

Chemical Carcinogens

The first report that cancer could be caused by environmental factors was by John Hill in 1761, who reported the association between nasal cancer and excessive use of tobacco snuff. Currently, approximately 60–90 percent of cancers are thought to be because of environmental factors. Any agent that can contribute to tumor formation is referred to as a carcinogen and can be chemical, physical, or viral agents. Chemicals are classified into three groups based on how they contribute to tumor formation. The first group of chemical agents, the genotoxins, can initiate carcinogenesis by causing a mutation. The second group, the co-carcinogens, by themselves cannot cause cancer, but potentiate carcinogenesis by enhancing the potency of genotoxins. The third group, tumor promoters, enhance tumor formation when given after exposure to genotoxins.

Physical Carcinogens

Physical carcinogenesis can occur through induction of inflammation and cell proliferation over a period of time or through exposure to physical agents that induce DNA damage. In humans, clinical scenarios associated with chronic irritation and inflammation such as chronic nonhealing wounds, burns, and inflammatory bowel syndrome have all been associated with an increased risk of cancer. *H. pylori* is associated with gastritis and gastric cancer; and the liver fluke Opisthorchis viverrini leads to local inflammation and cholangiocarcinoma. The induction of lung and mesothelial cancers from asbestos fibers and nonfibrous particles such as silica are other examples of foreign-body–induced physical carcinogenesis.

Radiation is the best known agent of physical carcinogenesis and is classified as ionizing radiation (x-rays, gamma rays, and α and β particles) or nonionizing radiation (UV). The carcinogenic potential of ionizing radiation was recognized soon after Roentgen's discovery of x-rays in 1895. Long-term follow-up of survivors of the Hiroshima and Nagasaki atom bombs revealed that virtually all tissues exposed to radiation are at risk for cancer.

Viral Carcinogens

One of the first observations that cancer may be caused by transmissible agents was by Peyton Rous in 1911 when he demonstrated that cell-free extracts from sarcomas in chickens could transmit sarcomas to other animals injected with these extracts. This was subsequently discovered to represent viral transmission of cancer by the Rous sarcoma virus (RSV). At present. It is estimated that 15 percent of all human tumors worldwide are caused by viruses.

Viruses may cause or increase the risk of malignancy through several mechanisms, including direct transformation, expression of oncogenes that interfere with cell-cycle checkpoints or DNA repair, expression of cytokines or other growth factors, and alteration of the immune system. Oncogenic viruses may be ribonucleic acid (RNA) or DNA viruses. Oncogenic RNA viruses are retroviruses and contain a reverse transcriptase. After the viral infection, the single-stranded RNA viral genome is transcribed into a double-stranded DNA copy, which is then integrated into the chromosomal DNA of the cell. Retroviral infection of the cell is permanent, thus integrated DNA sequences remain in the host chromosome. Oncogenic transforming retroviruses carry oncogenes derived from cellular genes. These cellular genes, referred to as protooncogenes, usually are involved in mitogenic signaling and growth control.

Unlike the oncogenes of the RNA viruses, those of the DNA tumor viruses are viral, not cellular in origin. These genes are required for viral replication using the host cell machinery. In permissive hosts, infection with an oncogenic DNA virus may result in a productive lytic infection, leading to cell death and the release of newly formed viruses. In nonpermissive cells, the viral DNA can be integrated into the cellular chromosomal DNA, and some of the early viral genes can be synthesized persistently, leading to transformation of cells to a neoplastic state.

Like other types of carcinogenesis, viral carcinogenesis is a multistep process. Although immunocompromised individuals are at elevated risk, most patients infected with oncogenic viruses do not develop cancer. When cancer does develop, it usually occurs several years after the viral infection. It is estimated, for example, that the risk of hepatocelluar carcinoma among hepatitis C virus–infected individuals is 1–3 percent after 30 years. There may be synergy between various environmental factors and viruses in carcinogenesis. Factors that predispose to hepatocellular carcinoma among hepatitis C virus–infected patients include heavy alcohol intake and hepatitis B co-infection.

CANCER RISK ASSESSMENT

Cancer risk assessment starts with a complete history that includes history of environmental exposures to potential carcinogens and a detailed family history. Risk assessment for breast cancer, for example, includes a family history to determine whether another member of the family is known to carry a breast cancer susceptibility gene; whether there is familial clustering of breast cancer, ovarian cancer, thyroid cancer, sarcoma, adrenocortical carcinoma, endometrial cancer, brain tumors, dermatologic manifestations, leukemia, or lymphoma; and whether the patient is from a population at increased risk such as individuals of Ashkenazi Jewish descent. Patients who have a family history suggestive of a cancer susceptibility syndrome would benefit from genetic counseling and possibly genetic testing.

Patients who do not seem to have a strong hereditary component of risk can be evaluated on the basis of their age, race, personal history, and exposures. One of the most commonly used models for risk assessment in breast cancer is the Gail model. The model uses risk factors such as an individual's age, age at menarche, age at first live birth, number of first-degree relatives with breast cancer, and number of previous breast biopsies and histology. This tool allows a health professional to project a woman's individualized estimated risk for invasive breast cancer over a 5-year period and over her lifetime (to age 90 years). These risk assessment tools have been validated and are now in widespread clinical use. Similar models are in development or being validated for other cancers.

CANCER SCREENING

Early detection is the key to success in cancer therapy. Screening for common cancers using relatively noninvasive tests is expected to lead to early diagnosis, allow more conservative surgical therapies with decreased morbidity, and potentially improve surgical cure rates and overall survival rates. Key factors that influence screening guidelines are the prevalence of the cancer in the population, the risk associated with the screening measure, and whether early diagnosis actually affects outcome. The value of a widespread screening mea-sure is likely to go up with the prevalence of the cancer in a population, often determining the age cutoffs for screening, and explaining why only common cancers are screened for. The risks involved with the screening measure are a significant consideration, especially with more invasive screening measures such as colonoscopy. The consequences of a false-positive screening test also need to be considered. For example, when 1000 screening mammograms are performed, only two to four new incidences of cancer will be identified; this number is slightly higher (6–10 prevalent cancers per 1000 mammograms) in the initial screening mammograms performed. However, as many as 10 per-cent of screening mammograms may be potentially suggestive of abnormality, requiring further imaging (i.e., a 10-percent recall rate). Of those women with abnormal mammograms, only 5–10 percent will be determined to have a breast cancer. Among women for whom biopsy is recommended, 25–40 percent will have a breast cancer. A false-positive screen is likely to induce significant emotional distress in patients, leads to unnecessary biopsies, and has cost im-plications for the health care system.

Screening guidelines are developed for the general baseline-risk population. These guidelines need to be modified for patients who are at high risk.

CANCER DIAGNOSIS

The definitive diagnosis of solid tumors is usually obtained with a biopsy of the lesion. Biopsy determines the tumor histology and grade and thus assists in definitive therapeutic planning. Biopsies of mucosal lesions usually are ob-tained endoscopically (e.g., via colonoscope). Lesions that are easily palpable, such as those of the skin, can either be excised or sampled by punch biopsy. Deep-seated lesions can be localized with CT scan or ultrasound guidance for biopsy.

A sample of a lesion can be obtained with a needle or with an open in-cisional or excisional biopsy. Fine-needle aspiration is easy and relatively safe, but has the disadvantage of not giving information on tissue architec-ture. For example, fine-needle aspiration biopsy of a breast mass can make the diagnosis of malignancy, but cannot differentiate between an invasive and noninvasive tumor. Therefore core-needle biopsy is more advantageous when the histology will affect the recommended therapy. Core biopsy, like fine-needle aspiration, is relatively safe and can be performed either by direct palpation (e.g., a soft-tissue mass) or can be guided by an imaging study. Core biopsies, like fine-needle aspirations, have the disadvantage of introducing sampling error. It is crucial to ensure that the histologic findings are consis-tent with the clinical scenario, and to know the appropriate interpretation of each histologic finding. A needle biopsy in which the report is inconsistent with the clinical scenario should be either repeated or followed by an open biopsy.

Open biopsies have the advantage of providing more tissue for histologic evaluation and the disadvantage of being an operative procedure. Incisional biopsies are reserved for very large lesions in which a definitive diagnosis cannot be made with needle biopsy.

Excisional biopsies are performed for lesions in which core biopsy is either not possible or is nondiagnostic. Excisional biopsies should be performed with curative intent, that is, by obtaining adequate tissue around the lesion to ensure negative surgical margins. Orientation of the margins by sutures or clips by the surgeon and inking of the specimen margins by the pathologist will allow for determination of the surgical margins and will guide surgical re-excision if one or more of the margins are positive for microscopic tumor or close. The biopsy incision should be oriented to allow for excision of the biopsy scar if repeat operation is necessary. The biopsy incision should directly overlie the area to be removed. Finally, meticulous hemostasis during a biopsy is essential.

CANCER STAGING

Cancer staging is a system used to describe the anatomic extent of a malignant process in an individual patient. Staging systems may incorporate relevant clinical prognostic factors such as tumor size, location, extent, grade, and dissemination to regional lymph nodes or distant sites.

Cancer patients who are considered to be at high risk for distant metastasis usually undergo a preoperative staging work-up. This involves a set of imaging studies of sites of preferential metastasis for a given cancer type. For example, for a patient with breast cancer, a staging work-up would include a chest radiograph, bone scan, and scan of the abdomen to evaluate for lung, bone, and liver metastases, respectively.

Standardization of staging systems is essential to allow for comparison of different studies worldwide. The staging systems proposed by the American Joint Committee on Cancer (AJCC) and the Union Internationale Contre Cancer (International Union Against Cancer, UICC) are among the most widely accepted staging systems. Both the AJCC and the UICC have adopted a shared TNM staging system that defines the cancer in terms of the anatomic extent of disease and is based on assessment of three components: the primary tumor (T), the presence (or absence) and extent of nodal metastases (N), and the presence (or absence) and extent of distant metastases (M).

The TNM staging applies only to cases that have been microscopically confirmed to be malignant. Standard TNM staging (clinical and pathologic) is completed at initial diagnosis. Clinical staging (cTNM or TNM) is based on information gained up until the initial definitive treatment. Pathologic staging (pTNM) includes clinical information and information obtained from pathologic examination of the resected primary tumor and regional lymph nodes.

The clinical measurement of tumor size (T) is the one judged to be the most accurate for each individual case based on physical examination and imaging studies. If even one lymph node is involved by tumor, the N component is at least N1. For many solid tumor types, simply the absence or presence of lymph node involvement is recorded and the tumor is categorized either as N0 or N1. For other tumor types, the number of lymph nodes involved, the size of the lymph nodes or the lymph node metastasis, or the regional lymph node basin involved also has been shown to have prognostic value. In these cancers, N1, N2, N3, or N4 suggests an increasing abnormality of lymph nodes based on size, characteristics, and location. NX indicates that the lymph nodes cannot be fully assessed.

Cases in which there is no distant metastasis are designated M0, cases in which one or more distant metastases are detected are designated M1, and cases in which the presence of distant metastasis cannot be assessed are designated MX.

The practice of dividing cancer cases into groups according to stage is based on the observation that the survival rates are higher for localized (lower stage) tumors than for tumors that have extended beyond the organ of origin. Therefore staging is used to analyze and compare groups of patients. Such staging assists in (1) selection of therapy, (2) estimation of prognosis, (3) evaluation of treatments, (4) exchange of information among treatment centers, and (5) continued investigation of human cancers. For example, melanoma staging system can distinguish different prognostic groups on the basis of 15-year survival curves. Notably, the AJCC regularly updates its staging system to incorporate advances in prognostic technology to improve the predictive accuracy of the TNM system. Therefore it is important to know which revision of a staging system is being used when evaluating studies.

TUMOR MARKERS

Prognostic and Predictive Tissue Markers

Tumor markers are substances that can be detected in higher than normal amounts in the serum, urine, or tissues of patients with certain types of cancer. Tumors markers are produced either by the cancer cells themselves or by the body as a response to the cancer.

Over the past decade, there has been an especially large interest in identifying tissue tumor markers that can be used as prognostic or predictive markers. Although the terms prognostic marker and predictive marker are sometimes used interchangeably, the term prognostic marker usually is used to describe molecular markers that predict disease-free survival, disease-specific survival, and overall survival, although the term predictive marker is often used in the context of predicting response to certain therapies.

The goal is to identify prognostic markers that can give information on prognosis independent of other clinical characteristics, and therefore can provide information in addition to what can be projected on the basis of clinical presentation. This would allow us to further classify patients as being at higher or lower risk within clinical subgroups and to identify patients who may benefit most from adjuvant therapy.

Predictive markers are markers that can prospectively identify patients who will benefit from a certain therapy. Some of the best predictive markers are estrogen receptor and HER2/neu, which can identify patients who can benefit from antiestrogen therapies (e.g., tamoxifen) and anti-HER2/neu therapies (e.g., trastuzumab), respectively. There is increasing interest in identifying predictive markers for chemotherapy so that patients can be given the regimens they are most likely to benefit from, although those who are not likely to benefit from existing conventional therapies can be spared the toxicity of the therapy and be offered investigational therapies.

Serum Markers

Serum markers are under active investigation as they may allow early diagnosis of a new cancer or may be used to follow a cancer's response to therapy or monitor for recurrence. Unfortunately, identification of serum markers of clinical value has been challenging. Many of the tumor markers proposed so far have had low sensitivities and specificities (Table 9-2).

Tumor markers may not be elevated in all patients with cancer, especially in the early stages, when a serum marker would be most useful for diagnosis. Therefore when using a tumor marker to monitor recurrence, it is important to be certain that the tumor marker was elevated prior to primary therapy.

TABLE 9-2 Sensitivity and Specificity of Some Common Tumor Markers

Marker	Cancer	Sensitivity	Specificity
Prostate-specific antigen (4 μg/L)	Prostate	57–93 percent	55–68 percent
Carcinoembryonic antigen	Colorectal	40–47 percent	90 percent
	Breast	45 percent	81 percent
	Recurrent disease	84 percent	100 percent
Alpha-fetoprotein	Hepatocellular	98 percent	65 percent
CA 19.9	Pancreatic	78–90 percent	95 percent
CA 27.29	Breast	62 percent	83 percent
CA 15.3	Breast	57 percent	87 percent

Source: Adapted from http://medicine.wust1.edu/~labmed/1996vol4no9.html Tumor Marker Overview, 1996, Laboratory Medicine Newsletter.

Moreover, tumor markers can be elevated in benign conditions. Many tumor markers are not specific for a certain type of cancer and can be elevated with more than one type of tumor. Because there may be significant laboratory variability, it is important to obtain serial results from the same laboratory. Despite these many clinical limitations, several serum markers are in clinical use. A few of the commonly measured serum tumor markers are discussed below.

Circulating Cancer Cells

It has been suggested that circulating cancer cells can be an effective tool in selecting patients who have a high risk of relapse. One methodology widely used to detect cancer cells in the peripheral blood is reverse transcriptase (RT)-PCR. The use of this methodology to detect circulating cancer cells as a prognostic marker is under active investigation by many groups; however, its high sensitivity and potential for contamination leading to false-positive results has made investigation especially challenging. A recent promising approach is the use of the number of circulating tumor cells as an early predictor of response to systemic therapy.

SURGICAL APPROACHES TO CANCER THERAPY

Multidisciplinary Approach to Cancer

Although surgery is the most effective therapy for most solid tumors, most patients die of metastatic disease. Therefore, to improve patient survival rates, a multimodality approach with systemic therapy and radiation therapy is key for most tumors. It is important that surgeons involved in cancer care know not only how to perform a cancer operation but also the alternatives to surgery and be well versed in reconstructive options. It is also crucial that the surgeon be familiar with the indications for and complications of preoperative and postoperative chemotherapy and radiation therapy. As such, the surgeon often is responsible for determining the most appropriate adjuvant therapy for a given patient, and the best sequence for therapy. In most instances, a multidisciplinary approach beginning at the patient's initial presentation is likely to yield the best result.

Surgical Management of Primary Tumors

The goal of surgical therapy for cancer is to achieve oncologic cure. A curative operation presupposes that the tumor is confined to the organ of origin, or to the organ and the regional lymph node basin. Patients in whom the primary tumor is not resectable with negative surgical margins are considered to have inoperable disease. The operability of primary tumors is best determined before surgery with appropriate imaging studies that can define the extent of local-regional disease. Disease involving multiple distant metastases is deemed inoperable because it is usually not curable with surgery of the primary tumor. Therefore patients who are at high risk of having distant metastasis should have a staging work-up prior to surgery for their primary tumor. On occasion, primary tumors are resected in these patients for palliative reasons, such as improving the quality of life by alleviating pain, infection, or bleeding. Patients with limited metastases from a primary tumor on occasion are considered surgical candidates if the natural history of isolated distant metastases for that cancer type is favorable, or the potential complications associated with leaving the primary tumor intact are significant.

In the past it was presumed that the more radical the surgery, the better the oncologic outcome would be. Over the past 20 years, this has been recognized as not necessarily being true, leading to more conservative operations, with wide local excisions replacing compartmental resections of sarcomas; and breast-conserving therapies replacing radical mastectomies for breast cancer. The uniform goal for all successful oncologic operations seems to be achieving widely negative margins with no evidence of macroscopic or microscopic tumor at the surgical margins. Inking of the margins, orientation of the specimen by the surgeon, and immediate gross evaluation of the margins by the pathologist with frozen section analysis where necessary may assist in achieving negative margins at the first operation. In the end, although radiation therapy and systemic therapy can assist in decreasing local recurrence rates in the setting of positive margins, adjuvant therapy cannot substitute for adequate surgery.

Surgical Management of the Regional Lymph Node Basin

Most neoplasms metastasize via the lymphatics. Therefore, most oncologic operations have been designed to remove the primary tumor and draining lymphatics en bloc. This type of operative approach is usually undertaken when the lymph nodes draining the primary tumor site lie adjacent to the tumor bed, as is the case for colorectal cancers and gastric cancers. For tumors where the regional lymph node basin is not immediately adjacent to the tumor (e.g., melanomas), lymph node surgery can be performed through a separate incision.

It is generally accepted that a formal lymphadenectomy is likely to minimize the risk of regional recurrence of most cancers. On the other hand, there have been two opposing views regarding the role of lymphadenectomy on survival of cancer patients. The traditional Halsted view states that lymphadenectomy is important for staging and survival. The opposing view counters that cancer is systemic at inception and that lymphadenectomy, although useful for staging, does not affect survival. For most cancers, involvement of the lymph nodes is one of the most significant prognostic factors. Interestingly, the number of lymph nodes removed has been found to have an inverse relationship with overall survival rate in many solid tumors, including breast cancer, colon cancer, and lung cancer. There may be alternate explanations for the same finding. For example, the surgeon who performs a more extensive lymphadenectomy may obtain wider margins around the tumor, or even provide better overall care such as ensuring that patients receive the appropriate adjuvant therapy or undergo a more thorough staging work-up.

Alternatively, the pathologist may perform a more thorough examination, identifying more nodes and more accurately staging the nodes. The effect of appropriate staging on survival is twofold. Patients with nodal metastases may be offered adjuvant therapy, improving their survival chances. Further, the improved staging can improve perceived survival rates through a "Will Rogers effect," meaning identification of metastases that had formerly been silent and unidentified leads to a stage migration and thus to a perceived improvement in chances of survival. Clearly the impact of lymphadenectomy on survival will not be easily resolved. Because minimizing regional recurrences as much as possible is a goal of cancer treatment, the standard of care remains lymphadenectomy for most tumors.

A relatively new development in the surgical management of the clinically negative regional lymph node basin is the introduction of lymphatic mapping technology. Lymphatic mapping and sentinel lymph node biopsy were first reported in 1977 by Cabanas for penile cancer. Now sentinel node biopsy is the standard of care for the management of melanoma and is rapidly becoming the standard of care in breast cancer. The first node to receive drainage from the tumor site is termed the sentinel node. This node is the node most likely to contain metastases, if metastases to that regional lymph node basin are present. The goal of lymphatic mapping and sentinel lymph node biopsy is to identify and remove the lymph node most likely to contain metastases in the least invasive fashion. The practice of sentinel lymph node biopsy followed by selective regional lymph node dissection for patients with a positive sentinel lymph node avoids the morbidity of lymph node dissections in patients with negative nodes. An additional advantage of the sentinel lymph node technique is that it directs attention to a single node, allowing more careful analysis of the lymph node most likely to have a positive yield and increasing the accuracy of nodal staging.

Two criteria are used to assess the efficacy of a sentinel lymph node biopsy: the sentinel lymph node identification rate and the false-negative rate. The sentinel lymph node identification rate is the proportion of patients in whom a sentinel lymph node was identified and removed among all patients undergoing an attempted sentinel lymph node biopsy. The false-negative rate is the proportion of patients with regional lymph node metastases in whom the sentinel lymph node was found to be negative. False-negative biopsies may be because of identification of the wrong node or to missing the sentinel node (i.e., surgical error), or they may be because of the cancer cells establishing metastases not in the first encountered node, but in a second echelon node (i.e., biologic variation). Alternatively, false-negative biopsies may be because of inadequate histologic evaluation of the lymph node.

Lymphatic mapping is performed by using isosulfan blue dye, technetium-labeled sulfur colloid or albumin, or a combination of both techniques to detect sentinel nodes. The combination of blue dye and technetium has been reported to improve the capability of detecting sentinel lymph nodes. The nodal drainage pattern usually is determined with a preoperative lymphoscintogram, and the "hot" and/or blue nodes are identified with the assistance of a gamma probe and careful nodal basin exploration. Careful manual palpation is a crucial part of the procedure to minimize the false-negative rate. The nodes are evaluated with serial sectioning, hematoxylin and eosin staining, and immunohistochemical staining with S-100 and HMB-45 for melanoma and cytokeratin for breast cancer.

Surgical Management of Distant Metastases

The treatment of a patient with distant metastases depends on the number and sites of metastases, the cancer type, the rate of tumor growth, the previous treatments delivered and the responses to these treatments, and the patient's age, physical condition, and desires. Although once a tumor has metastasized it is usually not curable with surgical therapy, such therapy has resulted in cure in selected cases with isolated metastases to the liver, lung, or brain.

Patient selection is the key to success of surgical therapy for distant metastases. The cancer type is a major determinant in surgical decision making. The growth rate of the tumor also plays an important role and can be determined in part by the disease-free interval and the time between treatment of the primary tumor and detection of the distant recurrence. Patients with longer disease-free intervals have a higher survival rate after surgical metastasectomy than those with a short disease-free interval. The natural history of metastatic disease is so poor in some tumors (e.g., pancreatic cancer) that there is no role at this time for surgical metastasectomy. In cancers with more favorable outlooks, observation for several weeks or months, potentially with initial treatment with systemic therapy, can allow the surgeon to monitor for metastases at other sites.

In curative surgery for distant metastases, as with surgery for primary tumors, the goal is to resect the metastases with negative margins. In patients with hepatic metastases that are unresectable because their location near intrahepatic blood vessels precludes a margin-negative resection, or because of multifocality or inadequate hepatic function, tumor ablation with cryotherapy or radiofrequency ablation is an alternative. Curative resections or ablative procedures should be attempted only if the lesions are accessible and the procedure can be performed safely.

CHEMOTHERAPY

Clinical Use of Chemotherapy

In patients with documented distant metastatic disease, chemotherapy is usually the primary modality of therapy. The goal of therapy in this setting is to decrease the tumor burden, thus prolonging survival. It is rare to achieve cure with chemotherapy for metastatic disease in most solid tumors. Chemotherapy administered to a patient who is at high risk for distant recurrence, but has no evidence of distant disease, is referred to as adjuvant chemotherapy. The goal of adjuvant chemotherapy is eradication of micrometastatic disease, with the intent of decreasing relapse rates and improving survival rates.

Adjuvant therapy can be given after surgery (postoperative chemotherapy) or before surgery (preoperative chemotherapy, neoadjuvant chemotherapy, or induction therapy). A portion or all of the planned adjuvant chemotherapy can be administered prior to the surgical removal of the primary tumor. Preoperative chemotherapy has three potential advantages. The first is that preoperative regression of tumor can facilitate resection of tumors that were initially inoperable or allow more conservative surgery for patients whose cancer was operable to begin with. The second advantage of preoperative chemotherapy is the treatment of micrometastases without the delay of postoperative recovery. The third goal is the ability to assess a cancer's response to treatment clinically, after a number of courses of chemotherapy, and pathologically, after surgical resection. This is especially important if alternative treatment regimens are available to be offered to patients whose disease responded inadequately.

Response to chemotherapy is monitored clinically with imaging studies and physical examinations. Response usually is defined as complete response, partial response, minimal response or stable disease, or progression. Complete response is defined as the disappearance of all evidence of disease and no evidence of new disease for a specified interval, usually 4 weeks. Partial response is defined as a 50 percent or more decrease of the product of the two largest perpendicular tumor diameters (relative to the initial product), determined by two observations not less than 4 weeks apart. Additionally, there can be no appearance of new lesions or progression of any lesion. Stable disease refers to the situation in which neither complete or partial response nor progression has been demonstrated. Progressive disease refers to a 25 percent or greater increase in the product of one or more measurable lesions (relative to the smallest size measured because treatment start) or the appearance of new lesions.

Cancer is usually not detectable until 10^9 cancer cells (1 g) are present. A 3-log increase in cancer cells produces 10^{12} cells (1 kg), which can be fatal. A clinical "complete response" (i.e., disappearance of all clinically detectable disease) can be achieved with millions of cancer cells still remaining.

Principles of Chemotherapy

Chemotherapy destroys cells by first-order kinetics, meaning that with the administration of a drug a constant percentage of cells are killed, not a constant number of cells. If a patient with 10^{12} tumor cells is treated with a dose that results in 99.9 percent cell kill (3-log cell kill), the tumor burden will be reduced from 10^{12} to 10^9 cells (or 1 kg to 1 g). If the patient is retreated with the same drug, which theoretically could result in another 3-log cell kill, the number of cells would decrease from 10^9 to 10^6 (1 g to 1 mg) rather than being eliminated totally.

Chemotherapeutic agents can be classified according to the phase of the cell cycle they are effective in. Cell-cycle phase–nonspecific agents (e.g., alkylating agents) have a linear dose-response curve, such that the fraction of cells killed increases with dose of the drug. In contrast, the cell-cycle phase–specific drugs have a plateau with respect to cell killing ability, and cell kill will not increase with further increases in drug dose.

Anticancer Agents

Alkylating Agents

Alkylating agents are cell-cycle–nonspecific agents, meaning that they are able to kill cells in any phase of the cell cycle. They act by cross-linking the two strands of the DNA helix or by other direct damage to the DNA. The damage to the DNA prevents cell division and, if severe enough, leads to apoptosis. The alkylating agents comprise three main subgroups: classic alkylators, nitrosoureas, and miscellaneous DNA-binding agents.

Antitumor Antibiotics

Antitumor antibiotics are the products of fermentation of microbial organisms. Like the alkylating agents, these agents are cell-cycle nonspecific. Antitumor antibiotics damage the cell by interfering with DNA or RNA synthesis, although the exact mechanism of action may differ by agent.

Antimetabolites

Antimetabolites are generally cell-cycle–specific agents that have their major activity during the S phase of the cell cycle and have little effect on cells in G0. These drugs are most effective, therefore, in tumors that have a high growth fraction. Antimetabolites are structural analogues of naturally occurring metabolites involved in DNA and RNA synthesis. Therefore, they interfere with normal synthesis of nucleic acids by substituting for purines or pyrimidines in the metabolic pathway to inhibit critical enzymes in nucleic acid synthesis. The antimetabolites include folate antagonists, purine antagonists, and pyrimidine antagonists.

Plant Alkaloids

Plant alkaloids are derived from plants such as the periwinkle plant, *Vinca rosea* (e.g., vincristine, a vinca alkaloid), or the root of mandrake, *Podophyllum peltatum* (e.g., etoposide, a podophyllotoxin). Vinca alkaloids affect the cell by binding to tubulin in the S phase. This blocks microtubule polymerization, resulting in impaired mitotic spindle formation in the M phase. Taxanes such a paclitaxel, on the other hand, cause excess polymerization and stability of microtubules, blocking the cell cycle in mitosis. The epipodophyllotoxins act to inhibit a DNA enzyme called topoisomerase II by stabilizing the DNA–topoisomerase II complex. This results in an inability to synthesize DNA, thus the cell cycle is stopped in G1 phase.

Combination Chemotherapy

Combination chemotherapy may provide greater efficacy than single-agent therapy by three mechanisms: (1) it provides maximum cell kill within the range of toxicity for each drug that can be tolerated by the host, (2) it offers a broader range of coverage of resistant cell lines in a heterogeneous population, and (3) it prevents or delays the emergence of drug-resistant cell lines. Drugs with different mechanisms of action are combined to allow for additive or synergistic effects. Combining cell-cycle–specific and cell-cycle–nonspecific agents may be especially advantageous. Drugs with differing dose-limiting toxic effects are combined to allow for each drug to be given at therapeutic doses. Drugs with different patterns of resistance are combined whenever possible to minimize cross-resistance. The treatment-free interval between cycles is kept at the shortest possible time that will allow for recovery of the most sensitive normal tissue.

Drug Resistance

Several tumor factors influence tumor cell kill. Tumors are heterogenous, and, according to the Goldie Coldman hypothesis, tumor cells are genetically unstable and tend to mutate to form different cell clones. This has been used as an argument for giving chemotherapy as soon as possible in treatment, to reduce the likelihood of resistant clones emerging. Tumor size is another important variable. The greater the tumor, the larger the heterogeneity. Because of the larger proportion of cells dividing, smaller tumors may be more chemosensitive.

Multiple mechanisms of chemotherapy resistance have been identified. Cells may exhibit reduced sensitivity to drugs by virtue of their cell-cycle distribution. For example, cells in G0 phase are resistant to drugs active in the S phase. Alternatively, tumor cells may exhibit "pharmacologic resistance," when the failure to kill cells is because of insufficient drug concentration. This may occur when tumor cells are located in sites where effective drug concentrations are difficult to achieve (such as the central nervous system), or can be because of enhanced metabolism of the drug after its administration, decreased conversion of the drug to active form, or a decrease in the intracellular drug level because of increased removal of the drug from the cell associated with enhanced expression of P-glycoprotein, the protein product of the multidrug resistance gene 1 (MDR-1). Other mechanisms of resistance include decreased affinity of the target enzyme for the drug, altered amount of the target enzyme, or enhanced repair of the drug-induced defect.

Drug Toxicity

Tumors are more susceptible than normal tissue to chemotherapeutic agents, in part because they have a higher proportion of dividing cells. Normal tissues with a high growth fraction, such as the bone marrow, oral and intestinal mucosa, and hair follicles are also sensitive to chemotherapeutic effects. Therefore, treatment with chemotherapeutic agents can produce toxic effects such as bone marrow suppression, stomatitis, ulceration of the gastrointestinal tract, and alopecia. Toxic effects are usually graded from 0 to 4 on the basis of World Health Organization (WHO) standard criteria. Significant drug toxicity may necessitate a dose reduction. A toxic effect requiring a dose modification or change in dose intensity is referred to as a dose-limiting toxic effect. As maintaining dose intensity is important to maintaining as high a tumor cell kill as possible, several supportive strategies have been developed, such as administration of colony-stimulating factors and erythropoietin for poor bone marrow reserve and administration of cytoprotectants such as sodium 2-mercaptoethane sulfonate (MESNA) and amifostine to prevent renal dysfunction.

Administration of Chemotherapy

Chemotherapy usually is administered systemically (intravenously, intramuscularly, subcutaneously, or orally). Systemic administration treats micrometastases at widespread sites and prevents systemic recurrence. However, it increases the drug's toxicity to a wide range of organs throughout the body. One method to minimize systemic toxicity while enhancing target organ delivery of chemotherapy is regional administration of chemotherapy. Many of these approaches require surgical access, such as intrahepatic delivery of chemotherapy for hepatic carcinomas or metastatic colorectal cancer with a hepatic artery infusion pump, limb perfusion for extremity melanoma and sarcoma, or intraperitoneal hyperthermic perfusion for pseudomyxoma peritonei.

HORMONAL THERAPY

Some tumors, most notably breast and prostate cancers, originate from tissues whose growth is under hormonal control. The first attempts at hormonal therapy were through surgical ablation of the organ producing the hormones of interest, such as oophorectomy for breast cancer. Hormones or hormone-like agents can be administered to inhibit tumor growth by blocking or antagonizing the naturally occurring substance, such as estrogen antagonist tamoxifen. Other substances that block the synthesis of the natural hormone can be administered as alternatives. Aromatase inhibitors, for example, block the peripheral conversion of endogenous androgens to estrogens in postmenopausal women.

BIOLOGIC THERAPY

Over the past decade, increasing understanding of cancer biology has fostered the emerging field of molecular therapeutics. The basic principle of molecular therapeutics is to exploit the molecular differences between normal cells and cancer cells to develop targeted therapies. The ideal molecular target would be exclusively expressed in the cancer cells, be the driving force of the proliferation of the cancer cells, and be critical to their survival. A large number of molecular targets are currently being explored, both preclinically and in clinical trials. The major groups of targeted therapies include inhibitors of growth factor receptors, inhibitors of intracellular signal transduction, cell-cycle inhibitors, apoptosis-based therapies, and antiangiogenic compounds.

Protein kinases have come to the forefront as attractive therapeutic targets with the success of STI571 (imitanib mesylate, Gleevec) in chronic myelogenous leukemia and gastrointestinal stromal tumors and trastuzumab (Herceptin) in breast cancer, which work by targeting bcr-abl, c-kit, and HER2/neu, respectively. Therefore, protein kinases involving these aberrantly activated pathways are being aggressively pursued in molecular therapeutics. Most of the compounds in development are monoclonal antibodies like trastuzumab or small-molecule kinase inhibitors like STI-571. Some of the kinase inhibitors in clinical development include inhibitors of EGFR, Ras, Raf, MEK, mammalian target of rapamycin (mTOR), CDK, PKC, and 3-phosphoinositide-dependent protein kinase 1 (PDK-1).

IMMUNOTHERAPY

The aim of immunotherapy is to induce or potentiate inherent antitumor immunity that can destroy cancer cells. Central to the process of antitumor immunity is the ability of the immune system to recognize tumor-associated antigens present on human cancers and to direct cytotoxic responses through humoral or T-cell–mediated immunity. Overall, T-cell–mediated immunity appears to have the greater potential of the two for eradicating tumor cells. T cells recognize antigens on the surfaces of target cells as small peptides presented by class I and class II major histocompatibility complex (MHC) molecules.

One approach to antitumor immunity is nonspecific immunotherapy, which stimulates the immune system as a whole by administering bacterial agents or their products, such as bacille Calmette-Guérin (BCG). This approach is thought to activate the effectors of antitumor response such as natural killer cells and macrophages, and polyclonal lymphocytes. Another approach to nonspecific immunotherapy is systemic administration of cytokines such as IL-2, interferon α, and interferon γ.

Antigen-specific immunotherapy can be active, achieved through antitumor vaccines, or passive. In passive immunotherapy, antibodies to specific tumor-associated antigens can be produced by hybridoma technique and then administered to patients whose cancers express these antigens, inducing antibody-dependent cellular cytotoxicity.

The early attempts at vaccination against cancers used allogeneic cultured cancer cells, including irradiated cells, cell lysates, or shed antigens isolated from tissue culture supernatants. An alternate strategy is the use of autologous tumor vaccines, which have the potential advantage of being more likely to contain antigens relevant for the individual patient, but have the disadvantage of needing a large amount of tumor tissue for preparation, which restricts eligibility of patients for this modality. Strategies to enhance immunogenicity of tumor cells include the introduction of genes encoding cytokines or chemokines, or fusion of the tumor cells to allogeneic MHC II–bearing cells.

Identification of tumor antigens has made it possible to perform antigen-specific vaccination. Vaccines directed at defined tumor antigens aim to combine selected tumor antigens and appropriate routes for delivering these antigens to the immune system to optimize antitumor immunity. Several different vaccination approaches are under study including tumor cell–based vaccines, peptide-based vaccines, recombinant virus–based vaccines, DNA-based vaccines, and dendritic cell vaccines.

In adoptive transfer, antigen-specific cytotoxic T lymphocytes or antigen-nonspecific natural killer cells can be transferred to a patient. These effector cells can be obtained from the tumor (tumor-infiltrating lymphocytes) or the peripheral blood.

Clinical experience in patients with metastatic disease has shown objective tumor responses to a variety of immunotherapeutic modalities. It is thought, however, that the immune system is overwhelmed with the tumor burden in this setting, and thus adjuvant therapy may be preferable, reserving immunotherapy for decreasing tumor recurrences. How to best integrate immunotherapy with other therapies are not well understood for most cancer types.

GENE THERAPY

Gene therapy is being pursued as a possible approach to modifying the genetic program of cancer cells and for treatment of metabolic diseases. The field of cancer gene therapy uses a variety of strategies, ranging from replacement of mutated or deleted tumor suppressor genes to enhancement of immune responses to cancer cells.

As the goal in cancer therapy is to eradicate systemic disease, optimization of delivery systems is the key to success for gene therapy strategies. Gene therapy is likely to be most successful when combined with standard therapies, but it will provide the advantage of customization of therapy based on the molecular status of an individual's tumor.

RADIATION THERAPY

Physical Basis of Radiation Therapy

Ionizing radiation is energy strong enough to remove an orbital electron from an atom. This radiation can be electromagnetic, such as a high-energy photon, or particulate, such as an electron, proton, neutron, or alpha particle. Radiation therapy is delivered primarily as high-energy photons (gamma rays and x-rays) and charged particles (electrons). Gamma rays are photons that are released from the nucleus of a radioactive atom. X-rays are photons that are created electronically, such as with a clinical linear accelerator. Currently, high-energy radiation is delivered to tumors primarily with linear accelerators. X-rays traverse the tissue, depositing the maximum dose beneath the surface, and thus spare the skin. Electrons are used to treat superficial skin lesions, superficial tumors, or surgical beds to a depth of 5 cm. Gamma rays typically are produced by radioactive sources used in brachytherapy.

The dose of radiation absorbed correlates with the energy of the beam. The basic unit is the amount of energy absorbed per unit of mass (joules per kilogram) and is known as a gray (Gy). One gray is equivalent to 100 rads, the unit of radiation measurement used in the past.

Biologic Basis of Radiation Therapy

Radiation deposition results in DNA damage manifested by single- and double-strand breaks in the sugar phosphate backbone of the DNA molecule. Cross-linking between the DNA strands and chromosomal proteins also occurs. The mechanism of DNA damage differs by the type of radiation delivered. Electromagnetic radiation is indirectly ionizing through short-lived hydroxyl radicals produced primarily by the ionization of cellular hydrogen peroxide (H_2O_2). Protons and other heavy particles are directly ionizing and directly damage DNA.

Radiation damage is manifested primarily by the loss of cellular reproductive integrity. Most cell types do not show signs of radiation damage until they attempt to divide, so slowly proliferating tumors may persist for months and appear viable. Some cell types, however, undergo apoptosis.

The extent of DNA damage following radiation is dependent on several factors. The most important of these is cellular oxygen. Hypoxic cells are significantly less radiosensitive than aerated cells.

The extent of DNA damage from indirectly ionizing radiation is also dependent on the phase of the cell cycle. The most radiation-sensitive phases are G2 and M, although G1 and late S phases are less sensitive. Thus irradiation of a population of tumor cells results in killing of a greater proportion of cells in G2 and M phases. However, delivery of radiation in divided doses, a concept referred to as fractionation, allows the surviving G1 and S phase cells to progress to more sensitive phases, a process referred to as reassortment. In contrast to DNA damage following indirectly ionizing radiation, that following exposure to directly ionizing radiation is less dependent on the cell-cycle phase.

Several chemicals can modify the effects of ionizing radiation. These include hypoxic cell sensitizers such as metronidazole and misonidazole, which mimic oxygen and increase cell kill of hypoxic cells. A second category of radiation sensitizers are thymidine analogues iododeoxyuridine and bromo-deoxyuridine. These molecules are incorporated into the DNA in place of thymidine and render the cells more susceptible to radiation damage. Furthermore, several chemotherapeutic agents sensitize cells to radiation through various mechanisms, including 5-fluorouracil, actinomycin D, gemcitabine, paclitaxel, topotecan, doxorubicin, and vinorelbine.

Radiation Therapy Planning

Radiation therapy is delivered in a homogeneous dose to a well-defined region that includes tumor and/or surrounding tissue at risk for subclinical disease. The first step in planning is to define the target to be irradiated and the dose-limiting organs in the vicinity. Treatment planning includes evaluation of alternative treatment techniques, which is done through a process referred to as simulation. Once the beam distribution is determined that will best achieve homogenous delivery to the target volume and minimize the dose to the normal tissue, immobilization devices and markings or tattoos on the patient's skin are used to ensure that each daily treatment is given in the same way. Conventional fractionation is 1.8–2 Gy per day, administered 5 days each week for 3–7 weeks.

Another mode of postoperative radiation therapy is brachytherapy. In brachytherapy, unlike external beam therapy, the radiation source is in contact with the tissue being irradiated. The radiation source may be cesium, gold, iridium, or radium. Brachytherapy is administered with temporary or permanent implants such as needles, seeds, or catheters. Temporary brachytherapy catheters are placed either during open surgery or percutaneously soon after surgery. The implants are loaded interstitially and treatment usually is given postoperatively for a short duration such as 1–3 days. Although brachytherapy has the advantage of patient convenience owing to the shorter treatment duration, it has the disadvantages of leaving scars at the catheter insertion site and requiring special facilities for inpatient brachytherapy therapy.

Side Effects

Both tumor and normal tissue have radiation dose-response relationships that can be plotted on a sigmoidal curve. A minimum dose of radiation must be given before any response is seen. The response to radiation then increases slowly with an increase in dose. At a certain dose level the curves become exponential, with increases in tumor response and normal tissue toxicity with each incremental dose increase. The side effects of radiation therapy can be acute, occurring during or 2–3 weeks after therapy, or chronic, occurring weeks to years after therapy. The side effects depend on the tissue included in the target volume.

CANCER PREVENTION

The old axiom "an ounce of prevention is worth a pound of cure" is being increasingly recognized in oncology. Cancer prevention can be divided into three categories: (1) primary prevention (i.e., preventing initial cancers in healthy individuals); (2) secondary prevention (i.e., preventing cancer in individuals with premalignant conditions); and (3) tertiary prevention (i.e., preventing second primary cancers in patients cured of their initial disease).

The administration of systemic or local therapies to prevent the development of cancer, called chemoprevention, is being actively explored for several cancer types. Tamoxifen reduces the risk of breast cancer by one half in high-risk patients. Therefore tamoxifen has been approved by the FDA for breast cancer chemoprevention. Celecoxib has been shown to reduce polyps in patients with familial adenomatous polyposis. In head and neck cancer, 13-cis-retinoic acid was shown to both reverse oral leukoplakia and reduce second primary tumor development. Thus the chemoprevention trials completed so far have demonstrated success in primary, secondary, and tertiary prevention. It is important for surgeons to be aware of these preventive options because they are likely to be involved in the diagnosis of premalignant and malignant conditions, and will be the ones to counsel patients about their chemopreventive options.

In selected scenarios, the risk of cancer is high enough to justify surgical prevention. These high-risk scenarios include hereditary cancer syndromes such as hereditary breast ovarian cancer syndrome, hereditary diffuse gastric cancer, multiple endocrine neoplasia type 2, FAP, and HNPCC, and some nonhereditary scenarios such as chronic ulcerative colitis. Most prophylactic surgeries are large ablative surgeries (e.g., bilateral risk-reducing mastectomy or total proctocolectomy). Therefore it is important that the patient be completely informed about potential surgical complications and long-term lifestyle consequences. Further, the conservative options of close surveillance and chemoprevention need to be discussed. The patient's cancer risk needs to be assessed accurately and implications for survival discussed. Ultimately, the decision to proceed with surgical prevention should be individualized and made with caution.

TRENDS AND EVOLVING TECHNOLOGIES IN ONCOLOGY

Cancer Screening and Diagnosis

It is clear that the practice of oncology will change dramatically over the next few decades as our understanding of the molecular basis of cancer and available technologies are evolving rapidly. One of the critical changes expected is earlier detection of cancers. With improvements in available imaging modalities and development of newer functional imaging technologies, it is likely that many tumors may be detected at earlier, more curable stages in the near future.

Another area of rapid development is the identification of serum markers. High-throughput technologies such as matrix-assisted laser-desorption-ionization time of flight (MALDI-TOF) mass spectroscopy and liquid chromatography-ion-spray tandem mass spectroscopy (LC-MS/MS) have revolutionized the field of proteomics and identification of unique proteins and unique proteomic profiles for most cancer types is being pursued actively by many researchers, which if successful, could dramatically enhance our ability to detect cancers early.

Surgical Therapy

The current trend in surgery is moving toward more conservative resections. With earlier identification of tumors, more conservative surgeries may be possible. The goal, however, is always to remove the tumor en bloc with wide negative margins. Another interesting area being explored is the destruction of tumors by such techniques as radiofrequency ablation, cryoablation, and heat-producing technologies such as lasers, microwaves, or focused ultrasound. Pilot studies have demonstrated that radiofrequency ablation is effective for destruction of small primary breast cancers. Although this approach remains experimental and potentially of limited applicability, with the development of imaging technologies that can accurately map the extent of cancer cells, these types of noninvasive interventions are likely to come to the forefront.

Systemic Therapy

The current trend in systemic therapy is moving toward individualized therapy. It now is presumed that all cancers of a certain cell origin are the same, thus all patients are offered the same systemic therapy. Not all patients respond to these therapies, however, emphasizing the biologic variability within the groups. Therefore the intent is to determine the underlying biology of each tumor to tailor therapy accordingly. The approaches used include high-throughput techniques such as proteomics, or more frequently, transcriptional profiling. It is likely that in the near future tumors can be tested and treatments individualized. Patients who will respond to conventional therapies can be given these regimens, although patients who will not respond are not, sparing them the toxicity. Instead, these patients can be offered novel therapies.

Furthermore, with emerging biologic therapies, it is likely that patients may be given a combination of biologic therapies specifically targeting the alterations in their own tumors. Finally, stratification of patients by gene expression profile for prognosis may assist in determining which patients are at higher risk of relapse, sparing patients whose tumors have less aggressive biologic characteristics further therapy.

Suggested Readings

Jemal A, Murray T, Samuels A, et al: Cancer statistics, 2003. CA Cancer J Clin 53:5, 2003.

Fearon ER, Vogelstein B: A genetic model for colorectal tumorigenesis. Cell 61:759, 1990.

Blume-Jensen P, Hunter T: Oncogenic kinase signaling. Nature 411: 355, 2001.

Chambers AF, Groom AC, MacDonald IC: Dissemination and growth of cancer cells in metastatic sites. Nat Rev Cancer 2:563, 2002.

Knudson AG: Two genetic hits (more or less) to cancer. Nat Rev Cancer 1:157, 2001.

King MC, Wieand S, Hale K, et al: Tamoxifen and breast cancer incidence among women with inherited mutations in BRCA1 and BRCA2: National Surgical Adjuvant Breast and Bowel Project (NSABP-P1) Breast Cancer Prevention Trial. JAMA 286:2251, 2001.

Little JB: Radiation carcinogenesis. Carcinogenesis 21:397, 2000.

Lehnert BE, Goodwin EH, Deshpande A: Extracellular factor(s) following exposure to alpha particles can cause sister chromatid exchanges in normal human cells. Cancer Res 57:2164, 1997.

Lists of IARC Evaluations, 2002, International Agency for Research on Cancer (IARC). Accessed April 15, 2003, from http://monographs.iarc.fr/monoeval/grlist.html.

Butel JS: Viral carcinogenesis: Revelation of molecular mechanisms and etiology of human disease. Carcinogenesis 21:405, 2000.

Smith RA, Cokkinides V, Eyre HJ: American Cancer Society guidelines for the early detection of cancer, 2003. CA Cancer J Clin 53:27, 2003.

Greene FL, Page DL, Fleming ID, et al (eds): AJCC Cancer Staging Manual, 6th ed. New York: Springer-Verlag, 2002, p 484.

10 | Transplantation

Abhinav Humar and David L. Dunn

The field of organ transplantation has made remarkable progress in a short period of time. From an experimental procedure just 50 years ago, transplantation has evolved to become the treatment of choice for end-stage organ failure resulting from almost any of a wide variety of causes. Transplantation of the kidney, liver, pancreas, intestine, heart, and lungs has now become commonplace in all parts of the world.

Definitions

Transplantation is the act of transferring an organ, tissue, or cell from one place to another. Broadly speaking, transplants are divided into three categories based on the similarity between the donor and the recipient: autotransplants, allotransplants, and xenotransplants. Autotransplants involve the transfer of tissue or organs from one part of an individual to another part of the same individual. They are the most common type of transplants and include skin grafts and vein grafts for bypasses. Because the donor and the recipient are the same person and no immunologic disparity exists, no immunosuppression is required. Allotransplants involve transfer from one individual to a different individual of the same species—the most common scenario for most solid organ transplants performed today. Immunosuppression is required for allograft recipients to prevent rejection. Finally, xenotransplants involve transfer across species barriers. Currently, xenotransplants are largely relegated to the laboratory, given the complex, potent immunologic barriers to success.

TRANSPLANT IMMUNOBIOLOGY

It was only after a basic understanding of transplant immunobiology was obtained could the obstacle of rejection posttransplant be overcome, thus making clinical transplants possible. The success of transplants today is due in large part to control of the rejection process, thanks to an ever-deepening understanding of the immune process triggered by a transplant.

The immune system is important not only in graft rejection, but also in the body's defense system against viral, bacterial, fungal, and other pathogens. It also helps prevent tumor growth and helps the body respond to shock and trauma. As with the body's reaction to an infection, graft rejection is triggered when specific cells of the transplant recipient, namely T and B lymphocytes, recognize foreign antigens.

Transplant Antigens

The main antigens involved in triggering rejection are coded for by a group of genes known as the major histocompatibility complex (MHC). These antigens and hence genes define the "foreign" nature of one individual to another within the same species. In humans, the MHC complex is known as the human leukocyte antigen (HLA) system. It comprises a series of genes located on chromosome 6.

In a nontransplant setting, the function of the HLA gene product is to present antigens as fragments of foreign proteins that can be recognized

216

by T lymphocytes. In the transplant setting, HLA molecules can initiate rejection and graft damage, via either humoral or cellular mechanisms. Humoral rejection occurs if the recipient has circulating antibodies specific to the donor's HLA from prior exposure (i.e., blood transfusion, previous transplant, or pregnancy), or if posttransplant, the recipient develops antibodies specific to the donor's HLA. The antibodies then bind to the donor's recognized foreign antigens, activating the complement cascade and leading to cell lysis. The blood group antigens of the ABO system, although not part of the HLA system, may also trigger this form of humoral rejection.

Cellular rejection is the more common type of rejection after organ transplants. Mediated by T lymphocytes, it results from their activation and proliferation after exposure to donor MHC molecules.

Allorecognition and Destruction

The recognition of foreign HLA antigens by the recipient T cells is referred to as allorecognition. This process may occur by either a direct or an indirect pathway. In the direct pathway, the recipient's T cells directly interact with donor HLA molecules, leading to the generation of activated cytotoxic T cells. In the indirect pathway, the recipient's own antigen-presenting cells (APCs) first process the donor's antigens (which may be shed from the parenchymal cells of the graft into the recipient's circulation, or alternatively may be encountered by the recipient's APCs in the graft itself); then the recipient's APCs present the donor's antigens to the recipient T cells, leading to the activation of those T cells.

Regardless of the method of presentation of foreign MHC, the subsequent steps are similar. Binding of the T cell to the foreign molecule occurs at the T-cell receptor (TCR)-CD3 complex on the surface of the lymphocyte. This binding leads to transduction of a signal to the cell, named signal 1. This signal by itself, however, is not sufficient to result in T-cell activation. Full activation requires transduction of a second signal that is not antigen-dependent. Signal 2 is provided by the binding of accessory molecules on the T cell to corresponding molecules (ligands) on the APC. An example is CD25 on the T lymphocytes binding with its ligand B7 on the surface of the APC. Transmission of signal 1 and 2 to the cell nucleus leads to interleukin-2 (IL-2) gene expression and to production of this important cytokine. IL-2 then permits the entire cascade of T-cell activation to proceed, leading to proliferation and differentiation of these cells into cells capable of causing damage to the graft.

T-cell activation is key in initiating the rejection process, but B-cell activation and antibody production also play a role. Foreign antigens are acquired by immunoglobulin receptors on the surface of B cells. These antigens are then processed similarly to the way that APCs process the donor's antigens. The antigen-presenting B cells can then interact with activated T-helper cells. This interaction leads to B-cell proliferation, differentiation into plasma cells, and to antibody production.

Clinical Rejection

Graft rejection is a complex process involving several components, including T lymphocytes, B lymphocytes, macrophages, and cytokines, with resultant local inflammatory injury and graft damage. Rejection can be classified into the following types based on timing and pathogenesis: hyperacute, acute, and chronic.

Hyperacute

This type of rejection, which usually occurs within min after the transplanted organ is reperfused, is because of the presence of preformed antibodies in the recipient, antibodies that are specific to the donor. These bind to the vascular endothelium in the graft and activate the complement cascade, leading to platelet activation and to diffuse intravascular coagulation. The result is a swollen, darkened graft, which undergoes ischemic necrosis.

Acute

This used to be the most common type of rejection, but with modern immunosuppression it is becoming less and less common. Acute rejection is usually seen within days to a few months posttransplant. It is predominantly a cell-mediated process, with lymphocytes being the main cells involved. With current immunosuppressive drugs, most acute rejection episodes are generally asymptomatic. They usually manifest with abnormal laboratory values (e.g., elevated creatinine in kidney transplant recipients, and elevated transaminase levels in liver transplant recipients).

Acute rejection episodes may also be mediated by a humoral, rather than cellular, immune response. B cells may generate antidonor antibodies, which can damage the graft. Establishing the diagnosis may be difficult, as biopsy may not demonstrate a significant cellular infiltrate; special immunologic stains may be necessary.

Chronic

This form of rejection occurs months to years posttransplant. Now that short-term graft survival rates have improved so markedly, chronic rejection is an increasingly common problem. Histologically, the process is characterized by atrophy, fibrosis, and arteriosclerosis. Both immune and nonimmune mechanisms are likely involved. Clinically, graft function slowly deteriorates over months to years.

CLINICAL IMMUNOSUPPRESSION

The success of modern transplantation is in large part because of the successful development of effective immunosuppressive agents. Over 15 agents are now approved in the United States by the Food and Drug Administration (FDA) for clinical immunosuppression (Table 10-1), with scores of others in various stages of clinical trials. Table 10-2 shows characteristics of some common immunosuppressive agents and their location of action.

Induction immunosuppression refers to the drugs administered immediately posttransplant to induce immunosuppression. Maintenance immunosuppression refers to the drugs administered to maintain immunosuppression once recipients have recovered from the operative procedure. Individual drugs can be categorized as either biologic or nonbiologic agents. Biologic agents consist of antibody preparations directed at various cells or receptors involved in the rejection process; they are generally used in induction (rather than maintenance) protocols. Nonbiologic agents form the mainstay of maintenance protocols.

TABLE 10-1 Immunosuppressive Drugs by Classification

Immunophilin binders
Calcineurin inhibitors Cyclosporine Tacrolimus (FK506) Noninhibitors of calcineurin Sirolimus (rapamycin)
Antimetabolites
Inhibitors of de novo purine synthesis Azathioprine Mycophenolate mofetil (MMF) Inhibitors of de novo pyrimidine synthesis Leflunomide
Biologic immunosuppression
Polyclonal antibodies ATGAM Thymoglobulin Monoclonal antibodies OKT3 IL-2R (humanized)
Others
Deoxyspergualin Corticosteroids FTY720

ATGAM = antithymocyte gamma-globulin; OKT3 = anti-CD3 monoclonal antibody; IL-2R = interleukin-2 receptor.

Nonbiologic Agents

Corticosteroids

Steroids have both antiinflammatory and immunosuppressive properties as the two are closely related. Their effects on the immune system are complex. Historically, corticosteroids represent the first family of drugs used for clinical immunosuppression. Today steroids remain an integral component of most immunosuppressive protocols, and often are the first-line agents in the treatment of acute rejection. Despite their proven benefit, steroids have significant side effects, especially with long-term use. Hence there has been considerable interest recently in withdrawing steroids from long-term maintenance protocols. The newer immunosuppressive agents may make doing so possible.

Azathioprine

An antimetabolite, azathioprine (AZA) is a derivative of 6-mercaptopurine, the active agent. Until the introduction of cyclosporine, it was the most widely used immunosuppressive drug, but now has become an adjunctive component of immunosuppressive drug regimens. With the introduction of newer agents, the use of AZA may be discontinued altogether.

AZA acts late in the immune process, affecting the cell cycle by interfering with DNA synthesis, thus suppressing proliferation of activated B and T lymphocytes. AZA is valuable in preventing the onset of acute rejection, but is not effective in the treatment of rejection episodes themselves.

TABLE 10-2 Characteristics of Common Immunosuppressive Drugs

Drug	Mechanism of action	Adverse effects	Clinical uses	Dosage
Cyclosporine	Binds to cyclophilin; inhibits calcineurin and IL-2 synthesis	Nephrotoxicity; tremor; hypertension; hirsutism	Improved bioavailability of microemulsion form; used as mainstay of maintenance protocols	Oral dose is 8 to 10 mg/kg/day (given in 2 divided doses)
Tacrolimus (FK506)	Binds to FKBPs; inhibits calcineurin and IL-2 synthesis	Nephrotoxicity; hypertension; neurotoxicity; GI toxicity (nausea, diarrhea)	Improved patient and graft survival in (liver) primary and rescue therapy; used as mainstay of maintenance, like cyclosporine	IV 0.05 to 0.1 mg/kg/day; PO 0.15 to 0.3 mg/kg/day (given q12h)
Mycophenolate mofetil (MMF)	Antimetabolite; inhibits enzyme necessary for de novo purine synthesis	Leukopenia; GI toxicity	Effective for primary and rescue therapy in kidney transplants; may replace azathioprine	1.0 g bid PO (may need 1.5 g in black recipients)
Sirolimus (rapamycin)	Inhibits lymphocyte effects driven by IL-2 receptor	Thrombocytopenia; increased serum cholesterol/LDL; vasculitis (animal studies)	May allow early withdrawal of steroids and decreased calcineurin doses	3 to 5 mg/day, adjusted to trough drug levels
Corticosteroids	Multiple actions; antiinflammatory; inhibit lympokine production	Cushingoid state; glucose intolerance; osteoporosis	Used in induction, maintenance, and treatment of acute rejection	Varies from milligrams to several grams per day; maintenance doses, 5 to 10 mg/day
Azathioprine (AZA)	Antimetabolite; interferes with DNA and RNA synthesis	Thrombocytopenia; neutropenia; liver dysfunction	Used in maintenance protocols	1 to 3 mg/kg/day for maintenance

bid = two times daily; FKBPs = FK506-binding proteins; GI = gastrointestinal; IL-2 = interleukin-2; LDL = low-density lipoproteins.

Cyclosporine

The introduction of cyclosporine in the early 1980s dramatically altered the field of transplantation. It significantly improved results after kidney transplants, but its greatest impact was on extrarenal transplants. When it was introduced, cyclosporine was the most specific immunosuppressive agent available. Currently, cyclosporine plays a central role in maintenance immunosuppression in almost all types of organ transplants.

Adverse effects of cyclosporine can be classified as renal or nonrenal. Nephrotoxicity is the most important and troubling adverse effect of cyclosporine. Cyclosporine has a vasoconstrictor effect on the renal vasculature. This vasoconstriction (likely a transient, reversible, and dose-dependent phenomenon) may cause early posttransplant graft dysfunction or may exaggerate existing poor graft function. Also, long-term cyclosporine use may result in interstitial fibrosis of the renal parenchyma, coupled with arteriolar lesions. The exact mechanism is unknown, but renal failure may eventually result.

A number of nonrenal side effects may also be seen with the use of cyclosporine. Cosmetic complications, most commonly hirsutism and gingival hyperplasia, may result in considerable distress, possibly leading to noncompliant behavior, especially in adolescents and women. Several neurologic complications, including headaches, tremor, and seizures, also have been reported. Other nonrenal side effects include hyperlipidemia, hepatotoxicity, and hyperuricemia.

Tacrolimus

Tacrolimus (FK506) is a metabolite of the soil fungus Streptomyces tsukubaensi, found in Japan. Released in the United States in April 1994 for use in liver transplantation, it is currently used in a fashion similar to cyclosporine. Tacrolimus, like cyclosporine, is a calcineurin inhibitor and has a very similar mechanism of action.

Adverse effects of tacrolimus and cyclosporine are similar. The most common problems include nephrotoxicity, neurotoxicity, impaired glucose metabolism, hypertension, infection, and gastrointestinal (GI) disturbances. Nephrotoxicity is dose-related and reversible with dose reduction. Neurotoxicity seen with tacrolimus ranges from mild symptoms (tremors, insomnia, and headaches) to more severe events (seizures and coma); it is usually related to high levels and resolves with dose reduction. These side effects are most common early posttransplant and subsequently tend to decrease in incidence.

Sirolimus

A macrolide antibiotic derived from a soil actinomycete originally found on Easter Island (Rapa Nui), sirolimus (previously known as rapamycin) is structurally similar to tacrolimus and binds to the same immunophilin (FKBP). Unlike tacrolimus, it does not affect calcineurin activity.

To date, sirolimus has been used in a variety of combinations and situations. It is most commonly used in conjunction with one of the calcineurin inhibitors. In such combinations, sirolimus is usually used to help withdraw or avoid the use of steroids completely in maintenance immunosuppressive regimens. It also has been used as an alternative to tacrolimus or cyclosporine, as part of a calcineurin-sparing protocol. The advantage of this type of protocol is that it is not associated with long-term nephrotoxicity (as may be seen with the calcineurin agents). Hence, sirolimus may prove to be better for long-term preservation of renal function in transplant recipients.

The major side effects of sirolimus include neutropenia, thrombocytopenia, and a significant elevation of the serum triglyceride and cholesterol levels. It also has been associated with impaired wound healing, leading to a higher incidence of wound-related complications.

Mycophenolate Mofetil

Mycophenolate mofetil (MMF) was approved in May 1995 by the FDA for use in the prevention of acute rejection after kidney transplants. It has since been rapidly incorporated into routine clinical practice at many centers as part of maintenance regimens. It works by inhibiting inosine monophosphate dehydrogenase, which is a crucial, rate-limiting enzyme in de novo synthesis of purines. The net result is a selective, reversible antiproliferative effect on T and B lymphocytes.

MMF differs from cyclosporine, tacrolimus, and sirolimus in that it does not affect cytokine production or the events immediately after antigen recognition. Rather, MMF works further distally in the chain of activation events to prevent proliferation of the stimulated T cell. Like AZA, it is an antimetabolite; unlike AZA, its impact is selective: it only affects lymphocytes, not neutrophils or platelets. In several clinical trials, it has proven to be more effective than AZA, and has largely replaced it.

The incidence and types of adverse events with MMF are similar to those seen with AZA. Notable exceptions are GI side effects (diarrhea, gastritis, and vomiting), which are more common with MMF. Clinically significant leukopenia also is more common, affecting about one third of recipients.

Biologic Agents

Polyclonal antibodies directed against lymphocytes have been used in clinical transplantation since the 1960s. Monoclonal antibody techniques, developed later, allowed in turn for the development of biologic agents (such as OKT3) targeted to specific subsets of cells. A number of different monoclonal antibodies (MABs) are currently under development or have been recently approved for use in clinical transplantation. Many are directed against functional secreted molecules of the immune system or their receptors, rather than against actual groups of cells.

Polyclonal Antibodies

Polyclonal antibodies are produced by immunizing animals (such as horses, goats, or rabbits) with human lymphoid tissue, allowing for an immune response, removing the resultant immune sera, and purifying the sera in an effort to remove unwanted antibodies. What remain are antibodies that will recognize human lymphocytes.

After administration of these antibodies into a transplant recipient, the total lymphocyte count should fall. Lymphocytes, especially T cells, are either lysed after antibody binding and complement deposition at the cell surface, inactivated by binding to T-cell receptors, or are cleared from the circulation and deposited into the reticuloendothelial system. Currently available polyclonal preparations include antithymocyte globulin (obtained by immunizing horses with human thymocytes) and thymoglobulin (obtained by immunizing rabbits with human thymocytes).

Monoclonal Antibodies

MABs are produced by the hybridization of murine antibody-secreting B lymphocytes with a nonantibody-secreting myeloma cell line. A number of MABs have been produced that are active against different stages of the immune response. OKT3 remains the most commonly used MAB, but the last few years have seen the introduction of a number of "humanized" MABs (genetically engineered to possess large domains of human antibody while retaining the murine antigen binding site), which have a significantly lower potential for toxicity than OKT3.

OKT3 is highly effective and versatile. Most commonly, it is used to treat severe acute rejection episodes (i.e., those resistant to steroids). OKT3 also has been used as prophylaxis against rejection, as induction therapy, and as primary rejection treatment.

Significant, even life-threatening adverse effects may be seen after OKT3 administration, most commonly immediately after one of the first several doses. Such effects may occur when cytokines (such as tumor necrosis factor, IL-2, and γ-interferon) are released by T cells from the circulation. The most common symptoms are fever, chills, and headaches. The most serious side effect of OKT3 is a rapidly developing, noncardiogenic pulmonary edema; the risk of this side effect significantly increases if the patient is fluid-overloaded at the time of OKT3 treatment. Other serious side effects include encephalopathy, aseptic meningitis, and nephrotoxicity.

Several other monoclonal antibodies (MABs) targeting different steps of the immune process are available for clinical use. As noted, IL-2 is an important cytokine necessary for the proliferation of cytotoxic T cells. Two MABs are currently approved to target the IL-2 receptor (IL-2R): basiliximab and dacluzimab. Both are humanized products and therefore are not associated with significant first-dose reactions or drug-specific adverse events. They have been proven effective as induction agents, decreasing the incidence of acute rejection in kidney transplant recipients when compared to placebo in clinical trials. They have not been used to treat established acute rejection. More recently, alemtuzumab, a MAB directed against the CD52 antigen found on B and T cells, has been used, usually as an induction agent.

Organ Procurement and Preservation

The biggest problem facing transplant centers today is the shortage of organ donors. Mechanisms that might increase the number of available organs include: (1) optimizing the current donor pool (e.g., the use of multiple organ donors or marginal donors); (2) increasing the number of living-donor transplants (e.g., the use of living unrelated donors); (3) using unconventional and controversial donor sources (e.g., using deceased donors without cardiac activity or anencephalic donors); and (4) performing xenotransplants.

Deceased Donors

Most extrarenal transplants performed today, and roughly one half of all renal transplants, are from deceased donors. These donors are deceased individuals who meet the criteria for brain death, but whose organs are being perfused by life-support measures, allowing adequate time for referral to an organ procurement organization. A member of that organization can then ascertain whether donation is possible, and if so, approach the potential donor's family and possibly obtain consent to procure suitable organs.

Once the diagnosis of brain death has been established, the process of organ donation can be initiated. The focus then switches from the treatment of elevated intracranial pressure to preserving organ function and optimizing peripheral oxygen delivery. It is important to keep in mind that management of the deceased organ donor is an active process, requiring aggressive monitoring and intervention to ensure that perfusion to the organs of interest is not compromised.

Living Donors

Living-donor transplantation is unique in that surgeons commonly operate on a healthy individual (i.e., a living donor) who has no medical disorders and does not require an operation. The use of living donors is an integral and important part of the field of transplantation today. But living-donor transplants pose a unique set of medical, ethical, financial, and psychosocial problems that must be dealt with by the transplant team.

The use of living donors offers numerous advantages. Primary is the availability of a life-saving organ. A certain percentage of transplant candidates die while waiting for a deceased donor organ as a direct result of a complication, or of progression of their underlying disease. For such ill candidates, the advantage of a living donor is obvious. Even for candidates who would receive a deceased donor organ, a living-donor transplant may significantly shorten the waiting time. A shorter waiting time generally implies a healthier candidate—one whose body has not been ravaged by prolonged end-stage organ failure. Lastly, long-term results may be superior with living-donor transplants, which is certainly the case with kidney transplants.

The disadvantages of a living-donor transplant for the potential recipient are minimal. With some organ transplants (e.g., living donor liver or lung) the procedure may be more technically complex, resulting in an increased incidence of surgical complications. However, this disadvantage is offset by numerous advantages. The major disadvantage is to the donor. Medically, there is no possibility of benefit for the donor, only potential for harm. The risk of death associated with donation depends on the organ being removed. For nephrectomy, the mortality risk is estimated to be less than 0.05 percent. However, for partial hepatectomy, it is about 0.5 percent. Risks for surgical and medical complications also depend on the procedure being performed. Additionally, long-term complications or problems may be associated with partial loss of organ function through donation.

The kidney, the first organ to be used for living-donor transplants, is the most common type of organ donated by living donors today. Potential donors are first evaluated to ensure that they have normal renal function with two equally functioning kidneys and that they do not have any significant risk factors for developing renal disease (e.g., hypertension or diabetes). The anatomy of their kidneys and the vasculature can be determined by using various radiologic imaging techniques. Nephrectomy can be performed through a flank incision, by an anterior retroperitoneal approach, or by a laparoscopic technique. With the laparoscopic technique, an intraperitoneal approach is used.

Living-donor liver transplants have been performed for almost 15 years. Initially, they involved adult donors and pediatric recipients. In such cases, the left lateral segment of the donor's liver is resected. Inflow to the graft occurs via the donor's left hepatic artery and left portal vein; outflow is via the left hepatic vein. For adult recipients, a larger piece of the liver is required; usually the right lobe is chosen. The risks for living liver donors are higher than those for living kidney donors. The risks are also generally higher for right lobe donors than for left lateral segment donors. The most worrisome complication for living liver donors is a bile leak, either from the cut surface of the liver or from the bile duct stump.

Living-donor transplants with organs besides the kidney and liver are not as common, but are performed at various centers. Living-donor pancreas transplants involve a distal pancreatectomy, with the graft consisting of the body and tail of the pancreas; vascular inflow and outflow are provided by the splenic artery and splenic vein. Living-donor intestinal transplants usually involve removal of about 200 cm of the donor's ileum, with inflow and outflow provided by the ileocolic vessels. Living-donor lung transplants involve removal of one lobe of one lung from each of two donors; both grafts are then transplanted into the recipient.

Preservation

Organ preservation methods have played an important role in the success of cadaver donor transplants. They have resulted in improved graft function immediately posttransplant and have diminished the incidence of primary nonfunction of organs. By prolonging the allowable cold ischemia times, they have also allowed for better organ allocation and for safer transplants.

The most common methods involve the use of hypothermia and pharmacologic inhibition to slow down metabolic processes in the organ once it has been removed from the deceased donor. Hypothermia very effectively slows down enzymatic reactions and metabolic activity, allowing the cell to make its limited energy reserves last much longer. Cold storage solutions have been developed to improve organ preservation by ameliorating some of the detrimental effects of hypothermia alone. Essentially, these solutions suppress hypothermia-induced cellular swelling and minimize the loss of potassium from the cell.

The most commonly used fluid worldwide is the University of Wisconsin solution. It contains lactobionate, raffinose, and hydroxyethyl starch. Lactobionate is impermeable and prevents intracellular swelling; it also lowers the concentration of intracellular calcineurin and free iron, which may be beneficial in reducing reperfusion injury. Hydroxyethyl starch, a synthetic colloid, may help decrease hypothermia-induced cell swelling of endothelial cells and reduce interstitial edema.

Although cold preservation has improved cadaver donor transplant results, the amount of time that an organ can be safely preserved is limited. After that, the incidence of organ nonfunction starts to increase. With kidneys, exceeding the preservation time limit results in delayed graft function, requiring dialysis support for the recipient until function improves. With livers, the result is primary nonfunction, requiring an urgent retransplant. How long an organ can be safely preserved depends on the type of organ and on the condition of the donor. With kidneys, cold ischemic times should be kept below 36–40 h; after that, delayed graft function significantly increases. With pancreata, more than 24 h of ischemia increases problems because of pancreatitis and duodenal leaks. With livers, more than 16 h of ischemia increases the risk for primary nonfunction and biliary complications. Hearts and lungs tolerate preservation poorly; ideally, ischemia times should be below 6 h. With marginal donors, all of these times should be adjusted further downward.

KIDNEY TRANSPLANTATION

A kidney transplant now represents the treatment of choice for patients with end-stage renal disease (ESRD). It offers the greatest potential for restoring a healthy, productive life in most such patients. Compared with dialysis, it is associated with better patient survival and superior quality of life, and is more cost-effective.

Preoperative Evaluation

Very few absolute contraindications to kidney transplants exist. Therefore, most patients with ESRD should be considered as potential transplant candidates. However, the surgery and general anesthesia impose a significant cardiovascular stress. Subsequent lifelong immunosuppression also is associated with some risk. Pretransplant evaluation should identify any factors that would contraindicate a transplant or any risk factors that could be minimized pretransplant.

The preoperative evaluation can be divided into four parts: medical, surgical, immunologic, and psychosocial. The purpose of the medical evaluation is to identify risk factors for the surgical procedure. Mortality posttransplant usually is because of underlying cardiovascular disease, so a detailed cardiac evaluation is necessary. Untreated malignancy and active infection are absolute contraindications to a transplant, because of the requisite lifelong immunosuppression. After curative treatment of malignancy, an interval of 2–5 years is recommended pretransplant. The medical evaluation also should concentrate on GI problems such as peptic ulcer disease, symptomatic cholelithiasis, and hepatitis. Patients who demonstrate serologic evidence of hepatitis C or B, but without evidence of active hepatic inflammation or cirrhosis, are acceptable transplant candidates.

The surgical evaluation should identify vascular or urologic abnormalities that may contraindicate or complicate a transplant. Evidence of vascular disease that is revealed by the history (claudication or rest pain) or the physical examination (diminished or absent pulse or bruit) should be evaluated further by Doppler studies or angiography. Urologic evaluation should exclude chronic infection in the native kidney, which may require nephrectomy pretransplant. Other indications for nephrectomy include huge polycystic kidneys, significant vesicoureteral reflux, or uncontrollable renovascular hypertension.

The immunologic evaluation involves determining blood type, tissue type (HLA-A, -B, or -DR antigens), and presence of any cytotoxic antibodies against HLA antigens (because of prior transplants, blood transfusions, or pregnancies). If a living-donor transplant is planned, a cross-match should be performed early on during the initial evaluation.

The psychosocial evaluation is necessary to ensure that transplant candidates understand the nature of the transplant procedure and its attendant risk. They must be capable of rigorously adhering to the medical regimen posttransplant. Patients who have not been compliant with their medical regimen in the past must demonstrate a willingness and capability to do so before they undergo the transplant.

One important aspect of the preoperative evaluation is the search for and evaluation of potential living donors. Living-donor kidney recipients enjoy improved long-term success, avoid a prolonged wait, and are able to plan the timing of their transplant in advance. Moreover, they have a significantly decreased incidence of ATN and increased potential for HLA matching. As a result, living-donor transplants generally have better short- and long-term results, as compared with cadaver donor transplants. Of course, the risks to the living donor must be acceptably low. The donor must be fully aware of potential risks and must freely give informed consent. The search for a living donor should not be restricted to immediate family members. Results with living, unrelated donors are comparable to those with living, related (non-HLA-identical) donors.

Surgical Procedure

The transplanted kidney is usually placed in a heterotopic position, with no need for native nephrectomy except in select circumstances. Retroperitoneal placement is preferred, to allow for easy access for percutaneous renal biopsy. With the standard approach, the dissection is extraperitoneal. The iliac vessels are identified and assessed for suitability for anastomosis. The internal iliac artery can be used as the inflow vessel, with an end-to-end anastomosis, or the external iliac artery can be used with an end-to-side anastomosis. To minimize the risk of lymphocele formation after surgery, only a modest length of artery is dissected free and the lymphatics overlying the artery are ligated. The donor renal vein is anastomosed end to side to the external iliac vein.

After the vascular anastomosis is completed and the kidney perfused, urinary continuity can be restored by a number of well-described techniques. The important principles are to attach the ureter to the bladder mucosa in a tension-free manner and to cover the distal 1 cm of the ureter with a submucosal tunnel, thus protecting against reflux during voiding.

Early Postoperative Care

The immediate postoperative care of all recipients involves (1) stabilizing the major organ systems (e.g., cardiovascular, pulmonary, and renal); (2) evaluating graft function; (3) achieving adequate immunosuppression; and (4) monitoring and treating complications directly and indirectly related to the transplant.

Careful attention to fluid and electrolyte management is crucial. In general, recipients should be kept euvolemic or slightly hypervolemic. If initial graft function is good, fluid replacement can be regulated by hourly replacement of urine. Half-normal saline is a good solution to use for urine replacement. Aggressive replacement of electrolytes, including calcium, magnesium, and potassium, may be necessary, especially for recipients undergoing brisk diuresis. Those with acute tubular necrosis (ATN) and fluid overload or hyperkalemia may need fluid restriction and even hemodialysis. Magnesium levels should be kept above 2 mEq/L to prevent seizures, and phosphate levels kept between 2 and 5 mEq/L for proper support of the respiratory and alimentary tracts.

A critical aspect of postoperative care is the repeated evaluation of graft function, which in fact begins intraoperatively, soon after the kidney is reperfused. Signs of good kidney function include appropriate color and texture, along with evidence of urine production. Postoperatively, urine output is the most readily available and easily measured indicator of graft function. Urine volume may range from none (anuria) to large quantities (polyuria). When using posttransplant urine volume to monitor graft function, the clinician must have at least some knowledge of the recipient's pretransplant urine volume, if any. Laboratory values of obvious use in assessing graft function include serum blood urea nitrogen (BUN) and creatinine levels.

Recipients can be divided into three groups (by initial graft function as indicated by their urine output and serum creatinine) as those with: (1) immediate graft function (IGF), characterized by a brisk diuresis posttransplant and rapidly falling serum creatinine level; (2) slow graft function (SGF), characterized by a moderate degree of kidney dysfunction posttransplant, with modest amounts of urine and a slowly falling creatinine level, but no need for dialysis at any time posttransplant; and (3) delayed graft function (DGF), which represents the far end of the spectrum of posttransplant graft dysfunction and is defined by the need for dialysis posttransplant.

Decreased or minimal urine output is a frequent concern posttransplant. Most commonly, it is because of an alteration in volume status. Other causes include a blocked urinary catheter, vascular thrombosis, a urinary leak or obstruction, early acute rejection, drug toxicity, or DGF. Early diagnosis is important, and begins with an assessment of the recipient's volume status. The urinary catheter is checked to exclude the presence of occlusion with clots or debris. Other diagnostic tests that may be warranted, on the suspected cause, include a Doppler ultrasound, nuclear medicine scan, or a biopsy.

Complications

Monitoring for potential surgical and medical complications is important. Early diagnosis and appropriate intervention can minimize the detrimental impact on the graft and recipient. Potential complications that may occur early after surgery include hemorrhage, vascular complications, urologic complications, lymphocele, and several others.

Bleeding is uncommon after a kidney transplant; it usually occurs from unligated vessels in the graft hilum or from the retroperitoneum of the recipient. A falling hematocrit level, hypotension, or tachycardia should all raise the possibility of bleeding. Surgical exploration is seldom required because bleeding often tamponades. Vascular complications can involve the donor vessels (renal artery thrombosis or stenosis, renal vein thrombosis), the recipient vessels (iliac artery thrombosis, pseudoaneurysms, and deep venous thrombosis), or both. Renal artery thrombosis usually occurs early posttransplant; it is uncommon, with an incidence of less than 1 percent. However, it is a devastating complication, usually resulting in graft loss. Diagnosis is easily made with color flow Doppler studies. Urgent thrombectomy is indicated, but most such grafts cannot be salvaged and require removal. Renal vein thrombosis is not as common as its arterial counterpart, but again, graft loss is the usual end result. Causes include angulation or torsion of the vein, compression by hematomas or lymphoceles, anastomotic stenosis, and extension of an underlying deep venous thrombosis. Again, Doppler studies are the best diagnostic test. Urgent thrombectomy is rarely successful, and nephrectomy is usually required.

Urinary tract complications, manifesting as leakage or obstruction, generally occur in 2–10 percent of kidney recipients. The underlying cause is often related to poor blood supply and ischemia of the transplant ureter. Leakage most commonly occurs from the anastomotic site. Causes other than ischemia include undue tension created by a short ureter, and direct surgical injury. Presentation is usually early (before the fifth posttransplant week); symptoms include fever, pain, swelling at the graft site, increased creatinine level, decreased urine output, and cutaneous urinary drainage. Early surgical explo-ration with ureteral re-implantation is usually indicated, although small leaks may be managed by percutaneous nephrostomy and stent placement with good results.

The reported incidence of lymphoceles (fluid collections of lymph that gen-erally result from cut lymphatic vessels in the recipient) is 0.6–18 percent. Lymphoceles usually do not occur until at least two weeks posttransplant. Symptoms are generally related to the mass effect and compression of nearby structures (e.g., ureter, iliac vein, allograft renal artery), and patients develop hypertension, unilateral leg swelling on the side of the transplant, and elevated serum creatinine. The standard surgical treatment is creation of a peritoneal window to allow for drainage of the lymphatic fluid into the peritoneal cavity where it can be absorbed. Either a laparoscopic or an open approach may be used. Another option is percutaneous insertion of a drainage catheter, with or without sclerotherapy.

Late Posttransplant Care

The goal of late posttransplant care of the kidney transplant recipient is to op-timize immunosuppression, carefully monitor graft function, and screen and monitor for complications that are directly or indirectly related to immunosup-pressive medications. Optimizing immunosuppression entails fitting it to the individual recipient's needs. Recipients at low risk for rejection should have their immunosuppression lowered to minimize side effects and complications. Careful attention should be paid to compliance; it is often easy for recipients to become less attentive to their medications as they progress through the post-transplant period. Monitoring kidney function may help detect noncompliance, but is also important to detect late rejection episodes, recurrence of disease, or late technical problems (such as renal artery stenosis or ureteric stricture). Other potential problems in these recipients include hypercholesterolemia, hypertriglyceridemia, and increased blood pressure, which may or may not be related to the immunosuppressive drugs. Screening for malignancy (especially skin, colorectal, breast, cervical, and prostate) is important, although the inci-dence of many of these malignancies is equivalent to those seen in the general population.

PANCREAS TRANSPLANTATION

Diabetes mellitus is a very common medical condition with immense med-ical, social, and financial costs. In North America, it is the leading cause of kidney failure, blindness, nontraumatic amputations, and impotence. A suc-cessful pancreas transplant can establish normoglycemia and insulin indepen-dence in diabetic recipients, with glucose control similar to that seen with a functioning native pancreas. A pancreas transplant also has the potential to halt progression of some secondary complications of diabetes. No current method of exogenous insulin administration can produce a euglycemic, insulin-independent state akin to that achievable with a technically successful pancreas graft.

Currently, the main drawback of a pancreas transplant is the need for im-munosuppression. Pancreas transplants are now preferentially performed in diabetic patients with kidney failure who also are candidates for a kidney transplant, as they already require immunosuppression to prevent kidney rejec-tion. However, a pancreas transplant alone (PTA) is appropriate for nonuremic diabetics if their day-to-day quality of life is so poor (e.g., labile serum glucose with ketoacidosis and/or hypoglycemic episodes, or progression of severe diabetic retinopathy, nephropathy, neuropathy, and/or enteropathy) that chronic immunosuppression is justified to achieve insulin independence.

Preoperative Evaluation

The preoperative evaluation for pancreas transplant recipients does not differ substantially from that for diabetic kidney transplant recipients. Examination of the cardiovascular system is most important because significant coronary artery disease may be present. Noninvasive testing may not identify coronary artery disease, so coronary angiography is routinely performed. Detailed neurologic, ophthalmologic, metabolic, and kidney function testing may be needed to assess the degree of progression of secondary complications. A thorough evaluation of the peripheral vascular system is essential, given the high incidence of peripheral vascular disease in diabetics.

Once a patient is determined to be a good candidate for a pancreas transplant, with no obvious contraindications, it is important to decide which type of pancreas transplant is best for that individual. First, the degree of kidney dysfunction and the need for a kidney transplant must be determined. Patients with stable kidney function (creatinine less than 2.0 mg/dL and minimal protein in the urine) are candidates for a PTA. However, patients with moderate kidney insufficiency will likely require a kidney transplant as well; further deterioration of kidney function often occurs once calcineurin inhibitors are started for immunosuppression.

For patients requiring both a kidney and a pancreas transplant, various options are available. The two transplants can be performed either simultaneously or sequentially. A living donor or a deceased donor can be used, or both. Which option is best for the individual patient depends on the degree of kidney dysfunction, the availability of donors, and personal preference. The following options are currently possible:

1. Deceased-donor, simultaneous pancreas-kidney transplant (SPK): The most common option worldwide, deceased-donor SPK transplants have well-documented long-term survival results for both the kidney and the pancreas grafts.
2. Living-donor kidney transplant, followed weeks to months later by a deceased-donor pancreas transplant (pancreas after kidney [PAK] transplant): If a living donor is available for the kidney transplant, then this is a good option for uremic diabetic patients. It offers the possibility of performing the kidney transplant as soon as the living-donor evaluation is complete, rendering the recipient dialysis-free within a short period.
3. Simultaneous deceased-donor pancreas and living-donor kidney (SPLK) transplant: Candidates with a suitable living donor for the kidney transplant who have not yet progressed to dialysis can be placed on the deceased-donor pancreas transplant waiting list. When a deceased-donor pancreas becomes available, the living donor for the kidney is called in at the same time, and both procedures are performed simultaneously.
4. Living-donor, simultaneous pancreas-kidney transplant: If a single individual is suitable to donate both a kidney and a hemipancreas, then this potential option exists.

Surgical Procedure

The initial preparation of the donor pancreas is a crucial component of a successful transplant. Direct physical examination of the pancreas often is the best or only way to confirm its suitability. If it is sclerotic, calcific, or markedly discolored, it should not be used. Before implantation, a surgical procedure is undertaken to remove the spleen and any excess duodenum and to ligate blood vessels at the root of the mesentery. The inflow vessels to the graft are the splenic and superior mesenteric arteries; outflow is via the portal vein. Arterial reconstruction is performed before implanting the graft in the recipient. The donor superior mesenteric and splenic arteries are connected, most commonly using a reversed segment of donor iliac artery as a Y-graft. The pancreas graft is then implanted via an anastomosis of the aforementioned arterial graft to the recipient common iliac artery or distal aorta, and, via a venous anastomosis of the donor portal vein to the recipient iliac vein (for systemic drainage), or to the superior mesenteric vein (for portal drainage).

Once the pancreas is revascularized, a drainage procedure must be performed to handle the pancreatic exocrine secretions. Options include anastomosing the donor duodenum to the recipient bladder or to the small bowel, with the small bowel either in continuity or connected to a Roux-en-Y limb. Both enteric drainage and bladder drainage now have a relatively low surgical risk. The main advantage of bladder drainage is the ability to directly measure enzyme activity in the pancreatic graft exocrine secretions by measuring the amount of amylase in the urine. The leak rate is the same whether the pancreas is drained to the bladder or to the bowel, but the consequences of a bladder leak are much less severe than those associated with a bowel leak. The disadvantages of bladder drainage include complications such as dehydration and acidosis (from loss of alkalotic pancreatic secretions in the urine), and local problems with the bladder such as infection, hematuria, stones, and urethritis.

Postoperative Care

In general, pancreas recipients do not require intensive care monitoring in the postoperative period. Laboratory values—serum glucose, hemoglobin, electrolytes, and amylase—are monitored daily. The serum glucose level is monitored even more frequently if normoglycemia is not immediately achieved. Nasogastric suction and IV fluids are continued for the first several days until bowel function returns. In the early postoperative period, regular insulin is infused to maintain plasma glucose levels less than 150 mg/dL, because chronic hyperglycemia may be detrimental to beta cells.

Complications

One crucial aspect of posttransplant care is monitoring for rejection and complications (both surgical and medical). Rejection episodes may be identified by an increase in serum creatinine (in SPK recipients), a decrease in urinary amylase (in recipients with bladder drainage), an increase in serum amylase, or by an increase in serum glucose levels. Unfortunately, complications are common after pancreas transplants. The pancreas graft is susceptible to a unique set of complications because of its exocrine secretions and low blood flow. Potential complications include:

Thrombosis

The incidence of thrombosis is approximately 6 percent for pancreas transplants reported to the UNOS registry. Low-dose heparin, dextran, or antiplatelet agents are administered routinely in the early postoperative period at many centers, although these agents slightly increase the risk of postoperative bleeding. Treatment consists of graft removal.

Hemorrhage

Postoperative bleeding may be minimized by meticulous intraoperative control of bleeding sites. Hemorrhage may be exacerbated by anticoagulants and antiplatelet drugs, but their benefits seem to outweigh the risks. Bleeding is a much less significant cause (<1 percent) of graft loss than is thrombosis, according to United Network for Organs Sharing (UNOS) registry data. Significant bleeding is treated by immediate re-exploration.

Pancreatitis

Most cases of graft pancreatitis occur early, tend to be self-limited, and are probably because of ischemic preservation injury. Clinical manifestations may include graft tenderness and fever, to hyperamylasemia. Treatment consists of intravenous (IV) fluid replacement and keeping the recipient fasting.

Urologic Complications

Urologic complications are almost exclusively limited to recipients with bladder drainage. Hematuria is not uncommon in the first several months posttransplant, but it is usually transient and self-limiting. Bladder calculi may develop because exposed sutures or staples along the duodenocystostomy serve as a nidus for stone formation. Recurrent urinary tract infections commonly occur concurrently. Urinary leaks, most commonly from the proximal duodenal cuff or from the duodenal anastomosis to the bladder, typically occur during the first several weeks posttransplant. Small leaks can be successfully managed by prolonged (at least 2 weeks) urinary catheter drainage; larger leaks require surgical intervention.

Infections

Infections remain a significant problem after pancreas transplants. Most common are superficial wound infections and intraabdominal infections, often related to graft complications such as leaks. Thanks to appropriate perioperative antimicrobial regimens (for prophylaxis against gram-positive bacteria, gram-negative bacteria, and yeast) the incidence of significant infections has decreased.

Results

The International Pancreas Transplant Registry (IPTR) maintains data on pancreas transplants. The results (particularly as measured by long-term insulin independence) have continually improved over time. Patient survival rates are not significantly different between the three main recipient categories and are greater than 90 percent at 3 years posttransplant. Most deaths are because of preexisting cardiovascular disease; the mortality risk of a pancreas transplant per se is extremely low (e.g., patient survival at 1 year for PTA recipients is >95 percent). Pancreas graft survival rates at 1 year remain higher in the SPK (approximately 90 percent) than in the PAK (approximately 85 percent) and PTA (approximately 75 percent) categories, according to IPTR data.

Islet Cell Transplantation

The pancreas consists of two separate functional systems (endocrine and exocrine), but it is only the endocrine component that is of use in the transplant process. However, many of the complications seen with whole-organ pancreas transplants are because of the exocrine component. Therefore, the concept of transplanting simply the cells responsible for the production of insulin is very logical and attractive.

Islet cell transplantation involves extracting islets of Langerhans from a donor's pancreas and then injecting them into a diabetic recipient. These islet cells then engraft into the recipient and secrete insulin, providing excellent moment-to-moment control of blood glucose, as is seen with a whole-organ pancreas transplant. Compared with exogenous insulin injections, an islet cell transplant offers advantages similar to those of a whole-organ pancreas transplant. A successful islet transplant provides perfect glucose homeostasis, freeing the diabetic patient from the burden of frequent glucose monitoring and insulin injections. It potentially prevents secondary complications of diabetes and significantly improves quality of life.

Unlike a whole-organ pancreas transplant, an islet cell transplant is not a major surgical procedure. It can generally be performed as an outpatient procedure, with minimal recovery time for the recipient. It avoids a major surgical procedure, with its associated mortality and morbidity. Given this significantly lower surgical risk, islet cell transplants could theoretically have much wider application than whole-organ transplants.

One major disadvantage of an islet cell transplant (similar to that of a whole-organ transplant) is the need for long-term immunosuppression. This disadvantage has limited the use of islet cell transplants to patients with kidney failure who require immunosuppression because of a kidney transplant.

Islet cell transplants have been a possibility for many years, but the results have generally been poor. In 1995, a report of the International Islet Transplant Registry indicated that of 270 recipients, only 5 percent were insulin-independent at 1 year posttransplant. Recently, however, significantly improved results have been reported by using steroid-free immunosuppression and islet injections from multiple donors. These recent successes have stimulated a flurry of islet transplant activity at centers across the world. As results are likely to continue to improve, it is possible that islet cell transplants may come to replace whole-organ pancreas transplants.

LIVER TRANSPLANTATION

The field of liver transplantation has undergone remarkable advances in the last two decades. An essentially experimental procedure in the early 1980s, a liver transplant is now the treatment of choice for patients with acute and chronic liver failure. Patient survival at 1 year posttransplant has increased from 30 percent in the early 1980s to more than 85 percent at present. The major reasons for this dramatic increase include refined surgical and preservation techniques, better immunosuppressive protocols, more effective treatment of infections, and improved care during the critical perioperative period. However, a liver transplant remains a major undertaking, with the potential for complications affecting every major organ system.

Preoperative Evaluation

A liver transplant is indicated for liver failure, whether acute or chronic. Liver failure is signaled by a number of clinical symptoms (e.g., ascites, variceal bleeding, hepatic encephalopathy, and malnutrition), and by biochemical liver test results that suggest impaired hepatic synthetic function (e.g., hypoalbuminemia, hyperbilirubinemia, and coagulopathy). The cause of liver failure often influences its presentation. For example, patients with acute liver failure generally have hepatic encephalopathy and coagulopathy, whereas patients with chronic liver disease most commonly have ascites, GI bleeding, and malnutrition.

A host of diseases are potentially treatable by a liver transplant. Broadly, they can be categorized as acute or chronic, and then subdivided by the cause of the liver disease. Chronic liver diseases account for the majority of liver transplants today. The most common cause in North America is chronic hepatitis, usually because of hepatitis C and less commonly to hepatitis B. Chronic alcohol abuse accelerates the process, especially with hepatitis C. Cholestatic disorders also account for a significant percentage of transplant candidates with chronic liver disease. In adults, the most common causes are primary biliary cirrhosis (PBC) and primary sclerosing cholangitis (PSC). A variety of metabolic diseases can result in progressive, chronic liver injury and cirrhosis, including hereditary hemochromatosis, alpha1-antitrypsin deficiency, and Wilson's disease. Hepatocellular carcinoma (HCC) may be a complication of cirrhosis from any cause, most commonly with hepatitis B, hepatitis C, hemochromatosis, and tyrosinemia.

Acute liver disease, more commonly termed fulminant hepatic failure (FHF), is defined as the development of hepatic encephalopathy and profound coagulopathy shortly after the onset of symptoms, such as jaundice, in patients without preexisting liver disease. The most common causes include acetaminophen overdose, acute hepatitis B infection, various drugs and hepatotoxins, and Wilson disease; often, however, no cause is identified.

Indications for Transplant

The presence of chronic liver disease alone with established cirrhosis is not an indication for a transplant. Some patients have well-compensated cirrhosis with a low expectant mortality. Patients with decompensated cirrhosis, however, have a poor prognosis without transplant. The signs and symptoms of decompensated cirrhosis include: hepatic encephalopathy (HE), ascites, spontaneous bacterial peritonitis (SBP), portal hypertensive bleeding, hepatorenal syndrome (HRS), and other signs and symptoms such as severe weakness and fatigue.

Generally, FHF patients are more acutely ill than chronic liver failure patients, and thus require more intensive care pretransplant. Indications for transplant include worsening coagulopathy and encephalopathy. Cerebral edema is substantially more common in FHF patients. As many as 80 percent of the patients who die secondary to FHF have evidence of cerebral edema. The pathogenesis is unclear, but it may be because of potential neurotoxins that are normally cleared by the liver.

Once the indications for a transplant and the absence of contraindications have been established, a careful search for underlying medical disorders must be made. Unique to patients with chronic liver disease, the pretransplant evaluation must assess for any evidence of hepatopulmonary syndrome, pulmonary hypertension, and hepatorenal syndrome. Hepatopulmonary syndrome is characterized by impaired gas exchange, resulting from intrapulmonary arteriovenous shunts. A transplant may be contraindicated if intrapulmonary shunting is severe, as manifested by hypoxemia that is only partially improved with high inspired oxygen concentrations. Pulmonary hypertension is seen in a small proportion of patients with established cirrhosis. Diagnosing pulmonary hypertension pretransplant is critical, because major surgical procedures in the presence of nonreversible pulmonary hypertension are associated with a very high risk of mortality.

Surgical Procedure

The surgical procedure is divided into three phases: preanhepatic, anhepatic, and postanhepatic. The preanhepatic phase involves mobilizing the recipient's diseased liver in preparation for its removal. The basic steps include isolating the supra- and infrahepatic vena cava, portal vein, and hepatic artery, and then dividing the bile duct. Once the above structures have been isolated, vascular clamps are applied. The recipient's liver is removed, thus beginning the anhepatic phase. With the recipient liver removed, the donor liver is anastomosed to the appropriate structures to place it in an orthotopic position. The suprahepatic caval anastomosis is performed first, followed by the infrahepatic cava and the portal vein. The portal and caval clamps may be removed at this time. The new liver is then allowed to reperfuse. Either before or after this step, the hepatic artery may be anastomosed.

With the clamps removed and the new liver reperfused, the postanhepatic phase begins, often characterized by marked changes in the recipient's status. The most dramatic changes in hemodynamic parameters usually occur on reperfusion, namely hypotension and the potential for serious cardiac arrhythmias. Severe coagulopathy may also develop because of the release of natural anticoagulants from the ischemic liver or because of active fibrinolysis.

Variations on the Standard Procedure

Several variations of the standard operation have been described. With the "piggyback technique," the recipient's inferior vena cava is preserved, the infrahepatic donor cava is oversewn, and the suprahepatic cava is anastomosed to the confluence of the recipient hepatic veins. With this technique, the recipient's vena cava does not have to be completely cross-clamped during anastomosis, thus allowing blood from the lower body to return to the heart uninterrupted, without the need for venovenous bypass (VVB).

Another important variation of the standard operation is a partial transplant, either a living-donor transplant or a deceased-donor split-liver transplant. Both have developed in response to the donor shortage and are gaining in popularity. Usually, in living-donor liver transplants for pediatric recipients, the left lateral segment or left lobe is used; for adult recipients, the right lobe is used. Split-liver transplants from deceased donors involve dividing the donor liver into two segments, each of which is subsequently transplanted.

Living-Donor Liver Transplant

The greatest advantage of a living-donor liver transplant is that it avoids the often lengthy waiting period experienced with deceased-donor organ transplants. A partial hepatectomy in an otherwise healthy donor is a significant undertaking, so all potential donors must be carefully evaluated. Detailed medical screening must ensure that the donor is medically healthy, radiologic evaluation must ensure that the anatomy of the donor's liver is suitable, and a psychosocial evaluation must ensure that the donor is mentally fit and not being coerced in any way. If the recipient is a child, the lateral segment of the donor's liver (about 25 percent of the total liver) is removed. If the recipient is an adult, a larger portion of the liver needs to be removed. Usually the right lobe of the liver, which comprises approximately 60 percent of the total liver, is used. The operative procedure involves isolating the blood vessels supplying the portion of the liver to be removed, transecting the hepatic parenchyma, and then removing the portion to be transplanted.

Split-Liver Transplants

Another method to increase the number of liver transplants is to split the liver from a deceased donor into two grafts, which are then transplanted into two recipients. Thus, a whole adult liver from such a donor can be divided into two functioning grafts. The vast majority of split-liver transplants have been between one adult and one pediatric recipient. Usually the liver is split into a smaller portion (the left lateral segment, which can be transplanted into a pediatric recipient) and a larger portion (the extended right lobe, which can be transplanted into a normal-sized adult recipient). With appropriate donor and recipient selection criteria, a small percentage of livers from deceased donors could be split and transplanted into two adult recipients also.

Postoperative Care

The immediate postoperative care for liver recipients involves: (1) stabilizing the major organ systems (e.g., cardiovascular, pulmonary, and renal); (2) evaluating graft function and achieving adequate immunosuppression; and (3) monitoring and treating complications directly and indirectly related to the transplant. This initial care should generally be performed in an intensive care unit (ICU) setting because recipients usually require mechanical ventilatory support for the first 12–24 h. The goal is to maintain adequate oxygen saturation, acid-base equilibrium, and stable hemodynamics.

A crucial aspect of postoperative care is to repeatedly evaluate graft function. In fact, doing so begins intraoperatively, soon after the liver is reperfused. Signs of hepatic function include good texture and good color of the graft, evidence of bile production, and restoration of hemodynamic stability. Postoperatively, hepatic function can be assessed using clinical signs and laboratory values. Patients who rapidly awaken from anesthesia and whose mental status progressively improves likely have a well-functioning graft. Laboratory indicators of good graft function include normalization of the coagulation profile, resolution of hypoglycemia and hyperbilirubinemia, and clearance of serum lactate. Adequate urine production and good output of bile through the biliary tube (if present) are also indicators of good graft function.

Another important aspect of postoperative care is to monitor for any surgical and medical complications. The incidence of complications tends to be high after liver transplants, especially in patients who were severely debilitated pretransplant. Surgical complications related directly to the operation include postoperative hemorrhage and anastomotic problems.

The incidence of vascular complications after liver transplants ranges from 8–12 percent. Thrombosis is the most common early event, with stenosis and pseudoaneurysm formation occurring later. Hepatic artery thrombosis (HAT) has a reported incidence of about 3 to 5 percent in adults and about 5–10 percent in children. The incidence tends to be higher in partial liver transplant recipients. After HAT, liver recipients may be asymptomatic or may develop severe liver failure secondary to extensive necrosis. Doppler ultrasound evaluation is the initial investigative method of choice, with more than 90 percent sensitivity and specificity. If HAT is suggested by radiologic imaging, urgent re-exploration is indicated, with thrombectomy and revision of the anastomosis. If hepatic necrosis is extensive, a retransplant is indicated.

Thrombosis of the portal vein is less common. Signs include liver dysfunction, tense ascites, and variceal bleeding. Doppler evaluation should be used to establish the diagnosis. If thrombosis is diagnosed early, operative thrombectomy and revision of the anastomosis may be successful. If thrombosis occurs late, liver function is usually preserved because of the presence of collaterals; a retransplant is then unnecessary and attention is directed toward relieving the left-sided portal hypertension.

Biliary complications remain a significant problem after liver transplants, affecting 10–35 percent of all recipients. A higher incidence generally is seen after partial liver transplants, in which bile leaks may occur from the anastomoses or from the cut surface of the liver. Biliary complications manifest either as leaks or as obstructions. Leaks tend to occur early postoperatively and often require surgical repair; obstructions usually occur later and can be managed with radiologic or endoscopic techniques.

One devastating complication posttransplant is primary nonfunction of the hepatic allograft, with an attendant mortality rate of greater than 80 percent without a retransplant. By definition, primary nonfunction results from poor or no hepatic function from the time of the transplant procedure. The incidence in most centers is about 3–5 percent. Factors associated with primary nonfunction include advanced donor age, increased fat content of the donor liver, prolonged donor hospitalization prior to organ procurement, prolonged cold ischemia time, and partial liver donation.

Infectious complications after liver transplant are common and can be devastating. Early infections (within the first month posttransplant) usually are related to surgical complications, initial graft function, or preexisting comorbid conditions. Risk factors include prolonged surgery, large-volume blood transfusions, primary nonfunction requiring a retransplant, and reoperations for bleeding or bile leaks. The most common early infections are intraabdominal and wound infections. Intraabdominal infections should always lead the surgeon to consider the possibility of a bile leak. If an intraabdominal infection is suspected, a CT scan should be performed, with aspiration and culture of any fluid collections that are identified. The biliary tree should be evaluated to exclude the presence of a bile leak. Patients with FHF are at high risk for fungal infections, usually secondary to Candida or Aspergillus species. Common sites include the abdomen, lungs, and central nervous system.

Disease recurrence is a significantly more important problem after liver transplants than with other solid organ transplants. Recurrence of hepatitis C is almost universal after transplants for this condition. Fortunately, only a minority of recipients experience aggressive recurrence leading to cirrhosis and liver failure. Ribavirin and α-interferon therapy should be considered in recipients with evidence of significant recurrence, as indicated by liver biopsy findings. Recurrence of hepatitis B has been significantly decreased by the routine use of hepatitis B immune globulin and the antiviral agent lamivudine posttransplant, but recurrence may still be seen with resistant viral strains. Other diseases that may recur posttransplant are primary sclerosing cholangitis, primary hepatic malignany, and autoimmune hepatitis.

Pediatric Liver Transplants

The clinical indications for a pediatric liver transplant are similar to those already mentioned for adults. Endpoints that require a transplant include evidence of portal hypertension as manifested by variceal bleeding and ascites, significant jaundice, intractable pruritus, encephalopathy, failing synthetic function (e.g., hypoalbuminemia or coagulopathy), poor quality of life, and failure to thrive (as manifested by poor weight gain or poor height increase).

Biliary atresia is the most common indication for a pediatric liver transplant. The incidence of biliary atresia is about 1 in 10,000 infant births. Once the diagnosis is established, a portoenterostomy, or Kasai procedure, is indicated to drain microscopic ducts within the porta hepatis. Successful bile flow can be achieved in 40–60 percent of patients whose Kasai procedure takes place early in their life. However, even with a Kasai procedure, 75 percent of children with biliary atresia eventually require a liver transplant because of progressive cholestasis followed by cirrhosis. Other cholestatic disorders that may eventually require a transplant include sclerosing cholangitis, familial cholestasis syndromes, and paucity of intrahepatic bile ducts (as seen with Alagille syndrome).

The surgical procedure for children does not differ significantly from that used in adults. The recipient's size is a more important variable in pediatric transplants, and it has an impact on both the donor and the recipient operations. For pediatric patients (especially infants and small children), the chance of finding a size-matched graft from a deceased donor may be very small, as the vast majority of such donors are adults. With adult grafts for pediatric patients, options include reduced-size liver transplants, in which a portion of the liver, such as the right lobe or extended right lobe, is resected and discarded; split-liver transplants in which a whole liver is divided into two functional grafts; and living-donor liver transplants in which a portion, usually the left lateral segment, is resected from a living donor. Graft implantation may be more demanding in pediatric patients, given the small caliber and delicate nature of the vessels. Use of venovenous bypass is usually not technically possible because of the small size of the vessels. For that reason, and given the increasing use of partial transplants, vena cava–sparing procedures are generally performed in children.

Surgical complications, especially those related to the vascular anastomoses, tend to be more frequent in pediatric recipients. HAT is three to four times more common in children. Factors associated with this increased risk include small recipient weight (less than 10 kg), use of just the left lateral segment (rather than the whole liver), and complex arterial reconstructions.

Patient survival rates have improved dramatically for pediatric liver recipients since the early 1990s. Most centers now report patient survival of close to 90 percent at 1 year posttransplant. Even for small recipients, patient survival rates at 1 year are 80–85 percent. Also, pediatric recipients enjoy close to normal growth and development posttransplant. Usually, growth accelerates immediately posttransplant.

Results

Patient and graft survival rates after liver transplants have improved significantly since the mid-1990s, with most centers now reporting graft survival rates of 85–90 percent at 1 year. The main factors affecting short-term (within the first year posttransplant) patient and graft survival are the medical condition of the patient at the time of transplant and the development of early postoperative surgical complications. Severely debilitated patients with numerous comorbid conditions such as kidney dysfunction, coagulopathy, and malnutrition, have a significantly higher risk of early posttransplant mortality. Such patients are more likely to develop surgical and medical complications (especially infections) and are unable to tolerate them. National U.S. data show that for 2001, patient survival at 1 year was 86.4 percent, although graft survival was 80.2 percent.

INTESTINAL TRANSPLANTATION

Intestinal transplants have been performed in the laboratory for years. The first human intestinal transplant was performed in 1966, but it remained essentially an experimental procedure, producing dismal results well into the 1980s. Newer immunosuppressive drugs have played a significant role in the success with the procedure since the mid-1990s. However, intestinal transplants remain the least frequently performed of all transplants, with the highest rejection rates and the lowest graft survival rates.

Preoperative Evaluation

Currently an intestinal transplant is indicated for irreversible intestinal failure that is not successfully managed by TPN (because of malnutrition and failure to thrive) or that has life-threatening complications (e.g., hepatic dysfunction, repeated episodes of sepsis secondary to central access, loss of central venous access sites).

The causes of intestinal failure are different in adult than in pediatric patients. Most commonly, although, the underlying disease results in extensive resection of the small bowel with resultant short bowel syndrome. The development of short bowel syndrome depends not only on the length of bowel resected, but also on the location of the resection, on the presence or absence of the ileocecal valve, and on the presence or absence of the colon. As a rough guideline, most patients can tolerate resection of 50 percent of their intestine with subsequent adaptation, avoiding the need for long-term parenteral nutritional support. Loss of greater than 75 percent of the intestine, however, usually necessitates some type of parenteral nutritional support. The most common causes of intestinal failure in children are necrotizing enterocolitis, gastroschisis, and volvulus. In adults, Crohn disease, massive resection of ischemic bowel because of mesenteric vascular thrombosis, and trauma are the most common causes.

The pretransplant evaluation does not differ greatly from that for other transplants. Absolute contraindications such as malignancy and active infection must be ruled out, and hepatic function should be evaluated carefully. If there is evidence of significant liver dysfunction and cirrhosis, a combined liver and intestinal transplant is indicated.

Surgical Procedure

The operative procedure varies, depending on whether or not a liver transplant is also performed. In the case of an isolated intestinal transplant, the graft may be from a living or deceased donor. With a living donor, about 200 cm of the distal small bowel is used; inflow to the graft is via the ileocolic artery, and outflow via the ileocolic vein. With a deceased donor, the graft is based on the superior mesenteric artery for inflow and on the superior mesenteric vein for outflow. For a combined liver and intestinal transplant, the graft is usually procured intact with an aortic conduit that contains both the celiac and superior mesenteric arteries. The common bile duct can be maintained intact in the hepatoduodenal ligament along with the first part of the duodenum and a small rim of the head of the pancreas. Doing so avoids a biliary reconstruction in the recipient.

Postoperative Care

The early posttransplant care for intestinal transplant patients is in many ways similar to that of other transplant recipients. Initial care should take place in an ICU so that fluid, electrolytes, and blood product replacement can be carefully monitored. Broad-spectrum antibiotics are routinely administered, given the high risk for infectious complications.

A number of different immunosuppressive protocols have been described. Many involve some form of induction therapy, followed by tacrolimus-based maintenance immunosuppression. Regardless of the protocol, intestinal transplants clearly have a high risk of rejection. Therefore, careful monitoring for rejection is imperative and involves endoscopy with biopsy of the graft mucosa. Acute rejection episodes are often associated with infections. Rejection results in damage to the intestinal mucosa, leading to impaired barrier function and bacterial translocation. Therefore, advanced rejection can be very difficult to treat as concurrent infection invariably is present.

HEART AND LUNG TRANSPLANTATION

Heart transplantation is a well-established therapy for end-stage heart failure, and is performed in age groups from neonates to senior citizens. Lung transplantation is a newer field than heart transplantation, and far fewer lung transplants (about 1000) are performed each year. Results have improved since the early 1990s, mainly because of improvements in immunosuppression and refinements in surgical techniques, in particular with modification of the airway anastomosis. A combined heart-lung transplant is usually reserved for patients who have pulmonary hypertension and obvious right-sided heart failure.

Preoperative Evaluation

A heart transplant is generally indicated in the presence of end-stage heart failure. The most common cause is ischemic or dilated cardiomyopathy, followed by intractable angina, valvular disease, congenital heart disease, life-threatening recurrent ventricular arrhythmias, and isolated intracardiac tumors. Isolated lung transplants are performed for a number of indications, including chronic obstructive pulmonary disease, idiopathic pulmonary fibrosis, cystic fibrosis, and pulmonary hypertension (without right-sided heart failure). Patients with chronic obstructive pulmonary disease or idiopathic pulmonary fibrosis generally are treated with a single-lung transplant; those with cystic fibrosis or pulmonary hypertension (without right-sided heart failure) usually require a bilateral single-lung transplant. Patients with pulmonary hypertension with significant right-sided heart failure, or those with Eisenmenger syndrome, usually require a combined heart-lung transplant.

Surgical Procedure

A heart transplant is an orthotopic procedure. Therefore the first step of the procedure for heart or heart-lung recipients is removal of their corresponding thoracic organs. The recipient's aorta and vena cava are cannulated, an aortic cross-clamp is applied, and the diseased heart is excised along the atrioventricular groove. The recipient is maintained on cardiopulmonary bypass during this time. The new heart is then placed in an orthotopic position, with anastomoses performed in the following order: left atrium, right atrium, pulmonary artery, and aorta. Several variations to the original technique have been described, such as performing the aortic anastomosis before the pulmonary artery anastomosis to allow reperfusion of the heart and to minimize the ischemic time. Another variation is to perform selective anastomoses of the inferior and superior vena cava (rather than just of the right atrium); doing so is believed to allow for better geometry of the right atrium and to decrease the incidence of posttransplant atrial arrhythmias.

In heart-lung transplants, the new organs are implanted en bloc. Right and left pneumonectomies are carried out, with isolation and division of the trachea just above the carina. Anastomoses are then performed between the donor and recipient trachea, right atrium, and aorta.

Single-lung transplants are performed through a standard posterolateral thoracotomy. The superior and inferior pulmonary veins, pulmonary artery, and main stem bronchus are dissected. The pulmonary artery is then clamped to assess the recipient's hemodynamic status; cardiopulmonary bypass is used if necessary, although most recipients do not require bypass support. The bronchus and appropriate vascular structures are then clamped and the pneumonectomy completed. The bronchial anastomosis is performed first, followed by the pulmonary arterial and left atrial anastomoses. A telescoped bronchial anastomosis reduces the incidence of complications, most notably leaks. A pedicle of vascularized omentum can also be wrapped around the anastomosis for further reinforcement. Bilateral single-lung transplants are performed in a similar fashion, each side sequentially.

Postoperative Care

The immediate postoperative care does not differ significantly from any other major cardiac or pulmonary procedure. However, heart or lung recipients are at greater risk for infections than their nontransplant counterparts, and require appropriate precautions and prophylaxis regimens. As with other transplant recipients, maintenance immunosuppressive therapy is started immediately posttransplant.

After heart or heart-lung transplants, cardiac output is sustained by establishing a heart rate of 90–110 beats per minute, using either temporary epicardial atrial pacing or low-dose isoproterenol. For recipients who may suffer transient right-sided heart failure, adequate preload is important. Use of an oximetric Swan-Ganz catheter can be helpful to monitor pulmonary artery pressure and measure cardiac output. Urine output and arterial blood gases must be carefully monitored. Hypotension and a low cardiac output usually respond to an infusion of volume and to minor adjustments in inotropic support.

Complications can be surgical or medical, and may occur early or late post-transplant. Many of the complications, especially those occurring late, are medical in nature and are similar to those seen after other types of transplants. Generally, they are related to the medications and to the immunosuppressed state. Examples include hypertension, hyperglycemia, osteoporosis, and malignancy. Certain complications, such as airway problems, are unique to lung and heart recipients. Rejection, both acute and chronic, can occur, but manifests in very different ways as compared with abdominal organ transplants.

Early attempts at lung transplantation were severely hampered by a high incidence of airway complications. This anastomosis is at high risk for problems because of the poor blood supply. However, increased experience and refinements in surgical technique have dramatically reduced airway complications. Nonetheless, about 10–15 percent of lung recipients develop some airway complication, often resulting in significant morbidity and occasional mortality.

INFECTION AND MALIGNANCY

Infections

Transplant recipients exhibit an increased risk for infectious complications posttransplant, which can lead to significant morbidity and mortality. Numerous risk factors include long-standing end-stage organ failure (which can lead to an immunosuppressed state even before any immunosuppressive drugs are begun), impaired tissue healing, and poor vascular flow because of coexisting illnesses such as diabetes. The transplant surgery itself, which may involve opening nonsterile viscera such as the bladder or bowel, and the posttransplant need for powerful immunosuppressive agents further increase the risk for infections.

The spectrum of possible infections in transplant recipients is wide. Infections are classified by the type of pathogen involved into bacterial, viral, or fungal infections. However, more than one type of pathogen may be involved in several different types of infections (e.g., pneumonia may be caused by a viral, bacterial, or fungal pathogen). Moreover, a number of different pathogens may be involved in a single infection (e.g., an intraabdominal abscess can be because of several different bacterial and fungal pathogens).

Infections can also be classified by the primary method of treatment into surgical or medical infections. Surgical infections require some surgical intervention as an integral part of their treatment. They generally occur soon after the transplant operation and are usually related directly to it, or to some complication occurring as a result of it. Surgical infections are less likely to be related to the recipient's overall immunosuppressed state, although obviously this plays some role. Typical examples of surgical infections include generalized peritonitis, intraabdominal abscesses, and wound infections. In contrast, medical infections do not generally require an invasive intervention for treatment, but rather are primarily treated with antiviral, antibacterial, or antifungal agents. They tend to occur later posttransplant and are usually related to the recipient's overall immunosuppressive state. Typical examples of medical infections include those secondary to cytolomegavirus (CMV), polyomavirus-induced nephropathy, pneumonias, and Epstein-Barr virus (EBV)-related problems.

The most common surgical infections, especially in liver and pancreas transplant recipients, are intraabdominal infections. They are also the most likely to be life-threatening. They may range from diffuse peritonitis to localized abscesses. Their presentation, management, and clinical course will in part depend on their underlying cause, their location, and on the recipient's overall medical condition. The clinical presentation of intraabdominal infections will depend on their severity and location. Generalized peritonitis is usually associated with some catastrophic event such as biliary disruption or graft duodenal leak with spillage of enteric contents or urine into the peritoneal cavity. It may also occur as a result of perforation of some other viscus, unrelated to the transplant (e.g., perforated gastric ulcer or perforated cecum). Fortunately, most intraabdominal infections do not fall into the generalized peritonitis category. Instead, most of them consist of localized fluid collections in and around the graft. Patients usually develop symptoms such as fever, nausea, vomiting, and abdominal distention, with localized pain and guarding over the region of the fluid collection. A computed tomography (CT) scan with contrast is the best diagnostic tool in this clinical situation. Treatment of localized intraabdominal infections involves adequate drainage and administration of appropriate antibacterial or antifungal agents.

Medical infections posttransplant tend to be more varied compared to surgical infections, and can involve bacterial, viral, or fungal pathogens. Bacterial infections primarily occur in the first few weeks posttransplant. The major sites are the incisional wound, respiratory tract, urinary tract, and bloodstream. Administration of perioperative systemic antibiotics decreases the risk and incidence of some infections. Viral infections in transplant recipients often involve the herpesvirus group; CMV is clinically the most important. Fungal infections are most commonly caused by Candida species; Aspergillus, Cryptococcus, Blastomyces, Mucor, Rhizopus, and other species account for a much smaller percentage of fungal infections, but are more serious.

Malignancy

Transplant recipients are at increased risk for developing certain types of de novo malignancies, including nonmelanomatous skin cancers (3–7-fold increased risk), lymphoproliferative disease (2–3-fold increased risk), gynecologic and urologic cancers, and Kaposi sarcoma. The risk ranges from 1 percent among renal allograft recipients to approximately 5–6 percent among recipients of small bowel and multivisceral transplants.

The most common malignancies in transplant recipients are skin cancers. They tend to be located on sun-exposed areas and are usually squamous or basal cell carcinomas. Often they are multiple and have an increased predilection to metastasize. Diagnosis and treatment are the same as for the general population. Patients are encouraged to use sunscreen liberally and avoid significant sun exposure.

Lymphomas constitute the largest group of noncutaneous neoplasms in transplant recipients. The vast majority (> 95 percent) of these lymphomas consist of a spectrum of B-cell proliferation disorders associated with EBV, known collectively as posttransplant lymphoproliferative disorder (PTLD). Risk factors include a high degree of immunosuppression, anti–T-cell antibody therapy, tacrolimus, and primary EBV infection posttransplant. A wide variety of clinical manifestations may be seen. Symptoms may be systemic and include fever, fatigue, weight loss, or progressive encephalopathy. Lymphadenopathy may be localized, diffuse, or absent.

A variety of other malignancies occur with increased incidence in transplant recipients. Conventional treatment is appropriate for most malignancies posttransplant. Immunosuppression should be reduced, particularly if bone marrow suppressive chemotherapeutic agents are administered. However, allograft function should be maintained for those organs that are critical to survival, such as the heart, liver, and lung. For other types of transplants with alternative therapies to fall back on if necessary (e.g., hemodialysis for kidney transplants, exogenous insulin for pancreas or islet cell transplants, and TPN for intestinal transplants), the risks of ongoing immunosuppression must be weighed against the benefits of organ function compared to the alternative therapies.

Suggested Readings

Burke JF, Pirsch JD, Ramos EL, et al: Long-term efficacy and safety of cyclosporine in renal transplant recipients. N Engl J Med 331:358, 1994.

Van Buren CT, Barakat O: Organ donation and retrieval. Surg Clin North Am 74:1055, 1994.

Friedman A: Strategies to improve outcomes after renal transplantation. N Engl J Med 346:2089, 2002.

Humar A, Kandaswamy R, Granger D, et al: Decreased surgical risks of pancreas transplantation in the modern era. Ann Surg 231:269, 2000.

Sutherland DE, Gruessner RW, Dunn DL, et al: Lessons learned from more than 1000 pancreas transplants at a single institution. Am Surg 233:463, 2001.

Trotter JF, Wachs M, Everson GT, et al: Adult-to-adult transplantation of the right hepatic lobe from a living donor. N Engl J Med 346:1074, 2002.

Marcos A, Fisher RA, Ham JM, et al: Right lobe living donor liver transplantation. Transplantation 68:798, 1999.

Rogiers X, Malago M, Gawad K, et al: In situ splitting of cadaveric livers. The ultimate expansion of a limited donor pool. Ann Surg 224:331, 1996.

Humar A, Ramcharan T, Sielaff T, et al: Split liver transplantation for 2 adult recipients: An initial experience. Am J Transplant 1:366, 2001.

Kato T, Ruiz P, Thompson JF, et al: Intestinal and multivisceral transplantation. World J Surg 26:226, 2002.

11 | Patient Safety, Errors, and Complications in Surgery

Mark L. Shapiro and Peter B. Angood

Surgical complications prolong the course of illness, lengthen hospital stay, and increase morbidity and mortality rates. Although complications occur that are caused by a surgical disease, complications also occur because of lapses in the processes of care of disease. The issue of medical errors has received much attention since the Institute of Medicine (IOM) issues its 2000 report stating that between 45,000 and 98,000 medical error–related deaths occur annually. It is the processes of care that are increasingly recognized as the etiology for complications and errors, not the diseases or treatments themselves.

ISSUES PERTINENT TO ERRORS AND COMPLICATIONS

Patient Safety Initiatives

Most surgical quality improvement (QI) programs have been oriented toward patient diseases and their complications (e.g., postoperative abscesses following perforated viscus repair), provider decisions (e.g., a delay in diagnosis or errors in decision making), and to a lesser extent, the system processes related to patient care. Recently, the focus of QI programs has begun to shift toward patient safety.

The increasing complexity of health care carries an inherent risk that system failures may occur. An improvement in patient safety, accomplished through stronger vigilance and refinement of the processes of care, is the primary thrust for current QI initiatives.

Processes of Care

The simplicity of the phrase "processes of care" belies the complex set of systems involved. Even the simplest of processes, when broken into component parts and analyzed, becomes complex. The root causes of process failures are notoriously difficult to identify and resolve.

Recently, groups such as The Joint Commission for Accreditation of Healthcare Organizations (JCAHO), The Leapfrog Group, and The Institute for Healthcare Improvement (IHI) have begun offering new QI approaches to health care, and a new culture of patient safety awareness is occurring.

Quality Improvement Processes

QI systems focus on the recognition of problems, errors, system inefficiency, or patient safety concerns. Most QI programs, however, are reactive in the analysis and management of problems that are identified. A shift toward a forward-thinking system of QI needs to occur in order for ongoing improvements in care to become an inherent goal for practitioners, and for the mentality in health care to move from one of satisfaction to one of continued improvement.

A strong QI program has the following characteristics: (1) any employee/caregiver can identify problems and issues, (2) reporting a problem does not threaten job or position security, (3) problems are recorded and feedback

245

is provided to the reporter and those affected by the reporting, (4) all problems are addressed after they are clarified, evaluated for significance, and prioritized, (5) databases are used to help analyze the identified problem, (6) organized discussion forums are held to evaluate the problem and to propose solutions, (7) the reporting system is integrated with other QI programs and process improvement initiatives, (8) there is an oversight committee for institutional QI programs, (9) institutional resources are available when solutions are beyond simple restructuring or behavior change, (10) the success or failure of solutions is monitored, and the entire QI process is documented and reviewed, (11) there is ongoing communication with the employees who are affected by the changes instituted by the QI program, and (12) an incentive or reward system exists to facilitate change in human behavior."

Communication Strategies and the Importance of Care Plans

Communication failures are the most frequent cause of errors and complications in health care. An integrated communication system is essential for high quality care to flourish.

Traditionally, individual surgeons have been able to establish their practice preferences, and institutions have attempted to cater to all surgeons on an individual basis. This often leads to a chaotic organizational environment in terms of how to best manage surgical patients as an overall group. Surgeons are taught to retain their individual preferences (i.e., adhering to their best-known and most successful technique), although all groups of practitioners remain untrained regarding how to work within an integrated structure. Therefore, it is not surprising that the net result is poor communication and subsequent system failures.

One of the basic tenets for minimizing communications errors is to "speak the same language" through the use of protocols or clinical care plans that are based on sound evidence and are used by everyone. Protocols of care reduce misunderstanding, incorrect assumptions, and communications errors. Although common problems, such as a fractured hip or cholelithiasis, lend themselves to the development of clinical protocols, other surgical problems do not. When clinical variability exists, or outcome data are equivocal, randomized trials of treatment options can and should be established. Although the physician's autonomy will suffer in these regimented approaches to care, patient safety will improve because of a lower potential for complications and medical errors.

Documentation of Care and Evolving Issues

Careful and complete documentation is the essence of high-quality patient care. Although at times documentation remains an arduous task, the medical record must be rigorously maintained; procedures should never be presumed to have been performed if they have not been documented properly. The medical record is the only legal document that maintains a long-term transcription of patient care activity, and as such its maintenance should be considered a priority. The confidentiality of each patient's medical information is also a priority. Optimal medical record keeping includes all patient interactions. For outpatient care, the office chart needs to document all patient visits and correspondence, examination results, laboratory and radiology investigations, and assessment of the medical problems with a proposed plan of care, and records of procedures, pathology results, and any complications encountered. Inpatient medical records need to be equally thorough, and need to document the interactions between all care providers with patients and their families.

Medical records are not the forum for open discussion, inflammatory remarks on care, or denigrating comments on the patient, their family, friends and/or other health care providers. The records should always be clear, objective, and up-to-date. All entries must be dated and timed, and should not be back-dated at a later review of the record. Discussions related to ethically sensitive issues must also be stated clearly and advanced care directives and do-not-resuscitate (DNR) status should be clearly documented.

Complications Related to Surgery and Anesthesia Relationships

The relationships between surgeons and anesthesiologists are critical for the quality of care received by surgical patients. Although the fund of knowledge and skill sets of anesthesiologists have dramatically expanded in recent decades, the interrelationship and communication between surgical and anesthesia teams is often deficient, because of radically different patterns of care continuity and on-call availability.

Peri-operative care should involve a continuous, inclusive knowledge of a patient's surgical and comorbid conditions such that all medical providers are cognizant of all issues throughout the management of a patient's surgical disease state. An open line of communication between surgeons and anesthesiologists needs to occur during the preoperative, intraoperative, and postoperative management of patients. When issues, errors, or complications are developing for any particular patient, communication and decision making should be simplified so a minimum of redundant discussion or relearning of data occurs.

Intraoperatively, an open and continuous dialogue between the surgical and anesthesia teams is essential for optimal care. The two teams should be mutually and concurrently aware of the physiologic status of the patient, the effects of surgical or anesthetic interventions, and the postoperative care plans including analgesia. This is well recognized for vascular and cardiothoracic operations, but is equally important for unstable trauma cases, septic shock cases, patients with metabolic or intravascular volume abnormalities, or for patients at either extreme of age.

Ethics of Reporting Your Complications (and Those of Others)

Because of the very personal nature of medical care, patients enter into a trust relationship (and an informal contract or covenant) with their surgeon (and the associated institution). Both parties should expect that open communication will occur so that this trust relationship is not violated at any time during the relationship. When problems or complications occur, open communication must be maintained as the only morally, ethically, and legally correct action.

The reporting of complications to one's peers is an important component of quality assurance and improvement. However, it is equally important that the patient and their family members are included in the dialogue related to complications. Similarly, to the extent that the reporting of complications of one's peers is important for the care of the patient, the patient is entitled to these details of their care. Minor errors and missteps are common but may have no impact or consequence on a patient's care; these are discussed, in detail, if the patient or their family inquires about them. Major complications should be discussed with the patient if they are clearly identified as complications or errors, and if they affect the patient's care or prognosis.

All procedures carry the potential for unforeseen difficulties or complications. Problems may arise as a result of a patient's primary surgical disease and their comorbid conditions, or may arise because of technical problems, medication delivery errors, system process errors, communication errors, or other unexpected developments.

During the process of obtaining informed consent for any procedure, it is always prudent to describe for the patient and their significant others potential complications that may occur. Although it is not necessary to detail all of the possible problems or difficulties that may arise, it is important to state that no procedure should be assumed to be risk-free.

In general, patients are fairly accepting of medical errors when they have been informed ahead of time that the possibility for errors and complications exists, and when open and direct communication is provided after a procedural complication or error.

COMPLICATIONS IN MINOR PROCEDURES

Central Venous Access Catheters

Complications of central venous access catheters are common. Steps to decrease complications include the following:

1. Ensure that central venous access is indicated.
2. Experienced (credentialed) personnel should insert the catheter, or should supervise the insertion.
3. Use proper positioning and sterile technique. Controversy exists regarding whether or not placing the patient in Trendelenburg position facilitates access.
4. Central venous catheters should be exchanged only for specific indications (not as a matter of routine) and should be removed as soon as possible.

Common complications of central venous access include:

Pneumothorax. Occurrence rates from both subclavian and internal jugular vein approaches are 1–6 percent. Pneumothorax rates appear to be higher among the inexperienced but occur with experienced operators as well. If the patient is stable, and the pneumothorax is small (<15 percent) close expectant observation may be adequate. If the patient is symptomatic, a thoracostomy tube should be placed. Occasionally, pneumothorax will occur as late as 48–72 h after central venous access attempts. This usually creates sufficient compromise that a tube thoracostomy is required. Prevention requires proper positioning of the patient and correct technique. A postprocedure chest radiograph is mandatory to confirm the presence or absence of a pneumothorax, regardless of whether a pneumothorax is suspected.

Arrhythmias. Arrhythmias result from myocardial irritability secondary to guidewire placement, and usually resolve when the catheter or guidewire is withdrawn from the right heart. Prevention requires electrocardiogram (EKG) monitoring whenever possible during catheter insertion.

Arterial puncture. The inadvertent puncture or laceration of an adjacent artery with bleeding can occur, but the majority will resolve with direct pressure on or near the arterial injury site. Rarely will angiography, stent placement, or surgery be required to repair the puncture site, but close observation and a chest radiograph are indicated. Prevention requires careful attention to insertion technique.

Lost guidewire. A guidewire or catheter that migrates into the vascular space completely can be readily retrieved with interventional angiography techniques. A prompt chest x-ray and close monitoring of the patient until retrieval is indicated.

Air embolus. Although estimated to occur in only 0.2–1 percent of patients, an air embolism can be dramatic and fatal. Treatment may prove futile if the air bolus is larger than 50 mL. Auscultation over the precordium may reveal a "crunching" noise, but a portable chest radiograph is required for diagnosis. If an embolus is suspected, the patient should immediately be placed into a left lateral decubitus Trendelenburg position, so the entrapped air can be stabilized within the right ventricle. Aspiration via a central venous line accessing the heart may decrease the volume of gas in the right side of the heart, and minimize the amount traversing into the pulmonary circulation. Subsequent recovery of intracardiac and intrapulmonary air may require open surgical or angiographic techniques. Prevention requires careful attention to technique.

Pulmonary artery rupture. Flow-directed, pulmonary artery ("Swan-Ganz") catheters can cause pulmonary artery rupture because of excessive advancement of the catheter into the pulmonary circulation. There usually is a sentinel bleed noted when a pulmonary artery catheter balloon is inflated, and then the patient begins to have uncontrolled hemoptysis. Reinflation of the catheter balloon is the initial step in management, followed by immediate airway intubation with mechanical ventilation, an urgent portable chest radiograph, and notification of the operating room that an emergent thoracotomy may be required. If there is no further bleeding after the balloon is reinflated, the radiograph shows no significant consolidation of lung fields from ongoing bleeding and the patient is easily ventilated, then a conservative nonoperative approach may be considered. This approach might include observation alone if the patient has no signs of bleeding or hemodynamic compromise; however, more typically a pulmonary angiogram with angioembolization or vascular stenting is required. Hemodynamically unstable patients rarely survive because of the time needed to perform the thoracotomy and identify the branch of the pulmonary artery that has ruptured.

Central venous line infection. The Centers for Disease Control and Prevention (CDC) reports mortality rates of 12–25 percent when a central venous line infection becomes systemic, and this carries a cost of approximately $25,000 per episode. The CDC does not recommend routine central line changes, but when the clinical suspicion is high, the site of venous access must be changed. Additionally, nearly 15 percent of hospitalized patients will acquire central venous line sepsis. In many instances, once an infection is recognized as central line sepsis, removing the line is adequate. *Staphylococcus aureus* infections, however, present a unique problem because of the potential for metastatic seeding of bacterial emboli. The required treatment is 4–6 weeks of tailored antibiotic therapy.

Arterial Lines

Arterial lines are placed to facilitate arterial blood gas sampling and hemodynamic monitoring. They are often left in place to make routine blood sampling easier, but this practice leads to higher complication rates.

Arterial access requires a sterile Seldinger technique, and a variety of arteries are used, such as the radial, femoral, brachial, axillary, dorsal pedis, or superficial temporal arteries. Although complications occur less than 1 percent of the time, they can be catastrophic. Complications include thrombosis, bleeding, hematoma, arterial spasm (nonthrombotic pulselessness), and infection. Thrombosis or embolization of an extremity arterial catheter can result in the loss of a digit, hand, or foot, and the risk is nearly the same for both femoral and radial cannulation. Thrombosis with distal tissue ischemia is treated with anticoagulation, but occasionally surgical intervention is required to reestablish adequate inflow. Pseudo-aneurysms and arteriovenous fistulae can also occur.

Endoscopy and Bronchoscopy

The principal risk of gastrointestinal endoscopy is perforation. Perforations occur in 1:10,000 patients with endoscopy alone, but have a higher incidence rate when biopsies are performed (up to 10 percent). This increased risk is because of complications of intubating a gastrointestinal diverticulum (either esophageal or colonic), or from the presence of weakened or inflamed tissue in the intestinal wall (e.g., diverticulitis, glucocorticoid use, or inflammatory bowel disease).

Patients will usually complain of diffuse abdominal pain shortly after the procedure, and then will quickly progress with worsening abdominal discomfort on examination. In obtunded or older adult patients, a change in clinical status may take several h, and occasionally as long as 24–48 h, to become manifest. Radiologic studies to look for free intraperitoneal air, retroperitoneal air, or a pneumothorax are diagnostic. A delay in diagnosis results in ongoing contamination and sepsis.

Open or laparoscopic exploration locates the perforation, and allows repair and local decontamination of the surrounding tissues. The patient who may be a candidate for nonoperative management is one in which perforation arises during an elective, bowel-prepped, endoscopy, and yet the patient does not have significant pain or clinical signs of infection. The patient may be closely observed in a monitored setting, on strict dietary restriction and broad-spectrum antibiotics.

The complications of bronchoscopy include bronchial plugging, hypoxemia, pneumothorax, lobar collapse, and bleeding. When diagnosed in a timely fashion, they are rarely life-threatening. Bleeding usually resolves and rarely requires surgery, but may require repeat endoscopy for thermocoagulation or fibrin glue application. The presence of a pneumothorax necessitates placement of a thoracostomy tube when significant deoxygenation occurs or the pulmonary mechanics are compromised. Lobar collapse or mucous plugging responds to aggressive pulmonary toilet, but occasionally requires repeat bronchoscopy.

Tracheostomy

Tracheostomy facilitates weaning from a ventilator, decreases length of intensive care unit (ICU) or hospital stay, and improves pulmonary toilet.

Tracheostomies are now performed open, percutaneously, with or without bronchoscopy, and with or without Doppler guidance, and yet complications still arise.

Recent studies do not support obtaining a routine posttracheostomy chest radiograph after either percutaneous or open tracheostomy. However, significant lobar collapse can occur from copious tracheal secretions or mechanical obstruction.

The most dramatic complication of tracheostomy is tracheoinnominate artery fistula (TIAF). These occur rarely (approximately 0.3 percent), but carry a 50–80 percent mortality rate. TIAFs can occur as early as 2 days or as late as 2 months after tracheostomy. The prototypical patient is a thin woman with a long, gracile neck. The patient may have a sentinel bleed, which occurs in 50 percent of TIAF cases, followed by a most spectacular bleed. Should a TIAF be suspected, the patient should be transported immediately to the operating room for fiberoptic evaluation. If needed, remove the tracheostomy, and place a finger through the tracheostomy site to apply direct pressure anteriorly for compression of the innominate artery.

Percutaneous Endogastrostomy

A misplaced percutaneous endogastrostomy (PEG) may create intraabdominal sepsis with peritonitis and/or an abdominal wall abscess with necrotizing fasciitis. As in other minor procedures, the initial placement technique must be fastidious to avoid complications. Transillumination of the abdomen may decrease the risk for error. Inadvertent colotomies, intraperitoneal leakage of tube feeds with peritonitis, and abdominal wall abscesses require surgery to correct the complications and to replace the PEG with an alternate feeding tube, usually a jejunostomy.

A dislodged or prematurely removed PEG tube must be replaced within 8 h of dislodgment, because the gastrostomy site closes rapidly. A contrast radiograph should be performed to confirm the tube's intragastric position prior to feeding.

Tube Thoracostomy

Tube thoracostomy (chest tube insertion) is performed for pneumothorax, hemothorax, pleural effusions or empyema. A chest tube can be easily placed with a combination of local analgesia and light conscious sedation. Common complications include inadequate analgesia or sedation, incomplete penetration of the pleura with formation of a subcutaneous track for the tube, lacerations to the lung or diaphragm, intraperitoneal placement of the tube through the diaphragm, and bleeding related to these various lacerations or injury to pleural adhesions. Additional problems include slippage of the tube out of position, or mechanical problems related to the drainage system. All of these complications can be avoided with proper initial insertion techniques, plus a daily review of the drainage system and follow-up radiographs. Tube removal can create a residual pneumothorax if the patient does not maintain positive intrapleural pressure by Valsalva maneuver during tube removal and dressing application.

Diagnostic Peritoneal Lavage

Diagnostic peritoneal lavage (DPL) is performed in the emergent trauma setting for the hemodynamically unstable patient with neurologic impairment and an uncertain etiology for blood loss, when an abdominal trauma ultrasound is not available or is unreliable. Nasogastric and bladder catheter decompression is mandatory prior to DPL to avoid injury during the procedure. The small or large bowel, or the major vessels of the retroperitoneum also can be punctured inadvertently, and these injuries require surgical exploration and repair.

Complications of Angiography

Intramural dissection of a cannulated artery can lead to complications such as ischemic stroke from a carotid artery dissection or occlusion, mesenteric ischemia from dissection of the superior mesenteric artery, or a more innocuous finding of "blue toe syndrome" from a dissected artery in a peripheral limb. Invasive or noninvasive imaging studies confirm the suspected problem. The severity of the ischemia and the extent of the dissection determine if anticoagulation therapy or urgent surgical exploration is indicated.

Bleeding from the vascular access site usually is obvious, but may not be visible when the blood loss is tracking into the retroperitoneal tissue planes after femoral artery cannulation. These patients can present with hemorrhagic shock; an abdominopelvic computed tomography (CT) scan delineates the extent of bleeding into the retroperitoneum. The initial management is direct compression at the access site and clinical observation with resuscitation as indicated. Urgent surgical exploration may be required to control the bleeding site.

Renal complications of angiography occur in 1–2 percent of patients. Contrast nephropathy is a temporary and preventable complication of radiologic studies such as CT, angiography, and/or venography. Some studies suggest a benefit of n-acetylcysteine for this condition. For the patient with impaired renal function or dehydration prior to contrast studies, twice-daily dosing 24 h before and on the day of the radiographic study is suggested. Nonionic contrast also may be of benefit in higher-risk patients. Intravenous hydration before and after the procedure is the most efficient method for preventing contrast nephropathy.

Complications of Biopsies

Lymph node biopsies have direct and indirect complications which include bleeding, infection, lymph leakage, and seromas. Measures to prevent direct complications include proper surgical hemostasis, proper skin preparation, and a single preoperative dose of antibiotic to cover skin flora 30–60 min before incision. Bleeding at a biopsy site usually can be controlled with direct pressure. Infection at a biopsy site will appear 5–10 days postoperatively, and may require opening of the wound to drain the infection. Seromas or lymphatic leaks resolve with aspiration of seromas and the application of pressure dressings, but may require repeated treatments.

ORGAN SYSTEM COMPLICATIONS

Neurologic System

Neurologic complications that occur after surgery include motor or sensory deficits and mental status changes. Peripheral motor and sensory deficits are often because of neurapraxia secondary to improper positioning and/or padding during operations. Treatment is largely clinical observation, and the majority will resolve spontaneously within 1–3 months.

Direct injury to nerves during a surgical intervention is a well-known complication of several specific operations, including superficial parotidectomy (facial nerve), carotid endarterectomy (hypoglossal nerve), prostatectomy (nervi erigentes) and inguinal herniorrhaphy (ilioinguinal nerve). The nerve injury may simply be a stretch injury, or an unintentionally severed nerve. In addition to loss of function, severed nerves can result in a painful neuroma, which may require subsequent surgery.

Mental status changes in the postoperative patient can have numerous causes (Table 11-1). Mental status changes must be carefully documented and continually assessed. CT scanning should be employed early to detect intracranial causes.

Atherosclerotic disease increases the risk for intraoperative and postoperative stroke (cerebrovascular accident or CVA). Postoperatively, hypotension and hypoxemia are the most likely causes of CVA. Management is largely supportive once the diagnosis is made, and includes adequate intravascular volume replacement plus optimal oxygen delivery. Neurologic consultation should be obtained so that decisions regarding thrombolysis or anticoagulation can be made in a timely fashion.

Eyes, Ears, and Nose

Corneal abrasions are unusual, but are due to inadequate protection of the eyes during anesthesia. Overlooked contact lenses in a trauma patient may cause conjunctivitis.

Persistent epistaxis can occur after nasogastric tube placement or removal, and nasal packing is the best treatment option if prolonged persistent direct pressure on the external nares fails. Anterior and posterior nasal gauze packing with balloon tamponade, angioembolization, and fibrin glue placement may be required in refractory cases. The use of antibiotics for posterior packing is controversial, but the incidence of toxic shock syndrome is documented at approximately 17:100,000 cases.

External otitis and otitis media occasionally occur postoperatively. Patients complain of ear pain or decreased hearing, and treatment includes topical antibiotics and nasal decongestion for symptomatic improvement.

Ototoxicity because of aminoglycoside administration occurs in up to 10 percent of patients, and is often irreversible. Recent data show that iron chelating agents and alpha-tocopherol may be protective against ototoxicity. Vancomycin-related ototoxicity occurs about 3 percent of the time when used alone, and as high as 6 percent when used with other ototoxic agents, but is self-limited.

Vascular Problems of the Neck

Complications of carotid endarterectomy include central or regional neurologic deficits or bleeding with an expanding neck hematoma. An acute change in mental status or the presence of localized neurologic deficit may require an immediate return to the operating room to correct an iatrogenic occlusion. An expanding hematoma may warrant emergent airway intubation and subsequent transfer to the operating room for control of hemorrhage. Intraoperative anticoagulation with heparin during carotid surgery makes bleeding

TABLE 11-1 Common Causes of Mental Status Changes

Electrolyte imbalance	Toxins	Trauma	Metabolic	Medications
Sodium	Ethanol	Closed head injury	Thyrotoxicosis	Aspirin
Magnesium	Methanol	Pain	Adrenal insufficiency	Beta blockers
Calcium	Venoms and poisons	Shock	Hypoxemia	Narcotics
Inflammation	Ethylene glycol	Psychiatric	Acidosis	Antiemetics
Sepsis	Carbon monoxide	Dementia	Severe Anemia	MAOIs
AIDS		Depression	Hyperammonemia	TCAs
Cerebral abscess		ICU psychosis	Poor glycemic control	Amphetamines
Meningitis		Schizophrenia	Hypothermia	Antiarrhythmics
Fever/hyperpyrexia			Hyperthermia	Corticosteroids
				Anabolic steroids

AIDS = acquired immunodeficiency syndrome; ICU = intensive care unit; MAOI = monoamine oxidase inhibitor; TCA = tricyclic antidepressant.

a postoperative risk. Other complications can arise, such as arteriovenous fistulae, pseudoaneurysms, and infection, all of which are treated surgically.

Intraoperative hypotension during manipulation of the carotid bifurcation can occur, and is related to increased tone from baroreceptors that reflexly cause bradycardia. Should hypotension occur when manipulating the carotid bifurcation, an injection of 1 percent lidocaine solution around this structure should attenuate this reflexive response.

The most common late complication following carotid endarterectomy is myocardial infarction. The possibility of a postoperative myocardial infarction should be considered as a cause of labile blood pressure and arrhythmias in high-risk patients.

Thyroid and Parathyroid Glands

Surgery of the thyroid and parathyroid glands can result in hypocalcemia in the immediate postoperative period. Manifestations include electrocardiogram changes (shortened PR interval), muscle spasm (tetany, Chvostek sign, and Trousseau sign), paresthesias, and laryngospasm. Treatment includes calcium gluconate infusion, and if tetany ensues, chemical paralysis with intubation. Maintenance treatment is thyroid hormone replacement (after thyroidectomy) in addition to calcium carbonate and vitamin D.

Recurrent laryngeal nerve (RLN) injury occurs in less than 5 percent of patients. Of those with injury, approximately 10 percent are permanent. As the thyroid gland is dissected from lateral to medial, the dissection near the inferior thyroid artery is a common area for RLN injury. At the conclusion of the operation direct laryngoscopy confirms normal vocal cord apposition. The cord on the affected side will be in the paramedian position. If bilateral RLN has occurred, the chance of a successful extubation is poor. The cords are found to be in the midline, and an early sign of respiratory distress is stridor with labored breathing. If paralysis of the cords is not permanent, function may return 1–2 months after injury. Permanent RLN injury can be treated by various techniques to stent the cords in a position of function.

Superior laryngeal nerve injury is less debilitating, as the common symptom is loss of projection of the voice. The glottic aperture is asymmetrical on direct laryngoscopy and management is limited to clinical observation.

Respiratory System

Surgical complications that put the respiratory system in jeopardy are not always confined to technical errors. Malnutrition, inadequate pain control, inadequate mechanical ventilation, inadequate pulmonary toilet, and aspiration can cause serious pulmonary problems.

Pneumothorax can occur from central line insertion during anesthesia or from a diaphragmatic injury during an abdominal procedure. Hypotension, hypoxemia, and tracheal deviation away from the affected side may be present. A tension pneumothorax can cause complete cardiovascular collapse. Treatment is by needle thoracostomy, followed by tube thoracostomy. A large-bore needle is placed either in the midclavicular line in the second rib interspace, or where the chest tube will be inserted, the fifth intercostal space in the anterior axillary line.

Hemothorax because of trauma or intrathoracic disease should be evacuated completely. A delay in evacuation of the hemothorax leaves the patient at risk for empyema and entrapped lung. If evacuation is incomplete with tube thoracostomy, video-assisted thoracoscopy or open evacuation and pleurodesis may be required.

Pulmonary atelectasis results in a loss of functional residual capacity (FRC) of the lung, and can predispose to pneumonia. Poor pain control in the postoperative period contributes to poor inspiratory effort and collapse of the lower lobes in particular. An increase in FRC by 700 mL or more can be accomplished by sitting patients up to greater than 45 degrees. For mechanically ventilated patients, simply placing the head of the bed at 30–45 degrees in elevation improves pulmonary outcomes. The prevention of atelectasis is facilitated by delivering adequate tidal volumes (8–10 mL/kg), preventing the abdominal domain from impinging on the thoracic cavity, and by sitting the patient up as much as possible. This includes having the ventilated patient out of bed and sitting in a chair if possible.

Aspiration complications include pneumonitis and pneumonia. The treatment of pneumonitis is similar to that for acute lung injury (see below), and includes oxygenation with general supportive care. Antibiotics are usually contraindicated unless known organisms are detected with bacteriologic analysis. Hospitalized patients who develop aspiration pneumonia carry a mortality rate as high as 70–80 percent. Early, aggressive, and repeated bronchoscopy for suctioning of aspirated material from the tracheobronchial tree will help to minimize the inflammatory reaction of pneumonitis and facilitate improved pulmonary toilet.

Patients with inadequate pulmonary toilet are at increased risk for bronchial plugging and lobar collapse. Patients with copious and tenacious secretions develop these plugs most often, but foreign bodies in the bronchus can be the cause of lobar collapse as well. The diagnosis of bronchial plugging is based on chest radiograph and clinical suspicion when there is acute pulmonary decompensation with increased work of breathing and hypoxemia. Fiberoptic bronchoscopy can be useful to clear mucous plugs and secretions.

Pneumonia is the second most common nosocomial infection and is the most common infection in ventilated patients. Ventilator-associated pneumonia (VAP) occurs in 15–40 percent of ventilated ICU patients, and accrues at a daily probability rate of 5 percent per day, up to 70 percent at 30 days. The 30-day mortality rate of nosocomial pneumonia can be as high as 40 percent, and depends on the microorganisms involved and the timeliness of initiating appropriate treatment.

Once the diagnosis of pneumonia is suspected (an abnormal chest radiograph, fever, productive cough with purulent sputum, and no other obvious fever sources), it is invariably necessary to initially begin treatment with broad-spectrum antibiotics until proper identification, colony count ($\geq 100,000$ colony-forming units [CFU]), and sensitivity of the microorganisms are determined. The spectrum of antibiotic coverage should be narrowed as soon as the culture sensitivities are determined. Double-coverage antibiotic strategy for the two pathogens, Pseudomonas and Acinetobacter species, may be appropriate if the local prevalence of these particularly virulent organisms is high. One of the most helpful tools in treating pneumonia and other infections is the tracking of a medical center's antibiogram every 6–12 months.

Epidural analgesia decreases the risk of perioperative pneumonia. This method of pain control improves pulmonary toilet and the early return of bowel function; both have a significant impact on the potential for aspiration and for acquiring pneumonia. The routine use of epidural analgesia has a lower incidence of pneumonia than patient-controlled analgesia.

Acute lung injury (ALI) is a diagnosis applied to patients with similar findings to those with acute respiratory distress syndrome (ARDS). These should be considered a spectrum of the same disease process, with the difference being in the degree of oxygenation deficits of patients. The pathology, pathophysiology, and the mechanism of lung injury for ALI are the same as for ARDS, except that the arterial oxygen to inspired oxygen (Pao_2-to-Fio_2) ratio is >200 for ALI and < 200 for ARDS. Both types of patients will require some form of positive pressure ventilatory assistance to improve the oxygenation deficits, although simultaneously treating the primary etiology of the initiating disease.

The definition of ARDS includes five criteria (see Table 11-2). The recent multicenter ARDS Research Network (ARDSnet) research trial demonstrated improved clinical outcomes for ARDS patients ventilated at tidal volumes of only 5–7 mL/kg. It is important to note that these ventilator setting recommendations are for patients with ARDS, and not for patients requiring ventilatory support for a variety of other reasons. The beneficial effects of positive end-expiratory pressure (PEEP) for ARDS were confirmed in this study as well. The maintenance of PEEP during ventilatory support is determined based on blood gas analysis, pulmonary mechanics, and requirements for supplemental oxygen. As gas exchange improves with resolving ARDS, the initial step in decreasing ventilatory support should be to decrease the levels of supplemental oxygen first, and then to slowly bring the PEEP levels back down to minimal levels. This is done to minimize the potential for recurrent alveolar collapse and a worsening gas exchange.

Not all patients can be weaned easily from mechanical ventilation. When the respiratory muscle energy demands are not balanced, or there is an ongoing active disease state external to the lungs, patients may require prolonged ventilatory support. Protocol-driven ventilator weaning strategies are successful and have become part of the standard of care. The use of a weaning protocol for patients on mechanical ventilation greater than 48 h reduces the incidence of VAP and the overall length of time on mechanical ventilation, when compared with nonprotocol managed ventilator weaning. Unfortunately there is still no reliable way of predicting which patient will be successfully extubated after a weaning program, and the decision for extubation is based on a combination of clinical parameters and measured pulmonary mechanics. The Tobin Index (frequency-to-tidal volume ratio), also known as the rapid shallow breathing index (RSBI), is perhaps the best negative predictive instrument. If the result equals <105, then there is nearly a 70 percent chance the patient will pass extubation. If the score is >105, the patient has an approximately 80 percent chance of failing extubation. Other parameters such as the negative inspiratory force, minute ventilation, and respiratory rate are used, but individually have no better predictive value than the RSBI.

TABLE 11-2 Definition of Adult Respiratory Distress Syndrome

1. A known etiology or disease exists that would predispose to ARDS
2. Pulmonary artery occlusion pressures are less than 18 mmHg
3. No clinical evidence exists for right heart failure, subsequent to left heart failure
4. Diffuse bilateral pulmonary infiltrates are found on chest radiograph
5. The Pao_2-to-Fio_2 ratio is less than 200

Malnutrition and poor nutritional support may adversely affect the respiratory system. The respiratory quotient (RQ), or respiratory exchange ratio (RER), is the ratio of the rate of carbon dioxide produced to the rate of oxygen uptake ($RQ = Vco_2/Vo_2$). Lipids, carbohydrates, and protein have differing effects on carbon dioxide production. Patients consuming a diet consisting mostly of carbohydrates would have an RQ of 1 or greater. The RQ for a diet mostly of lipids would be closer to 0.7, and that for a diet of mostly protein would be closer to 0.8. Ideally, an RQ of 0.75–0.85 suggests adequate balance and composition of nutrient intake. An excess of carbohydrate may negatively affect ventilator weaning because of the abnormal RQ because of higher CO_2 production and altered pulmonary gas exchange.

Although not without risk, tracheostomy will decrease the pulmonary dead space and provides for improved pulmonary toilet. When performed prior to the tenth day of ventilatory support, tracheostomy may decrease the incidence of VAP, the overall length of ventilator time, and the number of ICU patient days.

The occurrence of pulmonary embolism (PE) is probably underdiagnosed. Its etiology stems from deep vein thrombosis (DVT). The diagnosis of PE is made when a high degree of clinical suspicion for PE leads to imaging techniques such as ventilation-to-perfusion nuclear scans (VQ scans) or CT pulmonary angiogram. Clinical findings include elevated central venous pressure, hypoxemia, shortness of breath, hypocarbia secondary to tachypnea, and right heart strain noted on electrocardiogram. VQ scans are often indeterminate in patients who have an abnormal chest radiograph. The pulmonary angiogram remains the gold standard for diagnosing PE, but spiral CT angiogram has become an alternative method because of its relative ease of use and reasonable rates of diagnostic accuracy. For cases without clinical contraindications to therapeutic anticoagulation, patients should be empirically started on heparin infusion until the imaging studies are completed if the suspicion of a PE is strong.

Sequential compression devices on the lower extremities, and low-dose subcutaneous heparin administration are routinely used to prevent DVT, and, by inference, the risk of PE. Neurosurgical and orthopedic patients have higher rates of PE, as do obese patients and those at prolonged bed rest.

When anticoagulation is contraindicated, or when a known clot exists in the inferior vena cava (IVC), therapy for PE includes insertion of an IVC filter. The Greenfield filter has been most widely studied, and it has a failure rate of less than 4 percent. Newer devices include those with nitinol wire that expands with body temperature and retrievable filters. Patients with spinal cord injury and multiple long-bone or pelvic fractures frequently receive IVC filters, and there appears to be a low long-term complication rate with their use.

Cardiac System

Arrhythmias are often seen preoperatively in older adult patients, but may occur postoperatively in any age group. Atrial fibrillation is the most common arrhythmia and occurs between postoperative days 3 to 5 in high-risk patients. This is typically when patients begin to mobilize their interstitial fluid into the vascular fluid space. Contemporary evidence suggests that rate control is more important than rhythm control for atrial fibrillation. The first-line treatment includes beta blockade and/or calcium channel blockade. B blockade must be used judiciously, because hypotension, and withdrawal from β blockade with rebound hypertension, is possible. Calcium channel blockers are an option if β blockers are not tolerated by the patient, but caution must be exercised in those with a history of congestive heart failure. Although digoxin is still a faithful standby medication, it has limitations because of the need for optimal dosing levels. Cardioversion may be required if patients become hemodynamically unstable and the rhythm cannot be controlled.

Ventricular arrhythmias and other tachyarrhythmias may occur in surgical patients as well. Similar to atrial rhythm problems, these are best controlled with beta blockade, but the use of other antiarrhythmics or cardioversion may be required if patients become hemodynamically unstable. Formal cardiac electrophysiology studies may be needed to clarify the etiology of the arrhythmias so that medical or surgical treatment can be tailored.

Cardiac ischemia is a cause of postoperative mortality. Acute myocardial infarction (AMI) can present insidiously or it can be more dramatic with the classic presentation of shortness of breath (SOB), severe angina, and sudden cardiogenic shock. The work-up to rule out an AMI includes an EKG and cardiac enzyme measurements. The patient should be transferred to a monitored (telemetry) floor as soon as a bed is available. Morphine, supplemental Oxygen, Nitroglycerine, and Aspirin (MONA) are the initial therapeutic maneuvers for those who are being investigated for AMI.

Hypertension in the immediate postoperative period may be merely a failure of adequate pain control, but other causes include hypoxia, volume overload, and rebound hypertension from failure to resume β blockade and/or clonidine. Perioperative hypertension carries significant morbidity and aggressive control is warranted. Twenty to 50 percent of patients with chronic atherosclerotic disease present with hypertension, and causes of perioperative hypertension include cerebrovascular disease, renal artery stenosis, aorto-occlusive disease, and rarely pheochromocytoma. Routine perioperative cardiac protection with β blockade is the standard of care for patients with a history of cardiovascular disease.

Gastrointestinal System

Surgery of the esophagus is potentially complicated because of its anatomic location and blood supply. The two primary types of esophageal resection performed are the transhiatal resection and the transthoracic (Ivor-Lewis) resection. The transhiatal resection has the advantage that a formal thoracotomy incision is avoided. The dissection of the esophagus is blind, however, and an anastomotic leak occurs more than with other resections. However, when a leak does occur, simple opening of the cervical incision and draining the leak is all that is usually required.

The transthoracic Ivor-Lewis resection includes an esophageal anastomosis performed in the chest near the level of the azygos vein. These resections tend not to leak as often, but when they do, they can be difficult to control. The reported mortality is about 50 percent with an anastomotic leak, and the overall mortality is about 5 percent, which is similar to transhiatal resection. Nutritional support strategies must be considered for esophageal resection patients to maximize the potential for survival.

Nissen fundoplication is an operation that is fraught with possibilities for error. Bleeding is always a potential hazard, so dissection of the short gastric vessels must be done with care. Laparoscopic port site bleeding, injury to the aorta, and liver lacerations can also contribute to significant blood loss. The fundoplication may be too tightly wrapped or become unwrapped postoperatively. Postoperative edema and patient noncompliance will produce symptoms of odynophagia and dysphagia.

Postoperative ileus is related to dysfunction of the neural reflex axis of the intestine. Excessive narcotic use may delay return of bowel function. Epidural anesthesia results in better pain control, and there is an earlier return of bowel function, and a shorter length of hospital stay. The limited use of nasogastric tubes and the initiation of early postoperative feeding are associated with an earlier return of bowel function.

Numerous studies have shown a decreased length of stay and improved pain control when bowel surgery is performed laparoscopically. In one study, however, patients with open colon resection were fed at the same time as the laparoscopically treated patients and had no difference in hospital length of stay.

Pharmacologic agents commonly used to stimulate bowel function include metoclopramide and erythromycin. Metoclopramide's action is limited to the stomach, and it may help primarily with gastroparesis. Erythromycin is a motilin-agonist that works throughout the stomach and bowel. Several studies demonstrate significant benefit from the administration of erythromycin in those suffering from an ileus.

Small bowel obstruction occurs in less than 1 percent of early postoperative patients. When it does occur, adhesions are usually the cause. Internal and external hernias, technical errors, and infections or abscesses are also causative. No one can accurately predict which patients will form obstructive postoperative adhesions, because all patients who undergo surgery form adhesions to some extent, and there is little that can limit this natural healing process. Hyaluronidase is a mucolytic enzyme that degrades connective tissue, and the use of a methylcellulose form of hyaluronidase, Seprafilm, has been shown to result in a 50 percent decrease in adhesion formation in some patients. This should translate into a lower occurrence of postoperative bowel obstruction, but this has yet to be proven.

Fistulae are the abnormal communication of one structure to an adjacent structure or compartment, and are associated with extensive morbidity and mortality. Common causes for fistula formation are summarized in the pneumonic FRIENDS (Foreign body, Radiation, Ischemia/Inflammation/Infection, Epithelialization of a tract, Neoplasia, Distal obstruction, and Steroid use). The cause of the fistula must be recognized early, and treatment may include nonoperative management with observation and nutritional support, or a delayed operative management strategy that also includes nutritional support and wound care.

Gastrointestinal bleeding can occur perioperatively (Table 11-3). Technical errors such as a poorly tied suture, a nonhemostatic staple line, or a missed injury can all lead to postoperative intestinal bleeding. The source of bleeding is in the upper gastrointestinal tract about 85 percent of the time, and is usually detected and treated endoscopically. Surgical control of intestinal bleeding is required in up to 40 percent of patients.

When patients in the ICU have a major bleed from stress gastritis, the mortality risk is as high as 50 percent. It is important to keep the gastric pH greater than 4 to decrease the overall risk for stress gastritis, particularly in patients mechanically ventilated for 48 h or greater and patients who are coagulopathic.

TABLE 11-3 Common Causes of Upper and Lower Gastrointestinal Hemorrhage

Upper GI bleed	Lower GI bleed
Erosive esophagitis	Angiodysplasia
Gastric varices	Radiation proctitis
Esophageal varices	Hemangioma
Dieulafoy's lesion	Diverticulosis
Aortoduodenal fistula	Neoplastic diseases
Mallory-Weiss tear	Trauma
Peptic ulcer disease	Vasculitis
Trauma	Hemorrhoids
Neoplastic disease	Aortoenteric fistula
	Intussusception
	Ischemic colitis
	Inflammatory bowel disease
	Postprocedure bleeding

Proton pump inhibitors, H_2 receptor antagonists, and intragastric antacid installation are all effective measures.

Hepatobiliary-Pancreatic System

Complications involving the hepatobiliary tree are usually because of technical errors. Laparoscopic cholecystectomy has become the standard of care for cholecystectomy, but common bile duct injury remains a nemesis of this approach. Intraoperative cholangiography has not been shown to decrease the incidence of common bile duct injuries, because the injury to the bile duct usually occurs prior to the cholangiogram. Early recognition of an injury is important, because delayed bile duct leaks often require a more complex repair.

Ischemic injury due to devascularization of the common bile duct has a delayed presentation days to weeks after an operation. Endoscopic retrograde cholangiopancreatography (ERCP) demonstrates a stenotic, smooth common bile duct. Liver function studies are elevated. The recommended treatment is a Roux-en-Y hepaticojejunostomy.

A bile leak because of an unrecognized injury to the ducts may present after cholecystectomy as a biloma. These patients may present with abdominal pain and hyperbilirubinemia. The diagnosis of a biliary leak can be confirmed by CT scan, ERCP, or radionuclide (HIDA) scan. Once a leak is confirmed, a retrograde biliary stent and external drainage is the treatment of choice.

Hyperbilirubinemia in the surgical patient can be a complex problem. Cholestasis makes up the majority of causes for hyperbilirubinemia, but other mechanisms of hyperbilirubinemia include reabsorption of blood (e.g., hematoma from trauma), decreased bile excretion (e.g., sepsis), increased unconjugated bilirubin because of hemolysis, hyperthyroidism, and impaired excretion because of congenital abnormalities or acquired disease. Errors in surgery that cause hyperbilirubinemia largely involve missed or iatrogenic injuries.

The presence of cirrhosis predisposes to postoperative complications. Abdominal or hepatobiliary surgery is problematic in the cirrhotic patient. Ascites leak in the postoperative period can be an issue when any abdominal operation has been performed. Maintaining proper intravascular oncotic pressure in the immediate postoperative period can be difficult, and resuscitation should be maintained with crystalloid solutions. Prevention of renal failure and the management of the hepatorenal syndrome can be difficult, as the demands of fluid resuscitation and altered glomerular filtration become competitive. Spironolactone with other diuretic agents may be helpful in the postoperative care. These patients often have a labile course and bleeding complications because of coagulopathy is common. The operative mortality in cirrhotic patients is 10 percent for Child class A, 30 percent for Child class B, and 82 percent for Child class C patients.

Pyogenic liver abscess occurs in less than 0.5 percent of adult admissions, because of retained necrotic liver tissue, occult intestinal perforations, benign or malignant hepatobiliary obstruction, and hepatic arterial occlusion. The treatment is long-term antibiotics with percutaneous drainage of large abscesses.

Pancreatitis can occur following injection of contrast during cholangiography and ERCP. These episodes range from a mild elevation in amylase and lipase with abdominal pain, to a fulminant course of pancreatitis with necrosis requiring surgical débridement. Traumatic injuries to the pancreas during surgical procedures on the kidneys, gastrointestinal tract, or spleen comprise the most common causes. Treatment involves serial CT scans and percutaneous drainage to manage infected fluid and abscess collections. A pancreatic fistula may respond to antisecretory therapy with a somatostatin analog, Octreotide. Management of these fistulae initially includes ERCP with or without pancreatic stenting, percutaneous drainage of any fistula fluid collections, total parenteral nutrition with bowel rest, and repeated CT scans. The majority of pancreatic fistulae will eventually heal spontaneously.

Renal System

Renal failure can be classified as prerenal failure, intrinsic renal failure, and postrenal failure. Postrenal failure, or obstructive renal failure, should always be considered when low urine output (oliguria) or anuria occurs. The most common cause is a misplaced or clogged urinary catheter. Other, less-common causes to consider are unintentional ligation or transection of ureters during a difficult surgical dissection (e.g., colon resection for diverticular disease), or a large retroperitoneal hematoma (e.g., ruptured aortic aneurysm).

Oliguria is evaluated by flushing the Foley catheter using sterile technique. When this fails to produce the desired response, it is reasonable to administer an intravenous fluid challenge with a crystalloid fluid bolus of 500–1000 mL. However, the immediate postoperative patient must be examined and have recent vital signs recorded with total intake and output tabulated, and urinary electrolytes measured (Table 11-4). A hemoglobin and hematocrit level should be checked immediately. Patients in compensated shock from acute blood loss may manifest anemia and end-organ malperfusion as oliguria.

TABLE 11-4 Urinary Electrolytes Associated with Acute Renal Failure and Their Possible Etiologies

	FE_{Na}	Osmolarity	UR_{Na}	Etiology
Prerenal	< 1	> 500	< 20	CHF, cirrhosis
Intrinsic failure	> 1	< 350	> 40	Sepsis, shock

CHF = congestive heart failure; FE_{Na} = fractional excretion of sodium; UR_{Na} = urinary excretion of sodium.

Acute tubular necrosis (ATN) carries a mortality risk of 25–50 percent because of the many complications that can cause, or result from, this insult. When ATN is due to poor inflow (prerenal failure), the remedy begins with intravenous administration of crystalloid or colloid fluids as needed. If cardiac insufficiency is the problem, the optimization of vascular volume is achieved first, followed by inotropic agents as needed. Intrinsic renal failure and subsequent ATN are often the result of direct renal toxins. Aminoglycosides, vancomycin, and furosemide, among other commonly used agents, contribute directly to nephrotoxicity. Contrast-induced nephropathy usually leads to a subtle or transient rise in creatinine. In patients who are volume depleted or have poor cardiac function, contrast nephropathy may permanently impair renal function.

The treatment of renal failure because of myoglobinuria in severe trauma patients has shifted away from the use of sodium bicarbonate for alkalinizing the urine, to merely maintaining brisk urine output of 100 mL/h with crystalloid fluid infusion. Mannitol and furosemide are not recommended as long as the intravenous fluid achieves the goal rate of urinary output.

Musculoskeletal System

A compartment syndrome can develop in any compartment of the body. Compartment syndrome of the extremities generally occurs after a closed fracture. The injury alone may predispose the patient to compartment syndrome, but aggressive fluid resuscitation can exacerbate the problem. Pain with passive motion is the hallmark of compartment syndrome, and the anterior compartment of the leg is usually the first compartment to be involved. Confirmation of the diagnosis is obtained by direct pressure measurement of the individual compartments. If the pressures are greater than 20–25 mmHg in any of the compartments, then a four-compartment fasciotomy is considered. Compartment syndrome can be caused by ischemia-reperfusion injury, after an ischemic time of 4 to 6 h. Renal failure (because of myoglobinuria), foot drop, tissue loss, and a permanent loss of function are possible results of untreated compartment syndrome.

Decubitus ulcers are preventable complications of prolonged bedrest because of traumatic paralysis, dementia, chemical paralysis, or coma. Ischemic changes in the microcirculation of the skin can be significant after 2 h of sustained pressure. Routine skin care and turning of the patient helps ensure a reduction in skin ulceration. This can be labor intensive and special mattresses and beds are available to help with this ubiquitous problem. The treatment of a decubitus ulcer in the noncoagulopathic patient is surgical débridement. Once the wound bed has a viable granulation base without an excess of fibrinous debris, a vacuum-assisted closure (VAC) dressing can be applied. Wet to moist dressings with frequent dressing changes is the alternative, and is labor intensive. Expensive topical enzyme preparations are also available. If the wounds fail to respond to these measures, soft tissue coverage by flap is considered.

Contractures are the result of muscle disuse. Whether from trauma, amputation, or from vascular insufficiency, contractures can be prevented by physical therapy and splinting. If not attended to early, contractures will prolong rehabilitation and may lead to further wounds and wound healing issues. Depending on the functional status of the patient, contracture releases may be required for long-term care.

Hematologic System

The transfusion guideline of maintaining the hematocrit level in all patients at greater than 30 percent is no longer valid. Only those patients with symptomatic anemia, or those who have significant cardiac disease, or the critically ill patient who requires increased oxygen-carrying capacity to adequately perfuse end-organs, requires higher levels of hemoglobin. Other than these select patients, the decision to transfuse should generally not occur until the hemoglobin level reaches 7.0 mg/dL or the hematocrit reaches 21 percent.

Transfusion reactions are common complications of blood transfusion. These can be attenuated with a leukocyte filter, but not completely prevented. The manifestations of a transfusion reaction include simple fever, pruritus, chills, muscle rigidity, and renal failure because of myoglobinuria secondary to hemolysis. Discontinuing the transfusion and returning the blood products to the blood bank is an important first step, but administration of antihistamine and possibly steroids may be required to control the reaction symptoms. Severe transfusion reactions are rare but can be fatal.

Infectious complications in blood transfusion range from cytomegalovirus transmission, which is benign in the nontransplant patient, to human immunodeficiency virus (HIV) infection, to passage of the hepatitis viruses, which can lead to subsequent hepatocellular carcinoma. Although the efficiency of infectious agent screening in blood products has improved, universal precautions should be rigidly maintained for all patients (Table 11-5).

Patients on Coumadin (warfarin) who require surgery can have anticoagulation reversal by administration of fresh frozen plasma (FFP). Each unit of FFP contains 200–250 mL of plasma and includes 1 unit of coagulation factor per mL of plasma.

Thrombocytopenia may require platelet transfusion for a platelet count less than 20,000/mL when invasive procedures are performed, or when platelet counts are low and ongoing bleeding from raw surface areas persists. One unit of platelets will increase the platelet count by 5000–7500 per mL in adults. It is important to delineate the cause of the low platelet count. Usually there is a self-limiting or reversible condition such as sepsis. Rarely, it is because of heparin-induced thrombocytopenia (HIT I and HIT II). Complications of HIT II can be serious because of the diffuse thrombogenic nature of the disorder. Simple precautions to limit this hypercoagulable state include saline solution flushes instead of heparin solutions, and to limit the use of heparin-coated catheters. The treatment is anticoagulation with synthetic agents such as argatroban.

TABLE 11-5 Rate of Viral Transmission in Blood Product Transfusions[a]

HIV	1:1.9 million
HBV[b]	1:137,000
HCV	1:1 million

HBV = hepatitis B virus; HCV = hepatitis C virus; HIV = human immunodeficiency virus.
[a]Postnucleic acid amplification technology (1999). Earlier rates were erroneously reported higher due to lack of contemporary technology.
[b]HBV is reported with prenucleic acid amplification technology. Statistical information is unavailable in postnucleic acid amplification technology at this writing.
Note that bacterial transmission is 50–250 times higher than viral transmission per transfusion.

For patients with uncontrollable bleeding because of disseminated intravascular coagulopathy (DIC), an expensive but useful drug is factor VIIa. Largely used in hepatic trauma and obstetric emergencies, this agent may mean the difference between life or death in some circumstances. The combination of ongoing, nonsurgical bleeding and renal failure can sometimes be successfully treated with desmopressin (DDAVP).

In addition to classic hemophilia, other inherited coagulation factor deficiencies can be difficult to manage in surgery. When required, transfusion of appropriate replacement products is coordinated with the regional blood bank center prior to surgery. Other blood dyscrasias seen by surgeons include hypercoagulopathic patients. Those who carry congenital anomalies such as the most common, Factor V Leiden deficiency, and protein C and S deficiencies, are likely to form thromboses if inadequately anticoagulated.

Abdominal Compartment Syndrome

Abdominal compartment syndrome (ACS) and intraabdominal hypertension represent the same problem. Multi-system trauma, thermal burns, retroperitoneal injuries, and surgery related to the retroperitoneum are the major initial causative factors that may lead to ACS. Ruptured abdominal aortic aneurysm, major pancreatic injury and resection, or multiple intestinal injuries are also examples of clinical situations in which a large volume of IV fluid resuscitation puts these patients at risk for intraabdominal hypertension. Manifestations of ACS typically include progressive abdominal distention followed by increased peak airway ventilator pressures, oliguria followed by anuria, and an insidious development of intracranial hypertension. These findings are related to elevation of the diaphragm and inadequate venous return from the vena cava or renal veins secondary to the transmitted pressure on the venous system.

Measurement of abdominal pressures is easily accomplished by transducing bladder pressures from the urinary catheter after instilling 100 mL of sterile saline into the urinary bladder. A pressure greater than 20 mmHg constitutes intraabdominal hypertension, but the diagnosis of ACS requires intraabdominal pressure greater than 25–30 mmHg, with at least one of the following: compromised respiratory mechanics and ventilation, oliguria or anuria, or increasing intracranial pressures.

The treatment of ACS is to open any recent abdominal incision to release the abdominal fascia, or to open the fascia directly if no abdominal incision is present. Immediate improvement in mechanical ventilation pressures, intracranial pressures, and renal output is usually noted. When expectant management for ACS is considered in the operating room, the abdominal fascia should be left open and covered under sterile conditions with plans made for a second-look operation and delayed fascial closure. Patients with intraabdominal hypertension should be monitored closely with repeated examinations and measurements of bladder pressure, so that any further deterioration is detected and operative management can be initiated. Left untreated, ACS may lead to multiple system end-organ dysfunction or failure, and has a high mortality.

Abdominal wall closure should be attempted every 48–72 h until the fascia can be reapproximated. If the abdomen cannot be closed within 5–7 days following release of the abdominal fascia, a large incisional hernia is the net result.

WOUNDS, DRAINS, AND INFECTION

Wound (Surgical Site) Infection

There exist no prospective, randomized, double-blind, controlled studies that demonstrate that antibiotics used beyond 24 h in the perioperative period prevent infections. There is a general trend toward providing a single preoperative dose, as antibiotic prophylaxis may not impart any benefit at all beyond the initial dosing. Irrigation of the operative field and the surgical wound with saline solution has shown benefit in controlling wound inoculum. Irrigation with an antibiotic-based solution has not demonstrated significant benefit in controlling postoperative infection.

Antibacterial-impregnated polyvinyl placed over the operative wound area for the duration of the surgical procedure has not been shown to decrease the rate of wound infection. Although skin preparation with 70 percent isopropyl alcohol has the best bacteriocidal effect, it is flammable, and could be hazardous when electrocautery is used. The contemporary formulae of chlorhexidine gluconate with isopropyl alcohol or povidone-iodine and iodophor with alcohol are more advantageous.

There is a difference between wound colonization and infection. Overtreating colonization is just as injurious as undertreating infection (Table 11-6). The strict definition of wound (soft tissue) infection is more than 10^5 CFU per g of tissue. This warrants expeditious and proper antibiotic/antifungal treatment. Often, however, clinical signs raise enough suspicion that the patient is treated before a confirmatory culture is undertaken. The clinical signs of wound infection include rubor, tumor, calor, and dolor (redness, swelling, heat, and pain), and once the diagnosis of wound infection has been established, the most definitive treatment remains open drainage of the wound to facilitate wound dressing care. The use of antibiotics for wound infection treatment should be limited.

One type of wound dressing/drainage system that is gaining popularity is the VAC dressing. The principle of the system is to decrease local wound edema and to promote healing through the application of a sterile dressing that is then covered and placed under controlled suction for a period of 2–4 days at a time. Although costly, the benefits are frequently dramatic and may offset the costs of nursing care, frequent dressing changes, and operative wound débridement.

Drain Management

The indications for applying a surgical drain are:

1. To collapse surgical dead space in areas of redundant tissue (e.g., neck and axilla).
2. To provide focused drainage of an abscess or grossly infected surgical site.

TABLE 11-6 Common Causes of Leukocytosis

Infection
Systemic inflammatory response syndrome
Glucocorticoid administration
Splenectomy
Leukemia
Medications
Physiologic stress
Increases in interleukin-1 and tumor necrosis factor

3. To provide early warning notice of a surgical leak (either bowel contents, secretions, urine, air, or blood)—the so-called sentinel drain.
4. To control an established fistula leak.

Open drains are often used for large contaminated wounds such as perirectal or perianal fistulas and subcutaneous abscess cavities. They prevent premature closure of an abscess cavity in a contaminated wound, but do not address the fact that bacteria are free to travel in either direction along the drain tract. More commonly, surgical sites are drained by closed suction drainage systems, but data do not support closed suction drainage to "protect an anastomosis," or to "control a leak" when placed at the time of surgery. Closed suction devices can exert a negative pressure of 70–170 mmHg at the level of the drain, therefore the presence of this excess suction may call into question whether an anastomosis breaks down on its own, or if the drain creates a suction injury that promotes leakage.

On the other hand, CT- or ultrasound-guided placement of percutaneous drains is now the standard of care for abscesses, loculated infections, and other isolated fluid collections such as pancreatic leaks. The risk of surgery is far greater than the placement of an image-guided drain, and the risk can often be reduced in these instances by a brief course of antibiotics.

The use of antibiotics when drains are placed should be examined from a cost-benefit perspective. Antibiotics are rarely necessary when a wound is drained widely. Twenty-four to 48 h of antibiotic use after drain placement is prophylactic, and after this period only specific treatment of positive cultures should be performed, to avoid increased drug resistance and superinfection.

Urinary Catheters

Several complications of urinary (Foley) catheters can occur that lead to an increased length of hospital stay and morbidity. It is recommended that the catheter be inserted its full length up to the hub, and that urine flow is established before the balloon is inflated, because misplacement of the catheter in the urethra with premature inflation of the balloon can lead to tears and disruption of the urethra.

Enlarged prostatic tissue can make catheter insertion difficult, and a coudé catheter may be required. If this attempt is also unsuccessful, then a urologic consultation for endoscopic placement of the catheter may be required to prevent harm to the urethra. For patients with urethral strictures, filiform-tipped catheters and followers may be used, but these can potentially cause bladder injury. If endoscopic attempts fail, the patient may require a percutaneously placed suprapubic catheter to obtain decompression of the bladder. Follow-up investigations of these patients are recommended so definitive care of the urethral abnormalities can be pursued.

The most frequent nosocomial infection is urinary tract infection (UTI). These infections are classified into complicated and uncomplicated forms. The uncomplicated type is a UTI that can be treated with trimethoprim-sulfamethoxazole for 3 days. The complicated UTI usually involves the hospitalized patient with an indwelling catheter whose UTI is diagnosed as part of a fever work-up. The interpretation of urine culture results of less than 100,000 CFU/mL is controversial. Before treating such a patient, one should change the catheter and then repeat the culture to see if the catheter was simply colonized with organisms. On the other hand, an argument can be made that until the foreign body (catheter) is removed, the bladder will continue to be the nidus of infection, and antibiotics should be started. Cultures with more than 100,000 CFU/mL should be treated with the appropriate antibiotics and the catheter removed as soon as possible. Undertreatment or misdiagnosis of a UTI can lead to urosepsis and septic shock.

Recommendations are mixed on the proper way to treat *Candida albicans* fungal bladder infections. Continuous bladder washings with fungicidal solution for 72 h have been recommended, but this is not always effective. Replacement of the urinary catheter and a course of fluconazole are appropriate treatments, but some infectious disease specialists claim that *C. albicans* in the urine may serve as an indication of fungal infection elsewhere in the body. If this is the case, then screening cultures for other sources of fungal infection should be performed whenever a fungal UTI is found.

Empyema

One of the most debilitating infections is an empyema, or infection of the pleural space. Frequently, an overwhelming pneumonia is the source of an empyema, but a retained hemothorax, systemic sepsis, esophageal perforation from any cause, and infections with a predilection for the lung (e.g., tuberculosis) are potential etiologies as well. The diagnosis is confirmed by chest radiograph or CT scan, followed by aspiration of pleural fluid for bacteriologic analysis. Gram's stain, lactate dehydrogenase, protein, pH, and cell count are obtained, and broad-spectrum antibiotics are initiated while the laboratory studies are performed. Once the specific organisms are confirmed, antiinfective agents are tailored appropriately. Placement of a thoracostomy tube is needed to evacuate and drain the infected pleural fluid, but depending on the specific nidus of infection, video-assisted thoracoscopy (VATS) may also be helpful for irrigation and drainage of the infection.

Abdominal Abscesses

Postsurgical intraabdominal abscesses can present with vague complaints of intermittent abdominal pain, fever, leukocytosis, and a change in bowel habits. Depending on the type and timing of the original procedure, the clinical assessment of these complaints is sometimes difficult, and a CT scan is usually required. When a fluid collection within the peritoneal cavity is found on CT scan, antibiotics and percutaneous drainage of the collection is the treatment of choice. There should still be a determination regarding what the cause of the infection was, so tailored antibiotic therapy can be initiated. Initial antibiotic treatment is usually with broad-spectrum antibiotics such as piperacillin-tazobactam or imipenem. Should the patient exhibit signs of peritonitis and/or have free air on radiograph or CT scan, then reexploration should be considered.

For patients who present primarily (i.e., not postoperatively) with the clinical and radiologic findings of an abscess but are clinically stable, the etiology of the abscess must be determined. A plan for drainage of the abscess and decisions about further diagnostic studies with consideration of the timing of any definitive surgery all need to be balanced. This can be a complex set of decisions, depending on the etiology (e.g., appendicitis or diverticulitis); but if the patient exhibits signs of peritonitis, urgent surgical exploration should be performed.

Necrotizing Fasciitis

Postoperative infections that progress to the fulminant soft tissue infection known as necrotizing fasciitis are uncommon. Group A streptococcal (M types 1, 3, 12, and 28) soft tissue infections, and infections with Clostridium perfringens and C. septicum carry a mortality of 30–70 percent. Septic shock can be present and patients can become hypotensive less than 6 h following inoculation. Manifestations of a group A *Streptococcus pyogenes* infection in its most severe form include hypotension, renal insufficiency, coagulopathy, hepatic insufficiency, ARDS, tissue necrosis, and erythematous rash.

These findings constitute a surgical emergency and the mainstay of treatment remains wide débridement of the necrotic tissue to the level of bleeding, viable tissue. A grey serous fluid at the level of the necrotic tissue is usually noted, and as the infection spreads, thrombosed blood vessels are noted along the tissue planes involved with the infection. Typically, the patient requires serial trips to the operating room for wide débridement until the infection is under control. Antibiotics are an important adjunct to surgical débridement and broad-spectrum coverage should be used because these infections may be polymicrobial (i.e., so-called mixed-synergistic infections). *S. pyogenes* is eradicated with penicillin, and it should still be used as the initial drug of choice.

Systemic Inflammatory Response Syndrome, Sepsis, and Multiple-Organ Dysfunction Syndrome

The systemic inflammatory response syndrome (SIRS) and the multiple-organ dysfunction syndrome (MODS) carry significant mortality risks (Table 11-7). Specific criteria have been established for the diagnosis of SIRS (Table 11-8), but two criteria are not required for the diagnosis of SIRS: lowered blood pressure and blood cultures positive for infection. SIRS is the result of proinflammatory cytokines related to tissue malperfusion or injury. The dominant cytokines implicated in this process include interleukin (IL)-1, IL-6, and tissue necrosis factor (TNF). Other mediators include nitric oxide, inducible macrophage-type nitric oxide synthase (iNOS), and prostaglandin I_2 (PGI_2).

Sepsis is categorized as sepsis, severe sepsis, and septic shock. An oversimplification of sepsis would be to define it as SIRS plus infection. Severe sepsis is defined as sepsis plus signs of cellular hypoperfusion or end-organ dysfunction. Septic shock would then be sepsis associated with hypotension after adequate fluid resuscitation.

MODS is the culmination of septic shock and multiple end-organ failure. Usually there is an inciting event (e.g., perforated sigmoid diverticulitis), and as the patient undergoes resuscitation, he or she develops cardiac hypokinesis and oliguric or anuric renal failure, followed by the development of ARDS and eventually septic shock with death.

TABLE 11-7 Mortality Associated with Patients Exhibiting Two or More Criteria for Systemic Inflammatory Response Syndrome (SIRS)

Prognosis	Mortality
2 SIRS criteria	5 percent
3 SIRS criteria	10 percent
4 SIRS criteria	15–20 percent

TABLE 11-8 Inclusion Criteria for the Systemic Inflammatory Response Syndrome (SIRS)

Temperature >38 or <36°C
Heart rate >90 beats/min
Respiratory rate >20 breaths/min or $Paco_2$ <32 mm Hg
White blood cell count <4000 or >12,000 cells/mm^3 or >10% immature forms

Management of SIRS/MODS includes aggressive global resuscitation and support of end-organ perfusion, correction of the inciting etiology, control of infectious complications, and management of iatrogenic complications. Drotrecogin α, or recombinant activated protein C, appears to specifically counteract the cytokine cascade of SIRS/MODS, but its use is still limited. Other adjuncts for supportive therapy include tight glucose control, low tidal volumes in ARDS, vasopressin in septic shock, and steroid replacement therapy.

NUTRITIONAL AND METABOLIC SUPPORT COMPLICATIONS

Nutrition-Related Complications

A basic principle is to use enteral feeding whenever possible, but complications can intervene such as aspiration, ileus, and to a lesser extent, sinusitis. There is no difference in aspiration rates when a small-caliber feeding tube is placed transpylorically into the duodenum or if it remains in the stomach. Patients who are fed via nasogastric tubes are at risk for aspiration pneumonia, because these relatively large-bore tubes stent open the esophagus, creating the possibility of gastric reflux. The use of enteric and gastric feeding tubes obviates complications of total parenteral nutrition (TPN), such as pneumothorax, line sepsis, upper extremity deep venous thrombosis, and the related expense. There is growing evidence to support the initiation of enteral feeding in the early postoperative period, prior to the return of bowel function, where it is usually well tolerated.

In patients who have had any type of nasal intubation that are having high, unexplained fevers, sinusitis must be entertained as a diagnosis. CT scan of the sinuses is warranted, followed by aspiration of sinus contents so the organism(s) are appropriately treated.

Patients who have not been enterally fed for prolonged periods secondary to multiple operations, those who have had enteral feeds interrupted for any other reason, or those with poor enteral access are at risk for the refeeding syndrome, which is characterized by severe hypophosphatemia and respiratory failure. Slow progression of the enteral feeding administration rate can avoid this complication.

Common TPN problems are mostly related to electrolyte abnormalities that may develop. These electrolyte errors include deficits or excesses in sodium, potassium, calcium, magnesium, and phosphate. Acid-base abnormalities can also occur with the improper administration of acetate or bicarbonate solutions.

The most common cause for hypernatremia in hospitalized patients is underresuscitation, and conversely, hyponatremia is most often caused by fluid overload. Treatment for hyponatremia is fluid restriction in mild or moderate cases and the administration of hypertonic saline for severe cases. An overly rapid correction of the sodium abnormality may result in central pontine myelinolysis, which results in a severe neurologic deficit. Treatment for hyponatremic patients includes fluid restriction to correct the free water deficit by 50 percent in the first 24 h. An overcorrection of hyponatremia can result in severe cerebral edema, a neurologic deficit or seizures.

Glycemic Control

In 2001, Van den Berghe and associates demonstrated that tight glycemic control by insulin infusion is associated with a 50 percent reduction in mortality in the critical care setting. This prospective, randomized, controlled trial of 1500 patients had two study arms: the intensive-control arm, where the serum glucose was maintained between 80 and 110 mg/dL with insulin infusion; and the control arm, in which patients received an insulin infusion only if blood glucose was > 215 mg/dL, but serum glucose was then maintained at 180 to 200 mg/dL.

The tight glycemic control group had an average serum glucose level of 103 mg/dL, and the average glucose level in the control group was 153 mg/dL. Hypoglycemic episodes (glucose < 40 mg/dL) occurred in 39 patients in the tightly controlled group, although the control group had episodes in 6 patients. The overall mortality was reduced from 8 percent to 4.6 percent, but the mortality of those patients whose ICU stay lasted longer than 5 days was reduced from 20 percent to 10 percent. Secondary findings included an improvement in overall morbidity, a decreased percentage of ventilator days, less renal impairment, and a lower incidence of bloodstream infections. These finding have been corroborated by subsequent similar studies, and the principal benefit appears to be a greatly reduced incidence of nosocomial infections and sepsis. It is not known whether the benefits are because of strict euglycemia, to the anabolic properties of insulin, or both, but the maintenance of strict euglycemia appears to be a powerful therapeutic strategy.

Metabolism-Related Complications

"Stress dose steroids" have been advocated for the perioperative treatment of patients on corticosteroid therapy, but recent studies strongly discourage the use of supraphysiologic doses of steroids when patients are on low or maintenance doses (e.g., 5–15 mg) of prednisone daily. Parenteral glucocorticoid treatment need only replicate physiologic replacement steroids in the perioperative period. When patients are on steroid replacement doses equal to or greater than 20 mg per day of prednisone, it may be appropriate to administer additional glucocorticoid doses for no more than two perioperative days.

Adrenal insufficiency may be present in patients with a baseline serum cortisol less than 20 μg/dL. A rapid provocative test with synthetic adrenocorticotropic hormone (ACTH) may confirm the diagnosis. After a baseline serum cortisol level is drawn, 250 μg of cosyntropin is administered. At exactly 30 and 60 min following the dose of cosyntropin, serum cortisol levels are obtained. There should be an incremental increase in the cortisol level of between 7 and 10 μg/dL for each half hour. If the patient is below these levels, a diagnosis of adrenal insufficiency is made, and glucocorticoid and mineralocorticoid administration is then warranted. Mixed results are common, but the complication of performing major surgery on an adrenally insufficient patient is sudden or profound hypotension.

Thyroid hormone abnormalities usually consist of previously undiagnosed thyroid abnormalities. Hypothyroidism and the so-called "sick-euthyroid syndrome" are more commonly recognized in the critical care setting. When surgical patients are not progressing satisfactorily in the perioperative period, screening for thyroid abnormalities should be performed. If the results show mild to moderate hypothyroidism, then thyroid replacement should begin immediately and thyroid function studies monitored closely. All patients should be reassessed after the acute illness has subsided regarding the need for chronic thyroid replacement therapy.

PROBLEMS WITH THERMOREGULATION

Hypothermia

Hypothermia is defined as a core temperature less than 35°C (95°F), and is divided into subsets of mild (35–32°C [95–89.6°F]), moderate (32–28°C [89.6–82.4°F]), and severe (<28°C [82.4°F]) hypothermia. Shivering, the body's attempt to reverse the effects of hypothermia, occurs between 37 (98.6°F) and 31°C (87.8°F), but ceases at temperatures below 31°C (87.8°F). Patients who are moderately hypothermic are at higher risk for complications than are those who are more profoundly hypothermic.

Hypothermia creates a coagulopathy that is related to platelet and clotting cascade enzyme dysfunction. This triad of metabolic acidosis, coagulopathy, and hypothermia is commonly found in long operative cases, and in patients with blood dyscrasias. The enzymes that contribute to the clotting cascade and platelet activity are most efficient at normal body temperatures; therefore all measures must be used to reduce heat loss intraoperatively.

The most common cardiac abnormality is the development of arrhythmias when body temperature drops below 35°C (95°F). Bradycardia occurs with temperatures below 30°C (86°F). It is well known that hypothermia may induce carbon dioxide retention resulting in respiratory acidosis. Renal dysfunction of hypothermia manifests itself as a paradoxic polyuria, and is related to an increased glomerular filtration rate, as peripheral vascular constriction creates central shunting of blood. This is potentially perplexing in patients that are undergoing resuscitation for hemodynamic instability, because the brisk urine output provides a false sense of an adequate intravascular fluid volume.

Neurologic dysfunction is inconsistent in hypothermia, but a deterioration in reasoning and decision-making skills progresses as body temperature falls, and profound coma (and a flat EEG) occurs as the temperature drops below 30°C (86°F). The diagnosis of hypothermia is important, so accurate measurement techniques are required to get a true core temperature.

Methods used to warm patients include warm air circulation over the patient, and heated intravenous fluids, and more aggressive measures such as bilateral chest tubes with warm solution lavage, intraperitoneal rewarming lavage, and extracorporeal membrane oxygenation. A rate of temperature rise of 2–4°C (35.6–39.2°F)/h is considered adequate, but the most common complication for nonbypass rewarming is arrhythmia with ventricular arrest.

Hyperthermia

Hyperthermia is a core temperature greater than 38.6°C (101.48°F), and has a host of etiologies (Table 11-9). Hyperthermia can be environmentally induced (e.g., summer heat with inability to dissipate heat or control exposure), iatrogenically induced (e.g., heat lamps and medications), endocrine in origin (e.g., thyrotoxicosis), or neurologically induced (i.e., hypothalamic).

TABLE 11-9 Common Causes of Elevated Temperature in Surgical Patients

Hyperthermia	Hyperpyrexia
Environmental	Sepsis
Malignant hyperthermia	Infection
Neuroleptic malignant syndrome	Drug reaction
Thyrotoxicosis	Transfusion reaction
Pheochromocytoma	Collagen disorders
Carcinoid syndrome	Factitious syndrome
Iatrogenic	Neoplastic disorders
Central/hypothalamic responses	
Pulmonary embolism	
Adrenal insufficiency	

Malignant hyperthermia (MH) occurs after exposure to agents such as succinylcholine and some halothane-based inhalational anesthetics. The presentation is dramatic, with rapid onset of increased temperature, rigors, and myoglobinuria related to myonecrosis. Medications must be discontinued immediately and dantrolene administered (2.5 mg/kg every 5 min) until symptoms subside. Aggressive cooling methods are also implemented, such as an alcohol bath, or packing in ice. In cases of severe malignant hyperthermia, the mortality rate is nearly 30 percent.

Thyrotoxicosis can occur after surgery, because of undiagnosed Graves disease. Hyperthermia ($> 40°C [104°F]$), anxiety, copious diaphoresis, congestive heart failure (present in about one-fourth of episodes), tachycardia (most commonly atrial fibrillation), and hypokalemia (up to 50 percent of patients), are hallmarks of the disease. The treatment of thyrotoxicosis includes glucocorticoids, propylthiouracil, β blockade, and iodide (Lugol solution) delivered in an emergent fashion. As the name suggests, these patients are usually toxic and require supportive measures as well. Acetaminophen, cooling modalities noted above, and vasoactive agents are often indicated.

ISSUES IN CARING FOR OBESE PATIENTS AND PATIENTS AT THE EXTREMES OF AGE

Surgery in the obese patient has multiple risks, and it is important to optimize these patients before surgery to minimize these risks. Optimization begins preoperatively with teaching about dietary modifications, exercise and pulmonary toilet issues. Obese patients often have eccentric left ventricular hypertrophy, right ventricular hypertrophy, and congestive heart failure. Sleep studies and patient history may also reveal significant sleep apnea and gastroesophageal reflux disease. Glycemic control is often poor and contributes significantly to infection and diabetes. The obese patient has a decrease in antithrombin III levels, and a higher risk of DVT and pulmonary embolism (PE). Measures to optimize physiologic function in obese patients include keeping the head of the bed elevated at all times. This can improve the functional residual capacity of the lungs by almost a liter, thereby decreasing complications associated with atelectasis and pneumonia. Proper glycemic control via a tight insulin sliding scale is also recommended. Finally, the risk of DVT may be attenuated by immediate use of prophylactic doses of low molecular weight heparin (LMWH) and early ambulation.

Issues for surgery in the very young and the very old have many similarities when it comes to potential errors and complications. Perhaps the most notable similarity is the lack of physiologic reserve. The older adult may have end-organ insufficiency, although the young can have underdeveloped or anomalous organ function that may not yet have become manifest. Similarly, the immune responses at the extremes of age are often compromised. This makes diagnosing an infection difficult; older adults may not be capable of mounting a febrile response, and young children can often resolve fevers overnight, and the cause may remain undiagnosed.

Other alterations in these groups include the amount and distribution of total body water and total body fat. This is important to consider because some medications are predominantly distributed to fat stores, and this deposition may lead to altered drug clearance. Similarly, total body water is decreased and serum concentrations of medications may be higher than anticipated. In both groups there is a lower lean body mass, which may potentiate the adverse effects of some anesthetic agents. Metabolism of various analgesic and anesthetic agents can be protracted, leading to postoperative problems such as prolonged intubation and the need for the administration of reversal agents.

Other issues that can lead to complex decision making include those related to communication. Whether because of neurologic impairments, agitation, confusion, or an inability to comprehend a language, these factors associated with the extremes of age increase the potential for medical errors. Open and direct communication with the supporting family members is critical for optimal outcomes in these patient groups.

Suggested Readings

Kohn LT, Corrigan JM, Donaldson MS (eds): To Err Is Human: Building a Safer Health System. Committee on Quality of Health Care in America, Institute of Medicine. Washington, DC: National Academy Press, 2000.

Rybak MJ, Abate BJ, Kang SL, et al: Prospective evaluation of the effect of an aminoglycoside dosing regimen on rates of observed nephrotoxicity and ototoxicity. Antimicrob Agents Chemother 43:1549, 1999.

The Acute Respiratory Distress Syndrome Network: Ventilation with lower tidal volumes as compared with traditional tidal volumes for acute lung injury and the acute respiratory distress syndrome. N Engl J Med 342:1301, 2000.

Yang KL, Tobin MJ: A prospective study of indexes predicting the outcome of trials of weaning from mechanical ventilation. N Engl J Med 324:1445, 1991.

Stewart BT, Woods RJ, Collopy BT, et al: Early feeding after elective open colorectal resections: A prospective randomized trial. Aust N Z J Surg 68:125, 1998.

Domschke W, Lederer P, Lux G: The value of emergency endoscopy in upper gastrointestinal bleeding: Review and analysis of 2014 cases. Endoscopy 15:126, 1983.

Flum DR, Dellinger EP, Cheadle A, et al: Intraoperative cholangiography and risk of common bile duct injury during cholecystectomy. JAMA 289:1639, 2003.

Stevens MA, McCullough PA, Tobin KJ, et al: A prospective randomized trial of prevention measures in patients at high risk for contrast nephropathy: Results of the P.R.I.N.C.E. study. Prevention of radiocontrast induced nephropathy clinical evaluation. J Am Coll Cardiol 33:403, 1999.

Ivatury RR, Porter JM, Simon RJ, et al: Intra-abdominal hypertension after life-threatening penetrating abdominal trauma: Prophylaxis, incidence, and clinical relevance to gastric mucosal pH and abdominal compartment syndrome. J Trauma 44:1016, 1998.

Gorecki PJ, Schein M, Mehta V, et al: Surgeons and infectious disease specialists: Different attitudes towards antibiotic treatment and prophylaxis in common abdominal surgical infections. Surg Infect (Larchmt) 1:115, 2000; discussion 125.

Van den Berghe G, Wouters P, Weekers F, et al: Intensive insulin therapy in the critically ill patients. N Engl J Med 345:1359, 2001.

12 | Physiologic Monitoring of the Surgical Patient

Louis H. Alarcon and Mitchell P. Fink

Patients are monitored to detect alterations in various physiologic parameters, providing advanced warning of impending deterioration in organ function. With this knowledge, appropriate and timely intervention may be taken to prevent or ameliorate physiologic derangement.

Synthesis of adenosine triphosphate (ATP), the energy "currency" of cells, requires the continuous delivery of oxygen from hemoglobin in red blood cells to the oxidative machinery within mitochondria. In essence, the goal of hemodynamic monitoring is to ensure that the flow of oxygenated blood through the microcirculation is sufficient to support aerobic metabolism at the cellular level. Under normal conditions when the supply of oxygen is plentiful, aerobic metabolism is determined by factors other than the availability of oxygen. These factors include the hormonal milieu and mechanical workload of contractile tissue. However, in pathologic circumstances when oxygen availability is inadequate, oxygen utilization (Vo_2) becomes dependent on oxygen delivery (Do_2). This is the point of critical oxygen delivery (Do_2crit) in which the transition from supply independent to supply dependent oxygen uptake occurs, and is approximately 300 mL/min per square meter.

ARTERIAL BLOOD PRESSURE

Arterial blood pressure is a complex function of both cardiac output and vascular input impedance. Blood pressure can be determined directly by measuring the pressure within the arterial lumen or indirectly using a cuff around an extremity.

Noninvasive Measurement of Arterial Blood Pressure

Both manual and automated means for the noninvasive determination of blood pressure use an inflatable cuff to increase pressure around an extremity. Erroneous measurements can be obtained from inappropriate sized cuffs. Noninvasive measurement of blood pressure requires detection of the arterial pulsations. The auscultation of the Korotkoff sounds is a time-honored method. Systolic pressure is defined as the pressure in the cuff when tapping sounds are first audible. Diastolic pressure is the pressure in the cuff when audible pulsations first disappear.

Another means for pulse detection when measuring blood pressure noninvasively depends on the detection of oscillations in the pressure within the bladder of the cuff. This approach is simple and can be performed even in a noisy environment, however, it is neither accurate nor reliable. Other methods for pulse detection are use of a Doppler stethoscope (reappearance of the pulse produces an audible amplified signal) or a pulse oximeter (reappearance of the pulse is indicated by flashing of a light-emitting diode).

275

Invasive Monitoring of Arterial Blood Pressure

Direct monitoring of arterial pressure is performed by using fluid-filled tubing to connect an intraarterial catheter to a transducer. The signal generated by the transducer is amplified and displayed as a continuous waveform by an oscilloscope. Digital values for systolic, diastolic and mean pressure, calculated by averaging the amplitude of the pressure waveform, can be displayed.

The fidelity of the catheter-tubing-transducer system is determined by the compliance of the tubing, the surface area of the transducer diaphragm, and the compliance of the diaphragm. If the system is underdamped, the inertia of the system, which is a function of the mass of the fluid in the tubing and the mass of the diaphragm, causes overshoot of the points of maximum positive and negative displacement of the diaphragm. Thus in an underdamped system, systolic pressure will be overestimated and diastolic pressure will be underestimated. In an overdamped system, displacement of the diaphragm fails to track the rapidly changing pressure waveform, and systolic pressure will be underestimated and diastolic pressure will be overestimated. Even in an underdamped or overdamped system, mean pressure will be accurately recorded, provided the system has been properly calibrated.

The radial artery is the site most commonly used for intraarterial pressure monitoring. It should be noted that central (aortic) and peripheral (radial artery) pressures are different as a result of the impedance and inductance of the arterial tree. Systolic pressures typically are higher and diastolic pressures are lower in the periphery, whereas mean pressure is approximately the same in the aorta and distal sites. Complications of arterial cannulation include: distal ischemia, retrograde embolization of air bubbles or thrombi into the intracranial circulation, and catheter-related infections.

ELECTROCARDIOGRAPHIC MONITORING

The electrocardiogram (ECG) records the electrical activity associated with cardiac contraction by detecting voltages on the body surface. A standard 3-lead ECG is obtained by placing electrodes that correspond to the left arm (LA), right arm (RA), and left leg (LL). The ECG waveforms can be continuously displayed on a monitor, and an alarm sounds if an abnormality of rate or rhythm is detected. Monitoring of the ECG waveform is essential in patients with acute coronary syndromes or blunt myocardial injury, because dysrhythmias are the most common lethal complication. In patients with shock or sepsis, dysrhythmias can occur as a consequence of inadequate myocardial oxygen delivery or as a complication of vasoactive or inotropic drugs used to support blood pressure and cardiac output.

Additional information can be obtained from a 12-lead ECG, which is essential for patients with potential acute coronary syndromes or other cardiac complications in acutely ill patients. Continuous monitoring of the 12-lead ECG provides greater sensitivity than 3-lead ECG for the detection of acute myocardial ischemia.

CARDIAC OUTPUT AND RELATED PARAMETERS

Bedside catheterization of the pulmonary artery was introduced to manage patients with cardiogenic shock and other acute cardiac diseases. Indications for this form of invasive hemodynamic monitoring have expanded to encompass a wide variety of clinical conditions.

Determinants of Cardiac Performance

Preload

According to Starling's law the force of muscle contraction depends on the initial length of the cardiac fibers, which represents preload and is determined by end-diastolic volume (EDV). For the right ventricle, central venous pressure (CVP) approximates right ventricular end-diastolic pressure (EDP). For the left ventricle, pulmonary artery occlusion pressure (PAOP), which is measured by transiently inflating a balloon at the end of a pressure monitoring catheter positioned in a small branch of the pulmonary artery, approximates left ventricular end-diastolic pressure. The presence of atrioventricular valvular stenosis will alter this relationship.

EDP is used as a surrogate for EDV, but EDP is determined not only by volume but also by the diastolic compliance of the ventricular chamber. Ventricular compliance is altered by various pharmacologic agents and pathologic conditions. Furthermore, the relationship between EDP and true preload is not linear, but rather is exponential.

Afterload

Afterload is defined as the force resisting fiber shortening once systole begins. Several factors contribute to ventricular afterload, including ventricular intracavitary pressure, wall thickness, chamber radius, and chamber geometry. Because these factors are difficult to assess clinically, afterload is commonly approximated by calculating systemic vascular resistance (SVR), defined as mean arterial pressure (MAP) divided by cardiac output.

Contractility

Contractility is defined as the inotropic state of the myocardium. Contractility is said to increase when the force of ventricular contraction increases at constant preload and afterload. Contractility is difficult to quantify, because the available measures are dependent to a certain degree on preload and afterload. If pressure-volume loops are constructed for each cardiac cycle, small changes in preload and/or afterload will result in shifts of the point defining the end of systole. These end-systolic points on the pressure-versus-volume diagram describe a straight line, known as the isovolumic pressure line. A steeper slope of this line indicates greater contractility.

Placement of Pulmonary Artery Catheters

In its simplest form, the pulmonary artery catheter (PAC) has four channels. One channel terminates in a balloon at the tip of the catheter which permits inflation of the balloon with air. A second channel contains wires that are connected to a thermistor located near the tip of the catheter to permit calculation of cardiac output using the thermodilution technique (see below). The final two channels are used for pressure monitoring and the injection of the thermal indicator for determinations of cardiac output. One of these channels terminates at the tip of the catheter; the other terminates 20 cm proximal to the tip.

Placement of a PAC requires access to the central venous circulation (antecubital, femoral, jugular, and subclavian veins). Cannulation of the vein is normally performed percutaneously, using the Seldinger technique (described elsewhere). An introducer sheath is placed, which is equipped with a diaphragm that permits insertion of the PAC whereas preventing the backflow of blood.

The proximal terminus of the distal port of the PAC is connected to a strain-gauge transducer. Although constantly observing the pressure tracing on an oscilloscope, the PAC is advanced with the balloon deflated until respiratory excursions are observed. The balloon is then inflated, and the catheter advanced further, although monitoring pressures sequentially in the right atrium and right ventricle en route to the pulmonary artery. The catheter is advanced out the pulmonary artery until a damped tracing indicative of the "wedged" position is obtained. The balloon is then deflated, taking care to ensure that a normal pulmonary arterial tracing is again observed on the monitor; leaving the balloon inflated can increase the risk of pulmonary infarction or perforation of the pulmonary artery. Unnecessary measurements of the pulmonary artery occlusion pressure are discouraged as rupture of the pulmonary artery may occur.

Hemodynamic Measurements

The PAC is capable of providing a remarkable amount of information about the hemodynamic status of patients. Additional information may be obtained if various modifications of the standard PAC are employed. By combining data obtained through use of the PAC with results obtained by other means (i.e., blood hemoglobin concentration and oxyhemoglobin saturation), derived estimates of systemic oxygen transport and utilization can be calculated. Table 12-1 summarizes the equations used to calculate the derived parameters and Table 12-2 gives the normal ranges for the measured and calculated homodynamic values.

Measurement of Cardiac Output by Thermodilution

Measurement of cardiac output (QT) using the thermodilution technique is simple and reasonably accurate. If a bolus of an indicator is rapidly and thoroughly mixed with a moving fluid upstream from a detector, then the concentration of the indicator at the detector will increase sharply and then exponentially diminish back to zero. The area under the resulting time-concentration curve is a function of the volume of indicator injected and the flow rate of the moving stream of fluid. Larger volumes of indicator result in greater areas under the curve, and faster flow rates of the mixing fluid result in smaller areas under the curve. When QT is measured by thermodilution, the indicator is heat and the detector is a temperature-sensing thermistor at the distal end of the PAC. The relationship used for calculating QT is called the Stewart-Hamilton equation:

$$QT = [V \times (TB - TI) \times K1 \times K2] \times \int TB(t)dt$$

in which V is the volume of the indicator injected, TB is the temperature of blood (i.e., core body temperature), TI is the temperature of the indicator, K1 is a constant that is the function of the specific heats of blood and the indicator, K2 is an empirically derived constant that accounts for several factors (the dead space volume of the catheter, heat lost from the indicator as it traverses the catheter, and the injection rate of the indicator), and $\int TB(t)dt$ is the area under the time-temperature curve. In clinical practice, the Stewart-Hamilton equation is solved by a microprocessor.

Determination of cardiac output by the thermodilution method is generally quite accurate, although it tends to overestimate QT at low values. The results

TABLE 12-1 Formulas for Calculation of Hemodynamic Parameters That Can Be Derived by Using Data Obtained by Pulmonary Artery Catheterization

$Q_T{}^*$ (L · min^{-1} · m^{-2}) = Q_T/BSA, where BSA is body surface area (m^2)

SV (mL) = Q_T/HR, where HR is heart rate (min^{-1})

SVR (dyne · sec · cm^{-5}) = [(MAP – CVP) × 80] /Q_T, where MAP is mean arterial pressure (mmHg)

SVRI (dyne · sec · cm^{-5} · m^{-2}) = [(MAP – CVP) × 80] /$Q_T{}^*$

PVR (dyne · sec · cm^{-5}) = [(PAP – PAOP) × 80] /QT, where PPA is mean pulmonary artery pressure

PVRI (dyne · sec · cm^{-5} · m^{-2}) = [(PAP – PAOP) × 80] /$Q_T{}^*$

RVEDV (mL) = SV/RVEF

$\dot{D}o_2$ (mL · min^{-1} · m^{-2}) = $Q_T{}^*$ × Cao_2 × 10, where Cao_2 is arterial oxygen content (mL/dL)

$\dot{V}o_2$ (mL · min^{-1} · m^{-2}) = $Q_T{}^*$ × (Cao_2 – $C\bar{v}o_2$) × 10, where $C\bar{v}o_2$ is mixed venous oxygen content (mL/dL)

Cao_2 = (1.36 × Hgb × Sao_2) + (0.003 + Pao_2), where Hgb is hemoglobin concentration (g/dL), Sao_2 is fractional arterial hemoglobin saturation, and Pao_2 is the partial pressure of oxygen in arterial blood

$C\bar{v}o_2$ = (1.36 × Hgb × $S\bar{v}o_2$) + (0.003 + $P\bar{v}o_2$), where $P\bar{v}o_2$ is the partial pressure of oxygen in pulmonary arterial (mixed venous) blood

Q_S/Q_T = (Cco_2 – Cao_2)/ (Cco_2 – Cvo_2), where Cco_2 (mL/dL) is the content of oxygen in pulmonary end capillary blood

Cco_2 = (1.36 × Hgb) + (0.003 + P_{AO_2}), where P_{AO_2} is the alveolar partial pressure of oxygen

P_{AO_2} = [F_{IO_2} × (P_B – P_{H_2O})] – Pa_{CO_2}/RQ, where F_{IO_2} is the fractional concentration of inspired oxygen, P_B is the barometric pressure (mmHg), P_{H_2O} is the water vapor pressure (usually 47 mmHg), Pa_{CO_2} is the partial pressure of carbon dioxide in arterial blood (mmHg), and RQ is respiratory quotient (usually assumed to be 0.8)

$C\bar{v}o_2$ = central venous oxygen pressure; CVP = mean central venous pressure; $\dot{D}o_2$ = systemic oxygen delivery; PAOP = pulmonary artery occlusion (wedge) pressure; PVR = pulmonary vascular resistance; PVRI = pulmonary vascular resistance index; Q_S/Q_T = fractional pulmonary venous admixture (shunt fraction); Q_T = cardiac output; $Q_T{}^*$ = cardiac output indexed to body surface area (cardiac index); RVEDV = right ventricular end-diastolic volume; RVEF = right ventricular ejection fraction; SV = stroke volume; SVI = stroke volume index; $S\bar{v}o_2$ = fractional mixed venous (pulmonary artery) hemoglobin saturation; SVR = systemic vascular resistance; SVRI = systemic vascular resistance index; $\dot{V}o_2$ = systemic oxygen utilization. Hgb = concentration of hemoglobin in blood.

generally should be recorded as the mean of two or three determinations obtained at random points in the respiratory cycle. Using cold injectate widens the difference between TB and TI and thereby increases signal-to-noise ratio. Nevertheless, most authorities recommend using room temperature injectate (normal saline or 5 percent dextrose in water) to minimize errors resulting from warming of the fluid as it is transferred from its reservoir to a syringe for injection.

Continuous measurement of QT by thermodilution is possible using a PAC with a heating element that heats the passing blood located upstream from the thermistor. It is then possible to estimate the average blood flow across the

TABLE 12-2 Approximate Normal Ranges for Selected Hemodynamic Parameters in Adults

Parameter	Normal range
CVP	0–6 mmHg
Right ventricular systolic pressure	20–30 mmHg
Right ventricular diastolic pressure	0–6 mmHg
PAOP	6–12 mmHg
Systolic arterial pressure	100–130 mmHg
Diastolic arterial pressure	60–90 mmHg
MAP	75–100 mmHg
Q_T	4–6 L/min
Q_T^*	2.5–3.5 $L \cdot min^{-1} \cdot m^{-2}$
SV	40–80 mL
SVR	800–1400 $dyne \cdot sec \cdot cm^{-5}$
SVRI	1500–2400 $dyne \cdot sec \cdot cm^{-5} \cdot m^{-2}$
PVR	100–150 $dyne \cdot sec \cdot cm^{-5}$
PVRI	200–400 $dyne \cdot sec \cdot cm^{-5} \cdot m^{-2}$
Cao_2	16–22 mL/dL
Cvo_2	~15 mL 02 dL blood
$\dot{D}o_2$	400–660 $mL \cdot min^{-1} \cdot m^{-2}$
$\dot{V}o_2$	115–165 $mL \cdot min^{-1} \cdot m^{-2}$

Cao_2 = arterial oxygen content; Cvo_2 = central venous oxygen pressure; CVP = mean central venous pressure; $\dot{D}o_2$ = systemic oxygen delivery; MAP = mean arterial pressure; PAOP = pulmonary artery occlusion (wedge) pressure; PVR = pulmonary vascular resistance; PVRI = pulmonary vascular resistance index; Q_T = cardiac output; Q_T^* = cardiac output indexed to body surface area (cardiac index); SV = stroke volume; SVI = stroke volume index; SVR = systemic vascular resistance; SVRI = systemic vascular resistance index; $\dot{V}o_2$ = systemic oxygen utilization.

filament and thereby calculate QT. Continuous determinations of QT using this approach agree well with data generated by conventional measurements.

Mixed Venous Oximetry

The Fick equation can be written as $QT = VO_2/(Cao_2 - Cvo_2)$, in which Cao_2 is the content of oxygen in arterial blood and Cvo_2 is the content of oxygen in mixed venous blood. The Fick equation can be rearranged as: $C\bar{v}o_2 = Cao_2 - VO_2/QT$. If the small contribution of dissolved oxygen to $C\bar{v}o_2$ and Cao_2 is ignored, the equation can be rewritten as $S\bar{v}o_2 = Sao_2 - VO_2/(QT \times Hgb \times 1.36)$, in which $S\bar{v}o_2$ is the fractional saturation of hemoglobin in mixed venous blood, Sao_2 is the fractional saturation of hemoglobin in arterial blood, and Hgb is the concentration of hemoglobin in blood. Accordingly, low values of $S\bar{v}o_2$ can be caused by a decrease in QT (e.g., heart failure or hypovolemia), a decrease in Sao_2 (e.g., intrinsic pulmonary disease), a decrease in Hgb (i.e., anemia), or an increase in metabolic rate (e.g., seizures or fever). With a conventional PAC, intermittent measurements of $S\bar{v}o_2$ require aspirating a sample of blood from the distal (i.e., pulmonary arterial) port of the catheter and injecting the sample into a blood gas analyzer.

By adding a fifth channel to the PAC, it is possible to monitor $S\bar{v}o_2$ continuously. This channel contains two fiber-optic bundles, which are used to transmit and receive light of the appropriate wavelengths to permit measurements of hemoglobin saturation by reflectance spectrophotometry. The device provides measurements of $S\bar{v}o_2$ that agree quite closely with those obtained by conventional analyses of pulmonary arterial blood.

The saturation of oxygen in the right atrium or superior vena cava ($Sc\bar{v}o_2$) correlates closely with $S\bar{v}o_2$ over a wide range of conditions. Because measurement of $Sc\bar{v}o_2$ requires placement of a central venous catheter rather than a PAC, it is somewhat less invasive and easier to carry out. By using a central venous catheter equipped to permit fiber-optic monitoring of $Sc\bar{v}o_2$, it may be possible to improve the resuscitation of patients with shock during the first few critical h after presentation to the hospital.

Right Ventricular Ejection Fraction

Ejection fraction (EF) is calculated as (EDV − ESV)/EDV, in which ESV is end-systolic volume. EF is an ejection-phase measure of myocardial contractility. By equipping a PAC with a thermistor with a short time constant, the thermodilution method can be used to estimate right ventricular (RV) EF. Measurements of RVEF by thermodilution agree reasonably well with those obtained by other means. Stroke volume (SV) is calculated as EDV − ESV. Left ventricular (LV) SV also equals QT/HR, in which HR is heart rate. Because LVSV is equal to RVSV, it is possible to estimate right ventricular end-diastolic volume (RVEDV) by measuring RVEF, QT, and HR.

Effect of Pulmonary Artery Catheterization on Outcome

Connors and colleagues reported surprising results in a major observational study evaluating the value of pulmonary artery catheterization in critically ill patients. They compared two groups of patients: those who did and those who did not undergo placement of a PAC during their first 24 h of intensive care unit (ICU) care. A critical assessment of this study reveals that the groups were well-matched with respect to a large number of pertinent clinical parameters. They concluded that placement of a pulmonary artery catheter during the first 24 h of stay in an ICU is associated with a significant increase in the risk of mortality, even when statistical methods are used to account for severity of illness.

This study confirmed the results of two prior similar observational studies. The first of these studies used as a database 3263 patients with acute myocardial infarction. Hospital mortality was significantly greater for patients treated using a PAC, even when multivariate statistical methods were employed to control for key potential confounding factors such as age, peak circulating creatine kinase concentration, and presence or absence of new Q waves on the electrocardiogram. The second large observational study of patients with acute myocardial infarction also found that hospital mortality was significantly greater for patients managed with the assistance of a PAC, even when the presence or absence of "pump failure" was considered in the statistical analysis. In neither of these earlier reports did the authors conclude that placement of a PAC was truly the cause of worsened survival after myocardial infarction. As a result of the study by Connors and colleagues, experts in the field questioned the value of bedside pulmonary artery catheterization, and some even called for a moratorium on the use of the PAC. Relatively few prospective, randomized controlled trials of pulmonary artery catheterization have been performed. All of these studies are flawed in one or more ways.

In the largest randomized controlled trial of the PAC, Sandham and associates randomized American Society of Anesthesiologists (ASA) class III and IV patients undergoing major thoracic, abdominal, or orthopedic surgery to placement of a PAC or CVP catheter. In the patients assigned to receive a PAC, physiologic goal-directed therapy was implemented by protocol. There were no differences in mortality at 30 days, 6 months, or 12 months between the two groups, and ICU length of stay was similar. There was a significantly higher rate of pulmonary emboli in the PAC group (0.9 vs. 0 percent).

Thus, the weight of current evidence suggests that routine pulmonary artery catheterization is not useful for the vast majority of patients undergoing cardiac, major peripheral vascular, or ablative surgical procedures.

One of the reasons for using a PAC is to optimize cardiac output and systemic oxygen delivery. Defining what constitutes the optimum cardiac output, however, has proven to be difficult. Based on an extensive observational database and comparisons of the hemodynamic and oxygen transport values recorded in survivors and nonsurvivors, Bland and colleagues proposed that "goal-directed" hemodynamic resuscitation should aim to achieve a QT greater than 4.5 L/min per square meter and VO_2 greater than 600 mL/min per square meter. A number of investigators have conducted randomized trials designed to evaluate the effect on outcome of goal-directed as compared to conventional hemodynamic resuscitation. Some studies provide support for the notion that interventions designed to achieve supraphysiologic goals for DO_2, VO_2, and QT improve outcome. However, other published studies do not support this view, and a meta-analysis concluded that interventions designed to achieve supraphysiologic goals for oxygen transport do not significantly reduce mortality rates in critically ill patients. At this time, supraphysiologic resuscitation of patients in shock cannot be endorsed.

Connors has offered several explanations for the apparent lack of effectiveness of the PAC. First, even though bedside pulmonary artery catheterization is quite safe, the procedure is associated with a finite incidence of serious complications, including ventricular arrhythmias, catheter-related sepsis, central venous thrombosis, pulmonary arterial perforation and pulmonary embolism. The adverse effects of these complications on outcome may equal or even outweigh any benefits associated with using a PAC to guide therapy. Second, the data generated by the PAC may be inaccurate, leading to inappropriate therapeutic interventions. Third, the measurements, even if accurate, are often misinterpreted in practice. Even well-trained intensivists are capable of misinterpreting results provided by pulmonary artery catheterization. Furthermore, the current state of understanding is primitive when it comes to deciding what is the best management for certain hemodynamic disturbances. Taking all of this into consideration, it may be that interventions prompted by measurements obtained with a PAC are actually harmful to patients. As a result, the marginal benefit now available by placing a PAC may be quite small. Less invasive modalities are available that can provide clinically useful hemodynamic information.

Minimally Invasive Alternatives to the Pulmonary Artery Catheter

There has been increasing interest in the development of less invasive methods for monitoring of hemodynamic parameters. None of these methods render the standard thermodilution technique of the PAC obsolete. However, these strategies may contribute to improvements in the hemodynamic monitoring of critically ill patients.

Doppler Ultrasonography

When ultrasonic sound waves are reflected by moving erythrocytes in the bloodstream, the frequency of the reflected signal is increased or decreased, depending on whether the cells are moving toward or away from the ultrasonic source. This change in frequency is called the Doppler shift, and its magnitude is determined by the velocity of the moving red blood cells. Using the cross-sectional area of a vessel and the mean red blood cell velocity of the blood flowing through it, one can calculate blood flow rate. If the vessel in question is the aorta, then QT can be calculated as:

$$QT = HR \times A \times \int V(t)dt$$

in which A is the cross-sectional area of the aorta and $\int V(t)dt$ is the red blood cell velocity integrated over the cardiac cycle.

Two approaches have been developed for using Doppler ultrasonography to estimate QT. The first approach uses an ultrasonic transducer, which is manually positioned in the suprasternal notch and focused on the root of the aorta. Although this approach is completely noninvasive, it requires a highly skilled operator to obtain meaningful results. Moreover, unless QT measured using thermodilution is used to back-calculate aortic diameter, accuracy using the suprasternal notch approach is not acceptable. Accordingly, the method is useful only for obtaining very intermittent estimates of QT, and has not been widely adopted by clinicians.

In the other approach blood flow velocity is continuously monitored in the descending thoracic aorta using a transducer introduced into the esophagus. The device consists of a continuous-wave Doppler transducer mounted at the tip of a transesophageal probe, and continuously measures the blood flow velocity in the descending aorta and the calculated QT. Results using these methods appear to be reasonably accurate across a broad spectrum of patients and are clinically useful. In a multicenter study, good correlation was found between esophageal Doppler and thermodilution ($r = 0.95$), with a small systematic underestimation (bias 0.24 L/min) using esophageal Doppler.

Impedance Cardiography

The impedance to flow of alternating electrical current in regions of the body is commonly called bioimpedance. In the thorax, changes in the volume and velocity of blood in the thoracic aorta lead to detectable changes in bioimpedance. The first derivative of the oscillating component of thoracic bioimpedance (dZ/dt) is linearly related to aortic blood flow. Empirically derived formulas have been developed to estimate SV, and subsequently QT. The approach is attractive because it is noninvasive and provides a continuous readout of QT. However, measurements of QT obtained by impedance cardiography are not sufficiently reliable to be used for clinical decision-making and have poor correlation with standard methods such as thermodilution and ventricular angiography.

Pulse Contour Analysis

Pulse contour analysis was originally described for estimating SV on a beat-to-beat basis. The mechanical properties of the arterial tree and the SV determine the shape of the arterial pulse waveform. The pulse contour method of estimating QT uses the arterial pressure waveform as an input for a model of the systemic circulation to determine beat-to-beat flow through the circulatory system. The parameters of resistance, compliance, and impedance are initially estimated based on the patient's age and sex, and can be subsequently refined by using a reference standard measurement of QT.

Measurements of QT based on pulse contour monitoring are comparable in accuracy to standard PAC-thermodilution methods, but it uses an approach that is less invasive because arterial and central venous, but not transcardiac, catheterization is needed. Using on-line pressure waveform analysis, the computerized algorithms can calculate SV, QT, systemic vascular resistance, and an estimate of myocardial contractility, the rate of rise of the arterial systolic pressure (dP/dT).

The use of pulse contour analysis has been applied using an even less invasive technology based on totally noninvasive photoplethysmographic measurements of arterial pressure. However, the accuracy of this technique has been questioned and its clinical utility remains to be determined.

Partial Carbon Dioxide Rebreathing

Partial carbon dioxide (CO_2) rebreathing uses the Fick principle to estimate QT noninvasively. By intermittently altering the dead space within the ventilator circuit via a rebreathing valve, changes in CO2 production (Vco_2) and end-tidal CO_2 (etco$_2$) are used to determine cardiac output using a modified Fick equation ($QT = \Delta Vco_2/\Delta etco_2$). Changes in intrapulmonary shunt and hemodynamic instability impair the accuracy of QT estimated by partial CO_2 rebreathing. Continuous in-line pulse oximetry and inspired fraction of inspired O_2 (Fio_2) are used to estimate shunt fraction to correct QT. Some studies suggest that the partial CO_2 rebreathing method for determination of QT compares favorably to measurements made using a PAC in critically ill patients.

Transesophageal Echocardiography

Transesophageal echocardiography (TEE) has made the transition from operating room to intensive care unit. TEE requires that the patient be sedated and usually intubated for airway protection. Using this powerful technology, global assessments of LV and RV function can be made, including determinations of ventricular volume, EF, and QT. Segmental wall motion abnormalities, pericardial effusions, and tamponade can be readily identified with TEE. Doppler techniques allow estimation of atrial filling pressures. The technique is somewhat cumbersome and requires considerable training and skill to obtain reliable results.

Assessing Preload Responsiveness

Although pulse contour analysis or partial CO_2 rebreathing may be able to provide fairly reliable estimates regarding SV and QT, these approaches alone offer little or no information about the adequacy of preload. Most clinicians determine preload by measuring CVP or PAOP. However, neither CVP nor PAOP correlate well with the true parameter of interest, left ventricular end-diastolic volume (LVEDV). Extremely high or low CVP or PAOP results are informative, but readings in a large middle zone (i.e., 5–20 mmHg) are not very useful. Furthermore, changes in CVP or PAOP fail to correlate well with changes in stroke volume. Echocardiography can be used to estimate LVEDV, but this approach is dependent on the skill and training of the individual using it, and isolated measurements of LVEDV fail to predict the hemodynamic response to alterations in preload.

When intrathoracic pressure increases during the application of positive airway pressure in mechanically ventilated patients, venous return decreases, and as a consequence, left ventricular stroke volume (LVSV) also decreases. Therefore, pulse pressure variation (PPV) during a positive pressure episode can be used to predict the responsiveness of cardiac output to changes in preload. PPV is defined as the difference between the maximal pulse pressure and the minimum pulse pressure divided by the average of these two pressures. Patients are considered as being preload responsive if their cardiac index increases by at least 15 percent after rapid infusion of a standard volume of intravenous fluid. Although atrial arrhythmias can interfere with the usefulness of this technique, PPV remains a useful approach for assessing preload responsiveness in most patients because of its simplicity and reliability.

Tissue Capnometry

Global indices of QT, DO_2, or VO_2 provide little useful information regarding the adequacy of cellular oxygenation and mitochondrial function. In theory, measuring tissue pH to assess the adequacy of perfusion is an attractive concept because anaerobiosis is associated with the net accumulation of protons. The detection of tissue acidosis should alert the clinician to the possibility that perfusion is inadequate. Tonometric measurements of tissue Pco_2 in the stomach or sigmoid colon could be used to estimate mucosal pH (pHi) and thereby monitor visceral perfusion in critically ill patients.

Unfortunately, using tonometric estimates of gastrointestinal mucosal pHi for monitoring perfusion is predicated on a number of assumptions, some of which may be invalid. Furthermore, methods for performing measurements of gastric mucosal Pco_2 in the clinical setting remain rather cumbersome and expensive. For these reasons gastric tonometry has primarily been used as a research tool. Some recent developments in the field may change this situation, and monitoring tissue Pco_2 may become common in the near future.

Tonometric determination of mucosal carbon dioxide tension, Pco_2muc, can be used to calculate pHi by using the Henderson-Hasselbalch equation as follows: pHi $= \log ([HCO_3-]muc/0.03 \times Pco_2muc)$, in which $[HCO_3-]$muc is the concentration of bicarbonate anion in the mucosa. $[HCO_3-]$muc cannot be measured directly, but must be estimated by assuming that the concentration of bicarbonate anion in arterial blood, $[HCO_3-]$art, is approximately equal to $[HCO_3-]$muc. Under pathologic conditions, however, the assumption that $[HCO_3-]$art $\cong [HCO_3-]$muc is almost certainly invalid.

There is another inherent problem in using pHi as an index of perfusion. As noted above, pHi calculated using the Henderson-Hasselbalch equation is a function of both Pco_2muc and $[HCO_3-]art$. Under steady-state conditions Pco_2muc, reflects the balance between inflow of CO_2 into the interstitial space and outflow of CO_2 from the interstitial space. An increase in Pco_2muc can reflect a decrease in mucosal perfusion, but may also can be caused by arterial hypercarbia, leading to increased diffusion of CO_2 from arterial blood into the interstitium. Thus, tonometrically derived estimates of pHi are not a reliable way to assess mucosal perfusion.

Despite the problems noted above, measurements of gastric pHi and/or mucosal-arterial Pco_2 gap have been proven to be a reliable predictor of outcome in a wide variety of critically ill patients. Moreover, in a landmark prospective, randomized, multicentric clinical trial by Gutierrez and associates of monitoring in medical intensive care unit patients, titrating resuscitation to a gastric pHi endpoint rather than conventional hemodynamic indices resulted in higher 30-day survival rate. In trauma patients, it has been shown that failure to normalize gastric pHi within 24 h was associated with a high mortality rate.

Monitoring tissue Pco_2 (tissue capnometry) will play an increasingly important role in the management of critically ill patients because it provides more reliable information about perfusion than does the derived parameter, pHi. By eliminating the potentially confounding effects of systemic hypocarbia or hypercarbia, calculating and monitoring the gap between tissue Pco_2 and arterial Pco_2 may prove to be even more valuable than simply following changes in tissue Pco_2. Additionally, monitoring tissue Pco_2 in sites such as the space under the tongue may be as informative as measuring Pco_2 in the wall of the esophagus or the gut and less invasive.

Increased sublingual Pco_2 ($Pslco_2$) is associated with decreases in arterial blood pressure and QT in patients with shock because of hemorrhage or sepsis. In a study of critically ill patients with septic or cardiogenic shock, the $Pslco_2$-$Paco_2$ gradient was found to be a good prognostic indicator. This study also demonstrated that sublingual capnography was superior to gastric tonometry in predicting patient survival. The $Pslco_2$-$Paco_2$ gradient also correlated with the mixed venous-arterial Pco_2 gradient, but failed to correlate with blood lactate level, mixed venous O_2 saturation ($S\bar{v}o_2$), or systemic DO_2. These latter findings suggest that the $Pslco_2$-$Paco_2$ gradient may be a better marker of tissue hypoxia than are these other parameters.

RESPIRATORY MONITORING

The ability to monitor various parameters of respiratory function is important in critically ill patients, to assess the adequacy of oxygenation and ventilation, guide weaning and liberation from mechanical ventilation, and detect adverse events associated with respiratory failure and mechanical ventilation.

Arterial Blood Gases

Blood gas analysis provides useful information when caring for patients with respiratory failure and to detect alterations in acid-base balance because of low QT, sepsis, renal failure, severe trauma, medication or drug overdose, or altered mental status. Arterial blood can be analyzed for pH, Po_2, Pco_2, HCO_3-concentration and calculated base deficit. When indicated, carboxyhemoglobin and methemoglobin levels also can be measured. Efforts have been made to decrease the unnecessary use of arterial blood gas analysis. For example, arterial blood gas determinations are not necessary for routine weaning from mechanical ventilation in the majority of postoperative patients.

Blood gas analyses involve the removal of an aliquot of blood from the patient, although continuous bedside arterial blood gas determinations are now possible via an indwelling arterial catheter that contains a biosensor. Excellent agreement between the two methods has been demonstrated.

Determinants of Oxygen Delivery

The primary goal of the cardiovascular and respiratory systems is to deliver oxygenated blood to the tissues. DO_2 is dependent to a greater degree on the oxygen saturation of hemoglobin (Hgb) in arterial blood (Sao_2) than on the partial pressure of oxygen in arterial blood (Pao_2). DO_2 also is dependent on QT and Hgb. Dissolved oxygen in blood, which is proportional to the Pao_2, makes only a negligible contribution to DO_2, as is apparent from the equation: $DO_2 = QT \times [(Hgb \times Sao_2 \times 1.36) + (Pao_2 \times 0.0031)]$.

Sao_2 in mechanically ventilated patients depends on the mean airway pressure, the fraction of inspired oxygen (Fio_2), and SVO_2. Thus, when Sao_2 is low, the clinician has only a limited number of ways to improve this parameter. The clinician can increase mean airway pressure by increasing positive-end expiratory pressure (PEEP) or inspiratory time. Fio_2 can be increased to a maximum of 1.0 by decreasing the amount of room air mixed with the oxygen supplied to the ventilator.

Peak and Plateau Airway Pressure

Airway pressures are routinely monitored in mechanically ventilated patients. The peak airway pressure measured at the end of inspiration (Ppeak) is a function of the tidal volume, the resistance of the airways, lung/chest wall compliance, and peak inspiratory flow. The airway pressure measured at the end of inspiration when the inhaled volume is held in the lungs by briefly closing the expiratory valve is termed the plateau airway pressure (Pplateau). Plateau airway pressure is independent of the airways resistance, and is related to the lung/chest wall compliance and tidal volume. Mechanical ventilators monitor Ppeak with each breath and can be set to trigger an alarm if the Ppeak exceeds a predetermined threshold. Pplateau is not measured routinely with each delivered tidal volume, but rather is measured intermittently by setting the ventilator to close the exhalation circuit briefly at the end of inspiration and record the airway pressure when airflow is zero.

If both Ppeak and Pplateau are increased (and tidal volume is not excessive), then the problem is a decrease in the compliance in the lung/chest wall unit. Common causes of this problem include pneumothorax, lobar atelectasis, pulmonary edema, pneumonia, acute respiratory distress syndrome (ARDS), active contraction of the chest wall or diaphragmatic muscles, abdominal distention, and intrinsic PEEP, such as occurs in patients with bronchospasm and insufficient expiratory times. When Ppeak is increased but Pplateau is relatively normal, the primary problem is an increase in airway resistance, such as occurs with bronchospasm, use of a small-caliber endotracheal tube, or kinking or obstruction of the endotracheal tube. A low Ppeak also should trigger an alarm, as it suggests a discontinuity in the airway circuit involving the patient and the ventilator.

Ventilator-induced lung injury (VILI) is now an established clinical entity of great relevance to the care of critically ill patients. Excessive airway pressure and tidal volume adversely affect pulmonary and possibly systemic responses to critical illness. Subjecting the lung parenchyma to excessive pressure, known as barotrauma, can result in parenchymal lung injury, diffuse alveolar damage similar to ARDS, and pneumothorax, and can impair venous return and therefore limit cardiac output. Lung-protective ventilation strategies have been developed to prevent the development of VILI and improve patient outcomes. In a large, multicenter randomized trial of patients with ARDS from a variety of etiologies, limiting plateau airway pressure to less than 30 cm H_2O and tidal volume to less than 6 mL/kg of ideal body weight reduced 28-day mortality by 22 percent relative to a ventilator strategy that used a tidal volume of 12 mL/kg. For this reason, monitoring of plateau pressure and using a low tidal volume strategy in patients with ARDS is now the standard of care.

Pulse Oximetry

Continuous, noninvasive monitoring of arterial oxygen saturation is possible using light-emitting diodes and sensors placed on the skin. Pulse oximetry employs two wavelengths of light (i.e., 660 nm and 940 nm) to analyze the pulsatile component of blood flow between the light source and sensor. Because oxyhemoglobin and deoxyhemoglobin have different absorption spectra, differential absorption of light at these two wavelengths can be used to calculate the fraction of oxygen saturation of hemoglobin. Under normal circumstances, the contributions of carboxyhemoglobin and methemoglobin are minimal. However, if carboxyhemoglobin levels are elevated, the pulse oximeter will incorrectly interpret carboxyhemoglobin as oxyhemoglobin and the arterial saturation displayed will be falsely elevated. When the concentration of methemoglobin is markedly increased, the Sao_2 will be displayed as 85 percent, regardless of the true arterial saturation. The accuracy of pulse oximetry begins to decline at Sao_2 values less than 92 percent, and tends to be unreliable for values less than 85 percent.

Because of its clinical relevance, ease of use, noninvasive nature, and cost-effectiveness, pulse oximetry has become a routine monitoring strategy in patients with respiratory disease, intubated patients, and those undergoing surgical intervention under sedation or general anesthesia. Pulse oximetry is especially useful in the titration of Fio_2 and PEEP for patients receiving mechanical ventilation, and during weaning from mechanical ventilation. The widespread use of pulse oximetry has decreased the need for arterial blood gas determinations in critically ill patients.

Capnometry

Capnometry is the measurement of Pco_2 in the airway throughout the respiratory cycle. In healthy subjects, end-tidal Pco_2 ($Petco_2$) is about 1–5 mmHg less than $Paco_2$. Thus, $Petco_2$ can be used to estimate $Paco_2$ without the need for blood gas determination. However, changes in $Petco_2$ may not correlate with changes in $Paco_2$ during a number of pathologic conditions (see below).

Capnography allows the confirmation of endotracheal intubation and continuous assessment of ventilation, integrity of the airway, operation of the ventilator, and cardiopulmonary function. Continuous monitoring with capnography has become routine during surgery under general anesthesia and for some intensive care patients. A number of situations can be promptly detected with continuous capnography. A sudden reduction in Petco$_2$ suggests either obstruction of the sampling tubing with water or secretions, or a catastrophic event such as loss of the airway, airway disconnection or obstruction, ventilator malfunction, or a marked decrease in QT. If the airway is connected and patent and the ventilator is functioning properly, then a sudden decrease in Petco$_2$ should prompt efforts to rule out cardiac arrest, massive pulmonary embolism, or cardiogenic shock. Petco$_2$ can be persistently low during hyperventilation or with an increase in dead space such as occurs with pulmonary embolization (even in the absence of a change in QT). Causes of an increase in Petco$_2$ include reduced minute ventilation or increased metabolic rate.

RENAL MONITORING

Urine Output

Bladder catheterization allows the monitoring of urine output, usually recorded hourly. With a patent Foley catheter, urine output is a crude indicator of renal perfusion. The generally accepted normal urine output is 0.5 mL/kg per hour for adults and 1 to 2 mL/kg per hour for neonates and infants. Oliguria may reflect inadequate renal artery perfusion because of hypotension, hypovolemia, or low QT. Low urine flow also can be a sign of intrinsic renal dysfunction. It is important to recognize that normal urine output does not exclude the possibility of impending renal failure.

Bladder Pressure

The triad of oliguria, elevated peak airway pressures, and elevated intraabdominal pressure is known as the abdominal compartment syndrome (ACS). ACS is associated with interstitial edema of the abdominal organs, resulting in elevated intraabdominal pressure. When intraabdominal pressure exceeds venous or capillary pressures, perfusion of the kidneys and other intraabdominal viscera is impaired. Oliguria is a cardinal sign. Although the diagnosis of ACS is a clinical one, measuring intraabdominal pressure is useful to confirm the diagnosis. Ideally, a catheter inserted into the peritoneal cavity could measure intraabdominal pressure to substantiate the diagnosis. In practice, transurethral bladder pressure measurement reflects intraabdominal pressure and is most often used to confirm the presence of ACS. After instilling 50–100 mL of sterile saline into the bladder via a Foley catheter, the tubing is connected to a transducing system to measure bladder pressure. Most authorities agree that a bladder pressure greater than 20–25 mmHg confirms the diagnosis of ACS.

NEUROLOGIC MONITORING

Intracranial Pressure

Because the brain is rigidly confined within the bony skull, cerebral edema or mass lesions increase intracranial pressure (ICP). Monitoring of ICP is currently recommended in patients with severe traumatic brain injury (TBI), defined as a Glasgow Coma Scale (GCS) score ≤ 8 with an abnormal CT scan, and in patients with severe TBI and a normal CT scan if two or more of the following are present: age older than 40 years, unilateral or bilateral motor posturing, or systolic blood pressure less than 90 mmHg. ICP monitoring also is indicated in patients with acute subarachnoid hemorrhage with coma or neurologic deterioration, intracranial hemorrhage with intraventricular blood, ischemic middle cerebral artery stroke, fulminant hepatic failure with coma and cerebral edema on CT scan, and global cerebral ischemia or anoxia with cerebral edema on CT scan. The goal of ICP monitoring is to ensure that cerebral perfusion pressure (CPP) is adequate to support perfusion of the brain. CPP is equal to the difference between MAP and ICP: CPP = MAP − ICP.

Ventriculostomy catheters are one type of ICP measuring device which consist of a fluid-filled catheter inserted into a ventricle and connected to an external pressure transducer. This device permits measurement of ICP and allows drainage of cerebrospinal fluid (CSF) as a means to lower ICP and sample CSF for laboratory studies. Other devices locate the pressure transducer within the central nervous system and are used only to monitor ICP. These devices can be placed in the intraventricular, parenchymal, subdural, or epidural spaces. Ventriculostomy catheters are the accepted standard for monitoring ICP in patients with TBI because of their accuracy, ability to drain CSF, and low complication rate. The associated complications include infection (5 percent), hemorrhage (1.4 percent), catheter malfunction or obstruction (6.3–10.5 percent), and malposition with injury to cerebral tissue.

The purpose of ICP monitoring is to detect and treat abnormal elevations of ICP that may be detrimental to cerebral perfusion and function. In TBI patients, ICP greater than 20 mmHg is associated with unfavorable outcomes. In patients with low CPP, therapeutic strategies to correct CPP can be directed at increasing MAP or decreasing ICP. Although it often has been recommended that CPP be maintained above 70 mmHg, data to support this recommendation are not convincing.

Electroencephalogram and Evoked Potentials

Electroencephalography offers the capacity to monitor global neurologic electrical activity, although evoked potential monitoring can assess pathways not detected by the conventional EEG. Continuous EEG (CEEG) monitoring in the intensive care unit permits ongoing evaluation of cerebral cortical activity. It is especially useful in obtunded and comatose patients. CEEG also is useful for monitoring of therapy for status epilepticus and detecting early changes associated with cerebral ischemia. CEEG can be used to adjust the level of sedation, especially if high-dose barbiturate therapy is being used to manage elevated ICP. Somatosensory and brain stem evoked potentials are less affected by the administration of sedatives than is the EEG. Evoked potentials are useful for localizing brain stem lesions or proving the absence of such structural lesions in cases of metabolic or toxic coma. They also can provide prognostic data in posttraumatic coma.

A recent advance in EEG monitoring is the use of the bispectral index (BIS) to titrate the level of sedative medications. The BIS device is often used in the operating room to continuously monitor the depth of anesthesia. The BIS is an empiric measurement statistically derived from a database of bifrontal EEG recordings and analyzed for burst suppression ratio, relative alpha-to-beta ratio, and bicoherence. The BIS ranges from 0 (isoelectric EEG) to 100 (fully awake). Its use has been associated with lower consumption of anesthetics during surgery and earlier awakening and faster recovery from anesthesia. The BIS also has been validated as a useful approach for monitoring the level of sedation for ICU patients, using the revised Sedation-Agitation Scale as a gold standard.

Transcranial Doppler Ultrasonography

This modality provides a noninvasive method for evaluating cerebral hemodynamics. Transcranial Doppler (TCD) measurements of middle and anterior cerebral artery blood flow velocity are useful for the diagnosis of cerebral vasospasm after subarachnoid hemorrhage. Although some have proposed using TCD to estimate ICP, studies have shown that TCD is not a reliable method for estimating ICP and CPP. TCD is useful to confirm the clinical examination for determining brain death in patients with confounding factors such as the presence of CNS depressants or metabolic encephalopathy.

Jugular Venous Oximetry

When the arterial oxygen content, hemoglobin concentration, and the oxyhemoglobin dissociation curve are constant, changes in jugular venous oxygen saturation (Sjo_2) reflect changes in the difference between cerebral oxygen delivery and demand. Generally, a decrease in Sjo_2 reflects cerebral hypoperfusion, whereas an increase in Sjo_2 indicates the presence of hyperemia. Sjo_2 monitoring cannot detect decreases in regional cerebral blood flow if overall perfusion is normal or above normal. This technique requires the placement of a catheter in the jugular bulb, usually via the internal jugular vein. Catheters that permit intermittent aspiration of jugular venous blood for analysis or continuous oximetry catheters are available.

Low Sjo_2 is associated with poor outcomes after TBI. Nevertheless, the value of monitoring Sjo_2 remains unproven, and should be used in conjunction with ICP and CPP monitoring.

Transcranial Near-Infrared Spectroscopy

Transcranial near-infrared spectroscopy is a noninvasive continuous monitoring method to determine cerebral oxygenation. It employs technology similar to that of pulse oximetry to determine the concentrations of oxy- and deoxyhemoglobin with near-infrared light and sensors, and takes advantage of the relative transparency of the skull to light in the near-infrared region of the spectrum. This form of monitoring remains largely a research tool at the present time.

Suggested Readings

The Acute Respiratory Distress Syndrome Network: Ventilation with lower tidal volumes as compared with traditional tidal volumes for acute lung injury and the acute respiratory distress syndrome. The Acute Respiratory Distress Syndrome Network. N Engl J Med 342:1301, 2000.

Bland RD, Shoemaker WC, Abraham E, et al: Hemodynamic and oxygen transport patterns in surviving and nonsurviving postoperative patients. Crit Care Med 13:85, 1985.

Connors AF Jr.: Right heart catheterization: Is it effective? New Horiz 5:195, 1997.

Connors AF Jr., Speroff T, Dawson NV, et al: The effectiveness of right heart catheterization in the initial care of critically-ill patients. JAMA 276:889, 1996.

Gutierrez G, Palizas F, Doglio G, et al: Gastric intramucosal pH as a therapeutic index of tissue oxygenation in critically-ill patients. Lancet 339:195, 1992.

Rivers E, Nguyen B, Havstad S, et al: Early goal-directed therapy in the treatment of severe sepsis and septic shock. N Engl J Med 345:1368, 2001.

Sandham JD, Hull RD, Brant RF, et al: A randomized, controlled trial of the use of pulmonary-artery catheters in high-risk surgical patients. N Engl J Med 348:5, 2003.

Shoemaker WC, Appel PL, Kram HB, et al: Prospective trial of supranormal values of survivors as therapeutic goals in high risk surgical patients. Chest 94:1176, 1988.

13 | Minimally Invasive Surgery

Blair A. Jobe and John G. Hunter

Minimally invasive surgery (MIS) describes an area of surgery that crosses all traditional disciplines, from general surgery to neurosurgery. It is not a discipline unto itself, but more a philosophy of surgery, a way of thinking. Minimally invasive surgery is a means of performing major operations through small incisions, often using miniaturized, high-tech imaging systems, to minimize the trauma of surgical exposure.

HISTORICAL BACKGROUND

Although the term minimally invasive surgery is relatively recent, the history of its component parts is nearly 100 years old. What is considered the newest and most popular variety of MIS, laparoscopy, is in fact the oldest. Primitive laparoscopy, placing a cystoscope within an inflated abdomen, was first performed by Kelling in 1901. Illumination of the abdomen required hot elements at the tip of the scope and was dangerous. In the late 1950s, Hopkins described the rod lens, a method of transmitting light through a solid quartz rod with no heat and little light loss. Around the same time, thin quartz fibers were discovered to be capable of trapping light internally and conducting it around corners, opening the field of fiberoptics and allowing the rapid development of flexible endoscopes. In the 1970s, the application of flexible endoscopy grew faster than that of rigid endoscopy except in a few fields such as gynecology and orthopedics. By the mid-1970s, rigid and flexible endoscopes made a rapid transition from diagnostic instruments to therapeutic ones. The explosion of video-assisted surgery in the past 10 years was a result of the development of compact, high-resolution, charge-coupled devices which could be mounted on the internal end of flexible endoscopes or on the external end of a Hopkins telescope. Coupled with bright light sources, fiberoptic cables, and high-resolution video monitors, the videoendoscope has changed our understanding of surgical anatomy and reshaped surgical practice.

THE MINIMALLY INVASIVE TEAM

A typical MIS team may consist of a laparoscopic surgeon and an operating room nurse with an interest in laparoscopic surgery. Adding dedicated laparoscopic assistants and circulating staff with an intimate knowledge of the equipment will add to and enhance the team nucleus. Studies have demonstrated that having a designated laparoscopic team reduces the conversion rate and overall operative time, which is translated into a cost savings for patient and hospital.

PHYSIOLOGY

Even with the least invasive of the MIS procedures, physiologic changes occur. Many minimally invasive procedures require minimal or no sedation, and there are few alterations to the cardiovascular, endocrinologic, or immunologic systems. Minimally invasive procedures that require general anesthesia have a

293

greater physiologic impact because of the anesthetic agent, the incision (even if small), and the induced pneumoperitoneum.

Laparoscopy

Carbon dioxide and nitrous oxide are used for inflating the abdomen. N_2O had the advantage of being physiologically inert and rapidly absorbed. It also provided better analgesia for laparoscopy performed under local anesthesia when compared with CO_2 or air. Despite initial concerns that N_2O would not suppress combustion, controlled clinical trials have established its safety within the peritoneal cavity. Additionally, nitrous oxide has recently been shown to reduce the intraoperative end-tidal CO_2 and minute ventilation required to maintain homeostasis when compared to CO_2 pneumoperitoneum. The safety of N_2O pneumoperitoneum in pregnancy has yet to be elucidated.

The physiologic effects of CO_2 pneumoperitoneum can be divided into two areas: (1) gas-specific effects and (2) pressure-specific effects. CO_2 is rapidly absorbed across the peritoneal membrane into the circulation. In the circulation, CO_2 creates a respiratory acidosis by the generation of carbonic acid. Body buffers, the largest reserve of which lies in bone, absorb CO_2 (up to 120 L) and minimize the development of hypercarbia or respiratory acidosis during brief endoscopic procedures. Once the body buffers are saturated, respiratory acidosis develops rapidly, and the respiratory system assumes the burden of keeping up with the absorption of CO_2 and its release from these buffers.

In patients with normal respiratory function this is not difficult; the anesthesiologist increases the ventilatory rate or vital capacity on the ventilator. If the respiratory rate required exceeds 20 breaths per min, there may be less efficient gas exchange and increasing hypercarbia. Conversely, if vital capacity is increased substantially, there is a greater opportunity for barotrauma and greater respiratory motion–induced disruption of the upper abdominal operative field. In some situations it is advisable to evacuate the pneumoperitoneum or reduce the intraabdominal pressure to allow time for the anesthesiologist to adjust for hypercarbia. Hypercarbia also causes tachycardia and increased systemic vascular resistance, which elevates blood pressure and increases myocardial oxygen demand.

The pressure effects of the pneumoperitoneum on cardiovascular physiology also have been studied. In the hypovolemic individual, excessive pressure on the inferior vena cava and a reverse Trendelenburg position with loss of lower extremity muscle tone may cause decreased venous return and cardiac output. The most common arrhythmia created by laparoscopy is bradycardia. A rapid stretch of the peritoneal membrane often causes a vagovagal response with bradycardia and occasionally hypotension. With the increased intraabdominal pressure compressing the inferior vena cava, there is diminished venous return from the lower extremities. This has been well documented in the patient placed in the reverse Trendelenburg position for upper abdominal operations. Venous engorgement and decreased venous return promote venous thrombosis. Many series of advanced laparoscopic procedures in which deep venous thrombosis (DVT) prophylaxis was not used demonstrate the frequency of pulmonary embolus. This usually is an avoidable complication with the use of sequential compression stockings, subcutaneous heparin, or low-molecular-weight heparin. The direct effect of the pneumoperitoneum on increasing intrathoracic pressure increases peak inspiratory pressure, pressure across the chest wall, and also the likelihood of barotrauma. Despite these concerns, disruption of blebs and consequent pneumothoraces are rare after uncomplicated laparoscopic surgery.

Increased intraabdominal pressure decreases renal blood flow, glomerular filtration rate, and urine output. These effects may be mediated by direct pressure on the kidney and the renal vein. The secondary effect of decreased renal blood flow is to increase plasma renin release, thereby increasing sodium retention. Increased circulating antidiuretic hormone (ADH) levels also are found during the pneumoperitoneum, increasing free water reabsorption in the distal tubules. Although the effects of the pneumoperitoneum on renal blood flow are immediately reversible, the hormonally mediated changes, such as elevated ADH levels, decrease urine output for up to 1 h after the procedure has ended. Intraoperative oliguria is common during laparoscopy, but the urine output is not a reflection of intravascular volume status. Early it was predicted that the surgical stress response would be significantly lessened with laparoscopic surgery, but this is not always the case. Serum cortisol levels after laparoscopic operations are often higher than after the equivalent operation performed through an open incision. In terms of endocrine balance, the greatest difference between open and laparoscopic surgery is the more rapid equilibration of most stress-mediated hormone levels after laparoscopic surgery. Immune suppression also is less after laparoscopy than after open surgery. There is a trend toward more rapid normalization of cytokine levels after a laparoscopic procedure than after the equivalent procedure performed by celiotomy.

Thoracoscopy

The physiology of thoracic MIS (thoracoscopy) is different from that of laparoscopy. Because of the bony confines of the thorax it is unnecessary to use positive pressure when working in the thorax. The disadvantages of positive pressure in the chest include decreased venous return, mediastinal shift, and the need to keep a firm seal at all trocar sites. Without positive pressure, it is necessary to place a double-lumen endotracheal tube so that the ipsilateral lung can be deflated when the operation starts. By collapsing the ipsilateral lung, working space within the thorax is obtained. Because insufflation is unnecessary in thoracoscopic surgery, it can be beneficial to use standard instruments via extended port sites in conjunction with thoracoscopic instruments. This approach is particularly useful when performing advanced procedures such as thoracoscopic anatomic pulmonary resection.

Extracavitary Minimally Invasive Surgery

Many new MIS procedures are creating working spaces in extrathoracic and extraperitoneal locations. Laparoscopic inguinal hernia repair usually is performed in the anterior extraperitoneal Retzius space. Laparoscopic nephrectomy often is performed with retroperitoneal laparoscopy. Recently, an endoscopic retroperitoneal approach to pancreatic necrosectomy has been introduced. Lower extremity vascular procedures and plastic surgical endoscopic procedures require the development of working space in unconventional planes, often at the level of the fascia, sometimes below the fascia, and occasionally in nonanatomic regions. Some of these techniques use insufflation of gas, but many use balloon inflation to develop the space, followed by low-pressure gas insufflation or lift devices to maintain the space. These techniques produce fewer and less severe adverse physiologic consequences than does the pneumoperitoneum, but the insufflation of gas into extraperitoneal locations can spread widely, causing subcutaneous emphysema and metabolic acidosis.

Anesthesia

MIS procedures usually are outpatient procedures, and short-acting anesthetic agents are preferable. Because the factors that require hospitalization after laparoscopic procedures include the management of nausea, pain, and urinary retention, the anesthesiologist should minimize the use of agents that provoke these conditions and maximize the use of medications that prevent such problems. Critical to the anesthesia management of these patients is the use of nonnarcotic analgesics (e.g., ketorolac) and the liberal use of antiemetic agents.

GENERAL PRINCIPLES OF ACCESS AND EQUIPMENT

The most natural ports of access for MIS are the anatomic portals of entry and exit. The nares, mouth, urethra, and anus are used to access the respiratory, gastrointestinal, and urinary systems. The advantage of using these points of access is that no incision is required. The disadvantages lie in the long distances between the orifice and the region of interest.

Increasingly, vascular access is obtained with percutaneous techniques using a small incision, a needle, and a guidewire, over which are passed a variety of different sized access devices. This approach, known as the Seldinger technique, is most frequently used by general surgeons for placement of Hickman catheters, but also is used to gain access to the arterial and venous system for performance of minimally invasive procedures. Guidewire-assisted, Seldinger-type techniques also are helpful for gaining access to the gut for procedures such as percutaneous endoscopic gastrostomy, for gaining access to the biliary system through the liver, and for gaining access to the upper urinary tract.

In thoracoscopic surgery, the access technique is similar to that used for placement of a chest tube. In these procedures general anesthesia and split-lung ventilation are essential. A small incision is made over the top of a rib and, under direct vision, carried down through the pleura. The lung is collapsed, and a trocar is inserted across the chest wall to allow access with a telescope. Once the lung is completely collapsed, subsequent access may be obtained with direct puncture, viewing all entry sites through the videoendoscope. Because insufflation of the chest is unnecessary, simple ports that keep the small incisions open are all that is required to allow repeated access to the thorax.

Laparoscopic Access

The requirements for laparoscopy are more involved, because the creation of a pneumoperitoneum requires that instruments of access (trocars) contain valves to maintain abdominal inflation.

Two methods are used for establishing abdominal access during laparoscopic procedures. The first, direct puncture laparoscopy, begins with the elevation of the relaxed abdominal wall with two towel clips or a well-placed hand. A small incision is made in the umbilicus, and a specialized spring-loaded (Veress) needle is placed in the abdominal cavity. With the Veress needle, two distinct pops are felt as the surgeon passes the needle through the abdominal wall fascia and the peritoneum. The umbilicus usually is selected as the preferred point of access because in this location the abdominal wall is quite thin, even in obese patients. The abdomen is inflated with a pressure-limited insufflator. CO_2 gas is usually used, with maximal pressures in the range of 14–15 mmHg. During the process of insufflation it is essential that the surgeon observe the pressure and flow readings on the monitor to confirm an intraperitoneal location of the Veress needle tip. Laparoscopic surgery can be performed under local anesthesia, but general anesthesia is preferable. Under local anesthesia, N_2O is used as the insufflating agent, and insufflation is stopped after 2 L of gas is insufflated or when a pressure of 10 mmHg is reached.

After peritoneal insufflation, direct access to the abdomen is obtained with a 5- or 10-mm trocar. The critical issues for safe direct-puncture laparoscopy include the use of a vented stylet for the trocar, or a trocar with a safety shield or dilating tip. The trocar must be pointed away from the sacral promontory and the great vessels. Patient position should be surveyed prior to trocar placement to ensure a proper trajectory. For performance of laparoscopic cholecystectomy, the trocar is angled toward the right upper quadrant.

Occasionally the direct peritoneal access (Hasson) technique is advisable. With this technique, the surgeon makes a small incision just below the umbilicus and under direct vision locates the abdominal fascia. Two Kocher clamps are placed on the fascia, and with a curved Mayo scissors a small incision is made through the fascia and underlying peritoneum. A finger is placed into the abdomen to make sure that there is no adherent bowel. A sturdy suture is placed on each side of the fascia and secured to the wings of a specialized trocar, which is then passed directly into the abdominal cavity. For safe access to the abdominal cavity, it is critical to visualize all sites of trocar entry. At the completion of the operation, all trocars are removed under direct vision and the insertion sites are inspected for bleeding. If bleeding occurs, direct pressure with an instrument from another trocar site or balloon tamponade with a Foley catheter placed through the trocar site generally stops the bleeding within 3–5 min. It generally is agreed that 5-mm trocars need no site suturing. Ten-mm trocars placed off the midline and above the transverse mesocolon do not require repair. Conversely, if the fascia has been dilated to allow the passage of the gallbladder, all midline 10-mm trocar sites should be repaired at the fascial level with interrupted sutures.

Access for Subcutaneous and Extraperitoneal Surgery

There are two methods for gaining access to nonanatomic spaces. For retroperitoneal locations, balloon dissection is effective. This access technique is appropriate for the extraperitoneal repair of inguinal hernias and for retroperitoneal surgery for adrenalectomy, nephrectomy, lumbar discectomy, pancreatic necrosectomy, or para-aortic lymph node dissection. The initial access to the extraperitoneal space is performed in a way similar to direct puncture laparoscopy, except that the last layer (the peritoneum) is not traversed. Once the transversalis fascia has been punctured, a specialized trocar with a balloon on the end is introduced. The balloon is inflated in the extraperitoneal space to create a working chamber. The balloon then is deflated and a Hasson trocar is placed. An insufflation pressure of 10 mmHg usually is adequate to keep the extraperitoneal space open for dissection and will limit subcutaneous emphysema.

Hand-Assisted Laparoscopic Access

Hand-assisted laparoscopic surgery (HALS) is thought to combine the tactile advantages of open surgery with the minimal access of laparoscopy and thoracoscopy. This approach is commonly used to assist with difficult cases before conversion to celiotomy is necessary. Additionally, HALS is employed to help surgeons negotiate the steep learning curve associated with advanced laparoscopic procedures. This technology employs a "port" for the hand which preserves the pneumoperitoneum and enables endoscopic visualization in combination with the use of minimally invasive instruments.

Port Placement

Trocars for the surgeon's left and right hand should be placed at least 10 cm apart. For most operations it is possible to orient the telescope between these two trocars and slightly retract from them. The ideal trocar orientation creates an equilateral triangle between the surgeon's right hand, left hand, and the telescope, with 10–15 cm on each leg. If one imagines the target of the operation (e.g., the gallbladder or gastroesophageal junction) oriented at the apex of a second equilateral triangle built on the first, these four points of reference create a diamond. The surgeon stands behind the telescope, which provides optimal ergonomic orientation but frequently requires that a camera operator (or robotic arm) reach between the surgeon's hands to guide the telescope.

The position of the operating table should permit the surgeon to work with both elbows in at the sides, with arms bent 90 degrees at the elbow. It usually is necessary to alter the operating table position with left or right tilt with the patient in the Trendelenburg or reverse Trendelenburg position, depending on the operative field.

Imaging Systems

Two methods of videoendoscopic imaging are widely used. Both methods use a camera with a charge-coupled device (CCD), which is an array of photosensitive sensor elements (pixels) that convert the incoming light intensity to an electric charge. The electric charge is subsequently converted into a black-and-white image. The first of these is flexible videoendoscopy, in which the CCD camera is placed on the internal end of a long, flexible endoscope. In the second method, thin quartz fibers are packed together in a bundle, and the CCD camera is mounted on the external end of the endoscope. Most standard gastrointestinal endoscopes have the CCD chip at the distal end, but small, delicate choledochoscopes and nephroscopes are equipped with fiberoptic bundles. Distally mounted CCD chips were developed for laparoscopy, but are unpopular.

Video cameras come in two basic designs. The one-chip camera has a black-and-white video chip that has an internal processor capable of converting gray scales to approximate colors. Perfect color representation is not possible with a one-chip camera, but perfect color representation is rarely necessary for endosurgery. The most accurate color representation is obtained using a three-chip video camera. A three-chip camera has red, green, and blue (RGB) input, and is identical to the color cameras used for television production. RGB imaging provides the highest fidelity, but is probably not necessary for everyday use. Priorities in a video system for MIS are illumination first, resolution second, and color third. Without the first two attributes, video surgery is unsafe. Imaging for laparoscopy, thoracoscopy, and subcutaneous surgery uses a rigid metal telescope, usually 30 cm in length. This telescope contains a series of quartz optical rods with differing optical characteristics that provide a specific character to each telescope. These metal telescopes vary in size from 2–10 mm in diameter. Because light transmission is dependent on the cross-sectional area of the quartz rod, when the diameter of a rod/lens system is doubled, the illumination is quadrupled.

Rigid telescopes may have a flat or angled end. The flat end provides a straight view (0 degrees), and the angled end provides an oblique view (30 or 45 degrees). Angled scopes allow greater flexibility in viewing a wider operative field through a single trocar site; rotating an angled telescope changes the field of view. The use of an angled telescope has distinct advantages for most videoendoscopic procedures, particularly in visualizing the common bile duct during laparoscopic cholecystectomy or visualizing the posterior esophagus or the tip of the spleen during laparoscopic fundoplication.

Light is delivered to the endoscope through a fiberoptic light cable. These light cables are highly inefficient, losing more than 90 percent of the light delivered from the light source. Extremely bright light sources (300 watts) are necessary to provide adequate illumination for video endosurgery.

The quality of the videoendoscopic image is only as good as the weakest component in the imaging chain. Therefore it is important to use a video monitor that has a resolution equal to or greater than the camera being used. Resolution is the ability of the optical system to distinguish between line pairs. The larger the number of line pairs per millimeter, the sharper and more detailed the image. Most high-resolution monitors have up to 700 horizontal lines. High-definition television (HDTV) can deliver up to eight times more resolution than the standard NTSC/PAL monitors; when combined with digital enhancement, a very sharp and well-defined image can be achieved.

Energy Sources for Endoscopic and Endoluminal Surgery

MIS uses conventional energy sources, but the requirement of bloodless surgery to maintain optimal visualization has spawned new ways of applying energy. The most common energy source is radiofrequency (RF) electrosurgery using an alternating current with a frequency of 500,000 cycles/s (Hz). Tissue heating progresses through the well-known phases of coagulation (60°C [140°F]), vaporization and desiccation (100°C [212°F]), and carbonization (>200°C [392°F]).

The two most common methods of delivering RF electrosurgery are with monopolar and bipolar electrodes. With monopolar electrosurgery a remote ground plate on the patient's leg or back receives the flow of electrons that originate at a point source, the surgical electrode. A fine-tipped electrode causes a high current density at the site of application and rapid tissue heating. Monopolar electrosurgery is inexpensive and easy to modulate to achieve different tissue effects. A short-duration, high-voltage discharge of current (coagulation current) provides extremely rapid tissue heating. Lower-voltage, higher-wattage current (cutting current) is better for tissue desiccation and vaporization. When the surgeon desires tissue division with the least amount of thermal injury and least coagulation necrosis, a cutting current is used.

With bipolar electrosurgery the electrons flow between two adjacent electrodes. The tissue between the two electrodes is heated and desiccated. There is little opportunity for tissue cutting when bipolar current is used, but the ability to coapt the electrodes across a vessel provides the best method of small-vessel coagulation without thermal injury to adjacent tissues.

To avoid thermal injury to adjacent structures, the laparoscopic field of view must include all uninsulated portions of the electrosurgical electrode. Additionally, the integrity of the insulation must be maintained and assured. Capacitive coupling occurs when a plastic trocar insulates the abdominal wall from the current; in turn the current is bled off of a metal sleeve or laparoscope into the viscera. This may result in thermal necrosis and a delayed fecal fistula. Another potential mechanism for unrecognized visceral injury may occur with the direct coupling of current to the laparoscope and adjacent bowel.

With endoscopic endoluminal surgery, radiofrequency alternating current in the form of a monopolar circuit represents the mainstay for procedures such as snare polypectomy, sphincterotomy, lower esophageal sphincter ablation, and "hot" biopsy. A grounding ("return") electrode is necessary for this form of energy. Bipolar electrocoagulation is used primarily for thermal hemostasis. The electrosurgical generator is activated by a foot pedal so the endoscopist may keep both hands free during the endoscopic procedure.

Methods of producing shock waves or heat with ultrasonic energy are also of interest. Extracorporeal shockwave lithotripsy creates focused shock waves that intensify as the focal point of the discharge is approached. When the focal point is within the body, large amounts of energy are capable of fragmenting stones. Slightly different configurations of this energy can be used to provide focused internal heating of tissues. Potential applications of this technology include the ability to noninvasively produce sufficient internal heating to destroy tissue without an incision.

A third means of using ultrasonic energy is to create rapidly oscillating instruments that are capable of heating tissue with friction; this technology represents a major step forward in energy technology. An example of its application is the laparoscopic coagulation shears (LCS) device (Harmonic Scalpel), which is capable of coagulating and dividing blood vessels by first occluding them and then providing sufficient heat to weld the blood vessel walls together and to divide the vessel. This nonelectric method of coagulating and dividing tissue with a minimal amount of collateral damage has facilitated the performance of numerous endosurgical procedures. It is especially useful in the control of bleeding from medium-sized vessels that are too big to manage with monopolar electrocautery and require bipolar desiccation followed by cutting.

Instrumentation

Hand instruments for MIS usually are duplications of conventional surgical instruments made longer, thinner, and smaller at the tip. It is important to remember that when grasping tissue with laparoscopic instruments, a greater force is applied over a smaller surface area, which increases the risk for perforation or injury.

Certain conventional instruments such as scissors are easy to reproduce with a diameter of 3–5 mm and a length of 20–45 cm, but other instruments, such as forceps and clamps, cannot provide remote access. Different configurations of graspers were developed to replace the various configurations of surgical forceps and clamps. Standard hand instruments are 5 mm in diameter and 30 cm in length, but smaller and shorter hand instruments are now available for pediatric surgery, for microlaparoscopic surgery, and for arthroscopic procedures.

Robotic Assistance

The term "robot" defines a device that has been programmed to perform specific tasks in place of those usually performed by people. The equipment that has been introduced under the heading of robotic assistance would perhaps be more aptly termed computer-assisted surgery, as it is controlled entirely by the surgeon for the purpose of improving team performance. An example of computer-assisted surgery includes laparoscopic camera holders, which enable the surgeon to maneuver the laparoscope either with head movements or voice activation. Randomized studies with such camera holders have demonstrated a reduction in operative time, steadier image, and a reduction in the number of required laparoscope cleanings. This device has the advantage of eliminating the need for a human camera holder, which serves to free valuable operating room personnel for other duties.

Room Setup and the Minimally Invasive Suite

Nearly all MIS, whether using fluoroscopic, ultrasound, or optical imaging, incorporates a video monitor as a guide. Occasionally two images are necessary to adequately guide the operation, as in procedures such as endoscopic retrograde cholangiopancreatography (ERCP), laparoscopic common bile duct exploration, and laparoscopic ultrasonography. When two images are necessary, the images should be displayed on two adjacent video monitors or projected on a single screen with a picture-in-picture effect. The video monitor(s) should be set across the operating table from the surgeon. The patient should be interposed between the surgeon and the video monitor; ideally, the operative field also lies between the surgeon and the monitor. In pelviscopic surgery it is best to place the video monitor at the patient's feet, and in laparoscopic cholecystectomy, the monitor is placed at the 10 o'clock position (relative to the patient) while the surgeon stands on the patient's left at the 4 o'clock position. The insufflating and patient-monitoring equipment ideally also is placed across the table from the surgeon, so that the insufflating pressure and the patient's vital signs and end-tidal CO_2 tension can be monitored.

The development of the minimally invasive surgical suite has been a tremendous contribution to the field of laparoscopy in that it has facilitated the performance of advanced procedures and techniques. By having the core equipment (monitors, insufflators, and imaging equipment) located within mobile, ceiling-mounted consoles, the surgery team is able to accommodate and make small adjustments rapidly and continuously throughout the procedure. The specifically designed minimally invasive surgical suite serves to decrease equipment and cable disorganization, ease the movements of operative personnel around the room, improve ergonomics, and facilitate the use of advanced imaging equipment such laparoscopic ultrasound.

Patient Positioning

Patients usually are placed in the supine position for laparoscopic surgery. When the operative field is the gastroesophageal junction or the left lobe of the liver, it is easiest to operate from between the legs. The legs may be elevated in Allen stirrups or abducted on leg boards to achieve this position. When pelvic procedures are performed, it usually is necessary to place the legs in Allen stirrups to gain access to the perineum. A lateral decubitus position with the table flexed provides the best access to the retroperitoneum when performing nephrectomy or adrenalectomy. For laparoscopic splenectomy, a 45-degree tilt of the patient provides excellent access to the lesser sac and the lateral peritoneal attachments to the spleen. For thoracoscopic surgery, the patient is placed in the lateral position with table flexion to open the intercostal spaces and the distance between the iliac crest and costal margin.

SPECIAL CONSIDERATIONS

Pediatric Considerations

The advantages of MIS in children may be more significant than in the adult population. MIS in the adolescent is little different from that in the adult, and standard instrumentation and trocar positions can usually be used. However, laparoscopy in the infant and young child requires specialized instrumentation. The instruments are shorter (15–20 cm), and many are 3 mm in diameter rather than 5 mm. Because the abdomen of the child is much smaller than that of the adult, a 5-mm telescope provides sufficient illumination for most operations. The development of 5-mm clippers and bipolar devices has obviated the need for 10-mm trocars in pediatric laparoscopy.

Pregnancy

Concerns about the safety of laparoscopic cholecystectomy or appendectomy in the pregnant patient have been eliminated. The pH of the fetus follows the pH of the mother linearly, and therefore fetal acidosis may be prevented by avoiding a respiratory acidosis in the mother. Experience in well over 100 cases of laparoscopic cholecystectomy in pregnancy have been reported with uniformly good results. The operation should be performed during the second trimester if possible. Access to the abdomen in the pregnant patient should take into consideration the height of the uterine fundus, which reaches the umbilicus at 20 weeks. In order not to damage the uterus or its blood supply, most surgeons feel that the open (Hasson) approach should be used in favor of direct puncture laparoscopy. The patient should be positioned slightly on the left side to avoid compression of the vena cava by the uterus. Because pregnancy poses a risk for thromboembolism, sequential compression devices are essential for all procedures.

Cancer

MIS techniques have been used for many decades to provide palliation for the patient with an obstructive cancer. Laser treatment, intracavitary radiation, stenting, and dilation are outpatient techniques that can be used to reestablish the continuity of an obstructed esophagus, bile duct, ureter, or airway. Laparoscopy also is used to assess the liver in patients being evaluated for pancreatic, gastric, or hepatic resection.

The most controversial role of MIS techniques is that of providing potentially curative surgery to the patient with cancer. It is possible to perform laparoscopy-assisted colectomy, gastrectomy, pancreatectomy, and hepatectomy in patients with intraabdominal malignant disease, and thoracoscopic esophagectomy and pneumonectomy in patients with intrathoracic malignant disease. There are not yet enough data to indicate whether minimally invasive surgical techniques provide survival rates or disease-free intervals comparable to those of conventional surgical techniques. It has been proven that in laparoscopy-assisted colectomy and gastrectomy a number of lymph nodes equal to that of an open procedure can be removed without any compromise of resection margins. A second concern centers on excessive tumor manipulation and the possibility that cancer cells would be shed during the dissection.

Cirrhosis and Portal Hypertension

Patients with hepatic insufficiency pose a significant challenge for any type of surgical intervention. The ultimate surgical outcome in this population relates directly to the degree of underlying hepatic dysfunction. Often, this group of patients has minimal reserve, and the stress of an operation will trigger complete hepatic failure or hepatorenal syndrome. These patients are at risk for major hemorrhage at all levels, including trocar insertion, operative dissection in a field of dilated veins, and secondary to an underlying coagulopathy. Additionally, ascitic leak from a port site may occur, leading to bacterial peritonitis. Therefore a watertight port site closure should be carried out in all patients.

It is essential that the surgeon be aware of the Child class of severity of cirrhosis of the patient prior to intervening so that appropriate preoperative optimization can be completed. For example, if a patient has an eroding umbilical hernia and ascites, a preoperative paracentesis or transjugular intrahepatic portosystemic shunt (TIPS) procedure in conjunction with aggressive diuresis may be considered. Because these patients commonly are intravascularly depleted, insufflation pressures should be reduced to prevent a decrease in cardiac output and minimal amounts of low-salt intravenous fluids should be given.

ROBOTIC SURGERY

Computer-enhanced ("robotic") surgery was developed with the intent of circumventing the limitations of laparoscopy and thoracoscopy, and to make minimally invasive surgical techniques accessible to those without a laparoscopic background. Additionally, remote site surgery (telesurgery), in which the surgeon is a great distance from the patient (e.g., combat or space), has potential future applications. This was recently exemplified when a team of surgeons located in New York performed a cholecystectomy on a patient located in France.

These devices offer a three-dimensional view with hand- and wrist-controlled instruments that possess multiple degrees of freedom, thereby facilitating surgery with a one-to-one movement ratio that mimics open surgery. Additionally, computer-enhanced surgery also offers tremor control. The surgeon is physically separated from the operating table and the working arms of the device are placed over the patient. An assistant remains at the bedside and changes the instruments as needed.

Because this equipment is very costly, a primary limitation to its uniform acceptance has been attempting to achieve increased value in the form of improved clinical outcomes. There have been two randomized controlled trials that compared robotic and conventional laparoscopic approaches to Nissen fundoplication. Although there was a reduction in operative time, there was no difference in ultimate outcome. Similar results have been achieved for laparoscopic cholecystectomy. Finally, it may be too early in its development (because of bulky equipment, difficulty in accessing patients, and limited instrumentation) for widespread adoption of this technology.

ENDOLUMINAL SURGERY

The fields of vascular surgery, interventional radiology, neuroradiology, gastroenterology, general surgery, pulmonology, and urology all encounter clinical scenarios that require the urgent restoration of luminal patency of a "biologic cylinder." Based on this need, fundamental techniques have been pioneered that are applicable to all specialties and virtually every organ system. As a result, all minimally invasive surgical procedures, from coronary artery angioplasty to palliation of pancreatic malignancy, involve the use of an endoluminal balloon, dilator, prostheses, biopsy forceps, chemical agent, or thermal technique (Table 13-1). Endoluminal balloon dilators may be inserted through an endoscope, or they may be fluoroscopically guided. Balloon dilators all have low compliance—that is, the balloons do not stretch as the pressure within the balloon is increased. The high pressures achievable in the balloon create radial expansion of the narrowed vessel or orifice, usually disrupting the atherosclerotic plaque, the fibrotic stricture, or the muscular band (e.g., esophageal achalasia).

Once the dilation has been attained, it is frequently beneficial to hold the lumen open with a stent. Stenting is particularly valuable in treating malignant lesions and in endovascular procedures. Stenting usually is not applicable for long-term management of benign gastrointestinal strictures except in patients with limited life expectancy.

A variety of stents are available that are divided into two basic categories, plastic stents and expandable metal stents. Plastic stents came first and are used widely as endoprostheses for temporary bypass of obstructions in the

TABLE 13-1 Modalities and Techniques of Restoring Luminal Patency

Modality	Technique
Core out	Photodynamic Therapy
	Laser
	Coagulation
	Endoscopic biopsy forceps
	Chemical
	Ultrasound
Fracture	Ultrasound
	Endoscopic biopsy
	Balloon
Dilate	Balloon
	Bougie
	Angioplasty
	Endoscope
Bypass	Transvenous intrahepatic portosystemic shunt
	Surgical (synthetic or autologous conduit)
Stent	Self-expanding metal stent
	Plastic stent

biliary or urinary systems. Metal stents generally are delivered over a balloon and expanded with the balloon to the desired size. These metal stents usually are made of titanium or nitinol. Although great progress has been made with expandable metal stents, two problems remain: propensity for tissue ingrowth through the interstices of the stent and stent migration. Most recently, anticoagulant-eluding coronary artery stents have been placed in specialized centers. This exciting technological advance may dramatically increase the long-term patency rates of stents placed in patients with coronary artery disease and peripheral atherosclerosis.

Intraluminal Surgery

The successful application of minimally invasive surgical techniques to the lumen of the gastrointestinal tract has hinged on the development of a port that maintains access to the gastrointestinal lumen while preventing intraperitoneal leakage of intestinal contents and facilitating adequate insufflation.

Procedures that are gaining acceptance include resection of benign and early malignant gastric tumors, transanal resection of polyps (transanal endoscopic microsurgery), pancreatic cyst gastrostomy, and biliary sphincterotomy.

The location of the lesion within the gastrointestinal tract is of utmost importance when considering an intraluminal approach. For example, a leiomyoma that is located on the anterior gastric wall may not be amenable to intraluminal resection because the working ports must also penetrate the anterior surface of the stomach. Preoperative endoscopy and endoscopic ultrasound should be routinely employed to determine resectability.

EDUCATION AND SKILL ACQUISITION

Surgeons in Training and Skill Acquisition

Surgeons in training acquire their skills in minimally invasive techniques through a series of operative experiences of graded complexity. This training occurs on patients. With the recent constraints placed on resident work hours, providing adequate minimally invasive training to future surgeons within a relatively brief time frame has become of paramount importance.

Laparoscopic surgery demands a unique set of skills that require the surgeon to function at the limit of his or her psychomotor abilities. The introduction of virtual reality training devices presents a unique opportunity to improve and enhance experiential learning in endoscopy and laparoscopy for all surgeons. This technology has the advantage of enabling objective measurement of psychomotor skills, which can be used to determine progress in skill acquisition, and ultimately technical competency. This technology will most likely be used to create benchmarks for the performance of future minimally invasive techniques. Additionally, virtual reality training enables the surgeon to build an experience base prior to venturing into the operating room. Be that as it may, no studies have demonstrated that simulator training improves overall patient outcome.

Some hospitals and training programs have established virtual reality and laparoscopic training centers that are accessible at all hours for surgeons' use.

Telementoring

In response to the Institute of Medicine's call for the development of unique technologic solutions to deliver health care to rural and underserved areas, surgeons are beginning to explore the feasibility of telementoring. Teleconsultation or telementoring is two-way audio and visual communication between two geographically separated providers. This communication can take place in the office setting, or directly in the operating room when complex scenarios are encountered. Although local communication channels may limit its performance in rural areas, the technology is available and currently being employed.

INNOVATION AND INTRODUCTION OF NEW PROCEDURES

The revolution in minimally invasive general surgery, which occurred in 1990, created ethical challenges for the profession. The problem was: If competence is gained from experience, how was the surgeon to climb the competency curve (otherwise known as the learning curve) without injuring patients? If it was indeed impossible to achieve competence without making mistakes along the way, how should one effectively communicate this to patients such that they understand the weight of their decisions? Even more fundamentally important is determining the path that should be followed before one recruits the first patient for a new procedure.

Although procedure development is fundamentally different than drug development, adherence to a process similar to that used to develop a new drug is a reasonable path for a surgical innovator. At the outset the surgeon must identify the problem that is not solved with current surgical procedures. For example, although the removal of a gallbladder through a Kocher incision is certainly effective, it creates a great deal of disability, pain, and scarification. As a result of those issues, many patients with very symptomatic biliary colic delayed operation until life-threatening complications occurred. Clearly there was a need for developing a less invasive approach.

Once the opportunity has been established, the next step involves a search through other disciplines for technologies and techniques that might be applied. Again, this is analogous to the drug industry, in which secondary drug indications have often turned out to be more therapeutically important than the primary indication for drug development. The third step is in vivo studies in the most appropriate animal model. Certainly these types of studies are controversial because of the resistance to animal experimentation, and yet without such studies many humans would be injured or killed during the developmental phase of medical drugs, devices, and techniques. These steps are often called the preclinical phase of procedure development.

The decision regarding when such procedures are ready to come out of the lab is a difficult one. Put simply, the procedure should be reproducible, provide the desired effect, and not have serious side effects. Once these three criteria are reached, the time for human application has arrived. Before the surgeon discusses the new procedure with his patient, it is important to achieve full institutional support. The dialogue with the patient who is to be first must be thorough, brutally honest, and well documented. The psychology that allows a patient to decide to be first is quite interesting, and may under certain circumstances require psychiatric evaluation. Certainly if a dying cancer patient has a chance with a new drug, this makes sense. Similarly, if the standard surgical procedure has a high attendant morbidity and the new procedure offers a substantially better outcome, the decision to be first is understandable. On the other hand, when the benefits of the new approach are small and the risks are largely unknown, a more complete psychological profile may be necessary before proceeding.

For new surgical procedures, it is generally wise to assemble the best possible operative team, including a surgeon experienced with the old technique, and assistants who have participated in the earlier animal work. This initial team of experienced physicians and nurses should remain together until full competence with the procedure is attained. This may take 10 procedures, or it may take 50 procedures. The team will know that it has achieved competence when the majority of procedures take the same length of time, and the team is relaxed and sure of the flow of the operation. This will complete phase I of the procedure development.

In phase II, the efficacy of the procedure is tested in a nonrandomized fashion. Ideally, the outcome of new techniques must be as good or better than the procedure that is being replaced. This phase should occur at several medical centers to prove that good outcomes are achievable outside of the pioneering institution. These same requirements may be applied to the introduction of new technology into the operating room. The value equation requires that the additional measurable procedure quality exceeds the additional measurable cost to the patient or health care system. In phase III, a randomized trial pits the new procedure against the old.

Once the competence curve has been climbed, it is appropriate for the team to engage in the education of others. During the ascension of the competence curve, other learners in the institution (i.e., surgical residents) may not have the opportunity to participate in the first case series. The second stage of learning occurs when the new procedure has proven its value and a handful of experts exist, but the majority of surgeons have not been trained to perform the new procedure. In this setting, it is relatively unethical for surgeons to forge ahead with a new procedure in humans as if they had spent the same amount of time in intensive study that the first team did. The fact that one or several surgical teams were able to perform an operation does not ensure that all others with the same medical degrees can perform the operation with equal skill. It behooves the learners to contact the experts and request their assistance to ensure an optimal outcome at the new center. Although it is important that the learners contact the experts, it is equally important that the experts be willing to share their experience with their fellow professionals. As well, the experts should provide feedback to the learners regarding whether they feel the learners are equipped to forge ahead on their own. If not, further observation and assistance from the experts are required. Although this approach may sound obvious, it is fraught with difficulties. In many situations ego, competitiveness, and monetary concerns have short-circuited this process and led to poor patient outcomes. To a large extent, MIS has recovered from the black eye that it received early in development, when inadequately trained surgeons caused an excessive number of significant complications.

Suggested Readings

Callery MP, Soper NJ: Physiology of the pneumoperitoneum, in Hunter (ed): Baillière's Clinical Gastroenterology: Laparoscopic Surgery. London/Philadelphia: Baillière Tindall, 1993, p 757.

Catarci M, Carlini M, Gentileschi P, Santoro E: Major and minor injuries during the creation of pneumoperitoneum. A multicenter study on 12,919 cases. Surg Endosc 15:566, 2001.

Emam TA, Hanna G, Cuschieri A: Ergonomic principles of task alignment, visual display, and direction of execution of laparoscopic bowel suturing. Surg Endosc 16:267, 2002.

Blanc B, d'Ercole C, Gaiato ML, Boubli L: Cause and prevention of electrosurgical injuries in laparoscopy. J Am Coll Surg 179:161, 1994.

Herron DM, Gagner M, Kenyon TL, Swanstrom LL: The minimally-invasive surgical suite enters the 21st century. A discussion of critical design elements. Surg Endosc 15:415, 2001.

Morrell DG, Mullins JR, et al: Laparoscopic cholecystectomy during pregnancy in symptomatic patients. Surgery 112:856, 1992.

Litwin DWM, Pham Q: Laparoscopic surgery in the complicated patient, in Eubanks WS, Swanstrom LJ, Soper NJ (eds): Mastery of Endoscopic and Laparoscopic Surgery. Philadelphia: Lippincott Williams & Wilkins, 2000, p 57.

Costi R, Himpens J, Bruyns J, Cadiere GB: Robotic fundoplication: from theoretic advantages to real problems. J Am Coll Surg 197:500, 2003.

Fleischer DE: Stents, cloggology, and esophageal cancer. Gastrointest Endosc 43:258, 1996.

Gallagher AG, Smith CD, Bowers SP, et al: Psychomotor skills assessment in practicing surgeons experienced in performing advanced laparoscopic procedures. J Am Coll Surg 197:479, 2003.

14 | Cell, Genomics, and Molecular Surgery

Xin-Hua Feng, Jeffrey B. Matthews, Xia Lin, and F. Charles Brunicardi

Modern biology aims at the molecular interpretation and full understanding of how cells, organs, and entire organisms function, both in a normal state and under pathologic conditions. The advent of recombinant DNA technology, polymerase chain reaction (PCR) techniques, and completion of the Human Genome Project are positively affecting human society by not only broadening our knowledge and understanding of disease development but also by bringing about necessary changes in disease treatment. Today's practicing surgeons are becoming increasingly aware that many modern surgical procedures rely on the information gained through molecular research. Hence surgeons will benefit from a clear introduction to how basic biochemical and biologic principles relate to the developing area of molecular biology.

This chapter reviews the current information on modern molecular biology. First, it introduces or updates the readers about the general concepts of molecular cell biology, which are essential for comprehending the real power and potential of modern molecular technology. The second aim is to inform the reader about the modern molecular techniques commonly used for surgical research and to provide a fundamental introduction on how these techniques are developed and applied to benefit patients.

BASIC CONCEPTS OF MOLECULAR RESEARCH

The modern era of molecular biology began in 1953 when James D. Watson and Francis H. C. Crick discovered the double-helical structure of deoxyribonucleic acid, or DNA. Although DNA had been implicated as genetic material prior to 1953, it was the base-paired structure of DNA that provided a logical interpretation of how a "double helix" could "unzip" to make copies of itself. This DNA synthesis, termed replication, immediately gave rise to the notion that a template was involved in the transfer of information between generations.

Within cells DNA is packed into chromosomes. One important feature of DNA as genetic material is its ability to encode important information for all of a cell's functions. Based on the principles of base complementarity, scientists also discovered how information in DNA is accurately transferred into the protein structure. DNA serves as a template for ribonucleic acid (RNA) synthesis, termed transcription, including messenger RNA (mRNA, or the protein-encoding RNA), ribosomal RNA (rRNA), and transfer RNA (tRNA). mRNA carries the information from DNA to make proteins, termed translation, with the assistance of rRNA and tRNA. Each of these steps is precisely controlled in such a way that genes are properly expressed in each cell at a specific time and location. Thus the differential gene activity in a cell determines its actions, properties, and functions.

DNA and Heredity

DNA forms a right-handed, double-helical structure that is composed of two antiparallel strands of unbranched polymeric deoxyribonucleotides. DNA is composed of four types of deoxyribonucleotides: adenine (A), cytosine (C), guanine (G), and thymine (T). The deoxyribonucleotides are joined together by phosphodiester bonds between the 5' carbon of one deoxyribose moiety to the 3' carbon of the next. In the double-helical structure deduced by Watson and Crick, the two strands of DNA are complementary to each other. Because of size, shape, and chemical composition, A always pairs with T, and C with G, through the formation of hydrogen bonds between complementary bases that stabilize the double helix.

For cells to pass on the genetic material (DNA) to each progeny, the amount of DNA must be doubled. The complementary base-pair structure of DNA implies the existence of a template-like mechanism for the copying of genetic material. The transfer of DNA material from the mother cell to a daughter cell takes place during somatic cell division (also called mitosis). Before a cell divides, DNA must be precisely duplicated. During replication, the two strands of DNA separate and each strand creates a new complementary strand by precise base-pair matching. The two new double-stranded DNAs carry the same genetic information, which can then be passed on to two daughter cells. Proofreading mechanisms ensure that the replication process occurs in a highly accurate manner. The fidelity of DNA replication is absolutely crucial to maintaining the integrity of the genome from generation to generation. However, mistakes can still occur during this process, resulting in mutations, which may lead to a change of the DNA's encoded protein and, consequently, a change of the cell's behavior. For example, there are many mutations present in the genome of a cancer cell.

Gene Regulation

Living cells have the necessary machinery to enzymatically transcribe DNA into RNA and translate the mRNA into protein. This machinery accomplishes the two major steps required for gene expression in all organisms: transcription and translation. However, gene regulation is far more complex, particularly in eukaryotic organisms. For example, many gene transcripts must be spliced to remove the intervening sequences. The sequences that are spliced off are called introns, which appear to be useless, but in fact may carry some regulatory information. The sequences that are joined together, and are eventually translated into protein, are called exons. Additional regulation of gene expression includes modification of mRNA, control of mRNA stability, and its nuclear export into cytoplasm (where it is assembled into ribosomes for translation). After mRNA is translated into protein, the levels and functions of the proteins can be further regulated posttranslationally. However, the following sections will mainly focus on gene regulation at transcriptional and translational levels.

Transcription

Transcription is the enzymatic process of RNA synthesis from DNA. In bacteria, a single RNA polymerase carries out all RNA synthesis, including that of mRNA, rRNA, and tRNA. Transcription often is coupled with translation in such a way that an mRNA molecule is completely accessible to ribosomes, and bacterial protein synthesis begins on an mRNA molecule even while it is still being synthesized. Transcription mechanisms in eukaryotes differ from those in prokaryotes. The unique features of eukaryotic transcription are as follows: (1) Three separate RNA polymerases are involved in eukaryotes: RNA polymerase I transcribes the precursor of 5.8S, 18S, and 28S rRNAs; RNA polymerase II synthesizes the precursors of mRNA; RNA polymerase III makes tRNAs and 5S rRNAs. (2) In eukaryotes, the initial transcript is often the precursor to final mRNAs, tRNAs, and rRNAs. The precursor is then modified and/or processed into its final functional form. RNA splicing is one type of processing to remove the noncoding introns (the region between coding exons) on an mRNA. (3) In contrast to bacterial DNA, eukaryotic DNA often is packaged with histone and nonhistone proteins into chromatins. Transcription will only occur when the chromatin structure changes in such a way that DNA is accessible to the polymerase. (4) RNA is made in the nucleus and transported into cytoplasm, in which translation occurs. Therefore, unlike bacteria, eukaryotes undergo uncoupled transcription and translation.

Eukaryotic gene transcription also involves the recognition and binding of RNA polymerase to the promoter DNA. However, the interaction between the polymerase and DNA is far more complex in eukaryotes than in prokaryotes. Because the majority of studies have been focused on the regulation and functions of proteins, this chapter primarily focuses on how protein-encoding mRNA is made by RNA polymerase II.

Translation

DNA directs the synthesis of RNA; RNA in turn directs the synthesis of proteins. Proteins are variable-length polypeptide polymers composed of various combinations of 20 different amino acids and are the working molecules of the cell. The genetic information on mRNA is composed of arranged sequences of four bases that are transferred to the linear arrangement of 20 amino acids on a protein. The process of decoding information on mRNA to synthesize proteins is called translation. Translation takes place in ribosomes composed of rRNA and ribosomal proteins. Amino acids are characterized by a central carbon unit linked to four side chains: an amino group ($-NH_2$), a carboxy group ($-COOH$), a hydrogen, and a variable group. The amino acid chain is assembled via peptide bonds between the amino group of one amino acid and the carboxy group of the next. Translation involves all three RNAs. The precise transfer of information from mRNA to protein is governed by genetic code; the set of rules by which codons are translated into an amino acid (Table 14-1). A codon, a triplet of three bases, codes for one amino acid. The codons on mRNA are sequentially recognized by tRNA adaptor proteins. Specific enzymes termed aminoacyl-tRNA synthetases link a specific amino acid to a specific tRNA. The translation of mRNA to protein requires the ribosomal complex to move stepwise along the mRNA until the start codon (encoding initiator methionine) is identified. Each new amino acid is added sequentially by the appropriate tRNA in conjunction with proteins called elongation factors. Protein synthesis proceeds in the amino-to-carboxy-terminus direction.

The biologic versatility of proteins is astounding. Among many other functions, proteins serve as enzymes that catalyze critical biochemical reactions, carry signals to and from the extracellular environment, and mediate diverse signaling and regulatory functions in the intracellular environment. They also transport ions and various small molecules across plasma membranes. Proteins make up the key structural components of cells and the extracellular matrix and are responsible for cell motility. The unique functional properties of proteins are largely determined by their structure.

TABLE 14-1 The Genetic Code

First Base in Codon	Second Base in Codon				Third Base in Codon
	U	C	A	G	
U	UUU Phe [F]	UCU Ser [S]	UAU Tyr [Y]	UGU Cys [C]	U
	UUC Phe [F]	UCC Ser [S]	UAC Tyr [Y]	UGC Cys [C]	C
	UUA Leu [L]	UCA Ser [S]	UAA STOP	UGA STOP	A
	UUG Leu [L]	UCG Ser [S]	UAG STOP	UGG Trp [W]	G
C	CUU Leu [L]	CCU Pro [P]	CAU His [H]	CGU Arg [R]	U
	CUC Leu [L]	CCC Pro [P]	CAC His [H]	CGC Arg [R]	C
	CUA Leu [L]	CCA Pro [P]	CAA Gln [Q]	CGA Arg [R]	A
	CUG Leu [L]	CCG Pro [P]	CAG Gln [Q]	CGG Arg [R]	G
A	AUU Ile [I]	ACU Thr [T]	AAU Asn [N]	AGU Ser [S]	U
	AUC Ile [I]	ACC Thr [T]	AAC Asn [N]	AGC Ser [S]	C
	AUA Ile [I]	ACA Thr [T]	AAA Lys [K]	AGA Arg [R]	A
	AUG Met [M]	ACG Thr [T]	AAG Lys [K]	AGG Arg [R]	G
G	GUU Val [V]	GCU Ala [A]	GAU Asp [D]	GGU Gly [G]	U
	GUC Val [V]	GCC Ala [A]	GAC Asp [D]	GGC Gly [G]	C
	GUA Val [V]	GCA Ala [A]	GAA Glu [E]	GGA Gly [G]	A
	GUG Val [V]	GCG Ala [A]	GAG Glu [E]	GGG Gly [G]	G

A = adenine; C = cytosine; G = guanine; U = uracil; Ala = alanine; Arg = arginine; Asn = asparagine; Asp = aspartic acid; Cys = cysteine; Glu = glutamic acid; Gln = glutamine; Gly = glycine; His = histidine; Ile = isoleucine; Leu = leucine; Lys = lysine; Met = methionine; Phe = phenylalanine; Pro = proline; Ser = serine; Thr = threonine; Trp = tryptophan; Tyr = tyrosine; Val = valine. Letter in [ ] indicates single lettercode for amino acid.

Regulation of Gene Expression

The human organism is made up of a myriad of different cell types that, despite their vastly different characteristics, contain the same genetic material. This cellular diversity is controlled by the genome and accomplished by tight regulation of gene expression. This leads to the synthesis and accumulation of different complements of RNA and, ultimately, to the proteins found in different cell types. For example, muscle and bone express different genes or the same genes at different times. Moreover, the choice of which genes are expressed in a given cell at a given time depends on signals received from its environment. There are multiple levels at which gene expression can be controlled along the pathway from DNA to RNA to protein. Transcriptional control refers to the mechanism for regulating when and how often a gene is transcribed. Splicing of the primary RNA transcript (RNA processing control) and selection of which completed mRNAs undergo nuclear export (RNA transport control) represent additional potential regulatory steps. The mRNAs in the cytoplasm can be selectively translated by ribosomes (translational control), or selectively stabilized or degraded (mRNA degradation control). Finally, the resulting proteins can undergo selective activation, inactivation, or compartmentalization (protein activity control).

Because a large number of genes are regulated at the transcriptional level, regulation of gene transcripts (i.e., mRNA) often is referred to as gene regulation in a narrow definition. Each of the steps during transcription is properly regulated in eukaryotic cells. Because genes are differentially regulated from one another, one gene can be differentially regulated in different cell types or at different developmental stages. Therefore, gene regulation at the level of transcription is largely context-dependent. However, there is a common scheme that applies to transcription at the molecular level. Each gene promoter possesses unique sequences called TATA boxes that can be recognized and bound by a large complex containing RNA polymerase II, forming the basal transcription machinery. Usually located upstream of the TATA box (but sometimes longer distances) are a number of regulatory sequences referred to as enhancers that are recognized by regulatory proteins called transcription factors. These transcription factors specifically bind to the enhancers, often in response to environmental or developmental cues, and cooperate with each other and with basal transcription factors to initiate transcription. Regulatory sequences that negatively regulate the initiation of transcription also are present on the promoter DNA. The transcription factors that bind to these sites are called repressors, in contrast to the activators that activate transcription. The molecular interactions between transcription factors and promoter DNA, and between the cooperative transcription factors, are highly regulated. Specifically, the recruitment of transcription factors to the promoter DNA occurs in response to physiologic signals.

Human Genome

Genome is a collective term for all genes present in one organism. The human genome contains DNA sequences of 3 billion base pairs, carried by 23 pairs of chromosomes. The human genome has an estimated 25,000–30,000 genes, and overall it is 99.9 percent identical in all people. Approximately 3 million locations in which single-base DNA differences exist have been identified and termed single nucleotide polymorphisms (SNPs). SNPs may be critical determinants of human variation in disease susceptibility and responses to environmental factors.

The medical field is building on the knowledge, resources, and technologies emanating from the human genome to further the understanding of the relationship of the genes and their mutations to human health and disease. This expansion of genomics into human health applications resulted in the field of genomic medicine and will consequently transform the practice of medicine and surgery in this century. In the 21st century, the goal is to use this information embedded in the human genome sequence to develop new ways to treat, cure, or even prevent the thousands of diseases that afflict humankind. By doing so, the genomic information can be used for diagnosing and predicting diseases and disease susceptibility. Furthermore, exploration into the function of each human gene is now possible, which will shed light on how faulty genes play a role in disease causation. This knowledge also makes possible the development of a new generation of therapeutics based on genes. Drug design is being revolutionized as researchers create new classes of medicines based on a reasoned approach to the use of information on gene sequence and protein structure function rather than the traditional trial-and-error method. Drugs targeted to specific sites in the body promise to have fewer side effects than many of today's medicines. Finally, other applications of genomics will involve the transfer of genes to replace defective versions or the use of gene therapy to enhance normal functions such as immunity.

Proteomics refers to the study of the structure and expression of proteins and the interactions among proteins encoded by a human genome. A number of Internet-based repositories for protein sequences exist, including Swiss-Prot (http://www.expasy.ch). These databases allow comparisons of newly identified proteins with previously characterized sequences to allow prediction of similarities, identification of splice variants, and prediction of membrane topology and posttranslational modifications. Tools for proteomic profiling include two-dimensional gel electrophoresis, mass spectrometry, and protein microarrays.

It is anticipated that a genomic and proteomic approach to human disease will lead to a new understanding of pathogenesis that will aid in the development of effective strategies for early diagnosis and treatment. For example, identification of altered protein expression in organs, cells, subcellular structures, or protein complexes may lead to development of new biomarkers for disease detection. Moreover, improved understanding of how protein structure determines function will allow rational identification of therapeutic targets, and thereby not only accelerate drug development, but also lead to new strategies to evaluate therapeutic efficacy and potential toxicity.

Cell Cycle and Apoptosis

Every organism has many different cell types. Many cells grow, although some cells such as nerve cells and striated muscle cells do not. All growing cells have the ability to duplicate their genomic DNA and pass along identical copies of this genetic information to every daughter cell. Thus the cell cycle is the fundamental mechanism to maintain tissue homeostasis. After a full cycle, two daughter cells with identical DNA are generated. The machinery that drives cell cycle progression is made up of a group of enzymes called cyclin-dependent kinases (CDK). Cyclins are essential for CDK activities and form complexes with CDK, and their expression fluctuates during the cell cycle. There also are negative regulators for CDK termed CDK inhibitors (CKIs), which inhibit the assembly or activity of the cyclin-CDK complex. Expression of cyclins and CKIs often are regulated by developmental and environmental factors.

The cell cycle is connected with signal transduction pathways and gene expression. During the G1 phase (the phase before DNA duplication), cells receive signals to enter S phase (the phase of DNA duplication) or remain in G1, respectively. Growing cells proliferate only when supplied with appropriate mitogenic growth factors. Mitogenic signals stimulate the activity of CDKs. Meanwhile, cells also receive antiproliferative signals such as those from tumor suppressors. These antiproliferative signals stop cells progress into the S phase by inducing CKI production. For example, when DNA is damaged, cells will repair the damage before entering the S phase. Accelerated proliferation or improper cell cycle progression with damaged DNA would be disastrous. Genetic gain-of-function mutations in oncogenes or loss-of-function mutations in tumor suppressor are causal factors for malignant transformation.

In addition to cell cycle control, cells use genetically programmed mechanisms to kill cells. This cellular process, called apoptosis or programmed cell death, is essential for the maintenance of tissue homeostasis. Normal tissues undergo proper apoptosis to remove unwanted cells, those that have completed their jobs or have been damaged or improperly proliferated. Apoptosis can be activated by many physiologic stimuli such as death signals, growth factor deprivation, DNA damage, and stress signals. What is central to the apoptotic machinery is the activation of a cascade of proteinases called caspases. Similarly to CDK in the cell cycle, activities and expression of caspases are well controlled by positive and negative regulators. The complex machinery of apoptosis must be tightly controlled. Perturbations of this process can cause neoplastic transformation or other diseases.

Signal Transduction Pathways

Gene expression in a genome is controlled in a temporal and spatial manner, at least in part by signaling pathways. A signaling pathway generally begins at the cell surface and, after a signaling relay by a cascade of intracellular effectors, ends up in the nucleus. All cells have the ability to sense changes in their external environment. The bioactive substances to which cells can respond are many and include proteins, short peptides, amino acids, nucleotides/nucleosides, steroids, retinoids, fatty acids, and dissolved gases. Some of these substances are lipophilic and thereby can cross the plasma membrane by diffusion to bind to a specific target protein within the cytoplasm (intracellular receptor). Other substances bind directly with a transmembrane protein (cell-surface receptor). Binding of ligand to receptor initiates a series of biochemical reactions (signal transduction) typically involving protein-protein interactions, leading to various cellular end responses.

Control and specificity through simple protein-protein interactions is a common feature of signal transduction pathways in cells. Signaling also involves catalytic activities of signaling molecules such as protein kinases/phosphatases that modify the structures of key signaling proteins. On binding and/or modification by upstream signaling molecules, downstream effectors undergo a conformational (allosteric) change and, consequently, a change in function.

The signal that originates at the cell surface and is relayed by the cytoplasmic proteins often ultimately reaches the transcriptional apparatus in the nucleus. It alters the DNA binding and activities of transcription factors that directly turn genes on or off in response to the stimuli. Abnormal alterations in signaling activities and capacities in otherwise normal cells can lead to diseases such as cancer.

In a given cell, many signaling pathways operate simultaneously and cross-talk with one another. A cell generally may react to a hormonal signal in a variety of ways: (1) by changing its metabolite or protein, (2) by generating an electric current, or (3) by contracting. Cells are continually subject to multiple input signals that simultaneously and sequentially activate multiple receptor- and non–receptor-mediated signal transduction pathways. Although the regulators responsible for cell behavior are rapidly identified as a result of genomic and proteomic techniques, the specific functions of the individual proteins, how they assemble, and the networks that control cellular behavior remain to be defined. An increased understanding of cell regulatory pathways—and how they are disrupted in disease—will likely reveal common themes based on protein interaction domains that direct associations of proteins with other polypeptides, phospholipids, nucleic acids, and other regulatory molecules. Advances in the understanding of signaling networks will require multidisciplinary and transdisciplinary methodologies within the emerging disciplines of medical informatics and computational biology.

Signaling pathways often are grouped according to the properties of signaling receptors. Many hydrophobic signaling molecules are able to diffuse across plasma membranes and directly reach specific cytoplasmic targets. Steroid hormones, thyroid hormones, retinoids, and vitamin D are examples that exert their activity on binding to structurally related members of the nuclear hormone receptor superfamily. Ligand binding induces a conformational change that enhances transcriptional activity of these receptors.

Most extracellular signaling molecules interact with transmembrane protein receptors that couple ligand binding to intracellular signals, leading to biologic actions. There are three major classes of cell-surface receptors: transmitter-gated ion channels, seven-transmembrane G-protein coupled receptors (GPCRs), and enzyme-linked receptors. The superfamily of GPCRs is one of the largest families of proteins, representing over 800 genes of the human genome. Members of this superfamily share a characteristic seven-transmembrane configuration. The ligands for these receptors are diverse and include hormones, chemokines, neurotransmitters, proteinases, inflammatory mediators, and even sensory signals such as odorants and photons. Most GPCRs signal through heterotrimeric G-proteins, which are guanine-nucleotide regulatory complexes. Thus the receptor serves as the receiver, the G-protein serves as the transducer, and the enzyme serves as the effector arm. Enzyme-linked receptors possess an extracellular ligand-recognition domain and a cytosolic domain that either has intrinsic enzymatic activity or directly links with an enzyme. Structurally, these receptors usually have only one transmembrane-spanning domain. Of various classes of enzyme-linked receptors, the growth factor receptors such as tyrosine kinase receptor or serine/threonine kinase receptors mediate diverse cellular events including cell growth, differentiation, metabolism, and survival/apoptosis. Dysregulation (particularly mutations) of these receptors is thought to underlie conditions of abnormal cellular proliferation in the context of cancer. The following sections further review two examples of growth factor signaling pathways and their connection with human diseases.

Insulin Pathway and Diabetes

Insulin is required for the growth and metabolism of most mammalian cells, which contain cell-surface insulin receptors (InsR). Insulin binding to InsR activates the tyrosine kinase activity of InsR. InsR then activates its immediate intracellular effector, called insulin receptor substrate (IRS). IRS plays a central role in coordinating the signaling of insulin by activating distinct signaling pathways, the PI3K-Akt pathway and mitogen-activated protein kinase (MAPK) pathway, both of which possess multiple protein kinases that can control transcription, protein synthesis, and glycolysis.

The primary physiologic role of insulin is in glucose homeostasis, which is accomplished through the stimulation of glucose uptake into insulin-sensitive tissues such as fat and skeletal muscle. Defects in insulin synthesis/secretion and/or responsiveness are major causal factors in diabetes, one of the leading causes of death and disability in the United States. Type 2 diabetes accounts for about 90 percent of all cases of diabetes. Clustering of type 2 diabetes in certain families and ethnic populations points to a strong genetic background for the disease. More than 90 percent of affected individuals have insulin resistance. The majority of type 2 diabetes cases may result from defects in InsR, IRS or downstream-signaling components in the insulin-signaling pathway. Type 2 diabetes is also associated with declining β-cell function, resulting in reduced insulin secretion. A full understanding of the basis of insulin resistance is crucial for the development of new therapies for type 2 diabetes. Furthermore, apart from type 2 diabetes, insulin resistance is a central feature of several other common human disorders, including atherosclerosis and coronary artery disease, hypertension, and obesity.

TGF-β Pathway and Cancers

B growth factor signaling controls cell growth, differentiation, and apoptosis. Although insulin and many mitogenic growth factors promote cell proliferation, some growth factors and hormones inhibit cell proliferation. Transforming growth factor-β (TGF-β) is one of them. The balance between mitogens and TGF-β plays an important role in controlling the proper pace of cell cycle progression. The growth inhibition function of TGF-β signaling in epithelial cells plays a major role in maintaining tissue homeostasis.

The TGF-β superfamily comprises a large number of structurally related growth and differentiation factors that act through a receptor complex at the cell surface. The complex consists of transmembrane serine/threonine kinases. The receptor signals through activation of downstream intracellular effectors called SMADs. Activated SMAD complexes translocate into the nucleus, in which they bind to gene promoters and cooperate with specific transcription factors to regulate the expression of genes that control cell proliferation and differentiation. For example, TGF-β strongly induces the transcription of a gene called p15INK4B (a type of CKI) and, at the same time, reduces the expression of many oncogenes such as c-Myc. The outcome of the altered gene expression leads to the inhibition of cell cycle progression. Therefore, activation of TGF-β signaling is an intrinsic mechanism for cells to ensure controlled proliferation.

Resistance to TGF-β's anticancer action is one hallmark of human cancer cells. TGF-β receptors and SMADs are identified as tumor suppressors.

The TGF-β signaling circuit can be disrupted in different types of human tumors through various mechanisms such as downregulation or mutations of the TGF-β receptors or SMADs. In pancreatic and colorectal cancers, 100 percent of cells derived from these cancers carry genetic defects in the TGF-β signaling pathway. Therefore, the TGF-β antiproliferative pathway is disrupted in a majority of human cancer cells.

Gene Therapy and Molecular Drugs in Cancer

Human diseases arise from improper changes in the genome, thus the continuous understanding of how the genome functions will make it possible to tailor medicine on an individual basis. In this section, cancer is used as an example to elaborate some therapeutic applications of molecular biology.

Cancer is a complex disease, involving uncontrolled growth and spread of tumor cells. Cancer development depends on the acquisition and selection of specific characteristics that transform normal cells into cancerous ones by derailing a wide spectrum of regulatory pathways including signal transduction pathways, cell cycle machinery, or apoptotic pathways. The early notion that cancer was caused by mutations in genes critical for the control of cell growth implied that genome stability is important for preventing oncogenesis. There are two major classes of cancer genes in which alteration has been identified in human and animal cancer cells: oncogenes, with dominant gain-of-function mutations, and tumor suppressor genes, with recessive loss-of-function mutations. In normal cells, oncogenes promote cell growth by activating cell cycle progression, although tumor suppressors counteract oncogenes' functions. Therefore, the balance between oncogenes and tumor suppressors maintains a well-controlled state of cell growth.

During the development of most types of human cancer, cancer cells can break away from primary tumor masses, invade adjacent tissues, and hence travel to distant sites where they form new colonies. This spreading process of tumor cells, called metastasis, is the cause of 90 percent of human cancer deaths. Metastatic cancer cells that enter the blood stream can reach virtually all tissues of the body. Bones are one of the most common places for these cells to settle and start growing again. Bone metastasis is one of the most frequent causes of pain in people with cancer. It also can cause bones to break and create other symptoms and problems for patients.

As a result of explosive new discoveries, some modern treatments were developed. Understanding the biology of cancer cells has led to the development of designer therapies for cancer prevention and treatment. Gene therapy, immune system modulation, genetically engineered antibodies, and molecularly designed chemical drugs, are all promising fronts in the war against cancer.

Immunotherapy

The growth of the body is controlled by many natural signals through complex signaling pathways. Some of these natural agents have been used in cancer treatment and have proven effective for fighting several cancers through the clinical trial process. These naturally occurring biologic agents such as interferons are given to patients to influence the natural immune response agents either by directly altering the cancer cell growth, or by acting indirectly to help healthy cells control the cancer. One of the most exciting applications of immunotherapy has come from the generation of antibodies aimed at tumor antigens. This was first used as a means of localizing tumors in the body for diagnosis, and was more recently used to attack cancer cells. For example, Trastuzumab is a monoclonal antibody that neutralizes the mitogenic activity of cell-surface growth factor receptor HER-2, which is overexpressed in approximately 25 percent of breast cancers. These tumors tend to grow faster and are generally more likely to recur than tumors that do not overproduce HER-2. Trastuzumab slows or stops the growth of these cells and increases the survival of HER-2–positive breast cancer patients. Another significant example is the administration of interleukin-2 (IL-2) to patients with metastatic melanoma or kidney cancer, which has been shown to mediate the durable regression of metastatic cancer.

IL-2, a cytokine produced by human T-helper lymphocytes, has no direct impact on cancer cells, yet has a wide range of immune regulatory effects including the expansion of lymphocytes with antitumor activity. The expanded lymphocytes somehow recognize the antigen on cancer cells. Thus, the molecular identification of cancer antigens has opened new possibilities for the development of effective immunotherapies for patients with cancer. Clinical studies using immunization with peptides derived from cancer antigens have shown that high levels of lymphocytes with antitumor activity can be produced in cancer-bearing patients. Highly avid antitumor lymphocytes can be isolated from immunized patients and grown in vitro for use in cell-transfer therapies.

Chemotherapy

The primary function of anticancer chemicals is to block different steps involved in cell growth and replication. These chemicals often block a critical chemical reaction in a signal transduction pathway or during DNA replication or gene expression. For example, STI571, also known as Gleevec, is one of the first molecularly targeted drugs based on the changes that cancer causes in cells. STI571 offers promise for the treatment of chronic myeloid leukemia (CML) and may soon surpass αinterferon-α as the standard treatment for the disease. In CML, STI571 is targeted at the Bcr-Abl kinase, an activated oncogene product in CML. Bcr-Abl is an overly activated protein kinase resulting from a specific genetic abnormality generated by chromosomal translocation that is found in the cells of patients with CML. STI571-mediated inhibition of Bcr-Abl-kinase activity not only prevents cell growth of Bcr-Abl–transformed leukemic cells, but also induces apoptosis. Clinically, the drug quickly corrects the blood cell abnormalities caused by the leukemia in a majority of patients, achieving a complete disappearance of the leukemic blood cells and the return of normal blood cells. Additionally, the drug appears to have some effect on other cancers including certain brain tumors and gastrointestinal stromal tumors (GISTs), a very rare type of stomach cancer.

Gene Therapy

Gene therapy is an experimental treatment that involves genetically altering a patient's own tumor cells or lymphocytes. For years, the concept of gene therapy has held promise as a new, potentially potent weapon to attack cancer. Several problems must be resolved to transform it into a clinically relevant form of therapy. The major issues that limit its translation to the clinic are improving the selectivity of tumor targeting, improving the delivery to the tumor, and the enhancement of the transduction rate of the cells of interest. An important aspect of effective gene therapy involves the choice of appropriate genes for manipulation. Genes that promote the production of messenger chemicals or other immune-active substances can be transferred into the patient's cells. These include genes that inhibit cell cycle progression, induce apoptosis, enhance host immunity against cancer cells, and block the ability of cancer cells to metastasize. The mapping of genes responsible for human cancer is likely to provide new targets for gene therapy in the future. The preliminary results of gene therapy for cancer clinical trials are encouraging, and as advancements are made in the understanding of the molecular biology of human cancer, the future of this rapidly developing field holds great potential for treating cancer.

It is noteworthy that the use of multiple therapeutic methods has proven more powerful than a single method. The use of chemotherapy after surgery to destroy the few remaining cancerous cells in the body is called "adjuvant therapy." Adjuvant therapy was first tested and found to be effective in breast cancer. It was later adopted for use in other cancers. A major discovery in chemotherapy is the advantage of multiple chemotherapeutic agents (known as combination or cocktail chemotherapy) over single agents. Some types of fast-growing leukemias and lymphomas (tumors involving the cells of the bone marrow and lymph nodes) responded extremely well to combination chemotherapy, and clinical trials led to gradual improvement of the drug combinations used. Many of these tumors can be cured today by combination chemotherapy. As cancer cells carry multiple genetic defects, the use of combination chemotherapy, immunotherapy, and gene therapies may be more effective in treating cancers.

Stem Cell Research

Stem cell biology represents a cutting-edge scientific research field with potential clinical applications. It may have an enormous impact on human health by offering hope for curing human diseases such as diabetes mellitus, Parkinson disease, neurologic degeneration, and congenital heart disease. Stem cells are endowed with two remarkable properties. First, stem cells can self-renew. Second, they have the ability to differentiate into many specialized cell types. There are two groups of stem cells: embryonic stem (ES) cells and adult stem cells. Human ES cells are derived from early preimplantation embryos called blastocysts (5 days postfertilization), and are capable of generating all differentiated cell types in the body. Adult stem cells are present in adult tissues. They are often tissue-specific and can only generate the cell types comprising a particular tissue in the body; however, in some cases they can transdifferentiate into cell types found in other tissues. Hematopoietic stem cells are adult stem cells. They reside in bone marrow and are capable of generating all cell types of the blood and immune system.

With the recent and continually increasing improvement in culturing stem cells, scientists are beginning to understand the molecular mechanisms of stem cell self-renewal and differentiation in response to environmental cues. It is believed that discovery of the signals that control self-renewal versus differentiation will be extremely important for the therapeutic use of stem cells in treating disease. It is possible that success in the study of the changes in signal transduction pathways in stem cells will lead to the development of therapies to specifically differentiate stem cells into a particular cell type to replace diseased or damaged cells in the body.

MOLECULAR APPROACHES TO SURGICAL RESEARCH

Rapid advances in molecular and cellular biology over the past half-century have revolutionized the understanding of disease and will radically transform the practice of surgery. In the future, molecular techniques will be increasingly applied to surgical disease and will lead to new strategies for the selection and implementation of operative therapy. Surgeons should be familiar with the fundamental principles of molecular and cellular biology so that emerging scientific information can be incorporated into improved care of the surgical patient.

The basic molecular approaches for modern surgical research include DNA cloning, cell manipulation, disease modeling in animals, and clinical trials in human patients. The greatest advances in the field of molecular biology have been in the areas of analysis and manipulation of DNA. Recombinant DNA technology in particular has drastically changed the world of biology. DNA molecules can be cloned for a variety of purposes including safeguarding DNA samples, facilitating sequencing, generating probes, and expressing recombinant proteins. Expression of recombinant proteins provides a method for analyzing gene regulation, gene functions, and in recent years for gene therapy and biopharmaceuticals. The basic molecular approaches for modern surgical research include DNA cloning, cell manipulation, disease modeling in animals, and clinical trials in human patients.

DNA Cloning

Recombinant DNA technology is the technology that uses advanced enzymatic and microbiologic techniques to manipulate DNA. This technology, often referred to as DNA cloning, is the basis of all other DNA analysis methods. It is only with the awesome power of recombinant DNA technology that the completion of the Human Genome Project was possible. It also has led to the identification of the entire gene complements of organisms such as viruses, bacteria, worms, flies, and plants.

Molecular cloning refers to the process of cloning a DNA of interest into a DNA vector that is ultimately delivered into bacterial or mammalian cells or tissues. This represents a very basic technique that is widely used in almost all areas of biomedical research. The process of molecular cloning involves several steps of manipulation of DNA. First, the vector DNA is cleaved with a restriction enzyme to create compatible ends with the foreign DNA fragment to be cloned. The vector and the DNA fragment are then joined by a DNA ligase. Finally, the ligation product is introduced into competent host *Escherichia coli*; this procedure is called transformation. The resulting plasmid vector can be amplified in *E. coli* to prepare large quantities of DNA for its subsequent applications such as transfection, gene therapy, transgenics, and knockout mice.

Detection of Nucleic Acids and Proteins

Southern Blot Hybridization

Southern blotting refers to the technique of transferring DNA fragments from an electrophoresis gel to a membrane support, and the subsequent analysis of the fragments by hybridization with a radioactively labeled probe. Southern blotting normally begins with the digestion of the DNA samples with appropriate restriction enzymes and the separation of DNA samples in an agarose gel. The DNA is then denatured and transferred onto a nitrocellulose membrane. After immobilization, the DNA can be subjected to hybridization analysis, enabling bands with sequence similarity to a radioactively labeled probe to be identified.

The development of Southern transfer and the associated hybridization techniques made it possible to obtain information about the physical organization of genes in complex genomes. Its applications include genetic fingerprinting and prenatal diagnosis of genetic diseases.

Northern Blot Hybridization

Northern blotting refers to the technique of size fractionation of RNA in a gel and the transferring of an RNA sample to a membrane support. In principle, Northern blot hybridization is similar to Southern blot hybridization (and hence its name), with the exception that RNA, not DNA, is on the membrane. The membrane is then hybridized with a labeled probe complementary to the mRNA of interest. Signals generated from detection of the membrane can be used to determine the size and abundance of the target RNA. Although RT-PCR has been used in many applications (described below), Northern analysis is the only method that provides information regarding mRNA size. Thus, Northern blot analysis is commonly used in molecular biology studies relating to gene expression.

Polymerase Chain Reaction

PCR is a method for the polymerase-directed amplification of specific DNA sequences using two oligonucleotide primers that hybridize to opposite strands and flank the region of interest in the target DNA. One cycle of PCR reaction involves template denaturation, primer annealing, and the extension of the annealed primers by DNA polymerase. Because the primer extension products synthesized in one cycle can serve as a template in the next, the number of target DNA copies nearly doubles at each cycle. Thus a repeated series of cycles result in the exponential accumulation of a specific fragment defined by the primers. The introduction of the thermostable DNA polymerase (e.g., Taq polymerase) transforms the PCR into a simple and robust reaction.

The emergence of the PCR technique has dramatically altered the approach to both fundamental and applied biologic problems. The capability of amplifying a specific DNA fragment from a gene or the whole genome greatly advances the study of the gene and its function. It is simple, yet robust, speedy, and most of all, flexible. As a recombinant DNA tool, it underlies almost all of molecular biology. This revolutionary technique enabled the modern methods for the isolation of genes, construction of a DNA vector, introduction of alterations into DNA, and quantitation of gene expression, making it a fundamental cornerstone of genetic and molecular analysis.

Antibody-based Techniques

Analyses of proteins are primarily carried out by antibody-directed immunologic techniques. For example, Western blotting, also called immunoblotting, is performed to detect protein levels in a population of cells or tissues, whereas immunoprecipitation is used to concentrate proteins from a larger pool. Using specific antibodies, microscopic analysis called immunofluorescence and immunohistochemistry is possible for the subcellular localization and expression of proteins in cells or tissues, respectively.

Immunoblotting refers to the process of identifying a protein from a mixture of proteins using specific antibody. It consists of five steps: sample preparation, electrophoresis, transfer of proteins from gel onto membrane support, immunodetection of target proteins with specific antibody, and colorimetric or chemiluminescent visualization of the antibody-recognized protein. Immuno-blotting is a powerful tool used to determine the presence and the quantity of a protein in a given cellular condition and its relative molecular weight. Immunoblotting also can be used to determine whether posttranslational modification such as phosphorylation has occurred on a protein. Importantly, through immunoblotting analysis a comparison of the protein levels and modification states in normal versus diseased tissues is possible.

Immunoprecipitation, another widely used immunochemical technique, is a method which uses antibody to enrich a protein of interest and any other proteins that are associated with it. The principle of the technique lies in the property of a strong and specific affinity between antibodies and their antigens to pull down the antibody-antigen complexes in the solution. The purified protein can then be analyzed by a number of biochemical methods. When immunoprecipitation is combined with immunoblotting, it can be used for detecting proteins in low concentrations and for analyzing protein-protein interactions or determining posttranslational modifications of proteins.

DNA Microarray

With the tens of thousands of genes present in the genome, traditional methods in molecular biology, which generally work on a one-gene-in-one-experiment basis, cannot generate the "whole" picture of genome function. To this end, DNA microarray has attracted tremendous interest among biologists and clinicians. This technology promises to monitor the whole genome on a single chip so researchers can have a better picture of the interactions among thousands of genes simultaneously.

DNA microarray, also called gene chip, DNA chip, and gene array, refers to large sets of probes of known sequences orderly arranged on a small chip, enabling many hybridization reactions to be carried out in parallel in a small device. Like Southern and Northern hybridization, the underlying principle of this technology is the remarkable ability of nucleic acids to form a duplex between two strands with complementary base sequences. DNA microarray provides a medium for matching known and unknown DNA samples based on base-pairing rules, and automating the process of identifying the unknowns. Microarrays require specialized robotics and imaging equipment that spot the samples on a glass or nylon substrate, carry out the hybridization, and analyze the data generated. The massive scale of microarray experiments requires the aid of computers to quantitate the extent of hybridization, and to allow meaningful interpretation of the extent of hybridization.

DNA microarray technology has produced many significant results in quite different areas of application. There are two major application forms for the technology: identification of sequence (gene/gene mutation) and determination of expression level (abundance) of genes. For example, analysis of genomic DNA detects amplifications and deletions found in human tumors. Differential gene expression analysis also has uncovered networks of genes differentially present in cancers that cannot be distinguished by conventional means.

Cell Manipulations

Cell culture is used in a diversity of biologic fields ranging from traditional cell biology to modern medicine. Through their ability to be maintained in vitro, cells can be manipulated by the introduction of genes of interest (cell transfection) and can be transferred into in vivo biologic receivers (cell transplantation) to study the biologic effect of the interested genes. In transfection, the transfer of foreign macromolecules, such as DNA, into living cells provides an efficient method for studying a variety of cellular processes and functions at the molecular level. DNA transfection has become an important tool for studying the regulation and function of genes. Depending on the cell type, many ways of introducing DNA into mammalian cells have been developed. Commonly used approaches include calcium phosphate, electroporation, liposome-mediated transfection, the nonliposomal formulation, and the use of viral vectors. One application of DNA transfection is the generation of transgenic or knockout mouse models. Transfected cells also can be transplanted into host organs.

Genetic Manipulations

Understanding how genes control the growth and differentiation of the mammalian organism has been the most challenging topic of modern research. Genetically altered mice are powerful model systems in which to study the function and regulation of genes during mammalian development. A gene of interest can be introduced into the mouse (transgenic mouse) to study its effect on development or diseases. The gene function also can be studied by creating mutant mice through homologous recombination (gene knockout). As mouse models do not precisely represent human biology, genetic manipulations of human somatic or embryonic stem cells provide a great means for the understanding of the molecular networks in human cells.

Transgenic Mice

The transgenic technique has proven to be extremely important for basic investigations of gene regulation, creation of animal models of human disease, and genetic engineering of livestock. A transgenic mouse is created by the microinjection of DNA into the one-celled mouse embryo, allowing the efficient introduction of cloned genes into the developing mouse somatic tissues, and into the germline. Generation of transgenic mice generally is comprised of the following steps: (1) Designs of a transgene. A simple transgene construct consists of a protein-encoding gene and a promoter that precedes it. The most common applications for the use of transgenic mice are similar to those in the cell culture system to study the functions of proteins encoded by the transgene, and to analyze the tissue-specific and developmental-stage–specific activity of a gene promoter. (2) Production of transgenic mice. Pure DNA is microinjected into mouse embryos. Mice that develop from injected eggs are often termed "founder mice." (3) Genotyping of transgenic mice. The screening of "founder mice" and the transgenic lines derived from the founders is accomplished by determining the integration of the injected gene into the genome. This is normally achieved by performing PCR or Southern blot analysis. Once a given founder mouse is identified to be transgenic, it will be mated to begin establishing a transgenic line. (4) Analysis of phenotype of transgenic mice. Phenotypes of transgenic mice are dictated by both the expression pattern and biologic functions of the transgene. Elucidation of the functions of the transgene-encoded protein in vitro often offers some clue to what the protein might do in vivo.

Gene Knockout in Mice

The isolation and genetic manipulation of ES cells represents one of the most important milestones for modern genetic technologies. Several unique properties of these ES cells, such as the pluripotency to differentiate into different tissues in an embryo, make them an efficient vehicle for introducing genetic alterations into this species. Thus, this technology provides an important breakthrough, making it possible to genetically manipulate ES cells in a controlled way in the culture dish and then introduce the mutation into the germline. This not only makes mouse genetics a powerful approach for addressing important gene functions but also identifies the mouse as a great system to model human disease. Generation of gene knockout in mice includes the following steps: (1) Construction of targeting vector. Two segments of homologous sequence to a gene of interest that flank a part of the gene essential for functions (e.g., the coding region) are used as arms of the targeting vector. On the homologous recombination between the arms of the vector and the corresponding genomic regions of the gene of interest in ES cells, the positive selectable marker will replace the essential segment of the target gene, thus creating a null allele. To create a conditional knockout (i.e., gene knockout in a spatiotemporal fashion), site-specific recombinases such as the popular cre-loxP system are used. This method is markedly useful to prevent developmental compensations and to introduce null mutations in the adult mouse that would otherwise be lethal. (2) Introduction of the targeting vector into ES cells. To alter the genome of ES cells, the targeting vector DNA is then transfected into ES cells. Stable ES cells are selected in the presence of a positive selectable antibiotic drug. Before injecting the ES cells, DNA is prepared from ES colonies to screen for positive ES cells that exhibit the correct integration or homologous recombination of the targeting vector. Positive ES colonies are then expanded and used for creation of chimeras. (3) Creation of the chimera. A chimeric organism is one in which cells originate from more than one embryo. Here, chimeric mice are denoted as those that contain some tissues from the ES cells with an altered genome. When these ES cells give rise to the lineage of the germ layer, the germ cells carrying the altered genome can be passed on to the offspring, thus creating the germline transmission from ES cells. ES cells are introduced into preimplantation-stage embryos by injection of embryonic cells directly into the cavity of blastocysts. The mixture of recognizable markers (e.g., coat color) that are specific for the donor mouse and ES cells can be used to identify chimeric mice. (4) Genotyping and phenotyping of knockout animals. The next step is to analyze whether germline transmission of targeted mutation occurs in mice. DNA from a small amount of tissue from offspring of the chimera is extracted and subjected to genomic PCR or Southern blot DNA hybridization. Positive mice (i.e., those with properly integrated targeting vector into the genome) will be used for the propagation of more knockout mice for phenotype analysis. The phenotypic studies of these mice provide ample information on the functions of these genes in growth and differentiation of organs, and during development of human diseases.

RNA Interference

Although gene ablation in animal models provides an important means to understand the in vivo functions of genes of interest, animal models may not adequately represent human biology.

Development of RNA interference (RNAi) technology in the past few years has provided a promising approach to understanding the biologic functions of human genes in human cells. RNAi is an ancient natural mechanism by which small, double-stranded RNA (dsRNA) acts as a guide for an enzyme complex that destroys complementary RNA and downregulates gene expression in a sequence-specific manner. There are two ways to introduce RNAi to knock down gene expression in human cells: (1) RNA transfection: siRNA can be made chemically or using an in vitro transcription method. siRNA oligos or mixtures can be transfected into cell lines. (2) DNA transfection: Expression vectors for expressing siRNA have been made using RNA polymerase III promoters. These promoters precisely transcribe a hairpin structure of dsRNA, which will be processed into siRNA in the cell. siRNA expression vectors are advantageous over siRNA oligos for the long-term silencing of target genes to allow a wide spectrum of applications in gene therapy.

There has been a fast and fruitful development of RNAi tools for in vitro and in vivo use in mammals. These novel approaches, together with future developments, will be crucial to put RNAi technology to use for effective disease therapy or to exert the power of mammalian genetics. Therefore, the applications of RNAi to human health are enormous. With the availability of the human genome sequences, RNAi approaches hold tremendous promise for unleashing the dormant potential of sequenced genomes. Practical applications of RNAi possibly will result in new therapeutic interventions. The concept of using siRNA in battling infectious diseases and carcinogenesis was proven effective. These include notable successes in blocking replication of viruses, such as human immunodeficiency virus (HIV), hepatitis B virus (HBV), and hepatitis C virus (HCV). In cancers, silencing of oncogenes such as c-Myc or Ras can slow down the proliferation rate of cancer cells. Finally, siRNA also has potential applications for some dominant genetic disorders.

The 21st century, already heralded as the "century of the gene," carries great promise for alleviating suffering from disease and improving human health. On the whole, completion of the human genome blueprint, the promise of gene therapy and RNA interference, and the existence of stem cells has captured the imagination of the public and the biomedical community for good reason. Surgeons must take the opportunity to participate together with scientists to make realistic promises and to face the new era of modern medicine.

Suggested Readings

Alberts B, Johnson A, Lewis J, et al: Molecular Biology of the Cell, 4th ed. New York: Garland Science, 2002.

Wolfsberg TG, Wetterstrand KA, Guyer MS, et al: A User's Guide to the Human Genome. Nature Genetics Supplement, 2002. Accessed from http://www.nature.com/nature/focus/humangenome.

Ptashne M, Gann A: Genes & Signals. New York: Cold Spring Harbor Laboratory Press, 2002.

Hanahan D, Weinberg RA: The hallmarks of cancer. Cell 100:57, 2000.

Kiessling AA, Anderson SC: Human Embryonic Stem Cells: An Introduction to the Science and Therapeutic Potential. Boston: Jones & Bartlett Pub, 2003.

Sambrook J: Molecular Cloning, A Laboratory Manual, 3rd ed. New York: Cold Spring Harbor Laboratory Press, 2001.

Mullis K, Faloona F, Scharf S, et al: Specific enzymatic amplification of DNA in vitro: The polymerase chain reaction. Cold Spring Harb Symp Quant Biol 51:263, 1986.

Bowtell D, Sambrook J: DNA Microarrays, A Molecular Cloning Manual. New York: Cold Spring Harbor Laboratory Press, 2003.

Nagy A, Gertsenstein M, Vintersten K, et al: Manipulating The Mouse Embryo, A Laboratory Manual, 3rd ed. New York: Cold Spring Harbor Laboratory Press, 2003.

Hannon GJ: RNAi, A Guide To Gene Silencing. New York: Cold Spring Harbor Laboratory Press, 2003.

PART II | SPECIFIC CONSIDERATIONS

15 | Skin and Subcutaneous Tissue

Scott L. Hansen, Stephen J. Mathes, and David M. Young

The skin is the largest and among the most complex organs of the body. Although the skin functions simply as a protective barrier to interface with our environment, its structure and physiology are complex. The skin protects against most noxious agents, such as chemicals (by the impermeability of the epidermis), solar radiation (by means of pigmentation), infectious agents (through efficient immunosurveillance), and physically deforming forces (by the durability of the dermis). Its efficient ability to conserve or disperse heat makes the skin the major organ responsible for thermoregulation. To direct all these functions, the skin has a highly specialized nervous structure. The palms and soles are particularly thick to bear weight. The fingertips have the highest density of sensory innervation and allow for intricate tasks. Even the lines of the skin, first described by Langer, are oriented perpendicularly to the long axis of muscles to allow the greatest degree of stretching and contraction without deformity.

ANATOMY AND PHYSIOLOGY

The skin is divided into three layers: the epidermis, the basement membrane, and the dermis. The epidermis is composed mainly of cells (keratinocytes), with very little extracellular matrix. The deep, mitotically active, basal cells are a single-cell layer of the least-differentiated keratinocytes. Some multiplying cells leave the basal layer and begin to travel upward. In the spinous layer, they lose the ability to undergo mitosis. These differentiated cells start to accumulate keratohyalin granules in the granular layer. Finally, in the horny layer, the keratinocytes age, the once-numerous intercellular connections disappear, and the dead cells are shed. The keratinocyte transit time is between 40 and 56 days. The internal skeleton of cells (intermediate filaments), called keratins in epithelial cells, play an important role in the function of the epidermis. Intermediate filaments provide flexible scaffolding that enables the cell to resist external stress. Different keratins are expressed at different stages of keratinocyte maturation. In the mitotically active inner layer of the epidermis, the keratinocytes mainly express keratins 5 and 14. Patients with epidermolysis bullosa simplex, a blistering disease, were found to have a point mutation in one or the other keratin gene, thus revealing the etiology of one of the more baffling skin diseases.

Melanocytes migrate to the epidermis from precursor cells in the neural crest and provide a barrier to radiation. There are 35 keratinocytes for every melanocyte. The melanocytes produce the pigment melanin from tyrosine and cysteine. The pigment is packaged in melanosomes and transported to the tips of dendritic processes and phagocytized by the keratinocyte (apocopation), thus transferring the pigment to the keratinocyte. The melanin aggregates on the superficial side of the nucleus in an umbrella shape. The density of melanocytes is constant among individuals of different skin color. The rate of melanin production, transfer to keratinocytes, and melanosome degradation determine the degree of skin pigmentation. Genetically activated factors, as well as ultraviolet radiation, hormones such as estrogen, adrenocorticotropic hormone, and melanocyte-stimulating hormone, influence these activities.

The Langerhans cells migrate from the bone marrow and function as the skin's macrophages. The Langerhans cells constitutively express class II major histocompatibility antigens and have antigen-presenting capabilities. These cells play a crucial role in immunosurveillance against viral infections and neoplasms of the skin, and may initiate skin allograft rejection.

The dermis is mostly comprised of several structural proteins. Collagen constitutes 70 percent of the dry weight of dermis and is responsible for its remarkable tensile strength. Of the seven structurally distinct collagens, the skin contains mostly type I. Early fetal dermis contains mostly type III (reticulin fibers) collagen, but this remains only in the basement membrane zone and the perivascular regions in postnatal skin. Elastic fibers are highly branching proteins that are capable of being reversibly stretched to twice their resting length. This allows skin to return to its original form after stretching. Ground substance, consisting of various polysaccharide–polypeptide (glycosaminoglycans) complexes, is an amorphous material that fills the remaining spaces.

Fibroblasts are scattered throughout the dermis and are responsible for production and maintenance of the protein matrix. Recently, proteins that control the proliferation and migration of fibroblasts have been isolated. The study of fibroblast activity by these growth factor interactions is crucial to understanding wound healing and organogenesis.

The basement membrane zone of the dermoepidermal junction is a highly organized structure of proteins that anchors the epidermis to the dermis. Mechanical disruption or a genetic defect in the synthesis of this structure results in separation of the epidermis from the dermis.

The remaining structures of the skin are situated in the dermis. An intricate network of blood vessels regulates body temperature. Vertical vascular channels interconnect two horizontal plexuses, one at the dermal–subcutaneous junction and one in the papillary dermis. Glomus bodies are tortuous arteriovenous shunts that allow a tremendous increase in blood flow to the skin when open. This ability not only provides for the nutritional needs of the skin, but enables it to dissipate a vast amount of body heat when needed. Sensory innervation follows a dermatomal distribution from segments of the spinal cord. These fibers connect to corpuscular receptors (pacinian, Meissner, and Ruffini) that respond to pressure, vibration, and touch, and to "unspecialized" free nerve endings associated with Merkel cells of the basal epidermis, and to hair follicles. These nerves are stimulated by temperature, touch, pain, and itch. The skin has three main adnexal structures. The eccrine glands, which produce sweat, are located over the entire body but are concentrated on the palms, soles, axillae, and forehead. The apocrine glands are found primarily in the axillae and the anogenital region. In lower mammals, these glands produce scent hormones (pheromones).

INJURIES TO SKIN AND SUBCUTANEOUS TISSUE

Injuries that violate the continuity of the skin and subcutaneous tissue can occur as a result of trauma or from various environmental exposures. Environmental exposures that damage the skin and subcutaneous tissues include caustic substances, exposure to extreme temperatures (Chapter 7), prolonged or excessive pressure, and exposure to radiation. Disruption of the continuity of the skin allows the entry of organisms that can lead to local or systemic infection.

Traumatic Injuries

Traumatic wounds include penetrating, blunt, and shear forces (sliding against a fixed surface), bite, and degloving injuries. Sharp lacerations, bullet wounds, "road rash" (injury from scraping against road pavement), and degloving injuries should be treated by gentle cleansing, débridement of all foreign debris and necrotic tissue, and application of a proper dressing. Dirty or infected wounds should be left open to heal by secondary intention or delayed primary closure. Clean lacerations may be closed primarily. Road rash injuries are treated as second-degree burns and degloving injuries as third-degree or full-thickness burns. The degloved skin can be placed back on the wound like a skin graft and assessed daily for survival. If the skin becomes necrotic, it is débrided and the wound is covered with split-thickness skin grafts.

Radiation Exposure

Acute radiation injuries such as those that occur in an industrial accident are devastating. The dose of radiation exposure is oftentimes lethal. In addition to the development of skin lesions (cutaneous radiation syndrome), patients suffer from gastrointestinal hemorrhage, bone marrow suppression, and multi-organ system failure. The most notable industrial radiation exposure accident occurred in 1986 at the Chernobyl nuclear power plant. Of the 237 individuals initially suspected of being exposed, 54 suffered from cutaneous radiation syndrome. The severity of symptoms ranged widely and included xerosis (dry skin), cutaneous telangiectasias and subungual splinter hemorrhages, hemangiomas and lymphangiomas, epidermal atrophy, disseminated keratoses, extensive dermal and subcutaneous fibrosis with partial ulcerations, and pigment changes (radiation lentigo). To date, no cutaneous malignancies have been noted.

Solar or ultraviolet (UV) radiation represents the most common form of radiation exposure. The ultraviolet spectrum is divided into UVA (400–315 nm), UVB (315–290 nm), and UVC (290–200 nm). Regarding skin damage and development of skin cancers, the only significant wavelengths are in the ultraviolet spectrum. The ozone layer absorbs UV wavelengths below 290 nm, thus allowing only UVA and UVB to reach the earth. UVB is responsible for the acute sunburns and for the chronic skin damage leading to malignant degeneration, although it makes up less than 5 percent of the solar UV radiation that hits the earth.

The treatment of various malignancies oftentimes includes radiation therapy. Given the basis of this therapy to act on rapidly dividing cell types, the skin and subcutaneous tissue are significantly affected. Acute radiation changes include erythema and basal epithelial cellular death. Dry desquamation may proceed to moist desquamation. With cellular repair, permanent hyperpigmentation is observed in the field of radiation. Chronic radiation changes begin at 4–6 months and are characterized by a loss of capillaries as a result of thrombosis and fibrinoid necrosis of vessel walls. This fibrosis and hypovascularity are generally progressive, which eventually may lead to ulceration because of poor tissue perfusion.

Inflammatory Diseases

Pyoderma Gangrenosum

Pyoderma gangrenosum (PG) is a relatively uncommon destructive cutaneous lesion that is associated with an underlying systemic disease including inflammatory bowel disease, rheumatoid arthritis, hematologic malignancy, and monoclonal immunoglobulin A (IgA) gammopathy. Recognition of the underlying disease is of paramount importance in the management of skin ulceration because surgical treatment without medical management is fraught with complication. The majority of patients are treated with systemic steroids and cyclosporine. Control of the inflammatory phase, local wound care and coverage with a skin graft is efficacious.

Staphylococcal Scalded Skin Syndrome and Toxic Epidermal Necrolysis

Staphylococcal scalded skin syndrome and toxic epidermal necrolysis create a similar clinical picture, which includes erythema of the skin, bullae formation, and, eventually, wide areas of skin loss. Staphylococcal scalded skin syndrome (SSSS) is caused by an exotoxin produced during a staphylococcal infection of the nasopharynx or middle ear in the pediatric population. Toxic epidermal necrolysis (TEN) is thought to be an immunologic reaction to certain drugs, such as sulfonamides, phenytoin, barbiturates, and tetracycline. Diagnosis can be made with a skin biopsy examination because SSSS produces a cleavage plane in the granular layer of the epidermis, whereas TEN occurs at the dermoepidermal junction. The injury is similar to a second-degree burn. Treatment involves fluid and electrolyte replacement and wound care as in a burn injury. Patients with less than 10 percent of epidermal detachment are classified as Stevens-Johnson syndrome, whereas those with more than 30 percent of total body surface area involvement are classified as TEN. In Stevens-Johnson syndrome, epithelial sloughing of the respiratory and alimentary tracts occurs with resultant respiratory failure and intestinal malabsorption. Patients with TEN should be treated in burn units to decrease the morbidity from the wounds. The skin slough has been successfully treated with cadaveric or porcine skin or semisynthetic biologic dressings (Biobrane). Temporary coverage with a biologic dressing allows the underlying epidermis to regenerate spontaneously. Corticosteroid therapy has not been efficacious.

BENIGN TUMORS

Cysts (Epidermal, Dermoid, Trichilemmal)

Epidermal cysts are the most common type of cutaneous cyst and can occur anywhere on the body as a single, firm nodule. Trichilemmal (pilar) cysts, the next most common, occur more often in females and usually on the scalp. When ruptured, these cysts have a characteristic strong odor. Dermoid cysts are present at birth and may result from epithelium trapped during midline closure in fetal development. Dermoid cysts are most often found in the midline of the face (e.g., on the nose or forehead) and also are common on the lateral eyebrow.

The walls of all these cysts consist of a layer of epidermis oriented with the basal layer superficial and the more mature layers deep (i.e., with the epidermis growing into the center of the cyst). The desquamated cells (keratin) collect in the center and form the creamy substance of the cyst. Histologic examination is needed to differentiate the different types. Surgeons often refer to cutaneous cysts as sebaceous cysts because they appear to contain sebum; however, this is a misnomer because the substance is actually keratin.

Cysts usually are asymptomatic and ignored until they rupture and cause local inflammation. The area becomes infected and an abscess forms. Incision and drainage is recommended for an acutely infected cyst. After resolution of the abscess, the cyst wall must be excised or the cyst will recur. Similarly, when excising an unruptured cyst, care must be taken to remove the entire wall to prevent recurrence.

Nevi (Acquired, Congenital)

Acquired melanocytic nevi are classified as junctional, compound, or dermal, depending on the location of the nevus cells. This classification does not represent different types of nevi but rather different stages in the maturation of nevi. Initially, nevus cells accumulate in the epidermis (junctional), migrate partially into the dermis (compound), and finally rest completely in the dermis (dermal). Eventually most lesions undergo involution.

Congenital nevi are much rarer, occurring in only 1 percent of neonates. These lesions are larger and oftentimes contain hair. Histologically they appear similar to acquired nevi. Congenital giant lesions (giant hairy nevus) most often occur in a bathing trunk distribution or on the chest and back. These lesions are cosmetically unpleasant. Additionally, they may develop malignant melanoma in 1–5 percent of the cases. Excision of the nevus is the treatment of choice, but often the lesion is so large that closure of the wound with autologous skin grafts is not possible because of the lack of adequate donor sites. Serial excisions over several years with either primary closure or skin grafting and tissue expansion of the normal surrounding skin are the present modes of therapy.

Soft-Tissue Tumors (Acrochordons, Dermatofibromas, Lipomas)

Acrochordons (skin tags) are fleshy, pedunculated masses located on the axillae, trunk, and eyelids. They are composed of hyperplastic epidermis over a fibrous connective tissue stalk. These lesions are usually small and are always benign.

Dermatofibromas are usually solitary nodules measuring approximately 1–2 cm in diameter. They are found primarily on the legs and sides of the trunk. The lesions are composed of whorls of connective tissue containing fibroblasts. The mass is not encapsulated and vascularization is variable. Dermatofibromas can be diagnosed by clinical examination. When lesions enlarge to 2–3 cm, excisional biopsy is recommended to assess for malignancy. Lipomas are the most common subcutaneous neoplasm. They are found mostly on the trunk but may appear anywhere. They may sometimes grow to a large size. Microscopic examination reveals a lobulated tumor containing normal fat cells. Excision is performed for diagnosis and to restore normal skin contour.

MALIGNANT TUMORS

Epidemiology

Increased exposure to ultraviolet radiation is associated with an increased development of all three of the common skin malignancies; basal cell carcinoma, squamous cell carcinoma, and melanoma. Chemical carcinogens such as tar, arsenic, and nitrogen mustard are known carcinogens. Human papillomavirus has been found in certain squamous cell cancers and may be linked with onco-genesis. Radiation therapy in the past for skin lesions such as acne vulgaris, when it resulted in radiation dermatitis, is associated with an increased inci-dence of basal and squamous cell cancers in the treated areas. Any area of skin subjected to chronic irritation, such as burn scars (Marjolin ulcers), re-peated sloughing of skin from bullous diseases, and decubitus ulcers, all have an increased chance of developing squamous cell cancer.

Immunosuppressed patients receiving chemotherapy for other malignan-cies or immunosuppressants for organ transplants have an increased incidence of basal cell and squamous cell cancers and malignant melanoma. Acquired immune deficiency syndrome (AIDS) is associated with an increased risk of developing skin neoplasms.

Basal Cell Carcinoma

Basal cell carcinomas contain cells that resemble the basal cells of the epi-dermis. It is the most common type of skin cancer and is subdivided into several types by gross and histologic morphology. The nodulocystic or nodu-loulcerative type accounts for 70 percent of basal cell carcinomas. It is a waxy, cream-colored lesion with rolled, pearly borders. It often contains a central ulcer. When these lesions are large they are called "rodent ulcers." Pigmented basal cell carcinomas are tan to black in color and should be distinguished by biopsy examination from melanoma. Superficial basal cell cancers occur more commonly on the trunk and form a red, scaling lesion that is sometimes difficult to distinguish grossly from Bowen disease. A rare form of basal cell carcinoma is the basosquamous type, which contains elements of basal cell and squamous cell cancer. These lesions can metastasize more like a squa-mous cell carcinoma and should be treated aggressively. Other types include morpheaform, adenoid, and infiltrative carcinomas.

Basal cell carcinomas usually are slow growing, and patients often neglect these lesions for years. Metastasis and death from this disease are extremely rare, but these lesions can cause extensive local destruction. The majority of small (less than 2 mm), nodular lesions may be treated by dermatologists with curettage and electrodesiccation or laser vaporization. A drawback to these procedures is that no pathologic specimen is obtained to confirm the diagnosis or evaluate the tumor margins. Larger tumors, lesions that invade bone or surrounding structures, and more aggressive histologic types (morpheaform, infiltrative, and basosquamous) are best treated by surgical excision with a 2–4-mm margin of normal tissue. Histologic confirmation that the margins of resection do not contain tumor is required. Because nodular lesions are less likely to recur, the smaller margin may be used, whereas other types need a wider margin of resection.

Squamous Cell Carcinoma

Squamous cell carcinomas arise from keratinocytes of the epidermis. It is less common than basal cell carcinoma but is more devastating because it can invade surrounding tissue and metastasize more readily. In situ lesions have the eponym of Bowen disease, and in situ squamous cell carcinomas of the penis are referred to as erythroplasia of Queyrat. Contrary to previous reports, Bowen's disease is not a marker for other systemic malignancies.

Tumor thickness correlates well with its biologic behavior. Lesions that re-cur locally are more than 4 mm thick and lesions that metastasize are 10 mm or more. The location of the lesion also is important. Tumors arising in burn scars (Marjolin ulcer), areas of chronic osteomyelitis, and areas of previous injury metastasize early. Lesions on the external ear frequently recur and involve regional lymph node basins early. Squamous cell cancers in areas with solar damage behave less aggressively and usually require only local excision.

Lesions should be excised with a 1-cm margin if possible, and histologic confirmation that the margins are tumor-free is mandatory. Tumor-invading bone should be excised if recurrence is to be avoided. Regional lymph node excision is indicated for clinically palpable nodes (therapeutic lymph node dissection). Lesions arising in chronic wounds behave aggressively and are more likely to spread to regional lymph nodes. For these lesions lymphadenectomy before the development of palpable nodes is indicated (prophylactic lymph node dissection). Metastatic disease is a poor prognostic sign, with only 13 percent of patients surviving after 10 years.

Alternative Therapy

Alternatives to surgical therapy for squamous and basal cell cancers consist of radiation therapy or topical 5-fluorouracil for patients unable or unwilling to undergo surgery. Radiation therapy for small and superficial lesions obtains cure rates comparable to surgical excision. Radiation damage to surrounding normal skin with inflammation and scarring can be a problem. The development of cutaneous malignancies in irradiated skin also is a serious long-term risk with this treatment modality.

For lesions on the face or near the nose or eye, resection of a wide rim of normal tissue to remove the entire tumor can cause significant functional and cosmetic problems. These lesions can be removed by Mohs micrographic surgery. Mohs fresh tissue chemosurgery technique, developed in 1932, is a method to serially excise a tumor by taking small increments of tissue until the entire tumor is removed. Each piece of tissue removed is frozen and immediately examined microscopically to determine whether the entire lesion has been resected. The advantage of the Mohs fresh tissue chemosurgery technique is that the entire margin of resection is evaluated, although with wide excision and traditional histologic examination, only selected samples of the surgical margin are examined. The major benefit of Mohs fresh tissue chemosurgery technique is the ability to remove a tumor with the least sacrifice of uninvolved tissue. This technique is effective for treating carcinomas around the eyelids and nose, where tissue loss is most conspicuous. Cure rates are comparable to those of wide excision.

Patients with basal cell carcinomas have been treated with intralesional injection of interferon. The majority of the lesions were eliminated or controlled by the injections. The major disadvantages of this treatment are the need for multiple office visits over several weeks for injections, the systemic side effects of interferon, and a potential need for surgery if the lesions do not respond to injections. Clinical trials with combinations of retinoids (vitamin A derivatives) and interferon have demonstrated good response rates in patients with advanced, inoperable squamous cell carcinomas.

Malignant Melanoma

What was a relatively rare disease 50 years ago has now become alarmingly more common. The rise in the rate of melanoma is the highest of any cancer in the United States. In 1935, the annual incidence of the disease was 1 per

100,000 people. By 1991, the incidence had risen to 12.9 per 100,000 people. The 1998 age-adjusted rate for invasive melanoma is 18.3 per 100,000 for white males and 13.0 per 100,000 for white females in the United States.

Pathogenesis

Melanoma arises from transformed melanocytes and occur anywhere that melanocytes have migrated during embryogenesis. The eye, central nervous system, gastrointestinal tract, and even the gallbladder have been reported as primary sites of the disease. More than 90 percent of melanomas are found on the skin; however, 4 percent are discovered as metastases without an identifiable primary site.

Nevi are benign melanocytic neoplasms found on the skin of most people. Once the melanocyte has transformed into the malignant phenotype, the growth of the lesion is radial in the plane of the epidermis. Even though microinvasion of the dermis can be observed during this radial growth phase, metastases do not occur. Only when the melanoma cells form nests in the dermis are metastases observed.

Types

The most common type of melanoma, representing up to 70 percent of melanomas, is the superficial spreading type. These lesions occur anywhere on the skin except the hands and feet. They are flat, commonly contain areas of regression, and measure 1–2 cm in diameter at the time of diagnosis. There is a relatively long radial growth phase before vertical growth begins. The nodular type accounts for 15–30 percent of melanomas. These lesions are darker and raised. Nodular melanoma lack radial growth peripheral to the area of vertical growth; hence, all nodular melanomas are in the vertical growth phase at the time of diagnosis. Although it is an aggressive lesion, the prognosis for a patient with a nodular-type lesion is the same as that for a patient with a superficial spreading lesion of the same depth of invasion. The lentigo maligna type, accounting for 4–15 percent of melanomas, occurs mostly on the neck, the face, and the back of the hands of older adult people. These lesions are always surrounded by dermis with heavy solar degeneration. They tend to become quite large before a diagnosis is made, but also have the best prognosis because invasive growth occurs late. Only 5–8 percent of lentigo malignas are estimated to evolve to invasive melanoma. Acral lentiginous type is the least-common subtype, representing only 2–8 percent of melanoma in whites. It occurs on the palms and soles and in the subungual regions. Although melanoma among dark-skinned people is relatively rare, the acral lentiginous type accounts for 29–72 percent of all melanomas in dark-skinned people (African Americans, Asians, and Hispanics) than in people with less-pigmented skin. Subungual lesions appear as blue-black discolorations of the posterior nail fold and are most common on the great toe or thumb. The additional presence of pigmentation in the proximal or lateral nail folds (Hutchinson sign) is diagnostic of subungual melanoma.

Prognostic Factors

The most current staging system, from the American Joint Committee on Cancer (AJCC), contains the best method of interpreting clinical information in regard to prognosis of this disease (Table 15-1).

The T classification of lesions comes from the original observation by Clark that prognosis is directly related to the level of invasion of the skin by the melanoma. Whereas Clark used the histologic level (I, superficial to basement membrane [in situ]; II, papillary dermis; III, papillary/reticular dermal junction; IV, reticular dermis; and V, subcutaneous fat), Breslow modified the approach to obtain a more reproducible measure of invasion by the use of an ocular micrometer. The lesions were measured from the granular layer of the epidermis or the base of the ulcer to the greatest depth of the tumor (I, 0.75 mm or less; II, 0.76–1.5 mm; III, 1.51–4.0 mm; IV, 4.0 mm or more). These levels of invasion have been subsequently modified and incorporated in the AJCC staging system.

Evidence of tumor in regional lymph nodes is a poor prognostic sign. This is accounted for in the staging system by advancing any T classifications from stage I or II to stage III (Table 15-2). The 15-year survival rate drops precipitously with the presence of lymph node metastasis. The number of positive lymph nodes also is correlated with survival rates.

The presence of distant metastasis is a grave prognostic sign (stage IV). The median survival ranges from 2–7 months, depending on the number and site of metastases, but survival up to a few years has been reported.

TABLE 15-1 TNM Classification of Melanoma of the Skin

Primary tumor (T)	
T1	1.0 mm in thickness or less
T1a	Without ulceration and Clark level II/III
T1b	With ulceration or level IV/V
T2	1.01–2.0 mm in thickness
T2a	Without ulceration
T2b	With ulceration
T3	2.01–4.0 mm in thickness
T3a	Without ulceration
T3b	With ulceration
T4	4.01 mm or greater in thickness
T4a	Without ulceration
T4b	With ulceration
Nodal status (N)	
N1	1 node
N1a	Micrometastasis (as diagnoses after sentinel lymph node or lymphadenectomy)
N1b	Macrometastasis (clinically detectable, confirmed by pathology)
N2	2–3 nodes
N2a	Micrometastasis
N2b	Macrometastasis
N2c	In-transit met(s) without metastatic nodes
N3	4 or more metastatic nodes, or matted nodes, or in-transit met(s)/satellite(s) with metastatic node(s)
Metastasis (M)	
M1	Distant skin, subcutaneous or nodal matastasis, serum LDH normal
M2	Lung metastasis, normal LDH
M3	All other visceral metastasis with normal LDH or any distant mets with elevated LDH

LDH = lactic dehydrogenase.

TABLE 15-2 Stage Grouping

Stage IA	T1a	N0	M0
IB	T1b	N0	M0
	T2a	N0	M0
IIA	T2b	N0	M0
T3a	N0	M0	
IIB	T3b	N0	M0
T4a	N0	M0	
IIC	T4b	N0	M0
III	Any T	N1	M0
		N2	
		N3	
IV	Any T	Any N	Any M1

Source: From the American Joint Committee on Cancer Staging.

Other independent prognostic factors have been identified:

Anatomic location. People with lesions of the extremities have a better prognosis than people with melanomas of the head and neck or trunk (82 percent 10-year survival rate for localized disease of the extremity, compared to a 68 percent survival rate with a lesion of the face).

Ulceration. The 10-year survival rate for patients with local disease (stage I) and an ulcerated melanoma was 50 percent, compared to 78 percent for the same stage lesion without ulceration. Early studies identified that the incidence of ulceration increases with increasing thickness, from 12.5 percent in melanomas less than 0.75 mm–72.5 percent in melanomas greater than 4.0 mm.

Gender. Numerous studies demonstrate that females have an improved survival compared to males. After correcting for thickness, age, and location, females continue to have a higher survival rate than men (80 percent 10-year survival rate for women vs. 61 percent 10-year survival rate for men with stage I disease).

Histologic type. Nodular melanomas have the same prognosis as superficial spreading types when lesions are matched for depth of invasion. Lentigo maligna types, however, have a better prognosis even after correcting for thickness, and acral lentiginous lesions have a worse prognosis.

Treatment

The treatment of melanoma is primarily surgical. The indication for procedures such as lymph node dissection, sentinel lymphadenectomy, superficial parotidectomy, and resection of distant metastases have changed somewhat over time, but the only hope for cure and the best treatment for regional control and palliation remains surgery. Most cases of cutaneous melanoma are cured by excision of the primary tumor alone. Radiation therapy, regional and systemic chemotherapy, and immunotherapy are effective in a limited set of circumstances, but none are a first-line option.

All suspicious lesions should undergo biopsy. A 1-mm margin of normal skin is taken if the wound can be closed primarily. If removal of the entire lesion creates too large a defect, then an incisional biopsy of a representative part is recommended. Biopsy incisions should be made with the expectation that a subsequent wide excision of the biopsy site may be done. Once a diagnosis of melanoma is made, the biopsy scar and any remains of the lesion need to be removed to eradicate any remaining tumor. Four randomized prospective trials suggest that lesions 1 mm or less in thickness can be treated with a 1-cm margin. For lesions 1–4-mm thick, a 2-cm margin is recommended. There is little data to support the use of margins wider than 2 cm. The surrounding tissue should be removed down to the fascia to remove all lymphatic channels. If the deep fascia is not involved by the tumor, removing it does not affect recurrence or survival rates, so the fascia is left intact. If the defect cannot be closed primarily, a skin graft or local flap is used.

All clinically positive lymph nodes should be removed by regional nodal dissection. When groin lymph nodes are removed, the deep (iliac) nodes must be removed along with the superficial (inguinal) nodes. For axillary dissections the nodes medial to the pectoralis minor muscle must also be resected. For lesions on the face, anterior scalp, and ear, a superficial parotidectomy to remove parotid nodes and a modified neck dissection is recommended. Disruption of the lymphatic outflow does cause significant problems with chronic edema, especially of the lower extremity.

Treatment of regional lymph nodes that do not obviously contain tumor in patients without evidence of metastasis (stages I and II) is determined by considering the possible benefits of the procedure as weighed against the risks. In patients with thin lesions (less than 0.75 mm), the tumor cells are still localized in the surrounding tissue, and the cure rate is excellent with wide excision of the primary lesion; therefore treatment of regional lymph nodes is not beneficial. With very thick lesions (more than 4 mm), it is highly likely that the tumor cells have already spread to the regional lymph nodes and distant sites. Removal of the lymph nodes has no effect on survival. Most of these patients die of metastatic disease before developing problems in regional nodes. Because there are significant morbid effects of lymphadenectomy, most surgeons defer the procedure until clinically evident disease appears. Approximately 40 percent of these patients eventually develop disease in the lymph nodes and require a second palliative operation. Elective lymphadenectomy is sometimes performed in these patients as a staging procedure before entry into clinical trials.

In patients with intermediate-thickness tumors (T2 and T3, 0.76–4.0 mm) and no clinical evidence of nodal or metastatic disease, the use of prophylactic dissection (elective lymph node dissection on clinically negative nodes) is controversial. Numerous retrospective studies suggested that patients with primary melanoma who underwent elective lymph node dissection had improved survival. However, prospective, randomized studies have not demonstrated that elective lymph node dissection improves survival in patients with intermediate-thickness melanomas. Careful examination of specimens in patients undergoing elective lymph node dissection have found that, in 25–50 percent of the cases, specimens contain micrometastases. Among patients who do not have an elective lymph node dissection, 20–25 percent eventually develop clinically evident disease and require lymphadenectomy. More evidence suggests that there may be improved survival with elective lymph node dissection in patients with a higher risk of developing metastasis (i.e., lesions with ulceration or those located on the trunk, head, and neck). The most compelling argument for the potential benefits of elective lymph node dissection comes from evidence in large clinical trials; patients with intermediate-thickness melanomas without elective node dissection continue to die of the disease 10 years later, whereas patients who had an elective lymph node dissection do not. However, these differences are not statistically significant.

Sentinel lymphadenectomy for malignant melanoma is rapidly becoming the standard procedure. The sentinel node may be preoperatively located with the use of a gamma camera, or by intraoperative injection of 1 percent iso-sulfan blue dye into the site of the primary melanoma. These techniques enable the surgeon to identify the lymphatic drainage from the primary lesion and determine the first (sentinel) lymph node draining the tumor. The node is removed, and if micrometastases are identified in frozen-section examination, a complete lymph node dissection is performed. Whether this procedure actually improves survival in these patients awaits the results of clinical trials.

When patients develop distant metastases, surgical therapy may be indicated. Once melanoma has spread to a distant site, median survival is 7–8 months and the 5-year survival rate is less than 5 percent. Solitary lesions in the brain, gastrointestinal tract, or skin that are symptomatic should be excised when possible. Although cure is extremely rare, the degree of palliation can be high and asymptomatic survival prolonged. A decision to operate on metastatic lesions must be made after careful deliberation with the patient.

A promising area in the nonsurgical treatment of melanoma is the use of immunologic manipulation. Interferon-α (INF-α) 2b is the only Food and Drug Administration (FDA)-approved adjuvant treatment for AJCC stages IIB/III melanoma. Several randomized trials of INF-α adjuvant therapy have been conducted. In these patients, both the relapse-free interval and overall survival were improved with use of INF-α. Side effects were common and frequently severe.

Vaccines have been developed with the hope of stimulating the body's own immune system against the tumor. All treatments are currently investigational. One defined-antigen vaccine has entered clinical testing, the ganglioside GM2. Gangliosides are carbohydrate antigens found on the surface of melanomas and many other tumors.

Although initially thought to be ineffective in the treatment of melanoma, radiation therapy has been shown to be useful. High-dose-per-fraction radiation produces a better response rate than low-dose large-fraction therapy. It has been found that postoperative radiation to the neck or axilla after radical lymph node dissections decreases regional recurrence rates in node-positive patients. Radiation therapy is the treatment of choice for patients with symptomatic multiple brain metastases. Up to 70 percent of treated patients show measurable improvement in tumor size, symptomatology, or performance status.

Hyperthermic regional perfusion of the limb with a chemotherapeutic agent (e.g., melphalan) is the treatment of choice for patients with local recurrence or in-transit lesions (local disease in lymphatics) on an extremity that is not amenable to excision. In-transit metastases develop in 5–8 percent of melanoma patients with a high-risk primary melanoma (>1.5 mm). The goal of regional perfusion therapy is to increase the dosage of the chemotherapeutic agent to maximize tumor response while limiting systemic toxic effects. Prospective clinical trials are under way to evaluate the use of regional perfusion for melanoma of the limbs as adjuvant therapy for patients with stage I disease. Additionally, regional perfusion therapy for metastatic disease to the liver is under investigation.

OTHER MALIGNANCIES

Merkel Cell Carcinoma (Primary Neuroendocrine Carcinoma of the Skin)

Merkel cell carcinomas are of neuroepithelial differentiation. These tumors are associated with a synchronous or metasynchronous squamous cell carcinoma 25 percent of the time. These tumors are very aggressive, and wide local resection with 3-cm margins is recommended. Local recurrence rates are high, and distant metastases occur in one third of patients. Prophylactic regional lymph node dissection and adjuvant radiation therapy are recommended. Overall, the prognosis is worse than for malignant melanoma.

Extramammary Paget Disease

This tumor is histologically similar to the mammary type. It is a cutaneous lesion that appears as a pruritic red patch that does not resolve. Biopsy demonstrates classic Paget cells. Paget disease is thought to be a cutaneous extension of an underlying adenocarcinoma, although an associated tumor cannot always be demonstrated.

Adnexal Carcinomas

This group includes the rare-type tumors apocrine, eccrine, and sebaceous carcinomas. They are locally destructive and can cause death by distant metastasis.

Angiosarcomas

Angiosarcomas may arise spontaneously, mostly on the scalp, face, and neck. They usually appear as a bruise that spontaneously bleeds or enlarges without trauma. Tumors also may arise in areas of prior radiation therapy or in the setting of chronic lymphedema of the arm, such as after mastectomy (Stewart-Treves syndrome). The angiosarcomas that arise in these areas of chronic change occur decades later. The tumors consist of anaplastic endothelial cells surrounding vascular channels. Although total excision of early lesions can provide occasional cure, the prognosis usually is poor, with 5-year survival rates of less than 20 percent. Chemotherapy and radiation therapy are used for palliation.

Kaposi Sarcoma

Kaposi sarcoma (KS) appears as rubbery bluish nodules that occur primarily on the extremities but may appear anywhere on the skin and viscera. These lesions are usually multifocal rather than metastatic. Classic KS is seen in people of Eastern Europe or sub-Saharan Africa. The lesions are locally aggressive but undergo periods of remission. Visceral spread of the lesions is rare, but a subtype of the African variety has a predilection for spreading to lymph nodes. A different variety of KS has been described for people with AIDS or with immunosuppression from chemotherapy. In this form of the disease, the lesions spread rapidly to the nodes, and the gastrointestinal and respiratory tract often are involved. Development of AIDS-related KS may be associated with concurrent infection with a herpes-like virus.

Treatment for all types of KS consists of radiation to the lesions. Combination chemotherapy is effective in controlling the disease, although most patients develop an opportunistic infection during or shortly after treatment. Surgical treatment is reserved for lesions that interfere with vital functions, such as bowel obstruction or airway compromise.

Dermatofibrosarcoma Protuberans

Dermatofibrosarcoma protuberans consists of large nodular lesions located mainly on the trunk. They often ulcerate and become infected. With enlargement, the lesions become painful. Histologically, the lesions contain atypical spindle cells, probably of fibroblast origin, located around a core of collagen tissue. Sometimes they are mistaken for an infected keloid. Metastases are rare and surgical excision can be curative. Excision must be complete because local recurrences are common.

Fibrosarcoma

Fibrosarcomas are hard, irregular masses found in the subcutaneous fat. The fibroblasts appear markedly anaplastic with disorganized growth. If they are not excised completely, metastases usually develop. The 5-year survival rate after excision is approximately 60 percent.

Liposarcoma

Liposarcomas arise in the deep muscle planes and, rarely, from the subcutaneous tissue. They occur most commonly on the thigh. An enlarging lipoma should be excised and inspected to distinguish it from a liposarcoma. Wide excision is the treatment of choice, with radiation therapy reserved for metastatic disease.

FUTURE DEVELOPMENTS IN SKIN SURGERY

Despite three decades of effort, the major challenge in surgical therapy for diseases of the skin remains the lack of an optimum replacement for diseased or damaged tissue. Autologous skin grafts are still the best method to treat skin defects, but donor-site problems and limited availability of autologous skin remain problematic. Tissue expansion with subcutaneous balloon implants produces new epidermis; however, much of this tissue is rearrangement of the old tissue. Expansion of skin produces a limited amount of useful tissue. The future of surgical therapy for diseases of the skin lies in the development of engineered skin replacements. Current research is directed at identifying different materials and cells that can be used to replace both epidermis and dermis.

Suggested Readings

Fuchs E, Cleveland DW: A structural scaffolding of intermediate filaments in health and disease. Science 279:514, 1998.

Lako M, Armstrong L, Cairns PM, et al: Hair follicle dermal cells repopulate the mouse haematopoietic system. J Cell Sci 115:3967, 2002.

Brentjens MH, Yeung-Yue KA, Lee PC, et al: Human papillomavirus: A review. Dermatol Clin 20:315, 2002.

Spies M, Sanford AP, Aili Low JF, et al: Treatment of extensive toxic epidermal necrolysis in children. Pediatrics 108:1162, 2001.

Luce EA: Oncologic considerations in nonmelanotic skin cancer. Clin Plast Surg 22:39, 1995.

Desmond RA, Soong S-J: Epidemiology of malignant melanoma. Surg Clin North Am 83:1, 2003.

Zettersten E, Shaikh L, Ramirez R, et al: Prognostic factors in primary cutaneous melanoma. Surg Clin North Am 83:61, 2003.

Balch CM, Buzaid AC, Soong SJ, et al: Final version of the American Joint Committee on Cancer staging system for cutaneous melanoma. J Clin Oncol 19:3635, 2001.

Essner R: Surgical treatment of malignant melanoma. Surg Clin North Am 83:109, 2003.

Leong SPL: Selective lymphadenectomy for malignant melanoma. Surg Clin North Am 83:157, 2003.

Bianco P, Robey PG: Stem cells in tissue engineering. Nature 414:118, 2001.

16 | The Breast

*Kirby I. Bland, Samuel W. Beenken
and Edward E. Copeland, III*

HISTORY OF MODERN BREAST CANCER SURGERY

In 1894, Halsted and Meyer established the radical mastectomy as state-of-the-art breast cancer treatment. They advocated complete dissection of axillary lymph node levels I–III and routinely resected the long thoracic nerve and the thoracodorsal neurovascular bundle with the axillary contents. In 1948, to reduce the morbidity of breast cancer surgery, Patey and Dyson of the Middlesex Hospital, London, advocated a modified radical mastectomy for the management of advanced operable breast cancer. Their technique included preservation of the pectoralis major muscle, the long thoracic nerve, and the thoracodorsal neurovascular bundle. They showed that removal of only the pectoralis minor muscle allowed adequate access to and clearance of axillary lymph node levels I–III. Subsequently, Madden advocated a modified radical mastectomy that preserved both the pectoralis major and minor muscles even though this approach prevented dissection of the apical (level III) axillary lymph nodes.

The National Surgical Adjuvant Breast and Bowel Project B-04 (NSABP B-04) conducted by Fisher and colleagues compared local and regional treatments of breast cancer. Life table estimates were obtained for 1665 women enrolled and followed for a mean of 120 months. This study randomized clinically node-negative women into three groups: (1) Halsted radical mastectomy (RM); (2) total mastectomy plus radiation therapy (TM+RT); and (3) total mastectomy (TM) alone. Clinically node-positive women were treated with RM or TM+RT. There were no differences in survival between the three groups of node-negative women or between the 2 groups of node-positive women. Correspondingly, there were no differences in survival during the first and second 5-year follow-up periods.

FUNCTIONAL ANATOMY OF THE BREAST

The breast is composed of 15–20 lobes, which are each composed of several lobules. Each lobe of the breast terminates in a major (lactiferous) duct (2–4 mm in diameter), which opens through a constricted orifice (0.4–0.7 mm in diameter) into the ampulla of the nipple. Fibrous bands of connective tissue travel through the breast (suspensory ligaments of Cooper), which insert perpendicularly into the dermis and provide structural support. The axillary tail of Spence extends laterally across the anterior axillary fold. The upper outer quadrant of the breast contains a greater volume of tissue than do the other quadrants.

Blood supply, innervation, and lymphatics. The breast receives its blood supply from (1) perforating branches of the internal mammary artery; (2) lateral branches of the posterior intercostal arteries; and (3) branches from the axillary artery, including the highest thoracic, lateral thoracic, and pectoral branches of the thoracoacromial artery. The veins and lymph vessels of the breast follow the course of the arteries with venous drainage being toward the axilla. The vertebral venous plexus of Batson, which invests the vertebrae and

344

extends from the base of the skull to the sacrum, can provide a route for breast cancer metastases to the vertebrae, skull, pelvic bones, and central nervous system.

Lateral cutaneous branches of the third through sixth intercostal nerves provide sensory innervation of the breast (lateral mammary branches) and of the anterolateral chest wall. The intercostobrachial nerve is the lateral cutaneous branch of the second intercostal nerve and may be visualized during surgical dissection of the axilla. Resection of the intercostobrachial nerve causes loss of sensation over the medial aspect of the upper arm.

The boundaries for lymph drainage of the axilla are not well demarcated, and there is considerable variation in the position of the axillary lymph nodes. The 6 axillary lymph node groups recognized by surgeons are (1) the axillary vein group (lateral); (2) the external mammary group (anterior or pectoral); (3) the scapular group (posterior or subscapular); (4) the central group; (5) the subclavicular group (apical); and (6) the interpectoral group (Rotter's).

The lymph node groups are assigned levels according to their relationship to the pectoralis minor muscle. Lymph nodes located lateral to or below the lower border of the pectoralis minor muscle are referred to as level I lymph nodes, which include the axillary vein, external mammary, and scapular groups. Lymph nodes located superficial or deep to the pectoralis minor muscle are referred to as level II lymph nodes, which include the central and interpectoral groups. Lymph nodes located medial to or above the upper border of the pectoralis minor muscle are referred to as level III lymph nodes, which make up the subclavicular group. The axillary lymph nodes usually receive more than 75 percent of the lymph drainage from the breast.

PHYSIOLOGY OF THE BREAST

Breast development and function. Breast development and function are initiated by a variety of hormonal stimuli, including estrogen, progesterone, prolactin, oxytocin, thyroid hormone, cortisol, and growth hormone. Estrogen, progesterone, and prolactin especially have profound trophic effects that are essential to normal breast development and function. Estrogen initiates ductal development, although progesterone is responsible for differentiation of epithelium and for lobular development. Prolactin is the primary hormonal stimulus for lactogenesis in late pregnancy and the postpartum period. It upregulates hormone receptors and stimulates epithelial development. Secretion of neurotrophic hormones from the hypothalamus is responsible for regulation of the secretion of the hormones that affect the breast tissues. The gonadotropins luteinizing hormone (LH) and follicle-stimulating hormone (FSH) regulate the release of estrogen and progesterone from the ovaries. In turn, the release of LH and FSH from the basophilic cells of the anterior pituitary is regulated by the secretion of gonadotropin-releasing hormone (GnRH) from the hypothalamus. Positive and negative feedback effects of circulating estrogen and progesterone regulate the secretion of LH, FSH, and GnRH.

Gynecomastia. Gynecomastia refers to an enlarged breast in the male. Physiologic gynecomastia usually occurs during three phases of life: the neonatal period, adolescence, and senescence. Common to each of these phases is an excess of circulating estrogens in relation to circulating testosterone. Neonatal gynecomastia is caused by the action of placental estrogens on neonatal breast tissues, although in adolescence, there is an excess of estradiol relative to testosterone, and with senescence, the circulating testosterone level falls, resulting in relative hyperestrinism. In gynecomastia, the ductal structures of the male breast enlarge, elongate, and branch with a concomitant increase in epithelium. During puberty, the condition often is unilateral and typically occurs between ages 12 and 15 years. In contrast, senescent gynecomastia usually is bilateral. In the nonobese male, breast tissue measuring at least 2 cm in diameter must be present before a diagnosis of gynecomastia is made. Dominant masses or areas of firmness, irregularity, and asymmetry suggest the possibility of a breast cancer, particularly in the older male. Mammography and ultrasonography are employed for diagnostic purposes.

INFECTIOUS AND INFLAMMATORY DISORDERS OF THE BREAST

Bacterial infection. *Staphylococcus aureus* and Streptococcus species are the organisms most frequently recovered from nipple discharge from an infected breast. Breast abscesses are typically seen in staphylococcal infections and present with point tenderness, erythema, and hyperthermia. These abscesses are related to lactation and occur within the first few weeks of breast-feeding. Progression of a staphylococcal infection may result in subcutaneous, subareolar, interlobular (periductal), and retromammary abscesses (unicentric or multicentric), necessitating operative drainage of fluctuant areas. Preoperative ultrasonography is effective in delineating the extent of the needed drainage procedure, which is best accomplished via circumareolar incisions or incisions paralleling Langer lines. Although staphylococcal infections tend to be more localized and may be located deep in the breast tissues, streptococcal infections usually present with diffuse superficial involvement. They are treated with local wound care, including warm compresses, and the administration of intravenous antibiotics (penicillins or cephalosporins). Breast infections may be chronic, possibly with recurrent abscess formation. In this situation, cultures are taken to identify acid-fast bacilli, anaerobic and aerobic bacteria, and fungi. Uncommon organisms may be encountered and long-term antibiotic therapy may be required.

Hidradenitis suppurativa. Hidradenitis suppurativa of the nipple-areola complex or axilla is a chronic inflammatory condition that originates within the accessory areolar glands of Montgomery or within the axillary sebaceous glands. When located in and about the nipple-areola complex, this disease may mimic other chronic inflammatory states, Paget disease of the nipple, or invasive breast cancer. Involvement of the axillary skin is often multifocal and contiguous. Antibiotic therapy with incision and drainage of fluctuant areas is appropriate treatment. Complete excision of the involved areas may be required and may necessitate coverage with advancement flaps or split-thickness skin grafts.

Mondor's disease. This variant of thrombophlebitis involves the superficial veins of the anterior chest wall and breast. In 1939, Mondor described the condition as "string phlebitis," a thrombosed vein presenting as a tender, cord-like structure. Typically, a woman presents with acute pain in the lateral aspect of the breast or the anterior chest wall. A tender, firm cord is found to follow the distribution of one of the major superficial veins. Most women have no evidence of thrombophlebitis in other anatomic sites. When the diagnosis is uncertain, or when a mass is present near the tender cord, biopsy is indicated. Therapy for Mondor disease includes the liberal use of antiinflammatory medications and warm compresses that are applied along the symptomatic vein. Restriction of motion of the ipsilateral extremity and shoulder and brassiere support of the breast are important. The process usually resolves within 4–6 weeks. When symptoms persist or are refractory to therapy, excision of the involved vein segment is appropriate.

COMMON BENIGN DISORDERS AND DISEASES OF THE BREAST

Aberrations of normal development and involution. The basic principles underlying the aberrations of normal development and involution (ANDI) classification of benign breast conditions are (1) benign breast disorders and diseases are related to the normal processes of reproductive life and to involution; (2) there is a spectrum of breast conditions that ranges from normal to disorder to disease; and (3) the ANDI classification encompasses all aspects of the breast condition, including pathogenesis and the degree of abnormality. The horizontal component of Table 16-1 defines ANDI along a spectrum from normal, to mild abnormality (disorder), to severe abnormality (disease). The vertical component defines the period during which the condition develops.

Reproductive Years: Fibroadenomas are seen predominantly in younger women age 15–25 years. Fibroadenomas usually grow to 1 or 2 cm in diameter

TABLE 16-1 ANDI Classification of Benign Breast Disorders

	Normal →	Disorder →	Disease
Early reproductive years (age 15–25)	Lobular development	Fibroadenoma	Giant fibroadenoma
	Stromal development	Adolescent hypertrophy	Gigantomastia
	Nipple eversion	Nipple inversion	Subareolar abscess Mammary duct fistula
Later reproductive years (age 25–40)	Cyclical changes of menstruation	Cyclical mastalgia	Incapacitating mastalgia
	Epithelial hyperplasia of pregnancy	Nodularity Bloody nipple discharge	
Involution (age 35–55)	Lobular involution	Macrocysts	
	Duct involution	Sclerosing lesions	
	–Dilation	Duct ectasis	Periductal mastitis
	–Sclerosis	Nipple retraction	
	Epithelial turnover	Epithelial hyperplasia	Epithelial hyperplasia with atypia

ANDI = Aberrations of normal development and involution.
Modified with permission from Hughes LE: Aberrations of normal development and involution (ANDI): A concept of benign breast disorders based on pathogenesis. In Hughes LE, Mansel RE, Webster DJT (eds): *Benign Disorders and Diseases of the Breast: Concepts and Clinical Management.* London: WB Saunders, 2000, p 23.

and then are stable, but may grow to a larger size. Small fibroadenomas (1 cm in size or less) are considered normal, although larger fibroadenomas (up to 3 cm) are disorders and giant fibroadenomas (larger than 3 cm) are disease. Similarly, multiple fibroadenomas (more than 5 lesions in one breast) are very uncommon and are considered disease. The precise etiology of adolescent breast hypertrophy is unknown. A spectrum of changes from limited to massive stromal hyperplasia (gigantomastia) is seen. Nipple inversion is a disorder of development of the major ducts, which prevents normal protrusion of the nipple. Mammary duct fistulas arise when nipple inversion predisposes to major duct obstruction, leading to recurrent subareolar abscess and mammary duct fistula.

Later Reproductive Years: Cyclical mastalgia and nodularity are usually associated with premenstrual enlargement of the breast and are regarded as normal. Cyclical pronounced mastalgia and severe painful nodularity that persists for more than 1 week of the menstrual cycle is considered a disorder. In epithelial hyperplasia of pregnancy, papillary projections sometimes give rise to bilateral bloody nipple discharge. The term fibrocystic disease is nonspecific. Too frequently, it is used as a diagnostic term to describe symptoms, to rationalize the need for breast biopsy, and to explain biopsy results. Synonyms include fibrocystic changes, cystic mastopathy, chronic cystic disease, chronic cystic mastitis, Schimmelbusch disease, mazoplasia, Cooper disease, Reclus disease, and fibroadenomatosis. Fibrocystic disease refers to a spectrum of histopathologic changes that are best diagnosed and treated specifically.

Treatment of Selected Benign Breast Disorders and Diseases

Cysts: In practice, the first investigation of palpable breast masses is frequently needle biopsy, which allows for the early diagnosis of cysts. A 21-gauge needle attached to a 10-mL syringe is placed directly into the mass, which is fixed by fingers of the nondominant hand. The volume of a typical cyst is 5–10 mL, but it may be 75 mL or more. If the fluid that is aspirated is not bloodstained, then the cyst is aspirated to dryness, the needle is removed, and the fluid is discarded as cytologic examination of such fluid is not cost-effective. After aspiration, the breast is carefully palpated to exclude a residual mass. If one exists, ultrasound examination is performed to exclude a persistent cyst, which is reaspirated if present. If the mass is solid, a tissue specimen is obtained. When cystic fluid is bloodstained, 2 mL of fluid are taken for cytology. The mass is then imaged with ultrasound and any solid area on the cyst wall is biopsied by needle. The presence of blood usually is obvious, but in cysts with dark fluid, an occult blood test or microscopy examination will eliminate any doubt. The two cardinal rules of safe cyst aspiration are (1) the mass must disappear completely after aspiration, and (2) the fluid must not be bloodstained. If either of these conditions is not met, then ultrasound, needle biopsy, and perhaps excisional biopsy are recommended.

Fibroadenomas: Removal of all fibroadenomas has been advocated irrespective of patient age or other considerations, and solitary fibroadenomas in young women are frequently removed to alleviate patient concern. Yet most fibroadenomas are self-limiting and many go undiagnosed, so a more conservative approach is reasonable. Careful ultrasound examination with core-needle biopsy will provide for an accurate diagnosis. Subsequently, the patient is counseled concerning the biopsy results, and excision of the fibroadenoma may be avoided.

Sclerosing Disorders: The clinical significance of sclerosing adenosis lies in its mimicry of cancer. It may be confused with cancer on physical examination, by mammography, and at gross pathologic examination. Excisional biopsy and histologic examination are frequently necessary to exclude the diagnosis of cancer. The diagnostic work-up for radial scars and complex sclerosing lesions frequently involves stereoscopic biopsy. It is usually not possible to differentiate these lesions with certainty from cancer by mammography features, hence biopsy is recommended.

Periductal Mastitis: Painful and tender masses behind the nipple-areola complex are aspirated with a 21-gauge needle attached to a 10-mL syringe. Any fluid obtained is submitted for cytology and for culture using a transport medium appropriate for the detection of anaerobic organisms. Women are started on a combination of metronidazole and dicloxacillin while awaiting the results of culture. Antibiotics are then continued based on sensitivity tests. Many cases respond satisfactorily, but when there is considerable pus present, surgical treatment is recommended. A subareolar abscess usually is unilocular and often is associated with a single duct system. Preoperative ultrasound will accurately delineate its extent. The surgeon may either undertake simple drainage with a view toward formal surgery, should the problem recur, or proceed with definitive surgery. In a woman of childbearing age, simple drainage is preferred, but if there is an anaerobic infection, recurrent infection frequently develops. Recurrent abscess with fistula is a difficult problem and may be treated by fistulectomy or by major duct excision, depending on the circumstances. When a localized periareolar abscess recurs at the previous site and a fistula is present, the preferred operation is fistulectomy, which has minimal complications and a high degree of success. However, when subareolar sepsis is diffuse rather than localized to one segment or when more than one fistula is present, total duct excision is the preferred procedure. The first circumstance is seen in young women with squamous metaplasia of a single duct, although the latter circumstance is seen in older women with multiple ectatic ducts. However, age is not always a reliable guide, and fistula excision is the preferred initial procedure for localized sepsis irrespective of age. Antibiotic therapy is useful for recurrent infection after fistula excision, and a 2–4-week course is recommended prior to total duct excision.

Nipple Inversion: More women request correction of congenital nipple inversion than request correction for the nipple inversion that occurs secondary to duct ectasia. Although the results are usually satisfactory, women seeking correction for cosmetic reasons should always be made aware of the surgical complications of altered nipple sensation, nipple necrosis, and postoperative fibrosis with nipple retraction. Because nipple inversion is a result of shortening of the subareolar ducts, a complete division of these ducts is necessary for permanent correction of the disorder.

RISK FACTORS FOR BREAST CANCER

Increased exposure to estrogen is associated with an increased risk for developing breast cancer, whereas reducing exposure is thought to be protective. Correspondingly, factors that increase the number of menstrual cycles, such as early menarche, nulliparity, and late menopause, are associated with increased risk. Moderate levels of exercise and a longer lactation period, factors that decrease the total number of menstrual cycles, are protective. The terminal differentiation of breast epithelium associated with a full-term pregnancy is also protective, so older age at first live birth is associated with an increased risk of breast cancer.

Risk assessment. The average lifetime risk of breast cancer for newborn U.S. females is 12 percent. The longer a woman lives without cancer, the lower her risk of developing breast cancer. Thus, a woman age 50 years has an 11 percent lifetime risk of developing beast cancer, and a woman age 70 years has a 7 percent lifetime risk of developing breast cancer. As risk factors for breast cancer interact, evaluating the risk conferred by combinations of risk factors is difficult. From the Breast Cancer Detection Demonstration Project, a mammography screening program conducted in the 1970s, Gail and colleagues developed the most frequently used model, which incorporates age at menarche, the number of breast biopsies, age at first live birth and the number of first-degree relatives with breast cancer. It predicts the cumulative risk of breast cancer according to decade of life. To calculate breast cancer risk with the Gail model, a woman's risk factors are translated into an overall risk score by multiplying her relative risks from several categories. This risk score is then compared to an adjusted population risk of breast cancer to determine a woman's individual risk. A software program incorporating the Gail model is available from the National Cancer Institute at http://bcra.nci.nih.gov/brc.

Risk management. Several important medical decisions may be affected by a woman's underlying risk of breast cancer. These decisions include when to use postmenopausal hormone replacement therapy; at what age to begin mammography screening; when to use tamoxifen to prevent breast cancer; and when to perform prophylactic mastectomy to prevent breast cancer. Postmenopausal hormone replacement therapy reduces the risk of coronary artery disease and osteoporosis by 50 percent, but increases the risk of breast cancer by approximately 30 percent.

Routine use of screening mammography in women age 50 years and older reduces mortality from breast cancer by 33 percent. This reduction comes without substantial risks and at an acceptable economic cost. However, the use of screening mammography is more controversial in women younger than age 50 years for several reasons: (1) breast density is greater and screening mammography is less likely to detect early breast cancer; (2) screening mammography results in more false-positive tests, resulting in unnecessary biopsies; and (3) younger women are less likely to have breast cancer so fewer young women will benefit from screening. However, on a population basis, the benefits of screening mammography in women between the ages of 40 and 49 years still appear to outweigh the risks.

Tamoxifen, a selective estrogen receptor modulator, was the first drug shown to reduce the incidence of breast cancer in healthy women. The Breast Cancer Prevention Trial (NSABP P-01) randomly assigned more than 13,000 women, with a 5-year Gail relative risk of breast cancer of 1.70 or greater, to tamoxifen or placebo. After a mean follow-up period of 4 years, tamoxifen had reduced the incidence of breast cancer by 49 percent. Tamoxifen currently is only recommended for women who have a Gail relative risk of 1.70 or greater and it is unclear whether the benefits of tamoxifen apply to women at lower risk. Additionally, deep venous thrombosis occurs 1.6 times, pulmonary emboli 3.0 times, and endometrial cancer 2.5 times as often in women taking tamoxifen. The increased risk for endometrial cancer is restricted to early stage cancers in postmenopausal women. Cataract surgery is required almost twice as often among women taking tamoxifen. Although no formal risk-benefit analysis is currently available, the higher a woman's risk of breast cancer, the more likely it is that the reduction in the incidence of breast cancer conveyed by tamoxifen will outweigh the risk of serious side effects.

EPIDEMIOLOGY AND NATURAL HISTORY OF BREAST CANCER

Epidemiology. Breast cancer is the most common site-specific cancer in women and is the leading cause of death from cancer for women age 40–44 years. It accounts for 33 percent of all female cancers and is responsible for 20 percent of the cancer-related deaths in women. It is predicted that approximately 211,240 invasive breast cancers will be diagnosed in women in the United States in 2005 and 40,410 of those diagnosed will die from that cancer. Breast cancer was the leading cause of cancer-related mortality in women until 1985, when it was surpassed by lung cancer. In the 1970s, the probability of a woman in the United States developing breast cancer was estimated at one in 13, in 1980 it was 1:11, and in 2002 it was 1:8. Cancer registries in Connecticut and upper New York state document that the age-adjusted incidence of new breast cancer cases has steadily increased since the mid-1940s. This increase was about 1 percent per year from 1973–1980, and there was an additional increase in incidence to 4 percent between 1980 and 1987, which was characterized by frequent detection of small primary cancers. The increase in breast cancer incidence occurred primarily in women age 55 years or older and paralleled a marked increase in the percentage of older women who had mammograms. At the same time, incidence rates for regional metastatic disease dropped and breast cancer mortality declined. From 1960–1963, 5-year overall survival rates for breast cancer were 63 and 46 percent in white and African American women, respectively, although the rates for 1981–1987 were 78 and 63 percent, respectively.

Natural history. Bloom and colleagues described the natural history of breast cancer based on the records of 250 women with untreated breast cancers who were cared for on charity wards in Middlesex Hospital, London, between 1805 and 1933. The median survival of this population was 2.7 years after initial diagnosis. The 5- and 10-year survival rates for these women were 18.0 and 3.6 percent, respectively. Only 0.8 percent survived for 15 years or longer. Autopsy data confirmed that 95 percent of these women died of breast cancer, although the remaining 5 percent died of other causes. Almost 75 percent of the women developed ulceration of the breast during the course of the disease. The longest surviving patient died in the nineteenth year after diagnosis.

HISTOPATHOLOGY OF BREAST CANCER

Carcinoma in situ. Cancer cells are in situ or invasive depending on whether or not they invade through the basement membrane. Broder's original description of in situ breast cancer stressed the absence of invasion of cells into the surrounding stroma and their confinement within natural ductal and alveolar boundaries. As areas of invasion may be minute, the accurate diagnosis of in situ cancer necessitates the analysis of multiple microscopy sections to exclude invasion. In 1941, Foote and Stewart published a landmark description of lobular carcinoma in situ (LCIS), which distinguished it from ductal carcinoma in situ (DCIS). Multicentricity refers to the occurrence of a second in situ breast cancer outside the breast quadrant of the primary in situ cancer, whereas multifocality refers to the occurrence of a second in situ breast cancer within the same breast quadrant as the primary in situ cancer. Multicentricity occurs in 60–90 percent of women with LCIS, although the rate of multicentricity for DCIS is 40–80 percent. LCIS occurs bilaterally in 50–70 percent of cases, although DCIS occurs bilaterally in 10–20 percent of cases.

Lobular Carcinoma In Situ: LCIS originates from the terminal duct lobular units and only develops in the female breast. It is characterized by distention and distortion of the terminal duct lobular units by cancer cells, which are large but maintain a normal nuclear-to-cytoplasmic ratio. The frequency of LCIS in the general population cannot be reliably determined because it usually presents as an incidental finding. The age at diagnosis is 44–47 years, which is approximately 15–25 years younger than the age at diagnosis for invasive breast cancer. LCIS has a distinct racial predilection, occurring 12 times more frequently in white women than in African American women. Invasive breast cancer develops in 25–35 percent of women with LCIS. Invasive lobular cancer may develop in either breast, regardless of which breast harbored the initial focus of LCIS, and is detected synchronously with LCIS in 5 percent of cases. In women with a history of LCIS, up to 65 percent of subsequent invasive cancers are ductal, not lobular in origin. For these reasons, LCIS is regarded as a marker of increased risk for invasive breast cancer rather than an anatomic precursor.

Ductal Carcinoma In Situ: Although DCIS is predominantly seen in the female breast, it accounts for 5 percent of male breast cancers. Published series suggest a detection frequency of 7 percent in all biopsy tissue specimens. The term intraductal carcinoma is frequently applied to DCIS, which carries a high risk for progression to an invasive cancer. Histologically, DCIS is characterized by a proliferation of the epithelium that lines the minor breast ducts. DCIS is now frequently classified based on nuclear grade and the presence of necrosis. The risk for invasive breast cancer is increased nearly 5-fold in women with DCIS. The invasive cancers are observed in the ipsilateral breast, usually in the same quadrant as the DCIS that was originally detected, suggesting that DCIS is an anatomic precursor of invasive ductal carcinoma.

Invasive breast carcinoma. Invasive breast cancers are described as lobular or ductal in origin with histologic classifications recognizing special types of ductal breast cancers (10 percent of total cases), which are defined by specific histologic features. To qualify as a special-type cancer, at least 90 percent of the cancer must contain the defining histologic features. Eighty percent of invasive breast cancers are described as invasive ductal carcinoma of no special type (NST). These cancers generally have a worse prognosis than special-type cancers. Foote and Stewart originally proposed the following classification for invasive breast cancer:

I. Paget disease of the nipple
II. Invasive ductal carcinoma
    A. Adenocarcinoma with productive fibrosis (scirrhous, simplex, no special type (NST)) 80 percent
    B. Medullary carcinoma 4 percent
    C. Mucinous (colloid) carcinoma 2 percent
    D. Papillary carcinoma 2 percent
    E. Tubular carcinoma (and invasive cribriform carcinoma (ICC)) 2 percent
III. Invasive lobular carcinoma 10 percent
IV. Rare cancers (adenoid cystic, squamous cell, apocrine)

Paget disease of the nipple was described in 1874. It frequently presents as a chronic, eczematous eruption of the nipple, which may be subtle, but may progress to an ulcerated, weeping lesion. Paget disease usually is associated with extensive DCIS and may be associated with an invasive cancer. A palpable mass may or may not be present. Biopsy of the nipple will show a population of cells that are identical to the underlying DCIS cells (pagetoid features or pagetoid change). Pathognomonic of this cancer is the presence of large, pale, vacuolated cells (Paget cells) in the rete pegs of the epithelium. Surgical therapy for Paget disease may involve lumpectomy, mastectomy, or modified radical mastectomy, depending on the extent of involvement and the presence of invasive cancer.

Invasive ductal carcinoma of the breast with productive fibrosis (scirrhous, simplex, NST) accounts for 80 percent of breast cancers and presents with macroscopic or microscopic axillary lymph node metastases in 60 percent of cases. This cancer usually presents in perimenopausal or postmenopausal women in the fifth to sixth decades of life as a solitary, firm mass. It has poorly defined margins and its cut surfaces show a central stellate configuration with chalky white or yellow streaks extending into surrounding breast tissues. The cancer cells often are arranged in small clusters, and there is a broad spectrum of histologies with variable cellular and nuclear grades.

DIAGNOSING BREAST CANCER

In 33 percent of breast cancer cases, the woman discovers a lump in her breast. Other less frequent presenting signs and symptoms of breast cancer include (1) breast enlargement or asymmetry; (2) nipple changes, retraction, or discharge; (3) ulceration or erythema of the skin of the breast; (4) an axillary mass; and (5) musculoskeletal discomfort. However, up to 50 percent of women presenting with breast complaints have no physical signs of breast pathology. Breast pain usually is associated with benign disease.

Misdiagnosed breast cancer accounts for the greatest number of malpractice claims for errors in diagnosis and for the largest number of paid claims. Litigation often involves younger women whose physical examination and mammography may be misleading. If a young woman (age 45 years or younger) presents with a palpable breast mass and equivocal mammography finding, ultrasound examination and biopsy are used to avoid a delay in diagnosis.

Examination

Inspection: The surgeon inspects the woman's breast with her arms by her side, with her arms straight up in the air, and with her hands on her hips (with and without pectoral muscle contraction). Symmetry, size, and shape of the breast are recorded, and any evidence of edema (peau d'orange), nipple or skin retraction, and erythema. With the arms extended forward and in a sitting position, the women leans forward to accentuate any skin retraction.

As part of the physical examination, the breast is carefully palpated. Examination of the patient in the supine position is best performed with a pillow supporting the ipsilateral hemithorax. The surgeon gently palpates the breast from the ipsilateral side, making certain to examine all quadrants of the breast from the sternum laterally to the latissimus dorsi muscle, and from the clavicle inferiorly to the upper rectus sheath. The surgeon performs the examination with the palmar aspects of the fingers avoiding a grasping or pinching motion. The breast may be cupped or molded in the surgeon's hands to check for retraction. A systematic search for lymphadenopathy then is performed. By supporting the upper arm and elbow, the shoulder girdle is stabilized. Using gentle palpation, all three levels of possible axillary lymphadenopathy are assessed. Careful palpation of supraclavicular and parasternal sites also is performed. A diagram of the chest and contiguous lymph node sites is useful for recording location, size, consistency, shape, mobility, fixation, and other characteristics of any palpable breast mass or lymphadenopathy.

Imaging Techniques

Mammography: Mammography has been used in North America since the 1960s and the techniques used continue to be modified and improved to enhance image quality. Conventional mammography delivers a radiation dose of 0.1 centigray (cGy) per study. By comparison, a chest radiograph delivers 25 percent of this dose. However, there is no increased breast cancer risk associated with the radiation dose delivered with screening mammography. Screening mammography is used to detect unexpected breast cancer in asymptomatic women. In this regard, it supplements history and physical examination. With screening mammography, two views of the breast are obtained, the craniocaudal (CC) view and the mediolateral oblique (MLO) view. The MLO view images the greatest volume of breast tissue, including the upper outer quadrant and the axillary tail of Spence. Compared with the MLO view, the CC view provides better visualization of the medial aspect of the breast and permits greater breast compression. Diagnostic mammography is used to evaluate women with abnormal findings such as a breast mass or nipple discharge. In addition to the MLO and CC views, a diagnostic examination may use views that better define the nature of any abnormalities, such as the 90-degree lateral and spot compression views. The 90-degree lateral view is used along with the CC view to triangulate the exact location of an abnormality. Spot compression may be done in any projection by using a small compression device, which is placed directly over a mammography abnormality that is obscured by overlying tissues. The compression device minimizes motion artifact, improves definition, separates overlying tissues, and decreases the radiation dose needed to penetrate the breast. Magnification techniques ($\times 1.5$) often are combined with spot compression to better resolve calcifications and the margins of masses. Mammography also is used to guide interventional procedures, including needle localization and needle biopsy.

Specific mammography features that suggest a diagnosis of a breast cancer include a solid mass with or without stellate features, asymmetric thickening of breast tissues, and clustered microcalcifications. The presence of fine, stippled calcium in and around a suspicious lesion is suggestive of breast cancer and occurs in as many as 50 percent of nonpalpable cancers. These microcalcifications are an especially important sign of cancer in younger women, in whom it may be the only mammography abnormality. Current guidelines of the National Cancer Center Network (NCCN) suggest that normal-risk women age 20 years or older should have a breast exam at least every 3 years. At age 40 years, breast exams should be performed yearly along with a yearly mammogram. Prospective, randomized studies of mammography screening confirm a 40 percent reduction for stages II, III, and IV cancer in the screened population, with a 30 percent increase in overall survival.

Xeromammography: Xeromammography techniques are identical to those of mammography with the exception that the image is recorded on a xerography plate, which provides a positive rather than a negative image. Details of the entire breast and the soft tissues of the chest wall may be recorded with one exposure.

Ultrasonography: Ultrasonography is second only to mammography in frequency of use for breast imaging and is an important method of resolving equivocal mammography findings, defining cystic masses, and demonstrating the echogenic qualities of specific solid abnormalities. On ultrasound examination, breast cysts are well circumscribed, with smooth margins and an echo-free center. Benign breast masses usually show smooth contours, round or oval shapes, weak internal echoes, and well-defined anterior and posterior margins. Breast cancer characteristically has irregular walls, but may have smooth margins with acoustic enhancement. Ultrasonography is used to guide fine-needle aspiration biopsy, core-needle biopsy, and needle localization of breast lesions. It is highly reproducible and has a high patient acceptance rate, but does not reliably detect lesions that are 1 cm or less in diameter.

Breast Biopsy

Nonpalpable Lesions: Image-guided breast biopsies are frequently required to diagnose nonpalpable lesions. Ultrasound localization techniques are employed when a mass is present, although stereotactic techniques are used when no mass is present (microcalcifications only). The combination of diagnostic mammography, ultrasound or stereotactic localization, and fine-needle aspiration (FNA) biopsy is almost 100 percent accurate in the diagnosis of breast cancer. However, although FNA biopsy permits cytologic evaluation, core-needle or open biopsy also permits the analysis of breast tissue architecture and allows the pathologist to determine whether invasive cancer is present. This permits the surgeon and patient to discuss the specific management of a breast cancer before therapy begins. Core-needle biopsy is accepted as an alternative to open biopsy for nonpalpable breast lesions. The advantages of core-needle biopsy include a low complication rate, avoidance of scarring, and a lower cost.

Palpable Lesions: FNA biopsy of a palpable breast mass is performed in an outpatient setting. A 1.5-inch, 22-gauge needle attached to a 10-mL syringe is used. A syringe holder enables the surgeon performing the FNA biopsy to control the syringe and needle with one hand while positioning the breast mass with the opposite hand. After the needle is placed in the mass, suction is applied while the needle is moved back and forth within the mass. Once cellular material is seen at the hub of the needle, the suction is released and the needle is withdrawn. The cellular material is then expressed onto microscope slides. Both air-dried and 95 percent ethanol-fixed microscopy sections are prepared for analysis. When a breast mass is clinically and mammographically suspicious, the sensitivity and the specificity of FNA biopsy approaches 100 percent. Core-needle biopsy of palpable breast masses is performed using a 14-gauge needle, such as the Tru Cut needle. Automated devices also are available. Tissue specimens are placed in formalin and then processed to paraffin blocks. Although the false-negative rate for core-needle biopsy is very low, a tissue specimen that does not show breast cancer cannot conclusively rule out that diagnosis because a sampling error may have occurred.

BREAST CANCER PROGNOSIS

Breast cancer staging. The clinical stage of breast cancer is determined primarily through physical examination of the skin, breast tissue, and lymph nodes (axillary, supraclavicular, and cervical). However, clinical determination of axillary lymph node metastases has an accuracy of only 33 percent. Mammography, chest radiograph, and intraoperative findings (primary cancer size, chest wall invasion) also provide necessary staging information. Pathologic stage combines clinical stage data with findings from pathologic examination of the resected primary breast cancer and axillary lymph nodes. A frequently used staging system is the TNM (tumor, nodes, and metastasis) system. The American Joint Committee on Cancer (AJCC) has modified the TNM system for breast cancer. The single most important predictor of 10- and 20-year survival rates in breast cancer is the number of axillary lymph nodes involved with metastatic disease. Table 16-2 shows traditional prognostic and predictive biomarkers for breast cancer.

OVERVIEW OF BREAST CANCER THERAPY

In situ breast cancer (stage 0). Both LCIS and DCIS may be difficult to distinguish from atypical hyperplasia or from cancers with early invasion. Expert pathologic review is required in all cases. Bilateral mammography is performed to determine the extent of the in situ cancer and to exclude a second cancer. Because LCIS is considered a marker for increased risk rather than an inevitable precursor of invasive disease, the current treatment of LCIS is observation with or without tamoxifen. The goal of treatment is to prevent or detect at an early stage the invasive cancer that subsequently develops in 25–35 percent of these women. There is no benefit to excising LCIS, as the disease diffusely involves both breasts and the risk of invasive cancer is equal for both breasts. The use of tamoxifen as a risk-reduction strategy should be considered in women with a diagnosis of LCIS.

Women with DCIS and evidence of widespread disease (two or more quadrants) require mastectomy. For women with limited disease, lumpectomy and radiation therapy are recommended. Low-grade DCIS of the solid, cribriform, or papillary subtype, which is less than 0.5 cm in diameter, may be managed by

TABLE 16-2 Traditional Prognostic and Predictive Factors for Invasive Breast Cancer

Tumor factors	Host factors
Nodal status	Age
Tumor size	Menopausal status
Histologic/nuclear grade	Family history
Lymphatic/vascular invasion	Previous breast cancer
Pathologic stage	Immunosuppression
Hormone receptor status	Nutrition
DNA content (ploidy, S-phase Prior chemotherapy fraction)	
Extensive intraductal component	Prior radiation therapy

DNA = deoxyribonucleic acid. Reproduced with permission from Beenken SW, Bland KI: Breast cancer genetics, in Ellis N (ed): *Inherited Cancer Syndromes.* New York: Springer-Verlag, 2003, p 112.

lumpectomy alone. For nonpalpable DCIS, needle localization techniques are used to guide the surgical resection. Specimen mammography is performed to ensure that all visible evidence of cancer is excised. Adjuvant tamoxifen therapy is considered for all DCIS patients. The gold standard against which breast conservation therapy for DCIS is evaluated is mastectomy. Women treated with mastectomy have local recurrence and mortality rates of less than 2 percent. Women treated with lumpectomy and adjuvant radiation therapy have a similar mortality rate, but the local recurrence rate increases to 9 percent. Forty-five percent of these recurrences will be invasive cancer.

Early invasive breast cancer (stage I, IIa, or IIb). NSABP B-06 compared total mastectomy to lumpectomy with or without radiation therapy in the treatment of stages I and II breast cancer. After 12- and 20-year follow-up periods, the disease-free, distant disease-free, and overall survival rates for lumpectomy with or without radiation therapy remain similar to those observed after total mastectomy. However, the incidence of ipsilateral breast cancer recurrence (in-breast recurrence) continues higher in the lumpectomy group not receiving radiation therapy (35 percent) when compared to those receiving radiation therapy (10 percent). These findings support the use of lumpectomy and radiation in the treatment of stages I and II breast cancer.

Currently, mastectomy with assessment of axillary lymph node status and breast conservation (lumpectomy with assessment of axillary lymph node status and radiation therapy) are considered equivalent treatments for stages I and II breast cancer. Axillary lymphadenopathy or metastatic disease in a sentinel axillary lymph node (see below) necessitates an axillary lymph node dissection. Breast conservation is considered for all patients because of the important cosmetic advantages. Relative contraindications to breast conservation therapy include (1) prior radiation therapy to the breast or chest wall; (2) involved surgical margins or unknown margin status following re-excision; (3) multicentric disease; and (4) scleroderma or other connective-tissue disease.

Traditionally, dissection of axillary lymph node levels I and II has been performed in early invasive breast cancer. Sentinel lymph node biopsy is now being performed by many surgeons in the elective situation to assess axillary lymph nodes status. Candidates for this procedure have clinically uninvolved axillary lymph nodes, a T1 or T2 primary breast cancer, and have not had neoadjuvant chemotherapy. If the sentinel lymph node cannot be identified or is found to harbor metastatic disease, then an axillary lymph node dissection is performed. The performance of a sentinel lymph node biopsy is not warranted when the selection of adjuvant therapy will not be affected by the status of the axillary lymph nodes, such as in some older adult patients and in those with serious comorbid conditions.

Adjuvant chemotherapy for early invasive breast cancer is considered for all node-positive cancers, all cancers that are larger than 1 cm in size, and node-negative cancers larger than 0.5 cm in size when adverse prognostic features are present. Adverse prognostic factors include blood vessel or lymph vessel invasion, high nuclear grade, high histologic grade, human epidermal growth receptor 2 (HER-2)/neu overexpression, and negative hormone receptor status. Adjuvant endocrine therapy consisting of tamoxifen or an aromatase inhibitor is considered for hormone receptor-positive women with cancers that are larger than 1 cm in size. HER-2/neu expression is determined for all newly diagnosed patients with breast cancer and may be used to provide prognostic information in patients with node-negative breast cancer, predict the relative efficacy of various chemotherapy regimens, and predict benefit from Herceptin in women with metastatic or recurrent breast cancer.

Advanced locoregional regional breast cancer (stage IIIa or IIIb). Women with stages IIIa and IIIb breast cancer have advanced locoregional breast cancer but have no clinically detected distant metastases. In an effort to provide optimal locoregional disease-free survival, and distant disease-free survival for these women, surgery is integrated with radiation therapy and chemotherapy. Stage IIIa patients are divided into those who have operable disease and those who have inoperable disease.

Internal mammary lymph nodes. Metastatic disease to internal mammary lymph nodes may be occult, evident on chest radiograph or CT scan, or may present as a painless parasternal mass with or without skin involvement. There is no consensus regarding the need for internal mammary lymph node radiation therapy in women who are at increased risk for occult involvement (cancers involving the medial aspect of the breast, axillary lymph node involvement), but who show no signs of internal mammary lymph node involvement. Systemic chemotherapy and radiation therapy are used in the treatment of grossly involved internal mammary lymph nodes.

Distant metastases (stage IV). Treatment for stage IV breast cancer is not curative, but may prolong survival and enhance a woman's quality of life. Hormonal therapies that are associated with minimal toxicity are preferred to cytotoxic chemotherapy. Appropriate candidates for initial hormonal therapy include women with hormone receptor-positive cancers; women with bone or soft tissue metastases only; and women with limited and asymptomatic visceral metastases. Systemic chemotherapy is indicated for women with hormone receptor-negative cancers, symptomatic visceral metastases, and hormone refractory metastases. Women with stage IV breast cancer may develop anatomically localized problems, which will benefit from individualized surgical treatment, such as brain metastases; pleural effusion; pericardial effusion; biliary obstruction; ureteral obstruction; impending or existing pathologic fracture of a long bone; spinal cord compression; and painful bone or soft tissue metastases. Bisphosphonates, which may be given in addition to chemotherapy or hormone therapy, should be considered in women with bone metastases.

Locoregional recurrence. Women with locoregional recurrence of breast cancer may be separated into two groups: those having had mastectomy and those having had lumpectomy. Women with a previous mastectomy undergo surgical resection of the locoregional recurrence and appropriate reconstruction. Chemotherapy and antiestrogen therapy are considered and adjuvant radiation therapy is given if the chest wall has not previously received radiation therapy. Women with previous breast conservation undergo a mastectomy and appropriate reconstruction. Chemotherapy and antiestrogen therapy are considered.

Breast cancer prognosis. Survival rates for women diagnosed with breast cancer between 1983 and 1987 have been calculated based on Surveillance, Epidemiology, and End Results (SEER) program data. The 5-year survival rate for stage I patients is 94 percent; for stage IIa patients, 85 percent; and for stage IIb patients, 70 percent; although for stage IIIa patients the 5-year survival rate, 52 percent; for stage IIIb patients, 48 percent and for stage IV patients, 18 percent.

SURGICAL TECHNIQUES IN BREAST CANCER THERAPY

Excisional biopsy with needle localization. Excisional biopsy implies complete removal of a breast lesion with a margin of normal-appearing breast tissue. Excellent scars generally result from circumareolar incisions through which subareolar and centrally located breast lesions may be approached. Elsewhere, incisions that parallel Langer lines, which are lines of tension in the skin that are generally concentric with the nipple-areola complex, result in acceptable scars. It is important to keep biopsy incisions within the boundaries of the skin excision that may be required as part of a subsequent mastectomy. Radial incisions in the upper half of the breast are not recommended because of possible scar contracture resulting in displacement of the ipsilateral nipple-areola complex.

After excision of a suspicious breast lesion, the biopsy tissue specimen is orientated for the pathologist using sutures, clips, or dyes. Additional margins (superior, inferior, medial, lateral, superficial, and deep) may be taken from the surgical bed to confirm complete excision of the suspicious lesion. Electrocautery or absorbable ligatures are used to achieve wound hemostasis. Although approximation of the breast tissues in the excision bed is usually not necessary, cosmesis may occasionally be facilitated by approximation of the surgical defect using 3-0 absorbable sutures. A running subcuticular closure of the skin using 4-0 or 5-0 absorbable monofilament sutures is performed, followed by approximation of the skin edges with Steri-Strips. Wound drainage is avoided.

Excisional biopsy with needle localization requires a preoperative visit to the mammography suite for placement of a localization wire. The lesion to be excised is accurately localized by mammography, and the tip of a thin wire hook is positioned close to the lesion. Using the wire hook as a guide, the surgeon subsequently excises the suspicious breast lesion while removing a margin of normal-appearing breast tissue. Before the patient leaves the operating room, specimen radiography is performed to confirm complete excision of the suspicious lesion.

Sentinel lymph node biopsy. Sentinel lymph node biopsy is primarily used in women with early breast cancers (T1 and T2, N0). It also is accurate for T3 N0 cancers, but nearly 75 percent of these women will have nonpalpable axillary lymph node metastases. In women undergoing neoadjuvant chemotherapy to permit conservation surgery, sentinel lymph node biopsy may be used. Contraindications to the procedure include palpable lymphadenopathy, prior axillary surgery, chemotherapy or radiation therapy, and multifocal breast cancers.

Evidence from large prospective studies suggests that the combination of intraoperative gamma probe detection of radioactive colloid and intraoperative visualization of isosulfan blue dye (Lymphazurin) is more accurate than the use of either agent alone. Some surgeons employ preoperative lymphoscintigraphy, although it is not necessary. On the day prior to surgery, or on the morning of surgery, radioactive colloid is injected. Using a tuberculin syringe and a 25-gauge needle, 0.5 mCi of 0.2-micron technetium-99 sulfur colloid in a volume of 0.2–0.5 mL is injected (three to four separate injections) at the cancer site or subdermally. Subdermal injections are given in proximity to the cancer site or subareolar. Subsequently, in the operating room, 4 mL of isosulfan blue dye (Lymphazurin) is injected in a similar fashion, but with an additional 1 mL injected between the cancer site and the overlying skin. For nonpalpable cancers, the injection is guided by either intraoperative ultrasound or by a localization wire that is placed preoperatively under ultrasound or stereotactic guidance. It is helpful for the radiologist to mark the skin overlying the breast cancer at the time of needle localization using an indelible marker. In women who have undergone previous excisional biopsy, the injections are made around the biopsy cavity but not into it. Women are told preoperatively that the isosulfan blue dye injection will impart a change to the color of their urine and that there is a very small risk of allergic reaction to the dye (1 in 10,000). Anaphylactic reactions have been documented. The use of radioactive colloid is safe and radiation exposure is very low.

A hand-held gamma counter is then employed transcutaneously to identify the location of the sentinel lymph node. A 3–4-cm incision is made in line with that used for an axillary dissection, which is a curved transverse incision in the lower axilla just below the hairline. After dissecting through the subcutaneous tissue and identifying the lateral border of the pectoralis muscles, the clavipectoral fascia is divided to gain exposure to the axillary contents. The gamma counter is employed to pinpoint the location of the sentinel lymph node. As the dissection continues, the signal from the probe increases in intensity as the sentinel lymph node is approached. The sentinel lymph node also is identified by visualization of isosulfan blue dye in the afferent lymph vessel and in the lymph node itself. Before removing the sentinel lymph node, a 10-second in vivo radioactivity count is obtained. After removal of the sentinel lymph node, a 10-second ex vivo radioactive count is obtained, and the lymph node is then sent to pathology for either permanent or frozen section analysis. The lowest false-negative rates for sentinel lymph node biopsy have been obtained when all blue lymph nodes and all lymph nodes with radiation counts greater than 10 percent of the 10-second ex vivo count of the sentinel lymph node are harvested (10 percent rule). Based on this, the gamma counter is employed before closing the axillary wound to measure residual radioactivity in the surgical bed. When necessary, a search is made for a second sentinel lymph node. This procedure is repeated until residual radioactivity in the surgical bed is less that 10 percent of the 10-second ex vivo count of the most radioactive sentinel lymph node.

Breast Conservation

Breast conservation involves resection of the primary breast cancer with a margin of normal-appearing breast tissue, adjuvant radiation therapy, and assessment of axillary lymph node status. Resection of the primary breast cancer is alternatively called segmental resection, lumpectomy, partial mastectomy, and tylectomy. Conservation surgery is currently the standard treatment for women with stage I or II invasive breast cancer. Women with DCIS generally require only resection of the primary cancer and adjuvant radiation therapy. When a lumpectomy is performed, a curvilinear incision lying concentric to the nipple-areola complex is made in the skin overlying the breast cancer. Skin encompassing a prior biopsy site is excised, but is not otherwise necessary. The breast cancer is removed with an envelope of normal-appearing breast tissue that is adequate to achieve at least a 1-cm cancer-free margin. Specimen orientation is performed and additional margins from the surgical bed are taken as described previously. Requests for hormone receptor status and HER-2/neu expression are conveyed to the pathologist.

After closure of the breast wound, dissection of the ipsilateral axillary lymph nodes has traditionally been completed for cancer staging and for control of regional disease. Ten to 15 level I and level II axillary lymph nodes usually are considered adequate for staging purposes. Sentinel lymph node biopsy is now the preferred staging procedure in the clinically uninvolved axilla. When the sentinel lymph node does not contain metastatic disease, axillary lymph node dissection is avoided.

Mastectomy and axillary dissection. A skin-sparing mastectomy removes all breast tissue, the nipple-areola complex, and only 1 cm of skin around excised scars. There is a recurrence rate of less than 2 percent when skin-sparing mastectomy is used for T1–T3 cancers. A total (simple) mastectomy removes all breast tissue, the nipple-areola complex, and skin. An extended simple mastectomy removes all breast tissue, the nipple-areola complex, skin, and the level I axillary lymph nodes. A modified radical mastectomy removes all breast tissue, the nipple-areola complex, skin, and the level I and level II axillary lymph nodes. The Halstead radical mastectomy removes all breast tissue and skin, the nipple-areola complex, the pectoralis major and pectoralis minor muscles, and the level I, II, and III axillary lymph nodes. Chemotherapy, hormone therapy, and radiation therapy for breast cancer have nearly eliminated the need for the radical mastectomy.

For a variety of biologic, economic, and psychosocial reasons, some women desire mastectomy rather than breast conservation. Women who are less concerned about cosmesis may view mastectomy as the most expeditious and desirable therapeutic option because it avoids the cost and inconvenience of radiation therapy. Women whose primary breast cancers have an extensive intraductal component undergo mastectomy because of very high local failure rates in the ipsilateral breast after breast conservation. Women with large cancers that occupy the subareolar and central portions of the breast and women with multicentric primary cancers also undergo mastectomy.

Modified Radical Mastectomy: A modified radical mastectomy preserves both the pectoralis major and pectoralis minor muscles, allowing removal of level I and level II axillary lymph I nodes but not the level III (apical) axillary lymph nodes. The Patey modification removes the pectoralis minor muscle and allows complete dissection of the level III axillary lymph nodes. A modified radical mastectomy permits preservation of the medial (anterior thoracic) pectoral nerve, which courses in the lateral neurovascular bundle of the axilla and usually penetrates the pectoralis minor to supply the lateral border of the pectoralis major. Anatomic boundaries of the modified radical mastectomy are the anterior margin of the latissimus dorsi muscle laterally; the midline of the sternum medially; the subclavius muscle superiorly; and the caudal extension of the breast 2–3 cm inferior to the inframammary fold inferiorly. Skin-flap thickness, which is inclusive of skin and tela subcutanea, varies with body habitus. Once the skin flaps are fully developed, the fascia of the pectoralis major muscle and the overlying breast tissue are elevated off the underlying musculature, allowing for the complete removal of the breast.

Subsequently, an axillary lymph node dissection is performed. The most lateral extent of the axillary vein is identified and the areolar tissue of the lateral axillary space is elevated as the vein is cleared on its anterior and inferior surfaces. The areolar tissues at the junction of the axillary vein with the anterior edge of the latissimus dorsi muscle, which include the lateral and subscapular lymph node groups (level I), are cleared in an inferomedial direction. Care is taken to preserve the thoracodorsal neurovascular bundle. The dissection then continues medially with clearance of the central axillary lymph node group (level II). The long thoracic nerve of Bell is identified and preserved as it travels in the investing fascia of the serratus anterior muscle. Every effort is made to preserve this nerve because permanent disability with a winged scapula and shoulder weakness will follow denervation of the serratus anterior muscle. If there is palpable lymphadenopathy at the apex of the axilla, the tendinous portion of the pectoralis minor muscle is divided near its insertion onto the coracoid process, which allows dissection of the axillary vein medially to the costoclavicular (Halsted) ligament. Finally, the breast and axillary contents are removed from the surgical bed and are sent for pathologic assessment.

Seromas beneath the skin flaps or in the axilla represent the most frequent complication of mastectomy and axillary lymph node dissection, reportedly occurring in as many as 30 percent of cases. The use of closed-system suction drainage reduces the incidence of this complication. Catheters are retained in the wound until drainage diminishes to less than 30 mL per day. Wound infections occur infrequently after a mastectomy and the majority occur secondary to skin-flap necrosis. Culture of the infected wound for aerobic and anaerobic organisms, débridement, and antibiotics are effective management. Moderate or severe hemorrhage in the postoperative period is rare and is best managed with early wound exploration for control of hemorrhage and re-establishment of closed-system suction drainage. The incidence of functionally significant lymphedema after a modified radical mastectomy is 10 percent. Extensive axillary lymph node dissection, radiation therapy, the presence of pathologic lymph nodes, and obesity are predisposing factors. Individually fitted compressive sleeves and intermittent compression devices may be necessary.

Reconstruction of the breast and chest wall. The goals of reconstructive surgery following a mastectomy for breast cancer are wound closure and breast reconstruction, which is either immediate or delayed. For most women, wound closure after mastectomy is accomplished with simple approximation of the wound edges. However, if a more radical removal of skin and subcutaneous tissue is necessary, a skin graft provides functional coverage that will tolerate adjuvant radiation therapy. When soft-tissue defects are present that cannot be covered with a skin graft, myocutaneous flaps are employed. Breast reconstruction after prophylactic mastectomy or after mastectomy for early invasive breast cancer is performed immediately after surgery, although reconstruction following surgery for advanced breast cancer is delayed for 6 months after completion of adjuvant therapy to insure that locoregional control of disease is obtained. Many different types of myocutaneous flaps are employed for breast reconstruction, but the latissimus dorsi and the rectus abdominus myocutaneous flaps are most frequently used. The latissimus dorsi myocutaneous flap consists of a skin paddle based on the underlying latissimus dorsi muscle, which is supplied by the thoracodorsal artery with contributions from the posterior intercostal arteries. The transverse rectus abdominis myocutaneous (TRAM) flap consists of a skin paddle based on the underlying rectus abdominis muscle, which is supplied by vessels from the deep inferior epigastric artery. The free TRAM flap uses microvascular anastomoses to establish blood supply to the flap. When the bony chest wall is involved with cancer, resection of a portion of the bony chest wall is indicated. If only one or two ribs are resected and soft-tissue coverage is provided, reconstruction of the bony defect usually is not necessary as scar tissue will stabilize the chest wall. If more than two ribs are sacrificed, it is advisable to stabilize the chest wall with Marlex mesh, which is then covered with soft tissue by using a latissimus dorsi or TRAM flap.

NONSURGICAL BREAST CANCER THERAPIES

Radiation therapy. Radiation therapy is used for all stages of breast cancer. For women with limited DCIS (stage 0), in whom negative margins are achieved by lumpectomy or by re-excision, adjuvant radiation therapy is given to reduce the risk of local recurrence. For women with stage I, IIa, or IIb breast cancer in which negative margins are achieved by lumpectomy or by re-excision, adjuvant radiation therapy is given to reduce the risk of local recurrence. Those women treated with mastectomy who have cancer at the surgical margins are at sufficiently high risk for local recurrence to warrant the use of adjuvant radiation therapy to the chest wall and supraclavicular lymph nodes. Women with metastatic disease involving four or more axillary lymph nodes and premenopausal women with metastatic disease involving one to three lymph nodes also are at increased risk for recurrence and are candidates for the use of chest wall and supraclavicular lymph node radiation therapy. In advanced locoregional breast cancer (stage IIIa or IIIb), women are at high risk for recurrent disease following surgical therapy and adjuvant radiation therapy is employed to reduce the recurrence rate.

Chemotherapy

Adjuvant Chemotherapy: Adjuvant chemotherapy is of minimal benefit to node-negative women with cancers 0.5 cm or less in size and is not recommended. Node-negative women with cancers 0.6–1.0 cm are divided into those with a low risk of recurrence and those with unfavorable prognostic features that portend a higher risk of recurrence and a need for adjuvant chemotherapy. Adverse prognostic factors include blood vessel or lymph vessel invasion, high nuclear grade, high histologic grade, HER-2/neu overexpression, and negative hormone receptor status. Adjuvant chemotherapy is recommended for these women when unfavorable prognostic features are present.

For women with hormone receptor-negative cancers that are larger than 1 cm in size, adjuvant chemotherapy is appropriate. However, node-negative women with hormone receptor-positive cancers that are 1–3 cm in size are candidates for tamoxifen with or without chemotherapy. For special-type cancers (tubular, mucinous, medullary, etc.), adjuvant chemotherapy or tamoxifen for cancers smaller than 3 cm in size is controversial. For node-positive women or women with a special-type cancer that is larger than 3 cm in size, the use of chemotherapy with or without tamoxifen is appropriate. Current treatment recommendations for operable stage IIIa breast cancer are a modified radical mastectomy followed by adjuvant chemotherapy with a doxorubicin-containing regimen followed by adjuvant radiation therapy. These recommendations are based in part on the results of NSABP B-15. In this study, node-positive women with tamoxifen-nonresponsive cancers who were age 59 years or younger were randomized to 2 months of therapy with Adriamycin and cyclophosphamide versus 6 months of cyclophosphamide, methotrexate, and 5-fluorouracil (CMF). There was no difference in relapse-free survival or overall survival rates and women preferred the shorter regimen.

Neoadjuvant Chemotherapy: NSABP B-18 evaluated the role of neoadjuvant chemotherapy in women with operable stage III breast cancer. Women entered into this study were randomized to surgery followed by chemotherapy or neoadjuvant chemotherapy followed by surgery. There was no difference in the 5-year disease-free survival rate, but after neoadjuvant chemotherapy there was an increase in the number of lumpectomies performed. It was suggested that neoadjuvant chemotherapy be considered for the initial management of breast cancers judged too large for initial lumpectomy. Current recommendations for operable advanced locoregional breast cancer are neoadjuvant chemotherapy with an Adriamycin-containing regimen, followed by mastectomy or lumpectomy with axillary lymph node dissection if necessary, followed by adjuvant chemotherapy, followed by adjuvant radiation therapy. For inoperable stage IIIa and for stage IIIb breast cancer, neoadjuvant chemotherapy is used to decrease the locoregional cancer burden. This may then permit subsequent modified radical or radical mastectomy, which is followed by adjuvant chemotherapy and adjuvant radiation therapy.

Chemotherapy for Distant Metastases: For women with stage IV breast cancer, an antiestrogen (usually tamoxifen) is the preferred therapy. However, women with hormone receptor-negative cancers with symptomatic visceral metastasis or with hormone refractory cancer may receive systemic chemotherapy. Pamidronate may be given to women with osteolytic bone metastases in addition to hormonal therapy or chemotherapy. Women with metastatic breast cancer may also be enrolled into clinical trials of high-dose chemotherapy with bone marrow or peripheral blood stem cell transplantation. No survival benefit for transplantation therapy has yet been shown.

Antiestrogen therapy.   An overview analysis by the Early Breast Cancer Trialists' Collaborative Group showed that adjuvant therapy with tamoxifen produced a 25 percent reduction in the annual risk of breast cancer recurrence and a 7 percent reduction in annual breast cancer mortality. The analysis also showed a 39 percent reduction in the risk of cancer in the contralateral breast. The major advantage of tamoxifen over chemotherapy is the absence of severe toxicity. Bone pain, hot flashes, nausea, vomiting, and fluid retention may occur. Thrombotic events occur in less than 3 percent of treated women. Cataract surgery is more frequently performed in patients receiving tamoxifen. A rare long-term risk of tamoxifen use is endometrial cancer. Tamoxifen therapy usually is discontinued after 5 years.

Node-negative women with hormone receptor-positive breast cancers that are 1–3 cm in size are candidates for adjuvant tamoxifen with or without chemotherapy. For node-positive women and for all women with a cancer that is more than 3 cm in size, the use of tamoxifen in addition to adjuvant chemotherapy is appropriate. For women with stage IV breast cancer, an antiestrogen (usually tamoxifen), is the preferred initial therapy. For women with prior antiestrogen exposure, recommended second-line hormonal therapies include aromatase inhibitors in postmenopausal women and progestins, androgens, high-dose estrogen or oophorectomy (medical, surgical or radioablative) in premenopausal women. Women who respond to hormonal therapy with either shrinkage of their breast cancer or with long-term stabilization of disease receive additional hormonal therapy at the time of progression. Women with hormone receptor-negative cancers, with symptomatic visceral metastasis, or with hormone refractory disease receive systemic chemotherapy rather than hormone therapy.

Aromatase Inhibitors: In 2001, an analysis of the "Arimedex, Tamoxifen, Alone or in Combination (ATAC) Trial," showed that in postmenopausal women with estrogen receptor (ER) and/or progesterone receptor (PR) positive cancers, Anastrozole was superior to Tamoxifen for both 1) disease-free survival and 2) reduction of new primary cancers in the contralateral breast. Follow-up studies are ongoing.

Anti-HER-2/neu antibody therapy. The determination of HER-2/neu expression for all newly diagnosed patients with breast cancer is now recommended. It is used for prognostic purposes in node-negative patients; to assist in the selection of adjuvant chemotherapy because response rates appear to be better with Adriamycin-based adjuvant chemotherapy in patients with cancer that overexpress HER-2/neu; and baseline information for when the patient develops recurrent disease that may benefit from anti-HER-2/neu therapy (trastuzumab, Herceptin). Patients with cancers that overexpress HER-2/neu may benefit if trastuzumab is added to paclitaxel chemotherapy. Considerable cardiotoxicity may develop if trastuzumab is added to Adriamycin-based chemotherapy.

SPECIAL CLINICAL SITUATIONS

Nipple Discharge

Unilateral Nipple Discharge: Nipple discharge is suggestive of cancer if it is spontaneous, unilateral, localized to a single duct, occurs in women age 40 years or older, is bloody, or is associated with a mass. A trigger point on the breast may be present where pressure induces discharge from a single duct. In this circumstance, mammography is indicated. A ductogram is also useful and consists of the cannulation of a single duct with a small nylon catheter or needle and the injection of 1.0 mL of water-soluble contrast solution. Nipple discharge associated with a cancer is clear, bloody, or serous. Testing for the presence of hemoglobin is helpful, but hemoglobin may also be detected when only an intraductal papilloma or duct ectasia is present. Definitive diagnosis depends on excisional biopsy of the offending duct and any mass lesion. A 3.0 lacrimal duct probe is used to identify the duct that requires excision. Needle localization biopsy is performed when the questionable mass lies more than 3.0 cm from the nipple.

Bilateral Nipple Discharge: Nipple discharge is suggestive of a benign condition if it is bilateral and multiductal in origin, occurs in women age 39 years or younger, or is milky or blue green in color. Prolactin-secreting pituitary adenomas are responsible for bilateral nipple discharge in less than 2 percent of cases. If serum prolactin levels are repeatedly elevated, plain x-rays of the sella turcica are indicated and thin-section computed tomography (CT) scan is required. Optical nerve compression, visual field loss, and infertility are associated with large pituitary adenomas.

Axillary lymph node metastases with unknown primary cancer. A woman who presents with an axillary lymph node metastasis that is consistent with a breast cancer metastasis has a 90 percent probability of harboring an occult breast cancer. However, axillary lymphadenopathy is the initial presenting sign in only 1 percent of breast cancer patients. Fine-needle biopsy and/or open biopsy of an enlarged axillary lymph node is performed when metastatic disease cannot be excluded. When metastatic cancer is found, immunohistochemical analysis may classify the cancer as epithelial, melanocytic, or lymphoid in origin. The presence of hormone receptors suggests a breast cancer, but is not diagnostic. The search for a primary cancer includes careful examination of the thyroid, breast, and pelvis, including the rectum. Routine radiologic and laboratory studies include chest radiograph, liver function studies, and mammography. Chest, abdominal, and pelvic CT scans may be helpful. Positron emission tomography (PET) scans are also being employed. Suspicious mammography findings necessitate breast biopsy. When a breast cancer is found, treatment consists of an axillary lymph node dissection with a mastectomy or with whole-breast radiation therapy. Consideration is given to adjuvant chemotherapy and tamoxifen.

Breast cancer during pregnancy. Breast cancer occurs in 1 of every 3000 pregnant women and axillary lymph node metastases are present in up to 75 percent of these women. The average age of the pregnant woman with breast cancer is 34 years. Less than 25 percent of the breast nodules developing during pregnancy and lactation will be cancerous. Ultrasonography and needle biopsy are used in the diagnosis of these nodules. Open biopsy may be required. Mammography is rarely indicated because of its decreased sensitivity during pregnancy and lactation and because of the risk of radiation injury to the fetus. Approximately 30 percent of the benign conditions encountered will be unique to pregnancy and lactation (galactoceles, lobular hyperplasia, lactating adenoma and mastitis or abscess). Once a breast cancer is diagnosed, complete blood count (CBC), chest radiograph (with shielding of the abdomen), and liver function studies are performed.

Because of the deleterious effects of radiation therapy on the fetus, a modified radical mastectomy is the surgical procedure of choice during the first and second trimesters of pregnancy, even though there is an increased risk of spontaneous abortion following first trimester anesthesia. During the third trimester, lumpectomy with axillary node dissection is considered if adjuvant radiation therapy is deferred until after delivery. Lactation is suppressed. Chemotherapy administered during the first trimester carries a risk of spontaneous abortion and a 12 percent risk of birth defects. There is no evidence of teratogenicity resulting from administration of chemotherapeutic agents in the second and third trimesters. Pregnant women with breast cancer present at a later stage of disease because breast tissue changes that occur in the hormone-rich environment of pregnancy obscure early cancers. However, pregnant women with breast cancer have a prognosis, stage by stage, that is similar to that of nonpregnant women with breast cancer.

Male breast cancer. Less than 1 percent of all breast cancers occur in men. The incidence appears to be highest among North Americans and the British, in whom breast cancer constitutes as much as 1.5 percent of all male cancers. Jewish and African American males have the highest incidence. Male breast cancer is preceded by gynecomastia in 20 percent of men. It is associated with radiation exposure, estrogen therapy, testicular feminizing syndromes, and with Klinefelter syndrome (XXY). Breast cancer is rarely seen in young males and has a peak incidence in the sixth decade of life. A firm, nontender mass in the male breast requires investigation. Skin or chest wall fixation is particularly worrisome.

DCIS makes up less than 15 percent of male breast cancer, although infiltrating ductal carcinoma makes up more than 85 percent. Special-type cancers, including infiltrating lobular carcinoma, have only occasionally been reported. Male breast cancer is staged in an identical fashion to female breast cancer, and, stage by stage, men with breast cancer have the same survival rate as women. Overall, men do worse because of the advanced stage of their cancer (stage III or IV) at the time of diagnosis. The treatment of male breast cancer is surgical, with the most common procedure being a modified radical mastectomy. Adjuvant radiation therapy is appropriate in cases in which there is a high risk for local recurrence. Eighty percent of male breast cancers are hormone receptor-positive, and adjuvant tamoxifen is considered. Systemic chemotherapy is considered for men with hormone receptor-negative cancers and for men whose cancers relapse after tamoxifen therapy.

Phyllodes tumors. The nomenclature, presentation, and diagnosis of phyllodes tumors (including cystosarcoma phyllodes) have posed many problems for surgeons. These tumors are classified as benign, borderline, or malignant. Borderline tumors have a greater potential for local recurrence. Mammography evidence of calcifications and morphologic evidence of necrosis do not distinguish between benign, borderline, and malignant phyllodes tumors. Consequently, it is difficult to differentiate benign phyllodes tumors from the malignant variant and from fibroadenomas. Phyllodes tumors are usually sharply demarcated from the surrounding breast tissue, which is compressed and distorted. Connective tissue composes the bulk of these tumors, which have mixed gelatinous, solid, and cystic areas. Cystic areas represent sites of infarction and necrosis. These gross alterations give the gross cut tumor surface its classical leaf-like (phyllodes) appearance. The stroma of a phyllodes tumor generally has greater cellular activity than that of a fibroadenoma.

Most malignant phyllodes tumors contain liposarcomatous or rhabdomyosarcomatous elements rather than fibrosarcomatous elements. Evaluation of the number of mitoses and the presence or absence of invasive foci at the tumor margins may help to identify a malignant tumor. Small phyllodes tumors are excised with a 1-cm margin of normal-appearing breast tissue. When the diagnosis of a phyllodes tumor with suspicious malignant elements is made, re-excision of the biopsy site to insure complete excision of the tumor with a 1-cm margin of normal-appearing breast tissue is indicated. Large phyllodes tumors may require mastectomy. Axillary dissection is not recommended as axillary lymph node metastases rarely occur.

Inflammatory breast carcinoma. Inflammatory breast carcinoma (stage IIIb) accounts for less than 3 percent of breast cancers. This cancer is characterized by the skin changes of brawny induration, erythema with a raised edge, and edema (peau d'orange). Permeation of the dermal lymph vessels by cancer cells is seen in skin biopsies. There may be an associated breast mass. The clinical differentiation of inflammatory breast cancer may be extremely difficult, especially when a locally advanced scirrhous carcinoma invades dermal lymph vessels skin to produce peau d'orange and lymphangitis. Inflammatory breast cancer may also be mistaken for a bacterial infection of the breast. More than 75 percent of women afflicted with inflammatory breast cancer present with palpable axillary lymphadenopathy and frequently also have distant metastases. A report of the SEER program found distant metastases at diagnosis in 25 percent of white women with inflammatory breast carcinoma.

Surgery alone and surgery with adjuvant radiation therapy have produced disappointing results in women with inflammatory breast cancer. However, neoadjuvant chemotherapy with an Adriamycin-containing regimen may effect dramatic regressions in up to 75 percent of cases. In this setting, mastectomy, modified radical mastectomy, or radical mastectomy is performed to remove residual cancer from the chest wall and axilla. Adjuvant chemotherapy is then given. Finally, the chest wall and the supraclavicular, internal mammary, and axillary lymph node basins receive adjuvant radiation therapy. This multimodal approach results in 5-year survival rates that approach 30 percent.

Suggested Readings

The Breast: Comprehensive Management of Benign and Malignant Disorders. Bland KI, Copeland EM III (eds): Philadelphia: WB Saunders, 2004.

Beenken SW, Bland KI: Breast Cancer Genetics in C. Neal Ellis (ed) Inherited Cancer Syndromes: Current Clinical Management. New York: Springer-Verlag, 2004, p 91.

Carlson RW, Anderson BO, Bensinger W, et al: Breast cancer: Clinical practice guidelines in oncology. JNCCN 1:148, 2003.

Fletcher SW, Elmore JG: Clinical practice. Mammographic screening for breast cancer. N Engl J Med 348:1672, 2003.

Fisher B, Anderson S, Bryant J, et al: Twenty-year follow-up of a randomized trial comparing total mastectomy, lumpectomy, and lumpectomy plus irradiation for the treatment of invasive breast cancer. N Engl J Med 347:1233, 2002.

Cox CE: Lymphatic mapping in breast cancer: Combination technique. Ann Surg Oncol 8:678, 2001.

Hughes LE, Mansel RE, Webster DJT: Aberrations of normal development and involution (ANDI): A concept of benign breast disorders based on pathogenesis, in Hughes LE, Mansel RE, Webster DJT (eds): Benign Disorders and Diseases of the Breast Concepts and Clinical Management, 2nd ed. Philadelphia: WB Saunders, 2000, pp 21,73.

Fisher B, Costantino JP, Wickerham DL, et al: Tamoxifen for the prevention of breast cancer: Report of the national surgical adjuvant breast and bowel project P-1 study. J Natl Cancer Inst 90:1371, 1998.

Haagensen CD: Diseases of the Breast, 3rd ed., Philadelphia: WB Saunders, 1986.

Bloom HJG, Richardson WW, Harries EJ, et al: Natural history of untreated breast cancer (1805–1933): Comparison of untreated and treated cases according to histological grade of malignancy. Br Med J 5299:213, 1962.

17 | Disorders of the Head and Neck

Richard O. Wein, Rakesh K. Chandra, and Randal S. Weber

The head and neck is a complex anatomical region in which different pathologies may affect an individual's ability to see, smell, hear, speak, obtain nutrition and hydration, or breathe. A multidisciplinary approach to many of the disorders in this region is essential in an attempt to achieve the best functional results with care. This chapter is intended to review many of the common diagnoses encountered in the field of Otolaryngology-Head and Neck Surgery. The goal of this chapter is to provide an overview that the clinician could use as a foundation for understanding head and neck diseases. As is the case with every field of surgery, care for patients with disorders of the head and neck is constantly changing as issues of quality of life and the economics of medicine continue to evolve.

BENIGN CONDITIONS OF THE HEAD AND NECK

Ear Infections

Infections may involve the external, middle, and/or internal ear. In each of these scenarios, the infection may follow an acute or chronic course and may be associated with both otologic and intracranial complications. Note that typical pathogens of common head and neck infections are listed in Table 17-1.

Otitis externa (OE) typically refers to infection of the skin of the external auditory canal. Acute OE is commonly known as "swimmer's ear," as moisture that persists within the canal after swimming often initiates the process. This leads to skin maceration, itching, and erosion of the skin/cerumen barrier with microbial proliferation and tissue cellulitis. Infected, desquamated debris accumulates within the canal. In the chronic inflammatory stage of the infection, the pain subsides but profound itching occurs for prolonged periods with gradual thickening of the external canal skin. Standard treatment requires removal of debris under otomicroscopy and application of appropriate topical antimicrobials. Systemic antibiotics are reserved for those with severe infections, diabetics, and immunosuppressed patients. Diabetic, older adult, and immune deficient patients are susceptible to a condition called malignant OE, a fulminant necrotizing infection of the otologic soft tissues combined with osteomyelitis of the temporal bone and possible cranial neuropathies may be observed. The classic physical finding is granulation tissue along the floor of the external auditory canal. These patients require intravenous antiPseudomonas therapy and possibly surgical débridement.

Otitis media (OM), in its acute phase, typically implies a bacterial infection of the middle ear. This diagnosis accounts for 25 percent of all antibiotic prescriptions and is the most common bacterial infection of childhood. Most cases occur before age 2 years and are secondary to immaturity of the eustachian tube. Contributing factors include upper respiratory viral infection and day care attendance, and craniofacial conditions affecting eustachian tube function, such as cleft palate. Day care attendance has been further correlated with antibiotic resistant infecting organisms.

369

TABLE 17-1 Microbiology of Common Otolaryngologic Infections

Condition	Microbiology
OE and Malignant OE	*Pseudomonas aeruginosa,* fungi (aspergillus most common)
Acute OM	Pneumococcus, *Haemophilus influenzae, Moraxella catarrhalis*
Chronic OM	Bacteria of acute OM plus *Staphylococcus aureus* and epidermidis, other Streptococci. May be polymicrobial. Exact role of bacteria unclear
AS	Bacteria seen in acute OM plus viruses that cause URI
CS	Same as bacteria, of chronic OM. Some forms may also represent immune response to fungi.
Pharyngitis	Viruses of URI, *Streptococcus pyogenes,* Pneumococcus, group C and G streptococci, *Corynebacterium diptheriae, Bordatella pertussis,* syphilis, *Neisseria gonorrhea,* Candida, EBV (mononucleosis), HPV, CMV, HSV, HIV

AS = acute sinitus; CMV = cytomegalovirus; CS = coronary sinus; EBV = Epstein-Barr virus; HIV = human immunodeficiency virus; HPV = human papilloma virus; HSV = herpers simplex virus; OE = otitis externa; OM = otitis media; URI = upper respiratory infection.

Classification of the infection as acute is based on the duration of the process being less than 3 weeks. In this phase, otalgia and fever are the most common symptoms, and physical exam reveals a bulging, opaque tympanic membrane. If the process lasts 3–8 weeks, it is called subacute. Chronic OM, lasting more than 8 weeks, usually results from an unresolved acute OM. Twenty percent of patients demonstrate a persistent middle ear effusion 8 weeks after resolution of the acute phase.

Rather than a purely infectious process, however, it represents chronic inflammation and hypersecretion by the middle ear mucosa associated with eustachian tube dysfunction, viruses, allergy, ciliary dysfunction, and other factors. Physical exam reveals a retracted tympanic membrane that may exhibit an opaque character, bubbles, or an air-fluid level.

Treatment for uncomplicated OM is appropriate oral antibiotic therapy. OM following a chronic or recurrent acute pattern is frequently treated with myringotomy and tube placement to remove the effusion and ventilate the middle ear.

Tympanic membrane perforation during acute OM frequently results in resolution of severe pain and provides for drainage of purulent fluid and middle ear ventilation. These perforations usually heal spontaneously after the infection has resolved. Chronic OM, however, may be associated with nonhealing tympanic membrane perforations and persistent otorrhea. This requires surgical closure (tympanoplasty) after medical treatment (topical and/or oral antibiotics) for any residual acute infection. Chronic inflammation also may be associated with erosion of the ossicular chain and/or cholesteatoma, which is an expansile destructive epidermoid cyst of the middle ear and/or mastoid. Chronic OM also may be associated with chronic mastoiditis, which along with cholesteatoma, are indications for mastoidectomy.

Complications of OM may be grouped into two categories: intratemporal (otologic) and intracranial. Intratemporal complications include acute coalescent mastoiditis, petrositis, facial nerve paralysis, and labyrinthitis. In acute coalescing mastoiditis, destruction of the bony lamellae by an acute purulent process results in severe pain, fever, and swelling behind the ear. These diagnoses are confirmed by computed tomography (CT) scan. Facial nerve paralysis also may occur secondary to an acute inflammatory process in the middle ear or mastoid. Intratemporal complications are managed by myringotomy tube placement and appropriate intravenous (IV) antibiotics. Urgent mastoidectomy may also be necessary. Labyrinthitis refers to inflammation of the inner ear. Most cases are idiopathic or are secondary to viral infections of the endolymphatic space, but this may be bacterial (suppurative) when it complicates OM. The patient experiences vertigo with sensorineural hearing loss, and symptoms may smolder over several weeks. Acute suppurative labyrinthitis may hallmark impending meningitis and must be treated rapidly. The goal of management of inner ear infection that occurs secondary to middle ear infection is to "sterilize" the middle ear space with antibiotics and the placement of a myringotomy tube.

Meningitis is the most common intracranial complication. Otologic meningitis in children is most commonly associated with a *Haemophilus influenzae* type B infection. Other intracranial complications include epidural abscess, subdural abscess, brain abscess, otitic hydrocephalus (pseudotumor), and sigmoid sinus thrombophlebitis. The otogenic source must be urgently treated with antibiotics and myringotomy tube placement. Mastoidectomy and neurosurgical consultation may be necessary.

Bell palsy, or idiopathic facial paralysis, may be considered within the spectrum of otologic disease given the facial nerve's course through the temporal bone. This entity is the most common etiology of facial nerve paralysis and is clinically distinct from that occurring as a complication of OM in that the otologic exam is normal. Historically, Bell palsy was synonymous with "idiopathic" facial paralysis. It is now accepted, however, that the majority of these cases represent a viral neuropathy cased by herpes simplex. Treatment includes oral steroids plus antiviral therapy. Complete recovery is the norm, but does not occur universally, and selected cases may benefit from surgical decompression of the nerve within its bony canal. Varicella zoster virus may also cause facial nerve paralysis when the virus reactivates from dormancy in the nerve. This condition, known as Ramsey-Hunt syndrome, is characterized by severe otalgia followed by the eruption of vesicles of the external ear. Treatment is similar to Bell palsy, but full recovery is only seen in approximately two-thirds of cases.

Sinus Inflammatory Disease

Sinusitis is a clinical diagnosis based on patient signs and symptoms. The Task Force on Rhinosinusitis has established criteria to define "a history consistent with sinusitis." To qualify for the diagnosis, the patient must exhibit at least two major factors or one major and two minor factors. Major factors include congestion, nasal drainage, smell loss, and facial pressure, although minor factors include nonspecific symptoms such as headache, tooth pain, bad breath, and otalgia. The classification of sinusitis as acute, subacute, or chronic is based on the time course over which those criteria have been met. If signs and symptoms are present for 7–10 days but less than 4 weeks, the process is designated acute sinusitis (AS). Sub-AS has been present for 4–12 weeks, and chronic sinusitis (CS) is diagnosed when the patient has had signs and symptoms for at least 12 weeks. In the setting of the appropriate clinical signs/symptoms, the diagnosis may be confirmed by CT, which can demonstrate mucosal thickening and/or sinus opacification. The diagnosis should be established by history and endoscopy, rather than CT alone.

AS typically follows a viral upper respiratory infection (URI) whereby sinonasal mucosal inflammation results in closure of the sinus ostium. This results in stasis of secretions, tissue hypoxia, and ciliary dysfunction. These conditions promote bacterial proliferation and acute inflammation. The mainstay of treatment is oral antibiotics empirically directed toward the three most common organisms. Other treatments include topical and systemic decongestants, nasal saline spray, topical nasal steroids, and oral steroids in selected cases. In the acute setting, surgery is reserved for complications or pending complications, which may include extension to the eye (orbital cellulitis or abscess) or the intracranial space (meningitis, intracranial abscess). Strictly speaking, the viral URI induces acute sinus inflammation. As an effort to exclude common colds from receiving antibiotic therapy, the criteria for AS stipulate that symptoms be present for at least 7–10 days, by which time the common cold should be in a resolution phase.

CS represents a heterogeneous group of patients with multifactorial etiologies contributing to ostial obstruction, ciliary dysfunction, and inflammation. Components of genetic predisposition, allergy, anatomic obstruction, bacterial, fungal, and environmental factors play varying roles, depending on the individual patient. As of yet, no immunologic "final common pathway" has been defined, but the clinical picture is well described. CS also may be associated with nasal polyps, which are manifestations of longstanding mucosal inflammatory disease. Polyps themselves may block sinus outflow, further exacerbating microbial proliferation. Nasal endoscopy is a critical element of the diagnosis of CS. Anatomic abnormalities, such as septal deviation, nasal polyps, and purulence may be observed. Pus found on endoscopic exam is diagnostic alone. This may be cultured, and subsequent antibiotic therapy can be directed accordingly. The spectrum of bacteria found in CS is variable, and antibiotic resistance is rising. Medical management of CS includes a prolonged course of oral antibiotics (>3 weeks), oral steroids, and nasal irrigations with saline or antibiotic solutions. Underlying allergic disease is managed with antihistamines and possible allergy immunotherapy. Those failing medical management are candidates for elective endoscopic sinus surgery, in which the goals are to enlarge the natural sinus ostia and to remove chronically infected bone to promote both ventilation and drainage of the sinus cavities.

The role of fungi in sinusitis is an area of active investigation. Fungal sinusitis may take on both noninvasive and invasive forms. The former category includes fungal ball ("mycetoma") and allergic fungal sinusitis, both of which occur in immunocompetent patients. Fungal ball usually consists of Aspergillus and is associated with only scant inflammatory changes. In contrast allergic fungal sinusitis involves brisk chronic hypersensitivity reactions to fungal antigens within the nose and sinuses. The exact immunologic mechanisms involved are a matter of debate. Endoscopic evaluation reveals florid polyposis and inspissated mucin containing fungal debris and products of eosinophil breakdown. The implicated organisms are usually those of the Dematiaceae family, but Aspergillus species also are seen. These conditions are treated surgically, but systemic steroids and topical (and occasionally systemic) antifungals also are indicated in allergic fungal sinusitis. Rarely, immunocompetent patients also may develop an indolent form of invasive fungal sinusitis, but more commonly, invasive fungal sinusitis affects immunocompromised patients, diabetics, or the very older adult. Fungal invasion of the microvasculature causes ischemic necrosis and black, necrotic escharation of the sinonasal mucosa. Aspergillus and fungi of the Mucoreciae family are often implicated with the latter more common in diabetics. Treatment requires aggressive surgical débridement and IV antifungals, but the prognosis is nonetheless dismal.

Pharyngeal and Adenotonsillar Disease

Infectious pharyngitis, in the vast majority of cases, is viral rather than bacterial in origin. Most cases resolve, without complication, from supportive care and possibly antibiotics. Patients with tonsillitis present with sore throat, dysphagia, and fever. Tonsillar exudates and cervical adenitis may be seen when the etiology is bacterial. If adenoiditis is present, the symptoms may be similar to those of sinusitis, but visual evaluation of the adenoid, at least in children, requires endoscopy and/or imaging (lateral neck soft tissue radiograph). Tonsillitis and adenoiditis may follow acute, recurrent acute, and chronic temporal patterns. It should be noted, however, that clinical diagnosis is often inaccurate to determine whether the process is bacterially induced and thus requires antibiotics. When a bacterial cause is suspected, antibiotics should be initiated to cover the usual organisms, particularly group A beta hemolytic streptococci (Streptococcus pyogenes). Currently, rapid antigen assays for group A streptococci are available with sensitivity and specificity of approximately 85 and 90 percent, respectively. Complications of Streptococcus pyogenes pharyngitis may be systemic, including rheumatic fever (3 percent), poststreptococcal glomerulonephritis, and scarlet fever. Locoregional complications of include peritonsillar abscess, and rarely, deep neck space abscess. These conditions require surgical incision and drainage. Peritonsillar abscess may be drained transorally, and some report that needle aspiration without incision is sufficient. Deep neck space abscess, which more commonly is odontogenic in origin, usually requires external incision and drainage.

Obstructive adenotonsillar hyperplasia may present with nasal obstruction, rhinorrhea, voice changes, dysphagia, and sleep disordered breathing or obstructive sleep apnea, depending on the particular foci of lymphoid tissue involved. Adenotonsillar hypertrophy may be associated with sleep disorders, which exist on a continuum from simple snoring to upper airway resistance syndrome (UARS) to obstructive sleep apnea (OSA). UARS and OSA are associated with excessive daytime somnolence and frequent sleep arousals. Polysomnography to quantify the number of apneas, hypopneas, and oxygen desaturations can be used to grade the severity.

Tonsillectomy and adenoidectomy are indicated for chronic or recurrent acute infection and for obstructive hypertrophy. Multiple techniques have been described including electrocautery, sharp dissection, laser, and radiofrequency ablation. There is no consensus regarding the best method. In cases of chronic or recurrent infection, surgery is considered only after failure of medical therapy. Patients with recurrent peritonsillar abscess should undergo tonsillectomy when the acute inflammatory changes have resolved. Selected cases, however, require tonsillectomy in the acute setting for the management of severe inflammation, systemic toxicity, or impending airway compromise. Adenoidectomy may benefit selected children with chronic or recurrent OM to lower the bacterial burden and to decompress the eustachian tube. The primary complications of adenotonsillectomy include bleeding (3–5 percent), airway obstruction, velopharyngeal insufficiency, pharyngeal stenosis, death, and readmission for dehydration secondary to postoperative dysphagia.

In addition to adenotonsillectomy, surgery for sleep-disordered breathing may include uvulopalatopharyngoplasty, tongue base reduction, tongue advancement, hyoid suspension, and a variety of maxillomandibular advancement procedures, depending on the sites of airway collapse. Adults with significant nasal obstruction may benefit from septoplasty or sinus surgery. Patients with severe OSA with unfavorable anatomy or comorbid pulmonary disease may require tracheotomy. Prior to surgery, these patients should be given a trial of nocturnal continuous positive airway pressure (CPAP).

Benign Conditions of the Larynx

Disorders of voice may affect a wide array of patients with respect to age, gender, and socioeconomic status. The principal symptom of these disorders, at least when a mass lesion is present, is hoarseness. Other vocal manifestations include hypophonia or aphonia, breathiness, and pitch breaks. Benign laryngeal disorders also may be associated with airway obstruction, dysphagia, and reflux. Smoking also may be a risk factor for benign disease, but this element of the history should raise the index of suspicion for malignancy.

Recurrent respiratory papillomatosis (RRP) reflects involvement of human papilloma virus (HPV) within the mucosal epithelium of the upper aerodigestive tract. The larynx is the most frequently involved site, and subtypes 6 and 11 are the most often implicated. The disorder typically presents in the early childhood, secondary to viral acquisition during vaginal delivery. Many cases resolve after puberty, but the disorder may progresses into adulthood. The diagnosis can be established with office endoscopy. Currently, there is no "cure" for RRP. The treatment involves operative microlaryngoscopy with excision or laser ablation, and the natural history is eventual recurrence. Multiple procedures are typically required over the patient's lifetime.

Laryngeal granulomas typically occur in the posterior larynx on the arytenoid mucosa and develop secondary to multiple factors including reflux, voice abuse, chronic throat clearing, endotracheal intubation, and vocal fold paralysis. Effective management requires identification of the underlying cause(s). Patients report pain (often with swallowing) more commonly than vocal changes. In addition to fiberoptic laryngoscopy, workup may include voice analysis, laryngeal electromyography (EMG), and pH probe testing.

Edema in the superficial lamina propria of the vocal cord (VC) is known as polypoid corditis, polypoid laryngitis, polypoid degeneration of the VC, or Reinke edema. The superficial lamina propria just underlies the vibratory epithelial surface. Edema (usually bilateral) is thought to arise from injury to the capillaries that exist in this layer, with subsequent extravasation of fluid. Patients report progressive development of a rough, low-pitched voice. Females more commonly present for medical attention. The etiology is also multifactorial, and may involve smoking, laryngopharyngeal reflux, hypothyroidism, and vocal hyperfunction. Most of these patients are heavy smokers.

Focal, unilateral hemorrhagic VC polyps are more common in men. These occur secondary to capillary rupture within the mucosa by shearing forces during voice abuse. Use of anticoagulant or antiplatelet drugs may be a risk factor.

Cysts may occur under the laryngeal mucosa, particularly in regions containing mucous-secreting glands, such as the supraglottic larynx. Occasionally they derive from minor salivary glands, and congenital cysts may persist as remnants of the branchial arch. Cysts of the VC may be difficult to distinguish from vocal polyps, and video stroboscopic laryngoscopy may be necessary to help establish the diagnosis. Although benign VC lesions may be treated via microsurgical laryngoscopic techniques, first-line modalities that may be employed include voice rest, voice retraining, and antireflux therapy. When maximal reflux therapy has failed, fundoplication may be indicated.

Leukoplakia of the vocal fold represents a white patch (which cannot be wiped off) on the mucosal surface, usually on the superior surface of the true VC. Rather than a diagnosis per se, the term describes a clinical finding. The significance of leukoplakia is that it may represent squamous hyperplasia, dysplasia, and/or carcinoma. Lesions exhibiting hyperplasia have a 1–3 percent risk of progression to malignancy, although that risk is 10–30 percent for dysplastic lesions. Ulceration, erythroplasia, or a history of smoking/alcohol abuse suggests possible malignancy, and excision is indicated. In the absence of risk factors, conservative measures are employed for 1 month. Any lesions that progress, persist, or recur should be considered for excision.

VC paralysis is most commonly iatrogenic in origin, following surgery to the thyroid, parathyroid, carotid, or cardiothoracic structures. This may also be secondary to malignant processes in the lungs, thoracic cavity, skull base, or neck. In the pediatric population, up to one fourth of cases may be neurologic, with Arnold-Chiari malformation being the most common. Overall, the left VC is more commonly involved secondary to course of the left recurrent laryngeal nerve into the thoracic cavity. The cause remains idiopathic in up to 20 percent of adults and 35 percent of children. These cases should prompt an imaging work-up to examine the skull base to the aortic arch on the left and from skull base to the subclavian on the right to rule out neoplasms of the lung, thyroid, or esophagus. Adults typically present with hoarseness, and the voice may be breathy if the contralateral VC has not compensated to close the glottic valve, in which case aspiration also is possible. Children may have a weak cry. Flexible fiberoptic laryngoscopy usually confirms the diagnosis, but laryngeal EMG may be necessary. In bilateral VC paralysis, the cords often are paralyzed in a paramedian position, creating airway compromise that necessitates tracheotomy. Treatment of unilateral VC paralysis includes speech therapy, and some patients do well with this modality alone. Medialization of the paralyzed vocal fold is performed to provide a surface on which the contralateral normal fold may make contact. This can be accomplished via injection or implantation of a variety of autologous (fat, collagen) or alloplastic (hydroxylapatite, silicone, Gore-Tex) compounds. Autologous materials are preferred. This technique also is useful for VC atrophy, which may occur with aging.

Trauma of the Head and Neck

Management of soft tissue trauma in the head and neck has several salient features. Wound closure must be understood in the context of the cosmetic and functional anatomic landmarks of the head and neck. Management of injuries to the eyelid requires identification of the orbicularis oculi, which is closed in a separate layer. The gray line must be carefully approximated to avoid lid notching or height mismatch. Management of lip injuries follows the same principle. The orbicularis oris must be closed, and the vermilion border carefully approximated. Injuries involving one fourth of the width of the eyelid or one-third the width of the lip may be closed primarily. Otherwise, flap or grafting procedures may be required. With laceration of the auricle, key structures like the helical rim and antihelix must be carefully aligned with care to assure cartilage is covered. Cartilage has no intrinsic blood supply and thus is susceptible to ischemic necrosis following trauma. Thus auricular hematomas must be drained promptly, with placement of a bolster as a pressure dressing. Similarly, nasal septal hematomas require early drainage. The surgeon must avoid the temptation to perform aggressive débridement of facial soft tissues as many soft tissue components that appear devitalized will indeed survive secondary to healthy blood supply in this region.

Soft tissue injuries occurring in the midface may involve distal facial nerve branches. Those injured anterior to a vertical line dropped from the lateral canthus do not require repair secondary to collateral innervation in the anterior midface. Posterior to this line, the nerve should be repaired microscopically using 8-0–10-0 monofilament suture to approximate the epineurium. If neural segments are missing, cable grafting is performed using either the greater auricular (provides 7–8 cm) or sural nerve (up to 30 cm). Injuries to the buccal branch should alert the examiner to a possible parotid duct injury, which lies on a line drawn from the tragus to the midline upper lip. The duct should be repaired over a 22G stent or marsupialized into the oral cavity.

The mandible is the most commonly fractured facial bone. Fractures most often involve the angle, body, or condyle, and 2 or more sites are typically involved. Fractures are described as either favorable or unfavorable depending in whether or not the masticatory musculature tends to pull the fracture into reduction or distraction. The fracture is usually evaluated radiographically using a Panorex, but specialized plain film views and occasionally CT scan are necessary in selected cases. Classical management of mandible fractures dictated closed reduction and a 6-week period of intermaxillary fixation (IMF), with arch bars applied via circumdental wiring. Currently, arch bars and IMF are performed to establish occlusion. The fracture is then exposed and reduced, using transoral approaches where possible. Rigid fixation is then accomplished by the application of plates and screws. IMF has been associated with gingival and dental disease, and significant weight loss and malnutrition during the fixation period. Malocclusion is a longer-term complication. Edentulous patients may require refashioning of their dentures once healing in complete.

Classical signs of midface fractures in general include subconjunctival hemorrhage, malocclusion, midface numbness or hypesthesia (maxillary division of the trigeminal nerve), facial ecchymoses/hematoma, ocular signs/symptoms, and mobility of the maxillary complex. These fractures are classically described in three patterns: LeForte I, II, and III. Type I crosses the alveolus, type II passes obliquely through the maxillary sinus, and type III reflects craniofacial disjunction. Realistically, midface fractures comprise combinations of these three types. Zygoma fractures may involve the malar area and/or arch and may be associated with an orbital blowout fracture. Blowout may result in enophthalmos or entrapment of the inferior oblique muscle with diplopia on upward gaze. Fractures of the midface, zygoma, and orbital floor are best evaluated using CT scan, and repair requires a combination of transoral and external approaches to achieve at least two points of fixation for each fractured segment. Blowout fractures demonstrating significant entrapment or enophthalmos are treated by orbital exploration and reinforcement of the floor with mesh or bone grafting.

Temporal bone fractures occur in approximately one-fifth of skull fractures and blunt trauma is usually implicated. Fractures are divided into two patterns, longitudinal and transverse, but in practice, most are oblique. By classical descriptions, longitudinal fractures comprise 80 percent and are associated with lateral skull trauma. Signs and symptoms include conductive hearing loss, ossicular injury, bloody otorrhea, and labyrinthine concussion. The facial nerve is injured in approximately 20 percent of cases. In contrast, the transverse pattern comprises only 20 percent of temporal bone fractures and occurs secondary to fronto-occipital trauma. The facial nerve is injured in 50 percent of cases. Transverse injuries frequently involve the otic capsule to cause sensorineural hearing loss and loss of vestibular function. Hemotympanum may be observed. A cerebrospinal fluid (CSF) leak must be suspected in temporal bone trauma. This resolves with conservative measures in most cases. The most significant consideration in the management of temporal bone injuries is the status of the facial nerve. Delayed or partial paralysis will almost always resolve with conservative management. Patients with immediate complete paralysis or with unfavorable electrophysiologic testing should be considered for surgical decompression when medically stable. It is of paramount importance to protect the eye in patients with facial nerve paralysis of any etiology, as absence of an intact blink reflex will predispose to corneal drying and abrasion. This requires the placement of artificial tears throughout the day, with lubricant ointment, eye taping, and/or a humidity chamber at night.

TUMORS OF THE HEAD AND NECK

When a discussion of neoplasms of the upper aerodigestive tract is initiated frequently the conversation focuses on squamous cell carcinoma. This is justifiable because the majority of malignancies of this region are represented by this pathology. The evaluation of local, regional, and distant spread of tumor and the selection of treatment protocols vary for each site within the head and neck.

Etiology and Epidemiology

Abuse of tobacco and alcohol are the most common preventable risk factors associated with the development of head and neck cancers. Individuals who both smoke (2 packs per day) and drink (4 units of alcohol per day) had an odds ratio of 35 for the development of a carcinoma compared to controls. Users of smokeless tobacco have a four times increased risk of oral cavity carcinoma when compared to nonusers.

Tobacco is the leading preventable cause of death in the United States and is responsible for 1 out of every 5 deaths. Recent trends have demonstrated an increase in the use of tobacco products by women and the long-term affects have yet to be realized. The evidence supporting the need for head and neck cancer patients to pursue smoking cessation after treatment is compelling. Forty-percent of patients that continue to smoke after treatment went on to recur or develop a second head and neck malignancy. Induction of specific p53 mutations within upper aerodigestive tract tumors have been noted in patients with histories of tobacco and alcohol use.

In India and Southeast Asia the product of the Areca catechu tree, known as a betel nut, is chewed in a habitual manner in combination with lime and cured tobacco as a mixture known as a quid. The long-term use of the betel nut quid is destructive to oral mucosa and is highly carcinogenic.

Environmental ultraviolet light exposure has been associated with the development of lip cancer. The projection of the lower lip, as it relates to this solar exposure, has been used to explain why the majority of squamous cell carcinomas arise along the vermilion border of the lower lip.

TABLE 17-2 TNM Staging for Oral Cavity Carcinoma

Primary tumor	
TX	Unable to assess primary tumor
T0	No evidence of primary tumor
Tis	Carcinoma in situ
T1	Tumor is <2 cm in greatest dimension
T2	Tumor >2 cm and <4 cm in greatest dimension
T3	Tumor >4 cm in greatest dimension
T4 (lip)	Primary tumor invading cortical bone, inferior alveolar nerve, floor of mouth, or skin of face (e.g., nose or chin)
T4a (oral)	Tumor invades adjacent structures (e.g., cortical bone, into deep tongue musculature, maxillary sinus) or skin of face
T4b (oral)	Tumor invades masticator space, pterygoid plates, or skull base and/or encases the internal carotid artery

Regional lymphadenopathy	
NX	Unable to assess regional lymph nodes
N0	No evidence of regional metastasis
N1	Metastasis in a single ipsilateral lymph node, 3 cm or less in greatest dimension
N2a	Metastasis in single ipsilateral lymph node, >3 cm and <6 cm
N2b	Metastasis in multiple ipsilateral lymph nodes, all nodes <6 cm
N2c	Metastasis in bilateral or contralateral lymph nodes, all nodes <6 cm
N3	Metastasis in a lymph node >6 cm in greatest dimension

Distant metastases	
MX	Unable to assess for distant metastases
M0	No distant metastases
M1	Distant metastases

TMN staging			
Stage 0	Tis	N0	M0
Stage I	T1	N0	M0
Stage II	T2	N0	M0
Stage III	T3	N0	M0
	T1-3	N1	M0
Stage IVa	T4a	N0	M0
	T4a	N1	M0
	T1-4a	N2	M0
Stage IVb	Any T	N3	M0
	T4b	Any N	M0
Stage IVc	Any T	Any N	M1

Source: American Joint Committee on Cancer Staging Manual, 6th ed.[51]

Staging

Staging for upper aerodigestive tract malignancies is defined by the American Joint Committee on Cancer (AJCC) and follows TNM (primary Tumor, regional Nodal metastases, distant Metastasis) staging format. The T staging criteria for each site varies depending on the relevant anatomy. Table 17-2 demonstrates TNM staging for oral cavity lesions.

UPPER AERODIGESTIVE TRACT

Lip

The majority of lip malignancies present on the lower lip (88–98 percent), followed by the upper lip (2–7 percent) and oral commissure (1 percent). The histology of lip cancers is predominantly squamous cell carcinoma, however, other tumors such as keratoacanthoma, verrucous carcinoma, basal cell carcinoma, malignant melanoma, minor salivary gland malignancies and tumors of mesenchymal origin (e.g., malignant fibrous histiocytoma) also may present in this location. Basal cell carcinoma presents disproportionately more frequently on the upper lip than lower.

Clinical findings in lip cancer include an ulcerated lesion on the vermilion or cutaneous surface or, less commonly, on the mucosal surface. A nodular or sclerotic lesion may be palpable within the deeper tissues. The presence of paresthesias in the area adjacent to the lesion may indicate mental nerve involvement.

Small primary lesions may be treated with surgery or radiation with equal success and acceptable cosmetic results. However, surgical excision with histologic confirmation of tumor-free margins is the preferred modality. The overall 5-year cure rate of lip cancer approximates 90 percent and drops to 50 percent in the presence of neck metastases. Postoperative radiation is administered to the primary site and neck for patients with close or positive margins, lymph node metastases, or perineural invasion.

The reconstruction of lip defects after tumor excision requires innovative techniques to provide oral competence, maintenance of dynamic function, and acceptable cosmesis. The typical lip length is 6–7 cm. Resection with primary closure is possible with a defect of up to one-third of the lip. When the resection includes one third to one half of the lip, techniques such as Burow triangles in combination with advancement flaps or an Abbe-Estlander flap can be considered. For larger defects of up to 75 percent, the Karapandzic flap uses a sensate, neuromuscular flap that includes the remaining orbicularis oris muscle, conserving its blood supply from branches of the labial artery. Microstoma is a potential complication with these types of lip reconstruction. For very large defects, Webster or Bernard types of repair using lateral nasolabial flaps with buccal advancement have been described as well.

Oral Cavity

The oral cavity is composed of several sites with different anatomic relationships. The majority of tumors in the oral cavity are squamous cell carcinomas (>90 percent). Each site is briefly reviewed with emphasis placed on anatomy, diagnosis, and treatment options.

Oral Tongue

The oral tongue is a muscular structure with overlying nonkeratinizing squamous epithelium. The posterior limit of the oral tongue is the circumvallate papillae, whereas its ventral portion is contiguous with the anterior floor of mouth. Tumors of the tongue begin in the stratified epithelium of the surface and eventually invade into the deeper muscular structures. The presentation is commonly an ulcerated or exophytic mass. The lingual nerve and the hypoglossal nerve may be invaded directly by tumors. Their involvement produces the clinical findings of loss of sensation of the dorsal tongue surface, deviation on tongue protrusion, fasciculations, and atrophy.

Surgical treatment of small (T1–T2) primary tumors is wide local excision with either primary closure or healing by secondary intention. A partial glossectomy, which removes a significant portion of the lateral oral tongue, permits reasonably effective postoperative function. Resection of larger tumors of the tongue that invade deeply can result in significant functional impairment in speech and swallowing function. The use of soft pliable fasciocutaneous free flaps can provide intraoral bulk and preservation of tongue mobility. Treatment of the regional lymphatics is typically performed with the modality used to address the primary site, which most frequently is via modified radical or selective neck dissection. Depth of invasion of the primary tumor can direct the need for elective lymph node dissection with early stage lesions.

Floor of Mouth

The floor of mouth is the mucosally covered semilunar area that extends from the anterior tonsillar pillar posteriorly to the frenulum anteriorly and from the inner surface of the mandible to the ventral surface of the oral tongue. The ostia of the submandibular and sublingual glands are contained in the anterior floor of mouth.

Anterior or lateral extension of tumor to the mandibular periosteum is of primary importance in preoperative treatment planning for these lesions. Deep invasion into the intrinsic musculature of the tongue causes fixation and mandates a partial glossectomy in conjunction with resection of the floor of mouth. Lesions in the anterior floor of mouth may directly invade the sublingual gland or submandibular duct and require resection of either of these glands in continuity with the primary lesion.

The resection of large tumors of the floor of mouth may require a lip-splitting incision and usually require immediate reconstruction. The goals are to obtain watertight closure to avoid a salivary fistula and to avoid tongue tethering to maximize mobility. For small mucosal lesions, wide local excision can be followed by placement of a split-thickness skin graft over the muscular bed. Larger defects that require marginal or segmental mandibulectomy require complex reconstruction with a fasciocutaneous or a vascularized bone flap.

Alveolus/Gingiva

The alveolar mucosa overlies the bone of the mandible and maxilla. It extends from the gingivobuccal sulcus to the mucosa of the floor of mouth and hard palate. Because of the tight attachment of the alveolar mucosa to the mandibular and maxillary periosteum, treatment of lesions of the alveolar mucosa frequently require resection of the underlying bone.

Marginal resection of the mandible can be performed for tumors of the alveolar surface that are associated with minimal bone invasion. Access for such a procedure can be performed using an anterior mandibulotomy, however, use of transoral and pull-through procedures are preferred if a coronal or sagittal marginal mandibulotomy is performed. For more extensive tumors that invade into the medullary cavity, segmental mandibulectomy is necessary.

Preoperative radiographic evaluation of the mandible plays an important role in determining the type of bone resection required. Sectional CT scanning with bone settings is the optimum modality for imaging subtle cortical invasion.

Retromolar Trigone

The retromolar trigone is represented by tissue posterior to inferior alveolar ridge and ascends over the inner surface of the ramus of the mandible. Similar to alveolar lesions, early involvement of the mandible is common because of the lack of intervening soft tissue in the region. Presentation of trismus may indicate muscle of mastication involvement and potential spread to the skull base. Resection of retromolar trigone tumors usually requires a marginal or segmental mandibulectomy with a soft tissue and/or osseous reconstruction. Ipsilateral elective and therapeutic neck dissection is performed because of the risk of metastasis to the regional lymphatics.

Buccal Mucosa

The buccal mucosa includes all of the mucosal lining from the inner surface of the lips to the line of attachment of mucosa of the alveolar ridges and pterygo-mandibular raphe. Tumors in this area have a propensity to spread locally and to metastasize to regional lymphatics. Local intraoral spread may necessitate resection of the alveolar ridge of the mandible or maxilla. Lymphatic drainage is to the facial and the submandibular nodes (Level I). Small lesions can be excised surgically, but more advanced tumors require combined surgery and postoperative radiation. Deep invasion into the cheek may require through-and-through resection. Ideal reconstruction to provide both internal and external lining is best accomplished with a folded fasciocutaneous free flap.

Palate

The hard palate extends from the inner surface of the superior alveolar ridge to the posterior edge of the palatine bone. Inflammatory lesions arising on the palate may mimic malignancy and can be differentiated by biopsy. Necrotizing sialometaplasia appears on the palate as a butterfly shaped ulcer and mimics carcinoma. Treatment is symptomatic and biopsy confirms its benign nature.

Squamous cell carcinoma and minor salivary gland tumors are the most common malignancies of the palate. Minor salivary gland tumors tend to arise at the junction of the hard and soft palate.

Squamous carcinoma of the hard palate is treated surgically. Adjuvant radiation is indicated for advanced staged tumors. Because the periosteum of the palate bones acts as a barrier to spread, mucosal excision may be adequate for very superficial lesions. Involvement of the periosteum requires removal of a portion of the bony palate. Partial or subtotal maxillectomy is required for larger lesions or those involving the maxillary antrum. Malignancies may extend along the greater palatine nerve making biopsy important for identifying neurotropic spread. Through-and-through defects of the palate require a dental prosthesis for rehabilitation of swallowing and speech.

Oropharynx

The oropharynx extends from the soft palate to the superior surface of the hyoid bone (or floor of the vallecula) and includes the base of tongue, the inferior surface of the soft palate and uvula, the anterior and posterior tonsillar pillars, the pharyngeal tonsils, and the lateral and posterior pharyngeal walls.

The histology of the majority of tumors in this region is squamous cell carcinoma. Although less common, minor salivary gland tumors may present as submucosal masses in the tongue base and palate. The palatine and lingual tonsils of Waldeyer ring may be the presenting site of a lymphoma noted as an asymmetrically enlarged tonsil or tongue base mass.

Oropharyngeal cancer usually presents as an ulcerated, exophytic mass. Tumor fetor from tumor necrosis is common. A muffled or "hot potato" voice is seen with large tongue base tumors. Dysphagia and weight loss are common symptoms. Referred otalgia, mediated by the tympanic branches of CN IX and CN X, is a common complaint. The incidence of regional metastases from cancers of the tongue base and other oropharyngeal sites is high. Consequently, a neck metastasis is a frequent presenting sign.

The treatment goals for patients with oropharyngeal cancer include maximizing survival and preserving function. Management of squamous cancers of this region includes surgery alone, primary radiation alone, surgery with postoperative radiation, and combined chemotherapy with radiation therapy. Many tumors of the oropharynx are poorly differentiated squamous cell carcinoma and tend to be radiosensitive. Early stage lesions, T1 and T2, may be eradicated with radiation alone or combination chemoradiation.

Tumors of the soft palate and tonsil extending to the tongue base are associated with poorer survival. Extensive oropharyngeal cancers that are infiltrative usually are managed with surgical resection and postoperative radiotherapy. Lesions that involve the mandible or its periosteum require composite resections, such as the classic jaw-neck resection or "commando" procedure. Tongue base involvement requires at least partial glossectomy, with the possibility of total glossectomy for lesions crossing the midline. Preservation of the larynx after total glossectomy is associated with the risk of postoperative aspiration and dysphagia.

Hypopharynx and Cervical Esophagus

The hypopharynx extends from the vallecula to the lower border of the cricoid cartilage and includes the pyriform sinuses, the lateral and posterior pharyngeal walls, and the postcricoid region. Squamous cancers of the hypopharynx frequently present at an advanced stage. Clinical findings are similar to those of lower oropharyngeal lesions and include a neck mass, muffled or hoarse voice, referred otalgia, dysphagia, and weight loss. A common symptom is dysphagia, starting with solids and progressing to liquids, leaving patients malnourished and catabolic at the time of presentation. Invasion of the larynx by direct extension can result in vocal cord paresis or paralysis and potential airway compromise.

Routine office examination should include flexible fiberoptic laryngoscopy to properly assess the extent of tumor. Barium swallow can provide information regarding postcricoid and upper esophageal extension, potential multifocality within the esophagus, and document the presence of aspiration. CT or magnetic resonance imaging (MRI) should be obtained through the neck and upper chest to assess for invasion of the laryngeal framework and to identify for regional metastases with special attention given to the paratracheal and upper mediastinal nodes.

Tumors of the hypopharynx and cervical esophagus are associated with poorer survival than other sites in the head and neck because of advanced primary stage and lymph node metastasis at presentation. Definitive radiation therapy is effective for smaller T1–T2 tumors. Surgery with postoperative radiation therapy has been shown to improve locoregional control compared to single modality therapy in the treatment of advanced stage tumors. Surgical salvage after radiation failure has a success rate of less than 50 percent and can be associated with significant wound-healing complications. Because the majority of patients with tumors of the hypopharynx present with large lesions and significant submucosal spread, total laryngectomy often is required to achieve adequate margins.

When laryngopharyngectomy is performed for hypopharyngeal tumors the surgical defect is preferentially repaired by primary closure when possible. Generally, 4 cm or more of pharyngeal mucosa is necessary for primary closure to provide an adequate lumen for swallowing and to minimize the risk of stricture formation. Larger surgical defects require closure with the aid of pedicled myocutaneous flaps or microvascular reconstruction with radial forearm or jejunal free flap. When total laryngopharyngoesophagectomy is necessary, gastric pull-up reconstruction is performed.

Organ preservation for hypopharyngeal cancer using a platinum-based chemotherapy with radiation has resulted in a laryngeal preservation rate of 30 percent. Diminished locoregional control rates have been observed when compared to surgery and postoperative radiation. No decrease was noted in the rate distant metastases.

For the most part, cervical esophageal cancer is managed surgically. Preservation of the larynx has been described if the cricopharyngeus muscle is not involved. Unfortunately, this is not often the case and many patients with cervical esophageal cancer require a laryngectomy. Total esophagectomy is performed because of the tendency for multiple primary tumors and skip lesions seen with esophageal cancers. Recently, chemotherapy and external beam radiotherapy with and without surgery have been advocated.

Despite aggressive treatment strategies, 5-year survival for cervical esophageal cancer is less than 20 percent. Because of the presence of paratracheal lymphatic disease, surgical treatment for tumors of this area must include paratracheal lymph node dissection in addition to treatment of the lateral cervical lymphatics.

Larynx

Laryngeal carcinoma is a diagnosis typically entertained in individuals with prominent smoking histories and the complaint of a prolonged hoarse voice. The larynx is composed of three regions: the supraglottis, the glottis, and the subglottis.

The supraglottis includes the epiglottis, aryepiglottic folds, arytenoids, and ventricular bands (false vocal folds). The inferior boundary of the supraglottis is a horizontal plane passing through the lateral margin of the ventricle. The glottis is composed of the true vocal cords (superior and inferior surfaces) and includes the anterior and posterior commissures. The subglottis extends from the inferior surface of the glottis to the lower margin of the cricoid cartilage.

The normal functions of the larynx are airway patency, protection of the tracheobronchial tree during swallowing, and phonation. Patients with tumors of the supraglottic larynx may present with symptoms of chronic sore throat, dysphonia ("hot potato" voice), dysphagia, or a neck mass secondary to regional metastasis. Referred otalgia or odynophagia is encountered with advanced supraglottic cancers. Large bulky tumors of the supraglottis may result in airway compromise. In contrast to most supraglottic lesions, hoarseness is an early symptom in patients with tumors of the glottis. Airway obstruction from a glottic tumor is usually a late symptom and is the result of tumor bulk or impaired vocal cord mobility. Decreased vocal cord mobility may be caused by direct laryngeal muscle invasion or involvement of the recurrent laryngeal nerve. Superficial tumors that are bulky may appear to cause cord fixation through mass effect. Subglottic cancers are relatively uncommon and typically present with laryngeal paralysis (usually unilateral), stridor, and/or pain.

The staging classification for squamous cancers of the larynx includes assessment of vocal cord mobility and the sites of tumor extension. Accurate clinical staging of laryngeal tumors requires fiberoptic endoscopy in the office and direct laryngoscopy of the larynx under general anesthesia. Direct laryngoscopy, used to assess the extent of local spread, may be combined with esophagoscopy or bronchoscopy to adequately stage the primary tumor and to exclude the presence of a synchronous lesion.

Radiographic imaging by CT or MRI provides important staging information and is crucial for identifying cartilage erosion or invasion and extension into the preepiglottic and paraglottic spaces.

For severe dysplasia or carcinoma in situ of the vocal cord, stripping of the surface mucosa has been shown to be an effective treatment. Multiple procedures may be necessary to control the disease and to prevent progression to an invasive cancer. Close follow-up examinations and smoking cessation are mandatory adjuncts of therapy. For early tumors of the glottis and the supraglottis, radiation therapy is equally as effective in controlling disease as surgery. The critical factors in determining the appropriate treatment modality are the patient's wishes to preserve voice, comorbid conditions (chronic obstructive pulmonary disease, cardiovascular and renal disease), and tumor stage. Voice preservation and maintenance of quality of life are key issues and significantly impact therapeutic decisions. The use of radiation therapy for early stage disease of the glottis and supraglottis provides excellent disease control with reasonable if not excellent preservation of vocal quality. Partial laryngectomy for small glottic cancers provides excellent tumor control, but with some degree of voice impairment. For supraglottic cancers without arytenoid or vocal cord extension, standard supraglottic laryngectomy results in excellent disease control with good voice function. For advanced tumors with extension beyond the endolarynx or with cartilage destruction, total laryngectomy followed by postoperative radiation is still considered the standard of care. In this setting, pharyngeal reconstruction by means of a pectoralis major flap or free flap reconstruction is occasionally required.

Subglottic tumors are rare, constituting only 1 percent of laryngeal tumors, and are best treated by total laryngectomy. Because these tumors present with adenopathy in 40 percent of cases, special attention must be given to the treatment of paratracheal lymph nodes and removal of one or both lobes of the thyroid.

The approach to the treatment for patients with advanced tumors of the larynx and hypopharynx continues to evolve over time. Sequential and concomitant chemotherapy and radiation trials have demonstrated the feasibility of these approaches for organ preservation. The recently completed RTOG 91-11 trial for laryngeal preservation demonstrated a higher laryngeal preservation rate among patients receiving concomitant chemotherapy and radiotherapy as opposed to radiation alone or sequential chemotherapy followed by radiation therapy. A randomized laryngeal preservation trial of neoadjuvant induction chemotherapy followed by radiation therapy has yielded survival rates similar to those of laryngectomy with the benefit of preservation of the larynx in 65 percent of patients. Surgical salvage is available in cases of treatment failure or recurrent disease. The results of this study indicate that although overall survival rates are similar, patients who underwent total laryngectomy had better locoregional control, whereas those treated with chemotherapy and radiation therapy had lower rates of distant metastases.

Unknown Primary

When patients present with cervical nodal metastases without clinical or radiologic evidence of an upper aerodigestive tract primary tumor, they are referred to as having an unknown or occult primary. Given the difficulty in examining regions such as the base of tongue, crevices within the tonsillar fossa, and the nasopharynx, examination under anesthesia with directed tissue biopsies have been advocated. Ipsilateral tonsillectomy, direct laryngoscopy with base of tongue and piriform biopsies, examination of the nasopharynx, and bimanual examination can allow for identification of a primary site in a portion of patients. In those individuals in which a primary site cannot be ascertained, empiric treatment of the mucosal sources of the upper aerodigestive tract at risk and the cervical lymphatics with radiation therapy is performed.

NOSE AND PARANASAL SINUSES

As discussed previously, the nose and paranasal sinuses are the site of a great deal of infectious and inflammatory pathology. The diagnosis of tumors within this region is frequently made after a patient has been unsuccessfully treated for recurrent sinusitis and undergoes diagnostic imaging. Symptoms associated with sinonasal tumors are subtle and insidious. They include chronic nasal obstruction, facial pain, headache, epistaxis, and facial numbness. As such, tumors of the paranasal sinuses frequently present at an advanced stage. Orbital invasion can result in proptosis, diplopia, epiphora, and visual loss. Paresthesia within the distribution of CN V2 is suggestive of pterygopalatine fossa or skull base invasion and is generally a poor prognostic factor. Maxillary sinus tumors can present with loose dentition indicating erosion of the alveolar and palatal bones.

A variety of benign tumors arise in the nasal cavity and paranasal sinuses and include inverted papillomas, hemangiomas, hemangiopericytoma, angiofibroma, minor salivary tumors, and benign fibrous histiocytoma. Fibro-osseous and osseous lesions, such as fibrous dysplasia, ossifying fibroma, osteoma, and myxomas, also can arise in this region.

Malignant tumors of the sinuses are predominantly squamous cell carcinomas. Sinonasal undifferentiated carcinoma (SNUC), adenocarcinoma, mucosal melanoma, lymphoma, and olfactory neuroblastoma are some of the malignancies that have been described. Metastases from the kidney, breast, lung, and thyroid may also present as an intranasal mass.

The diagnosis of intranasal tumors is made with the assistance of a headlight and nasal speculum or nasal endoscope. The site of origin, involved bony structures, and the presence of pulsations or hypervascularity should be assessed. For paranasal sinus tumors MRI and CT scanning often are complimentary studies in determining orbital and intracranial invasion.

The standard treatment for most malignant tumors of the paranasal sinuses is surgical resection with postoperative adjuvant radiation therapy. The extent of surgery is determined by the preoperative evaluation of disease spread. Tumors arising along the medial wall of the maxillary sinus may be treated by means of a medial maxillectomy. The treatment of advanced tumors of the paranasal sinuses frequently involves a multispecialty approach including the head and neck surgeon, neurosurgeon, prosthodontist, ophthalmologist, and reconstructive surgeon. When craniofacial resection is necessary for intracranial spread, cerebrospinal fluid decompression is performed through a lumbar drain.

NASOPHARYNX AND MEDIAN SKULL BASE

The nasopharynx extends in a plane superior to the hard plate from the choana, of the posterior nasal cavity, to the posterior pharyngeal wall. It includes the fossa of Rosenmüller, the eustachian tube orifices (torus tubarius) and the site of the adenoid pad. Tumors arising in the nasopharynx are usually of squamous cell origin and range from lymphoepithelioma to well-differentiated carcinoma. However, the differential diagnosis for nasopharyngeal tumors is broad and also includes lymphoma, chordoma, nasopharyngeal cysts, angiofibroma, minor salivary gland tumors, paraganglioma, rhabdomyosarcoma, extramedullary plasmacytoma, and neuroblastoma.

Risk factors for nasopharyngeal carcinoma include area of habitation, ethnicity, environment, and tobacco use. There is a high incidence of nasopharyngeal cancer in southern China, Africa, Alaska, and in Greenland Eskimos. A strong correlation exists between nasopharyngeal cancer and the presence of Epstein-Barr virus (EBV) infection, such that EBV titers may be used as a means to follow a patient's response to treatment.

The symptoms associated with presentation of nasopharyngeal tumors include nasal obstruction, posterior (Level V) neck mass, epistaxis, headache, serous otitis media with hearing loss, and otalgia. Cranial nerve involvement is indicative of skull base extension and advanced disease.

Examination of the nasopharynx is facilitated by the use of the flexible or rigid fiberoptic endoscope. Evaluation with imaging studies is important for staging and treatment planning. CT with contrast is best for determining bone destruction, and MRI is important for determining intracranial and soft tissue extension. The status of the cavernous sinus and optic chiasm should also be evaluated when reviewing imaging to determine the potential for treatment related morbidities.

For squamous cell carcinoma and undifferentiated nasopharyngeal carcinoma, the standard treatment is a combination of chemotherapy and radiation therapy. Combination therapy has been shown to produce superior rates over radiation alone for nasopharyngeal carcinoma. Surgical treatment for nasopharyngeal carcinoma is rarely feasible, but may occasionally be considered as salvage therapy for patients with localized recurrences.

EAR AND TEMPORAL BONE

Tumors of the ear and temporal bone are uncommon and account for less than 1 percent of all head and neck malignancies. Primary sites can include the external ear (pinna), external auditory canal (EAC), middle ear, mastoid, or petrous portion of the temporal bone. The most common site is the EAC and the most common histology is squamous cell carcinoma. Minor salivary gland tumors, including adenoid cystic carcinoma and adenocarcinoma, may also present in this region. The pinna, because of its exposure to ultraviolet light, is a site for basal cell and squamous cell carcinoma to arise. In the middle ear, squamous cell carcinoma related to the presence of chronic otitis media is a typical feature. In the pediatric population, tumors of the temporal bone are most commonly soft tissue sarcomas. For advanced stage tumors with extensive temporal bone extension, the complex anatomy of the temporal bone makes removal of tumors with functional preservation challenging.

The diagnosis of tumors of the ear and temporal bone is frequently delayed because the initial presentation of these patients appears consistent with benign infectious disease. When patients fail to improve with conservative care and symptoms evolve to include a facial nerve paralysis or worsening hearing loss, the need for imaging and biopsy are considered. Granulation tissue in the external auditory canal or middle ear should always be biopsied in patients with atypical presentations or histories consistent with chronic otologic disease. The complexity of the temporal bone anatomy makes the use of imaging studies of paramount importance in the diagnosis, staging, and treatment of tumors of the temporal bone. Temporal bone CT scans (thin cuts with axial and coronal planes), MRI imaging, and angiography can allow for assessment of tumor extension of the skull base and involvement of the carotid.

Small skin cancers on the helix of the ear can be readily treated with simple excision and primary closure. Mohs microsurgery with frozen section margin control may also be used for cancer of the external ear. In lesions that are recurrent or invade the underlying perichondrium and cartilage, rapid spread through tissue planes can occur. Tumors may extend from the cartilaginous external canal to the bony canal and invade the parotid, temporomandibular joint, and the skull base. For extensive pinna-based lesions more radical procedures, such as auriculectomy, may be required in combination with additional procedures. Radiation therapy is combined with surgery for advanced skin cancer or in the context of positive margins or perineural spread.

The optimal treatment for tumors of the middle ear and bony external canal is en bloc resection followed by radiation therapy. Management of the regional lymphatics is determined by the site and stage of the tumor at presentation.

NECK

The diagnostic evaluation of a neck mass requires a planned approach that does not compromise the effectiveness of future treatment options. A neck mass in a 50-year-old smoker/drinker with a synchronous oral ulcer is different than a cystic neck mass in an 18-year-old that enlarges with an upper respiratory infection. As with all diagnoses, a complete history with full head and neck exam, including flexible laryngoscopy, are the core to this work-up. The differential diagnosis of a neck mass is dependent on its location and the patient's age. In children, most neck masses are inflammatory or congenital. However, in the adult population a neck mass greater than 2 cm in diameter has a greater than 80 percent probability of being malignant. Once the physician has developed a differential diagnosis, interventions to confirm or dispute diagnoses are initiated. Fine needle aspiration, with or without the assistance of ultrasound or CT guidance, can provide a valuable tool for early treatment planning that provides less oncologic disruption to a tissue mass than an open biopsy. The use of CT scanning and/or MRI imaging is dictated by the patient's presentation. Imaging allows the physician the ability to evaluate the anatomic relationships of the mass to the surrounding neck, and as such, sharpen the differential. A cystic lesion may represent benign pathology such a branchial cleft cyst, however, it may also represent a regional metastasis of a tonsil/base of tongue squamous cell carcinoma or a papillary thyroid carcinoma. In this circumstance, evaluation of these potential primary sites, in addition to the characteristics of the neck mass, can alter the planned operative intervention such that a "lumpectomy" can be spared with the need for definitive surgery in a previously operated field.

Patterns of Lymph Node Metastasis

The regional lymphatic drainage of the neck is divided into seven levels. The levels allow for a standardized format for radiologists, surgeons, pathologists, and radiation oncologists to communicate concerning specific sites within the neck and does not represent regions isolated by fascial planes. The levels are defined as the following:

- Level I – the submental and submandibular nodes
  - Level Ia – the submental nodes; medial to the anterior belly of the digastric muscle bilaterally, symphysis of mandible superiorly, and hyoid inferiorly
  - Level Ib – the submandibular nodes and gland; posterior to the anterior belly of digastric, anterior to the posterior belly of digastric and inferior to the body of the mandible
- Level II – upper jugular chain nodes
  - Level IIa – jugulodigastric nodes; deep to sternocleidomastoid (SCM), anterior to the posterior border of the muscle, posterior to the posterior aspect of the posterior belly of digastric, superior to the level of the hyoid, inferior to spinal accessory nerve (CN XI)
  - Level IIb – submuscular recess; superior to spinal accessory nerve to the level of the skull base
- Level III – middle jugular chain nodes; inferior to the hyoid, superior to the level of the hyoid, deep to SCM from posterior border of the muscle to the strap muscles medially
- Level IV – lower jugular chain nodes; inferior to the level of the cricoid, superior to the clavicle, deep to SCM from posterior border of the muscle to the strap muscles medially
- Level V – posterior triangle nodes
  - Level Va – lateral to the posterior aspect of the SCM, inferior and medial to splenius capitis and trapezius, superior to the spinal accessory nerve
  - Level Vb – lateral to the posterior aspect of SCM, medial to trapezius, inferior to the spinal accessory nerve, superior to the clavicle
- Level VI – anterior compartment nodes; inferior to the hyoid, superior to suprasternal notch, medial to the lateral extent of the strap muscles bilaterally
- Level VII – paratracheal nodes; inferior to the suprasternal notch in the upper mediastinum.

Patterns of spread from primary tumor sites in the head and neck to cervical lymphatics are well described. The location and incidence of metastasis vary according to the primary site. Primary tumors within the oral cavity and lip metastasize to the nodes in Levels I, II, and III. The occurrence of skip metastases with oral tongue lesions makes possible the involvement of nodes in Level III or IV without involvement of higher echelon nodes. Tumors arising in the oropharynx, hypopharynx, and larynx most commonly spread to the lymph nodes in Levels II, III, and IV. Isolated Level V nodes are uncommon with oral cavity, pharyngeal and laryngeal primaries, however, Level V adenopathy may be seen with concomitant involvement of higher echelon nodes. Malignancies of the nasopharynx and thyroid commonly spread to posterior lymph nodes in addition to the jugular chain nodes. Retropharyngeal nodes are sites for metastasis from tumors of the nasopharynx, soft palate, and lateral and posterior walls of the oropharynx and hypopharynx. Tumors of the hypopharynx, cervical esophagus, and thyroid frequently involve the paratracheal nodal compartment and may extend to the lymphatics in the upper mediastinum (Level VII). The Delphian node, a pretracheal lymph node, may become involved by advanced tumors of the glottis with subglottic spread.

Selective neck dissection options have become increasingly popular given the benefits of improved shoulder function and cosmetic impact on neck contour when compared to modified radical neck dissection (MRND). The principle behind preservation of certain nodal groups is that specific primary sites preferentially drain their lymphatics in a predictable pattern, as mentioned previously. Types of selective neck dissections include the supraomohyoid neck dissection, the lateral neck dissection, and the posterolateral neck dissection. The supraomohyoid dissection, typically used with oral cavity primaries, removes lymph nodes in levels I–III. The lateral neck dissection, frequently used for laryngeal malignancies, removes those nodes in levels II–IV. The posterolateral neck dissection, used with thyroid cancer, removes the lymphatics in levels II–V. In the clinically negative neck (N0), if the risk for occult metastasis is greater than 20 percent, an elective treatment of the nodes at risk is advocated. This may be in the form of elective neck irradiation or elective neck dissection, typically using a selective neck dissection option.

For clinically N+ necks, frequently the surgical treatment of choice is the MRND or radical neck dissection (RND). Selective neck dissection (SND) options have been advocated by some authors for treatment of limited N1 disease, however, do not have a role in the treatment of advanced N-stage disease. When negative prognostic factors such as extracapsular spread, perineural invasion, vascular invasion, and the presence of multiple positive node surgical management of the neck alone is not adequate. Adjuvant radiation therapy is indicated in these cases.

Benign Neck Masses

A number of benign masses of the neck occur that require surgical management. Many of these masses are seen in the pediatric population. The differential diagnosis includes thyroglossal duct cyst, branchial cleft cyst, lymphangioma (cystic hygroma), hemangioma, and dermoid cyst.

Thyroglossal duct cysts represent the vestigial remainder of the tract of the descending thyroid gland from the foramen cecum, at the tongue base, into the lower anterior neck during fetal development. They present as a midline or paramedian cystic mass adjacent to the hyoid bone. After an upper respiratory infection, the cyst may enlarge or even suppurate. Surgical management of a thyroglossal duct cyst requires removal of the cyst, the tract, and the central portion of the hyoid bone (Sistrunk procedure), and a portion of the tongue base up to the foramen cecum.

Congenital branchial cleft remnants are derived from the branchial cleft apparatus that persists after fetal development. There are several types, numbered according to their corresponding embryologic branchial cleft. First branchial cleft cysts and sinuses are associated intimately with the external auditory canal and the parotid gland. Second and third branchial cleft cysts are found along the anterior border of the sternocleidomastoid muscle and can produce drainage via a sinus tract to the neck skin. Secondary infections can occur, producing enlargement, cellulitis, and neck abscess that requires operative drainage. The removal of branchial cleft cysts and fistula requires removal of the fistula tract to the point of origin to decrease the risk of recurrence. The second branchial cleft remnant tract courses between the internal and external carotid arteries and proceeds into the tonsillar fossa. The third branchial cleft remnant courses posterior to the common carotid artery, ending in the pyriform sinus region. Surgical excision is preferred to establish the definitive diagnosis of a branchial cleft cyst and avoid nontreatment of a masquerading head and neck regional metastasis. Cystic metastasis from squamous cell carcinoma of the tonsil or tongue base to a cervical lymph node can be confused for a branchial cleft cyst in an otherwise asymptomatic patient. Dermoid cysts tend to present as midline masses and represent trapped epithelium originating from the timing embryonic closure of the midline.

Lymphatic malformations such as lymphangiomas and cystic hygromas can be difficult management problems. They typically present as mobile, fluid-filled masses with either firm or doughy consistency. Because of their predisposition to track extensively into the surrounding soft tissues, complete removal to these lesions often is difficult. Recurrence and regrowth occur with incomplete removal, and cosmetic deformity or nerve damage can result when extensive surgical dissection is performed for large lesions. In newborns and infants, there is higher associated morbidity when cystic hygromas and lymphangiomas become massive, require tracheostomy, and involve the deep neck and mediastinum.

SALIVARY GLAND TUMORS OF THE HEAD AND NECK

Tumors of the salivary gland are relatively uncommon and represent less than 2 percent of all head and neck neoplasms. The major salivary glands are the parotid, submandibular, and sublingual glands. Minor salivary glands are found throughout the submucosa of the upper aerodigestive tract with the highest density found within palate. Eighty-five percent of salivary gland neoplasms arise in the parotid gland. The majority of these neoplasms are benign with the most common histology being pleomorphic adenoma (benign mixed tumor). In contrast, approximately 50 percent of tumors arising in the submandibular and sublingual glands are malignant. Tumors arising from minor salivary gland tissue carry an even higher risk for malignancy (75 percent).

Salivary gland tumors are usually slow growing and well-circumscribed. Patients with a mass and findings of rapid growth, pain, paresthesias, and facial weakness are at increased risk of harboring a malignancy. The facial nerve, which separates the superficial and deep lobes of the parotid, may be directly involved by tumors in 10–15 percent of patients. Additional findings ominous for malignancy include skin invasion and fixation to the mastoid tip. Trismus suggests invasion of the masseter or pterygoid muscles.

Submandibular and sublingual gland tumors present as a neck mass or floor of mouth swelling, respectively. Malignant tumors of the sublingual or submandibular gland may invade the lingual or hypoglossal nerves, causing paresthesias or paralysis. Bimanual examination is important for determining the size of the tumor and possible fixation to the mandible or involvement of the tongue.

Minor salivary gland tumors present as painless submucosal masses and most frequently are seen at the junction of the hard and soft palate, but can occur throughout the upper aerodigestive tract. Minor salivary gland tumors arising in the prestyloid parapharyngeal space may produce medial displacement of the lateral oropharyngeal wall and tonsil.

Benign and malignant tumors of the salivary glands are divided into epithelial, nonepithelial, and metastatic neoplasms. Benign epithelial tumors include pleomorphic adenoma (80 percent), monomorphic adenoma, Warthin tumor, oncocytoma, or sebaceous neoplasms. Nonepithelial benign lesions include hemangioma, neural sheath tumors, and lipoma. Treatment of benign neoplasms is surgical excision of the affected gland or, in the case of the parotid, excision of the superficial lobe with facial nerve dissection and preservation. The minimal surgical procedure for neoplasms of the parotid is superficial parotidectomy with preservation of the facial nerve. "Shelling out" of the tumor mass is not recommended because of the risk of incomplete excision and tumor spillage.

Tumor spillage of a pleomorphic adenoma during removal can lead to recurrences and should be avoided.

The primary treatment of salivary malignancies is surgical excision. In this setting, basic surgical principles include the en bloc removal of the involved gland with preservation of all nerves unless invaded directly by tumor. For parotid tumors that arise in the lateral lobe, superficial parotidectomy with preservation of CN VII is indicated. If the tumor extends into the deep lobe of the parotid, a total parotidectomy with nerve preservation is performed. Although malignant tumors may abut the facial nerve, if a plane of dissection can be developed without leaving gross tumor, it is preferable to preserve the nerve. If the nerve is encased by tumor and preservation would mean leaving gross residual disease, the nerve is sacrificed. Sacrifice of the facial nerve and temporal bone resection are a component of the surgical removal of advanced tumors with direct extension into the facial nerve or temporal bone. Radiation therapy is used as adjuvant treatment in the postoperative setting for specific indications.

The removal of submandibular malignancies includes en bloc resection of the gland and submental and submandibular lymph nodes. Radical resection is indicated with tumors that invade the mandible, tongue or floor of mouth. Therapeutic removal of the regional lymphatics is indicated for clinical adenopathy or when the risk of regional metastasis exceeds 20 percent based on tumor characteristics.

Postoperative radiation treatment plays an important role in the treatment of salivary malignancies. The presence of extraglandular disease, perineural invasion, direct invasion of regional structures, regional metastasis, and high-grade histology are all indications for radiation treatment.

RECONSTRUCTION IN HEAD AND NECK SURGERY

Defects of soft tissue and bony anatomy of the head and neck can occur after oncologic resection. Tumor surgery frequently necessitates removal of structures related to speech and swallowing. Loss of sensation and motor function can produce dysphagia through impairment of food bolus formation, manipulation, and propulsion. Cosmetic deformities that result from surgery also can significantly impact the quality of life of cancer survivors.

Basic principles of reconstruction typically include attempting to replace resected tissue components (bone, skin, soft tissue) with like tissue. The head and neck reconstructive surgeon must take into consideration a patient's preoperative comorbidities and anatomy when constructing a care plan.

A stepladder analogy has been used to describe the escalation in complexity of reconstructive options in the repair of head and neck defects. It is important to remember that the most complex is not always the most appropriate. Progression for closure by secondary intention, primary closure, skin grafts, local flaps, regional flaps, and free-tissue transfer flaps (free flaps) run the gamut of options available. The most appropriate reconstructive technique used is based on the medical condition of the patient, the location and size of the defect to be repaired, and the functional impairment associated with the defect.

Skin Grafts

Split- and full-thickness skin grafts are used in the head and neck for a variety of defects. Following oral cavity resections, split-thickness grafts can provide adequate reconstruction of the mucosal surface if an adequate soft tissue bed is available to support the blood supply needed for survival. These grafts incorporate into the recipient site at around 5 days and do not provide replacement of absent soft tissue, but are expeditious for covering mucosal defects and provide for ease of monitoring for recurrences of the primary tumor. Full-thickness grafts are used on the face when local rotational flaps are not available. These grafts have far less contracture than split-thickness grafts and also can provide a good color match for the defect area. Grafts can be harvested from the postauricular or supraclavicular areas to maximize the match of skin characteristics.

Local Flaps

Local flaps encompass a large number of mainly random pattern flaps used to reconstruct defects in adjacent areas. It is beyond the scope of this chapter to enumerate all of these flaps, but they should be designed according to the relaxed skin tension lines of the face and neck skin. These lines are tension lines inherent in the facial regions and caused in part by the insertions of muscles of facial animation. Incisions paralleling the relaxed skin tension lines that respect the aesthetic subunits of the face heal with the least amount of tension and camouflage into a more appealing result. Poorly designed incisions or flaps result in widened scars and distortion of important aesthetic units. Flaps have many different configurations and sizes, with the most common being the rotation and transposition flaps.

Regional Flaps

Regional flaps are those that are available as pedicled transfer of soft tissue or bone from areas adjacent to the defect. These flaps have an axial blood supply that traverses the flap longitudinally from proximal to distal between the fascia and subcutaneous tissue. Single-stage reconstruction is possible and harvest can occur simultaneously with the resection of primary disease, thus decreasing operative time.

The deltopectoral fasciocutaneous flap is a medially based flap from the anterior chest wall reliant on the perforators of the internal mammary artery. The flap provides a fair color match for surface defects. Its pliability permits folding, making it useful for reconstruction of pharyngoesophageal defects. Use of the flap requires a second stage for insetting approximately 2 weeks after the original procedure.

The pectoralis myocutaneous flap is based on the pectoral branch of the thoracoacromial artery (medial) and the lateral thoracic artery (lateral). The latter vessel may be sacrificed to increase the arc of rotation. This flap includes the pectoralis major muscle, either alone or with overlying anterior chest skin. The pectoralis myocutaneous flap has enjoyed tremendous popularity because of its ease of harvest, the ability to tailor its thickness to the defect, and minimal donor site morbidity. It can be used for many reconstructive needs in the oropharynx, oral cavity, and the hypopharynx and can be tubed in some cases to replace cervical esophageal defects. Bulk associated with this flap may make certain applications less practical and this problem is exacerbated in obese patients. The arc of rotation limits the superior extent of this flap to the zygomatic arch externally and the superior pole of the tonsil internally. It should be remembered that the least reliable portion of this flap is that portion furthest from the blood supply: the skin. When portions of the flap are extended into regions beyond the underlying muscle, relying on random blood supply, healing at the primary site may be adversely affected. For patients that require expeditious recovery to initiate postoperative radiation therapy this can be a significant problem. This flap is still frequently used but has been replaced in many instances by free-tissue transfer for oral cavity and oropharyngeal defects because of its greater reliability and pliability.

Free-Tissue Transfer

Free-tissue transfer with microvascular anastomosis (free flaps) affords the reconstructive surgeon unparalleled ability to replace tissue loss with tissues of similar characteristics. There are a number of donor sites available for various types of flaps, including osteomyocutaneous, myocutaneous, fasciocutaneous, fascial, and myoosseous flaps. The flaps most popular in head and neck reconstructive armamentarium are those with ease of harvesting from a standpoint of patient positioning and those that allow for a two-teamed approach for simultaneous flap harvesting and oncologic resection.

The radial forearm fasciocutaneous flap is a hardy flap with constant vascular anatomy and a potentially long vascular pedicle, allowing for ease of insetting and choice in anastomotic vascular recipient sites. It is pliable and can be reinnervated as a sensate flap, making it ideal for repair of oral cavity and oropharyngeal defects. It can be tubed to repair hypopharyngeal and upper esophageal defects.

The lateral thigh flap, based on perforators of the profunda femoris artery, provides relatively pliable tissue that can be tubed and is used to reconstruct similar defects as that of the radial forearm flap, and pharyngoesophageal defects extending from the thoracic inlet to the nasopharynx.

The fibular osteocutaneous or osteomyocutaneous flap allows for one-stage reconstruction of resected mandible. In the adult, 25 cm of bone can be harvested, and a cuff of soleus and flexor hallucis longus muscles can be included for additional soft tissue bulk. The pedicle length can be extended by harvesting a long segment of bone; the donor site defect is well tolerated as long as approximately 6 cm of bone is retained proximally and distally for knee and ankle stability.

Iliac crest osteocutaneous flaps are frequently used for mandible defects involving the angle; the natural shape of this donor site bone is similar to the mandibular angle and eliminates the need for shaping of the bone flap prior to insetting into the defect.

Large soft tissue defects can result from trauma, excision of skull base tumors, and tumors involving large segments of skin. Furthermore, after extensive skull base resections in the anterior and lateral skull base, the need for separation of the oropharyngeal and sinonasal tracts from the dura requires soft tissue interposition between the dura and the contaminated upper aerodigestive tract. The rectus abdominis myocutaneous flap provides a large amount of soft tissue and is ideal for closure of wounds of the lateral skull base and dura.

For reconstruction of defects of the hypopharynx and cervical esophagus, both free flaps and regional pedicled flaps are available. The free transfer of a jejunal segment can be performed based on branches of the superior mesenteric artery. Other free flaps used in this area include fasciocutaneous flaps, such as tubed radial forearm, lateral thigh, and lateral arm flap. The gastric pull-up is a regional flap that also is in use for reconstruction of cervical esophageal defects. The stomach is mobilized and pedicled on the right gastric and gastroepiploic vessels into the defect via tunneling through the anterior mediastinum.

TRACHEOSTOMY

Tracheostomy is indicated in the management of patients who require prolonged intubation, assisted ventilation, pulmonary toilet, and in those patients with neurologic deficits that impair protective airway reflexes. Its use in head and neck surgery often is for the temporary management of the airway in the perioperative period. After surgical resection of oral cavity and oropharyngeal cancers, bleeding into the sublingual and submaxillary soft tissue spaces may result in airway compromise, and elective tracheostomy is indicated to prevent loss of the airway.

The avoidance of prolonged orotracheal and nasotracheal intubation decreases the risk of laryngeal damage and subglottic stenosis, facilitates oral and pulmonary toilet, and decreases patient discomfort. When the tracheostomy is no longer needed, the tube is removed and prompt closure of the opening usually occurs. Complications of tracheostomy include pneumothorax or pneumomediastinum, recurrent laryngeal nerve injury, formation of granulation tissue, tracheal stenosis, wound infection with large vessel erosion, and failure to close after decannulation. The use of cricothyroidotomy as an alternative to tracheostomy for patients who require prolonged intubation has been associated with a higher incidence of vocal cord dysfunction and subglottic stenosis. When cricothyroidotomy is used in the setting of establishing an emergency airway, conversion to a standard tracheostomy should be considered if decannulation is not anticipated within 5–7 days.

Placement of a tracheostomy does not obligate a patient to loss of speech. When a large cuffed tracheostomy tube is in place, expecting a patient to be capable of normal speech is impractical. However, after a patient is downsized to an uncuffed tracheostomy tube, intermittent finger occlusion or Passy-Muir valve placement will allow a patient to communicate while still using the tracheostomy to bypass the upper airway for inhalation. When a patient no longer has the original indication for the tracheostomy (secretion management, need for ventilatory support, upper airway edema) and can tolerate capping of the trach tube for greater than 24 h, decannulation is considered safe. If an upper airway mass or tissue reconstruction was the indication for the tracheostomy, predecannulation flexible laryngoscopic examination of the airway is recommended.

Suggested Readings

Lanza DC, Kennedy DW: Adult rhinosinusitis defined. Otolaryngol Head Neck Surg 117:S1, 1997.

Paradise J, Bluestone C, Bachman R, et al: Efficacy of tonsillectomy in recurrent throat infections in severely affected children. N Engl J Med 310:674,1984.

Gates G, Cooper J, Avery C et al: Chronic secretory OM: effects of surgical management. Ann Otol Rhinol Laryngol Suppl 98:2,1989.

Zeitels SM, Casiano RR, Gardner GM, et al: Management of common voice problems: Committee report. Otolaryngol Head Neck Surg 126:333,2002.

Shumrick K, Kersten R, Kulwin D, et al: Extended access/internal approaches for the management of facial trauma. Arch Otolaryngol Head Neck Surg 118:1105, 1992.

Peters LJ, Weber RS, Morrison WH, et al: Neck surgery in patients with primary oropharyngeal cancer treated by radiotherapy. Head Neck 18:552, 1996.

Lefebve JL, Chevalier D, Luboinski B, et al: Larynx preservation in piriform sinus cancer: Preliminary results of a European organization for research and treatment of cancer phase III trial. J Natl Cancer Inst 88:890, 1996.

Weber RS, Berket BA, Forastiere A, et al: Outcome of salvage total laryngectomy following organ preservation therapy: the Radiation Therapy Oncology Group trial 91-11. Arch Otolaryngol Head Neck Surg 129:44–9, 2003.

Eicher SA, Weber RS: Surgical management of cervical lymph node metastases Curr Opin Oncol. 8:215, 1996.

Urken ML, Buchbinder D, Costantino PD, et al: Oromandibular reconstruction using microvascular composite flaps: Report of 210 cases. Arch Otolaryngol Head Neck Surg, 124:46, 1998.

Chest Wall, Lung, Mediastinum, and Pleura

Michael A. Maddaus and James D. Luketich

LUNG

Anatomy

Lymphatic Drainage

Lymph nodes draining the lungs are divided into two groups according to the tumor-node-metastasis (TNM) staging system for lung cancer: the pulmonary lymph nodes, N1, and the mediastinal nodes, N2.

Thoracic Surgical Approaches

Mediastinoscopy is used for diagnostic assessment of mediastinal lymph-adenopathy and staging of lung cancer and is performed through 2–3-cm suprasternal notch incision. Blunt dissection along the anterior trachea is performed to the level of the carina. The mediastinoscope is insegted, and anatomic definition of the trachea, carina, and lateral aspect of both proximal main bronchi is achieved with blunt dissection using a long suction catheter. Long biopsy forceps can be inserted through the scope for sampling. The standard staging procedure for lung cancer includes biopsies of the paratracheal (stations 4R and 4L) and subcarinal lymph nodes (station 7).

In patients with left upper lobe tumors, lymph node spread is often to the regional aortopulmonary and preaortic lymph nodes (station 5 and 6). These nodes can be sampled via a modified Chamberlain procedure through a 4–5-cm incision over the left second costal cartilage, which on occasion is excised. This approach also may be used to biopsy anterior masses.

The posterolateral thoracotomy incision is the most common incision for the majority of pulmonary resections, esophageal operations, and for access to the posterior mediastinum and vertebral column. The skin incision typically starts at the anterior axillary line just below the nipple level and extends posteriorly below the tip of the scapula. The latissimus dorsi is divided and the serratus anterior is retracted. Typically the fifth interspace is entered and a rib spreader is used to separate the rib space.

The anterolateral thoracotomy has traditionally been used in trauma victims. This approach allows quick entry into the chest with the patient supine. In the face of hemodynamic instability, this approach is better than the lateral decubitus position, and gives the anesthesiologist control over the patient's cardiopulmonary system and resuscitation efforts. The incision is submammary, beginning at the sternal border overlying the fourth intercostal space and extending to the midaxillary line. Should more exposure be necessary, the sternum can be transected and the incision carried to the contralateral thoracic cavity ("clamshell" thoracotomy). A bilateral anterior thoracotomy incision with transection of the sternum ("clamshell" thoracotomy) is a standard operative approach to the heart and mediastinum in certain elective circumstances such as double-lung transplantation. A median sternotomy also can be added to an anterior thoracotomy ("trap-door" thoracotomy) for access to mediastinal structures.

The median sternotomy incision allows exposure of anterior mediastinal structures and is principally used for cardiac operations and for anterior and middle mediastinal tumors. Either pleural cavity may be entered, and if indicated, formal pulmonary resection can be performed. Sternotomy is associated with less pain and less compromise of pulmonary function than a lateral thoracotomy.

Video-Assisted Thoracoscopic Surgery

Video-assisted thoracoscopic surgery (VATS) is a common approach to the diagnosis and treatment of pleural effusions, recurrent pneumothoraces, lung biopsies, lobectomy, resection of bronchogenic and mediastinal cysts, esophageal myotomy, and intrathoracic esophageal mobilization for esophagectomy. VATS is performed via two to four incisions measuring 0.5–1.2 cm in length to allow insertion of the thoracoscope and instruments. The incision location varies according to the procedure. Formal VATS lobectomy for cancer is now accepted as equivalent to the open procedure for lung cancer. It is performed with and a 6-cm access incision without rib spreading and two to three additional 1-cm ports. The specimen is removed via the access incision. Endoscopic staplers are used to divide the major vascular structures and bronchus.

Postoperatively, the pleural cavity typically is drained with a chest tube(s). Each chest tube is brought out through a separate stab incision in the chest wall below the level of the thoracotomy, or through a VATS port site. If the pleura has not been violated and no drainage is expected (i.e., after VATS sympathectomies), no chest tube is necessary. The lung is then ventilated and placed under positive pressure ventilation to assist with reexpansion of atelectatic segments.

Postoperative Care

Chest Tube Management

Pleural tubes are left for two reasons: to drain fluid, thereby preventing pleural fluid accumulation, and to evacuate air if an air leak is present. The volume of drainage over 24 h predicting safe chest tube removal is unknown. The ability of the pleural lymphatics to absorb fluid is substantial. It can be as high as 0.40 mL/kg per hour in a healthy individual, resulting in absorption of up to 500 mL of fluid over 24 h. The capacity of the pleural space to manage and absorb fluid is high if the pleural lining and lymphatics are healthy.

A drainage volume of 150 mL or less over 24 h has been thought necessary to safely remove a chest tube. Recently, it has been shown that pleural tubes can be removed after VATS lobectomy with 24-hour drainage volumes as high as 400 mL, without subsequent development of pleural effusions. Currently, it is the practice of these authors to remove chest tubes with 24-h outputs of 400 mL or less after lobectomy or lesser pulmonary resections.

If the pleural space is altered (e.g., malignant pleural effusion, pleural space infections or inflammation, and pleurodesis), strict adherence to a volume requirement before tube removal is appropriate (typically 100–150 mL over 24 h). Such circumstances alter normal pleural fluid dynamics.

The use of suction and the management of air leaks vary. Suction levels of 20 cm H_2O have been routinely used after pulmonary surgery in an effort to eradicate residual air spaces and to control postoperative parenchymal air leaks. Recently it has been shown that the routine use of a water seal (with the patient off suction) actually promotes more rapid healing of parenchymal air leaks. The main guidelines for the use of a water seal are the degree of air leakage and the degree of expansion of the remaining lung. If the leak is significant enough to induce atelectasis or collapse during use of water seal (off suction), suction should be used to achieve lung reexpansion.

It is important to remember the process of assessing an air leak. The chest tube and its attached tubing should be examined and the lack of kinks or external mechanical obstruction (e.g., patient lying on the tube) verified. The patient is asked to voluntarily cough. During the cough, the water seal chamber is observed. If bubbles pass through the water seal chamber, an air leak is presumed. Occasionally, if the chest tube is not secured snugly at the skin surface, air can entrain around the tube into the patient with respiration; thus an air leak will be present, although not emanating from the lung itself. During the voluntary cough, the fluid level in the water seal chamber should move up and down with the cough and with deep respiration, reflecting the pleural pressure changes occurring with these maneuvers. A stationary fluid level implies a mechanical blockage, either because of external tube compression or a clot or debris within the tube.

Pain Control

Good pain control permits the patient to actively participate in breathing maneuvers designed to clear and manage secretions, and promotes ambulation and a feeling of well being. The two most common techniques of pain management are epidural and intravenous. To maximize efficacy, epidural catheters should be inserted at about the T6 level, roughly at the level of the scapular tip. Lower placement risks inadequate pain control and higher placement may provoke hand and arm numbness. Typically, combinations of fentanyl at 0.3 μg/mL, combined with either bupivacaine (0.125 percent) or ropivacaine (0.1 percent) are used. Ropivacaine has less cardiotoxicity than bupivacaine; thus in the case of inadvertent intravenous injection, the potential for refractory complete heart block that is seen with bupivacaine is significantly less.

When properly placed, a well-managed epidural can provide outstanding pain control without significant systemic sedation. Urinary retention is a frequent side effect, particularly in males who require an indwelling urinary catheter. Additionally, the use of local anesthetics may cause sympathetic outflow blockade, leading to vasodilation and hypotension often requiring intravenous vasoconstrictors (an alpha agonist such as phenylephrine) and/or fluid administration. In such circumstances, fluid administration for hypotension may be undesirable in pulmonary surgery patients, particularly after pneumonectomy.

Alternatively, intravenous narcotics via patient-controlled analgesia can be used, often in conjunction with ketorolac. Titration of basal and intermittent dosing is often necessary to balance the degree of pain relief with the degree of sedation. Oversedated, narcotized patients are as ominous as patients without adequate pain control, because of the significant risk of secretion retention and development of atelectasis or pneumonia. Proper pain control with intravenous narcotics is a balance of pain relief and sedation. An alternative to epidural is the intraoperatively placed intercostal nerve catheter. A recent randomized trial demonstrated that a catheter placed along the intercostal nerves with infusion of local anesthetic yielded equivalent pain control to epidural catheter in a postthoracotomy study.

Respiratory Care

The best respiratory care is an effective cough to clear secretions. The process ideally begins preoperatively, with clear instructions on using pillows (or other support techniques) over the wound and then applying pressure. Postoperatively, proper pain control is essential, without oversedation. Adjunctive respiratory care techniques (e.g., intermittent positive pressure breathing and incentive spirometry)has been shown to be of limited benefit, consistent with our impression that respiratory care is best accomplished by a dedicated team and educated patients.

In patients whose pulmonary function preoperatively is significantly impaired, generating an effective cough postoperatively may be nearly impossible. Here routine nasotracheal suctioning can be employed, but is uncomfortable for the patient. A better alternative is placement at the time of surgery of a percutaneous transtracheal suction catheter which is comfortable and allows suctioning.

Postoperative Complications

Postpneumonectomy pulmonary edema occurs in 1–5 percent of patients undergoing pneumonectomy, with a higher incidence after right pneumonectomy. Clinically, symptoms of respiratory distress manifest hours to days after surgery. Radiographically, diffuse interstitial infiltration or frank alveolar edema is seen. The syndrome reportedly has a nearly 100 percent mortality rate despite aggressive therapy. Treatment consists of ventilatory support, fluid restriction, and diuretics.

Postoperative air leak and bronchopleural fistula are two different problems, but distinguishing the two may be difficult. Postoperative air leaks are common after pulmonary resection. They occur more often and last longer in patients with emphysematous changes because the fibrotic changes and destroyed blood supply impairs healing of surface injuries. Prolonged air leaks—those lasting over 7 days—may be treated by diminishing or discontinuing suction (if used), by continuing chest drainage, or by instilling a pleurodesis agent, usually talcum powder.

If the leak is moderate to large and if a bronchopleural fistula from the resected bronchial stump is possible, flexible bronchoscopy is performed. Management options include continued prolonged chest tube drainage; reoperation and reclosure (with stump reinforcement with intercostals or a serratus muscle pedicle flap); or, for fistulas less than 4 mm, bronchoscopic fibrin glue application. Patients often have concomitant empyemas and open drainage may be necessary.

Solitary Pulmonary Nodule

A solitary pulmonary nodule or "coin lesion" is typically recognized as a single, well-circumscribed, spherical lesion less than 3 cm in diameter and completely surrounded by normal lung parenchyma. About 150,000 solitary nodules are found incidentally each year. The clinical significance of such a lesion depends on whether or not it represents a malignancy.

Differential Diagnosis

In nonselected patient populations, a new solitary pulmonary nodule has a 20–40 percent likelihood of being malignant, with the risk approximating 50 percent or higher for smokers. The remaining causes of pulmonary nodules are numerous benign conditions. Infectious granulomas arising from a variety of organisms account for 70–80 percent of this type of solitary nodule; hamartomas are the next most common single cause, accounting for about 10 percent. The initial assessment of a pulmonary nodule should proceed from a clinical history and physical examination. Risk factors for malignancy include a history of smoking, prior neoplastic disease, hemoptysis, and age over 35 years.

Imaging

Chest thin-section computed tomography (CT) scan is critical in characterizing nodule location, size, margin morphology, calcification pattern, and growth rate. Lesions larger than 3 cm are regarded as masses and are more likely malignant. Irregular, lobulated, or spiculated edges strongly suggest malignancy. The corona radiata sign (consisting of fine linear strands extending 4–5 mm outward and appearing spiculated on radiographs) is highly cancer-specific.

Calcification within a nodule suggests a benign lesion. Four patterns of benign calcification are common: diffuse, solid, central, and laminated or "popcorn." Granulomatous infections such as tuberculosis can demonstrate the first three patterns, whereas the popcorn pattern is most common in hamartomas.

Calcification that is stippled, amorphous, or eccentric is usually associated with cancer. Characteristically neoplasms grow, and several studies have confirmed that lung cancers have volume-doubling times from 20–400 days. Lesions with shorter doubling times are likely because of infection, as longer doubling times suggest benign tumors. Traditionally, 2-year size stability per chest radiography has been considered a sign of a benign tumor. This long-held notion has been challenged by recent investigations, which demonstrated only a 65 percent positive predictive value for chest radiographs. Thus size stability of a pulmonary mass on chest films is a relatively unreliable benign indicator that must be interpreted with caution.

PET is used to help differentiate benign from malignant nodules. One metaanalysis estimated its sensitivity for identifying neoplasms as 97 percent and its specificity as 78 percent. False-negative results can occur (especially in patients who have bronchoalveolar carcinomas, carcinoids, and tumors less than 1 cm in diameter), and false-positive results (because of confusion with other infectious or inflammatory processes).

Biopsy versus Resection

Only a biopsy can definitively diagnose a pulmonary nodule. Bronchoscopy has a 20–80 percent sensitivity for detecting a neoplastic process within a solitary pulmonary nodule, depending on the nodule size, its proximity to the bronchial tree, and the prevalence of cancer in the population being sampled. Transthoracic fine-needle aspiration (FNA) biopsy can accurately identify the status of peripheral pulmonary lesions in up to 95 percent of patients; the false-negative rate ranges from 3–29 percent.

VATS is often used for excising and diagnosing indeterminate pulmonary nodules. Lesions most suitable for VATS are those that are located in the outer one third of the lung and those that are less than 3 cm in diameter. Certain principles must be followed when excising potentially malignant lesions via VATS. The nodule must not be directly manipulated with instruments, the visceral pleura overlying the nodule must not be violated, and the excised nodule must be extracted from the chest within a bag to prevent seeding of the chest wall.

TABLE 18-1 Cumulative Percentage of Survival by Stage After Treatment for Lung Cancer

	Time after treatment	
Pathologic stage	24 Months	60 Months
pT1N0M0 ($n = 511$)	86 percent	67 percent
pT2N0M0 ($n = 549$)	76 percent	57 percent
pT1N1M0 ($n = 76$)	70 percent	55 percent
pT2N1M0 ($n = 288$)	56 percent	39 percent
pT3N0M0 ($n = 87$)	55 percent	38 percent

Lung Neoplasms

Lung cancer is the leading cancer killer in the United States accounting for 30 percent of all cancer deaths—more than cancers of the breast, prostate, and ovary combined. It is the third most frequently diagnosed cancer in the United States, behind prostate cancer in men and breast cancer in women. Most patients are diagnosed at an advanced stage of disease, so therapy is rarely curative. The overall 5-year survival for all patients with lung cancer is 15 percent, making lung cancer the most lethal of the leading four cancers (Table 18-1).

Epidemiology

Cigarette smoking is the primary cause of lung cancer. Two lung cancer cell types, squamous cell carcinoma and small cell carcinoma, are extraordinarily rare in the absence of cigarette smoking. The risk of developing lung cancer escalates with the number of cigarettes smoked, the number of years smoked, and the use of unfiltered cigarettes. Conversely, the risk of lung cancer declines with smoking cessation. Only 15 percent of lung cancers are not related to smoking, and the majority of these are adenocarcinomas.

Lung Cancer Histology

The term bronchial carcinoma is synonymous with lung cancer in general. Both terms refer to any epithelial carcinoma occurring in the bronchopulmonary tree. Lung cancer is broadly divided into two main groups based primarily on light microscopic observations: non–small-cell lung carcinoma and neuroendocrine tumors (typical carcinoid, atypical carcinoid, large-cell neuroendocrine carcinoma, and small-cell carcinoma).

Non–small-cell lung carcinoma. The term non–small-cell lung carcinoma (NSCLC) is used to distinguish a group of tumors from small-cell carcinoma. Tumors in the NSCLC group include squamous cell carcinoma, adenocarcinoma (including bronchoalveolar carcinoma), and large-cell carcinoma. Although they differ in appearance histologically, their clinical behavior and treatment is similar. As such, they are usefully thought of as a uniform group. However, each type has unique features that affect their clinical presentation and findings.

Squamous cell carcinoma. Squamous cell carcinoma accounts for 30–40 percent of lung cancers. It is the cancer most frequently found in men and is highly correlated with cigarette smoking. Importantly, squamous cell carcinoma is primarily located centrally and arises in the major bronchi, often causing the typical symptoms of centrally located tumors, such as hemoptysis, bronchial obstruction with atelectasis, dyspnea, and pneumonia. Central necrosis is frequent and may lead to the radiographic findings of a cavity (possibly with an air-fluid level). Such cavities may become infected, with resultant abscess formation.

Adenocarcinoma.   The incidence of adenocarcinoma has increased over the last several decades, and it now accounts for 25–40 percent of all lung cancers. It occurs with equal frequency in males and females. In contradistinction to squamous cell carcinoma, adenocarcinoma is most often a peripherally based tumor, thus it is frequently discovered incidentally on routine chest radiographs. Symptoms of chest wall invasion or malignant pleural effusions dominate.

Bronchoalveolar carcinoma.   Bronchoalveolar carcinoma (BAC) is a relatively unusual (5 percent of all lung cancers) subtype of adenocarcinoma that has a unique growth pattern that differs from adenocarcinoma. Rather than invading and destroying contiguous lung parenchyma, tumor cells multiply and fill the alveolar spaces. To be classified as a pure BAC, no evidence of destruction of surrounding lung parenchyma should be seen. Because of their growth within alveoli, BAC tumor cells from one site can aerogenously seed other parts of the same lobe or lung, or the contralateral lung. This growth pattern and tendency to seed can produce three radiographic presentations: a single nodule, multiple nodules (in single or multiple lobes), or a diffuse form with an appearance mimicking that of a lobar pneumonia. Because tumor cells fill the alveolar spaces and envelop small airways rather than destroying them, air bronchograms can be seen, unlike with other carcinomas.

Large-cell carcinoma.   Large-cell carcinoma accounts for 10–20 percent of lung cancers and may be located centrally or peripherally.

Neuroendocrine neoplasms.   Recently, neuroendocrine lung tumors have been reclassified into neuroendocrine hyperplasia and three separate grades of neuroendocrine carcinoma (NEC). Listed below is the grading system now applied to NEC (left column), with the previously used common name (right column):

Grade I NEC	Classic or typical carcinoid
Grade II NEC	Atypical carcinoid
Grade III NEC	Large-cell type or small-cell type

Grade I NEC (classic or typical carcinoid) is a low-grade NEC. An epithelial tumor, it arises primarily in the central airways, although 20 percent of the time it occurs peripherally. It occurs primarily in younger patients. Because of the central location, it classically presents with hemoptysis, with or without airway obstruction and pneumonia. These tumors are very vascular which can predispose to life-threatening hemorrhage with even simple bronchoscopic biopsy maneuvers. Regional lymph node metastases are seen in 15 percent of patients, but rarely spread systemically or cause death.

Grade II NEC (atypical carcinoid) describes a group of tumors with a degree of aggressive clinical behavior. Unlike Grade I NEC, these tumors are etiologically linked to cigarette smoking and are more likely to be peripherally located. These tumors have a much higher malignant potential. Lymph node metastases are found in 30–50 percent of patients. At the time of their diagnosis, 25 percent of patients already have remote metastases.

Grade III NEC large-cell type tumors occur primarily in heavy smokers. These tumors tend to occur in the middle to peripheral lung fields. Their neuroendocrine nature is revealed by positive immunohistochemical staining for at least one neuroendocrine marker. Grade III NEC small-cell type (small-cell lung carcinoma [SCLC]) is the most malignant NEC, and accounts for 25 percent of all lung cancers. These tumors are centrally located and consist of smaller cells with a diameter of 10–20 μm that have little cytoplasm and very dark nuclei. They also have a high mitotic rate and areas of extensive necrosis. Multiple mitoses are easily seen. Importantly, very small bronchoscopic biopsies can distinguish NSCLC from SCLC, but crush artifact may make NSCLC appear similar to SCLC. These tumors are the leading producer of paraneoplastic syndromes.

Clinical Presentation

Lung cancer displays one of the most diverse presentation patterns of all human maladies. The wide variety of symptoms and signs is related to (1) histologic features, which often help determine the anatomic site of origin in the lung; (2) the specific tumor location in the lung and its relationship to surrounding structures; (3) biologic features, and the production of a variety of paraneoplastic syndromes; and (4) the presence or absence of metastatic disease.

Tumor Histology

Squamous cell and small-cell carcinomas frequently arise in centrally located main, lobar, and first segmental bronchi. Symptoms of airway irritation or obstruction are common, and include cough, hemoptysis, wheezing (because of high-grade airway obstruction), dyspnea (because of bronchial obstruction with or without postobstructive atelectasis), and pneumonia (caused by airway obstruction with secretion retention and atelectasis).

In contrast, adenocarcinomas are often located peripherally and are often discovered incidentally as an asymptomatic lesion on chest radiograph. When symptoms occur, they are because of pleural or chest wall invasion (pleuritic or chest wall pain) or pleural seeding with malignant pleural effusion. Bronchoalveolar carcinoma (a variant of adenocarcinoma) may present as a solitary nodule, as multifocal nodules, or as a diffuse infiltrate mimicking an infectious pneumonia (pneumonic form).

Tumor Location

Symptoms related to the local intrathoracic effect of the primary tumor can be conveniently divided into two groups: pulmonary and nonpulmonary thoracic.

Pulmonary symptoms. Pulmonary symptoms result from the direct effect of the tumor on the bronchus or lung tissue. Symptoms (in order of frequency) include cough (secondary to irritation or compression of a bronchus), dyspnea (usually because of central airway obstruction or compression, with or without atelectasis), wheezing (with narrowing of a central airway of greater than 50 percent), hemoptysis (typically, blood streaking of mucus that rarely is massive, and indicates a central airway location), pneumonia (usually because of airway obstruction by the tumor), and lung abscess (because of necrosis and cavitation, with subsequent infection).

Nonpulmonary thoracic symptoms. Nonpulmonary thoracic symptoms result from invasion of the primary tumor directly into a contiguous structure (e.g., chest wall, diaphragm, pericardium, phrenic nerve, recurrent laryngeal nerve, superior vena cava, and esophagus), or from mechanical compression of a structure (e.g., esophagus or superior vena cava) by enlarged tumor-bearing lymph nodes.

Peripherally located tumors (often adenocarcinomas) extending through the visceral pleura lead to irritation or growth into the parietal pleura, and potentially to continued growth into the chest wall structures. Three types of symptoms, depending on the extent of chest wall involvement, are possible: (1) pleuritic pain, from noninvasive contact of the parietal pleura with inflammatory irritation and from direct parietal pleural invasion, (2) localized chest wall pain, with deeper invasion and involvement of the rib and/or intercostal muscles, and (3) radicular pain, from involvement of the intercostal nerve(s).

Superior sulcus tumors (usually adenocarcinomas), may produce the Pancoast syndrome. Depending on the exact tumor location, symptoms can include apical chest wall and/or shoulder pain (from involvement of the first rib and chest wall), Horner syndrome (unilateral enophthalmos, ptosis, miosis, and facial anhidrosis from invasion of the stellate sympathetic ganglion), and radicular arm pain (from invasion of T1, and occasionally C8, brachial plexus nerve roots).

Invasion of the primary tumor into the mediastinum may lead to involvement of the phrenic or recurrent laryngeal nerves. Direct invasion of the phrenic nerve occurs with tumors of the medial surface of the lung, or with anterior hilar tumors. Symptoms may include shoulder pain (referred), hiccups, and dyspnea with exertion because of diaphragm paralysis. Radiographically, the diagnosis is suggested by unilateral diaphragm elevation on chest radiograph, and can be confirmed by fluoroscopic examination of the diaphragm with breathing and sniffing (the "sniff" test).

Recurrent laryngeal nerve (RLN) involvement most commonly occurs on the left side, given the hilar location of the left RLN as it passes under the aortic arch. Paralysis may occur from invasion of the vagus nerve above the aortic arch by a medially based left upper lobe (LUL) tumor, from invasion of the RLN directly by a hilar tumor, or from invasion by hilar or aortopulmonary lymph nodes involved with metastatic tumor. Symptoms include voice change, often referred to as hoarseness, but more typically a loss of tone associated with a breathy quality, and coughing, particularly when drinking liquids.

Superior vena cava (SVC) syndrome most frequently occurs with small-cell carcinoma, with bulky enlargement of involved mediastinal lymph nodes and compression of the SVC. Symptoms include variable degrees of swelling of the head, neck, and arms; headache; and conjunctival edema.

Direct invasion of a vertebral body produces symptoms of back pain, which is often localized and severe. If the neural foramina are involved, radicular pain may also be present.

Tumor Biology

Lung cancers, both non–small-cell and small-cell, are capable of producing a variety of paraneoplastic syndromes, most often from tumor production and release of biologically active materials systemically. The majority of such syndromes are caused by small-cell carcinomas, including many endocrinopathies. Paraneoplastic syndromes may produce symptoms even before symptoms are produced by the primary tumor, thereby leading to early diagnosis. Their presence does not influence resectability or the potential to successfully treat the tumor. Symptoms of the syndrome often will abate with successful treatment, and recurrence may be heralded by recurrent paraneoplastic symptoms.

One of the more common paraneoplastic syndromes in patients with SCLC is hypertrophic pulmonary osteoarthropathy (HPO). Clinically, the syndrome is characterized by tenderness and swelling of the ankles, feet, forearms, and hands. It is because of periostitis of the fibula, tibia, radius, metacarpals, and metatarsals.

Hypercalcemia occurs in up to 10 percent of patients with lung cancer and is most often because of metastatic disease. However, 15 percent of cases are because of secretion of ectopic parathyroid hormone–related peptide, most often with squamous cell carcinoma. A diagnosis of ectopic parathyroid hormone secretion can be made by measuring elevated serum levels of parathyroid hormone; however, the clinician must also rule out concurrent metastatic bone disease by a bone scan. Symptoms of hypercalcemia include lethargy, depressed level of consciousness, nausea, vomiting, and dehydration. Most patients have resectable tumors, and following complete resection the calcium level will normalize. Endocrinopathies are caused by the release of hormones or hormone analogues into the systemic circulation. Most occur with SCLCs.

Metastatic Symptoms

Metastases occur most commonly in the central nervous system (CNS), vertebral bodies, bones, liver, adrenal glands, lungs, and skin and soft tissues. At diagnosis, 10 percent of patients with lung cancer have CNS metastases; another 10–15 percent will develop CNS metastases. Symptoms are often focal and include headache, nausea and vomiting, seizures, hemiplegia, and speech difficulty.

Nonspecific Symptoms

Lung cancer often produces a variety of nonspecific symptoms such as anorexia, weight loss, fatigue, and malaise. The cause of these symptoms is often unclear, but should raise concern about possible metastatic disease.

Diagnosis, Evaluation, and Staging

In a patient with either a histologically confirmed lung cancer or a pulmonary lesion suspected to be a lung cancer, assessment encompasses three areas: the primary tumor, presence of metastatic disease, and functional status (the patient's ability to tolerate a pulmonary resection).

Assessment of the primary tumor.   Assessment includes questions regarding the presence or absence of pulmonary, nonpulmonary, thoracic, and paraneoplastic symptoms. Patients often have already undergone a chest radiograph or CT scan before their initial visit with the surgeon; the location of the tumor can then help direct the history.

A routine chest CT should include intravenous contrast for delineation of mediastinal lymph nodes relative to normal mediastinal structures. Chest CT allows assessment of the primary tumor and its relationship to surrounding and contiguous structures and may demonstrate invasion of contiguous structures. Thoracotomy should not be denied because of presumptive evidence of invasion of the chest wall, vertebral body, or mediastinal structures; proof of invasion may require thoracoscopy or even thoracotomy. Magnetic resonance imaging (MRI), because of its excellent imaging of vascular structures, may be of value primarily to define a tumor's relationship to a major vessel.

Tissue diagnosis of the primary tumor can be obtained through bronchoscopy or needle biopsy. Bronchoscopy is particularly useful for centrally located tumors with a higher probability of being visualized and biopsied and may discover additional unsuspected endobronchial lesions. Diagnostic tissue from bronchoscopy can be obtained by one of four methods: (1) brushings and washings for cytology, (2) direct forceps biopsy of a visualized lesion, (3) FNA with a Wang needle of an externally compressing lesion without visualized endobronchial tumor, and (4) transbronchial biopsy with the use of forceps guided to the lesion by fluoroscopy.

Transthoracic needle aspiration is ideally suited for peripheral lesions not easily accessible by bronchoscopy. Using image guidance (fluoroscopy or CT), either an FNA or core-needle biopsy is performed. The primary complication is pneumothorax (in up to 50 percent of patients) usually is minor and requires no treatment. Three biopsy results are possible: malignant, a specific benign process, or indeterminate. The overall false-negative rate is 20–30 percent, therefore unless a specific benign diagnosis (such as granulomatous inflammation or hamartoma) is made, malignancy is not ruled out and further efforts at diagnosis are warranted.

A thoracotomy occasionally is necessary to diagnose and stage a primary tumor. Although this occurs in fewer than 5 percent of patients, two circumstances may require such an approach: (1) a deep-seated lesion that yielded an indeterminate needle biopsy result or that could not be biopsied for technical reasons, or (2) inability to determine invasion of a mediastinal structure by any method short of palpation. In the circumstance of a deep-seated lesion without a diagnosis, FNA, a Tru-Cut biopsy, or preferably an excisional biopsy, can be performed with frozen-section analysis. If the biopsy result is indeterminate, a lobectomy may instead be necessary. When a pneumonectomy is required, a tissue diagnosis of cancer must be made before excision.

Assessment of metastatic disease. Distant metastases are found in about 40 percent of patients with newly diagnosed lung cancer. As with the primary tumor, assessment for the presence of metastatic disease should begin with the history and physical examination, focusing on the presence or absence of new bone pain, neurologic symptoms, and new skin lesions. Additionally, constitutional symptoms (e.g., anorexia, malaise, and unintentional weight loss of greater than 5 percent of body weight) suggest either a large tumor burden or the presence of metastases. Physical examination should focus on the patient's overall appearance, noting any evidence of weight loss with muscle wasting. The appearance of cervical and supraclavicular lymph nodes and that of the oropharynx should also be examined for tobacco-associated tumors. Routine laboratory studies include serum glutamic oxaloacetic transaminase and alkaline phosphatase and serum calcium (to detect bone metastases or the ectopic parathyroid syndrome). Elevation of either hepatic enzymes or serum calcium levels typically occurs with extensive metastases.

Mediastinal lymph nodes. Chest CT is the most effective noninvasive method available to assess the mediastinal and hilar nodes for enlargement. However, a positive CT result (i.e., nodal diameter more than 1.0 cm) predicts actual metastatic involvement in only about 70 percent of patients. Thus, up to 30 percent of such nodes are enlarged from inflammation because of atelectasis or pneumonia secondary to the tumor. Therefore, no patient should be denied an attempt at curative resection just because of a positive CT result for mediastinal lymph node enlargement. Any CT finding of metastatic nodal involvement must be confirmed histologically.

Positron emission tomography (PET) scanning for metastatic disease is now routine and allows whole body imaging permiting simultaneous evaluation of the primary lung lesion, mediastinal lymph nodes, and distant organs.

Cervical mediastinoscopy is commonly employed to evaluate mediastinal lymph nodes. It has several advantages over other techniques of mediastinal lymph node staging. It can provide a tissue diagnosis, allows sampling of all paratracheal and subcarinal lymph nodes, and permits visual determination of the presence of extracapsular extension of nodal metastasis. An absolute indication for mediastinoscopy is mediastinal lymph node enlargement greater than 1.0 cm by CT scan. When the size of mediastinal lymph nodes is normal, mediastinoscopy is generally recommended for centrally located tumors, for T2 and T3 primary tumors, and occasionally for T1 adenocarcinomas.

Pleural effusion. The presence of pleural effusion on a CT scan (or chest radiograph) is not synonymous with a malignant effusion. Malignant pleural effusion can only be diagnosed by finding malignant cells in a sample of pleural fluid examined microscopically. Pleural effusion is often secondary to the atelectasis or consolidation seen with central tumors. However, pleural effusion associated with a peripherally based tumor, particularly one that abuts the visceral or parietal pleural surface, does have a higher probability of being malignant. Regardless, no pleural effusion should be assumed to be malignant.

Distant metastases. Until recently, detection of distant metastases outside the thorax was performed with a combination of chest CT scan and multiorgan scanning (e.g., brain CT or MRI, abdominal CT, and bone scan). Chest CT scans always include the upper abdomen and allow visualization of the liver and adrenal glands. Routine preoperative multiorgan scanning is not recommended for patients with a negative clinical evaluation and clinical stage I disease. However, it is recommended for patients with regionally advanced (clinical stage II, IIIA, and IIIB) disease. Any patient, regardless of clinical stage who has a positive clinical evaluation should also undergo radiographic evaluation for metastatic disease.

PET scanning has supplanted multiorgan scanning in the search for distant metastases to the liver, adrenal glands, and bones. Currently, chest CT and PET are routine in the evaluation of patients with lung cancer. Brain MRI should be performed when the suspicion or risk of brain metastases is increased. Several reports show that PET scanning appears to detect an additional 10–15 percent of distant metastases not detected by routine chest or abdominal CT and bone scans.

Assessment of functional status. For patients with a potentially resectable primary tumor, their functional status and ability to tolerate either lobectomy or pneumonectomy needs to be carefully assessed. The surgeon should first estimate the likelihood of pneumonectomy, lobectomy, or possibly sleeve resection, given the CT scan results. A sequential process of evaluation then unfolds.

A patient's history is the most important tool for gauging risk. It must be emphasized that numbers alone (e.g., forced expiratory volume in 1 second [FEV-1] and carbon monoxide diffusion capacity [DLCO]) do not supplant the clinician's assessment. The clinical assessment entails the observation of the patient's general vigor and attitude.

When obtaining the patient's history, specific questions should be routinely asked that help determine the amount of lung that the patient will likely tolerate having resected. Can the patient walk on a flat surface indefinitely, without oxygen and without having to stop and rest secondary to dyspnea? If so, the patient will be very likely to tolerate thoracotomy and lobectomy. Can the patient walk up two flights of stairs (up two standard levels), without having to stop and rest secondary to dyspnea? If so, the patient will likely tolerate pneumonectomy. Finally, nearly all patients, except those with CO_2 retention on arterial blood gas analysis, will be able to tolerate periods of single-lung ventilation and wedge resection.

Other pertinent elements of the history are current smoking status and sputum production. Current smokers have a significantly increased risk of postoperative complications. To diminish the risk significantly requires cessation of smoking at least 8 weeks preoperatively, a requirement that is often not feasible in a cancer patient. Nevertheless, efforts to abstain should be encouraged, ideally for 2 weeks before surgery. Sputum culture, antibiotic administration, and bronchodilators may be warranted preoperatively.

Pulmonary function studies are routinely performed when any resection greater than a wedge resection will be performed. The two most valuable measurements are FEV-1 and DLco. General guidelines for the use of FEV-1 in assessing the patient's ability to tolerate pulmonary resection are as follows: greater than 2.0 L can tolerate pneumonectomy, and greater than 1.2 L can tolerate lobectomy. It must be emphasized that these are guidelines only. It is also important to note that the raw value is often imprecise because normal values are reported as "percent predicted" based on corrections made for age, height, and gender. For example, a raw FEV-1 value of 1.3 L in a 62-year-old, 6-foot 3-inch male has a percent predicted value of 30 percent (because the normal expected value is 4.31 L); in a 62-year-old, 5-foot 2-inch female, the predicted value is 59 percent (normal expected value 2.21 L). The male patient is at high risk for lobectomy, although the female could potentially tolerate pneumonectomy.

The percent predicted value of both FEV-1 and DLco correlates with the risk of development of complications postoperatively, particularly pulmonary complications. Patients with predicted values of less than 50 percent show a significant increase in complication rates, with the risk of complications increasing in a stepwise fashion for each 10 percent decline.

Quantitative perfusion scanning is used in select circumstances to help estimate the functional contribution of a lobe or whole lung. Such perfusion scanning is most useful when the impact of a tumor on pulmonary physiology is difficult to discern. With complete collapse of a lobe or whole lung, the impact is apparent, and perfusion scanning is usually unnecessary. However, with centrally located tumors associated with partial obstruction of a lobar or main bronchus or of the pulmonary artery, perfusion scanning may be valuable in predicting the postoperative result of resection. Exercise testing that yields maximal oxygen consumption (VO_2max) has emerged as a valuable decision-making technique for patients with abnormal FEV-1 and DLco. In these circumstances, and in other situations in which decision making is difficult, the VO_2max should be measured. Values of less than 10 mL/kg per min generally prohibit any major pulmonary resection, although those greater than 15 mL/kg per min generally indicate the patient's potential ability to tolerate pneumonectomy.

The risk assessment of a patient is an amalgam of clinical judgment and data. Commonly, there are gray areas in which data such as that described above can provide more accurate assessment of the risk. This risk must be integrated with the experienced clinician's sense of the patient, and with the patient's attitude toward the disease and toward life.

Lung Cancer Staging

The staging of any tumor is an attempt to measure or estimate the extent of disease present and in turn use that information to help determine the patient's prognosis. The staging of solid epithelial tumors is based on the tumor-node-metastasis (TNM) staging system. The "T" status provides information about the primary tumor itself, such as its size and relationship to surrounding structures; the "N" status provides information about regional lymph nodes; and the "M" status provides information about the presence or absence of metastatic disease. Table 18-2 lists the TNM descriptors that have been developed for use in NSCLC.

The designation of lymph nodes as N1, N2, or N3 requires familiarity with the mediastinal lymph node map, which places lymph nodes in stations defined by clearly delineated anatomic boundaries. A tumor in a given patient is typically classified into a clinical stage and a pathologic stage. The clinical stage (cTNM) is derived from an assessment of all data short of surgical resection of the primary tumor and lymph nodes. Thus clinical staging information would include the history and physical examination, radiographic test results, and diagnostic biopsy information. A therapeutic plan is then generated based on the clinical stage. After surgical resection of the tumor and lymph nodes, a postoperative pathologic stage (pTNM) is determined, providing further prognostic information.

Treatment

Early stage disease.   Early stage disease is typically defined as stages I and II. In this group are T1 and T2 tumors (with or without local N1 nodal involvement), and T3 tumors (without N1 nodal involvement). This group represents a small proportion of the total number of patients diagnosed with lung cancer each year (about 15 percent of 150,000 patients).

The current standard of treatment is surgical resection, accomplished by lobectomy or pneumonectomy, depending on the tumor location. Despite the term "early stage," surgery as a single treatment modality remains disappointing. After surgical resection of postoperative pathologic stage IA disease, 5-year survival is only 67 percent as reported by Mountain in 1997. The figures decline with higher stages. The overall 5-year survival rate for stage I disease as a group is about 65 percent; for stage II disease it is about 41 percent.

Appropriate surgical procedures for patients with early stage disease include lobectomy, sleeve lobectomy, and occasionally pneumonectomy with mediastinal lymph node dissection or sampling. Sleeve resection is performed for tumors located at airway bifurcations when an acceptable length bronchial margin cannot be obtained by standard lobectomy. Pneumonectomy is rarely performed; it is indicated primarily for larger central tumors involving the distal main stem bronchus when a bronchial sleeve resection is not possible, and when resection of involved N1 lymph nodes cannot be achieved short of pneumonectomy. The latter circumstance occurs with bulky adenopathy or with extracapsular nodal spread.

Pancoast tumor (apical tumor) resection should always be preceded by mediastinoscopy. In general, the treatment of these tumors has evolved to a multimodal approach in which radiation plays a constant role. Typically, an induction radiation dose of 30–35 Gy is administered to enhance the probability of

TABLE 18-2 American Joint Committee on Cancer Staging System for Lung Cancer

	Stage	TNM
	IA	T1N0M0
	IB	T2N0M0
	IIA	T1N1M0
	IIB	T2N1M0
		T3N0M0
	IIIA	T3N1M0
		T1–3N2M0
	IIIB	T4 Any N M0
		Any T N3 M0
	IV	Any T Any N M1

TNM Definitions

T	TX	Positive malignant cell, but primary tumor not visualized by imaging or bronchoscopy
	T0	No evidence of primary tumor
	Tis	Carcinoma in situ
	T1	Tumor $\leq$ 3 cm, surrounded by lung or visceral pleura, without bronchoscopic evidence of invasion more proximal than the lobar bronchus
	T2	Tumor with any of the following features of size or extent:

- $>$ 3 cm in greatest dimension
- $>$ Involves main bronchus, $\geq$ 2 cm distal to the carina
- $>$ Invades the visceral pleura
- $>$ Associated with atelectasis or obstructive pneumonitis that extends to the hilar region but does not involve the entire lung

	T3	Tumor of any size that directly invades any of the following: chest wall (including superior sulcus tumors), diaphragm, mediastinal pleura, parietal pericardium; or tumor in the main bronchus < 2 cm distal to the carina, but without involvement of the carina; or associated atelectasis or obstructive pneumonitis of the entire lung
	T4	Tumor of any size that invades any of the following: mediastinum, heart, great vessels, trachea, esophagus, vertebral body, carina; or tumor with a malignant pleural or pericardial effusion, or with satellite tumor nodule(s) within the ipsilateral primary-tumor lobe of the lung
N	NX	Regional lymph nodes cannot be assessed
	N0	No regional lymph node metastasis
	N1	Metastasis to ipsilateral peribronchial and/or ipsilateral hilar lymph nodes, and intrapulmonary nodes involved by direct extension of the primary tumor
	N2	Metastasis to ipsilateral mediastinal and/or subcarinal lymph node(s)
	N3	Metastasis to contralateral mediastinal, contralateral hilar, ipsilateral or contralateral scalene, or supraclavicular lymph node(s)

TABLE 18-2 *(Continued)*

M	MX	Presence of distant metastasis cannot be assessed
	M0	No distant metastasis
	M1	Distant metastasis present (including metastatic tumor nodule[s] in the ipsilateral nonprimary tumor lobe[s] of the lung)

Summary of Staging Definitions

Occult stage	Microscopically identified cancer cells in lung secretions on multiple occasions (or multiple daily collections); no discernible primary cancer in the lung
Stage 0	Carcinoma in situ
Stage IA	Tumor surrounded by lung or visceral pleura $\leq$ 3 cm arising more than 2 cm distal to the carina (T1 N0)
Stage IB	Tumor surrounded by lung > 3 cm, or tumor of any size with visceral pleura involved arising more than 2 cm distal to the carina (T2 N0)
Stage IIA	Tumor $\leq$ 3 cm not extended to adjacent organs, with ipsilateral peribronchial and hilar lymph node involvement (T1 N1)
Stage IIB	Tumor > 3 cm not extended to adjacent organs, with ipsilateral peribronchial and hilar lymph node involvement (T2 N1)
	Tumor invading chest wall, pleura, or pericardium but not involving carina, nodes negative (T3 N0)
Stage IIIA	Tumor invading chest wall, pleura, or pericardium and nodes in hilum or ipsilateral mediastinum (T3, N1–2) or tumor of any size invading ipsilateral mediastinal or subcarinal nodes (T1–3, N2)
Stage IIIB	Direct extension to adjacent organs (esophagus, aorta, heart, cava, diaphragm, or spine); satellite nodule same lobe, or any tumor associated with contralateral mediastinal or supraclavicular lymph-node involvement (T4 or N3)
Stage IV	Separate nodule in different lobes or any tumor with distant metastases (M1)

complete resection, followed by surgery 4–5 weeks later. With this approach, 5-year survival rates of 35 percent have been achieved. Surgical excision usually includes a portion of the lower trunk of the brachial plexus, the stellate ganglion, and the chest wall, along with lobectomy.

With chest wall involvement, en bloc chest wall resection, along with lobectomy, is performed, with or without chest wall reconstruction. For small rib resections or those posterior to the scapula, chest wall reconstruction is usually unnecessary. Larger defects (two rib segments or more) are usually reconstructed with Gore-Tex to provide chest wall contour and stability.

If a patient is deemed medically unfit for major pulmonary resection because of inadequate pulmonary reserve or other medical conditions, then options include limited surgical resection or radiotherapy. Limited resection, defined as segmentectomy or wedge resection, can only be applied to more peripheral T1 or T2 tumors. Moreover, limited resection is associated with an increased rate of local recurrence and a decreased long-term survival rate, probably because of incomplete resection of occult intrapulmonary lymphatic tumor spread. Alternatively, definitive radiotherapy consisting of a total dose of 60–65 Gy has resulted in a 5-year survival rate of about 30 percent for patients with stage I disease.

The role of chemotherapy in early stage NSCLC is evolving. Postoperative adjuvant chemotherapy previously was of no benefit in multiple prospective randomized trials; however, newer, more effective agents have been of benefit, although the final results of current trials are pending.

Locoregional advanced disease. Surgical resection as sole therapy has a limited role in stage III disease. T3N1 tumors can be treated with surgery alone and have a 5-year survival rate of approximately 25 percent. Patients with N2 disease are a heterogeneous group. Patients with clinically evident N2 disease (i.e., bulky adenopathy present on CT scan or mediastinoscopy, with lymph nodes often replaced by tumor) have a 5-year survival rate of 5–10 percent with surgery alone. In contrast, patients with microscopic N2 disease discovered incidentally in one lymph node station after surgical resection have a 5-year survival rate that may be as high as 30 percent. Surgery generally does not play a role in the care of patients with N3 disease (IIIB); however, it is occasionally appropriate in select patients with a T4 primary tumor (superior vena caval, carinal, or vertebral body involvement) and no N2 or N3 disease. Survival rates remain low for these patients.

Definitive radiotherapy as a single modality can cure patients with N2 or N3 disease, albeit in less than 10 percent. Recent improvement has been seen with three-dimensional conformal radiotherapy and altered fractionation. Such poor results are reflective of the facts that radiotherapy is a locoregional treatment, and that most stage III patients die of systemic disease. Therefore, definitive treatment of stage III disease (when surgery is not felt to be feasible at any time) is usually a combination of chemotherapy and radiation.

Small-cell lung carcinoma. Small-cell lung carcinoma (SCLC) accounts for about 20 percent of primary lung cancers and is not generally treated surgically. These aggressive neoplasms have early widespread metastases. Histologically, they can be difficult to distinguish from lymphoproliferative lesions and atypical carcinoid tumors. Therefore a definitive diagnosis must be established with adequate tissue samples.

Unlike NSCLC, clinical staging of SCLC is broadly defined by the presence of local or distant disease. Patients present without evidence of distant metastatic disease, but often have bulky locoregional disease, termed "limited" SCLC. Most often, the primary tumor is large and associated with bulky mediastinal adenopathy, which may lead to obstruction of the superior vena cava. The other clinical stage, disseminated, usually presents with widely disseminated metastatic disease. Patients in either stage are treated primarily with chemotherapy and radiation.

Metastatic lesions to the lung. Surgical resection of pulmonary metastases has a role in properly selected patients. General principles of selection include the following: (1) the primary tumor must already be controlled; (2) the patient must be able to tolerate general anesthesia, potential single-lung ventilation, and the planned pulmonary resection; (3) the metastases must be completely resectable according to CT imaging; (4) there must be no evidence of extrapulmonary tumor burden; and (5) alternative superior therapy must be unavailable.

The technical aim of pulmonary metastasis resections is complete resection of all macroscopic tumor. Additionally, any adjacent structure involved should be resected en bloc (i.e., chest wall, diaphragm, and pericardium). Multiple lesions and/or hilar lesions may require lobectomy. Pneumonectomy is rarely justified or employed. In general the best prognosis is seen with germ-cell tumors, osteosarcomas, a disease-free interval over 36 months, and a single metastasis.

Pulmonary Infections

Lung Abscess

A lung abscess is a localized area of pulmonary parenchymal necrosis caused by an infectious organism; tissue destruction results in a solitary or dominant cavity measuring at least 2 cm in diameter. Based on this lung abscesses are classified as primary or secondary. A primary lung abscess occurs, for example, in immunocompromised patients (as a result of malignancy, chemotherapy, or an organ transplant, etc.), in patients as a result of highly virulent organisms inciting a necrotizing pulmonary infection, or in patients who have a predisposition to aspirate oropharyngeal or gastrointestinal secretions. A secondary lung abscess occurs in patients with an underlying condition such as a partial bronchial obstruction, a lung infarct, or adjacent suppurative infections (subphrenic or hepatic abscesses).

Microbiology. In community-acquired pneumonia, the causative bacteria are predominantly gram-positive; in hospital-acquired pneumonia, 60–70 percent of the organisms are gram-negative. Gram-negative bacteria associated with nosocomial pneumonia include *Klebsiella pneumoniae*, *Haemophilus influenzae*, Proteus species, *Pseudomonas aeruginosa*, *Escherichia coli*, *Enterobacter cloacae*, and *Eikenella corrodens*. Normal oropharyngeal secretions contain many more Streptococcus species and more anaerobes (about 108 organisms/mL) than aerobes (about 107 organisms/mL Overall, at least 50 percent of these infections are caused by purely anaerobic bacteria, 25 percent are caused by mixed aerobes and anaerobes, and 25 percent or fewer are caused by aerobes only.

Clinical features and diagnosis. Typical symptoms include productive cough, fever, chills, leukocytosis ($>15,000$ cells/mm^3), weight loss, fatigue, malaise, pleuritic chest pain, and dyspnea. Lung abscesses may also present in a more indolent fashion, with weeks to months of cough, malaise, weight loss, low-grade fever, night sweats, leukocytosis, and anemia. After aspiration pneumonia, 1–2 weeks typically elapse before cavitation occurs; 40–75 percent of such patients produce a putrid, foul-smelling sputum. Severe complications such as massive hemoptysis, endobronchial spread to other portions of the lungs, rupture into the pleural space and development of pyopneumothorax, or septic shock and respiratory failure are rare in the modern antibiotic era. The mortality rate is about 5–10 percent, except in the presence of immunosuppression, in which rates range from 9–28 percent.

Chest radiograph shows a density or mass with a relatively thin-walled cavity and air-fluid level, indicating a communication with the tracheobronchial tree. CT scan is useful to clarify the diagnosis when the radiograph is equivocal, to help rule out endobronchial obstruction, and to look for an associated mass or other pathologic anomalies. A cavitating lung carcinoma is frequently mistaken for a lung abscess.

Bronchoscopy is essential to rule out endobronchial obstruction, which is usually because of tumor or foreign body, and to obtain uncontaminated cultures by bronchoalveolar lavage. Cultures can also be obtained by percutaneous, transthoracic FNA under ultrasound or CT guidance.

Management. Systemic antibiotics are the mainstay of therapy. For community-acquired infections secondary to aspiration, likely pathogens are oropharyngeal streptococci and anaerobes. Penicillin G, ampicillin, or amoxicillin are the main therapeutic agents, but a β-lactamase inhibitor or metronidazole should be added to cover the increasing prevalence of gram-negative anaerobes that produce β-lactamase. Clindamycin is also a primary therapeutic agent. For hospital-acquired infections, Staphylococcus aureus and aerobic gram-negative bacilli are common organisms of the oropharyngeal flora. Piperacillin or ticarcillin with a β-lactamase inhibitor (or equivalent alternatives) provide better coverage of likely pathogens. The duration of antimicrobial therapy is variable: 1–2 weeks for simple aspiration pneumonia and 3–12 weeks for necrotizing pneumonia and lung abscess.

Surgical drainage of lung abscesses is uncommon because drainage usually occurs spontaneously via the tracheobronchial tree. Indications for intervention include failure of medical therapy; an abscess under tension; an abscess increasing in size during appropriate treatment; contralateral lung contamination; an abscess larger than 4–6 cm in diameter; necrotizing infection with multiple abscesses, hemoptysis, abscess rupture, or pyopneumothorax; and inability to exclude a cavitating carcinoma. External drainage may be accomplished with tube thoracostomy, percutaneous drainage, or surgical cavernostomy. Surgical resection is required in fewer than 10 percent of lung abscess patients.

Mycobacterial Infections

Microbiology. Mycobacterium tuberculosis is the highly virulent bacillus of this species that produces invasive infection among humans, principally pulmonary tuberculosis. Because of improper application of antimycobacterial drugs and multifactorial interactions, MDRTB organisms have emerged that are defined by their resistance to two or more first-line antimycobacterial drugs. Approximately 10 percent of new tuberculosis cases, and as many as 40 percent of recurrent cases, are attributed to MDRTB organisms. The more important NTM organisms include *M. kansasii*, *M. avium*, and *M. intracellulare* complex (MAC), and *M. fortuitum*. The highest incidence of *M. kansasii* infection is in midwestern U.S. cities among middle-aged males from good socioeconomic surroundings. MAC organisms are important infections in older adult and immunocompromised patient groups. *M. fortuitum* infections are common complications of underlying severe debilitating disease. None of these organisms are as contagious as *M. tuberculosis*.

Pathogenesis and pathology. The main route of transmission is via airborne inhalation of viable mycobacteria. Three stages of primary infection have been described. In the first stage, alveolar macrophages ingest the bacilli. In the second stage, from days –21, the bacteria continue to multiply in macrophages. The patient is often asymptomatic. The third stage is characterized by the onset of cell-mediated immunity (CD4 + helper T cells) and delayed-type hypersensitivity. Activated macrophages acquire an increased capacity for bacterial killing. Macrophage death increases, resulting in the formation of a granuloma, the characteristic lesion found on pathologic examination.

Clinical presentation and diagnosis. About 80–90 percent of tuberculosis patients present with clinical disease in the lungs. In 85–90 percent of these patients, involution and healing occur, leading to a dormant phase that may last a lifetime. The only evidence of tuberculosis infection may be a positive skin reaction to tuberculin challenge or a Ghon complex observed on chest radiograph. Within the first 2 years of primary infection, reactivation may occur in up to 10–15 percent of infected patients. In 80 percent, reactivation occurs in the lungs; other reactivation sites include the lymph nodes, pleura, and the musculoskeletal system.

After primary infection, pulmonary tuberculosis is frequently asymptomatic. Systemic symptoms of low-grade fever, malaise, and weight loss are subtle and may go unnoticed. A productive cough may develop, usually after tubercle cavitation. Hemoptysis often develops from complications of disease such as bronchiectasis or erosion into vascular malformations associated with cavitation. Extrapulmonary involvement is because of hematogenous or lymphatic spread from pulmonary lesions. Virtually any organ can become infected, giving rise to the protean manifestations of tuberculosis. Of note to the thoracic surgeon, the pleura, chest wall, and mediastinal organs may all be involved. More than one third of immunocompromised patients have disseminated disease, with hepatomegaly, diarrhea, splenomegaly, and abdominal pain.

The definitive diagnosis of tuberculosis requires identification of the mycobacterium in a patient's bodily fluids or involved tissues. Skin testing using purified protein derivative is important for epidemiologic purposes, and can help exclude infection in uncomplicated cases. For pulmonary tuberculosis, sputum examination is inexpensive and has a high diagnostic yield. Bronchoscopy with alveolar lavage has high diagnostic accuracy. Chest CT scan can delineate the extent of parenchymal disease.

Management. Medical therapy is the primary treatment of pulmonary tuberculosis and is often initiated before a mycobacterial pathogen is definitively identified. Combinations of two or more drugs are routinely used to minimize resistance, which inevitably develops with only single-agent therapy. First-line drugs include isonicotinic acid hydrazine (isoniazid; INH), ethambutol, rifampin, and pyrazinamide. Second-line drugs include cycloserine, ethionamide, kanamycin, ciprofloxacin, and amikacin, among others.

The initial therapy for patients with active pulmonary tuberculosis consists of various drug regimens lasting from 6–9 months. Bacterial sensitivity profiles help to tailor drug therapy. In the case of MDRTB organisms, four or more antimycobacterial drugs are often used, generally for 18–24 months. Rifampin and INH augmented with one or more second-line drugs are most commonly used to treat NTM infections. Generally, therapy lasts about 18 months. The overall response rate is unsatisfactory in 20–30 percent of patients with *M. kansasii* infection, although most such patients do not require surgical intervention. In contrast, pulmonary MAC infections respond poorly, even to combinations of four or more drugs, thus most such patients become surgical candidates. Overall, sputum conversion is achieved in only 50–80 percent of NTM infections, and relapses occur in up to 20 percent of patients.

In the United States, surgical intervention for MDRTB is necessary when lung tissue has been destroyed and with persistent thick-walled cavitation. Indications for surgery are: (1) complications of previous surgery for tuberculosis; (2) failure of optimum medical therapy (e.g., progressive disease, lung gangrene, intracavitary aspergillosis superinfection); (3) biopsy for definitive diagnosis; (4) complications of pulmonary scarring (e.g., massive hemoptysis, cavernomas, bronchiectasis, or bronchostenosis); (5) extrapulmonary thoracic involvement; (6) pleural tuberculosis; and (7) NTM infections. The goal of surgery generally is removal of all gross disease with preservation of uninvolved lung tissue. Scattered nodular disease may be left, given its low mycobacterial burden. Antimycobacterial medications are given preoperatively (for about 3 months) and postoperatively for 12–24 months. Overall, 90 percent of patients are cured with appropriate medical and surgical therapy.

Pulmonary Mycoses

Mycotic lung infections can often mimic bronchial carcinoma or tuberculosis. Most fungal infections occur as opportunistic. Examples include Aspergillus, Cryptococcus, Candida, and Mucor. However, some fungi are primary or true pathogens including Histoplasma, Coccidioides, and Blastomyces.

Fungal infections are definitively diagnosed by directly identifying the organism in body exudates or tissues, preferably grown in culture. Serologic testing to identify mycotic-specific antibodies may be useful.

Aspergillosis. Three species of Aspergillus most commonly cause clinical disease: *A. fumigatus*, *A. flavus*, and *A. niger*. Aspergillus is a saprophytic, filamentous fungus with septate hyphae. Spores (2.5–3 μm in diameter) are inhaled and then reach the distal bronchi and alveoli. Three syndromes may occur: Aspergillus hypersensitivity lung disease, aspergilloma, or invasive pulmonary aspergillosis. Overlap occurs between these syndromes, depending on the patient's immune status. Hypersensitivity leads to cough, fever, infiltrates, eosinophilia, and elevation of immunoglobulin (Ig)E antibodies to Aspergillus.

Aspergilloma (fungal ball) results from colonization of preexisting cavities. Fungal balls are the most common presentation of (noninvasive) pulmonary aspergillosis. Clinical features vary from asymptomatic, to hemoptysis (sometimes life threatening), to a chronic process of productive cough, clubbing, malaise, and weight loss. Chest radiograph can show a crescentic radiolucency above a rounded radiopaque lesion (Monad sign). Asymptomatic aspergilloma do not require treatment. For mild, non–life-threatening hemoptysis, initial treatment is medical management with Amphotericin B. Indications for surgery include recurrent or massive hemoptysis, chronic cough with systemic symptoms, progressive infiltrate around the mycetoma, and a pulmonary mass of unknown cause. The postresectional residual space in the thorax should be obliterated. Techniques to do so include pleural tent, pneumoperitoneum, decortication, muscle flap, omental transposition, and thoracoplasty.

Invasive pulmonary aspergillosis usually affects immunocompromised patients and is an invasive and often necrotizing bronchopneumonia. Presentation is fever unresponsive to antibiotic therapy in the setting of neutropenia. A chest CT scan shows infiltrate and consolidation and occasional characteristic signs (e.g., halo sign and cavitary lesions). Empiric antifungal therapy (using amphotericin B) should be started in these high-risk patients. The mortality rate is high, from 90 percent in bone marrow transplantion and up to 40 percent in kidney transplantion. Surgical removal of the infectious nidus is advocated by some groups because medical treatment has such poor outcomes.

Cryptococcosis. Cryptococci are present in soil and dust contaminated by pigeon droppings. When inhaled, a nonfatal pulmonary and central nervous system infection may occur. Cryptococcosis is the fourth most common opportunistic infection in patients with HIV infection, affecting 6–10 percent of that population. Four pathologic patterns are seen: granulomas; granulomatous pneumonia; diffuse alveolar or interstitial involvement; and proliferation of fungi in alveoli and lung vasculature. Symptoms and radiographic findings are nonspecific. Cryptococcus may be isolated from sputum, bronchial washings, percutaneous needle aspiration of the lung, or cerebrospinal fluid. Multiple antifungal agents are effective against *C. neoformans*, including amphotericin B and the azoles.

Candidiasis. Candida organisms are oval, budding cells (with or without mycelial elements) that colonize the oropharynx of many healthy individuals and are common hospital and laboratory contaminants. Usually, *Candida albicans* causes disease in the oral or bronchial mucosa, among other anatomic sites. Other potentially pathogenic Candida species include *C. tropicalis*, *C. glabrata*, and *C. krusei*.

Candida infections are no longer confined to immunocompromised patients, but now affect those who are critically ill, are taking multiple antibiotics longterm, have indwelling vascular catheters (or urinary catheters), sustain recurrent gastrointestinal perforations, or have burn wounds. With respect to the thorax, such patients commonly have candidal pneumonia, pulmonary abscess, esophagitis, and mediastinitis. Amphotericin B, often in combination with 5-fluorocytosine, is a proven therapeutic treatment for Candida tissue infections.

Primary fungal pathogens. Histoplasmosis primarily affects the respiratory system after spore inhalation. It is the most common of all fungal pulmonary infections. In the United States this disease is endemic in the Midwest and Mississippi River Valley, where about 500,000 new cases arise each year. Active, symptomatic disease is uncommon. Acute forms present as primary or disseminated pulmonary histoplasmosis; chronic forms present as pulmonary granulomas (histoplasmomas), chronic cavitary histoplasmosis, mediastinal granulomas, fibrosing mediastinitis, or broncholithiasis. In immunocompromised patients, the infection may become systemic and more virulent. Diagnosis is by fungal smear, culture, direct biopsy of infected tissues, or serologic testing.

Acute pulmonary histoplasmosis commonly presents with fever, chills, headache, chest pain, and nonproductive cough. Chest radiographs may be normal or may show mediastinal lymphadenopathy and patchy parenchymal infiltrates. Most patients improve in a few weeks and do not require antifungal therapy. Amphotericin B is the treatment of choice if moderate symptoms persist for 2–4 weeks; if the illness is extensive, including dyspnea and hypoxia; and if patients are immunosuppressed.

With healing the infiltrate will consolidate into a solitary nodule (histoplasmoma). This condition is asymptomatic and usually is seen incidentally on radiographs as a coin-shaped lesion with central calcification.

When lymph nodes and pulmonary granulomas calcify over time, pressure atrophy on the bronchial wall may result in erosion and migration of the granulomatous mass into the bronchus, causing broncholithiasis. Typical symptoms include cough, hemoptysis, and dyspnea. Life-threatening complications include massive hemoptysis or bronchoesophageal fistula. Treatment is surgical removal of the bronchial mass repair of associated complications.

Coccidioides immitis is an endemic fungus found in soil and dust of the southwestern United States. Acute pulmonary coccidioidomycosis occurs in about 40 percent of people who inhale spores. Symptoms consist of fever, sweating, anorexia, weakness, arthralgia, cough, sputum, and chest pain. When symptoms and radiographic findings persist for more than 6–8 weeks, the disease is considered to be persistent coccidioidal pneumonia. Immunocompromised patients are susceptible to disseminated coccidioidomycosis, which carries a mortality rate over 40 percent. Treatment is with itraconazole and fluconazole for mild to moderate disease and amphotericin B for disseminated disease and immunocompromised patients. Surgical resection is considered if cavities persist for more than 2 years; are larger than 2 cm in diameter; rapidly enlarge, rupture, are thick-walled; or are associated with severe or recurrent hemoptysis.

Blastomyces dermatitidis is a round, single-budding yeast with a characteristic thick, refractile cell wall. It primarily infects the lungs of people who inhale contaminated soil that has been disturbed. *B. dermatitidis* has a worldwide distribution; in the United States it is endemic in the central states. Symptoms include cough, sputum production, fever, weight loss, and hemoptysis. In acute disease, consolidation is seen on radiographs; in chronic disease, fibronodular lesions (with or without cavitation) similar to tuberculosis are noted. Oral itraconazole for 6 months is the treatment of choice. Amphotericin B is warranted for patients with cavitary blastomycosis, disseminated disease, or extensive lung involvement and immunocompromised patients. After adequate drug therapy, surgical resection of cavitary lesions is considered because viable organisms can persist.

Antifungals. Amphotericin B has been the mainstay for systemic fungal infections. A lipophilic organic compound leads to binding ergosterol in the fungal cell membrane with disruption and ion leakage. Nephrotoxicity limits its applicability. Three lipid-based formulations of amphotericin B have shown decreased nephrotoxicity and higher drug-dose delivery but higher costs and limited data concerning better efficacy have tempered widespread adoption. The azoles include miconazole, ketoconazole, fluconazole, and itraconazole. This drug class inhibitscytochrome P450, interfering with fungal cell membrane synthesis.

Massive Hemoptysis

Massive hemoptysis is generally defined as expectoration of over 600 mL of blood within a 24-hour period. It is a medical emergency associated with a mortality rate of 30–50 percent. One should be aware, however, that the volume of hemoptysis that is life-threatening is highly dependent on the individual's respiratory status.

Anatomy

Most cases of massive hemoptysis involve bleeding from the bronchial artery circulation or from the pulmonary circulation pathologically exposed to the high pressures of the bronchial circulation. In many cases of hemoptysis, particularly those because of inflammatory disorders, the bronchial arterial tree becomes hyperplastic and tortuous. The systemic pressures within these arteries, combined with a disease process within the airway and erosion, lead to bleeding.

Causes

Most common causes of massive hemoptysis are secondary to inflammation. Chronic inflammatory disorders (i.e., bronchiectasis, cystic fibrosis, tuberculosis) lead to localized bronchial arterial proliferation, and with erosion, bleeding of these hypervascular areas occurs.

Tuberculosis can cause hemoptysis by erosion of a broncholith (a calcified tuberculous lymph node) into a vessel, or when a tuberculous cavity is present, by erosion of a blood vessel within the cavity. Within such cavities, aneurysms of the pulmonary artery (referred to as Rasmussen aneurysm) can erode with subsequent massive bleeding.

Hemoptysis because of lung cancer usually is mild, resulting in blood-streaked sputum. When massive, bleeding hemoptysis usually is because of malignant invasion of pulmonary artery vessels by large central tumors and is often a terminal event.

Management

Treatment involves a multidisciplinary team of intensive care physicians, interventional radiologists, and thoracic surgeons. Treatment priorities are: (1) respiratory stabilization and prevention of asphyxiation, (2) localize the bleeding site, (3) stop the hemorrhage, (4) determine the cause, and (5) definitively prevent recurrence. The clinically pragmatic definition of massive hemoptysis is a degree of bleeding that threatens respiratory stability. Therefore clinical judgment of the risk of respiratory compromise is the first step in evaluating a patient. Two scenarios are possible: (1) bleeding is significant and persistent, but its rate allows a rapid but sequential diagnostic and therapeutic approach, and (2) bleeding is so rapid that emergency airway control and therapy are necessary.

Scenario 1: significant, persistent, but nonmassive bleeding. Although bleeding is brisk in scenario 1, the patient may be able to maintain clearance of the blood and secretions with his or her own respiratory reflexes. Immediate measures are admission to an intensive care unit, strict bedrest, Trendelenburg positioning with the affected side down (if known), administration of humidified oxygen, monitoring of oxygen saturation and arterial blood gases, and insertion of large-bore intravenous catheters. Strict bedrest with sedation may lead to slowing or cessation of bleeding, and the judicious use of intravenous narcotics or other relaxants to mildly sedate the patient and diminish some of the reflexive airway activity often is necessary. Also recommended are administration of aerosolized adrenaline, intravenous antibiotic therapy if needed, and correction of abnormal blood coagulation study results. Finally, unless contraindicated, intravenous vasopressin (20 U over 15 min, followed by an infusion of 0.2 U/min) can be given.

A chest radiograph may reveal a localized lesion but the effects of blood soiling of other areas of the lungs may predominate, obscuring the area of pathology. Chest CT scan provides more detail and is nearly always performed if the patient is stable.

Some clinicians argue that rigid bronchoscopy should always be performed. However, if clinically stable and the ongoing bleeding is not imminently threatening, flexible bronchoscopy is appropriate. It allows diagnosis of airway abnormalities and will usually permit localization of the bleeding site to either a lobe or even a segment.

Because most cases of massive hemoptysis arise from the bronchial arterial tree selective bronchial arteriography and embolization is next. Prearteriogram bronchoscopy is extremely useful to direct the angiographer. However, if bronchoscopy fails to localize the bleeding site, then bilateral bronchial arteriograms can be performed. Typically, the abnormal vascularity is visualized, rather than extravasation of the contrast dye.

Embolization will acutely arrest the bleeding in 80–90 percent of patients. However, 30–60 percent of patients will have recurrences. Therefore, embolization should be viewed as an immediate but likely temporizing measure to acutely control bleeding. Subsequently, definitive treatment of the underlying pathologic process is appropriate. If bleeding persists after embolization, a pulmonary artery source should be suspected and a pulmonary angiogram performed.

If respiratory compromise is impending, orotracheal intubation should be performed. After intubation, flexible bronchoscopy should be performed to clear blood and secretions and to attempt localization of the bleeding site. Depending on the possible causes of the bleeding, bronchial artery embolization or (if appropriate) surgery can be considered.

Scenario 2: significant, persistent, and massive bleeding. Life-threatening bleeding requires emergency airway control and preparation for potential surgery. Such patients are best cared for in an operating room equipped with rigid bronchoscopy. Immediate orotracheal intubation may be necessary to gain control of ventilation and suctioning. However, rapid transport to the operating room with rigid bronchoscopy should be facilitated. Rigid bronchoscopy allows adequate suctioning of bleeding with visualization of the bleeding site; the nonbleeding side can be cannulated with the rigid scope and the patient ventilated. After stabilization, ice-saline lavage of the bleeding site can then be performed (up to 1 L in 50-mL aliquots); bleeding stops in up to 90 percent of patients.

Alternatively, blockade of the main stem bronchus of the affected side can be accomplished with a double-lumen endotracheal tube, with a bronchial blocker, or by intubation of the nonaffected side by an uncut standard endotracheal tube. Placement of a double-lumen endotracheal tube is challenging in these circumstances, given the bleeding and secretions. Proper placement and suctioning may be difficult, and attempts could compromise the patient's ventilation. The best option is to place a bronchial blocker in the affected bronchus with inflation. The blocker is left in place for 24 h and the area is reexamined bronchoscopically. After this 24-h period, bronchial artery embolization can be performed.

Surgical intervention. In most patients, bleeding can be stopped, recovery can occur, and plans to definitively treat the underlying cause can be made. In scenario 1 (significant, persistent, but nonmassive bleeding), the patient may undergo further evaluation as an inpatient or outpatient. A chest CT scan and pulmonary function studies should be obtained preoperatively. In scenario 2 (patients with significant, persistent, and massive bleeding), surgery, if appropriate, usually will be performed during the same hospitalization as the rigid bronchoscopy or main stem bronchus blockade. In less than 10 percent of patients, emergency surgery will be necessary, delayed only by efforts to localize the bleeding site by rigid bronchoscopy.

Surgical treatment is individualized according to the source of bleeding and the patient's medical condition, prognosis, and pulmonary reserve. General indications for urgent surgery include (1) presence of a fungus ball, (2) a lung abscess, (3) significant cavitary disease, or (4) failure to control the bleeding.

Spontaneous Pneumothorax

Spontaneous pneumothorax is most commonly because of rupture of an apical subpleural bleb which occurs most frequently in young postadolescent males with a tall thin body habitus. Treatment is generally chest tube insertion with water seal. If a leak is present and it persists for greater than 3 days, thoracoscopic management (i.e., bleb resection with pleurodesis by talc or pleural abrasion) is performed. Recurrences or complete lung collapse with the first episode are generally indications for thoracoscopic intervention.

Other causes of spontaneous pneumothorax are emphysema (rupture of a bleb or bulla), cystic fibrosis, acquired immune deficiency syndrome [AIDS], metastatic cancer (especially sarcoma), asthma, lung abscess, and occasionally lung cancer. Management of pneumothorax in these circumstances is often tied to therapy of the specific disease process and may involve tumor resection, thoracoscopic pleurectomy, or talc pleurodesis.

CHEST WALL

Chest Wall Mass

Clinical Approach

All chest wall tumors should be considered malignant until proven otherwise. Patients with either a benign or malignant chest wall tumor typically present with a slowly enlarging palpable mass (50–70 percent), chest wall pain (25–50 percent), or both.

Pain is typically localized to the area of the tumor, and although more often present (and more intense) with malignant tumors, it also can be present in one-third of benign tumors. With Ewing sarcoma, fever and malaise may also be present. Age can provide guidance regarding the possibility of malignancy. Patients with benign chest wall tumors are on average 26 years old; the average age for patients with malignant tumors is 40 years old. Overall, the probability of a chest wall tumor being malignant is 50–80 percent.

Evaluation and Management

Radiography. Chest radiograph may reveal evidence of rib destruction and calcification within the lesion. CT scan is routinely performed done to evaluate the primary lesion and to determine its relationship to contiguous structures and to search for pulmonary metastases. Contiguous involvement of underlying lung or other soft tissues or the presence of pulmonary metastases does not preclude successful surgery.

MRI is valuable for evaluating tumors contiguous to or near neurovascular structures or spine and can potentially enhance the ability to distinguish benign from malignant sarcomas.

Biopsy. Inappropriate or misguided attempts at tissue diagnosis through casual open biopsy techniques have the potential (if the lesion is a sarcoma) to seed surrounding tissues and contiguous body cavities (e.g., the pleural space) with tumor cells, potentially compromising local tumor control and patient survival. Accurately typing chest wall sarcomas has a profound impact on their management.

Tissue diagnosis can be made by one of three methods: a needle biopsy (typically CT-guided, FNA or a core biopsy), incisional biopsy, or excisional biopsy.

An excisional biopsy should be done when the initial radiographic diagnosis indicates that it is a benign lesion, or when the lesion has the classic appearance of a chondrosarcoma (in which case definitive surgical resection can be undertaken). Any lesion less than 2.0 cm can be excised as long as the resulting wound is small enough to close primarily. When the diagnosis cannot be made by radiographic evaluation, a needle biopsy (FNA or core) should be done. Needle biopsy has the advantage of avoiding wound and body cavity contamination (a potential complication with an incisional biopsy).

If a needle biopsy is nondiagnostic, an incisional biopsy may be performed, with caveats. When performing an incisional biopsy, the skin incision must be placed directly over the mass and oriented to allow subsequent excision of the scar. Development of skin flaps must be avoided, and in general no drains are used. A drain may be placed if a hematoma is likely to develop, as this can potentially limit soft tissue contamination by tumor cells. Subsequently, if definitive surgical resection is undertaken, the entire area of the biopsy (including skin) must be excised en bloc with the tumor.

CHEST WALL NEOPLASMS

Benign

Chondroma. Chondromas are one of the more common benign tumors of the chest wall. They are primarily seen in children and young adults and occur at the costochondral junction anteriorly. Clinically, a painless mass is present. Chondromas may grow to huge sizes if left untreated. Treatment is surgical resection with a 2-cm margin. One must be certain, however, that the lesion is not a well-differentiated chondrosarcoma. In this case, a wider 4-cm margin is required to prevent local recurrence. Therefore, large chondromas should be treated surgically as low-grade chondrosarcomas.

Osteochondroma. Osteochondromas are the most common benign bone tumor and are often detected as incidental radiographic findings. Most are solitary; however, patients with multiple osteochondromas have a higher incidence of malignancy.

Osteochondromas occur in the first two decades of life and they arise at or near the growth plate of bones. The lesions are benign during youth or adolescence. Osteochondromas that enlarge after completion of skeletal growth have the potential to develop into chondrosarcomas.

Desmoid tumors. Desmoid tumors are unusual soft tissue neoplasms that arise from fascial or musculoaponeurotic structures. Some authorities consider desmoid tumors to be a form of fibrosarcoma. Clinically, patients are usually in the third to fourth decade, and have pain, a fixed chest wall mass, or both. No radiographic findings are typical. Histologic diagnosis may not be possible by a needle biopsy because of low cellularity. An open incisional biopsy for lesions over 3–4 cm often is necessary, following the caveats listed above.

Desmoid tumors do not metastasize, but they have a significant propensity to recur locally, with local recurrence rates as high as 5–50 percent, sometimes despite complete initial resection with histologically negative margins. Such locally aggressive behavior is secondary to microscopic tumor infiltration of muscle and surrounding soft tissues.

Surgery consists of wide local excision with a margin of 2–4 cm, and with intraoperative assessment of resection margins by frozen section. Survival after wide local excision with negative margins is 90 percent at 10 years.

Primary Malignant Chest Wall Tumors

Sarcomas can be divided into two broad groups by potential chemotherapeutic responsiveness. Preoperative (neoadjuvant) chemotherapy offers the ability to (1) assess tumor chemosensitivity by the degree of tumor size reduction and microscopic necrosis, (2) determine which chemotherapeutic agents the tumor is sensitive to, and (3) lessen the extent of surgical resection by reducing tumor size. Patients whose tumors are responsive to preoperative chemotherapy (as judged by the reduction in the size of the primary tumor and/or by the degree of necrosis seen histologically following resection) have a much better prognosis than those with a poor response.

Given the tumor's potential response to chemotherapy or the presence of metastatic disease, the initial treatment is either (1) preoperative chemotherapy (for patients with osteosarcoma, rhabdomyosarcoma, primitive neuroectodermal tumor [PNET], or Ewingsarcoma) followed by surgery and postoperative chemotherapy, (2) primary surgical resection and reconstruction (for patients with nonmetastatic malignant fibrous histiocytoma, fibrosarcoma, liposarcoma, or synovial sarcoma), or (3) neoadjuvant chemotherapy followed by surgical resection if indicated in patients presenting with metastatic soft tissue sarcomas.

Malignant Chest Wall Bone Tumors

Chondrosarcoma. Chondrosarcomas are the most common primary chest wall malignancy. As with chondromas, they usually arise anteriorly from the costochondral arches. These slowly enlarging, often painful masses of the anterior chest wall can reach massive proportions. CT scan shows a radiolucent lesion often with stippled calcifications pathognomonic for chondrosarcomas.

Most chondrosarcomas are slow growing, low-grade tumors. For this reason, any lesion in the anterior chest wall likely to be a chondroma or a low-grade chondrosarcoma should be treated with wide (4-cm) resection. Chondrosarcomas are not sensitive to chemotherapy or radiation therapy. Prognosis is determined by tumor grade and extent of resection.

Osteosarcoma. Osteosarcomas are the most common bone malignancy, but they are an uncommon malignancy of the chest wall, representing only 10 percent of all malignant chest wall tumors. They present as rapidly enlarging, painful masses. Although they primarily occur in young adults, osteosarcomas can occur in patients older than the age of 40 years, sometimes in association with previous radiation, Paget disease, or chemotherapy.

As with chondrosarcomas, careful CT assessment of the pulmonary parenchyma for metastasis is necessary. Osteosarcomas have a propensity to spread to the lungs and up to one third of patients present with metastatic disease.

Osteosarcomas are potentially sensitive to chemotherapy. Currently, preoperative chemotherapy before surgical resection is common. After chemotherapy, complete resection is performed with wide (4-cm) margins, followed by reconstruction. In patients presenting with lung metastases that are potentially amenable to surgical resection, induction chemotherapy may be given, followed by surgical resection of the primary tumor and of the pulmonary metastases. Following surgical treatment of known disease, additional maintenance chemotherapy is usually recommended.

Other Tumors

Ewing's Sarcoma

Ewing sarcomas occur in adolescents and young adults who present with progressive chest wall pain, but without the presence of a mass. Systemic symptoms of malaise and fever often are present with elevation of the erythrocyte sedimentation rate and white blood cell count.

Radiographically, the characteristic onion peel appearance is produced by multiple layers of periosteum in the bone formation. The diagnosis can be made by a percutaneous needle biopsy or an incisional biopsy.

These tumors have a strong propensity to spread to the lungs and skeleton. Their aggressive behavior produces patient survival rates of only 50 percent or less at 3 years. Increasing tumor size is associated with decreasing survival. Treatment has improved significantly, now consisting of multiagent chemotherapy, radiation therapy, and surgery.

Malignant Chest Soft Tissue Sarcomas

Soft tissue sarcomas of the chest wall are uncommon and include fibrosarcomas, liposarcomas, malignant fibrous histiocytomas (MFHs), rhabdomyosarcomas, angiosarcomas, and other extremely rare lesions. With the exception of rhabdomyosarcomas, the primary treatment of these lesions is wide surgical resection with 4-cm margins and reconstruction. Rhabdomyosarcomas are sensitive to chemotherapy and are often treated with preoperative chemotherapy. As with all sarcomas, soft tissue sarcomas of the chest wall have a propensity to spread to the lungs. The prognosis of such tumors heavily depends on their grade and stage.

Chest Wall Reconstruction

The principles of surgery for any malignant chest wall tumor are to strategically plan the anatomy of resection and to carefully assess what structures will need to be sacrificed to obtain a 4-cm margin. Prosthetic reconstruction is usually with 2-mm Gore-Tex, and with appropriate soft-tissue coverage to obtain good coverage of a potentially large defect and to achieve an acceptable cosmetic result.

The extent of resection depends on the tumor's location and on any involvement of contiguous structures. Laterally based lesions often require simple wide excision, with resection of any contiguously involved lung, pleura, muscle, or skin. Anteriorly based lesions contiguous with the sternum require partial sternectomy. Primary malignant tumors of the sternum may require complete sternectomy. Posterior lesions involving the rib heads over their articulations with the vertebral bodies may, depending on the extent of rib involvement, require partial en bloc vertebrectomy.

Reconstruction of the chest wall can always be accomplished with the use of 2-mm Gore-Tex, attached to the surrounding bony structures with stout sutures of Gore-Tex or polypropylene. Gore-Tex is impervious to fluid, thus preventing pleural fluid from entering the chest wall; it is firm and provides excellent rigidity and stability when secured taut to the surrounding bony structures; and it provides a good platform for myocutaneous flap reconstruction.

Tissue coverage, except for smaller lesions, invariably involves the use of myocutaneous flaps using the latissimus dorsi, serratus anterior, rectus abdominis, or pectoralis major muscles.

MEDIASTINUM

General Concepts

Anatomy and Pathologic Entities

The mediastinum, the central part of the thoracic cavity, can be divided into three compartments for classification of anatomic components and disease processes: the anterior, middle, and posterior mediastinum. The anterior mediastinum lies between the sternum and the anterior surface of the heart and great vessels. The middle mediastinum is located between the great vessels and the trachea. Posterior to this is the posterior mediastinum.

The anterior compartment includes the thymus gland or its remnant, the internal mammary artery and vein, lymph nodes, and fat. The middle mediastinum contains the pericardium and its contents, the ascending and transverse aorta, the superior and inferior venae cavae, the brachiocephalic artery and vein, the phrenic nerves, the upper vagus nerve trunks, the trachea, the main bronchi and their associated lymph nodes, and the central portions of the pulmonary arteries and veins. The posterior mediastinum contains the descending aorta, esophagus, thoracic duct, azygos and hemiazygos veins, and lymph nodes.

History and Physical Examination

The type of mediastinal pathology encountered varies significantly by age of the patient. In adults, the most common tumors include neurogenic tumors of the posterior compartment, benign cysts occurring in any compartment, and thymomas of the anterior mediastinum. In children, neurogenic tumors of the posterior mediastinum are also common; lymphoma is the second most common mediastinal tumor, usually located in the anterior or middle mediastinum; and thymoma is rare. In both age groups, about 25 percent of mediastinal tumors are malignant.

Up to two thirds of mediastinal tumors in adults are incidental findings radiologic studies ordered for other problems. Benign masses are even more likely to be asymptomatic. Local symptoms usually arise from larger, bulky tumors, expanding cysts, and teratomas which can cause compression of mediastinal structures, in particular the trachea, leading to cough, dyspnea on exertion, or stridor. Chest pain or dyspnea may be reported secondary to associated pleural effusions, cardiac tamponade, or phrenic nerve involvement.

The history and physical examination in conjunction with the imaging findings may suggest a specific diagnosis. The association of a mediastinal mass, enlarged lymph nodes, and a constitutional symptom such as night sweats or weight loss suggests a lymphoma. An anterior mediastinal mass in the setting of a history of fluctuating weakness and early fatigue or ptosis suggests a thymoma and myasthenia gravis.

Diagnostic Evaluation

Imaging and Serum Markers

Discovery of a mediastinal mass on chest radiograph is followed by contrast-enhanced CT scan. MRI often is performed for posterior mediastinal masses to delineate the relationship of the mass to the spinal column and to assess the possibility of neural foraminal invasion.

The use of serum markers to evaluate a mediastinal mass is important in the diagnosis and therapeutic monitoring of patients with mediastinal germ cell tumors. For example, seminomatous and nonseminomatous germ cell tumors can frequently be diagnosed and often distinguished from one another by the levels of alpha-fetoprotein (AFP) and human chorionic gonadotropin (hCG). In over 90 percent of nonseminomatous germ cell tumors, either the AFP or the hCG level will be elevated. Results are close to 100 percent specific if the level of either AFP or hCG is greater than 500 ng/mL. Some centers institute chemotherapy based on this result alone, without a biopsy. In contrast, the AFP level is always normal in patients with mediastinal seminomas; only 10 percent will have an elevated hCG, which is usually less than 100 ng/mL.

Diagnostic Nonsurgical Biopsies of the Mediastinum

The indications and decision-making steps for performing a diagnostic biopsy of a mediastinal mass remain somewhat controversial. In some patients, given noninvasive imaging results and the history, surgical removal may be the obvious choice; preoperative biopsy may be unnecessary and even hazardous. In other patients whose primary treatment is likely to be nonsurgical, a biopsy is essential.

Percutaneous biopsy may be technically difficult because of the overlying bony thoracic cavity and the proximity to lung tissue, the heart, and great vessels. FNA biopsy minimizes some of these potential hazards and may be effective in diagnosing mediastinal thyroid tissue, cancers, carcinomas, seminomas, inflammatory processes, and cysts. Other noncarcinomatous malignancies such as lymphoproliferative disorders, thymomas, and benign tumors may require larger pieces of tissue. Such biopsies may be obtained by a core-needle technique or by surgically performed open biopsy. In general, if the clinical and radiographic features suggest a lymphoproliferative lesionsurgical biopsy is indicated because a larger volume of tissue is often required to both diagnose and type the lymphoma. However, if a nonlymphoproliferative diagnosis was suggested, FNA has a high yield and is recommended.

If an anterior mediastinal mass appears localized and consistent with a thymoma, surgical resection is performed. Surgical resection without biopsies for most localized tumors of the posterior mediastinum suspected to be neurogenic in origin also appropriate.

Surgical Biopsies and Resection of Mediastinal Masses

For mediastinal tumors not amenable to CT-guided needle biopsy or needle biopsy has not yielded sufficient tissue for diagnosis, surgical biopsy is indicated. Masses in the paratracheal region are easily biopsied by mediastinoscopy. For tumors of the anterior or posterior mediastinum, a left or right VATS approach often allows safe and adequate surgical biopsies. In some patients, an anterior mediastinotomy (i.e., Chamberlain procedure) may be ideal for an anterior tumor or a tumor with significant parasternal extension. Before a surgical biopsy is pursued, a discussion should be held with the pathologist regarding routine histologic assessment, special stains and markers, and requirements for lymphoma work-up.

The gold standard for the resection of most anterior and middle mediastinal masses is through a median sternotomy or lateral thoracotomy. In some cases, a lateral thoracotomy with sternal extension (hemi-clamshell) provides excellent exposure for extensive mediastinal tumors that have a lateral component. Alternatively, a right or left VATS approach can be used for resection of the thymus gland and for resection of small (1–2 cm) encapsulated thymomas. Most would agree that if a larger anterior mediastinal tumor is seen or malignancy is suspected, a median sternotomy with a more radical resection should be performed.

Neoplasms

Thymus

Thymic Tumors

Thymoma. Thymoma is the most frequently encountered neoplasm of the anterior mediastinum in adults (seen most frequently between 40 and 60 years of age). They are rare in children. Most thymomas are asymptomatic. However, between 10 and 50 percent have symptoms suggestive of myasthenia gravis or have circulating antibodies to acetylcholine receptor. However, less than 10 percent of patients with myasthenia gravis are found to have a thymoma on CT. Thymectomy leads to improvement or resolution of symptoms of myasthenia gravis in only about 25 percent of patients with thymomas. In contrast, in patients with myasthenia gravis and no thymoma, thymectomy results are superior: up to 50 percent of patients have a complete remission and 90 percent improve. In 5 percent of patients with thymomas, other paraneoplastic syndromes, including red cell aplasia, hypogammaglobulinemia, systemic lupus erythematosus, Cushing syndrome, or syndrome of inappropriate antidiuretic hormone (SIADH) may be present. Large thymic tumors may present with symptoms related to a mass effect, which may include cough, chest pain, dyspnea, or superior vena cava syndrome.

The diagnosis may be suspected based on CT scan and history, but imaging alone is not diagnostic. CT-guided FNA biopsy has a diagnostic sensitivity of 85 percent and a specificity of 95 percent in specialized centers. Cytokeratin is the marker that best distinguishes thymomas from lymphomas. In most patients, the distinction between lymphomas and thymomas can be made on CT scan, because most lymphomas have marked lymphadenopathy and thymomas most frequently appear as a solitary encapsulated mass.

The most commonly accepted staging system for thymomas is that of Masaoka. It is based on the presence or absence of gross or microscopic invasion of the capsule and of surrounding structures, and on the presence or absence of metastases.

The definitive treatment for thymomas is complete surgical removal for all resectable tumors; local recurrence rates and survival vary according to stage. Resection is generally accomplished by median sternotomy with extension to hemi-clamshell in more advanced cases. Even advanced tumors with local invasion of resectable structures such as the pericardium, superior vena cava, or innominate vessels should be considered for resection with reconstruction.

Currently, chemotherapy is being offered preoperatively and postoperatively to select patients with advanced stage thymomas.

Common Adult Neurogenic Tumors

Nerve sheath tumors.   Nerve sheath tumors account for 20 percent of all mediastinal tumors. More than 95 percent of nerve sheath tumors are benign neurilemomas or neurofibromas. Malignant neurosarcomas are much less common.

Neurilemoma.   Neurilemomas, also called schwannomas, arise from Schwann cells in intercostal nerves. They are firm, well-encapsulated, and generally benign. If routine CT scan suggests extension of a neurilemoma into the intervertebral foramen, MRI is suggested to evaluate the extent of this "dumbbell" configuration. Such a configuration may lead to cord compression and paralysis, and requires a more complex surgical approach. It is recommended that most nerve sheath tumors be resected. Traditionally, this has been performed by open thoracotomy but more recently, a VATS approach has been established as safe and effective for simple operations. It is reasonable to follow small, asymptomatic paravertebral tumors in older patients or in patients at high risk for surgery.

In children, ganglioneuroblastomas or neuroblastomas are more common; therefore all neurogenic tumors should be completely resected.

Neurofibroma.   Neurofibromas have components of both nerve sheaths and nerve cells and account for up to 25 percent of nerve sheath tumors. Up to 40 percent of patients with mediastinal fibromas have generalized neurofibromatosis (von Recklinghausen's disease). About 70 percent of neurofibromas are benign. Malignant degeneration to a neurofibrosarcoma may occur in 25–30 percent of patients.

Neurofibrosarcomas carry a poor prognosis because of rapid growth and aggressive local invasion along nerve bundles. Complete surgical resection is the mainstay of treatment.

Ganglion cell tumors.   Ganglion cell tumors arise from the sympathetic chain or from the adrenal medulla and include ganglioneuromas, ganglioneuroblastomas, and neuroblastomas.

Lymphoma

Overall, lymphomas are the most common malignancy of the mediastinum. In about 50 percent of patients who have both Hodgkin and non-Hodgkin lymphoma, the mediastinum may be the primary site. The anterior compartment is most commonly involved, with occasional involvement of the middle compartment and hilar nodes. The posterior compartment is rarely involved. Chemotherapy and/or radiation results in a cure rate of up to 90 percent for patients with early stage Hodgkin disease, and up to 60 percent with more advanced stages.

Mediastinal Germ Cell Tumors

Germ cell tumors are uncommon neoplasms, with only about 7000 diagnosed each year. However, they are the most common malignancy in young men between age 15 and 35 years. Most germ cell tumors are gonadal in origin. Those with the mediastinum as the primary site are rare, constituting less than 5 percent of all germ cell tumors, and less than 1 percent of all mediastinal tumors (usually occurring in the anterior compartment). If a malignant mediastinal germ cell tumor is found, it is important to exclude a gonadal primary tumor. Primary mediastinal germ cell tumors (including teratomas, seminomas, and nonseminomatous malignant germ cell tumors) are a heterogeneous group of benign and malignant neoplasms thought to originate from primitive pluripotent germ cells "misplaced" in the mediastinum during embryonic development.

About one-third of all primary mediastinal germ cell tumors are seminomatous. Two thirds are nonseminomatous tumors or teratomas. Treatment and prognosis vary considerably within these two groups. FNA biopsy alone may be diagnostic for seminomas, usually with normal serum markers, including hCG and AFP. In 10 percent of seminomas, hCG levels may be slightly elevated. FNA findings, along with high hCG and AFP levels, can accurately diagnose nonseminomatous tumors. If the diagnosis remains uncertain after assessment of FNA findings and serum marker levels, then core-needle biopsies or surgical biopsies may be required. An anterior mediastinotomy (Chamberlain procedure) or a thoracoscopy is the most frequent diagnostic surgical approach.

Teratoma. Teratomas are the most common type of mediastinal germ cell tumors, accounting for 60–70 percent of mediastinal germ cell tumors. They contain two or three embryonic layers that may include teeth, skin, hair (ectodermal), cartilage and bone (mesodermal), or bronchial, intestinal, or pancreatic tissue (endodermal). Therapy for mature, benign teratomas is surgical resection, which confers an excellent prognosis.

Seminoma. Most patients with seminomas have advanced disease at the time of diagnosis and present with symptoms of local compression, including superior vena caval syndrome, dyspnea, or chest discomfort. With advanced disease, the preferred treatment is combination cisplatin-based chemotherapy regimens with bleomycin and either etoposide or vinblastine. Complete responses have been reported in over 75 percent of patients treated with these regimens. Surgical resection may be curative for small asymptomatic seminomas that are found incidentally with screening CT scans. Surgical resection of residual masses after chemotherapy may be indicated.

Nonseminomatous germ cell tumors. Nonseminomatous germ cell tumors include embryonal cell carcinomas, choriocarcinomas, endodermal sinus tumors, and mixed types. They are often bulky, irregular tumors of the anterior mediastinum with areas of low attenuation on CT scan because of necrosis, hemorrhage, or cyst formation. Frequently, adjacent structures have been involved, with metastases to regional lymph nodes, pleura, and lungs. Lactate dehydrogenase (LDH), AFP, and hCG levels are frequently elevated. Chemotherapy is the preferred treatment and includes combination therapy with cisplatin, bleomycin, and etoposide. With this regimen, survival at 2 years is 67 percent and at 5 years is 60 percent. Surgical resection of residual masses is indicated, as it may guide further therapy. Up to 20 percent of residual masses contain additional tumors; in another 40 percent, mature teratomas; and the remaining 40 percent, fibrotic tissue.

Mediastinitis

Acute Mediastinitis

Acute mediastinitis is a fulminant infectious process that spreads along the fascial planes of the mediastinum. Infections originate most commonly from esophageal perforations, sternal infections, and oropharyngeal or neck infections, but a number of less common etiologic factors can lead to this deadly process. As infections from any of these sources enter the mediastinum, spread may be rapid along the continuous fascial planes connecting the cervical and mediastinal compartments. Clinical signs and symptoms include fever, chest pain, dysphagia, respiratory distress, and cervical and upper thoracic subcutaneous crepitus. In severe cases, the clinical course can rapidly deteriorate to florid sepsis, hemodynamic instability, and death. Thus, a high index of suspicion is required in the context of any infection with access to the mediastinal compartments.

A chest CT scan can be particularly helpful in determining the extent of spread and the best approach to surgical drainage. Acute mediastinitis is a true surgical emergency and treatment must be instituted immediately and must be aimed at correcting the primary problem, such as the esophageal perforation or oropharyngeal abscess. Another major concern is débridement and drainage of the spreading infectious process within the mediastinum, neck, pleura, and other tissue planes. Antibiotics, fluid resuscitation, and other supportive measures are important, but surgical correction of the problem at its source and open débridement of infected areas are critical measures. Surgical débridement may need to be repeated, and other planes and cavities explored depending on the patient's clinical status. Persistent sepsis or collections on CT scan may require further radical surgical débridement.

Chronic Mediastinitis

Sclerosing or fibrosing mediastinitis is a result of chronic inflammation of the mediastinum, most frequently as a result of granulomatous infections such as histoplasmosis or tuberculosis. The process begins in lymph nodes and continues as a chronic, low-grade inflammation leading to fibrosis and scarring. In many patients, the clinical manifestations are silent. However, if the fibrosis is progressive and severe, it may lead to encasement of the mediastinal structures, causing entrapment and compression of the low-pressure veins (including the superior vena cava and innominate and azygos veins). This fibrotic process can compromise other structures such as the esophagus and pulmonary arteries. There is no definitive treatment. Surgery is indicated only for diagnosis or in specific patients to relieve airway or esophageal obstruction or to achieve vascular reconstruction.

DISEASES OF THE PLEURA AND PLEURAL SPACE

Pleural Effusion

Pleural effusion refers to any significant collection of fluid within the pleural space. Normally, there is an ongoing balance between the lubricating fluid flowing into the pleural space and its continuous absorption. Between 5 and 10 L of fluid normally enters the pleural space daily by filtration through microvessels supplying the parietal pleura. The net balance of pressures in these capillaries leads to fluid flow from the parietal pleural surface into the pleural space, and the net balance of forces in the pulmonary circulation leads to absorption through the visceral pleura. Normally, 15–20 mL of pleural fluid is present at any given time. Any disturbance in these forces can lead to imbalance and accumulation of pleural fluid. Common pathologic conditions in North America that lead to pleural effusion include congestive heart failure, bacterial pneumonia, malignancy, and pulmonary emboli.

Diagnostic Work-Up

The initial evaluation of a pleural effusion is guided by the history and physical examination. Bilateral pleural effusions are because of congestive heart failure in over 80 percent of patients.

The presence of a unilateral effusion in a patient with cough, fever, leukocytosis, and unilateral infiltrate is likely to be a parapneumonic process. If the effusion is small and the patient responds to antibiotics, a diagnostic thoracentesis may be unnecessary. However, a patient who has an obvious pneumonia and a large pleural effusion that is purulent and foul-smelling has an empyema. Aggressive drainage with chest tubes is required, possibly with surgical intervention. Outside of the setting of congestive heart failure or small effusions associated with an improving pneumonia, most patients with pleural effusions of unknown cause should undergo thoracentesis.

A general classification of pleural fluid collections into transudates and exudates is helpful in understanding the various causes. Transudates are protein-poor ultrafiltrates of plasma that occur because of alterations in the systemic hydrostatic pressures or colloid osmotic pressures (for example, with congestive heart failure or cirrhosis). On gross visual inspection, a transudative effusion is generally clear or straw-colored. Exudates are protein-rich pleural fluid collections that generally occur because of inflammation or invasion of the pleura by tumors. Grossly, they are often turbid, bloody, or purulent. Grossly bloody effusions in the absence of trauma are frequently malignant, but may also occur in the setting of a pulmonary embolism or pneumonia. Several criteria have been traditionally used to differentiate transudates from exudates. An effusion is considered exudative if the pleural fluid to serum ratio of protein is greater than 0.5 and the LDH ratio is greater than 0.6 or the absolute pleural LDH level is greater than two-thirds of the normal upper limit for serum. If these criteria suggest a transudate, the patient should be carefully evaluated for congestive heart failure, cirrhosis, or conditions associated with transudates.

If an exudative effusion is suggested, further diagnostic studies may be helpful. If total and differential cell counts reveal a predominance of neutrophils ($>$ 50 percent of cells), the effusion is likely to be associated with an acute inflammatory process (such as a parapneumonic effusion or empyema, pulmonary embolus, or pancreatitis). A predominance of mononuclear cells suggests a more chronic inflammatory process (such as cancer or tuberculosis). Gram's stains and cultures should be obtained, if possible with inoculation into culture bottles at the bedside. Pleural fluid glucose levels are frequently decreased ($<$ 60 mg/dL) with complex parapneumonic effusions or malignant effusions.

Cytologic testing should be done on exudative effusions to rule out an associated malignancy. Cytologic diagnosis is accurate in diagnosing over 70 percent of malignant effusions associated with adenocarcinomas, but is less sensitive for mesotheliomas ($<$ 10 percent), squamous cell carcinomas (20 percent), or lymphomas (25–50 percent). If the diagnosis remains uncertain after drainage and fluid analysis, thoracoscopy and direct biopsies are indicated. Tuberculous effusions can now be diagnosed accurately by increased levels of pleural fluid adenosine deaminase (above 40 U per L). Pulmonary embolism should be suspected in a patient with a pleural effusion occurring in association with pleuritic chest pain, hemoptysis, or dyspnea out of proportion to the size of the effusion. These effusions may be transudative, but if an associated infarct near the pleural surface occurs, an exudate may be seen. If a pulmonary embolism is suspected in a postoperative patient, most clinicians would obtain a spiral CT scan.

Malignant Pleural Effusion

Malignant pleural effusions may occur in association with a variety malignancies, most commonly lung cancer, breast cancer, and lymphomas, depending on the patient's age and gender. Malignant effusions are exudative and often tinged with blood. An effusion in the setting of a malignancy means a more advanced stage; it generally indicates an unresectable tumor, with a mean survival of 3–11 months. Occasionally, benign pleural effusions may be associated with a bronchogenic NSCLC, and surgical resection may still be indicated if the cytology of the effusions is negative for malignancy. An important issue is the size of the effusion and the degree of dyspnea that results. Symptomatic, moderate to large effusions should be drained by chest tube, pigtail catheter, or VATS, followed by instillation of a sclerosing agent. Before sclerosing the pleural cavity, whether by chest tube or VATS, the lung should be nearly fully expanded. Poor expansion of the lung (because of entrapment by tumor or adhesions) generally predicts a poor result. The choice of sclerosant includes talc, bleomycin, or doxycycline. Success rates of controlling the effusion range from 60–90 percent, depending on the exact scope of the clinical study, the degree of lung expansion after the pleural fluid is drained, and the care with which the outcomes were reported.

Empyema

Thoracic empyema is defined by a purulent pleural effusion. The most common causes are parapneumonic, but postsurgical or posttraumatic empyema is also common. Grossly purulent, foul-smelling pleural fluid makes the diagnosis of empyema obvious on visual examination at the bedside. Diagnosis is confirmed by a combination of clinical scenario with positive pleural fluid cultures.

Pathophysiology

The spectrum of organisms involved in the development of a parapneumonic empyema is changing. Pneumococci and staphylococci continue to be the most common, but gram-negative aerobic bacteria and anaerobes are becoming more prevalent. Cases involving mycobacteria or fungi are rare. Multiple organisms may be found in up to 50 percent of patients, but cultures may be sterile if antibiotics were initiated before the culture or if the culture process was not efficient. Therefore, it is imperative that the choice of antibiotics be guided by the clinical scenario and not just the organisms found on culture. Broad spectrum coverage may be still required even when cultures have failed to grow out an organism or if a single organism is grown when the clinical picture is more consistent with a multiorganism process. Common gram-negative organisms include *Escherichia coli*, Klebsiella, Pseudomonas, and Enterobacteriaceae. Anaerobic organisms may be fastidious and difficult to document by culture and are associated with periodontal diseases, aspiration syndromes, alcoholism, general anesthesia, drug abuse, or other functional associations with gastroesophageal reflux.

The route of organism entry into the pleural cavity may be by contiguous spread from pneumonia, lung abscess, liver abscess, or another infectious process with contact with the pleural space. Organisms may also enter the pleural cavity by direct contamination from thoracentesis, thoracic surgical procedures, esophageal injuries, or trauma.

In the early stage of an empyema the effusion is watery and free-flowing in the pleural cavity. Thoracentesis at this stage yields fluid with a pH typically above 7.3, a glucose level greater than 60 mg/dL, and a low LDH level (< 500 U/L). At this stage, the decision to use antibiotics alone or perform a repeat thoracentesis, chest tube drainage, thoracoscopy, or open thoracotomy depends on the amount of pleural fluid, its consistency, the clinical status of the patient, the degree of expansion of the lung after drainage, and the presence of loculated fluid in the pleural space (versus free-flowing purulent fluid). If relatively thin, purulent pleural fluid is diagnosed early in the setting of a pneumonic process, the fluid often can be completely drained with simple large-bore thoracentesis. If complete lung expansion is obtained and the pneumonic process is responding to antibiotics, no further drainage may be necessary. Pleural fluid with a pH lower than 7.2 and with a low glucose level means that a more aggressive approach to drainage should be pursued.

The pleural fluid may become thick and loculated over the course of h to days, and may be associated with fibrinous adhesions (the fibrinopurulent stage). At this stage, chest tube insertion with closed-system drainage or drainage with thoracoscopy may be necessary to remove the fluid and adhesions and to allow complete lung expansion. Further progression of the inflammatory process leads to the formation of a pleural peel, which may be flimsy and easy to remove early on. However, as the process progresses, a thick pleural rind may develop, leaving a trapped lung; complete lung decortication by thoracotomy would then be necessary, or in some patients, thoracoscopy.

Management

If there is a residual space, persistent pleural infection is likely to occur. A persistent pleural space may be secondary to contracted, but intact, underlying lung; or it may be secondary to surgical lung resection. If the space is small and well-drained by a chest tube, a conservative approach may be possible. This requires leaving the chest tubes in place and attached to closed-system drainage until symphysis of the visceral and parietal surfaces takes place. At this point, the chest tubes can be removed from suction; if the residual pleural space remains stable, the tubes can be cut and advanced out of the chest over the course of several weeks. If the patient is stable, tube removal can frequently be done in the outpatient setting, guided by the degree of drainage and the size of the residual space visualized on serial CT scans. Larger spaces may require open thoracotomy and decortication in an attempt to reexpand the lung to fill this residual space. If reexpansion has failed or appears too high risk, then open drainage, rib resection, and prolonged packing may be required, with delayed closure with muscle flaps or thoracoplasty. Most chronic pleural space problems can be avoided by early specialized thoracic surgical consultation and complete drainage of empyemas, allowing space obliteration by the reinflated lung.

Chylothorax

Chylothorax develops most commonly after surgical trauma to the thoracic duct or a major branch, but may be also associated with a number of other conditions. It is generally unilateral; for example, it may occur on the right after esophagectomy in which the duct is most frequently injured during dissection of the distal esophagus. The esophagus comes into close proximity to the thoracic duct as it enters the chest from its origin in the abdomen at the cisterna chyli. If the mediastinal pleura is disrupted on both sides, bilateral chylothoraces may occur. Left-sided chylothoraces may develop after a left-sided neck dissection, especially in the region of the confluence of the subclavian and internal jugular veins. It may be seen in association with a variety of benign and malignant diseases that generally involve the lymphatic system of the mediastinum or neck.

Pathophysiology

Most commonly, the thoracic duct originates in the abdomen from the cisterna chyli, which is located in the midline, near the level of the second lumbar vertebra. From this origin, the thoracic duct ascends into the chest through the aortic hiatus at the level of T10 to T12, and courses just to the right of the aorta. As the thoracic duct courses cephalad above the diaphragm, it most commonly remains in the right chest, lying just behind the esophagus, between the aorta and azygos vein. At about the level of the fifth or sixth thoracic vertebra, it crosses behind the aorta and the aortic arch into the left posterior mediastinum. From this location, it again courses superiorly, staying near the esophagus and mediastinal pleura as it exits the thoracic inlet. As it exits the thoracic inlet, it passes just to the left, just behind the carotid sheath and anterior to the inferior thyroid and vertebral bodies. Just medial to the anterior scalene muscle, it courses inferiorly and drains into the union of the internal jugular and subclavian veins.

The treatment plan for any chylothorax depends on its cause, the amount of drainage, and the clinical status of the patient. In general, most patients are treated with a short period of chest tube drainage, nothing by mouth (NPO) orders, total parenteral nutrition (TPN), and observation. Chest cavity drainage must be adequate to allow complete lung expansion. Somatostatin has been advocated by some authors, with variable results. If significant chyle drainage (> 500 mL per day in an adult, > 100 mL in an infant) continues despite TPN and good lung expansion, early surgical ligation of the duct is recommended.

Chylothoraces because of malignant conditions often respond to radiation and/or chemotherapy, so less commonly require surgical ligation. Untreated chylothoraces are associated with significant nutritional and immunologic depletion that leads to significant mortality. Before the introduction of surgical ligation of the thoracic duct, the mortality rate from chylothorax exceeded 50 percent. With the availability of TPN for nutritional supplementation and surgical ligation for persistent leaks, the mortality rate of chylothorax is less than 10 percent.

Tumors of the Pleura

Malignant Mesothelioma

Malignant mesothelioma is the most common pleural tumor, with an annual incidence in the United States of 3000 cases. Asbestos exposure is the only known risk factor; it can be established in over 50 percent of patients. Malignant mesotheliomas have a male predominance of 2:1, and are most common after the age of 40.

Clinical presentation. Most patients present with dyspnea and chest pain. Over 90 percent have a pleural effusion. Thoracentesis is diagnostic in less than 10 percent of patients. Frequently, a thoracoscopy or open pleural biopsy with special stains is required to differentiate mesotheliomas from adenocarcinomas. Once the diagnosis is confirmed, cell types can be distinguished (e.g., epithelial, sarcomatous, and mixed). Epithelial types are associated with a more favorable prognosis, and in some patients long-term survival may be seen with no treatment. Sarcomatous and mixed tumors share a more aggressive course.

Surgical Management

Surgical options include palliative pleurectomy or talc pleurodesis with improved local control and a modest improvement in short-term survival. More radical surgical approaches (such as extrapleural pneumonectomy followed by adjuvant chemotherapy and radiation) have an increased morbidity rate; moreover, the mortality rate exceeds 10 percent in all but the most experienced centers.

Suggested Readings

Dewey TM, Mack MJ: Lung cancer. Surgical approaches and incisions. Chest Surg Clin North Am 10:803, 2000.

Ost D, Fein AM, Feinsilver SH: Clinical practice. The solitary pulmonary nodule. N Engl J Med 348:2535, 2003.

Mountain CF: Revisions in the international system for staging lung cancer. Chest 111:1710, 1997.

Pastorino U, Buyse M, Friedel G, et al: Long-term results of lung metastasectomy: Prognostic analyses based on 5206 cases. J Thorac Cardiovasc Surg 113:27, 1997.

Frieden TR, Sterling TR, Munsiff SS, et al: Tuberculosis. Lancet 362:887, 2003.

Wheat LJ, Goldman M, Sarosi G: State-of-the-art review of pulmonary fungal infections. Semin Respir Infect 17:158, 2002.

Walsh GL, Davis BM, Swisher SG, et al: A single-institutional, multidisciplinary approach to primary sarcomas involving the chest wall requiring full-thickness resections. J Thorac Cardiovasc Surg 121:48, 2001.

Nichols CR, Saxman S, Williams SD, et al: Primary mediastinal nongerminomatous germ cell tumors: A modern single institute experience. Cancer 65:1641, 1989.

Light RW: Parapneumonic effusion and empyema. Clin Chest Med 6:55, 1985.

Miller JI Jr.: The history of surgery of empyema, thoracoplasty, eloesser flap, and muscle flap transposition. Chest Surg Clin North Am 10:45, viii, 2000.

19 | Congenital Heart Disease

Tara B. Karamlou, Irving Shen,
and Ross M. Ungerleider

In the modern era, the goal in most cases of congenital heart disease (CHD) is early definitive repair. Therefore, a more clinically relevant classification scheme divides particular defects into three categories based on the feasibility of achieving this goal: (1) defects that have no reasonable palliation and for which repair is the only option; (2) defects for which repair is not possible and for which palliation is the only option; and (3) defects that can either be repaired or palliated in infancy. It bears mentioning that all defects in the second category are those in which the appropriate anatomic components either are not present, as in hypoplastic left-heart syndrome, or cannot be created from existing structures.

DEFECTS IN WHICH REPAIR IS THE ONLY OR BEST OPTION

Atrial Septal Defect

An atrial septal defect (ASD) is defined as an opening in the interatrial septum that enables the mixing of blood from the systemic venous and pulmonary venous circulations.

Anatomy

ASDs can be classified into three different types: (1) sinus venosus defects, comprising approximately 5–10 percent of all ASDs; (2) ostium primum defects, which are more correctly described as partial atrioventricular canal defects; and (3) ostium secundum defects, which are the most prevalent subtype, comprising 80 percent of all ASDs.

Pathophysiology

ASDs result in an increase in pulmonary blood flow secondary to left-to-right shunting through the defect. The direction of the intracardiac shunt is predominantly determined by the compliance of the respective ventricles. In utero, the distensibility, or compliance, of the right and left ventricles is equal, but postnatally the left ventricle (LV) becomes less compliant than the right ventricle (RV).

A minority of patients with ASDs develop progressive pulmonary vascular changes as a result of chronic overcirculation. The increased pulmonary vascular resistance in these patients leads to an equalization of left and right ventricular pressures, and their ratio of pulmonary (Qp) to systemic flow (Qs), Qp:Qs, will approach 1. This does not mean, however, that there is no intracardiac shunting, only that the ratio between the left-to-right component and the right-to-left component is equal.

The ability of the right ventricle to recover normal function is related to the duration of chronic overload, because those undergoing ASD closure before age 10 years have a better likelihood of achieving normal RV function in the postoperative period.

The physiology of sinus venosus ASDs is similar to that discussed above except that these are frequently accompanied by anomalous pulmonary venous drainage. This often results in significant hemodynamic derangements that accelerate the clinical course of these infants.

The same increase in symptoms is true for those with ostium primum defects because the associated mitral insufficiency from the "cleft" mitral valve can lead to more atrial volume load and increased atrial level shunting.

Diagnosis

Patients with ASDs may present with few physical findings. Auscultation may reveal prominence of the first heart sound with fixed splitting of the second heart sound. This results from the relatively fixed left-to-right shunt throughout all phases of the cardiac cycle. A diastolic flow murmur indicating increased flow across the tricuspid valve may be discerned, and, frequently, an ejection flow murmur can be heard across the pulmonary valve. A right ventricular heave and increased intensity of the pulmonary component of the second heart sound indicate pulmonary hypertension and possible unrepairability.

Chest radiographs in the patient with an ASD may show evidence of increased pulmonary vascularity, with prominent hilar markings and cardiomegaly. The electrocardiogram (ECG) shows right axis deviation with an incomplete bundle-branch block. When right bundle-branch block is associated with a leftward or superior axis, an AV canal defect should be strongly suspected.

Diagnosis is clarified by two-dimensional echocardiography, and use of color-flow mapping facilitates an understanding of the physiologic derangements created by the defects. Echocardiography also enables the clinician to estimate the amount of intracardiac shunting, can demonstrate the degree of mitral regurgitation in patients with ostium primum defects, and with the addition of microcavitation, can assist in the detection of sinus venosus defects.

The advent of two-dimensional echocardiography with color-flow Doppler has largely obviated the need for cardiac catheterization because the exact nature of the ASD can be precisely defined by echo alone. However, in cases in which the patient is older than age 40 years, catheterization can quantify the degree of pulmonary hypertension present, because those with a pulmonary vascular resistance (PVR) greater than 12 U/mL are considered inoperable. Cardiac catheterization also can be useful in that it provides data that enable the calculation of Qp and Qs so that the magnitude of the intracardiac shunt can be determined. The ratio (Qp:Qs) can then be used to determine whether closure is indicated in equivocal cases, because a Qp:Qs greater than 1.5:1 is generally accepted as the threshold for surgical intervention. Finally, in patients older than age 40 years, cardiac catheterization can be important to disclose the presence of coronary artery disease.

In general, ASDs are closed when patients are between 4 and 5 years of age. Children of this size can usually be operated on without the use of blood transfusion and generally have excellent outcomes. Patients who are symptomatic may require repair earlier, even in infancy. Some surgeons, however, advocate routine repair in infants and children, as even smaller defects are associated with the risk of paradoxical embolism, particularly during pregnancy. In a recent review by Reddy and colleagues, 116 neonates weighing less than 2500 g who underwent repair of simple and complex cardiac defects with the use of cardiopulmonary bypass were found to have no intracerebral hemorrhages, no long-term neurologic sequelae, and a low operative-mortality rate (10 percent). These results correlated with the length of cardiopulmonary bypass and the complexity of repair. These investigators also found an 80 percent actuarial survival at 1 year and, more importantly, that growth following complete repair was equivalent to weight-matched neonates free from cardiac defects.

Treatment

ASDs can be repaired in a facile manner using standard cardiopulmonary bypass (CPB) techniques through a midline sternotomy approach. The details of the repair itself are generally straightforward. An oblique atriotomy is made, the position of the coronary sinus and all systemic and pulmonary veins are determined, and the rim of the defect is completely visualized. Closure of ostium secundum defects is accomplished either by direct suture or by insertion of a patch. The decision of whether patch closure is necessary can be determined by the size and shape of the defect and by the quality of the edges.

Sinus venosus ASDs associated with partial anomalous pulmonary venous connection are repaired by inserting a patch, with redirection of the pulmonary veins behind the patch to the left atrium. Care must be taken with this approach to avoid obstruction of the pulmonary veins or the superior vena cava, although usually the superior vena cava is dilated and provides ample room for patch insertion.

These operative strategies have been well established, with a low complication rate and a mortality rate approaching zero. As such, attention has shifted to improving the cosmetic result and minimizing hospital stay and convalescence. Multiple new strategies have been described to achieve these aims, including the right submammary incision with anterior thoracotomy, limited bilateral submammary incision with partial sternal split, transxiphoid window, and limited midline incision with partial sternal split. Some centers use video-assisted thoracic surgery (VATS) in the submammary and transxiphoid approaches to facilitate closure within a constricted operative field. The morbidity and mortality of all of these approaches are comparable to those of the traditional median sternotomy; however, each has technical drawbacks. The main concern is that operative precision be maintained with limited exposure. Luo and associates recently described a prospective randomized study comparing ministernotomy (division of the upper sternum for aortic and pulmonary lesions, and the lower sternum for septal lesions) to full sternotomy in 100 consecutive patients undergoing repair of septal lesions. The patients in the ministernotomy group had longer procedure times (by 15–20 min), less bleeding, and shorter hospital stays. These results have been echoed by other investigators from Boston who maintain that ministernotomy provides a cosmetically acceptable scar without compromising aortic cannulation or limiting the exposure of crucial mediastinal structures. This approach also can be easily extended to a full sternotomy should difficulty or unexpected anomalies be encountered.

First performed in 1976, transcatheter closure of ASDs with the use of various occlusion devices is gaining widespread acceptance. Certain types of ASDs, including patent foramen ovale, secundum defects, and some fenestrated secundum defects, are amenable to device closure. Complications reported to occur with transcatheter closure include air embolism (1–3 percent); thromboembolism from the device (1–2 percent); disturbed atrioventricular valve function (1–2 percent); systemic/pulmonary venous obstruction (1 percent); perforation of the atrium or aorta with hemopericardium (1–2 percent); atrial arrhythmias (1–3 percent); and malpositioning/embolization of the device requiring intervention (2–15 percent). Thus, although percutaneous approaches are cosmetic and often translate into shorter periods of convalescence, their attendant risks are considerable, especially because their use may not result in complete closure of the septal defect.

Results

Surgical repair of ASDs should be associated with a mortality rate near zero. Early repairs in neonates weighing less than 1000 g have been increasingly reported with excellent results. Uncommonly, atrial arrhythmias or significant left atrial hypertension may occur soon after repair. The latter is caused by the noncompliant small, left atrial chamber and generally resolves rapidly.

AORTIC STENOSIS

Anatomy and Classification

The spectrum of aortic valve abnormality represents the most common form of CHD, with the great majority of patients being asymptomatic until midlife. Obstruction of the left ventricular outflow tract (LVOT) occurs at multiple levels: subvalvular, valvular, and supravalvular. The critically stenotic aortic valve in the neonate or infant is commonly unicommissural or bicommissural, with thickened, dysmorphic, and myxomatous leaflet tissue and a reduced cross-sectional area at the valve level. Associated left-sided lesions are often present. Endocardial fibroelastosis also is common among infants with critical aortic stenosis (AS). In this condition, the LV is largely nonfunctional, and these patients are not candidates for simple valve replacement or repair, because the LV is incapable of supporting the systemic circulation. Often, the LV is markedly hypertrophic with a reduced cavity size, but on rare occasion, a dilated LV, reminiscent of overt heart failure, is encountered.

Pathophysiology

The unique intracardiac and extracardiac shunts present in fetal life allow even neonates with critical aortic stenosis (AS) to survive. In utero, left ventricular hypertrophy and ischemia cause left atrial hypertension, which reduces the right-to-left flow across the foramen ovale. In severe cases, a reversal of flow may occur, causing right ventricular volume loading. The RV then provides the entire systemic output via the patent ductus arteriosus. Although cardiac output is maintained, the LV suffers continued damage as the intracavitary pressure precludes adequate coronary perfusion, resulting in LV infarction and subendocardial fibroelastosis. The presentation of the neonate with critical AS is then determined by both the degree of left ventricular dysfunction and on the completeness of the transition from a parallel circulation to an in-series circulation on closure of the foramen ovale and the ductus arteriosus. Those infants with mild-to-moderate AS in which LV function is preserved are asymptomatic at birth. The only abnormalities may be a systolic ejection murmur and ECG evidence of left ventricular hypertrophy. However, those neonates with severe AS and compromised LV function are unable to provide adequate cardiac output at birth, and will present in circulatory collapse once the ductus closes, with dyspnea, tachypnea, irritability, narrowed pulse pressure, oliguria, and profound metabolic acidosis. If ductal patency is maintained, systemic perfusion will be provided by the RV via ductal flow, and cyanosis may be the only finding.

Diagnosis

Neonates and infants with severe valvular AS may have a relatively nonspecific history of irritability and failure to thrive. Angina, if present, is usually manifested by episodic, inconsolable crying that coincides with feeding. As discussed previously, evidence of poor peripheral perfusion, such as extreme pallor, indicates severe LVOT obstruction. Differential cyanosis is an uncommon finding, but is present when enough antegrade flow occurs only to maintain normal upper body perfusion, although a large patent ductus arteriosus produces blue discoloration of the abdomen and legs.

Physical findings include a systolic ejection murmur, although a quiet murmur may paradoxically indicate a more severe condition with reduced cardiac output. A systolic click correlates with a valvular etiology of obstruction. As LV dysfunction progresses, evidence of congestive heart failure occurs.

The chest radiograph is variable, but may show dilatation of the aortic root, and the ECG often demonstrates LV hypertrophy. Echocardiography with Doppler flow is extremely useful in establishing the diagnosis, and quantifying the transvalvular gradient. Furthermore, echocardiography can facilitate evaluation for the several associated defects that can be present in critical neonatal AS, including mitral stenosis, LV hypoplasia, LV endocardial fibroelastosis, subaortic stenosis, VSD, or coarctation. The presence of any or several of these defects has important implications related to treatment options for these patients. Although cardiac catheterization is not routinely performed for diagnostic purposes, it can be invaluable as part of the treatment algorithm if the lesion is amenable to balloon valvotomy.

Treatment

The infant with severe AS may require urgent intervention. Preoperative stabilization, however, has dramatically altered the clinical algorithm and outcomes for this patient population. The preoperative strategy begins with endotracheal intubation and inotropic support. Prostaglandin infusion is initiated to maintain ductal patency, and confirmatory studies are performed prior to operative intervention.

Therapy is generally indicated in the presence of a transvalvular gradient of 50 mm Hg with associated symptoms including syncope, congestive heart failure (CHF), or angina, or if a gradient of 50–75 mmHg exists with concomitant ECG evidence of LV strain or ischemia. In the critically ill neonate, there may be little gradient across the aortic valve because of poor LV function. These patients depend on patency of the ductus arteriosus to provide systemic perfusion from the RV, and all ductal-dependent patients with critical AS require treatment. However, the decision regarding treatment options must be based on a complete understanding of associated defects. For example, in the presence of a hypoplastic LV (left ventricular) end-diastolic volume < 20 mL/m^2, isolated aortic valvotomy should not be performed because studies have demonstrated high mortality in this population following isolated valvotomy.

Relief of valvular AS in infants and children can be accomplished with standard techniques of CPB and direct exposure to the aortic valve. A transverse incision is made in the ascending aorta above the sinus of Valsalva, extending close to, but not into, the noncoronary sinus. Exposure is attained with placement of a retractor into the right coronary sinus. After inspection of the valve, the chosen commissure is incised to within 1–2 mm of the aortic wall.

Balloon valvotomy performed in the cath lab has gained widespread acceptance as the procedure of choice for reduction of transvalvular gradients in symptomatic infants and children. This procedure is an ideal palliative option because mortality from surgical valvotomy can be high because of the critical nature of these patients' condition. Furthermore, balloon valvotomy provides relief of the valvular gradient by opening the valve leaflets without the trauma created by open surgery, and allows future surgical intervention to be performed on an unscarred chest. In general, most surgical groups have abandoned open surgical valvotomy and favor catheter-based balloon valvotomy. The decision regarding the most appropriate method to use depends on several crucial factors including the available medical expertise, the patient's overall status and hemodynamics, and the presence of associated cardiac defects requiring repair. Although recent evidence is emerging to the contrary, simple valvotomy, whether performed percutaneously or open, is generally considered a palliative procedure. The goal is to relieve LVOT obstruction without producing clinically significant regurgitation, to allow sufficient annular growth for eventual aortic valve replacement. The majority of survivors of valvotomy performed during infancy will require further intervention on the aortic valve in 10 years.

Valvotomy may result in aortic insufficiency. Eventually, the combination of aortic stenosis and/or insufficiency may result in the need for an aortic valve replacement. Neonates with severely hypoplastic LVs or significant LV endocardial fibroelastosis may not be candidates for two-ventricle repair and are treated the same as infants with the hypoplastic left-heart syndrome (HLHS), which is discussed later (see Hypoplastic Left-Heart Syndrome below).

Many surgeons previously avoided aortic valve replacement for aortic stenosis in early childhood because the more commonly used mechanical valves would be outgrown and require replacement later, and the obligatory anticoagulation for mechanical valves resulted in a substantial risk for complications. Additionally, mechanical valves had an important incidence of bacterial endocarditis or perivalvular leak requiring re-intervention.

The use of allografts and the advent of the Ross procedure have largely obviated these issues and made early definitive correction of critical AS a viable option. Donald Ross first described transposition of the pulmonary valve into the aortic position with allograft reconstruction of the pulmonary outflow tract in 1967, in which a normal trileaflet semilunar valve made of a patient's native tissue was used to replace the damaged aortic valve. Since then, the Ross procedure has become the optimal choice for aortic valve replacement in children, because it has improved durability and can be performed with acceptable morbidity and mortality rates. Lupinetti and Jones compared allograft aortic valve replacement with the Ross procedure and found a more significant transvalvular gradient reduction and regression of left ventricular hypertrophy in those patients who underwent the Ross procedure. In some cases, the pulmonary valve may not be usable because of associated defects or congenital absence. These children are not candidates for the Ross procedure and are now most frequently treated with cryopreserved allografts (cadaveric human aortic valves). At times, there may be a size discrepancy between the RVOT and the LVOT, especially in cases of severe critical AS in infancy. For these cases, the pulmonary autograft is placed in a manner that also provides enlargement of the aortic annulus (Ross/Konno).

Subvalvular AS occurs beneath the aortic valve and may be classified as discrete or tunnel-like (diffuse). A thin, fibromuscular diaphragm immediately proximal to the aortic valve characterizes discrete subaortic stenosis. This diaphragm typically extends for 180 degrees or more in a crescentic or circular fashion, often attaching to the mitral valve and the interventricular septum. The aortic valve itself is usually normal in this condition, although the turbulence imparted by the subvalvular stenosis may affect leaflet morphology and valve competence.

Diffuse subvalvular AS results in a long, tunnel-like obstruction that may extend to the left ventricular apex. In some individuals, there may be difficulty in distinguishing between hypertrophic cardiomyopathy and diffuse subaortic stenosis. Operation for subvalvular AS is indicated with a gradient exceeding 30 mmHg or when symptoms indicating LVOT obstruction are present. Some surgeons advocate repair in all cases of discrete AS, because it entails only simple membrane excision, to avoid aortic insufficiency, which often occurs with this lesion. Diffuse AS oftentimes requires aortoventriculoplasty as previously described. Results are generally excellent, with operative mortality less than 5 percent.

Supravalvular AS occurs more rarely, and also can be classified into a discrete type, which produces an hourglass deformity of the aorta, and a diffuse form that can involve the entire arch and brachiocephalic arteries. The aortic valve leaflets are usually normal, but in some cases, the leaflets may adhere to the supravalvular stenosis, thereby narrowing the sinuses of Valsalva in diastole and restricting coronary artery perfusion. Additionally, accelerated intimal hyperplastic changes in the coronary arteries can be demonstrated in these patients because the proximal position of the coronary arteries subjects them to abnormally high perfusion pressures.

The signs and symptoms of supravalvular AS are similar to other forms of LVOT obstruction. An asymptomatic murmur is the presenting manifestation in approximately half these patients. Syncope, poor exercise tolerance, and angina may all occur with nearly equal frequency. Occasionally, supravalvular AS is associated with Williams syndrome, a constellation of elfin facies, mental retardation, and hypercalcemia. Following routine evaluation, cardiac catheterization should be performed to delineate coronary anatomy, and to delineate the degree of obstruction. A gradient of 50 mmHg or greater is an indication for operation. However, the clinician must be cognizant of any coexistent lesions, most commonly pulmonic stenosis, which may add complexity to the repair.

The localized form of supravalvular AS is treated by creating an inverted Y-shaped aortotomy across the area of stenosis, straddling the right coronary artery. The obstructing shelf is then excised and a pantaloon-shaped patch is used to close the incision.

The diffuse form of supravalvular stenosis is more variable, and the particular operative approach must be tailored to each specific patient's anatomy. In general, either an aortic endarterectomy with patch augmentation can be performed, or if the narrowing extends past the aorta arch, a prosthetic graft can be placed between the ascending and descending aorta. Operative results for discrete supravalvular AS are generally good, with a hospital mortality of less than 1 percent and an actuarial survival rate exceeding 90 percent at 20 years. In contrast, however, the diffuse form is more hazardous to repair, and carried a mortality of 15 percent in a recent series.

Patent Ductus Arteriosus

Anatomy

The ductus arteriosus is derived from the sixth aortic arch and normally extends from the main or left pulmonary artery to the upper descending thoracic aorta, distal to the left subclavian artery.

Delayed closure of the ductus is termed prolonged patency, whereas failure of closure causes persistent patency, which may occur as an isolated lesion or in association with more complex congenital heart defects. In many of these infants with more complex congenital heart defects, either pulmonary or systemic perfusion may depend on ductal flow, and these infants may decompensate if exogenous PGE is not administered to maintain ductal patency.

Natural History

The incidence of patent ductus arteriosus (PDA) is approximately 1 in every 2000 births; however, it increases dramatically with increasing prematurity. In some series, PDAs have been noted in 75 percent of infants of 28–30 weeks gestation. Persistent patency occurs more commonly in females, with a 2:1 ratio.

PDA is not a benign entity, although prolonged survival has been reported. The estimated death rate for infants with isolated, untreated PDA is approximately 30 percent. The leading cause of death is congestive heart failure, with respiratory infection as a secondary cause. Endocarditis is more likely to occur with a small ductus and is rarely fatal if aggressive antibiotic therapy is initiated early.

Clinical Manifestations and Diagnosis

After birth, in an otherwise normal cardiovascular system, a PDA results in a left-to-right shunt that depends on both the size of the ductal lumen and its total length. As the pulmonary vascular resistance falls 16–18 weeks postnatally, the shunt will increase, and its flow will ultimately be determined by the relative resistances of the pulmonary and systemic circulations.

The hemodynamic consequences of an unrestrictive ductal shunt are left ventricular volume overload with increased left atrial and pulmonary artery pressures, and right ventricular strain from the augmented afterload. These changes result in increased sympathetic discharge, tachycardia, tachypnea, and ventricular hypertrophy. The diastolic shunt results in lower aortic diastolic pressure and increases the potential for myocardial ischemia and underperfusion of other systemic organs, although the increased pulmonary flow leads to increased work of breathing and decreased gas exchange. Unrestrictive ductal flow may lead to pulmonary hypertension within the first year of life. These changes will be significantly attenuated if the size of the ductus is only moderate, and completely absent if the ductus is small.

Physical examination of the afflicted infant will reveal evidence of a hyperdynamic circulation with a widened pulse pressure and a hyperactive precordium. Auscultation demonstrates a systolic or continuous murmur, often termed a machinery murmur. Cyanosis is not present in uncomplicated isolated PDA.

The chest radiograph may reveal increased pulmonary vascularity or cardiomegaly, and the ECG may show LV strain, left atrial enlargement, and possibly RV hypertrophy. Echochardiogram with color mapping reliably demonstrates the patency of the ductus and estimates the shunt size. Cardiac catheterization is necessary only when pulmonary hypertension is suspected.

Therapy

The presence of a persistent PDA is sufficient indication for closure because of the increased mortality and risk of endocarditis. In older patients with pulmonary hypertension, closure may not improve symptoms and is associated with much higher mortality.

In premature infants, aggressive intervention with indomethacin to achieve early closure of the PDA is beneficial. Term infants, however, are generally unresponsive to pharmacologic therapy with indomethacin, so mechanical closure must be undertaken once the diagnosis is established. This can be accomplished either surgically or with catheter-based therapy. Currently, transluminal placement of various occlusive devices, such as the Rashkind double-umbrella device or embolization with Gianturco coils, are in widespread use. However, there are a number of complications inherent with the use of percutaneous devices, such as thromboembolism, endocarditis, incomplete occlusion, vascular injury, and hemorrhage secondary to perforation. Additionally, these techniques may not be applicable in very young infants, as the peripheral vessels do not provide adequate access for the delivery devices.

Video-assisted thoracoscopic occlusion, using metal clips, also has been described, although it offers few advantages over the standard surgical approach. Preterm newborns and children, however, may do well with the thoracoscopic technique, although older patients (older than age 5 years) and those with smaller ducts (< 3 mm) do well with coil occlusion. In fact, Moore and colleagues recently concluded from their series that coil occlusion is the procedure of choice for ducts smaller than 4 mm. Complete closure rates using catheter-based techniques have steadily improved. Comparative studies of cost and outcome between open surgery and transcatheter duct closure, however, have shown no overwhelming choice between the two modalities. Burke prospectively reviewed coil occlusion and VATS at Miami Children's Hospital, and found both options to be effective and less morbid than traditional thoracotomy.

Standard surgical approach involves triple ligation of the ductus with permanent suture through either a left anterior or a posterior thoracotomy. Occasionally, a short, broad ductus, in which the dimension of its width approaches that of its length, will be encountered. In this case, division between vascular clamps with oversewing of both ends is advisable. In extreme cases, the use of CPB to decompress the large ductus during ligation is an option.

Outcomes

In premature infants, the surgical mortality is very low, although the overall hospital death rate is significant as a consequence of other complications of prematurity. In older infants and children, mortality is less than 1 percent. Bleeding, chylothorax, vocal cord paralysis, and the need for reoperation occur infrequently. With the advent of muscle-sparing thoracotomy, the risk of subsequent arm dysfunction or breast abnormalities is virtually eliminated.

Aortic Coarctation

Anatomy

Coarctation of the aorta (COA) is defined as a luminal narrowing in the aorta that causes an obstruction to blood flow. This narrowing is most commonly located distal to the left subclavian artery. Extensive collateral circulation develops, predominantly involving the intercostals and mammary arteries as a direct result of aortic flow obstruction. This translates into the well-known finding of "rib-notching" on chest radiograph, and a prominent pulsation underneath the ribs.

Other associated anomalies, such as ventricular septal defect, patent ductus arteriosus, and atrial septal defect, may be seen with COA, but the most common is that of a bicuspid aortic valve, which can be demonstrated in 25–42 percent of cases.

Pathophysiology

Infants with COA develop symptoms consistent with left ventricular outflow obstruction, including pulmonary overcirculation and, later, biventricular failure. Additionally, proximal systemic hypertension develops as a result of mechanical obstruction to ventricular ejection, and hypoperfusion-induced activation of the renin–angiotensin–aldosterone system. Interestingly, hypertension is often persistent after surgical correction despite complete amelioration of the mechanical obstruction and pressure gradient. It has been shown that early surgical correction may prevent the development of long-term hypertension, which undoubtedly contributes to many of the adverse sequelae of COA, including the development of circle of Willis aneurysms, aortic dissection and rupture, and an increased incidence of coronary arteriopathy with resulting myocardial infarction.

Diagnosis

COA is likely to become symptomatic either in the newborn period if other anomalies are present or in the late adolescent period with the onset of left ventricular failure.

Physical examination will demonstrate a hyperdynamic precordium with a harsh murmur localized to the left chest and back. Femoral pulses will be dramatically decreased when compared to upper extremity pulses, and differential cyanosis may be apparent until ductal closure.

Echocardiography will reliably demonstrate the narrowed aortic segment, and define the pressure gradient across the stenotic segment. Additionally, detailed information regarding other associated anomalies can be gleaned. Aortography is reserved for those cases in which the echocardiographic findings are equivocal.

Therapy

The routine management of hemodynamically significant COA in all age groups has traditionally been surgical. The most common technique in current use is resection with end-to-end anastomosis or extended end-to-end anastomosis, taking care to remove all residual ductal tissue. The subclavian flap aortoplasty is another frequently used repair. In this method, the left subclavian artery is transected and brought down over the coarcted segment as a vascularized patch. The main benefit of these techniques is that they do not involve the use of prosthetic materials.

However, end-to-end anastomosis may not be feasible when there is a long segment of coarctation, because sufficient mobilization of the aorta above and below the lesion may not be possible. In this instance, prosthetic materials, such as a patch aortoplasty, in which a prosthetic patch is used to enlarge the coarcted segment, or an interposition tube graft must be employed.

The most common complications after COA repair are late restenosis and aneurysm formation at the repair site. Aneurysm formation is particularly common after patch aortoplasty when using Dacron material. In a large series of 891 patients, aneurysms occurred in 5.4 percent of the total, with 89 percent occurring in the group who received Dacron-patch aortoplasty, compared to 8 percent in those who received resection with primary end-to-end anastomosis. A further complication, although uncommon, is lower-body paralysis resulting from ischemic spinal cord injury during the repair. This unfortunate outcome complicates 0.5 percent of all surgical repairs, but its incidence can be lessened with the use of some form of distal perfusion, preferably left-heart bypass with the use of femoral arterial or distal thoracic aorta for arterial inflow and the femoral vein or left atrium for venous return.

Although operative repair is still the gold standard, treatment of COA by catheter-based intervention has become more widespread. Both balloon dilatation and primary stent implantation have been used successfully. The most extensive study of the results of balloon angioplasty reported on 970 procedures: 422 native and 548 recurrent COAs. Mean gradient reduction was 74 ± 24 percent for native and 70 ± 31 percent for recurrent COA. This demonstrated that catheter-based therapy could produce equally effective results both in recurrent and in primary COA, a finding with far-reaching implications in the new paradigm of multidisciplinary treatment algorithms for CHD. In the valvuloplasty and angioplasty of congenital anomalies (VACA) report, higher preangioplasty gradient, earlier procedure date, older patient age, and the presence of recurrent COA were independent risk factors for suboptimal procedural outcome.

The gradient after balloon dilatation in most series is generally acceptable. However, there is a significant minority (0–26 percent) for whom the procedural outcome is suboptimal, with a postprocedure gradient of 20 mmHg or greater. These patients may be ideal candidates for primary stent placement. Restenosis is much less common in children, presumably reflecting the influence of vessel wall scarring and growth in the pediatric age group.

Deaths from the procedure also are infrequent (less than 1 percent of cases), and the main major complication is aneurysm formation, which occurs in 7 percent of patients. With stent implantation, many authors have demonstrated improved resolution of stenosis compared with balloon dilatation alone, yet the long-term complications on vessel wall compliance remain largely unknown because only mid-term data are widely available.

In summary, children younger than age 6 months with native COA should be treated with surgical repair, although those requiring intervention at later ages may be ideal candidates for balloon dilatation or primary stent implantation. Additionally, catheter-based therapy should be employed for those cases of restenosis following either surgical or primary endovascular management.

Total Anomalous Pulmonary Venous Connection

Total anomalous pulmonary venous connection (TAPVC) occurs in 1–2 percent of all cardiac malformations and is characterized by abnormal drainage of the pulmonary veins into the right heart, whether through connections into the right atrium or into its tributaries. Accordingly, the only mechanism by which oxygenated blood can return to the left heart is through an ASD, which is almost uniformly present with TAPVC.

Unique to this lesion is the absence of a definitive form of palliation. Thus, TAPVC represents one of the only true surgical emergencies across the entire spectrum of congenital heart surgery.

Anatomy and Embryology

The lungs develop from an outpouching of the foregut, and their venous plexus arises as part of the splanchnic venous system. TAPVC arises when the pulmonary vein evagination from the posterior surface of the left atrium fails to fuse with the pulmonary venous plexus surrounding the lung buds. In place of the usual connection to the left atrium, at least one connection of the pulmonary plexus to the splanchnic plexus persists. Accordingly, the pulmonary veins drain to the heart through a systemic vein.

Darling and colleagues classified TAPVC according to the site or level of connection of the pulmonary veins to the systemic venous system: type I (45 percent), anomalous connection at the supracardiac level; type II (25 percent), anomalous connection at the cardiac level; type III (25 percent), anomalous connection at the infracardiac level; and type IV (5 percent), anomalous connection at multiple levels. Within each category, further subdivisions can be implemented, depending on whether pulmonary venous obstruction exists. Obstruction to pulmonary venous drainage is a powerful predictor of adverse natural outcome and occurs most frequently with the infracardiac type, especially when the pattern of infracardiac connection prevents the ductus venosus from bypassing the liver.

Pathophysiology and Diagnosis

Because both pulmonary and systemic venous blood return to the right atrium in all forms of TAPVC, a right-to-left intracardiac shunt must be present in order for the afflicted infant to survive. This invariably occurs via a nonrestrictive patent foramen ovale. Because of this obligatory mixing, cyanosis is usually present, and its degree depends on the ratio of pulmonary to systemic blood flow. Decreased pulmonary blood flow is a consequence of pulmonary venous obstruction, the presence of which is unlikely if the right ventricular pressure is less than 85 percent of systemic pressure.

The child with TAPVC may present with severe cyanosis and respiratory distress necessitating urgent surgical intervention if a severe degree of pulmonary venous obstruction is present. However, in cases in which there is no obstructive component, the clinical picture is usually one of pulmonary overcirculation, hepatomegaly, tachycardia, and tachypnea with feeding. In a child with serious obstruction, arterial blood gas analysis reveals severe hypoxemia (Po_2 less than 20 mmHg), with metabolic acidosis.

Chest radiography will show normal heart size with generalized pulmonary edema. Two-dimensional echocardiography is very useful in establishing the diagnosis, and also can assess ventricular septal position, which may be leftward secondary to small left ventricular volumes, and estimate the right ventricular pressure based on the height of the tricuspid regurgitant jet. Echocardiography can usually identify the pulmonary venous connections (types I–IV), and it is rarely necessary to perform other diagnostic tests.

Cardiac catheterization is not recommended in these patients because the osmotic load from the intravenous contrast can exacerbate the degree of pulmonary edema. When cardiac catheterization is performed, equalization of oxygen saturations in all four heart chambers is a hallmark finding in this disease because the mixed blood returned to the right atrium gets distributed throughout the heart.

Therapy

Operative correction of TAPVC requires anastomosis of the common pulmonary venous channel to the left atrium, obliteration of the anomalous venous connection, and closure of the atrial septal defect.

All types of TAPVC are approached through a median sternotomy, and most surgeons use deep hypothermic circulatory arrest to achieve an accurate and widely patent anastomosis. The technique for supracardiac TAPVC includes early division of the vertical vein, retraction of the aorta and the superior vena cava laterally to expose the posterior aspect of the left atrium and the pulmonary venous confluence, and a side-to-side anastomosis between a long, horizontal biatrial incision and a longitudinal incision within the pulmonary venous confluence. The ASD can then be closed with an autologous pericardial patch.

In patients with TAPVC to the coronary sinus without obstruction, a simple unroofing of the coronary sinus can be performed through a single right atriotomy. If pulmonary venous obstruction is present, the repair should include generous resection of roof of the coronary sinus.

Repair of infracardiac TAPVC entails ligation of the vertical vein at the diaphragm, followed by construction of a proximal, patulous longitudinal venotomy. This repair is usually performed by "rolling" the heart toward the left, thus exposing the left atrium where it usually overlies the descending vertical vein.

The perioperative care of these infants is crucial because episodes of pulmonary hypertension can occur within the first 48 h, which contribute significantly to mortality following repair. Muscle relaxants and narcotics should be administered during this period to maintain a constant state of anesthesia. Arterial Pco_2 should be maintained at 30 mmHg with use of a volume ventilator and the FiO_2 should be increased to keep the pulmonary arterial pressure at less than two-thirds of the systemic pressure.

Results

Results of TAPVC in infancy have markedly improved in recent years, with an operative mortality of 5 percent or less in some series. This improvement is probably multifactorial, mainly as a consequence of early noninvasive diagnosis and aggressive perioperative management. The routine use of echocardiography; improvements in myocardial protection with specific attention to the right ventricle; creation of a large, tension-free anastomosis with maximal use of the venous confluence and atrial tissue; careful geometric alignment of the pulmonary venous sinus with the body of the left atrium avoiding tension and rotation of the pulmonary veins; and prevention of pulmonary hypertensive events have likely played a major role in reducing operative mortality. Risk factors such as venous obstruction at presentation, urgency of operative repair, and infradiaphragmatic anatomic type are no longer correlated with early mortality.

The most significant postoperative complication of TAPVC repair is pulmonary venous obstruction, which occurs 9–11 percent of the time, regardless of the surgical technique employed. Mortality varies between 30 and 45 percent and alternative catheter interventions do not offer definitive solutions. Recurrent pulmonary venous obstruction can be localized at the site of the pulmonary venous anastomosis (extrinsic), which can usually be cured with patch enlargement or balloon dilatation, or it may be secondary to endocardial thickening of the pulmonary venous ostia frequently resulting in diffuse pulmonary venous sclerosis (intrinsic), which carries a 66 percent mortality rate because few good solutions exist. More commonly, postrepair left ventricular dysfunction can occur as the noncompliant left ventricle suddenly is required to handle an increased volume load from redirected pulmonary venous return. This can manifest as an increase in pulmonary artery pressure but is distinguishable from primary pulmonary hypertension (another possible postoperative complication following repair of TAPVC) from the elevated left atrial pressure found in LV dysfunction along with echocardiographic evidence of poor LV contractility. In pulmonary hypertension, the left atrial (LA) pressure may be low, the LV may appear "underfilled" (by echocardiography), and the RV may appear dilated. In either case, postoperative support for a few days with extracorporeal membrane oxygenation (ECMO) may be life-saving, and TAPVC should be repaired in centers that have this capacity.

Some investigators have speculated that preoperative pulmonary venous obstruction is associated with increased medial thickness within the pulmonary vasculature, which may predispose these infants to intrinsic pulmonary venous stenosis despite adequate pulmonary venous decompression. Another complication following repair of TAPVC is the development of atrial arrhythmias secondary to altered atrial geometry and left atrial enlargement procedures. These arrhythmias may be asymptomatic, and certain surgeons therefore advocate routine long-term follow-up with 24-h ECG monitoring to facilitate their detection and treatment.

DEFECTS REQUIRING PALLIATION

Hypoplastic Left-Heart Syndrome (HLHS)

Hypoplastic Left-Heart Syndrome (HLHS) comprises a wide spectrum of cardiac malformations, including hypoplasia or atresia of the aortic and mitral valves and hypoplasia of the left ventricle and ascending aorta. HLHS has a reported prevalence of 0.2 per 1000 live births and occurs twice as often in boys as in girls. Left untreated, HLHS is invariably fatal and is responsible for 25 percent of early cardiac deaths in neonates. However, the recent evolution of palliative surgical procedures has dramatically improved the outlook for patients with HLHS, and an improved understanding of anatomic and physiologic alterations have spurred advances in parallel arenas such as intrauterine diagnosis and fetal intervention, echocardiographic imaging, and neonatal critical care.

Anatomy

As implied by its name, HLHS involves varying degrees of underdevelopment of left-sided structures, including the left ventricle and the aortic and mitral valves. Thus, HLHS can be classified into four anatomic subtypes based on the valvular morphology: (1) aortic and mitral stenosis; (2) aortic and mitral atresia; (3) aortic atresia and mitral stenosis; and (4) aortic stenosis and mitral atresia. Aortic atresia tends to be associated with more-severe degrees of hypoplasia of the ascending aorta than does aortic stenosis.

Even in cases without frank aortic atresia, however, the aortic arch is generally hypoplastic and, in severe cases, may even be interrupted. There is an associated coarctation shelf in 80 percent of patients with HLHS, and the ductus itself is usually quite large, as is the main pulmonary artery. The segmental pulmonary arteries, however, are small, secondary to reduced intrauterine pulmonary blood flow, which is itself a consequence of the left-sided outflow obstruction. The left atrial cavity is generally smaller than normal, and is accentuated because of the leftward displacement of the septum primum. There is almost always an interatrial communication via the foramen ovale, which can be large, but more commonly restricts right-to-left flow. In rare cases, there is no atrial-level communication, which can be lethal for these infants because there is no way for pulmonary venous return to cross over to the right ventricle.

Associated defects can occur with HLHS, and many of them have importance with respect to operative repair. For example, if a ventricular septal defect is present, the left ventricle can retain its normal size during development even in the presence of mitral atresia. This is because a right-to-left shunt through the defect impels growth of the left ventricle. This introduces the feasibility of biventricular repair for this subset of patients.

Although HLHS undoubtedly results from a complex interplay of developmental errors in the early stages of cardiogenesis, many investigators have hypothesized that the altered blood flow is responsible for the structural underdevelopment that characterizes HLHS. In other words, if the stimulus for normal development of the ascending aorta from the primordial aortic sac is high-pressure systemic blood flow from the left ventricle through the aortic valve, then an atretic or stenotic aortic valve, which impedes flow and leads to only low-pressure diastolic retrograde flow via the ductus, will change the developmental signals and result in hypoplasia of the downstream structures. Normal growth and development of the left ventricle and mitral valve can be secondarily affected, resulting in hypoplasia or atresia of these structures.

Pathophysiology and Diagnosis

Neonates with severe HLHS receive all pulmonary, systemic, and coronary blood flow from the right ventricle. Generally, a child with HLHS will present with respiratory distress within the first day of life, and mild cyanosis may be noted. These infants must be rapidly triaged to a tertiary center, and echocardiography should be performed to confirm the diagnosis. Prostaglandin E1 must be administered to maintain ductal patency, and the ventilatory settings adjusted to avoid excessive oxygenation and increase carbon dioxide tension. These maneuvers will maintain pulmonary vascular resistance and promote improved systemic perfusion. Cardiac catheterization should generally be avoided because it is not usually helpful and might result in injury to the ductus and compromised renal function secondary to the osmotic dye load.

Treatment

In 1983, Norwood and colleagues described a two-stage palliative surgical procedure for relief of HLHS that was later modified to the currently used three-stage method of palliation. Stage 1 palliation, also known as the modified Norwood procedure, bypasses the left ventricle by creating a single outflow vessel, the neoaorta, which arises from the right ventricle.

The current technique of arch reconstruction involves completion of a connection between the pulmonary root, the native ascending aorta, and a piece of pulmonary homograft used to augment the diminutive native aorta. There are several modifications of this anastomosis, most notably the

Damus-Kaye-Stansel (DKS) anastomosis, which involves dividing both the aorta and the pulmonary artery at the sinotubular junction. The proximal aorta is anastomosed to the proximal pulmonary artery creating a "double-barreled" outlet from the heart. This outlet is anastomosed to the distal aorta, which can be augmented with homograft material if there is an associated coarctation. At the completion of arch reconstruction, a 3.5- or 4-mm shunt is placed from the innominate artery to the right pulmonary artery. The interatrial septum is then widely excised, thereby creating a large interatrial communication and preventing pulmonary venous hypertension.

The DKS connection, as described above, might avoid postoperative distortion of the tripartite connection in the neoaorta, and thus decrease the risk of coronary insufficiency. It can be used when the aorta is 4 mm or larger. Unfortunately, in many infants with HLHS; especially if there is aortic atresia; the aorta is diminutive and often less than 2 mm in diameter.

Following stage 1 palliation, the second surgical procedure is the creation of a bidirectional cavopulmonary shunt, generally at 3–6 months of life when the pulmonary vascular resistance has decreased to normal levels. This is the first step in separating the pulmonary and systemic circulations, and it decreases the volume load on the single ventricle. The existing innominate artery-to-pulmonary shunt (or RV-pulmonary shunt) is eliminated during the same operation.

The third stage of surgical palliation, known as the modified Fontan procedure, completes the separation of the systemic and pulmonary circulations and is performed between 18 months and 3 years of age, or when the patient has outgrown the capacity to perfuse the systemic circulation with adequately oxygenated blood and becomes progressively cyanotic. This has traditionally required a lateral tunnel within the right atrium to direct blood from the inferior vena cava to the pulmonary artery, allowing further relief of the volume load on the right ventricle, and providing increased pulmonary blood flow to alleviate cyanosis. More recently, many favor using an extracardiac conduit (e.g., 20-mm tube graft) to connect the inferior vena cava to the pulmonary artery.

Not all patients with HLHS require this three-stage palliative repair. Some infants afflicted with a milder form of HLHS, recently described as hypoplastic left-heart complex (HLHC), have aortic or mitral hypoplasia without intrinsic valve stenosis and antegrade flow in the ascending aorta. In this group, a two-ventricle repair can be achieved with reasonable outcome.

Transplantation can be used as a first-line therapy or when anatomic or physiologic considerations exist that preclude a favorable outcome with palliative repair. Significant tricuspid regurgitation, intractable pulmonary artery hypertension, or progressive right ventricular failure, are cases in which cardiac replacement may be advantageous. The local probability of organ availability should be considered prior to electing transplantation, as 24 percent of infants died awaiting transplantation in the largest series to date.

Results

Outcomes for HLHS are still significantly worse than those for other complex cardiac defects. However, with improvements in perioperative care and modifications in surgical technique, the survival following the Norwood procedure now exceeds 80 percent in experienced centers. The outcome for low-birth-weight infants has improved, but low weight still remains a major predictor of adverse survival, especially when accompanied by additional cardiac defects, such as systemic outflow obstruction, or extracardiac anomalies.

DEFECTS THAT MAY BE PALLIATED OR REPAIRED

Transposition of the Great Arteries

Anatomy

Complete transposition is characterized by connection of the atria to their appropriate ventricles with inappropriate ventriculoarterial connections. Thus, the aorta arises anteriorly from the right ventricle, although the pulmonary artery arises posteriorly from the left ventricle. Van Praagh and coworkers introduced the term D-transposition of the great arteries (D-TGA) to describe this defect, although L-TGA describes a form of corrected transposition in which there is concomitant atrioventricular discordance.

D-TGA requires an obligatory intracardiac mixing of blood, which usually occurs at both the atrial and the ventricular levels or via a patent ductus.

Pathophysiology

D-TGA results in parallel pulmonary and systemic circulations, with patient survival dependent on intracardiac mixing of blood. Postnatally, the left ventricle does not hypertrophy because it is not subjected to systemic afterload. The lack of normal extrauterine left ventricular maturation has important implications for the timing of surgical repair because the LV must be converted to the systemic ventricle early enough to allow adaptation, usually within a few weeks after birth.

Clinical Manifestations and Diagnosis

Infants with D-TGA and an IVS are usually cyanotic at birth, with an arterial Po_2 between 25 and 40 mm Hg. If ductal patency is not maintained, deterioration will be rapid with ensuing metabolic acidosis and death. Conversely, those infants with a coexisting VSD may be only mildly hypoxemic and may come to medical attention after 2–3 weeks, when the falling PVR leads to symptoms of CHF.

The ECG will reveal right ventricular hypertrophy, and the chest radiograph will reveal the classic egg-shaped configuration. Definitive diagnosis is made by echocardiography, which reliably demonstrates ventriculoarterial discordance and any associated lesions. Cardiac catheterization is rarely necessary, except in those infants requiring surgery after the neonatal period to assess the suitability of the LV to support the systemic circulation. Limited catherization, however, is useful for performance of atrial septostomy in those neonates with inadequate intracardiac mixing.

Surgical Repair

Blalock and Hanlon introduced the first operative intervention for D-TGA with the creation of an atrial septectomy to enhance intracardiac mixing. This initial procedure was feasible in the precardiopulmonary bypass era, but carried a high mortality rate. Later, Rashkind and Causo developed a catheter-based balloon septostomy, which largely obviated the need for open septectomy.

These early palliative maneuvers, however, met with limited success, and it was not until the late 1950s, when Senning and Mustard developed the first "atrial repair," that outcomes improved. The Senning operation consisted of rerouting venous flow at the atrial level by incising and realigning the atrial septum over the pulmonary veins and using the right atrial free wall to create a pulmonary venous baffle.

Although the Mustard repair was similar, it made use of either autologous pericardium or synthetic material to create the interatrial baffle. These atrial switch procedures resulted in a physiologic correction, but not an anatomic one, as the systemic circulation is still based on the right ventricle. Still, survival rose to 95 percent in most centers by using an early balloon septostomy followed by an atrial switch procedure at 3–8 months of age.

Despite the improved early survival rates, long-term problems, such as superior vena cava or pulmonary venous obstruction, baffle leak, arrhythmias, tricuspid valve regurgitation, and right ventricular failure, prompted the development of the arterial switch procedure by Jatene in 1975. The arterial switch procedure involves the division of the aorta and the pulmonary artery, posterior translocation of the aorta (LeCompte maneuver), mobilization of the coronary arteries, placement of a pantaloon-shaped pericardial patch, and proper alignment of the coronary arteries on the neoaorta.

The most important consideration is the timing of surgical repair, because arterial switch should be performed within 2 weeks after birth, before the left ventricle loses its ability to pump against systemic afterload. In patients presenting later than 2 weeks, the left ventricle can be retrained with preliminary pulmonary artery banding and aortopulmonary shunt followed by definitive repair. Alternatively, the unprepared left ventricle can be supported following arterial switch with a mechanical assist device for a few days although it recovers ability to manage systemic pressures. Echocardiography can be used to assess left ventricular performance and guide operative planning in these circumstances.

For patients with D-TGA, IVS, and VSD the arterial switch operation provides excellent long-term results with a mortality rate of less than 5 percent. Operative risk is increased when unfavorable coronary anatomic configurations are present, or when augmentation of the aortic arch is required. The most common complication is supravalvular pulmonary stenosis, occurring 10 percent of the time, which may require reoperation.

Results of the Rastelli operation have improved substantially, with an early mortality rate of 5 percent in a recent review. Late mortality rate results were less favorable because conduit failure requiring reoperation, pacemaker insertion, or relief of left ventricular outflow obstruction were frequent.

Tetralogy of Fallot

Anatomy

The four features of tetralogy of Fallot (TOF) are (1) malalignment ventricular septal defect, (2) dextroposition of the aorta, (3) right ventricular outflow tract obstruction, and (4) right ventricular hypertrophy. This combination of defects arises as a result of underdevelopment and anteroleftward malalignment of the infundibular septum.

Anomalous coronary artery patterns, related to either origin or distribution, have been described in TOF. However, the most surgically important coronary anomaly occurs when the left anterior descending artery arises as a branch of the right coronary artery. This occurs in approximately 3 percent of cases of

TOF and may preclude placement of a transannular patch, as the left anterior descending coronary artery crosses the RVOT at varying distances from the pulmonary valve annulus.

Coexisting lesions are uncommon in TOF, but the most frequently associated lesions are atrial septal defect, patent ductus arteriosus, complete atrioventricular septal defect, and multiple VSDs.

Pathophysiology and Clinical Presentation

The initial presentation of a child afflicted with TOF depends on the degree of RVOT obstruction. Those children with cyanosis at birth usually have severe pulmonary annular hypoplasia with concomitant hypoplasia of the peripheral pulmonary arteries. Most children, however, present with mild cyanosis at birth, which then progresses as the right ventricular hypertrophy further compromises the RVOT. Cyanosis usually becomes significant within the first 6–12 months of life, and the child may develop characteristic "tet" spells, which are periods of extreme hypoxemia. These spells are characterized by decreased pulmonary blood flow and an increase in aortic flow. They can be triggered by any stimulus that decreases systemic vascular resistance, such as fever or vigorous physical activity. Cyanotic spells increase in severity and frequency as the child grows, and older patients with uncorrected TOF may often squat, which increases peripheral vascular resistance and relieves the cyanosis.

Physical examination in the older patient with TOF may demonstrate clubbing, polycythemia, or brain abscesses. Chest radiography will demonstrate a boot-shaped heart, and ECG will show the normal pattern of right ventricular hypertrophy. Echocardiography confirms the diagnosis because it demonstrates the position and nature of the VSD, defines the character of the RVOT obstruction, and often visualizes the branch pulmonary arteries and the proximal coronary arteries. Cardiac catheterization is rarely necessary and is actually risky in TOF because it can create spasm of the RVOT muscle and result in a hypercyanotic episode (tet spell). Occasionally, aortography is necessary to delineate the coronary artery anatomy.

Treatment

The optimal age and surgical approach of repair of TOF have been debated for several decades. Currently, most centers favor primary elective repair in infancy, as contemporary perioperative techniques have improved outcomes substantially in this population. Additionally, definitive repair protects the heart and other organs from the pathophysiology inherent in the defect, and its palliated state.

However, systemic-to-pulmonary shunts, generally a B-T shunt, may still be preferred with an unstable neonate younger than 6 months of age, when an extracardiac conduit is required because of an anomalous left anterior descending coronary artery, or when pulmonary atresia, significant branch pulmonary artery hypoplasia, or severe noncardiac anomalies coexist with TOF.

Traditionally, TOF was repaired through a right ventriculotomy, providing excellent exposure for closure of the VSD and relief of the RVOT obstruction, but concerns that the resultant scar would significantly impair right ventricular function or lead to lethal arrhythmias led to the development of a transatrial approach. Transatrial repair, except in cases when the presence of diffuse RVOT hypoplasia requires insertion of a transannular patch, is now being increasingly advocated by many, although its superiority has not been conclusively demonstrated.

Results

Operative mortality for primary repair of TOF in infancy is less than 5 percent in most series. Previously reported risk factors such as transannular patch insertion or younger age at time of repair have been eliminated secondary to improved intraoperative and postoperative care.

A major complication of repaired TOF is the development of pulmonary insufficiency, which subjects the RV to the adverse effects of acute and chronic volume overload. This is especially problematic if residual lesions such as a VSD or peripheral pulmonary stenosis exists. When significant deterioration of ventricular function occurs, insertion of a pulmonary valve may be required, although this is rarely necessary in infants.

Ventricular Septal Defect

Anatomy

VSD refers to a hole between the left and right ventricles. These defects are common, comprising 20–30 percent of all cases of congenital heart disease, and may occur as an isolated lesion or as part of a more complex malformation. VSDs vary in size from 3–4 mm to more than 3 cm, and are classified into four types based on their location in the ventricular septum: perimembranous, atrioventricular canal, outlet or supracristal, and muscular.

Perimembranous VSDs are the most common type requiring surgical intervention, comprising approximately 80 percent of cases. These defects involve the membranous septum and include the malalignment defects seen in tetralogy of Fallot. In rare instances, the anterior and septal leaflets of the tricuspid valve adhere to the edges of the perimembranous defect, forming a channel between the left ventricle and the right atrium. These defects result in a large left-to-right shunt owing to the large pressure differential between the two chambers.

Atrioventricular canal defects, also known as inlet defects, occur when part or all of the septum of the AV canal is absent. The VSD lies beneath the tricuspid valve and is limited upstream by the tricuspid annulus, without intervening muscle.

The supracristal or outlet VSD results from a defect within the conal septum. Characteristically, these defects are limited upstream by the pulmonary valve and are otherwise surrounded by the muscle of the infundibular septum.

Muscular VSDs are the most common type, and may lie in four locations: anterior, midventricular, posterior, or apical. These are surrounded by muscle, and can occur anywhere along the trabecular portion of the septum. The rare "Swiss-cheese" type of muscular VSD consists of multiple communications between the right and left ventricles, complicating operative repair.

Pathophysiology and Clinical Presentation

The size of the VSD determines the initial pathophysiology of the disease. Large VSDs are classified as nonrestrictive, and are at least equal in diameter to the aortic annulus. These defects allow free flow of blood from the left ventricle to the right ventricle, elevating right ventricular pressures to the same level as systemic pressure. Consequently, Qp:Qs is inversely dependent on the ratio of pulmonary vascular resistance to systemic vascular resistance.

Nonrestrictive VSDs produce a large increase in pulmonary blood flow, and the afflicted infant will present with symptoms of congestive heart failure. However, if untreated, these defects will cause pulmonary hypertension with a corresponding increase in pulmonary vascular resistance. This will lead to a reversal of flow (a right-to-left shunt), which is known as Eisenmenger's syndrome.

Small restrictive VSDs offer significant resistance to the passage of blood across the defect, and therefore right ventricular pressure is either normal or only minimally elevated and Qp:Qs rarely exceeds 1.5. These defects are generally asymptomatic because there are few physiologic consequences. However, there is a long-term risk of endocarditis, because endocardial damage from the jet of blood through the defect may serve as a possible nidus for colonization.

Diagnosis

The child with a large VSD will present with severe congestive heart failure and frequent respiratory tract infections. Those children with Eisenmenger syndrome may be deceptively asymptomatic until frank cyanosis develops.

The chest radiograph will show cardiomegaly and pulmonary overcirculation and the ECG will show signs of left ventricular or biventricular hypertrophy. Echocardiography provides definitive diagnosis, and can estimate the degree of shunting and pulmonary arterial pressures. Cardiac catheterization has largely been supplanted by echocardiography, except in older children in which measurement of pulmonary resistance is necessary prior to recommending closure of the defect.

Treatment

VSDs may close or narrow spontaneously, and the probability of closure is inversely related to the age at which the defect is observed. Thus, infants at 1 month of age have an 80 percent incidence of spontaneous closure, whereas a child at 12 months of age has only a 25 percent chance of closure. This has an important impact on operative decision making, because a small or moderate-size VSD may be observed for a period of time in the absence of symptoms. Large defects and those in severely symptomatic neonates should be repaired during infancy to relieve symptoms and because irreversible changes in pulmonary vascular resistance may develop during the first year of life.

Repair of isolated VSDs requires the use of cardiopulmonary bypass with moderate hypothermia and cardioplegic arrest. The right atrial approach is preferable for most defects, except apical muscular defects, which often require a left ventriculotomy for adequate exposure. Supracristal defects may alternatively be exposed via a longitudinal incision in the pulmonary artery a transverse incision in the right ventricle below the pulmonary valve. Regardless of the type of defect present, a right atrial approach can be used initially to inspect the anatomy, as this may be abandoned should it offer inadequate exposure for repair. After careful inspection of the heart for any associated malformations, a patch repair is employed, taking care to avoid the conduction system. Routine use of intraoperative transesophageal echocardiography should be used to assess for any residual defects.

Successful percutaneous device closure of VSDs using the Amplatzer muscular VSD was recently described. The device has demonstrated a 100 percent closure rate in a small series of patients with isolated or residual VSDs, or as a collaborative treatment strategy for the VSD component in more complex congenital lesions. Proponents of device closure argue that their use can decrease the complexity of surgical repair, avoid reoperation for a small residual lesion, or avoid the need for a ventriculotomy.

Multiple or "Swiss-cheese" VSDs represent a special case, and many cannot be repaired during infancy. In those patients in whom definitive VSD closure cannot be accomplished, temporary placement of a pulmonary artery band can be employed to control pulmonary flow. This allows time for spontaneous closure of many of the smaller defects, thus simplifying surgical repair.

Some centers, however, have advocated early definitive repair of the Swiss-cheese septum, by using oversize patches, fibrin glue, and combined intraoperative device closure, and techniques to complete the repair transatrially. At the UCSF, 69 percent of patients with multiple VSDs underwent single-stage correction, and the repaired group had improved outcome as compared to the palliated group.

Results

Even in very small infants, closure of VSDs can be safely performed with hospital mortality near 0 percent. The main risk factor remains the presence of other associated lesions, especially when present in symptomatic neonates with large VSDs.

Selected Readings

Peterson GE, Brickner ME, Reimold SC: Transesophageal echocardiography: Clinical indications and applications. Circulation 107:2398, 2003.

Reddy VM: Cardiac surgery for premature and low birth weight neonates. Semin Thorac Cardiovasc Surg Pediatr Card Surg Annu 4:271, 2001.

Jones TK, Lupinetti FM: Comparison of Ross procedures and aortic valve allografts in children. Ann Thorac Surg 66:S170, 1998.

Mavroudis, C, Backer CL, Gevitz M: Forty-six years of patent ductus arteriosus division at Children's Memorial Hospital of Chicago. Standards for comparison. Ann Thorac Surg 220:402, 1994.

McCrindle BW, Jones TK, Morrow WR, et al: Acute results of balloon angioplasty of native coarctation versus recurrent aortic obstruction are equivalent. Valvuloplasty and Angioplasty of Congenital Anomalies (VACA) Registry Investigators. J Am Coll Cardiol 28:1810, 1996.

de Leval MR, Kilner P, Gerwillig M, et al: Total cavopulmonary connection: A logical alternative to atriopulmonary connection for complex Fontan operations. J Thorac Cardiovasc Surg 96:682, 1988.

Jacobs ML, Norwood WI: Fontan operation: Influence of modifications on morbidity and mortality. Ann Thorac Surg 58:945, 1994.

Culbert EL, Ashburn DA, Cullen-Dean G, et al: Quality of life after repair of transposition of the great arteries. Circulation 108:857, 2003.

Mahle WT, McBride MG, Paridon SM: Exercise performance in tetralogy of Fallot: The impact of primary complete repair in infancy. Pediatr Cardiol 23:224, 2002.

Roussin R, Belli E, Lacour-Gayet F, et al: Aortic arch reconstruction with pulmonary autograft patch aortoplasty. J Thorac Cardiovasc Surg 123:443, 2002.

20 | Acquired Heart Disease

Charles F. Schwartz, Aubrey C. Galloway,
Ram Sharony, Paul C. Saunders, Eugene
A. Grossi, and Stephen B. Colvin

Clinical Evaluation

The importance of the history and physical examination when evaluating a patient with acquired heart disease for potential surgery cannot be overemphasized. It is imperative that the surgeon be well aware of the functional status of the patient and the clinical relevance of each symptom because operative decisions depend on the accurate assessment of the significance of a particular pathologic finding. Associated risk factors and coexisting conditions must be identified, as they significantly influence a patient's operative risk for cardiac or noncardiac surgery.

Symptoms

The classic symptoms of heart disease are fatigue, angina, dyspnea, edema, cough or hemoptysis, palpitations, and syncope as outlined by Braunwald. An important feature of cardiac disease is that myocardial function or coronary blood supply that may be adequate at rest may become inadequate with exercise or exertion. Thus chest pain or dyspnea that occurs primarily during exertion is frequently cardiac in origin, although symptoms that occur at rest often are not.

In addition to evaluating the patient's primary symptoms, the history should include a family history, past medical history (prior surgery or myocardial infarction [MI], concomitant hypertension, diabetes, and other associated diseases), personal habits (smoking, alcohol or drug use), functional capacity, and a detailed review of systems.

Easy fatigability is a frequent but nonspecific symptom of cardiac disease that can arise from many causes. In some patients, easy fatigability reflects a generalized decrease in cardiac output or low-grade heart failure. The significance of subjective easy fatigability is vague and nonspecific.

Angina pectoris is the hallmark of myocardial ischemia secondary to coronary artery disease, although a variety of other conditions can produce chest pain. Classic angina is precordial pain described as squeezing, heavy, or burning in nature, lasting from 2–10 min. Angina usually is provoked by exercise, emotion, sexual activity, or eating, and is relieved by rest or nitroglycerin. Angina is present in its classic form in 75 percent of patients with coronary disease, although atypical symptoms occur in 25 percent of patients and more frequently in women. A small but significant number of patients have "silent" ischemia, most typically occurring in diabetics. Angina also is a classic symptom of aortic stenosis.

Noncardiac causes of chest pain that may be confused with angina include gastroesophageal reflux disease, musculoskeletal pain, peptic ulcer disease, costochondritis, biliary tract disease, pleuritis, pulmonary embolus, pulmonary hypertension, pericarditis, and aortic dissection. Dyspnea appears as an early sign in patients with mitral stenosis because of restriction of flow from the left atrium into the left ventricle. However, with other forms of heart disease dyspnea is a late sign, as it develops only after the left ventricle has failed and

458

the end-diastolic pressure rises significantly. Dyspnea associated with mitral insufficiency, aortic valve disease, or coronary disease represents relatively advanced pathophysiology.

A number of other respiratory symptoms represent different degrees of pulmonary congestion. These include orthopnea, paroxysmal nocturnal dyspnea, cough, hemoptysis, and pulmonary edema. Occasionally dyspnea represents an "angina equivalent," occurring secondary to ischemia-related left ventricular dysfunction. This finding is more common in women and in diabetic patients.

Left-sided heart failure may result in fluid retention and pulmonary congestion, subsequently leading to pulmonary hypertension and progressive right-sided heart failure. A history of exertional dyspnea with associated edema is frequently because of heart failure.

Palpitations are secondary to rapid, forceful, ectopic, or irregular heartbeats. These should not be ignored, as occasionally they represent significant or potentially life-threatening arrhythmias. The underlying cardiac arrhythmia may range from premature atrial or ventricular contractions to atrial fibrillation, atrial flutter, paroxysmal atrial or junctional tachycardia, or sustained ventricular tachycardia.

Atrial fibrillation is one of the most common causes of palpitations. It is a common arrhythmia in patients with mitral stenosis, and results from left atrial hypertrophy that evolves from sustained elevation in left atrial pressure. Palpitations caused by a slow heart rate are frequently because of complete or intermittent atrioventricular nodal block.

Severe, life-threatening forms of ventricular tachycardia or ventricular fibrillation may occur in any patient with ischemic disease, either from ongoing ischemia or from prior infarction and myocardial scarring.

Syncope, or sudden loss of consciousness, is usually a result of sudden decreased perfusion of the brain. The differential diagnosis includes: (1) third-degree heart block with bradycardia or asystole, (2) malignant ventricular tachyarrhythmias or ventricular fibrillation, (3) aortic stenosis, (4) hypertrophic cardiomyopathy, (5) carotid artery disease, (6) seizure disorders, and (7) vasovagal reaction. Many of these conditions can result in sudden death.

Functional Disability and Angina

An important part of the history is the assessment of the patient's overall cardiac functional disability, which is a good approximation of the severity of the patient's underlying disease. The New York Heart Association (NYHA) has developed a classification of patients with heart disease based on symptoms and functional disability (Table 20-1). A different grading system for patients with ischemic disease, developed by the Canadian Cardiovascular Society (CCS), is used to assess the severity of angina (Table 20-2).

Cardiac Risk Assessment in General Surgery Patients

Cardiac risk stratification for patients undergoing noncardiac surgery is an important part of the preoperative evaluation of the general surgery patient. The joint American College of Cardiology/American Heart Association (ACC/AHA) task force, chaired by Eagle, recently reported guidelines and recommendations. In general, the preoperative cardiovascular evaluation involves an assessment of clinical markers, the patient's underlying functional capacity, and various surgery-specific risk factors.

TABLE 20-1 New York Heart Association Functional Classification

Class I: Patients with cardiac disease but without resulting limitation of physical activity. Ordinary physical activity does not cause undue fatigue, palpitation, dyspnea, or angina pain.

Class II: Patients with cardiac disease resulting in slight limitation of physical activity. They are comfortable at rest. Ordinary physical activity results in fatigue, palpitation, dyspnea, or angina pain.

Class III: Patients with cardiac disease resulting in marked limitation of physical activity. They are comfortable at rest. Less than ordinary physical activity causes fatigue, palpitation, dyspnea, or anginal pain.

Class IV: Patients with cardiac disease resulting in an inability to carry on any physical activity without discomfort. Symptoms of cardiac insufficiency or of the anginal syndrome may be present even at rest. If any physical activity is undertaken, discomfort is increased.

Based on the clinical markers, the functional class of the patient, and the proposed surgical procedure, the patient is assigned a high, intermediate, or low cardiac risk, and then managed appropriately. In patients who are considered high cardiac risk because of clinical markers or by virtue of noninvasive testing, coronary angiography may be recommended prior to surgery. Because of the common atherosclerotic etiology and the close association between clinically relevant coronary artery disease and peripheral vascular disease, patients undergoing major vascular surgery should be screened closely. Any significant underlying coronary disease should be aggressively treated, either with intensive perioperative management or with coronary revascularization prior to surgery, using standard indications.

Diagnostic Studies

Electrocardiogram and Chest Radiograph

The electrocardiogram (ECG) and the chest radiograph are the two classic diagnostic studies. The electrocardiogram is used to detect rhythm disturbances, heart block, atrial or ventricular hypertrophy, ventricular strain, myocardial ischemia, and MI. The chest radiograph is excellent for determining cardiac enlargement and pulmonary congestion, and for assessing associated pulmonary pathology.

TABLE 20-2 Canadian Cardiovascular Society

Class I: Ordinary physical activity, such as walking or climbing stairs, does not cause angina. Angina may occur with strenuous, rapid, or prolonged exertion at work or recreation.

Class II: There is slight limitation of ordinary activity. Angina may occur with walking or climbing stairs rapidly, walking uphill, walking or stair climbing after meals or in the cold, in the wind, or under emotional stress, or walking more than two blocks on the level, or climbing more than one flight of stairs under normal conditions at a normal pace.

Class III: There is marked limitation of ordinary physical activity. Angina may occur after walking one or more blocks on the level or climbing one flight of stairs under normal conditions at a normal pace.

Class IV: There is inability to carry on any physical activity without discomfort; angina may be present at rest.

Echocardiography

Echocardiography has become the most widely used cardiac diagnostic study. It incorporates the use of ultrasound and reflected acoustic waves for cardiac imaging. Intracardiac pressures, valvular insufficiency, and transvalvular gradients can be estimated from Doppler measurements. Transthoracic echocardiography has become an excellent noninvasive screening test for evaluating cardiac size and wall motion and for assessing valvular pathology.

Transesophageal echocardiography (TEE), which is done by placement of the two-dimensional transducer in a flexible endoscope is particularly useful in evaluation of the left atrium, the mitral valve, and the aortic arch. TEE studies are used when more precise imaging is required or when the diagnosis is uncertain after the transthoracic study. Dobutamine stress echocardiography has evolved as an important noninvasive provocative study and is used to assess cardiac wall motion in response to inotropic stimulation.

Radionuclide Studies

Currently the most widely used myocardial perfusion screening study is the thallium scan, which uses the nucleide thallium-201. Initial uptake of thallium-201 into myocardial cells is dependent on myocardial perfusion, although delayed uptake depends on myocardial viability. Thus, reversible defects occur in underperfused, ischemic, but viable zones, although fixed defects occur in areas of infarction.

The exercise thallium test is widely used to identify inducible areas of ischemia and is 95 percent sensitive in detecting multivessel coronary disease. This is the best overall test to detect myocardial ischemia, but it requires the patient to exercise on the treadmill. The dipyridamole thallium study is a provocative study using intravenous dipyridamole, which induces vasodilation and consequently unmasks myocardial ischemia in response to stress. This is the most widely used provocative study for risk stratification for patients who cannot exercise. Global myocardial function frequently is evaluated by the gated blood pool scan (equilibrium radionuclide angiocardiography) using technetium-99m (99mTc). This study can detect areas of hypokinesis and measure left ventricular ejection fraction, end-systolic volume, and end-diastolic volume. An exercise-gated blood pool scan is an excellent method for assessing a patient's global cardiac response to stress.

Positron Emission Tomography Scan

The positron emission tomography (PET) scan is a special radionuclide imaging technique used to assess myocardial viability in underperfused areas of the heart. PET allows the noninvasive functional assessment of perfusion, substrate metabolism, and cardiac innervation in vivo. The PET scan may be most useful in determining whether an area of apparently infarcted myocardium may in fact be hibernating and capable of responding to revascularization.

Magnetic Resonance Imaging Viability Studies

Magnetic resonance imaging (MRI) may be used to delineate the transmural extent of MI and to distinguish between reversible and irreversible myocardial ischemic injury.

Cardiac Catheterization

The cardiac catheterization study remains an important part of cardiac diagnosis. Complete cardiac catheterization includes the measurement of intracardiac pressures, cardiac output, localization of intracardiac shunts, determination of internal cardiac anatomy, ventricular wall motion by cineradiography, and determination of coronary anatomy by coronary angiography. During cardiac catheterization the cardiac output can be calculated using the Fick oxygen method, in which cardiac index (1/min per square meter) = oxygen consumption (mL/min per square meter)/ arteriovenous oxygen content difference (mL/min).

The area of a cardiac valve can be determined from measured cardiac output and intracardiac pressures using Gorlin formula. This formula relates the valve area to the flow across the valve divided by the square root of the transvalvular pressure gradient. The significance of valvular stenosis should be based on the calculated valve area (the normal mitral valve area is 4 to 6 cm^2 and the normal aortic valve area is 2.5–3.5 cm^2 in adults).

Coronary angiography is currently the primary diagnostic procedure for determining the degree of coronary artery disease. The left coronary system supplies the major portion of the left ventricular myocardium, through the left main, left anterior descending, and circumflex coronary arteries. The right coronary artery supplies the right ventricle, and the posterior descending artery supplies the inferior wall of the left ventricle. The atrioventricular (AV) nodal artery arises from the right coronary artery in 80–85 percent of patients, termed right dominant circulation. In 15–20 percent of cases the circumflex branch of the left coronary system supplies the posterior descending branch and the AV nodal artery, termed left dominant, although 5 percent are codominant.

Computed Tomography Coronary Angiography

Technologic advances in computed tomography (CT) now allow less invasive imaging of the coronary anatomy. Newer rapid CT coronary angiography has been shown to be extremely sensitive in detecting coronary stenoses, comparable to traditional angiography in some recent studies.

Extracorporeal Perfusion

The pioneering imagination and efforts of Gibbon were largely responsible for the development of extracorporeal circulation (cardiopulmonary bypass [CPB] with pump-oxygenators). Subsequently, bubble oxygenators were developed, using a blood-gas interface, although membrane oxygenators now widely used use a blood-membrane-gas interface for oxygenation and gas exchange. In addition to the oxygenator, the initial heart-lung machine used a simple roller pump, developed by DeBakey, for perfusion. A variety of other pumps have subsequently been used, such as the centrifugal pump, which minimizes trauma to blood elements.

Technique

Heparin is given to elevate the activated clotting time (ACT) above 500 seconds starting with a heparin dose of 3–4 mg/kg. At New York University (NYU), a centrifugal pump is used for arterial perfusion, in combination with vacuum-assisted venous drainage and a membrane oxygenator. Venous blood was traditionally drained by gravity through large cannulae, but more recently vacuum-assisted venous drainage has been used. Flow rates during extracorporeal perfusion depend on the body oxygen consumption requirements of the patient, which vary based on the patient's body temperature. Normothermic perfusion is done at a flow rate of about 2.5–3.5 L/min per square meter, which is the normal cardiac index. Because hypothermia decreases the metabolic rate (approximately 50 percent for each 7°C [44.6°F]), flow rates can be diminished as the patient is cooled. Oxygen flow through the oxygenator is adjusted to produce an arterial oxygen tension above 150 mm Hg. Systemic temperature is controlled with a heat exchanger in the circuit; the temperature is usually lowered to 25–32°C (77–89.6°F), although colder temperatures are necessary for more complex procedures. Spilled intracardiac blood is aspirated with a suction apparatus, filtered, and returned to the oxygenator. A cell-saving device is routinely used to aspirate spilled blood before and after bypass.

Once the operation is completed and the patient is systemically rewarmed to normothermic levels, perfusion is slowed and then stopped. Prior to discontinuing bypass, the surgeon checks the ECG, potassium level, hematocrit, and hemostasis of the suture lines. Both visual inspection and TEE are used to assess myocardial contractility. As the perfusion flow rate is slowed, the patient's blood is returned from the pump to the patient, restoring normal intracardiac pressures. After discontinuing bypass, heparin is neutralized with protamine, which is given to achieve the baseline ACT.

Systemic Response

Significant changes in bodily functions occur during extracorporeal perfusion. These changes mainly involve platelet dysfunction and a generalized systemic inflammatory response syndrome (SIRS), because of the activation of complement and other acute phase inflammatory components by extracorporeal circuits. Aprotinin and steroids may attenuate the inflammatory response to bypass, although aprotinin and ε-aminocaproic acid diminish coagulopathy. Zero-balance ultrafiltration (Z-BUF) is a method of ultrafiltration during CPB. This technique removes significant amounts of inflammatory mediators associated with CPB, and potentially attenuates the adverse effects of bypass although maintaining the patient's volume status.

Myocardial Protection

The development of a myocardial protective solution (cardioplegia) to induce asystolic cardiac arrest and protect the heart muscle during cardiac surgery was a major advance. The primary theory is that when infused through the coronary circulation, cold, high-potassium cardioplegic solution produces diastolic arrest, slowing the metabolic rate and protecting the heart from ischemia. The arrested heart allows the surgeon to work precisely on the heart in a bloodless field.

CORONARY ARTERY DISEASE

History

Starting in the late 1930s, different investigators attempted to increase the blood supply to the ischemic heart by developing collateral circulation with vascular adhesions. In 1946, Vineberg developed implantation of the internal mammary artery into a tunnel in the myocardium. Coronary artery endarterectomy for coronary revascularization was attempted by Longmire. Late results were poor, however, because of progressive restenosis and occlusion. Shortly thereafter, CPB was used to facilitate coronary revascularization.

The development of the coronary artery bypass operation in the 1960s was a dramatic medical milestone. In the United States, the principal credit belongs to Favalaro and Effler from the Cleveland Clinic, who did the first series of coronary bypass grafts beginning in 1967, using CPB and saphenous vein grafts, launching the modern era of coronary bypass surgery. An additional breakthrough came in 1968 when Green and colleagues performed the first left internal mammary artery to left anterior descending artery bypass.

Etiology and Pathogenesis

The etiology of coronary artery disease is atherosclerosis. The disease is multifactorial, with the primary risk factors being hyperlipidemia, smoking, diabetes, hypertension, obesity, sedentary lifestyle, and male gender. Newly identified risk factors include elevated levels of C-reactive protein, lipoprotein (a), and homocysteine. Atherosclerosis is the leading cause of death in the Western world, and acute MI alone accounts for 25 percent of the deaths in the United States each year.

Among the three major coronary arteries, the proximal anterior descending artery frequently is stenosed or occluded, with the distal half of the artery remaining patent. The right coronary artery often is stenotic or occluded throughout its course, but the posterior descending and left atrioventricular groove branches almost always are patent. The circumflex artery often is diseased proximally, but one or more distal marginal branches usually are patent.

Clinical Manifestations

Myocardial ischemia from coronary artery disease may result in angina pectoris, MI, congestive heart failure, or cardiac arrhythmias and sudden death. Angina is the most frequent symptom, but MI may appear without prior warning. Congestive heart failure usually results as a sequela of MI, with significant muscular injury resulting in ischemic myopathy.

Angina pectoris, the most common manifestation, manifests by periodic chest discomfort, usually substernal, and typically appearing with exertion. Establishing a diagnosis of myocardial ischemia in these patients is difficult and perhaps impossible without provocative diagnostic studies. The differential diagnosis in patients with atypical symptoms includes aortic stenosis, hypertrophic cardiomyopathy, musculoskeletal disorders, pulmonary disease, gastritis or peptic ulcer disease, gastroesophageal reflux, and anxiety.

Myocardial infarction is the most common serious complication of coronary artery disease, with 900,000 occurring in the United States annually. Modern therapy, which involves early reperfusion with either thrombolytic therapy or emergent angioplasty, has lowered the mortality to less than 5 percent. MI may result in acute pump failure and cardiogenic shock, or in mechanical rupture of infarcted zones of the heart.

Preoperative Evaluation

A complete history and physical examination should be performed in every patient with suspected coronary artery disease, along with a chest radiograph, ECG, and baseline echocardiogram. In patients with atypical symptoms, provocative stress tests, such as adenosine thallium or dobutamine echocardiography, may also be beneficial in deciding if cardiac catheterization is indicated. Cardiac catheterization remains the gold standard of evaluation, as it outlines the location and severity of the coronary disease and accurately assesses cardiac function. "Angiographically significant" coronary stenosis is considered to be present when the diameter is reduced by more than 50 percent, corresponding to a reduction in cross-sectional area greater than 75 percent.

Ventricular function is expressed as the left ventricular ejection fraction, with 0.55–0.70 considered as normal, 0.40–0.55 as mildly depressed, less than 0.40 as moderately depressed, and below 0.25 as severely depressed. The left ventricular ejection fraction is used to determine operative risk and the long-term prognosis.

Studies such as the PET scan, thallium scan, dobutamine echocardiogram, or MRI viability scan may be used to determine myocardial viability and the reversibility of ischemia in areas of the heart that might benefit from revascularization.

Coronary Artery Bypass Grafting

Indications

Coronary artery bypass grafting (CABG) may be indicated in patients with chronic angina, unstable angina, or postinfarction angina, and in asymptomatic patients or patients with atypical symptoms who have easily provoked ischemia during stress testing.

Chronic angina. In some patients with chronic angina, CABG is associated with improved survival and improved complication-free survival when compared to medical management. In general, patients with more severe angina (Canadian Cardiovascular Society (CCS) class III or IV symptoms) are most likely to benefit from bypass. For patients with less severe angina (CCS class I or II), other factors, such as the anatomic distribution of disease (left main disease or triple-vessel disease versus single-vessel disease) and the degree of left ventricular dysfunction, are used to determine which patients will most benefit from operative revascularization.

Unstable angina. Unstable angina exists when angina is persistent or rapidly progressive despite optimal medical therapy. Patients with unstable angina should be promptly hospitalized for intensive medical therapy and undergo prompt cardiac catheterization. Most patients with unstable angina will require urgent revascularization with either percutaneous coronary intervention (PCI) or coronary bypass grafting.

Acute myocardial infarction. CABG generally does not have a primary role in the treatment of uncomplicated acute MI, as PCI or thrombolysis is the preferred method of emergent revascularization in these patients. However, patients with subendocardial MI and underlying left main disease or postinfarction angina and multivessel involvement may require surgery.

The primary indication for surgery after acute transmural MI is in patients who develop late complications, such as postinfarction ventricular septal defect, papillary muscle rupture with mitral insufficiency, or left ventricular rupture. Postinfarction ventricular septal defect (VSD) typically occurs 4–5 days after MI, in approximately 1 percent of patients. These patients usually present with congestive heart failure and pulmonary edema, and a new systolic murmur. Once recognized, patients with postinfarction VSD should have an intraaortic balloon pump placed and undergo emergent repair. Papillary muscle rupture with acute mitral insufficiency also typically presents 4–5 days postinfarction and prompt valve repair or replacement offers the only meaningful chance for survival. Operative risk is 10–20 percent. Left ventricular free wall rupture presents with cardiogenic shock, often with acute tamponade. Emergent surgery has a success rate of approximately 50 percent.

Percutaneous Coronary Intervention Versus Coronary Artery Bypass Grafting

PCI, or angioplasty, has significantly changed the treatment of patients with coronary artery disease. The indications for PCI have continually expanded as the technology has advanced. Most recently, stents coated with pharmacologic agents (such as paclitaxel or sirolimus) aimed at reducing in-stent restenosis have been introduced. A number of large, randomized studies have compared outcomes of patients with coronary disease treated with PCI and CABG. These studies have attempted to identify the optimal therapy for patients with coronary disease, based on their anatomy and risk stratification.

Results demonstrate that with appropriate patient selection both procedures are safe and effective, with little difference in mortality. PCI is associated with less short-term morbidity, decreased cost, and shorter hospital stay, but requires more late reinterventions. CABG provides more complete relief of angina, requires fewer reinterventions, and is more durable. CABG appears to offer a survival advantage in diabetic patients with multivessel disease.

Operative Techniques and Results

Conventional coronary artery bypass grafting. Conventional CABG is performed through a median sternotomy incision using cardiopulmonary bypass for extracorporeal perfusion and cold cardioplegia for intraoperative myocardial protection of the heart.

In the vast majority of patients the left internal mammary artery (IMA) is used as the primary conduit for bypassing the left anterior descending artery. The left IMA has a 10-year patency rate of approximately 95 percent when used as an in situ graft to the left anterior descending artery. The excellent results obtained with in situ left IMA grafts prompted other centers to use the right IMA in coronary revascularization. The right IMA can be used to provide a second arterial conduit as either an in situ or a free graft. Even when the IMA is used as a "free" graft, patency rates are approximately 70–80 percent at 10 years.

Saphenous vein grafts, which were initially the primary conduits used for CABG, continue to be used widely, usually for grafting secondary targets on the side and back of the heart. Once CPB has been established and the heart arrested, a small arteriotomy is performed in the coronary artery, and the distal anastomosis is performed between the saphenous vein and the coronary artery. The proximal anastomosis then connects each vein graft to the ascending aorta. The 10-year patency of saphenous vein grafts is approximately 65 percent.

Surgeons have explored the use of other arterial conduits. The most widely used has been the radial artery graft. Other alternative arterial grafts include the right gastroepiploic artery and the inferior epigastric artery. Reports are mixed regarding late patency rates, however. Although the expanded use of arterial grafts is appealing, improved patency of alternative arterial conduits compared to vein grafts has yet to be verified.

Results. The operative mortality for coronary artery bypass is 1–3 percent, depending on the number of risk factors present. Both the Society of Thoracic Surgeons (STS) and New York State have established large databases to establish risk factors and report outcomes. Variables that have been identified as influencing operative risk according to STS risk modeling include: female gender, age, race, body surface area, NYHA class IV status, low ejection fraction, hypertension, peripheral vascular disease, prior stroke, diabetes, renal failure, chronic obstructive pulmonary disease, immunosuppressive therapy, prior cardiac surgery, recent MI, urgent or emergent presentation, cardiogenic shock, left main disease, and concomitant valvular disease. Late results demonstrate that relief of angina is striking after CABG. Angina is completely relieved or markedly decreased in over 98 percent of patients, and recurrent angina is rare in the first 5–7 years. Reintervention is required in less than 10 percent of patients within 5 years.

Late survival is similarly excellent after CABG, with a 5-year survival of over 90 percent and a 10-year survival of 75–90 percent, depending on the number of comorbidities present. Late survival is influenced by age, diabetes, left ventricular function, NYHA class, congestive heart failure, associated valvular insufficiency, completeness of revascularization, and nonuse of an IMA graft. Intense medical therapy for control of diabetes, hypercholesterolemia, and hypertension, and cessation of smoking significantly improves late survival.

Off-pump coronary artery bypass. One of the most significant developments in cardiac surgery in the last 15–20 years has been the introduction of off-pump coronary artery bypass (OPCAB). The main concept driving this approach is the elimination of the deleterious consequences of cardiopulmonary bypass. During OPCAB surgery the coronary artery is temporarily snared or occluded to provide a relatively bloodless field for the creation of the anastomosis.

Results. The OPCAB technique has been extensively studied and results compared to conventional surgery. Initial attention was given to assessing the accuracy of graft placement with the OPCAB approach, which required grafting onto the beating heart. Results were equivalent to those published for conventional CABG. A prospective randomized comparison between OPCAB and conventional CABG, reported by Puskas, demonstrated equivalent operative mortality and risk of stroke in each group, but less myocardial injury, fewer blood transfusions, earlier postoperative extubation, and earlier hospital discharge in OPCAB patients.

A study performed at NYU in high-risk patients with severe atheromatous aortic arch disease who required CABG compared outcomes in 245 OPCAB patients with outcomes in 245 conventional patients. In this high-risk patient population OPCAB was associated with a decreased risk of death (6.5 vs. 11.4 percent), stroke (1.6 vs. 5.7 percent), and all perioperative complications.

Minimally invasive direct coronary artery bypass. An even less invasive off-pump approach for CABG, termed minimally invasive direct coronary artery bypass (MIDCAB), uses a small left anterior minithoracotomy incision to perform bypass grafting on the beating heart, without cardiopulmonary bypass. The technique uses a mechanical stabilizer to isolate the coronary artery and facilitate the anastomosis and an in situ left IMA graft. The technique is mainly useful in performing bypass to the anterior wall of the heart, primarily to the left anterior descending artery or to the diagonal branches.

Results. The operative mortality for MIDCAB has been less than 2 percent, and the patency rate of the IMA graft has been approximately 98 percent. MIDCAB patients have less pain and blood loss, fewer perioperative complications, and a shorter recovery time than conventional CABG patients.

New Developments

Total endoscopic coronary artery bypass. Minimal access coronary artery bypass performed using endoscopic instrumentation is facilitated with the latest generation of surgical robotic technology. Total endoscopic coronary artery bypass (TECAB) has been reported on both the arrested and beating heart. Robotic instrumentation also has been described to perform internal mammary artery harvests as part of the MIDCAB technique.

Transmyocardial laser revascularization. Transmyocardial laser revascularization (TMR) uses a high-powered carbon dioxide laser or holmium:yttrium-aluminum-garnet laser to drill multiple holes (1 cm^2) through the myocardium into the ventricular cavity. The procedure is performed on the beating heart with the laser pulses gated to the R wave on the ECG. The TMR procedure has been used primarily for patients with refractory angina who are unsuitable candidates for standard CABG because of poor distal coronary artery anatomy. The mechanism of benefit of TMR remains uncertain. The most likely possibility is that TMR works by stimulating angiogenesis in the area of injury. Despite subjective reports of improvement, however, the results of objective cardiac perfusion measurements after TMR have been inconclusive.

Facilitated anastomotic devices. Significant technologic progress has led to the development of devices that mechanically construct proximal and distal vascular anastomoses, without the need for sutures or knot tying. The goals for these devices are to provide safe, rapid, and reproducible anastomoses; reduce operative time; limit anastomotic variability between surgeons; and improve graft patency.

VENTRICULAR ANEURYSMS

Pathophysiology

Approximately 5–10 percent of transmural myocardial infarctions result in left ventricular aneurysms, which develop 4–8 weeks following a transmural infarct as necrotic myocardium is replaced by fibrous tissue.

The classic aneurysm is an avascular thin scar, 4–6-mm thick, which bulges outward when the remaining left ventricular muscle contracts in systole. Left ventricular aneurysms generally do not rupture, but manifest clinically as progressive heart failure, often with associated malignant ventricular arrhythmias. Over 80 percent of aneurysms are in the anteroapical portion of the left ventricle, resulting from occlusion of the left anterior descending coronary artery. Posterior ventricular aneurysms are less common (15–20 percent) and lateral wall aneurysms are rare.

Diagnostic Evaluation

The diagnostic workup generally begins with echocardiography to assess wall motion in the various zones of the heart, to determine left ventricular end-systolic and end-diastolic size, and to assess for any associated mitral valve insufficiency. Cardiac MRI may also be useful. Cardiac catheterization is performed preoperatively to assess for the severity of coronary artery disease, and to determine the anatomic extent of the aneurysm and the areas of myocardium that still have good function. Workup of arrhythmias may include electrophysiologic studies.

Operative Treatment

Operative treatment requires excision or exclusion of the aneurysm and by-pass grafting of diseased coronary arteries. The classic repair was performed by excision of the aneurysm and linear closure of the ventricle. However, this technique had a geometrically deforming effect on the remaining left ventricle, and did not address aneurysmal deformity of the septum. Therefore, a more physiologic technique of intracavitary endoventricular patch reconstruction, or left ventricular restoration, was proposed by Jatene, Cooley, and Dor. Endoventricular patch reconstruction involves placement of a Dacron patch to obliterate the aneurysmal ventricle and septum. This repair remodels the ventricular cavity and obliterates the septal component of the aneurysm.

Results

Doss and colleagues compared the long-term results of linear closure and endoventricular patch reconstruction with 8 years follow up. The left ventricular ejection fraction increased significantly in patients who underwent endoventricular reconstruction, but decreased in those who underwent linear closure. The operative mortality was 1.9 percent, with an 8-year survival of 85.6 percent. In general, the published data suggest better results with the endoventricular patch reconstruction technique.

ISCHEMIC CARDIOMYOPATHY

Patients with ischemic cardiomyopathy and heart failure are being evaluated and treated by surgeons with increasing frequency, as surgical options for the failing heart have expanded considerably over the last 10–20 years. Anatomically, ischemic cardiomyopathy results from multiple myocardial infarctions, which produce extensive myocardial scarring with decreased left ventricular systolic function. These patients may have a definable left ventricular aneurysm, but more commonly have diffuse myocardial scarring with large, nonfunctioning, akinetic zones of the heart.

Ventricular Restoration Surgery

Left ventricular surgical restoration for ischemic cardiomyopathy is performed similarly to the endoventricular patch reconstruction described above for repair of anteroapical left ventricular aneurysms. The goal of ventricular restoration is to restore the normal left ventricular size and shape, thus improving the efficiency of left ventricular ejection.

Results

A large international study (reconstructive endoventricular surgery returning torsion original radius elliptical shape to the LV (RESTORE)) investigated outcomes after surgical anterior ventricular endocardial restoration (SAVER). They found an overall hospital mortality of 6.6 percent, with an increase in ejection fraction from 29.7–40 percent and a 3-year survival rate approaching 90 percent.

MECHANICAL CIRCULATORY SUPPORT AND MYOCARDIAL REGENERATION

IntraAortic Balloon Pump

The intraaortic balloon pump (IABP) is the most common and effective technique for assisted circulation. The most frequent indications for use of IABP are to provide hemodynamic support during or after cardiac catheterization, cardiogenic shock, weaning from cardiopulmonary bypass, and for preoperative use in high-risk patients and refractory unstable angina. A balloon catheter is inserted through the femoral artery and advanced into the thoracic aorta. With electronic synchronization, the balloon is inflated during diastole and deflated during systole. Coronary blood flow is increased by improved diastolic perfusion, and afterload is reduced. The cardiac index typically improves after insertion, and the preload decreases.

Limb ischemia on the side of insertion is the most serious complication, and the extremity must be examined frequently for viability. Studies have shown major IABP complications (limb ischemia, bleeding, balloon leakage, or death directly because of IABP insertion) occur in 2.6 percent of cases.

Ventricular Assist Devices

Mechanical circulatory support systems (ventricular assist devices; VADs) are designed for temporary assisted circulation ("bridge to recovery"), for long-term treatment ("bridge to transplantation"), or as a permanent substitute for the heart ("artificial heart" or "destination therapy"). Temporary assisted circulation is a valuable clinical modality in the treatment of transient cardiac injury. The most common indication for temporary assisted circulation is cardiac failure after cardiac surgery. Inflow for these devices is through either the left atrium or the apex of the left ventricle, and outflow is into the aorta. External pulsatile assist devices deliver blood flow in synchrony with the native heart and are used for short-term support after cardiac surgery or as a long-term bridge to cardiac transplantation.

A definitive solution for heart failure may be a permanent artificial heart. Total cardiac replacement with an artificial heart, however, is still in the experimental arena. Long-term risks include thromboembolic complications, the risk of infection, and trauma to blood elements.

VALVULAR HEART DISEASE

General Principles

According to the STS database, valve operations accounted for 14.0 percent of all classified procedures performed in 1996. By 2002, that percentage had increased by 45 percent of all classified procedures. Although CABG volume declined by 15.3 percent between 1996 and 1999, aortic valve replacements increased by 11.7 percent and mitral valve operations increased by 58 percent during the same period.

Valvular heart disease can result in a pressure load (valvular stenosis), a volume load (valvular insufficiency), or both (mixed stenosis and insufficiency). Demonstration of a decreased ejection fraction at rest (or a rise in the end-systolic volume by echocardiography) or a fall in the ejection fraction during exercise are probably the best signs that the systolic function of the heart is beginning to deteriorate and that surgery should be performed promptly.

Postoperative cardiac function generally returns to normal if the operation is performed at an early phase of ventricular dysfunction. Even with impaired left ventricular function, NYHA class IV disability, and pulmonary hypertension, patients with valvular heart disease are rarely inoperable. Except in the rare case of advanced cardiomyopathy combined with other systemic disease, surgery should not be denied to patients. The typical valve-related complications from valvular surgery include thromboembolic events, anticoagulant-related hemorrhage, prosthetic valve failure, endocarditis, prosthetic paravalvular leakage, and failure of valve repair.

Surgical Options

Two basic types of prosthetic valves are available: mechanical valves and tissue valves (xenografts). Valve replacement, in particular aortic valve replacement, also can be performed using human homografts or autografts. Finally, valve repair is increasingly an option, as opposed to valve replacement. The recommendations for valve repair or replacement, type of prosthesis, and operative approach are based on multiple factors, such as the patient's age, lifestyle, associated medical conditions, access to follow-up health care, desire for future pregnancy, and experience of the surgeon.

Mechanical prostheses are highly durable but require permanent anticoagulation therapy to minimize the risk of valve thrombosis and thromboembolic complications. Lifelong anticoagulation therapy carries the risk of hemorrhagic complications and may dictate lifestyle changes.

Tissue valves are more natural and less thrombogenic, and therefore generally do not require anticoagulation therapy. Consequently, tissue valves have lower risks of thromboembolic and anticoagulant-related complications, with the total yearly risk of all valve-related complications being considerably less than with mechanical valves. Unfortunately, tissue valves are more prone to structural failure because of late calcification of the xenograft tissue. However, it is anticipated that it may take 15–20 years before structural failure will occur in these prostheses.

For aortic valve replacement, a mechanical prosthesis, a newer-generation tissue valve (either stented or nonstented), a homograft, or a pulmonary autograft (Ross procedure) may be recommended. Some type of tissue valve usually is recommended for patients older than 65 years of age because anticoagulation therapy may be hazardous and valve durability is better in older patients.

Although valve repair can be performed in the vast majority of patients with mitral insufficiency, valve replacement may still be required in certain patients, and in the vast majority with rheumatic disease and valvular stenosis. When valve replacement is necessary, a tissue valve is an appropriate choice in women planning pregnancy or in patients over 60–65 years of age. A mechanical prosthesis is recommended for younger patients, especially if the patient is in atrial fibrillation, because anticoagulation therapy is already required in this group.

Mechanical Valves

A common mechanical valve used in the United States is the St. Jude Medical bileaflet prosthesis. Mechanical (disk) valves have excellent flow characteristics, acceptable low risk of late valve-related complications, and an extremely low risk of mechanical valve failure. With proper anticoagulation and keeping the international normalized ratio (INR) at 2–3 times the normal for mechanical aortic valves and 2.5–3.5 times the normal for mechanical mitral valves, the incidence of thromboembolism is approximately 1–2 percent per patient per year, and the risk of anticoagulant-related hemorrhage is 0.5–2 percent per patient per year.

Tissue Valves·

Several types of xenograft tissue valves are available and widely used. The stented valves are most common (either porcine or bovine pericardial), although stentless valves are being increasingly used by some groups. Stented tissue valves have the drawback of having higher gradients across the valve, particularly in smaller sizes. The limitations in flow characteristics observed in small sizes of stented tissue valves led to the development of stentless valves in an attempt to maximize the effective valve orifice area. Although the long-term durability of stentless valves has not yet been established, these valves offer excellent hemodynamics.

Homografts

Surgical alternatives to prosthetic valve replacement have been developed in an attempt to use the body's natural tissue and lower the incidence of valve-related complications. In the 1960s, Ross in England and Barrett-Boyes in New Zealand described a procedure for aortic valve replacement using antibiotic-preserved aortic homograft (allograft) valves. The main disadvantage of a homograft valve is its uncertain durability, especially in young patients, as structural degeneration of the valve tissue leads to graft dysfunction and valve failure.

Autografts

Ross described a potentially durable but more complicated alternative for aortic valve replacement with natural autologous tissue, using the patient's native pulmonary valve as an autograft for aortic valve replacement and replacing the pulmonary valve with a homograft. This operation, referred to as the Ross procedure, has the advantage of placing an autologous valve into the aortic position, which functions physiologically and does not require anticoagulation therapy. The Ross procedure may be indicated for younger patients who require aortic valve replacement and want to avoid the need for anticoagulation.

Valve Repair

Valve repair has become the procedure of choice for most patients with mitral valve insufficiency, although repair of the aortic valve is feasible in certain situations. The primary advance in mitral valve repair resulted from work by Carpentier in the 1970s. Valve repair has subsequently proved to be highly reproducible for correction of mitral insufficiency, with excellent durability and freedom from late valve-related complications. Repair lowers the risk of thromboembolic- and anticoagulant-related complications. Survival may also be improved in certain groups of patients after valve repair.

Mitral Valve Disease

Mitral Stenosis

Etiology. Mitral valve stenosis or mixed mitral stenosis and insufficiency almost always are caused by rheumatic heart disease, although a definite clinical history can be obtained in only 50 percent of patients. Congenital mitral stenosis is rarely seen in adults. Occasionally, intracardiac tumors such as left atrial myxoma may obstruct the mitral orifice and cause symptoms that mimic mitral stenosis.

Pathology. Rheumatic valvulitis produces three distinct degrees of pathologic change: fusion of the commissures alone, commissural fusion plus subvalvular shortening of the chordae tendineae, and extensive fixation of the valve and subvalvular apparatus with calcification and scarring of both leaflets and chordae.

Pathophysiology. Mitral stenosis usually has a prolonged course after the initial rheumatic infection, and symptoms may not appear for 10–20 years. The progression to valvular fibrosis and calcification may be related to repeated episodes of rheumatic fever, or may result from scarring produced by inflammation and turbulent blood flow. The normal cross-sectional area of the mitral valve is 4–6 cm^2. Symptoms may progressively develop with moderate stenosis, defined as a cross-sectional area 1.0–1.5 cm^2. Severe symptomatic stenosis occurs when the mitral valve area is less than 0.8–1.0 cm^2.

The pathophysiology associated with mitral stenosis results from an elevation in left atrial pressure, producing pulmonary venous congestion and pulmonary hypertension. Left ventricular function usually remains normal because the ventricle is protected by the stenotic valve.

Clinical manifestations. The main symptoms of mitral stenosis are exertional dyspnea and decreased exercise capacity. Dyspnea occurs when the left atrial pressure becomes elevated because of the stenotic valve, resulting in pulmonary congestion. Orthopnea and paroxysmal nocturnal dyspnea may also occur, or in advanced cases, hemoptysis. The most serious development is pulmonary edema. Atrial fibrillation develops in a significant number of patients with chronic mitral stenosis. Atrial thrombi result from dilation and stasis of the left atrium, with the left atrial appendage being especially susceptible to clot formation.

The characteristic auscultatory findings of mitral stenosis, called the auscultatory triad, are an increased first heart sound, an opening snap, and an apical diastolic rumble. A loud pansystolic murmur transmitted to the axilla usually indicates associated mitral insufficiency.

Diagnostic studies. The electrocardiogram may show atrial fibrillation, left atrial enlargement (P mitrale), and right-axis deviation, or it may be normal. On chest radiograph, enlargement of the left atrium typically is seen on the posteroanterior film as a double contour visible behind the right atrial shadow. Calcifications of the mitral valve also may be seen.

The Doppler echocardiogram is diagnostic. Transesophageal echocardiography provides enhanced resolution of the mitral valve and the posterior cardiac structures, including the left atrium and the atrial appendage. Echocardiography gives a very accurate measurement of the transvalvular gradient and the cross-sectional area of the mitral valve.

Indications for valvuloplasty or commissurotomy. Although percutaneous balloon valvuloplasty has become an acceptable alternative for many patients with uncomplicated mitral stenosis, open mitral commissurotomy remains a reproducible and durable option. Commissurotomy has the advantage of addressing nonpliable or calcified mitral valves, mobilize fused subvalvular restrictive disease, repair patients with mixed stenosis and insufficiency, and remove left atrial clot. Either balloon valvuloplasty or open surgical commissurotomy is indicated for symptomatic patients with moderate (mitral valve area <1.5 cm^2) or severe (mitral valve area <1.0 cm^2) mitral stenosis.

Mitral Insufficiency

Etiology. Degenerative disease is the most common cause of mitral insufficiency in the United States, accounting for 50–60 percent of the patients requiring surgery. Other causes include rheumatic fever (15–20 percent), ischemic disease (15–20 percent), endocarditis, congenital abnormalities, and cardiomyopathy.

Pathology. The major structural components of the mitral valve are the annulus, the leaflets, the chordae tendinae, and the papillary muscles. A defect in any of these components may create mitral insufficiency. A functional classification for mitral insufficiency was proposed by Carpentier, who characterized three basic types of functionally diseased valves. Degenerative causes include myxomatous degeneration and fibroelastic deficiency. In patients with rheumatic disease, the chordae tendinae are thickened and foreshortened, producing restrictive leaflet motion. Posterior dilatation of the mitral annulus also usually is present. With ischemic insufficiency, ventricular injury results in tethering of the mitral leaflets, producing restrictive leaflet motion, and central insufficiency, often with secondary annular dilation.

Pathophysiology. The basic physiologic abnormality in patients with mitral insufficiency is regurgitation of a portion of the left ventricular stroke volume into the left atrium. This results in decreased forward blood flow and an elevated left atrial pressure, producing pulmonary congestion and volume overload of the left ventricle. However, decreased systolic function of the heart is a relatively late finding, because the ventricle is "unloaded" as a result of the valvular insufficiency. Once left ventricular dysfunction and heart failure develop, the left ventricle usually has been significantly and often irreversibly injured.

Clinical manifestations. In patients with acute mitral regurgitation, congestive heart failure develops suddenly, although in patients with chronic mitral insufficiency, the left atrium and ventricle become compliant, and symptoms do not develop until later in the course of the disease.

On physical examination the characteristic findings of mitral insufficiency are an apical holosystolic murmur and a forceful apical impulse. The apical murmur usually is harsh and transmitted to the axilla or to the left sternal border.

Diagnostic studies. The severity of mitral insufficiency can be determined accurately with echocardiography, along with the site of valvular prolapse or restriction, and the level of left ventricular function. An important measurement is the size of the cardiac chambers. If there is uncertainty about the physiologic significance of mitral insufficiency, exercise stress-echocardiography may be used. Normally the ejection fraction rises with exercise, but a fall in ejection fraction with exercise is an early sign of left ventricular systolic dysfunction.

Indications for operation. Delaying operation until the patient is severely symptomatic and the heart is markedly dilated often results in a certain degree of irreversible ventricular injury. According to ACC/AHA guidelines, mitral valve repair or replacement is recommended in any symptomatic patient with mitral insufficiency, even with normal left ventricular function (defined as ejection fraction > 60 percent and end-systolic dimension <45 mm). Surgery also is currently recommended in asymptomatic patients with severe mitral insufficiency if there are signs of left ventricular systolic. Recent onset of atrial fibrillation, pulmonary hypertension, or an abnormal response to exercise testing are considered relative indications for surgery.

Operative Techniques

The traditional approach for mitral valve surgery is through a median sternotomy incision with cardiopulmonary bypass and cardioplegic arrest. The mitral valve is exposed through a left atrial incision, made posterior and parallel to the intraatrial groove. Alternative incisions for exposing the difficult mitral valve include a right atriotomy with transseptal incision, a superior approach through the dome of the atrium, and the biatrial transseptal approach.

Commissurotomy. Initially the atrial cavity is examined for thrombi, especially within the atrial appendage. The mitral valve is assessed by evaluating leaflet mobility, commissural fusion, and the degree of fibrosis in the subvalvular apparatus.

Once the commissure has been accurately identified and the chordae noted, a right-angle clamp is introduced beneath the fused commissure, stretching the adjacent chordae and leaflets, after which the commissure is carefully incised. The incision is made 2–3 mm at a time, serially confirming that the separated margins of the commissural leaflet remain attached to chordae tendineae. Once the commissurotomy is completed, any fused papillary muscle is incised as necessary to minimize restriction and improve mobility of the attached leaflet.

Mitral valve replacement. Mitral valve replacement is necessary when the extent of disease precludes commissurotomy or valve reconstruction. Valve replacement is most likely in patients with long-standing rheumatic disease. Once the valve is exposed and the need for valve replacement is determined, an incision is made in the anterior mitral leaflet, and most of the anterior leaflet is resected. The posterior leaflet is preserved whenever possible, and the chordal attachments to both leaflets are preserved or reattached to the annulus, as this has been shown to improve left ventricular function and lower the risk of posterior left ventricular free wall rupture.

Mitral valve reconstruction. The basic techniques of mitral valve reconstruction include resection of the posterior leaflet, chordal shortening, chordal transposition, artificial chordal replacement, and triangular resection for repair of the anterior leaflet disease. An annuloplasty to correct associated annular dilation also is recommended in most cases.

The intraoperative assessment of the valvular pathology is an important step in valve reconstruction. A localized roughened area of atrial endocardium, termed a jet lesion, may be present from regurgitant blood striking the endocardium, providing a guide to the location of the insufficiency. Subsequently the commissures are examined, noting whether these are prolapsed, fused, or malformed. The closing plane of the leaflets in the area supported by commissural chordae is determined next, and the anterior and posterior leaflets are then examined, noting areas of prolapse or restriction.

Posterior leaflet procedures. Quadrangular resection of the posterior leaflet has become the mainstay of mitral valve reconstruction. A rectangular excision is performed, cutting directly down to, but not through, the mitral annulus. Diseased tissue in the posterior leaflet is excised with a quadrangular excision, usually removing 1–2 cm of tissue. Strong chordae of proper length are identified on each side of the excised leaflet and encircled with retraction sutures. Once the quadrangular excision has been performed, the annulus of the excised segment of leaflet is corrected either by simple annular plication, folding plasty, or sliding plasty.

The folding plasty technique, described by the group from NYU, involves folding down the cut vertical edges of the posterior leaflet to the annulus and closing the ensuing cleft. The sliding plasty technique reported by Carpentier also is successful in reducing posterior leaflet height and moving the edge of leaflet coaptation posteriorly.

Anterior leaflet procedures. Four primary techniques are used for anterior leaflet reconstruction: chordal shortening, chordal transposition, artificial chordal replacement, and triangular resection of anterior leaflet tissue with primary repair. With chordal shortening, the elongated chord is imbricated either onto the free edge of the leaflet or onto the papillary muscle. In contrast, the chordal transposition technique uses a segment of structurally intact posterior leaflet directly opposite the prolapsed anterior leaflet. Artificial chordae replacement has been used by some groups as an alternative for anterior leaflet repair. Finally, triangular resection and primary repair has been increasingly used at NYU for treatment of anterior leaflet prolapse.

Repair of leaflet perforation. Leaflet perforations can be repaired by primary suture closure or by closure with a pericardial patch. Extensive leaflet destruction is best managed with mitral valve replacement.

Annuloplasty. Use of a mitral valve annuloplasty device (ring or partial band) to correct annular dilation during valve repair decreases the risk of late repair failure. The primary purpose of an annuloplasty device is to correct the associated annular dilation that invariably occurs in patients with chronic mitral insufficiency. Various types of annuloplasty devices are available. The relative advantages of the different types of devices remain under investigation, but it is widely accepted that use of an annuloplasty device to correct annular dilation improves long-term repair durability.

Results

Commissurotomy. The operative risk for open mitral commissurotomy is less than 1 percent, and long-term results have been excellent. Antunes and colleagues reported 9-year actuarial freedom from reoperation was 98 percent, and 93 percent were in NYHA functional class I or II.

Balloon valvuloplasty. The choice between surgical commissurotomy and balloon valvuloplasty varies widely among centers. The main advantages of commissurotomy over balloon valvuloplasty are that during surgery the fused chordae can be surgically divided and mobility restored.

Valve replacement. The operative mortality rate for mitral valve replacement is 2–6 percent, depending on the number of comorbidities present. The major predictors of increased operative risk after mitral valve replacement are age, left ventricular function, emergency operation, NYHA functional status, previous cardiac surgery, associated coronary artery disease, and concomitant disease in another valve. The major factors influencing long-term survival are age, urgency of operation, NYHA functional status, mitral insufficiency (versus stenosis), ischemic etiology, pulmonary hypertension, and the need for concomitant coronary bypass or procedures on another valve.

Studies have shown freedom from reoperation at 15 years was 98 percent with mechanical valves and 79 percent with tissue valves. Thus whereas mechanical valves and tissue valves result in similar long-term survival, there is an increased risk of late reoperation in patients receiving tissue valves.

Valve repair. The operative risk for mitral valve repair is less than 1–2 percent, and late results have demonstrated that compared to replacement, repair is associated with improved survival and better freedom from valve-related complications.

Minimally invasive mitral valve surgery. Newer techniques which allow mitral valve repair or replacement to be performed with a minimally invasive incision have been increasingly used over the last decade. At NYU minimally invasive mitral valve surgery has been performed through a small right anterior thoracotomy incision, entering the chest through the third or fourth intercostal space. Others have used partial upper sternotomy, partial lower sternotomy, or parasternal incisions.

Galloway and colleagues reported late results after minimally invasive valve repair, demonstrating that repair durability, freedom from valve-related complications, and survival were equivalent to results achieved with the traditional sternotomy approach. Thus the results after minimally invasive valve surgery are encouraging, and more widespread utilization of minimally invasive techniques is likely in the future.

New Developments

Edge-to-edge repair. In 1995, Alfieri described the "double-orifice" or "edge-to-edge" repair as an alternative technique for repair for mitral insufficiency. With this technique the free edge of the anterior leaflet is sutured to the opposing free edge of the posterior leaflet, converting the valve into a double-orifice "bow tie."

Robotic mitral valve surgery. Recent technological achievements in optics and computerized telemanipulation have enabled robotically assisted mitral valve operations. It has been reported that the articulated wrist-like instruments and three-dimensional visualization enable precise tissue telemanipulation. These systems still have significant limitations, however, and may not be readily adaptable to performing the multiple complex tasks necessary for valve surgery.

Aortic Valve Disease

Effective surgical treatment of aortic valve disease became possible in 1960 with the development of satisfactory prosthetic valves by Starr and Edwards and by Harken and associates.

Aortic Stenosis

Etiology. In the adult North American population the primary causes of aortic stenosis include acquired calcific disease, bicuspid aortic valve, and rheumatic disease. Acquired calcific aortic stenosis typically occurs in the seventh or eighth decade of life, and is the most frequent etiology, accounting for over half of the cases. Biscuspid aortic valve accounts for approximately one third of the cases of aortic stenosis in adults, typically presenting in the fourth or fifth decade of life, after years of turbulent flow through the bicuspid valve results in damage and calcification.

The third major cause of aortic stenosis, rheumatic heart disease, accounts for approximately 10–15 percent of patients in North America, but is more common in underdeveloped countries. Concomitant mitral valve disease almost always is present, although not always clinically significant.

Pathophysiology. Generally, the aortic valve must be reduced to one third its normal cross-sectional area before significant hemodynamic changes occur. A normal aortic valve has a cross-sectional area of 2.5–3.5 cm^2. Moderate aortic stenosis is defined as an aortic valve area between 0.8 and 1.2 cm^2, although severe stenosis is defined as a valve area less than 0.8 cm^2. Once the valve area is less than 0.5 cm^2, with a transvalvular gradient of 100 mm Hg or greater, the degree of stenosis is considered critical.

Myocardial ischemia develops in some patients with severe aortic stenosis, usually in response to exercise. The left ventricular mass and left ventricular systolic wall tension are increased, resulting in increased oxygen demand. Simultaneously, the cardiac output often is low and does not increase in response to exercise.

Clinical manifestations. The classic symptoms of aortic stenosis include exertional dyspnea, decreased exercise capacity, heart failure, angina, and syncope. Once the patient becomes symptomatic, prompt operation is indicated. If heart failure, angina, or syncope is present, the need for surgery is more urgent, as the risk of death exceeds 30–50 percent over the next 5 years. Sudden death, which accounts for a significant number of fatalities from aortic stenosis, possibly because of arrhythmias, becomes a more likely threat once the patient becomes severely symptomatic.

With auscultation the principal finding is a harsh, diamond-shaped (crescendo-decrescendo) systolic murmur at the base of the heart with radiation to the carotid arteries. The two components of the S2 may become synchronous, or aortic valve closure may even follow pulmonic valve closure, causing paradoxical splitting of the S2. The apical impulse has been described as a "prolonged heave," although the pulse pressure in the peripheral circulation is usually narrow and sustained (pulsus parvus et tardus).

Diagnostic studies. On radiograph the heart size may be either normal or enlarged because of left ventricular hypertrophy. Calcification of the valve often is visible in older patients. The ECG may demonstrate left ventricular hypertrophy, but may also be normal. Atrial fibrillation generally indicates the presence of advanced disease with a prolonged elevation of intracardiac pressures. The diagnosis of aortic stenosis is now most frequently made by echocardiography, which provides an accurate estimate of the peak and mean systolic transvalvular gradients. The echocardiogram also can demonstrate the amount of calcium in the leaflets, the degree of leaflet immobility, the left atrial size, the degree of left ventricular hypertrophy, the end-systolic and end-diastolic dimensions of the left ventricle, and the left ventricular function. Cardiac catheterization readily confirms the diagnosis by measuring the aortic transvalvular gradient and permitting calculation of the cross-sectional area of the valve.

Operative indications. Patients with aortic stenosis typically respond well to aortic valve replacement, which immediately relieves the increased afterload. A special subgroup of patients includes those with critical aortic stenosis and advanced left ventricular systolic dysfunction. These patients have an increased operative risk, but may still have significant improvement after valve replacement as long as the ventricle is not irreversibly damaged.

Aortic valve replacement is indicated for virtually all symptomatic patients with aortic stenosis. In asymptomatic patients with moderate to severe stenosis, periodic echocardiographic studies are performed to assess the transvalvular gradient, valve area, left ventricular size, and left ventricular function. Surgery is indicated with the first sign of left ventricular systolic dysfunction.

Aortic Insufficiency

Etiology and pathology. A variety of diseases can produce aortic valve insufficiency, including degenerative diseases, inflammatory or infectious diseases (endocarditis, rheumatic fever), congenital diseases, aortoannular ectasia or aneurysm of the aortic root, and aortic dissection. Mixed valvular stenosis and insufficiency can develop in any patient with aortic stenosis, regardless of etiology.

Degenerative valvular disease is a manifestation of fibroelastic deficiency or myxomatous degeneration that produces thin and elongated valvular tissue. The aortic valve leaflets sag into the ventricular lumen, often with no other tissue abnormality, producing central aortic insufficiency. Infectious and inflammatory etiologies of aortic insufficiency include bacterial endocarditis and rheumatic fever. Streptococci, staphylococci, or enterococci are the most common bacteria involved, in decreasing order of frequency.

Patients who have a congenitally bicuspid aortic valve rarely become symptomatic during childhood, but prolonged turbulence may lead to aortic stenosis, mixed stenosis and insufficiency, or pure insufficiency later in life. Congenital causes of aortic insufficiency account for 10–15 percent of the patients operated on for aortic insufficiency as adults.

Aneurysmal dilation of the aortic root is thought to be secondary to idiopathic or known connective tissue disorders, with the idiopathic variety seen with increasing frequency as the average age of the population increases. Aortoannular ectasia with aneurysm of the aortic root occurs in its most extreme form in patients with Marfan syndrome or Ehlers-Danlos syndrome. Valvular insufficiency results from dilatation of both the aortic sinotubular junction and the aortic valve annulus. Acute aortic dissection may produce aortic valve insufficiency by detachment of the commissures and prolapse of the valve cusps, usually involving the noncoronary cusp and the commissure between the left and right cusps.

Pathophysiology. With aortic valve insufficiency, blood regurgitates into the left ventricle during diastole, producing left ventricular volume overload. A widened pulse pressure and low diastolic pressure result in diminished coronary perfusion. Because ventricular compliance is normal, the left ventricular diastolic pressure does not increase initially, and the patient usually remains asymptomatic. As the heart continues to dilate, however, the ventricular muscle can no longer compensate and the ratio of wall thickness to cavity size decreases. Further progression leads to left ventricular failure and pulmonary hypertension.

Clinical manifestations. Symptoms develop at variable rates in patients with aortic insufficiency. Frequently the patient who gradually develops moderate to severe insufficiency remains asymptomatic for many years, often 10 or more. Once symptoms appear, however, ventricular function usually is significantly depressed and rapid clinical deterioration occurs over the next 4–5 years. The terminal illness usually is progressive heart failure and arrhythmias.

The most common symptoms are dyspnea on exertion and decreased exercise capacity. These symptoms gradually increase in severity as the ventricle deteriorates. Palpitations also are common. NYHA class IV symptoms, angina, and right heart failure occur with advanced disease or with severe incompetence in which the regurgitant flow exceeds 50 percent of forward flow.

Palpation reveals an enlarged heart and a prominent cardiac impulse. The hallmark of aortic insufficiency is a high-pitched decrescendo diastolic murmur. A light systolic ejection murmur because of increased flow across the aortic valve may also be present. A mid-diastolic rumble at the apex that simulates mitral stenosis has been described, the Austin Flint murmur, produced by the aortic insufficiency impeding the opening of the mitral valve during diastole. The pulse pressure is widened, partly from an increase in systolic pressure, but principally from a decrease in diastolic pressure, which may be in the range of 30–40 mm Hg.

Diagnostic studies. The chest radiograph usually shows impressive cardiac enlargement, with the apex displaced downward and to the left. The ECG is normal early in the disease, but with cardiac enlargement, signs of left ventricular hypertrophy become prominent. Sinus rhythm usually is present initially, although atrial fibrillation is common later in the course of the disease.

Echocardiography is the primary diagnostic tool. The classic finding on cardiac catheterization is the reflux of contrast material from the aortic root into the ventricle with aortic root angiography, graded from 1+ to 4+. Aortic root angiography or MRI studies may be performed if aneurysmal disease is suspected.

Operative indications. The development of symptoms is an absolute indication for surgery in patients with aortic insufficiency. However, postponing surgery until the patient becomes severely symptomatic is potentially dangerous, as many patients will have already developed substantial ventricular enlargement and cardiac dysfunction by that time. Therefore, echocardiographic studies are routinely used to determine the appropriate timing for surgical intervention. Asymptomatic patients with severe aortic insufficiency should be referred for surgery at the first sign of deteriorating left ventricular systolic function on echocardiography. Operative results indicate that cardiac function will return to normal and long-term survival will be improved significantly if an operation is done at this stage.

In the authors' experience valve replacement should be performed even in patients with low ejection fractions and advanced NYHA class IV symptoms, especially if recruitable ventricular wall motion is present with inotropic stimuli. Most class IV patients will improve significantly after surgery, although the degree of improvement may be uncertain for 6–12 months. Evidence supports routine electrophysiologic testing and implantation of an automatic internal cardiac defibrillator (AICD) if inducible arrhythmias are present.

Operative Techniques

Aortic valve replacement. Aortic valve replacement has traditionally been performed through a median sternotomy incision, and this approach remains the standard in most cardiac centers. Cardiopulmonary bypass with moderate systemic hypothermia is used, the aorta is cross-clamped, and the heart is protected by cardioplegia delivered antegrade into the aortic root, directly into the coronary ostia by hand-held cannulae, or retrograde through the coronary sinus.

After the heart has been arrested, an oblique or hockey stick–shaped aortotomy incision is made, beginning approximately 1 cm above the right coronary artery and extending medially toward the pulmonary artery and inferiorly into the noncoronary sinus. The aortic valve is excised totally, removing all leaflets and any fragments of calcium present in the annulus.

At NYU, pledgeted horizontal mattress sutures are routinely used, as this technique is thought to minimize the risk of paravalvular leakage. Care is taken to avoid damage to the coronary ostia, to the conduction bundle adjacent to the membranous septum between the right and the noncoronary valve cusps, and to the mitral valve posteriorly. The valve may be seated on the annulus in either of two ways.

Mechanical valves are widely used in younger patients. Two configurations are available, a single tilting disk and a bileaflet disk. The flow characteristics of the valve become important when the aortic annulus is small, to minimize the postoperative gradient across the smaller prosthesis. Patients with mechanical valves routinely require lifelong anticoagulation with warfarin to minimize the risk of thromboembolic complications. Tissue valves are most commonly used in older patients, although they now are increasingly used in younger patients who want to avoid the need for long-term anticoagulation therapy. Tissue valves may be either stented or stentless, with the traditional stented valves being easier to implant, and the stentless valves having better flow characteristics, particularly in smaller valve sizes. Current tissue valves have a projected durability of 15 years or longer and do not require long-term anticoagulation.

Results. The operative risk for aortic valve replacement is 1–5 percent for most patients, but may be considerably higher in elderly patients with multiple comorbidities and in patients with severely depressed left ventricular function. Chaliki and associates reported that aortic valve replacement in patients with aortic insufficiency and poor left ventricular function (ejection fraction less than 35 percent) resulted in increased operative risk, 14 percent compared to 3.7 percent in patients with ejection fractions above 50 percent. Ten-year survival was 70 percent in patients with good ventricular function, but only 42 percent in patients with ejection fractions less than 35 percent.

Postoperative care. Postoperative care is usually uneventful after aortic valve replacement in patients with normal left ventricular function. However, patients with significantly reduced left ventricular function may have a complicated postoperative course. Arrhythmias are relatively common, and continuous ECG monitoring is required for the first 48 h. Anticoagulation therapy is started 1 day after mechanical valve replacement, targeting an INR of 2.5–3 times normal. Antiplatelet therapy with aspirin is used in patients with tissue valves, homografts, or autografts.

Except for patients with severe ventricular dysfunction, most patients become asymptomatic and regain a normal range of physical activity within 1–2 months after operation. Thromboembolism, anticoagulant-related hemorrhage, endocarditis, and prosthetic valve failure are the principal late complications. Both thromboembolism and anticoagulant-related hemorrhage occur with incidences of 1–2 percent per year after mechanical valve replacement, despite careful anticoagulation therapy and monitoring. Patients with tissue valves have a risk of thromboembolism of 0.5–1 percent per year. Endocarditis remains an infrequent but serious late hazard after valve replacement, and routine antibiotic prophylaxis is recommended lifelong for any invasive procedure that might produce a transient bacteremia.

Aortic valve repair. David and Yacoub independently described different techniques for valve repair in patients with aortic insufficiency, with encouraging results. David's approach is based on the principle that aortic insufficiency in patients with aortoannular ectasia is secondary to annular dilatation and distortion of the sinotubular junction. David's approach involved excising the aneurysmal portion of the aortic root and reimplanting the aortic valve inside a tubular Dacron graft. Yacoub reported a similar valve-sparing technique for patients with annuloaortic ectasia. With Yacoub's technique the aortic wall and sinuses of Valsalva are excised down to the anatomic annulus. The Dacron graft is sutured to the annulus, the valve is resuspended, and the coronary buttons are reimplanted.

Ross procedure. The Ross procedure involves replacement of the aortic valve with an autograft from the patient's native pulmonary valve. The resected pulmonary valve is then replaced with a pulmonary homograft. Variations of the technique of implantation of the autograft for the aortic valve replacement include free-hand replacement with resuspension of the valve commissures, and cylinder root replacement with reimplantation of the coronary artery ostia.

The Ross procedure has risks similar to those associated with standard aortic valve replacement, although the risk of bleeding may be slightly higher. The primary benefit is that patients do not require long-term anticoagulation and the risk of thromboembolism is negligible. However, progressive late aortic insufficiency has been described in a number of patients, along with calcification of the pulmonary homograft and pulmonary stenosis. The risk of late reoperation ranges from 30–50 percent at 15–20 years.

Minimally invasive aortic valve surgery. Minimally invasive approaches for aortic valve surgery have recently become an acceptable alternative to conventional median sternotomy. Both ministernotomy and minithoracotomy approaches have been used with excellent success. Several centers have reported results that are at least comparable to standard surgery, but with less need for blood transfusions and shorter hospital stays. At NYU, minimally invasive aortic valve replacement is performed through a right anterior minithoracotomy incision. A report by Grossi and colleagues demonstrated that patients treated with the minimally invasive approach had less need for blood transfusions, fewer infections, and a shorter hospital stay than matched patients receiving traditional surgery. Thus, minimally invasive approaches for aortic valve replacement appear promising and deserve further investigation.

Idiopathic Hypertrophic Subaortic Stenosis

Patients with hypertrophic subaortic stenosis or idiopathic hypertrophic cardiomyopathy (IHSS) have varying degrees of subaortic left ventricular outflow tract obstruction, usually associated with systolic anterior motion of the mitral valve. The degree of left ventricular outflow tract obstruction at rest is a strong predictor of progression to severe symptoms of heart failure and death. However, most patients with hypertrophic cardiomyopathy and subaortic obstruction will respond to medical therapy, and only a minority will require surgical intervention.

Operative Techniques

Surgical septal myotomy and myectomy, developed by Morrow, has shown consistent results and remains the primary technique for treatment of IHSS. This approach requires resection of a trough of muscle from the subaortic outflow tract. Typically the resection is 1 cm wide and 1 cm deep, and extends the length of the septum to below the lower edge of the anterior leaflet of the mitral valve.

Tricuspid Stenosis and Insufficiency

Acquired tricuspid valve disease can be classified as organic or functional. Organic disease is almost always a result of either rheumatic fever or endocarditis. In patients with rheumatic disease, tricuspid stenosis or insufficiency virtually never occurs as an isolated lesion, but only in association with extensive disease of the mitral valve. Rarely, blunt trauma produces rupture of a papillary muscle or chordae tendineae with resultant tricuspid insufficiency.

Functional tricuspid regurgitation is much more common than insufficiency from organic disease. Functional tricuspid regurgitation develops from dilatation of the tricuspid annulus and right ventricle as a result of pulmonary hypertension and right ventricular failure. These abnormalities usually result from mitral valve disease or from other conditions that result in left ventricular failure and pulmonary hypertension.

With tricuspid stenosis the pathologic changes are similar to those found with the more familiar mitral stenosis, with fusion of the commissures. With rheumatic disease, mixed tricuspid stenosis and insufficiency or pure insufficiency may result from fibrosis and contraction of the valve leaflets, often in association with shortening and fusion of chordae tendineae. Calcification is rare.

Pathophysiology

With tricuspid stenosis or severe insufficiency, the mean right atrial pressure becomes elevated to 10–20 mm Hg or higher. The higher pressures are found with a tricuspid valve orifice smaller than 1.5 cm^2 and a mean diastolic gradient between the atrium and ventricle of 5–15 mm Hg or in patients with pulmonary hypertension and severe insufficiency. When the mean right atrial pressure remains above 15 mm Hg, hepatomegaly, ascites, and leg edema usually appear.

Clinical Manifestations

The symptoms and signs of tricuspid valve disease are similar to those of right heart failure resulting from mitral valve disease. They result from chronic elevation of right atrial pressure above the range of 15–20 mm Hg. Clinical manifestations include jugulovenous distention, hepatomegaly, pedal edema, and ascites. The characteristic murmur of tricuspid stenosis is best heard as a diastolic murmur at the lower end of the sternum. Tricuspid insufficiency produces a prominent systolic murmur heard best at the left lower sternal border. The murmur often is found in association with an enlarged, pulsating liver and prominent and engorged jugular veins.

Diagnostic Studies

The x-ray shows enlargement of the right atrium and right ventricle. Echocardiography confirms the diagnosis and differentiates stenosis from insufficiency. Cardiac catheterization is no longer necessary in most cases.

Indications for Surgery

Indications for surgery are based primarily on clinical findings, which are correlated with echocardiographic findings and hemodynamics. Severe insufficiency is indicated by echocardiography when the area of the regurgitant jet occupies a large part of the atrium, the effective regurgitant orifice is greater than 40 mm^2. Severe tricuspid regurgitation should clearly be repaired because it has been widely demonstrated that annuloplasty provides excellent late results with little added morbidity.

Operative Techniques

In the small minority of patients whose tricuspid stenosis is secondary to pure commissural fusion, a commissurotomy may be performed, usually combined with an annuloplasty. More commonly, valve replacement is necessary when significant tricuspid stenosis is present, because the entire valve and subvalvular apparatus are damaged. When a prosthetic valve is inserted, care is required in suture placement along the septal leaflet in which the conduction bundle is located, and sutures should be placed more superficially in this area.

In patients with functional tricuspid insufficiency the annulus is markedly dilated, although the leaflets appear entirely normal. Virtually all such patients can be treated by annuloplasty. Alternatively, a flexible or rigid annuloplasty device may be used.

Results

Data on more than 300 patients from the authors' institution show that the suture annuloplasty repair for functional tricuspid insufficiency is reproducible in the absence of significant intrinsic leaflet disease. Other centers prefer the use of rigid or flexible annuloplasty devices for correction of tricuspid insufficiency. When tricuspid valve replacement is required, the options include use of either a tissue valve or a mechanical valve. Data suggest that the risk of valve thrombosis is increased in mechanical valves placed in the tricuspid position. Bioprostheses are therefore preferred for most patients requiring tricuspid valve replacement.

Multivalve Disease

Disease involving multiple valves is relatively common, particularly in patients with rheumatic disease. Prominent signs in one valve can readily mask disease in others. With aortic valve disease, functional mitral insufficiency can result from a progressive rise in the left ventricular end-diastolic pressure and volume. Similarly, mitral valve disease may result in pulmonary hypertension, right heart failure, and functional tricuspid insufficiency. Often these secondary functional changes resolve without treatment if the primary pathology is corrected in a timely fashion.

Aortic and Mitral Valve Disease

Nine combinations of valvular pathology can produce aortic and mitral valve disease (AV + MV), because each valve can be stenotic, insufficient, or both. Stenosis in both valves may lead to underestimation of the degree of aortic stenosis, because return of blood to the left ventricle is limited as a result of mitral stenosis. Aortic insufficiency, which produces the Austin Flint murmur, might overshadow and mask true mitral stenosis. With functional mitral insufficiency resulting from severe aortic disease, aortic valve replacement can lead to resolution of insufficiency in some patients, but patients with more severe mitral insufficiency may require mitral repair or replacement.

Mitral and Tricuspid Valve Disease

Multiple combinations of valvular pathology are possible with mitral and tricuspid disease, but mitral disease with functional tricuspid insufficiency is the most common scenario, resulting from chronic pulmonary hypertension and right heart failure. The presence of associated tricuspid insufficiency increases the operative risk for patients undergoing mitral valve surgery. The risk for isolated mitral and tricuspid valve disease (MV + TV) is approximately 6 percent.

Triple-Valve Disease

Triple-valve surgery can be challenging because the clinical condition usually is a result of chronic aortic and mitral disease with severe pulmonary hypertension, biventricular failure, and functional tricuspid insufficiency. The degree of pulmonary hypertension is the most significant predictor of survival in patients with triple-valve disease.

PERICARDIAL DISEASES

Acute Pericarditis

Pericarditis results from acute inflammation of the pericardial space, resulting in substernal chest pain, ECG changes, and a pericardial friction rub on physical examination. Associated ECG changes frequently occur, most commonly sinus tachycardia with concave upward ST-segment elevation throughout the precordium. The ECG typically progresses to T-wave inversion, followed by the total resolution of all changes. The cause of acute pericarditis is variable, including infection, myocardial infarction, trauma, neoplasm, radiation, autoimmune diseases, drugs, nonspecific causes, and others.

Diagnosis

The diagnostic workup should attempt to determine the underlying cause of the pericarditis. Blood tests should include erythrocyte sedimentation rate, hematocrit level, white blood cell count, bacterial cultures, viral titers, blood urea nitrogen, T3, T4, thyroid-stimulating hormone, antinuclear antibody, rheumatoid factor, and myocardial enzyme levels. The ECG may be typical or nonspecific. The chest radiograph may be normal or may demonstrate an enlarged cardiac silhouette or a pleural effusion. An echocardiogram to evaluate the degree of pericardial effusion is essential. A pericardiocentesis or pericardial biopsy may be necessary when the diagnosis is uncertain.

Treatment

The preferred treatment depends on the underlying cause. Purulent pyogenic pericarditis requires drainage and prolonged intravenous antibiotic therapy. Postpericardiotomy syndrome, post–myocardial infarction syndrome, viral pericarditis, and idiopathic pericarditis often are self-limiting, but can require a short course of treatment with nonsteroidal antiinflammatory agents. If a significant pericardial effusion is present, surgical drainage is indicated if tamponade is suspected or if resolution is not prompt with antiinflammatory agents. A 5–7-day course of steroids is occasionally necessary.

Chronic Constrictive Pericarditis

Etiology

In the majority of patients, the cause of chronic constrictive pericarditis is unknown and probably is the end stage of an undiagnosed viral pericarditis. Tuberculosis is a rarity. Intensive radiation is a significant cause in some series. Constrictive pericarditis may develop after an open-heart operation. Previous cardiac surgery was reported to be the cause in 39 percent of the patients treated surgically for constrictive pericarditis at the authors' institution.

Pathology and Pathophysiology

The pericardial cavity is obliterated by fusion of the parietal pericardium to the epicardium, forming dense scar tissue that encases and constricts the heart. The physiologic handicap is limitation of diastolic filling of the ventricles. This results in a decrease in cardiac output from a decrease in stroke volume.

Clinical Manifestations

The disease is slowly progressive with increasing ascites and edema. Fatigability and dyspnea on exertion are common, but dyspnea at rest is unusual. Hepatomegaly and ascites often are the most prominent physical abnormalities. The heart size remains normal without murmurs or abnormal sounds.

Laboratory Findings

Venous pressure is elevated, often to 15–20 mm Hg or higher. The ECG, although not diagnostic, usually is abnormal with a low voltage and inverted T waves. The chest radiograph usually shows a heart of normal size, but pericardial calcification may be seen in a significant proportion of cases and often is the first clue to the diagnosis. Echocardiogram, MRI, or CT scan may demonstrate a thickened pericardium.

Findings on cardiac catheterization are highly characteristic. There is elevation of the right ventricular diastolic pressure with a change in contour, showing an early filling with a subsequent plateau, called the "square root" sign. There also is "equalization" of pressures in the different cardiac chambers. The one condition that cannot be excluded without myocardial biopsy is a restrictive cardiomyopathy.

Treatment

When the diagnosis has been made, pericardiectomy should be done promptly, because the disease relentlessly progresses. Operation can be done through a sternotomy incision or a long left anterolateral thoracotomy. The constricting pericardium should be removed from all surfaces of the ventricle. Cardiopulmonary bypass is not usually necessary, but may be needed in the event of significant hemorrhage. The pericardium is removed from the pulmonary veins on the right to the pulmonary veins on the left. Both phrenic nerves are mobilized and protected. Intracardiac pressures should be measured by direct needle puncture before and after pericardiectomy. Often with a complete pericardiectomy the characteristic pressure abnormalities are eliminated or greatly improved.

Results

After a radical pericardiectomy that corrects the hemodynamic abnormalities, patients improve promptly with a massive diuresis. The risk of operation varies with the age of the patient and the severity of the disease; the mortality rate usually is less than 5 percent. A good result can be anticipated for more than 95 percent of the patients.

CARDIAC NEOPLASMS

Primary cardiac neoplasms are rare, reported to occur with incidences ranging from 0.001–0.3 percent in autopsy series. Benign tumors account for 75 percent of primary neoplasms and malignant tumors account for 25 percent. The most frequent primary cardiac neoplasm is myxoma, comprising 30–50 percent. Other benign neoplasms, in decreasing order of occurrence, include lipoma, papillary fibroelastoma, rhabdomyoma, fibroma, hemangioma, teratoma, lymphangioma, and others. Most primary malignant neoplasms are sarcomas (angiosarcoma, rhabdomyosarcoma, fibrosarcoma, leiomyosarcoma, and liposarcoma), with malignant lymphomas accounting for 1–2 percent.

Metastatic cardiac neoplasms are more common than primary neoplasms, occurring in 4–12 percent of patients dying of cancer. Symptoms include dyspnea, fever, malaise, weight loss, arthralgias, and dizziness. Clinical findings may include murmurs of mitral stenosis or insufficiency, heart failure, pulmonary hypertension, and systemic embolization.

Usually, the diagnosis is readily established by two-dimensional echocardiography. Transesophageal echocardiography may be useful when transthoracic findings are equivocal or confusing. MRI has been of value in diagnosis, providing excellent cardiac definition. Cardiac catheterization may be necessary when other cardiac disease is suspected or if other diagnostic studies are equivocal.

Excision is the treatment of choice for most benign tumors. Care is taken to avoid deformity or destruction of adjacent cardiac structures, and reconstruction of the involved cardiac chamber is sometimes necessary. Total excision of metastatic or primary malignant neoplasms is less frequently possible but should be attempted. Otherwise incisional diagnostic biopsy is performed. Multimodality therapy with excision, chemotherapy, and radiotherapy is indicated for most malignant cardiac neoplasms.

Myxomas

Sixty to 75 percent of cardiac myxomas develop in the left atrium, almost always from the atrial septum near the fossa ovalis. Most other myxomas develop in the right atrium. Myxomas are true neoplasms, although their similarity to an organized atrial thrombus has led to considerable debate. Although they can recur locally, they do not invade or metastasize and are considered benign.

Pathology

The tumors usually are polypoid, projecting into the atrial cavity from a 1–2-cm stalk attached to the atrial septum. The size ranges from 0.5 cm to larger than 10.0 cm. Some myxomas grow slowly; a few patients have symptoms for many years. The friable consistency of a myxoma is of particular significance because fatal emboli have occurred after digital manipulation of the tumor at operation.

Pathophysiology

A myxoma may be completely asymptomatic until it grows large enough to obstruct the mitral or tricuspid valve or fragments to produce emboli. Embolization has been estimated to occur in 40–50 percent of patients. Intermittent acute obstruction of the mitral orifice has been reported to produce syncope and even sudden death. Some myxomas produce generalized symptoms resembling an autoimmune disorder, including fever, weight loss, digital clubbing, myalgia, and arthralgia.

Clinical Manifestations

Symptoms may include those of mitral valve obstruction that resemble mitral stenosis; peripheral embolization; or generalized autoimmune symptoms. The diagnosis often is made after an embolic episode from histologic examination of the surgically removed embolus, or as a result of subsequent diagnostic studies to determine the reason for embolism. The precision and reliability of two-dimensional echocardiography has greatly simplified diagnosis. Angiography is optional unless additional disease is suspected. CT scan has been reported to be helpful with small tumors, but MRI is more definitive.

Treatment

Surgery should be performed as soon as possible after the diagnosis has been established, because of the inherent risk of a disabling or fatal cerebral embolus. Either a sternotomy or a minimally invasive approach can be used. Palpation is avoided. The right atrium is opened and the fossa ovalis incised to expose the stalk of the myxoma. The left atrium is then opened in the interatrial groove. With the tumor visualized, the segment of atrial septum from which the tumor arises is excised, after which the tumor is removed through the left atrium. The defect in the atrial septum is closed primarily or with a small patch.

Metastatic Neoplasms

Cardiac metastases have been found in 4–12 percent of autopsies performed for neoplastic disease. Although they have occurred from primary neoplasms developing in almost every known site of the body, the most common have been carcinoma of the lung or breast, melanoma, and lymphoma. Cardiac metastases involving only the heart are very unusual. Similarly, a solitary cardiac metastasis is rare; usually there are multiple areas of involvement. The diagnosis of a primary cardiac malignant tumor may be suspected in a patient in whom an unexplained hemorrhagic pericardial effusion develops, especially in association with a bizarre cardiac shadow on the radiograph. Echocardiography should confirm the presence of an abnormal cardiac mass. Thoracotomy or sternotomy usually is required to establish the diagnosis. Combined chemotherapy and radiation is indicated, but only rarely is effective therapy possible.

Miscellaneous Tumors

Unusual benign lesions of the heart include fibromas, lipomas, angiomas, teratomas, and cysts. Fewer than 50 of each of these types of lesion have been reported. Fibromas have been found most frequently in the left ventricle, often as 2–5-cm nodules within the muscle. Sudden death, probably from a cardiac arrhythmia, has been reported with these tumors, and may be the reason that only 18 percent of tumors that have been reported have been found in adults.

Lipomas are rare asymptomatic tumors found projecting from the epicardial or endocardial surface of the heart in older patients. Angiomas are small, focal, vascular malformations of no clinical significance, although may be associated with heart block. Pericardial teratomas and bronchogenic cysts are rare lesions that can cause symptoms from compression of the right atrium and obstruction of venous return. Most of these occur in children.

Renal cell carcinoma, Wilms tumor, uterine tumors, and adrenal tumors may have intracardiac extension. Excision of these infradiaphragmatic tumors by radical surgery associated with cavoatrial thrombectomy has been suggested, and extracorporeal circulation and deep circulatory arrest provide an optimal technique for removing the tumor thrombus, even in the presence of metastatic disease, and have good early and long-term results.

POSTOPERATIVE CARE AND COMPLICATIONS

General Considerations

Postoperative care of cardiac surgical patients involves prevention, recognition, and correction of the metabolic and hemodynamic derangements that are frequently seen after cardiac surgery. Important areas include myocardial and pulmonary support, fluid and electrolyte management, and control of bleeding and coagulopathy. All patients are observed in a specialized recovery room or intensive care unit after cardiac surgery, in which hemodynamic data are continuously analyzed using both invasive and noninvasive monitoring. Additionally, important laboratory parameters, including arterial blood gases, enzymatic markers of cardiac injury, and mixed venous O_2 saturation, are measured serially.

Early postoperative complications include bleeding, cardiac tamponade, arrhythmias, myocardial infarction, graft occlusion, coronary spasm, low cardiac output syndrome, cardiac arrest, and stroke. Later complications include delayed bleeding, postpericardiotomy syndrome with pericardial effusion, renal dysfunction, ileus, mesenteric ischemia, gastrointestinal hemorrhage, pneumothorax, respiratory insufficiency, pneumonia, wound infection, and wound dehiscence. Although the incidence of serious complications is relatively low (3–6 percent), each complication is potentially life-threatening and can be associated with significant morbidity.

Hemodynamics

Maintenance of cardiac function is critical in any patient following heart surgery. Although adequate cardiac output may be reflected in the blood pressure and the urine output, exact determination may be obtained with invasive monitoring equipment. A cardiac index less than 2 L/min per square meter is an ominous finding, and should prompt immediate investigation into possible causes of decreased cardiac performance. The classic clinical findings of low cardiac output with inadequate oxygen transport include hypotension, vasoconstriction, oliguria, and metabolic acidosis. Untreated low cardiac output is ultimately fatal from either progressive renal failure or arrhythmias.

When evaluating low cardiac output in the postoperative setting, the first consideration is to exclude cardiac tamponade or hypovolemia because of intrathoracic bleeding. Once these have been excluded, the physiologic causes of low output should be reviewed in terms of preload, afterload, and intrinsic contractility of the heart.

Afterload reduction consists of reduction in peripheral vascular resistance with specific drugs that cause vasodilatation. If peripheral vascular resistance is elevated above the normal 1200 dynes/s/cm^2, afterload reduction should be one of the initial forms of therapy. The most popular drugs for intravenous infusion are nitroprussride or nitroglycerin. Vasodilation, or decreased peripheral resistance, should be treated with vasoconstrictors such as phenylephrine to maintain an adequate perfusion pressure.

Once bleeding and tamponade are excluded and preload and afterload have been optimized, inotropic agents may be used to augment myocardial contractility. First-line medications include milrinone and dobutamine, which may be augmented with nor-epinephrine or phenylephrine when the peripheral vascular resistance is low. Dopamine and epinephrine are useful second-line inotropic agents.

If the intrinsic cardiac rhythm is not sufficient to maintain optimal hemodynamics, cardiac pacing should be used to maintain both an adequate rate and rhythm. Optimal heart rate to maximize cardiac output without unduly increasing myocardial oxygen consumption generally is 80–90 beats per min.

If low cardiac output persists despite optimizing preload, afterload, and inotropic support, an intraaortic balloon pump (IABP) may be useful.

Electrocardiogram and Arrhythmias

The postoperative ECG is important for determining heart block, bundle-branch block, infarction (Q waves), ischemia (ST-segment elevation, T-wave inversion), and other signs of intraoperative injury. Acute ischemia or evolving infarction should be treated initially with nitrates and beta blockade. If ECG changes do not resolve promptly, acute graft occlusion should be considered, particularly if the patient is hemodynamically unstable.

In addition to serial 12-lead ECGs, continuous monitoring of the cardiac rhythm remains important in the postoperative setting. Life-threatening arrhythmias may develop unexpectedly despite the presence of a normal cardiac output and without any other signs of circulatory failure. Postoperative bradyarrhythmias and heart block are not uncommon, and for this reason temporary cardiac pacing wires are routinely placed in the right ventricle and right atrium at operation.

Other arrhythmias, including ventricular extrasystoles and ventricular tachycardia, may herald the development of ventricular fibrillation. Hypokalemia is an important cause of ventricular arrhythmias, as many patients undergoing cardiac surgery may have significant depletion of total body potassium stores from chronic diuretic therapy. Postoperatively serum potassium should be kept above 4.0 mEq/L. Continuous intravenous lidocaine or amiodarone has proven to be effective in controlling postoperative ventricular arrhythmias.

Atrial fibrillation remains the most common postoperative arrhythmia. Beta blockers should be initiated early postoperatively unless contraindicated, as this has been found to lower the risk of developing postoperative atrial fibrillation. If atrial fibrillation does develop, initial treatment involves heart rate control with beta blockers and intravenous digitalis. If atrial fibrillation persists, anticoagulation with heparin is indicated, followed by an attempt at cardioversion, usually pharmacologically. Amiodarone is effective in converting postoperative patients to sinus rhythm. If atrial fibrillation results in hemodynamic instability, the patient should be cardioverted with 50–100 J.

Cardiac Arrest and Resuscitation

Complete circulatory collapse in the postoperative cardiac surgical patient can occur without warning. Circulation must be restored within min or the brain and myocardium may suffer irreversible injury. Frequent causes of postoperative cardiac arrest include cardiac tamponade, arrhythmias, ischemia or graft occlusion, hypoxia, and drug toxicity.

Cardiac tamponade is a serious complication following cardiac surgery. It may occur early in the postoperative period from the accumulation of intrapericardial blood or later from a pericardial effusion. The classic findings of tamponade include: (1) elevation of central venous pressure; (2) equalization of central venous pressure, pulmonary artery diastolic pressure, and left atrial pressure; and (3) pulsus paradoxus of more than 10 mm Hg during inspiration. Clinical signs may include distended neck veins, muffled heart sounds, and hypotension. Extreme cases of tamponade may present with life-threatening hypotension or sudden circulatory collapse. A widening of the mediastinal shadow on chest radiograph or detection of significant pericardial effusion by echocardiography is suggestive of the diagnosis. No single test can exclude tamponade short of surgical exploration. Therefore any patient with suspected tamponade should be promptly returned to the operating room for definitive diagnosis and treatment. Moreover, any postoperative patient in extremis with suspected tamponade should undergo emergent re-exploration or subxiphoid drainage performed at the bedside to rule out tamponade.

Electrolyte imbalance, such as a deficiency of potassium or magnesium, also can cause serious arrhythmias leading to cardiac arrest or ventricular fibrillation. A serum potassium level below 3.0 mEq can produce severe cardiac irritability postoperatively. Difficulties with ventilation and hypoxia may lead to cardiac arrhythmias from low arterial oxygen tension and progressive metabolic acidosis. Common causes include inadequate ventilation from pneumothorax, dislodgment of the endotracheal tube, and plugging of the airway with secretions.

Drugs may induce bradycardia, heart block, ventricular fibrillation, or cardiac arrest, either from toxicity or from an idiosyncratic reaction. Digitalis is a common example because of its widespread use. The sensitivity of the myocardium to digitalis varies with a number of factors, one of the most important of which is the concentration of potassium. Procainamide and quinidine are examples of drugs with known proarrhythmic effects.

Profound bradycardia (heart rate < 60 beats per min) from any cause may result in escape beats leading to ventricular fibrillation and cardiac arrest. Ventricular arrhythmias may progress to bigeminy, ventricular tachycardia, and ventricular fibrillation.

Treatment

Advanced Cardiac Life Support (ACLS) guidelines include specific algorithms for the treatment of cardiac arrest and other causes of circulatory arrest. The immediate first steps in CPR are to secure an adequate airway and provide prompt ventilation. Effective perfusion with closed-chest massage or with inotropes or pressors may then be necessary. Effective CPR depends on adequate intermittent compression of the heart between the sternum and the vertebral column. The patient must be placed on a firm surface, usually by placing a board behind the back. The heel of the hand should be applied over the lower third of the sternum with the other hand above it to depress the sternum intermittently for 3–4 cm. Massage should be at a rate of about 60/min.

In the postoperative cardiac surgery patient with cardiac arrest, closed-chest massage may be initiated immediately as part of a resuscitative effort that may also include defibrillation and the administration of pharmacologic agents. If cardiac activity is not quickly restored or if the cardiac arrest is thought to be because of a mechanical cause such as tamponade or hemorrhage, the sternotomy incision is reopened immediately at the bedside and internal cardiac massage is instituted. The patient may then be returned to the operating room once the chest is opened, and CPB is initiated for support. After the patient is resuscitated the surgeon must determine if further therapy such as mechanical support or additional bypass grafting is indicated.

Drugs and Fluids

Epinephrine, sodium bicarbonate, and calcium are the most useful pharmacologic agents. Again, the protocols suggested by the ACLS program are followed. Epinephrine, 1 mg, may be given intravenously or alternately by direct intracardiac injection. Calcium, 3–4 mL of a 10 percent solution, is another powerful stimulant of myocardial contraction. Lidocaine is given primarily for ventricular arrhythmias, followed by amiodarone for refractory ventricular tachycardia. Medications are usually ineffective if severe myocardial anoxia or significant acidosis is present. Small amounts of fluid should be rapidly infused because vasodilatation is usually present. An intravenous infusion of a vasoconstrictor, norepinephrine or phenylephrine, is often helpful to maintain perfusion pressure. Blood transfusion may be required in the postoperative patient for volume resuscitation and improved oxygen-carrying capacity.

Defibrillation

Ventricular fibrillation can be differentiated from asystole only by the electrocardiogram or by direct inspection of the myocardium. Intravenous lidocaine is promptly administered. If this is not quickly effective and an electrocardiogram is not available, empiric defibrillation may be tried briefly because most resuscitations are effective when defibrillation is done promptly. Asystole is treated by pacing the heart with a transcutaneous pacemaker, a transvenous pacemaker if access is readily available, or a temporary pacing lead that can be placed directly on the myocardium if the chest is open.

Closed-chest defibrillation is usually done by applying electrodes over the base and apex of the heart. Defibrillation is best done with a direct current of 200–360 J. When open-chest defibrillation is used, the electrodes are applied directly to the heart and an impulse of 20–40 J is delivered. Vigorous cardiac massage should precede defibrillation to oxygenate the myocardium sufficiently.

Following restoration of an adequate heart beat and blood pressure, the critical question is the extent of injury to the heart and to the central nervous system. A thorough search for reversible causes of the arrhythmia is undertaken immediately. If ischemia or graft occlusion is suspected, the patient is taken for cardiac catheterization or back to the operating room.

Blood Loss

Blood conservation and minimization of bleeding associated with cardiac surgery begin preoperatively. Preoperative workup routinely includes a prothrombin time (PT), partial thromboplastin time (PTT), and platelet count. Patients with a history of abnormal bleeding or with chronic passive congestion of the liver receive full coagulation profiles and evaluation by a hematologist. Patients taking warfarin are instructed to discontinue the drug 3 to 4 days preoperatively so the PT can return to normal.

Because blood conservation is highly desirable, many patients operated on electively are able to donate autologous blood 1–3 weeks before surgery. Often erythropoietin is used after autologous donation to enhance the patient's red blood cell mass. Donor-directed blood units are solicited from family and friends.

Postoperative Bleeding

For most open heart cases coagulopathy is nonexistent and the postoperative blood loss is low. The normal total postoperative blood loss should range from 300 to 800 mL. Blood loss in excess of 300–500 mL/h or over 1–1.5 L total usually indicates active surgical bleeding, and is associated with a high incidence of hemodynamic compromise or cardiac tamponade.

The diagnosis of coagulopathy is made by the operating surgeon with the observation of abnormal bleeding from the operative field in the absence of a surgical source. Laboratory tests can confirm the diagnosis, but treatment should not be delayed until test results return, as this might further worsen the coagulation deficit, with fatal consequences.

Treatment of coagulopathy is urgent. Hypothermia should be corrected and extra protamine should be given until the activated clotting time returns to normal or until no further drop is seen in the activated clotting time. If abnormal bleeding persists, transfusion of platelets, fresh-frozen plasma, and cryoprecipitate is given until the clotting deficit is corrected. Antifibrinolytic agents such as ε-aminocaproic acid may be given to correct fibrinolysis. The pharmacologic prevention of coagulopathy is more effective if the protease inhibitor aprotonin is given preoperatively.

Ventilatory Support and Pulmonary Care

Nearly all cardiac surgical patients return to the recovery room intubated. Tidal volumes on the respirator are usually set at 10–15 mL/kg. Weaning the patient is done via the intermittent mandatory ventilation (IMV) mode or via progressive continuous positive airway pressure (CPAP) trials. With current preoperative preparation and intraoperative management, significant postoperative impairment of pulmonary function is uncommon, except in patients with preexisting pulmonary disease or advanced cardiac failure. If periods of ventilation longer than 3–4 days are anticipated, a cricothyroidotomy or tracheostomy should be considered.

General Care

Nutrition

The need for adequate postoperative nutrition cannot be overemphasized, particularly in elderly or chronically ill patients. The sick postoperative heart patient may require approximately 25–kcal/kg per day. Care should be taken to give adequate protein to patients with normal renal and hepatic function, although special formulas are available for patients with kidney or liver failure.

Wound Care

Early postoperative care of the surgical wound consists of the use of a sterile occlusive dressing for the first 24 h. Prophylactic antibiotics are started preoperatively and continued for 24–48 h postoperatively, usually until indwelling catheters and chest tubes are removed.

Fever

A moderate fever of 37.8–38.3°C (100–101°F) is common in the first 1–2 days, usually resulting from the systemic inflammatory response induced by the extracorporeal circulation and the stress of major surgery or from atelectasis. A fever occurring from 3–7 days postoperatively with a normal white blood cell count is frequently because of postpericardiotomy syndrome. The syndrome can be treated with nonsteroidal antiinflammatory agents or occasionally with a short course of steroids. Significant fevers should be evaluated with a chest radiograph and blood and urine cultures.

A serious sternal wound infection occurs in 1–2 percent of all open heart operations. Risk factors include diabetes, obesity, impaired nutrition, COPD, prolonged ventilatory support, harvest of bilateral internal mammary arteries, older age, low cardiac output, excessive mediastinal bleeding, re-exploration for bleeding, multiple transfusions, and prolonged CPB. *Staphylococcus aureus* and *Staphylococcus epidermidis* are the most common organisms isolated. Treatment requires prompt operation with either débridement and closure over antibiotic irrigation/drainage catheters or débridement followed by immediate or delayed closure with muscle flaps. The mortality rate from a sternal infection after cardiac surgery is 10–20 percent.

Rehabilitation

Most patients will benefit from early initiation of physical therapy and a cardiac rehabilitation program, but these treatments are especially important in elderly and debilitated patients. Physical therapy should begin early during the hospital stay and continue with a formalized rehabilitation program for an additional 1–2 weeks. Formal cardiac rehabilitation is usually available as either an inpatient or an outpatient program, depending on the patient's age and physical condition.

Suggested Readings

Eagle KA, Berger PB, Calkins H, et al: ACC/AHA guideline update for perioperative cardiovascular evaluation for noncardiac surgery—executive summary report of the American College of Cardiology/ American Heart Association Task Force on Practice Guidelines (Committee to Update the 1996 Guidelines on Perioperative Cardiovascular Evaluation for Noncardiac Surgery). Circulation 105:1257, 2002.

Coronary artery bypass surgery versus percutaneous coronary intervention with stent implantation in patients with multivessel coronary artery disease (the Stent or Surgery Trial): A randomised controlled trial. Lancet 360:965, 2002.

Puskas JD, Williams WH, Duke PG, et al: Off-pump coronary artery bypass grafting provides complete revascularization with reduced myocardial injury, transfusion requirements, and length of stay: A prospective randomized comparison of two hundred unselected patients undergoing off-pump versus conventional coronary artery bypass grafting. J Thorac Cardiovasc Surg 125:797, 2003.

Loop FD, Lytle BW, Cosgrove DM, et al: Influence of the internal mammary artery graft on 10-year survival and other cardiac events. N Engl J Med 314:1, 1986.

Dor V, Di Donato M, Sabatier M, et al: Left ventricular reconstruction by endoventricular circular patch plasty repair: A 17-year experience. Semin Thorac Cardiovasc Surg 13:435, 2001.

Athanasuleas CL, Stanley AW Jr., Buckberg GD, et al: Surgical anterior ventricular endocardial restoration (SAVER) in the dilated remodeled ventricle after anterior myocardial infarction. RESTORE group. Reconstructive Endoventricular Surgery, returning Torsion Original Radius Elliptical Shape to the LV. J Am Coll Cardiol 37:1199, 2001.

Bonow RO, Carabello B, de Leon AC Jr., et al: Guidelines for the management of patients with valvular heart disease: Executive summary. A report of the American College of Cardiology/American Heart Association Task Force on Practice Guidelines (Committee on Management of Patients with Valvular Heart Disease). Circulation 98:1949, 1998.

Carpentier A: Cardiac valve surgery—the "French correction." J Thorac Cardiovasc Surg 86:323, 1983.

Galloway AC, Grossi EA, Bizekis CS, et al: Evolving techniques for mitral valve reconstruction. Ann Surg 236:288, 2002; discussion 293.

David TE, Ivanov J, Armstrong S, et al: Aortic valve-sparing operations in patients with aneurysms of the aortic root or ascending aorta. Ann Thorac Surg 74:S1758, 2002; discussion S1792.

21 | Thoracic Aortic Aneurysms and Aortic Dissection

Joseph S. Coselli and Scott A. LeMaire

THORACIC AORTIC DISEASE

The aorta consists of two major segments—the proximal aorta and the distal aorta—each of which has anatomic characteristics that impact clinical manifestations and treatment strategies. The proximal aortic segment includes the ascending aorta and the transverse aortic arch. The ascending aorta begins at the aortic valve and ends at the origin of the innominate artery. The first portion of the ascending aorta is the aortic root, which includes the aortic valve annulus and the three sinuses of Valsalva and joins the tubular portion of the ascending aorta at the sinotubular ridge. The transverse aortic arch is the segment from which the brachiocephalic branches arise. The distal aorta includes the descending thoracic aorta and the abdominal aorta. The descending thoracic aorta begins distal to the origin of the left subclavian artery and extends to the diaphragmatic hiatus, in which it joins the abdominal aorta. The descending thoracic segment gives rise to multiple bronchial and esophageal branches and the segmental intercostal arteries, which provide circulation to the spinal cord.

Conditions that disrupt the integrity of the aorta (i.e., aortic dissection, aneurysm rupture, or traumatic injury) have catastrophic consequences.

THORACIC AORTIC ANEURYSMS

Aortic aneurysm is defined as a permanent dilatation resulting in at least a 50 percent increase in diameter. The incidence of thoracic aortic aneurysms is estimated to be 5.9 per 100,000 persons annually. Causes of thoracic aortic aneurysms include degenerative disease of the aortic wall, aortic dissection, aortitis, infection, and trauma. Thoracoabdominal aortic aneurysms, for example, involve both the descending thoracic aorta and abdominal aorta. In the most extreme, the entire aorta is aneurysmal; this often is described as "mega-aorta."

Aneurysms of the thoracic aorta consistently increase in size and progress to rupture, which is usually a fatal event. Aggressive treatment is indicated in all but the poorest surgical candidates. Small asymptomatic thoracic aortic aneurysms can be followed. Meticulous control of hypertension is the primary medical treatment.

Elective resection with graft replacement is indicated in asymptomatic patients with an aortic diameter of at least twice the normal diameter for the involved segment (5–6 cm in most thoracic segments). Contraindications to elective repair include severe coexisting cardiac or pulmonary disease, or a limited life expectancy. An emergency operation is required for any patient in whom a ruptured aneurysm is suspected.

Etiology and Pathogenesis

General Considerations

Table 21-1 lists causes of thoracic aortic aneurysms. These disparate pathologic processes share the final common pathway of progressive aortic expansion and

496

TABLE 21-1 Causes of Thoracic Aortic Aneurysms

Nonspecific medial degeneration
Aortic dissection
Genetic disorders
Marfan syndrome
Ehlers-Danlos syndrome
Familial aortic aneurysms
Bicuspid aortic valves
Poststenotic dilatation
Infection
Aortitis
Takayasu arteritis
Giant cell arteritis
Rheumatoid aortitis
Trauma

rupture. Hemodynamic factors clearly contribute to the process. The vicious cycle between increasing diameter and increasing wall tension, as characterized by the Laplace law (tension = pressure × radius), is well established. Turbulent blood flow also is recognized as a factor. Poststenotic aortic dilatation, for example, occurs in some patients with aortic valve stenosis or coarctation of the descending thoracic aorta.

Atherosclerosis is commonly cited as a cause of thoracic aortic aneurysms. Although atherosclerotic disease often is found in conjunction with aortic aneurysms, the notion that atherosclerosis is a distinct cause of aneurysm formation has been challenged. Imbalances between proteolytic enzymes (e.g., matrix metalloproteinases) and their inhibitors contribute to abdominal aortic aneurysm formation.

Nonspecific Medial Degeneration

Nonspecific medial degeneration is the most common cause of thoracic aortic disease. Histologic findings of mild medial degeneration, including fragmentation of elastic fibers and loss of smooth muscle cells, are expected in the aging aorta. An advanced, accelerated form of medial degeneration leads to progressive weakening of the aortic wall, aneurysm formation, and eventual rupture and/or dissection.

Aortic Dissection

Aortic dissections usually begin as a tear in the inner aortic wall, which initiates a progressive separation of the medial layers, creating two channels within the aorta and a profoundly weakened outer wall. As the most common catastrophe involving the aorta, dissection represents a major, distinct cause of thoracic aortic aneurysms.

Genetic Disorders

Marfan syndrome. Marfan syndrome is an autosomal dominant genetic disorder characterized by a specific connective tissue defect that leads to aneurysm formation. The phenotype of patients with Marfan syndrome typically includes a tall stature, high palate, joint hypermobility, lens disorders, mitral valve prolapse, and aortic aneurysms. The aortic wall is weakened by fragmentation of elastic fibers and deposition of extensive amounts of mucopolysaccharides (cystic medial degeneration). Patients with Marfan syndrome have a mutation involving the fibrillin gene located on the long arm of the chromosome 15. Abnormal fibrillin in the extracellular matrix decreases connective tissue strength in the aortic wall and produces abnormal elastic properties that predispose the aorta to dilatation from wall tension resulting from left ventricular ejection impulses. Seventy-five to 85 percent of patients with Marfan syndrome exhibit dilation of the ascending aorta with dilation of the aortic sinuses and annulus.

Ehlers-Danlos syndrome. Ehlers-Danlos syndrome includes a spectrum of inherited connective tissue disorders of collagen synthesis. Type IV Ehlers-Danlos syndrome is characterized by an autosomal dominant defect in type III collagen synthesis, and may produce life-threatening cardiovascular manifestations including aortic aneurysms. Spontaneous arterial rupture, usually involving the mesenteric vessels, is the most common cause of death in these patients.

Familial aortic aneurysms. Guo and colleagues demonstrated a linkage to the 5q locus in nine of 15 families with strong family histories (i.e., autosomal dominant transmission) of ascending aortic aneurysms and dissections. Similar studies have found linkages to chromosomes 3 and 11.

Congenital bicuspid aortic valve. Bicuspid aortic valve is the most common congenital malformation of the heart or great vessels, affecting nearly 1–2 percent of Americans. Patients with bicuspid aortic valves have an increased incidence of ascending aortic aneurysm formation and exhibit a more rapid rate of aortic enlargement. Aortic dissection occurs 10 times more often in patients with bicuspid valves. Patients with bicuspid aortic valves may have a congenital connective tissue abnormality that predisposes them to aneurysm formation in the setting of chronic turbulent flow through a deformed valve.

Infection

Primary infection of the aortic wall resulting in aneurysm formation is rare. Although termed mycotic aneurysms, the responsible pathogens are usually bacteria rather than fungi. Bacterial invasion of the aortic wall may result from bacterial endocarditis, endothelial trauma caused by an aortic jet lesion, or extension from an infected laminar clot within a preexisting aneurysm. The most common organisms include *Staphylococcus aureus*, *S. epidermidis*, Salmonella, and Streptococcus species. Infection often produces saccular aneurysms localized in areas destroyed by the infectious process.

Aortitis

Patients with preexisting degenerative thoracic aortic aneurysms can develop localized transmural inflammation and subsequent fibrosis. Although the severe inflammation is a superimposed problem rather than a primary cause, its onset within an aneurysm can further weaken the aortic wall and precipitate expansion.

Systemic autoimmune disorders also cause thoracic aortitis. Although Takayasu arteritis generally produces obstructive lesions related to severe intimal thickening, associated medial necrosis can lead to aneurysm formation. Patients with giant cell arteritis (temporal arteritis) may develop granulomatous inflammation involving the entire thickness of the aortic wall, causing intimal thickening and medial destruction. Rheumatoid aortitis, with medial inflammation and fibrosis, can affect the aortic root, causing ascending aortic aneurysm.

Pseudoaneurysms

Pseudoaneurysms, or false aneurysms, of the thoracic aorta usually represent chronic leaks that are contained by surrounding tissue and fibrosis. By definition, the wall of a pseudoaneurysm is not formed by intact aortic tissue; rather, the wall develops from organized thrombus and associated fibrosis. Pseudoaneurysms arise from primary defects in the aortic wall or anastomotic leaks after cardiovascular surgery.

Natural History

Classically, the natural history is characterized as progressive aortic dilatation and eventual rupture and/or dissection. Average expansion rates are 0.07 cm per year in ascending aortic aneurysms and 0.19 cm per year for descending thoracic aortic aneurysms. Aortic diameter is a strong predictor of rupture, dissection, and mortality. For thoracic aortic aneurysms greater than 6 cm in diameter, annual rates of catastrophic complications are 3.6 percent for rupture, 3.7 percent for dissection, and 10.8 percent for death. Critical diameters, at which the incidences of complications are significantly increased, are 6.0 cm for aneurysms of the ascending aorta and 7.0 cm for aneurysms of the descending thoracic aorta.

Patients with Marfan syndrome have aneurysms that dilate at an accelerated rate and rupture or dissect at smaller diameters.

Clinical Manifestations

In many patients with thoracic aortic aneurysms, the aneurysm is discovered incidentally when imaging studies are obtained for unrelated reasons. Therefore patients often are asymptomatic at the time of diagnosis. When thoracic aortic aneurysms go undetected, they ultimately create symptoms and signs that correspond with the segment of aorta. These aneurysms produce a wide variety of manifestations, including compression or erosion of adjacent structures, aortic valve insufficiency, distal embolism, and rupture.

Local Compression and Erosion

Initially, expansion and impingement on adjacent structures causes mild chronic pain. The most common symptom in patients with ascending aortic aneurysms is anterior chest discomfort, frequently precordial in location, but may radiate to the neck and jaw, mimicking angina. Aneurysms of the ascending and transverse aortic arch can cause symptoms related to compression of the superior vena cava, the pulmonary artery, the airway, or the sternum. Expansion of the distal aortic arch can stretch the recurrent laryngeal nerve, resulting in left vocal cord paralysis and hoarseness. Descending thoracic and thoracoabdominal aneurysms cause back pain localized between the scapulae. Descending thoracic aortic aneurysms may cause varying degrees of airway obstruction, manifested as cough, wheezing, stridor, or pneumonitis. Compression or erosion of the esophagus creates dysphagia and hematemesis, respectively.

Aortic Valve Insufficiency

Ascending aortic aneurysms that involve the aortic root cause commissural displacement and annular dilatation, resulting in progressive aortic valve insufficiency, a widened pulse pressure and a diastolic murmur. These patients may present with progressive heart failure.

Distal Embolization

Thoracic aortic aneurysms are commonly lined with atheromatous plaque and mural thrombus. This debris may embolize distally, causing occlusion and thrombosis of the intercostals, visceral, renal, or lower-extremity branches.

Rupture

Patients with ruptured thoracic aortic aneurysms often experience sudden, severe pain in the anterior chest (ascending aorta), upper back or left chest (descending thoracic aorta), or left flank or abdomen (thoracoabdominal aorta). When ascending aortic aneurysms rupture, they usually bleed into the pericardial space, producing acute cardiac tamponade and death. Descending thoracic aortic aneurysms rupture into the pleural cavity, producing a combination of severe hemorrhagic shock and respiratory compromise.

Diagnostic Evaluation

Plain Radiographs

Plain radiographs of the chest, abdomen, or spine often provide enough information to support the initial diagnosis of thoracic aortic aneurysm. It is important to recognize that chest radiographs are commonly normal. Aortic root aneurysms, for example, are often hidden within the cardiac silhouette. Ascending aortic aneurysms produce a convex shadow to the right of the cardiac silhouette. Plain chest radiographs may demonstrate convexity in the right superior mediastinum, loss of the retrosternal space, or widening of the descending thoracic aortic shadow, which may be highlighted by a rim of calcification outlining the dilated aneurysmal aortic wall. Aortic calcification may also be seen in the upper abdomen on a standard roentgenogram made in the anteroposterior or lateral projections.

Echocardiography

Both transthoracic and transesophageal echocardiography provide excellent visualization of the ascending aorta, including the aortic root.

Computed Tomography

Computed tomographic (CT) scanning is widely available and provides visualization of the entire thoracic and abdominal aorta. Consequently, it is the most common—and arguably the most useful—imaging modality for evaluating thoracic aortic aneurysms. In addition to establishing the diagnosis, CT provides information regarding location, extent, anatomic anomalies, and relationship to major branch vessels. Contrast-enhanced CT provides information regarding the aortic lumen, and can detect mural thrombus, aortic dissection, inflammatory periaortic fibrosis, and mediastinal or retroperitoneal hematoma because of contained aortic rupture. It is particularly useful in determining the absolute diameter of the aorta.

Magnetic Resonance Angiography

Magnetic resonance angiography (MRA) has become widely available and has the capability of assessing the entire aorta. MRA offers the advantage of avoiding exposure to nephrotoxic contrast and ionizing radiation. MRA offers excellent visualization of branch vessel details. The MRA environment is not appropriate for critically ill patients.

Aortography and Cardiac Catheterization

Diagnostic aortography was considered the standard criterion for evaluating thoracic aortic disease; CT and MRA have largely replaced this modality. Technologic improvements in CT and MRA provide excellent aortic imaging with less morbidity than catheter-based studies. If other imaging studies have not provided adequate detail, aortography can be obtained in patients with suspected branch vessel occlusive disease.

Cardiac catheterization continues to play a major role in diagnosis and preoperative planning, especially in patients with ascending aortic involvement. In addition to assessing the status of the coronary arteries and left ventricular function, proximal aortography evaluates the degree of aortic valve insufficiency, the extent of aortic root involvement, coronary ostial displacement, and the relationship of the aneurysm to the arch vessels.

The benefits of obtaining information from catheter-based diagnostic studies should be weighed against the established limitations and potential complications. Aortography only images the lumen, and may underestimate the size of large aneurysms that contain laminated thrombus. Manipulation of intraluminal catheters can result in embolization. Proximal aortography carries a 0.6–1.2 percent risk of stroke. Other risks include allergic reaction to contrast, iatrogenic aortic dissection, and bleeding at the arterial access site.

Management

Indications for Surgery

Thoracic aortic aneurysms are repaired to prevent fatal rupture. Therefore, elective operation is recommended when the diameter exceeds 5–6 cm, or when the rate of dilatation exceeds 1 cm/y. In patients with connective tissue disorders, such as Marfan and Ehlers-Danlos syndromes, the threshold for operation is lower for both absolute size and rate of growth. Smaller ascending aortic aneurysms (4–5 cm) also are considered for repair when they are associated with aortic valve insufficiency.

Many patients are asymptomatic at presentation and can undergo thorough preoperative evaluation and optimization. Symptomatic patients are at increased risk and warrant expeditious evaluation. The onset of new pain in patients with known aneurysms is especially concerning, and may herald significant expansion, leakage, or impending rupture. Emergent intervention is reserved for patients presenting with rupture or superimposed acute dissection.

Preoperative Assessment and Preparation

Cardiac evaluation. Coronary artery disease is common in patients with thoracic aortic aneurysms and is responsible for a substantial proportion of early and late postoperative deaths. Similarly, valvular pathology and myocardial dysfunction have important implications. Transthoracic echocardiography is a satisfactory noninvasive method for evaluating both valvular and biventricular function. Dipyridamole-thallium myocardial scanning identifies regions of myocardium that have reversible ischemia. Cardiac catheterization with coronary arteriography is obtained in patients with evidence of coronary disease—based on history or noninvasive studies—or an ejection fraction of 30 percent or less. Patients who have asymptomatic distal aortic aneurysms and severe coronary artery occlusive disease undergo percutaneous transluminal angioplasty or surgical revascularization prior to aneurysm replacement.

Pulmonary evaluation. Pulmonary function screening with arterial blood gases and spirometry are routinely obtained. Patients with a forced expiratory volume in 1 second (FEV-1) greater than 1.0 L and a partial pressure of carbon dioxide (Pco_2) less than 45 mm Hg are considered surgical candidates. In suitable patients, borderline pulmonary function can be improved by implementing smoking cessation, weight loss, exercise, and treatment of bronchitis for 1–3 months before surgery.

Renal evaluation. Renal function is assessed preoperatively via serum electrolytes, blood urea nitrogen, and creatinine measurements. Information regarding kidney size and perfusion are obtained from a CT scan or aortogram. Perfusion strategies and perioperative medications are adjusted based on renal function. Patients with thoracoabdominal aortic aneurysms and severe proximal renal occlusive disease undergo renal artery endarterectomy, stenting, or bypass grafting.

Operative Repair

Proximal thoracic aortic aneurysms. Operations for proximal aortic aneurysms—which involve the ascending aorta and/or transverse arch—are performed through a midsternal incision and require cardiopulmonary bypass. The spectrum of operations ranges from simple graft replacement of the tubular portion of the ascending aorta to graft replacement of the entire proximal aorta, including the aortic root, with reattachment of the coronary arteries and brachiocephalic branches. Options for managing aortic valve pathology, the aneurysm, and perfusion deserve detailed consideration (Table 21-2).

When aortic valvular disease is present and the sinus segment is normal, separate repair or replacement of the aortic valve and graft replacement of the tubular segment of the ascending aorta are carried out. Mild-to-moderate valve insufficiency with annular dilatation can be addressed by plicating the annulus with mattress sutures placed below each commissure. Valve replacement with a biologic or mechanical prosthesis is performed in patients with more severe valvular insufficiency or with valvular stenosis. Patients with Marfan syndrome or annuloaortic ectasia require full aortic root replacement.

In most cases, aortic root replacement employs a mechanical or biologic graft that has both a valve and aortic conduit. There are currently three commercially available graft options: (1) composite valve grafts, which consist of a mechanical valve attached to a polyester tube graft; (2) aortic root homografts, from cadavers and cryopreserved; and (3) stentless porcine aortic root grafts. A final option is valve-sparing aortic root replacement, which has evolved during the past decade. The valve-sparing technique that is currently favored is called aortic root reimplantation, and involves excision of the aortic sinuses, attachment of a prosthetic graft to the patient's annulus, and resuspension of the native aortic valve inside the graft. The avoidance of anticoagulation is a major advantage.

TABLE 21-2 Surgical Options During Proximal Aortic Surgery

Options for treating aortic valve pathology
   Aortic valve annuloplasty (annular plication)
   Aortic valve replacement with mechanical or biologic prosthesis
   Aortic root replacement
      Composite valve graft
      Aortic homograft
      Stentless porcine root
      Valve-sparing techniques
      Pulmonary autograft (Ross procedure)

Options for graft repair of the aortic aneurysm
   Patch aortoplasty
   Ascending replacement only
   Beveled hemiarch replacement
   Total arch replacement with reattachment of brachiocephalic branches
   Total arch replacement with separate grafts to each brachiocephalic branch
   Elephant trunk technique

Perfusion options
   Standard cardiopulmonary bypass
   Profound hypothermic circulatory arrest without adjuncts
   Profound hypothermic circulatory arrest with adjuncts
      Retrograde cerebral perfusion
      Selective antegrade cerebral perfusion
      Combined antegrade and retrograde cerebral perfusion

Regardless of the type of conduit used, aortic root replacement requires reattachment of the coronary arteries to openings in the graft. As originally described by Bentall and DeBono, this was accomplished by suturing the intact aortic wall surrounding each coronary artery to the openings in the graft. The aortic wall was then wrapped around the graft to create hemostasis. However, this technique frequently resulted in pseudoaneurysm formation originating from leaks at the coronary reattachment sites. The Cabrol modification—in which a separate, small tube graft is sutured to the coronary ostia and the main aortic graft—achieves tension-free coronary anastomoses and reduces the risk of pseudoaneurysm formation. The Kochoucous button modification of the Bentall procedure is currently the most widely used technique. The aneurysmal aorta is excised, leaving buttons of aortic wall surrounding both coronary arteries, which are then mobilized and sutured to the aortic graft. The coronary suture lines may be reinforced with polytetrafluoroethylene (PTFE) felt or pericardium to enhance hemostasis. When adequate mobilization of the coronary arteries is not feasible because of extremely large aneurysms or scarring from previous surgery, the Cabrol technique or bypass using interposition saphenous vein grafts can be used.

Saccular aneurysms arising from the lesser curvature of the distal transverse arch, less than 50 percent of the aortic circumference, are treated by patch graft aortoplasty. For fusiform aneurysms, when the distal portion of the arch is a reasonable size, a single beveled replacement of the lower curvature (hemiarch) is performed. More extensive arch aneurysms require total replacement, with a distal anastomosis to the proximal descending thoracic aorta and separate reattachment of the brachiocephalic branches. In extreme cases, the aneurysm will involve the entire arch and extend into the descending thoracic aorta, and is approached using the Borst elephant trunk technique of total arch replacement.

The distal anastomosis is constructed with a portion of the graft left suspended within the proximal descending thoracic aorta. During a subsequent distal operation, this "trunk" is used to facilitate repair.

Aneurysms that are isolated to the ascending segment can be replaced using cardiopulmonary bypass and distal ascending aortic clamping. Aneurysms involving the transverse aortic arch cannot be clamped during the repair, and require a period without cardiopulmonary bypass support called circulatory arrest. To protect the brain and other vital organs during the circulatory arrest period, the patient undergoes profound cooling prior to stopping pump flow. An electroencephalogram is monitored during cooling. Once electrocerebral silence is achieved—indicating cessation of brain activity and minimization of metabolic requirements—the pump flow is stopped and the arch is repaired. Electrocerebral silence usually occurs when nasopharyngeal temperature falls below 20°C (68°F).

Two perfusion strategies have been developed to reduce the risks of circulatory arrest: retrograde cerebral perfusion and selective antegrade cerebral perfusion. Retrograde cerebral perfusion delivers cold, oxygenated blood from the pump into a cannula placed in the superior vena cava. The apparent benefits of this technique are likely because of maintenance of cerebral hypothermia and retrograde flushing of air and debris. Selective antegrade cerebral perfusion delivers blood directly into the brachiocephalic arteries while circulatory arrest is maintained in the rest of the body. Small, flexible, balloon perfusion catheters are inserted into one or more of the branch arteries. A method, rapidly gaining popularity because of its relative simplicity, involves cannulation of the right axillary artery. On initiating circulatory arrest and occluding the proximal innominate artery, the axillary artery cannula delivers blood flow into the cerebral circulation via the right common carotid artery. In the combined approach, antegrade perfusion is delivered during the arch reconstruction, and a brief period of retrograde perfusion is used to provide flushing immediately prior to resuming full cardiopulmonary bypass.

Many patients require staged operative procedures to achieve complete repair of extensive aneurysms. When the descending segment is not disproportionately large (compared to the proximal aorta) and is not causing symptoms, the proximal aortic repair is carried out first. An important benefit of this approach is that it allows treatment of valvular and coronary artery occlusive disease at the first operation. The elephant trunk technique is used to perform the aortic arch repair in these patients. This technique permits access to the distal portion of the graft at the second operation, without the need to dissect around the distal transverse aortic arch, reducing the risk of injuring the left recurrent laryngeal nerve, esophagus, and pulmonary artery.

Distal thoracic aortic aneurysms. Descending thoracic aortic aneurysms involve the aorta in between the left subclavian artery and the diaphragm. Thoracoabdominal aneurysms can involve the entire thoracoabdominal aorta, from the origin of the left subclavian artery to the aortic bifurcation, and are categorized based on the Crawford classification. Extent I thoracoabdominal aortic aneurysms involve most of the descending thoracic aorta, usually beginning near the left subclavian artery, and extend down to encompass the aorta at the origins of the celiac axis and superior mesenteric arteries; the renal arteries may also be involved. Extent II aneurysms also arise near the left subclavian artery, but extend distally into the infrarenal abdominal aorta and often reach the aortic bifurcation. Extent III aneurysms originate in the lower descending thoracic aorta (below the sixth rib) and extend into the abdomen. Extent IV aneurysms begin within the diaphragmatic hiatus and often involve the entire abdominal aorta.

Descending thoracic aortic aneurysms are repaired through a left thoracotomy. In patients with thoracoabdominal aortic aneurysms, the thoracotomy is extended across the costal margin and into the abdomen. A double-lumen endobronchial tube allows selective ventilation of the right lung and deflation of the left lung. Transperitoneal exposure of the thoracoabdominal aorta is achieved by performing medial visceral rotation and circumferential division of the diaphragm. During a period of aortic clamping, the diseased segment is replaced with a polyester tube graft. Important branch arteries—including intercostal, celiac, superior mesenteric, and renal arteries—are reattached to openings made in the side of the graft. Options for correcting branch vessel stenosis include endarterectomy, direct arterial stenting, and bypass grafting.

Clamping the descending thoracic aorta creates ischemia of the spinal cord and abdominal viscera. Clinically significant manifestations of hepatic, pancreatic, and bowel ischemia are relatively uncommon. Spinal cord injury resulting in paraplegia or paraparesis and acute renal failure remain major causes of morbidity and mortality after these operations. Therefore several aspects of the operation are devoted to minimizing spinal and renal ischemia. The authors multimodality approach to spinal cord protection includes expeditious repair to minimize aortic clamping time, moderate systemic heparinization (1.0 mg/kg) to prevent small-vessel thrombosis, mild permissive hypothermia (32–34°C [89.6–93.2°F] nasopharyngeal temperature), and reattachment of segmental intercostal and lumbar arteries. During extensive thoracoabdominal aortic repairs (i.e., Crawford extents I and II), cerebrospinal fluid drainage and left heart bypass, which provides perfusion of the distal aorta and its branches during the clamping period, are used. Balloon perfusion cannulas connected to the left heart bypass circuit can be used to deliver blood directly to the celiac axis and superior mesenteric artery during their reattachment. Renal protection is achieved by perfusing the kidneys with cold (4°C [39.2°F]) crystalloid.

As discussed above, patients with extensive aneurysms involving the ascending, transverse arch, and descending thoracic aorta generally undergo staged operations to achieve complete repair. In this setting, when the descending or thoracoabdominal component is symptomatic (e.g., back pain or rupture) or disproportionately large (compared to the ascending aorta), the distal segment is treated during the initial operation, and repair of the ascending aorta and transverse aortic arch is performed as a second procedure. A reversed elephant trunk repair—in which a portion of the proximal end of the aortic graft is inverted down into the lumen—can be employed during the first operation; this facilitates the second-stage repair of the proximal aorta.

Recent Results

Improvements in anesthesia, surgical technique, and perioperative care have led to improvements in outcome. Tables 21-3 and 21-4 display the authors' results with surgical repair of proximal and distal aortic aneurysms, respectively.

Postoperative Considerations

During the initial 24 to 48 h, meticulous blood pressure control is maintained to protect the integrity of the anastomoses. Generally, the authors liberally use nitroprusside, beta antagonists, and calcium channel blockers to maintain the mean arterial blood pressure between 80 and 90 mm Hg. In patients with

TABLE 21-3 Results of Surgical Repair of Proximal Thoracic Aortic Aneurysms (Without Dissection)

No. of patients	30-Day mortality	Stroke	Bleeding[a]	Renal failure[b]	Paraplegia or paraparesis
784	49 (6.3%)	23 (2.9%)	18 (2.3%)	14 (1.8%)	6 (0.8%)

[a]Bleeding requiring reoperation.
[b]Acute renal failure requiring hemodialysis.

friable aortic tissue, i.e., Marfan syndrome, we lower the target range to 70 to 80 mm Hg.

AORTIC DISSECTION

Pathology and Classification

Aortic dissection—the most common catastrophic event involving the aorta—is the progressive separation of the aortic wall layers that usually occurs after a tear forms in the intima and inner media. Propagation of the separation within the layers of the media results in the formation of two or more channels. The original lumen, which remains lined by the intima, is called the true lumen. The newly formed channel within the layers of the media is called the false lumen. Additional tears allow communication between the two channels and are called re-entry sites.

In most cases, dissection occurs in patients without aneurysms. The subsequent progressive dilatation of the weakened outer aortic wall results in an aneurysm. Alternatively, in patients with degenerative aneurysms, the ongoing deterioration of the aortic wall can lead to a superimposed dissection; the overused term "dissecting aneurysm" should be reserved for this specific situation.

The extensive disruption of the aortic wall has severe anatomic consequences. The outer wall of the false lumen is extremely thin and fragile, making it prone to expansion or rupture in the face of ongoing hemodynamic stresses. The expanding false lumen can compress the true lumen and interfere with blood flow in the aorta or any of the aortic branch vessels, including the coronary, carotid, intercostal, visceral, renal, and iliac arteries. When the separation

TABLE 21-4 Results of Surgical Repair of Distal Thoracic Aortic Aneurysms (Without Dissection)

Extent[a]	No. of patients	30-day mortality	Stroke	Bleeding[b]	Renal failure[c]	Paraplegia or paraparesis
DTAA	282	12 (4.3%)	9 (3.2%)	6 (2.1%)	6 (2.1%)	6 (2.1%)
TAAA I	436	21 (4.8%)	7 (1.6%)	7 (1.6%)	7 (1.6%)	17 (3.9%)
TAAA II	411	36 (8.8%)	9 (2.2%)	19 (4.6%)	44 (10.7%)	33 (8.0%)
TAAA III	283	16 (5.7%)	2 (0.7%)	5 (1.8%)	20 (7.1%)	7 (2.5%)
TAAA IV	337	10 (3.0%)	1 (0.3%)	10 (3.0%)	25 (7.4%)	5 (1.5%)
Total	1749	95 (5.4%)	28 (1.6%)	47 (2.7%)	102 (5.8%)	68 (3.9%)

[a]Thoracoabdominal aortic aneurysm extents I–IV based on Crawford's classification.
[b]Bleeding requiring reoperation.
[c]Acute renal failure requiring hemodialysis.
DTAA = descending thoracic aortic aneurysm; TAAA = thoracoabdominal aortic aneurysm.

of layers occurs within the aortic root, the aortic valve commissures can become unhinged, resulting in an acutely incompetent valve.

Dissections are categorized based on anatomic location and extent. There are two traditional classification schemes: the DeBakey classification and the Stanford classification. Both of these methods describe the segments of aorta that are involved, rather than the site of the initial intimal tear.

Dissection is considered acute within the first 14 days. After 14 days, the dissection is described as chronic. The distinction between acute and chronic dissections has important implications in perioperative management strategies, techniques, and results.

Penetrating aortic ulcers are essentially disrupted atherosclerotic plaques. Eventually the ulcer can penetrate through the aortic wall, leading to dissection or rupture. An intramural hematoma is a collection of blood within the aortic wall without an intimal tear; accumulation of the hematoma ultimately results in dissection. The current consensus is that these variants of dissection should be treated identically to classic dissection.

Etiology and Natural History

Aortic dissection occurs in approximately 5–10 patients per million population per year. Without treatment, nearly one half of patients with acute proximal aortic dissection die within 24 h, and 60 percent of patients with acute distal aortic dissections die within 1 month.

Common general cardiovascular risk factors, such as smoking, hypertension, atherosclerosis, and hypercholesterolemia, are associated with aortic dissection. Patients with connective tissue disorders, aortitis, bicuspid aortic valve, or preexisting medial degenerative disease are at risk for dissection.

Clinical Manifestations

The onset of dissection often is associated with severe chest or back pain—classically described as "tearing"—that migrates distally as the dissection progresses along the length of the aorta. Pain in the anterior chest suggests involvement of the proximal aorta, although pain in the back and abdomen indicates involvement of the distal segment.

Proximal aortic dissection can directly injure the aortic valve. The severity of aortic valve insufficiency varies with the degree of commissural disruption. Patients with acute aortic valve regurgitation may complain of severe acute heart failure and worsening dyspnea.

Proximal dissections can extend into the coronary arteries creating acute coronary occlusion, most often the right coronary artery. By producing symptoms and signs consistent with myocardial ischemia, this presentation can mask the presence of aortic dissection, resulting in delayed diagnosis and treatment.

The thin and inflamed outer wall of a dissected ascending aorta often will produce a serosanguineous pericardial effusion that can accumulate and cause tamponade. Suggestive signs include jugular venous distention, muffled heart tones, pulsus paradoxus, and low-voltage electrocardiogram (ECG) tracings. Free rupture into the pericardial space produces rapid tamponade and generally is fatal.

Any branch vessel from the aorta can be compromised during progression of the dissection. Depending on which arteries are involved, dissection can produce acute stroke, paraplegia, hepatic failure, bowel infarction, renal failure, or a threatened ischemic limb.

Diagnostic Evaluation

Because of variations in severity and the wide variety of potential clinical manifestations, the diagnosis of acute aortic dissection can be challenging. Diagnostic delays are common; delays beyond 24 h after hospitalization occur in up to 39 percent of cases. A high index of suspicion is critical.

Most patients with acute aortic dissection (80–90 percent) experience severe pain in the chest, back, or abdomen. Classically, the pain occurs suddenly, has a "tearing" quality, and migrates distally as the dissection progresses along the aorta. For classification purposes (acute vs. subacute vs. chronic), the onset of pain is generally considered to represent the beginning of the dissection process. Most of the other common symptoms are nonspecific (Table 21-5).

A discrepancy in extremity pulse and/or blood pressure is the classic physical finding in patients with aortic dissection. This often occurs because of changes in flow in the true and false lumens. Involvement of the proximal aorta often creates differences between the right and left arms, although distal aortic dissection often causes differences between the upper and lower extremities.

Laboratory studies are of little help in diagnosing acute aortic dissection. Normal ECGs and serum markers in the setting of acute chest pain should

TABLE 21-5 Anatomic Complications of Aortic Dissection and Their Associated Symptoms and Signs

Anatomic manifestation	Symptoms and signs
Aortic valve insufficiency	Dyspnea
	Murmur
	Pulmonary rales
	Shock
Coronary malperfusion	Chest pain with characteristics of angina
	Nausea/vomiting
	Shock
	Ischemic changes on electrocardiogram
	Elevated cardiac enzymes
Pericardial tamponade	Dyspnea
	Jugular venous distention
	Pulsus paradoxus
	Muffled cardiac tones
	Shock
	Low-voltage electrocardiogram
Subclavian or iliofemoral artery malperfusion	Cold, painful extremity
	Extremity sensory and motor deficits
	Peripheral pulse deficit
Carotid artery malperfusion	Syncope
	Focal neurologic deficit (transient or persistent)
	Carotid pulse deficit
	Coma
Spinal malperfusion	Paraplegia
	Incontinence
Visceral malperfusion	Nausea/vomiting
	Abdominal pain
Renal malperfusion	Oliguria or anuria
	Hematuria

raise suspicion regarding the presence of aortic dissection. It is important to remember that when ECG changes and elevated serum markers indicate a myocardial infarction, they do not exclude the diagnosis of aortic dissection. Although chest radiographs may demonstrate a widened mediastinum or abnormal aortic contour, up to 16 percent of patients have a normal-appearing chest radiograph.

Once the diagnosis of dissection is considered, the thoracic aorta should be imaged with CT, MRA, or echocardiography. The diagnosis is usually established via contrast-enhanced CT. The classic diagnostic feature is a double-lumen aorta. Additionally, CT scans provide essential information regarding the segments of the aorta involved; the acuity of the dissection; aortic dilatation, including the presence of preexisting degenerative aneurysms; and the development of threatening sequelae, including pericardial effusion, early aortic rupture, and branch vessel compromise. The MRI suite is not well-suited for critically ill patients. In patients who cannot undergo contrast-enhanced CT or MRA, transthoracic echocardiography can be used to establish the diagnosis. Transesophageal echocardiography is excellent for determining and distinguishing the presence of dissection, aneurysm, and intramural hematoma in the ascending aorta.

In patients with proximal aortic dissection, coronary angiography is obtained prior to surgery in selected patients (i.e., those who have evidence of preexisting coronary artery disease).

Management

Initial Assessment and Management

Regardless of the location of the dissection, the initial management is the same for all patients with suspected or confirmed acute aortic dissection. Aggressive pharmacologic management is started once there is clinical suspicion of dissection, and is continued during the diagnostic evaluation. The goals of pharmacologic treatment are to stabilize the dissection and prevent rupture.

Patients are monitored closely in an intensive care unit. Indwelling radial arterial catheters are used to monitor blood pressure and optimize titration of antihypertensive agents. Pulmonary artery catheters are reserved for patients with severe cardiopulmonary dysfunction.

The initial evaluation focuses on whether any life-threatening complications are present. Particular attention is paid to changes in neurologic status, peripheral pulses, and urine output. Serial laboratory studies—including arterial blood gases, complete blood cell count, prothrombin and partial thromboplastin times, serum electrolytes, creatinine, blood urea nitrogen, and liver enzymes—are useful for determining the presence of organ ischemia.

The initial management strategy—commonly described as "antihypertensive therapy" or "blood pressure control"—focuses on reducing aortic wall stress, the force of left ventricular ejection, and the rate of change in blood pressure (dP/dT). Reductions in dP/dT are achieved by lowering both cardiac contractility and blood pressure. The drugs initially used to accomplish these goals include intravenous beta adrenergic blockers, direct vasodilators, calcium channel blockers, and angiotensin-converting enzyme inhibitors. These agents are used to achieve a heart rate between 60 and 80 beats/min, a systolic blood pressure between 100 and 110 mm Hg, and a mean arterial blood pressure between 60 and 75 mm Hg. These hemodynamic targets are maintained as long as urine output remains adequate and neurologic function is not impaired.

Adequate pain control with intravenous opiates such as morphine or fentanyl is important.

Beta antagonists are administered to all patients with acute aortic dissections, unless there are contraindications such as severe heart failure, bradyarrhythmia, high-grade atrioventricular conduction block, or bronchospastic disease. The dose of β antagonists is titrated to achieve a heart rate of 60–80 beats/min. In patients who cannot receive beta antagonists, calcium channel blockers such as diltiazem are an alternative. Nitroprusside, a direct vasodilator, can be administered once beta blockade is adequate. Enalapril and other angiotensin-converting enzyme inhibitors are useful in patients with renal malperfusion; the decrease in rennin release may improve renal blood flow.

Management of Proximal Aortic Dissection

Acute proximal dissection. The presence of an acute proximal aortic dissection has traditionally been an absolute indication for emergency surgical repair. However, specific patient groups may benefit from nonoperative management or delayed operation. Situations that warrant consideration of delayed repair include: (1) patients presenting with acute stroke or mesenteric ischemia; (2) older adult patients with substantial comorbidity; (3) stable patients who may benefit from transfer to specialized centers; and (4) patients who have undergone a cardiac operation in the remote past.

In the absence of the circumstances listed above, most patients with acute proximal aortic dissection undergo urgent graft replacement of the ascending aorta. The operation is conducted in a manner similar to that described for aneurysms of the transverse aortic arch. Intraoperative transesophageal echocardiography is commonly performed before beginning the operation to further assess baseline myocardial and valvular function and, if necessary, to confirm the diagnosis. The operation is performed via a median sternotomy with cardiopulmonary bypass and hypothermic circulatory arrest. The patient is cooled until monitoring demonstrates electrocerebral silence. Cardiopulmonary bypass is then stopped and the ascending aorta is opened. The dissecting membrane that separates the true and false lumens is completely excised. After occluding the innominate artery with a clamp or balloon catheter, flow from the axillary artery cannula is used to provide selective antegrade cerebral perfusion. The transverse aortic arch is carefully inspected. Replacement of the entire arch is performed only if a primary tear is located in the arch or if the arch is aneurysmal; in most cases, a less extensive beveled "hemiarch" repair is adequate. The distal aortic cuff is prepared by tacking the inner and outer walls together and using surgical adhesive to obliterate the false lumen and strengthen the tissue. A polyester tube graft is sutured to the distal aortic cuff. The anastomosis between the graft and the aorta is fashioned so that blood flow will be directed into the true lumen. In the absence of annuloaortic ectasia or Marfan syndrome—which generally require aortic root replacement—aortic valve insufficiency can be corrected by resuspending the commissures onto the outer aortic wall. The proximal aortic cuff is prepared with tacking sutures and surgical adhesive prior to performing the proximal aortic anastomosis.

In the majority of patients, the dissection persists distal to the site of the operative repair. Extensive dilatation of the distal aortic segment develops in 16 percent of the survivors, and rupture of the dilated distal aorta is the most common cause of late death. Following proximal repair, patients require aggressive management of the remaining acute distal aortic dissection.

Management of Distal Aortic Dissection

Nonoperative management. Nonoperative management of acute distal aortic dissection results in lower morbidity and mortality rates than those achieved with surgical treatment. These patients are primarily managed with pharmacologic treatment. However, the most common causes of death during nonoperative treatment are aortic rupture and end-organ malperfusion. Therefore, patients are continually reassessed for the development of complications. Serial CT scans are compared to the initial scan to rule out significant aortic expansion.

Once the patient has been stabilized, pharmacologic management is shifted from intravenous to oral. Oral therapy, including a beta antagonist, is initiated when systolic pressure is consistently 100–110 mm Hg and the neurologic, renal, and cardiovascular systems are stable.

Long-term pharmacologic therapy is important with chronic aortic dissection. Beta blockers remain the drugs of choice. In a 20-year follow-up study, DeBakey and colleagues reported that inadequate blood pressure control was associated with late aneurysm formation. Aneurysms developed in only 17 percent with "good" blood pressure control and 45 percent with "poor" control.

Contrast-enhanced CT and MRA scans provide excellent aortic imaging and facilitate serial comparisons to detect progressive aortic expansion. The first surveillance scan is obtained approximately 6 weeks after the onset of dissection. Subsequent scans are obtained at least every 3 months for the first year, every 6 months for the second year, and annually thereafter. Patients who have undergone graft repair also are evaluated with annual CT or MRA.

Indications for surgery. Surgery is reserved for patients who experience complications. Surgical intervention for acute distal aortic dissection is directed toward prevention or repair of rupture and relief of ischemic manifestations.

During the acute phase, the specific indications for operative intervention include (1) aortic rupture, (2) increasing periaortic or pleural fluid, (3) rapidly expanding aortic diameter, (4) uncontrolled hypertension, and (5) persistent pain despite adequate medical therapy. Acute dissection superimposed on a preexisting aneurysm is considered a life-threatening condition.

Acute malperfusion syndromes warrant intervention. In the recent past, visceral and renal malperfusion were considered indications for operation. Advances in percutaneous interventions have largely replaced open surgery for these complications. Percutaneous fenestration of the dissecting membrane or placement of branch artery stents can restore organ perfusion. When unsuccessful, surgical options—which include graft replacement of the aorta, open aortic fenestration, and visceral/renal artery bypass—can be employed. Lower extremity ischemia usually is addressed surgically via extra-anatomic revascularization.

In the chronic phase, the indications for operative intervention are similar to those for degenerative thoracic aortic aneurysms. Operation is considered when the affected segment has reached 5–6 cm, or when an aneurysm has enlarged more than 1 cm during a 1-year period.

Operative repair. Surgical repair of the descending thoracic or thoracoabdominal aorta in the setting of acute aortic dissection is associated with high morbidity and mortality. Therefore, the primary goals of surgery are to prevent fatal rupture and restore branch vessel perfusion. A limited graft repair of the symptomatic segment achieves these goals while minimizing risks. Because the most common site of rupture in distal aortic dissection is in the proximal third of the descending thoracic aorta, the upper descending thoracic aorta usually is repaired.

In patients with acute dissection, adjuncts that provide spinal cord protection are used liberally because of the increased risk of paraplegia. Cerebrospinal fluid drainage and left heart bypass often are employed. Proximal control is usually obtained between the left common carotid and left subclavian artery. The proximal and distal anastomoses use all layers of aortic wall, thereby excluding the false lumen.

A more aggressive replacement usually is performed during elective aortic repairs in patients with chronic dissection. In many regards, the operative approach in these patients is identical to that used for descending thoracic and thoracoabdominal aortic aneurysms. One key difference is the need to excise as much dissecting membrane as possible to clearly identify the true and false lumens and locate all important branch vessels. When the dissection extends into the visceral or renal arteries, the membrane can be fenestrated or the false lumen can be obliterated using sutures or intraluminal stents. When a distal dissection has progressed retrograde into the transverse aortic arch and placement of the proximal clamp is not technically feasible, hypothermic circulatory arrest can be used to facilitate the proximal portion of the repair.

Recent Results

Proximal aortic dissection. Table 21-6 displays these authors' results with proximal aortic dissection repair in 489 patients. Over 40 percent of repairs were performed in the acute setting. Compared to the lethality of unrepaired acute proximal aortic dissection, contemporary results of surgical treatment are excellent.

Distal aortic dissection. Despite aggressive pharmacologic management, 10–20 percent of patients die during the initial treatment phase. The primary causes of death during nonoperative management include rupture, malperfusion and cardiac failure. Risk factors associated with treatment failure—defined as death or need for surgery—include an enlarged aorta, persistent hypertension despitemaximal treatment, oliguria and peripheral ischemia. Table 21-7 displays the results of these authors with distal aortic dissection repair in 714 patients.

ENDOVASCULAR TREATMENT OF THORACIC AORTIC DISEASE

Although not yet considered standard therapy, endovascular stent-graft repairs are poised to play a major role in the armamentarium for treating thoracic aortic

TABLE 21-6 Results of Surgical Repair of Proximal Thoracic Aortic Dissection

Dissection	No. of patients	30-day mortality	Stroke	Bleeding[a]	Renal failure[b]	Paraplegia or paraparesis
Acute	209	23 (11.0%)	13 (6.2%)	8 (3.8%)	4 (1.9%)	2 (1.0%)
Chronic	280	12 (4.3%)	9 (3.2%)	11 (3.9%)	2 (0.7%)	2 (0.7%)
Total	489	35 (7.2%)	22 (4.5%)	19 (3.9%)	6 (1.2%)	4 (0.8%)

[a]Bleeding requiring reoperation.
[b]Acute renal failure requiring hemodialysis.

TABLE 21-7 Results of Surgical Repair of Distal Thoracic Aortic Dissection

Extent[a]	No. of patients	30-day mortality	Stroke	Bleeding[b]	Renal failure[c]	Paraplegia or paraparesis
DTAA	146	3 (2.1%)	1 (0.7%)	6 (4.1%)	3 (2.1%)	5 (3.4%)
TAAA I	218	13 (6.0%)	9 (4.1%)	2 (0.9%)	7 (3.2%)	6 (2.8%)
TAAA II	273	10 (3.7%)	6 (2.2%)	5 (1.8%)	13 (4.8%)	17 (6.2%)
TAAA III	44	3 (6.8%)	1 (2.3%)	1 (2.3%)	1 (2.3%)	1 (2.3%)
TAAA IV	33	2 (6.1%)	1 (3.0%)	0 (0.0%)	1 (3.0%)	1 (3.0%)
Total	714	31 (4.3%)	18 (2.5%)	14 (2.0%)	25 (3.5%)	30 (4.2%)

[a]Thoracoabdominal aortic aneurysm extents I–IV based on Crawford's classification.
[b]Bleeding requiring reoperation.
[c]Acute renal failure requiring hemodialysis.
DTAA = descending thoracic aortic aneurysm; TAAA = thoracoabdominal aortic aneurysm.

disease. In 1991, Parodi reported using stent-grafts for repair of abdominal aortic aneurysms. Three years after this seminal report, Dake and colleagues reported endovascular descending thoracic aortic repair using "home-made" stent-grafts in 13 patients. Subsequent reports have applied this new, less-invasive option in patients with aortic dissection and traumatic, mycotic, and ruptured aneurysms of the descending thoracic aorta. Data demonstrating long-term effectiveness currently are not available.

General mortality and morbidity following endovascular repair of descending thoracic aortic aneurysms is currently difficult to assess. For example, in the Stanford experience with "first generation" stent grafts in 103 patients with descending thoracic aortic aneurysms, the operative mortality rate was 9 percent, stroke occurred in 7 percent, paraplegia/paraparesis occurred in 3 percent, and actuarial survival was only 73 ± 5 percent at 2 years. However, 62 (60 percent) patients were not considered candidates for thoracotomy and open surgical repair; as expected, this group experienced the majority of the morbidity and mortality.

As the experience with descending thoracic aortic stent grafts continues to increase, reports regarding complications specifically related to device deployment are emerging in the literature. Many of these complications are directly related to manipulation of the delivery system within the iliac arteries and aorta. Patients with small, calcified, tortuous iliofemoral arteries are at particular risk for life-threatening iliac artery rupture. A more common complication is acute iatrogenic aortic dissection into the aortic arch and ascending aorta. There are several reports of this complication, most involving "new generation" devices and requiring emergency repair of the ascending aorta and aortic arch via sternotomy and cardiopulmonary bypass. Such a dissection converts a localized descending thoracic aortic disease into an acute problem involving the entire thoracic aorta. Early reports have documented a 20–25 percent incidence of endoleak, this is expected to decline. Early type I endoleaks—which result from an incomplete seal between the graft and aorta at attachment sites—can precipitate aortic rupture. Therefore, aggressive intervention is recommended, if feasible, when type I endoleaks develop within weeks after the initial procedure. Other device-related problems include stent graft misdeployment, device migration, and endograft kinking.

In contrast to endovascular repair of descending thoracic aortic aneurysms, experience with endovascular treatment of proximal aortic disease remains limited and purely experimental. The unique anatomy of the aortic arch and need for uninterrupted cerebral perfusion pose difficult challenges. Similarly, the experience with endovascular thoracoabdominal aortic aneurysm repair remains anecdotal. Thoracoabdominal aortic aneurysms have been repaired using hybrid approaches, with stent graft coverage of the entire aneurysm including branch vessel ostia, followed by open visceral bypass grafting to restore organ perfusion.

Acknowledgment

The authors gratefully acknowledge Autumn Jamison and Stacey Carter for their invaluable assistance while preparing this manuscript.

Suggested Readings

Coselli JS, LeMaire SA, Büket S: Marfan syndrome: The variability and outcome of operative management. J Vasc Surg 21:432, 1995.

Coselli JS, LeMaire SA, Conklin LD, et al: Left heart bypass during descending thoracic aortic aneurysm repair does not prevent paraplegia. Ann Thorac Surg 77:1298, 2004.

Coselli JS, LeMaire SA, Conklin LD, et al: Morbidity and mortality after extent II thoracoabdominal aortic aneurysm repair. Ann Thorac Surg 73:1107, 2002.

Coselli JS, LeMaire SA, Köksoy C, et al: Cerebrospinal fluid drainage reduces paraplegia after thoracoabdominal aortic aneurysm repair: Results of a randomized clinical trial. J Vasc Surg 35:635, 2002.

Coselli JS, LeMaire SA: Left heart bypass reduces paraplegia rates following thoracoabdominal aortic aneurysm repair. Ann Thorac Surg 67:1931, 1999.

Coselli JS, LeMaire SA, Miller CC III, et al: Mortality and paraplegia after thoracoabdominal aortic aneurysm repair: A risk factor analysis. Ann Thorac Surg 69:404, 2000.

LeMaire SA, Miller CC III, Conklin LD, et al: A new predictive model for adverse outcomes after elective thoracoabdominal aortic aneurysm repair. Ann Thorac Surg 71:1233, 2001.

LeMaire SA, Miller CC III, Conklin LD, et al: Estimating group mortality and paraplegia rates after thoracoabdominal aortic aneurysm repair. Ann Thorac Surg 75:508, 2003.

Coselli JS, LeMaire SA, Poli de Figueiredo L, et al: Paraplegia following thoracoabdominal aortic aneurysm repair: Is dissection a risk factor? Ann Thorac Surg 63:28, 1997.

Coselli JS, LeMaire SA, Walkes JC: Surgery for acute type A dissection. Operative Tech Thorac Cardiovasc Surg 4:13, 1999.

22 | Arterial Disease

Alan B. Lumsden, Peter H. Lin,
Ruth L. Bush, and Changyi Chen

EPIDEMIOLOGY

Peripheral arterial disease occurs in 12 percent of the adult population, affecting 8–10 million people in the United States. The most common symptomatic manifestation is intermittent claudication, which occurs at an annual incidence of 2 percent in people over the age of 65. These patients are at a significantly higher risk of death compared with healthy controls of similar age.

Clinical Manifestations of Vascular Disease

The Vascular History

Symptoms are elicited based on the presenting complaint. The patient with lower extremity pain on ambulation has intermittent claudication that occurs in certain muscle groups; for example, calf pain on exercise usually reflects superficial femoral artery disease, although pain in the buttocks reflects iliac disease. In most cases, the pain manifests in one muscle group below the level of the affected artery, occurs only with exercise, and is relieved with rest only to recur at the same location, hence the term "window-gazers disease." Rest pain (a manifestation of severe underlying occlusive disease) is constant and occurs in the foot (not the muscle groups), typically at the metatarsophalangeal junction, and is relieved by dependency. Often the patient is prompted to sleep with their foot hanging off one side of the bed to increase the hydrostatic pressure.

The patient with carotid disease in most cases is totally asymptomatic, having been referred based on the finding of a cervical bruit or duplex finding of stenosis. Symptoms of carotid territory TIAs include transient monocular blindness (amaurosis), contralateral weakness or numbness, and dysphasia. Symptoms persisting longer than 24 h constitute a stroke.

Chronic mesenteric ischemia presents with postprandial abdominal pain and weight loss. The patient fears eating because of the pain, avoids food, and loses weight. It is very unlikely that a patient with abdominal pain who has not lost weight has chronic mesenteric ischemia.

Of particular importance in the previous medical history is noting prior vascular interventions (endovascular or open surgical), and all vascular patients should have inquiry made about their prior cardiac history and current cardiac symptoms. Approximately 30 percent of vascular patients will be diabetic. A smoking history should be elicited.

The Vascular Examination

Specific vascular examination includes pulse examination (femoral, popliteal, posterior tibial, and dorsalis pedis) of the lower extremity. The femoral pulse is located at the midinguinal point (midway between the anterior superior iliac spine and the pubic tubercle). The popliteal artery is best palpated with the knee flexed to 45 degrees and the foot flat and supported on the examination table to relax the calf muscles. Palpation of the popliteal artery is a bimanual technique.

515

Both thumbs are placed on the tibial tuberosity anteriorly and the fingers are placed into the popliteal fossa between the two heads of the gastrocnemius muscle. The popliteal artery is palpated by compressing it against the posterior aspect of the tibia just below the knee. The posterior tibial pulse is detected by palpation 2 cm posterior to the medial malleolus. The dorsalis pedis is detected 1 cm lateral to the hallucis longus extensor tendon (which dorsiflexes the great toe and is clearly visible) on the dorsum of the foot. Pulses are graded using a four-point scale: 2+ is normal; 1+ palpable, but reduced; 0 is absent to palpation (Doppler signals should be noted); and 3+ indicates aneurysmal enlargement. The foot should be carefully examined for pallor on elevation and rubor on dependency, as these findings are indicative of chronic ischemia. Ulceration and other findings specific to disease states are described in relevant sections below.

Upper extremity examination is necessary when an arteriovenous graft is to be inserted in patients who have symptoms of arm pain with exercise. Thoracic outlet syndrome (TOS) can result in occlusion or aneurysm formation of the subclavian artery. Distal embolization is a manifestation of TOS; consequently, the fingers should be examined for signs of ischemia and ulceration. The axillary artery enters the limb below the middle of the clavicle, where it can be palpated in thin patients. It is usually easily palpable in the axilla and medial upper arm. The brachial artery is most easily located at the antecubital fossa immediately medial to the biceps tendon. The radial artery is palpable at the wrist anterior to the radius. The ulnar is palpable or present on Doppler examination on the medial side of the wrist. Doppler signals, particularly in the thumb, are usually detectable on either side of the digits. Digital Doppler signals also frequently can be detected in the fingers. The Allen test is a test of patency of the palmar arch. The radial and ulnar pulses are localized at the wrist, and the examiner occludes both by digital pressure. Then after the patient opens and closes the hand, pressure over one artery is released. Failure in hand reperfusion from one side indicates an incomplete palmar arch and indicates that occlusion of one artery (by catheter placement or by using it for an anastomosis) may be more likely to result in hand ischemia.

There is increasing interest in the use of the ankle-brachial index (ABI) to evaluate patients at risk for cardiovascular events. An ABI less than 0.9 correlates with increased risk of myocardial infarction and indicates significant, although perhaps asymptomatic, underlying peripheral vascular disease. The ankle-brachial index is determined in the following ways. Blood pressure (BP) is measured in both upper extremities using the highest systolic BP as the denominator for the ABI. The ankle pressure is determined by placing a blood pressure cuff above the ankle and measuring the return to flow of the posterior tibial and dorsalis pedis arteries using a pencil Doppler over each artery. The ratio of the systolic pressure in each vessel divided by the highest arm systolic pressure can be used to express the ABI in both the posterior tibial and dorsalis pedis arteries. Normal is more than 1. Claudicants are in the 0.6–0.9 range, with rest pain and gangrene occurring at less than 0.3. The test is less reliable in patients with heavily calcified vessels because of noncompressibility (i.e., diabetes and end-stage renal disease).

Aortic Examination

The abdomen should be palpated for an abdominal aortic aneurysm, detected as an expansile pulse above the level of the umbilicus. Because the aorta typically divides at the level of the umbilicus, an aortic aneurysm is most frequently palpable in the epigastrium. In thin individuals a normal aortic pulsation is palpable, although in obese patients even large aortic aneurysms may not be detectable. Suspicion of a clinically enlarged aorta should lead to the performance of an ultrasound scan for a more accurate definition of aortic diameter.

Carotid Examination

The carotids should be auscultated for the presence of bruits. A bruit at the angle of the mandible is a significant finding, leading to follow-up duplex scanning. Differential diagnosis is a transmitted murmur from a sclerotic or stenotic aortic valve. The carotid is palpable deep to the sternocleidomastoid muscle in the neck. Palpation, however, should be gentle and rarely yields clinically useful information. A prominent pulsation usually reflects tortuosity, although aneurysms occasionally occur.

The Vascular Graft Examination

The in situ lower extremity graft runs in the subcutaneous fat and can be palpated along most of its length. A change in pulse quality, aneurysmal enlargement, or a new bruit should be carefully noted and may represent development of stenoses or aneurysmal enlargement. Axillofemoral grafts, femoral-to-femoral grafts, and arteriovenous access grafts can usually be easily palpated as well.

The Noninvasive Vascular Laboratory and Vascular Testing

This includes duplex scanning, and measurement of segmental arterial pressures with pulse volume recordings (PVRs).

Duplex Scanning

Duplex implies two forms of ultrasound: B-mode, which is typically used to create a gray-scale anatomic image, and Doppler ultrasound. The latter allows moving structures to be imaged. Most physicians use the traditional pencil Doppler to detect nonpalpable blood vessels by sound. The more sophisticated duplex scanners display moving structures (in most cases red blood cells moving within a vascular structure) as a color map proportional to the flow velocity and as an auditory signal. Furthermore, the scanner permits an accurate graphical depiction of the velocity of the moving red blood cells, and this permits measurement of peak systolic velocity and end-diastolic velocity. It is the measurement of the end-diastolic flow velocity that is used to determine the degree of narrowing of a carotid artery.

Duplex scanning has become the first-line tool for imaging carotid arteries, lower extremity bypass grafts, the abdominal aorta, and for diagnosis of deep venous thrombosis.

For diagnosis of deep vein thrombosis (DVT), the B mode component of the scanner is of more importance. An occluded vein typically is larger than normal, not completely compressible, lacks respiratory variation, does not show flow augmentation with calf compression, and may have collateral flow.

Segmental Pressures

By placing serial blood pressure cuffs down the lower extremity and then measuring the pressure with a Doppler probe as flow returns to the artery below the cuff, it is possible to determine segmental pressures down the leg. This data can then be used to infer the level of the occlusion. The systolic pressure at each level is expressed as a ratio, with the highest systolic pressure in the upper extremities as the denominator. A pressure gradient of 20 mmHg between two subsequent levels is usually indicative of occlusive disease at that level. The most frequently used index is the ratio of the ankle pressure to the brachial pressure, the ABI. Normally the ABI is greater than 1.0, and a value less than 0.9 indicates some degree of arterial obstruction and has been shown to be correlated with an increased risk of coronary heart disease. Patients with claudication typically have an ABI in the 0.5–0.7 range, and those with rest pain are in the 0.3–0.5 range. Those with gangrene have an ABI less than 0.3. However, these ranges can vary depending on the degree of compressibility of the vessel.

In those patients with noncompressible vessels, segmental plethysmography can be useful. Cuffs placed at different levels on the leg detect changes in leg volume, which also can be used to localize levels of occlusion.

Angiography

Essential components to angiography are vascular access and catheter placement in the vascular bed to be imaged. The imaging system and the contrast agent are used to opacify the target vessel.

The preangiography checklist includes serum creatinine; medications such as anticoagulants and oral hypoglycemics, specifically metformin (which can cause lactic acidosis when combined with contrast agents); history of dye allergy; and hydration status. Contrast angiography should be avoided if possible in all patients with a serum creatinine level greater than 3.0. It should be performed only if it is truly necessary, and other imaging modalities cannot provide equivalent information in patients with a serum creatinine level greater than 2.0. All patients with a serum creatinine level greater than 1.7 mg/dL are premedicated with acetylcysteine 600 mg by mouth twice daily on the day before and the day of angiography.

Many patients give a history of dye allergy, which may vary from trivial to life-threatening. In those with a history of anaphylaxis, contrast is best avoided. However, most patients can be safely given contrast after appropriate preparation. The usual prophylactic treatment is oral prednisone 40 mg 12 h and 1 h prior to the procedure, and oral diphenhydramine hydrochloride 50 mg 1 hour prior to the procedure.

For angiography, the right femoral artery is most commonly accessed. The puncture should be over the femoral head and its position should be determined fluoroscopically (not estimated using skin landmarks). The artery is entered with an 18-gauge Seldinger needle. Good pulsatile flow confirms arterial access. A Bentsen wire is then inserted up into the aorta under fluoroscopic guidance. After removing the needle, a catheter is inserted over the wire. The catheter and wire can be steered to the target vascular bed and dye injected to opacify the vessels. Contrast angiography provides a lumenogram, so thrombus-filled aneurysms can be easily missed. Digital subtraction angiography (in which bony landmarks are electronically removed) provides the best delineation of vascular pathology. Once the procedure is complete, the catheter is removed from the femoral artery and pressure applied. This technique forms the basis for all interventional procedures.

Brachial artery access is another option, but carries a significantly higher incidence of complications, mainly thrombosis and median nerve compression, and potential damage from extravasation.

Computed Tomographic Angiography

CTA is a noninvasive, contrast-dependent method for imaging the arterial system. It depends on intravenous infusion of iodine-based contrast agents. The patient is advanced through a rotating gantry, which images serial transverse slices. The contrast-filled vessels can be extracted from the slices and rendered in three-dimensional format. The extracted image can be rotated and viewed from several different directions.

Magnetic Resonance Angiography

MRA has the advantage of not requiring iodinated contrast agents to provide vessel opacification. Gadolinium is used as a contrast agent for MRA studies, and as it is generally not nephrotoxic, it can be used in patients with elevated creatinine.

MEDICAL MANAGEMENT OF PERIPHERAL ARTERIAL DISEASE

The cornerstone of medical management is reduction of vascular risk factors such as smoking cessation, control of blood pressure, reduction of blood lipid levels including statin therapy, correction of elevated homocysteine levels, and tight control of blood sugar in diabetics. Smoking cessation has been shown to result in a reduction of the 10-year mortality rate from 54 down to 18 percent. In one clinical trial, at 7 years, 16 percent of smokers compared to 0 percent of quitters had progressed to rest pain.

It has been well established that the treatment of hypertension reduces the risk of stroke and coronary events. However, lowering of blood pressure may worsen intermittent claudication.

Multiple studies have proven that lowering total cholesterol and low-density lipoprotein (LDL) levels reduces mortality and morbidity in patients with peripheral arterial disease (PAD), regardless of their baseline cholesterol or LDL levels.

Statin therapy is effective in the treatment of elevated LDL cholesterol, but has little effect on high-density lipoprotein (HDL), triglycerides, or Lp(a). Fibrates effectively lower triglycerides and raise HDL cholesterol. Niacin therapy has beneficial effects on all lipid parameters and is the only drug known to lower Lp(a). It is also the most effective agent for elevating HDL cholesterol. Slow-release niacin has increased tolerability and compliance and is emerging as an important therapy in patients with dyslipidemia.

Hyperhomocysteinemia

The incidence of hyperhomocysteinemia is as high as 60 percent in patients with vascular disease, compared with 1 percent in the general population. Elevated homocysteine levels can be treated with folic acid supplementation of 0.5–1.0 mg/day.

Diabetes Mellitus and Impaired Glucose Tolerance

Many studies have shown an association between diabetes mellitus and the development of vascular disease. Over the last decade, the importance and prevalence of the metabolic syndrome, which is characterized by obesity, non–insulin-dependent diabetes mellitus, hyperinsulinemia, hyperlipidemia, hypertension, hyperuricemia, and cardiovascular disease has become evident. Recognition of patients with metabolic syndrome is important so that they may be treated.

Exercise Programs

Exercise has been shown to improve function, reduce symptoms, and possibly prolong survival. It can produce an increase in walking distance of up to 150 percent—a clinically meaningful improvement—and has been associated with a 24 percent reduction in cardiovascular mortality. Exercise programs that consist of exercise for more than 30 min and more frequently than 3 times per week are most effective.

Specific Medical Therapy for Claudication

Other medical therapies directed specifically at peripheral disease rather than its risk factors include pentoxifylline and cilostazol.

Cilostazol is the more effective of the two, has been shown to significantly increase walking distance in patients with claudication in several randomized trials and to result in improvement in physical functioning and quality of life. Improvement has ranged from 35–100 percent. A trial of the drug is indicated in symptomatic patients. It should be continued for at least 3 months before a decision is made about efficacy. The most common adverse effects are headache, transient diarrhea, palpitations, and dizziness. It is contraindicated in patients with congestive heart failure because of its effects on phosphodiesterase.

Antiplatelet medications should be started on all patients with peripheral vascular disease (PVD). Aspirin has been found to reduce the vascular death rate by about 25 percent. Clopidogrel is more effective than aspirin in reducing cardiovascular outcome events, especially in the patient with lower extremity occlusive disease, but is much more expensive.

Because of the systemic nature of atherosclerosis, all patients with PAD, whether they have a history of coronary disease or not, should benefit from medical prevention strategies. These include aggressive management of smoking, statin therapy with a goal of lowering LDL cholesterol to at least 100 mg/dL, treatment of blood pressure to attain 130/85 mmHg, and management of diabetes mellitus to a glycohemoglobin level of 7 percent. Drugs shown to have particular benefit in these patients include the statins for LDL reduction, angiotensin-converting enzyme (ACE) inhibitors to treat blood pressure, and beta blockers for their cardioprotective effects. Additionally, all patients should be given a trial of cilostazol, clopidogrel, or aspirin. Patients should also be investigated for other dyslipidemias and hyperhomocysteinemia and treated accordingly.

ANEURYSMAL DISEASE

An aneurysm is defined as a dilation of an artery greater than 1.5 times its normal diameter. They can occur in almost any artery in the body, but the most common locations are in the abdominal aorta, thoracic aorta, cerebral vessels, and iliac, popliteal, and femoral arteries.

Classification of Aneurysms

Aneurysms are classified in a variety of ways based on their shape, wall constituents, and etiology.

Shape

Fusiform, or spindle-shaped aneurysms Saccular, excentric with protrusion of one wall.

Wall Constituents

True Aneurysms: entirely contained by dilated arterial wall. Pseudoaneurysms or false aneurysms is composed partly of arterial wall and partly of adjacent structures.

Etiology

Dissecting Aneurysms: occur when the vessel wall is split and the vessel enlarged. Mycotic: vessel wall is infected leading to aneurysm formation. Traumatic: wall disrupted by trauma leading to aneurysm.

Abdominal Aortic Aneurysms

Natural History

Abdominal aortic aneurysms grow on average 0.4 cm/year. Risk of rupture is exponentially related to aneurysm diameter. Aneurysms 5.0 cm in diameter have an average yearly rupture rate of 3–5 percent. However, a 7-cm aneurysm carries a rupture rate of 19 percent per year. Currently, with perioperative mortality rates 3–5 percent, intervention is recommended for all aneurysms greater than 5 cm.

Epidemiology

AAA occur three times as frequently in males as in females and increase with age.

Etiology and Pathology

Although referred to as atherosclerotic aneurysms, the etiology is more complex. There is progressive loss of elastin in aortic aneurysms along with increased metalloprotease activity. Proteolysis and inflammation are the driving forces in abdominal aortic aneurysm (AAA) expansion. Normal aortic tissue contains 12 percent elastin, whereas aneurysmal tissue has only 1 percent elastin. There is a clear familial trend that is sex-linked and autosomally recessive. Presence of an aneurysm in a female usually is associated with aneurysms in family members. Estimated risk for first-degree relatives of affected family members is 11.6 times that of the rest of the population. Screening of siblings (over age 50) of patients with aneurysms revealed an aneurysm in 29 percent of brothers and 6 percent of sisters.

Clinical Manifestations

Symptoms. Most are asymptomatic, often being an incidental finding during evaluation of a concurrent condition. Calcified outer wall or a large soft tissue shadow is noted on an abdominal radiograph, or they are detected during performance of an ultrasound or CT scan, of the abdomen. The most common symptoms are new-onset low-back pain and abdominal pain, which are occasionally because of compression/erosion of adjacent structures such as an aortocaval fistula, a ureteric obstruction, gastrointestinal (GI) bleeding from a primary aortoduodenal fistula, or rarely, they can be because of lower extremity embolization. When symptomatic, expeditious evaluation and treatment is indicated.

Examination. In a thin patient may show prominent epigastric/umbilical pulsatility. Careful palpation reveals expansile pulsatility. In large patients they may not be palpable. Examination of the femoral and distal pulses is mandatory for concurrent femoral or popliteal aneurysms.

Testing is dictated by aneurysm size. Aneurysms in the 4.5–5-cm range, observation is reasonable, although recent expansion or high anxiety on the patient's part should lead to intervention. Aneurysms greater than 5.0 cm should be repaired unless the patient is very high risk. Ultrasound is the most cost efficient screening tool. For preoperative evaluation, computed tomography (CT scan) is best.

Preoperative Preparation

All patients should have preoperative cardiac clearance. Risk factors for open aneurysm repair include myocardial infarction in the last 6 months without revascularization, congestive heart failure, and angina. A forced expiratory volume in 1 second (FEV-1) of less than 1 L and creatinine levels greater than 2.0 mg/dL are also risk factors. Preoperative pulmonary evaluation, with optimization of pulmonary function and renal protection with fenoldopam mesylate are used in patients with elevated creatinine levels. Epidural anesthesia is a useful supplement for postoperative pain control.

Surgery

The open approach can be accomplished through either a mid-line transperitoneal abdominal incision or via a retroperitoneal approach. The latter is preferred in patients with adhesions, abdominal stoma, and with severe chronic obstructive pulmonary disorder (COPD). Limitation include: inability to reach the right renal distal right common iliac artery. Most surgeons prefer a midline incision. The peritoneum over the aorta is incised from the iliac bifurcation superiorly, around the duodenum, and up to the level of the left renal vein. The duodenum is mobilized to the patient's right, exposing the underlying aorta. Rarely does aneurysmal disease extend beyond the common iliac bifurcation. After anticoagulation, the iliac arteries are clamped, followed by the aorta. The aneurysm is opened longitudinally and thrombus evacuated. A tube or bifurcated graft is sewn end-to-end inside the aneurysm using 3-0 polypropylene suture for the aortic anastomoses. The retroperitoneum is then also closed over the aneurysmal sac.

Postoperative Course

Patients are observed in the intensive care unit (ICU) overnight and are hospitalized for 4–5 days.

The mortality rate in large institutions is 2–4 percent with a morbidity rate of 20 percent.

Complications

Pneumonia, ileus, renal failure, lower extremity ischemia, colonic ischemia, spinal cord ischemia, aortoenteric fistula, graft infection, and anastomotic pseudoaneurysm are all complications of abdominal aortic aneurysm.

Aortic Endografting

Thirty to 50 percent of aneurysms are currently treated with endografts. Endografts are inserted via a cutdown on each common femoral artery. A transverse arteriotomy is made to permit insertion of the main body endografts over a previously inserted guide wire. This is advanced up through the ipsilateral iliac system under fluoroscopic control. The proximal markers are placed immediately below the lowest renal arteries and the device appropriately oriented, then deployed. The contralateral gate is then cannulated with a guidewire and its intragraft position confirmed by reconforming a pigtail catheter and ensuring that it spins freely within the lumen of the grafts. A stiff wire is reinserted although the pigtail catheter and the contralateral limb advanced into the gate and deployed. Rapid changes in the type of endograft available and the options for the surgeon are presently occurring. Devices are now available for aortounilateral iliac aneurysms and for treatment of thoracic aortic aneurysms. Iliac artery injuries can occur from insertion of the device, which may manifest as rupture, dissection, or limb occlusion postendografting. Renal dysfunction can occur form dye toxicity, embolization, and occasionally inadvertent coverage of the renal artery by the device.

Complications: type I–IV endoleak, sac expansion, graft infection, migration of device, modular disconnection, limb occlusion.

Patients with endografts must be followed for life. Follow-up includes abdominal radiographs (e.g., anteroposterior [AP], lateral, and obliques), duplex ultrasound, and contrast-enhanced CT scanning. Endografts have significant advantages in high risk patients, permit a shorter hospital stay and earlier return to function than does open repair.

Juxtarenal Aneurysms

These extend to the renal arteries, thus requiring a suprarenal cross-clamp. Technical maneuvers that facilitate this are division of the left renal vein and a left retroperitoneal approach. Suprarenal clamping clearly increases the risk of renal dysfunction postprocedure. The graft can be sutured incorporating the inferior margin of the renal orifices.

Ruptured Abdominal Aortic Aneurysm

Fear of rupture is the driving force behind the elective repair of aneurysms. There has been almost no change in the mortality rate from ruptured AAAs in the last 20 years. Most patients die before reaching the hospital, and of those who do, the mortality remains close to 50 percent. This has led to some serious re-evaluation of the management of ruptured aneurysms, with increasing interest in the use of permissive hypotension and the use of emergent stent graft placement. These developments, however, remain to be validated.

Most patients with a ruptured aneurysm are often unaware of the presence of an aneurysm. Sudden-onset, severe abdominal pain and/or back pain are the principal presenting symptoms. Often there is a fainting episode that correlates with the initial aneurysm sac rupture, which is followed by a period of cardiovascular stability. Consequently the patient arrives in the emergency room with little to distinguish a ruptured AAA from other intraabdominal catastrophes. Palpation of a pulsatile mass, the outline of a calcified AAA or soft tissue mass on abdominal x-rays (i.e., Kidney, ureter and bladder (KUB)) or a known history of AAA greatly facilitates the diagnosis. Where the diagnosis is clear-cut, the patient should go directly to the operating room for emergent repair. Often, however, the diagnosis is uncertain and established by CT scanning. As in shock resuscitation for trauma, current thinking is to avoid aggressive resuscitation and infuse fluids or blood only to keep the patient stable and cerebrating, without creating hypertension that may accelerate additional bleeding. A systolic pressure of 70 mmHg with a cerebrating patient is tolerable while preparations are made to go to the operating room.

In the operating room, the abdomen is prepped and draped with the patient awake. Decompensation can occur with the induction of anesthesia and loss of abdominal wall splinting. Once the patient is anesthetized, a long midline abdominal incision is created. Usually a large hematoma contained within the retroperitoneum is apparent. The surgeon decides based on the extent and location of the hematoma whether to gain infrarenal control or supraceliac aortic control at the diaphragm. In the unstable patient, an aortic compressor can be used.

Several complications occur more frequently in ruptured than elective aneurysm repair, including venous injury (i.e., renal, iliac or inferior vena cava [IVC]), ureteral injury, and injury to the duodenum. Multisystem organ failure is common in survivors who have suffered significant blood loss.

The emerging endovascular approach involves placement of a descending aortic occlusion balloon that is inflated only if the patient's blood pressure cannot be maintained in the range of the low 70s of systolic pressure. A CT scan is rapidly performed or intravascular ultrasound and angiography are done in the operating room to allow appropriate endoluminal graft selection. The device is then placed as expeditiously as possible.

Mycotic Aortic Aneurysm

They are most frequently found in the aorta, most common organisms being staphylococci, followed by Salmonella. These aneurysms develop as a consequence of the infection, not as a result of infection in a preexisting aneurysm. Mycotic aneurysms can occur as a result of infected emboli that lodge in the artery and spread in the wall. Most commonly they arise from infected aortic and mitral valves. Other mycotic aneurysms occur from direct extension of an area of infection into the adjacent arterial wall. Because patients who are immunosuppressed (i.e., acquired immunodeficiency syndrome [AIDS] or organ transplant patients) are predisposed to infection, they are at an increased risk of developing mycotic aneurysms. Mycotic aneurysms often present with pain, are more rapidly progressive than degenerative aneurysms, and have a higher rupture rate.

Treatment is determined by location. Those arising within the visceral aortic segment have to be treated by débridement and in situ reconstruction. Cryopreserved aorta has been widely used for this purpose. Expanded polytetrafluoroethylene (ePTFE) grafts may also be more infection resistant than Dacron grafts, although antibiotic-impregnated Dacron grafts are being increasingly used. Aneurysms that occur in the infrarenal aorta can be treated by several techniques. The traditional approach is to revascularize the lower extremities via an extra-anatomic approach (axillobifemoral bypass), followed by aortic excision and oversewing of the aortic stump. This is associated with a 5 percent risk of aortic stump blow-out, which is usually fatal. Rifampin-soaked Dacron grafts have been placed into the aortic bed after excision, débridement, and irrigation. More recently, Clagett has popularized the use of bilateral superficial femoral vein to replace infected aortic grafts. Antibiotic therapy is used as directed by culture results, and long-term antibiotic therapy for 3–6 months is warranted.

Para-Anastomotic Aneurysms

Definition. Aneurysmal disease after bypass grafting of the abdominal aorta is defined radiographically as a focal dilatation juxtaposed to the aortic suture line or an adjacent aortic diameter that is greater than or equal to 4 cm. It is important to distinguish true versus false aneurysms and to identify early versus late aneurysmal development. True aneurysms are a dilation of the remaining infrarenal aorta. False aneurysms occur because of degeneration of the old suture line and separation of the graft from the aortic wall.

Management. Elective surgical management of para-anastomotic aortic aneurysm (PAAA) lesions is the treatment of choice because these lesions progressively increase in size and may rupture with time. Morbidity and mortality rates are acceptable in asymptomatic patients undergoing elective repair, as reported in these authors' series and by others. The operative repair most frequently involves excising the diseased segment of the artery and graft and placement of an interposition prosthesis.

More recently, use of endografts has become an increasingly popular method for treating anastomotic pseudoaneurysms. They are most easily used when the initial graft has been implanted well below the renal arteries such that a suitable landing and seal zone is available for positioning the device. In patients who are at high risk, stent grafting across the renal arteries with revascularization from the visceral or iliac vessels will avoid aortic cross-clamping.

Other Anastomotic Aneurysms

The most common location for an aneurysm that develops at a suture line is at the femoral anastomosis of an aortobifemoral graft. They are detected by the presence of an enlarging pulsatile mass in the groin. Ultrasound confirms the diagnosis. Both groins should always be examined, and treatment is by surgical repair. The groin is entered via a vertical incision, and control of the inflow graft is necessary. Once this has been controlled, the patient is anticoagulated and the aneurysm opened. Fogarty catheters are used endoluminally to control the profunda femoris, the superficial femoral artery, and the native common femoral artery if it remains open. An interposition piece of Dacron or ePTFE is used to restore continuity. Proximally, it is sewn end-to-end to the previous graft. Distally, the graft usually has to be tailored around both the superficial femoral and profunda femoris arteries.

Iliac Artery Aneurysms

Occasionally isolated common iliac aneurysms are encountered. Internal iliac aneurysm may also be diagnosed, although isolated aneurysms of the external iliac artery are rare. Treatment options include open surgical replacement with prosthetic graft or endovascular stent grafting. In patients with suitable anatomy, namely the presence of proximal and distal landing zones, stent grafting has become the treatment of choice.

Internal iliac artery aneurysms are treated by proximal ligation with opening of the aneurysm and oversewing of the distal branches. Because the distal end of the aneurysm may be located deep in the pelvis, an emerging approach is embolization and stent grafting across the orifice of the hypogastric. Although unilateral sacrifice of a hypogastric is well tolerated, bilateral ligation can result in pelvic ischemia. Consequently, an attempt should be made to revascularize one hypogastric.

Popliteal Artery Aneurysms

Popliteal arterial aneurysms are the most common peripheral arterial aneurysms, accounting for 70 percent, and are commonly bilateral in 50–75 percent. Finding one popliteal aneurysm mandates evaluation of the contralateral popliteal artery, usually with ultrasound. They are more common in males. These aneurysms present by a process of chronic distal embolization or sudden-onset acute occlusion of the popliteal artery. Consequently the clinical presentation is by development of claudication; chronic foot ischemia; or sudden-onset, limb-threatening, acute ischemia below the knee. Rupture is rare. Frequently a pattern of acute or chronic ischemia occurs, and the presence of chronic embolization of the infrapopliteal vessels can markedly complicate revascularization.

Examination reveals a pulsatile mass, which can be massive, in the popliteal fossa. Smaller aneurysms may not be palpable. Foot pulses may be diminished if embolization has been occurring. In patients with acute occlusion of the aneurysm or with embolization, many have all the clinical features of acute ischemia. A thrombosed aneurysm may be palpated as a hard mass, and pulsation is absent. Occasionally these aneurysms can be massive, filling the entire popliteal fossa. Large aneurysms compress the adjacent popliteal vein and occasionally present with acute deep venous thrombosis. Diagnosis is by ultrasound aneurysms greater than 2 cm should be treated. Preoperative angiography is usually performed in both the acute and elective situation to demonstrate the run off vessels. In the presence of limb-threatening ischemia, revascularization is undertaken emergently.

Choice of treatment is based on degree of ischemia and the ability to demonstrate distal target vessels for revascularization. Where no run-off is identifiable, the approach is to attempt thrombolysis via a catheter placed into, and ideally through, the aneurysm. Lytic agents are then infused in an attempt to open up the tibial vessels and permit a bypass graft to be created. Alternately, surgical exploration is performed of the distal popliteal artery, and all three trifurcation vessels should be dissected and controlled. Fogarty embolectomy catheters (no 3) are gently passed down each artery, inflated, and the thrombus removed. Once outflow is established, revascularization is performed as described for elective popliteal arterial aneurysms below.

In the elective situation in which target outflow vessels are evident, two approaches are open to the surgeon: medial and posterior. For the medial approach, reversed saphenous vein is tunneled from the superior to the inferior incision, and end-to-side anastomoses are created. The popliteal artery is then ligated distal and proximal to the bypass graft.

The posterior approach (e.g., patient prone, foot supported on a pillow) is useful for smaller aneurysms limited to the midpopliteal artery or for exploring aneurysms which have continued to expand after ligation and bypass. A Z-type incision is made centered on the skin crease. An endoaneurysmorrhaphy is easily performed by opening the aneurysm, oversewing tributaries, and placing an interposition reversed saphenous vein graft.

Femoral Artery Aneurysms

Femoral arterial aneurysms (FAAs) present as a pulsatile mass in the groin. They occur in older adult men, often with other manifestations of atherosclerosis. One third are bilateral and nearly two thirds are associated with aneurysms elsewhere (e.g., popliteal and aortic). Ultrasound is used to confirm the diagnosis, and although most are considered atherosclerotic in etiology, mycotic femoral arterial aneurysms are encountered, particularly in intravenous drug abusers. Femoral aneurysms can reach a large size and via thrombosis can create symptoms such as limb-threatening ischemia, embolization, or skin erosion; however, rupture is rarely encountered. FAAs are often asymptomatic, but local pain, distal embolization, rupture, and venous compression may all be presenting features.

Treatment. All aneurysms greater than 2.5 cm should be treated with resection and interposition grafting.

Hepatic Artery Aneurysms

Hepatic arterial aneurysms (HAAs) comprise 20 percent of splanchnic arterial aneurysms. Although not well-defined, the natural history of HAAs typically results in enlargement, rupture, and life-threatening hemorrhage. Hence, heightened clinical suspicion with conclusive diagnosis and effective treatment are imperative in the successful management of patients with these aneurysms.

Pseudoaneurysms typically affect younger male individuals and often reflect a traumatic etiology.

Plain abdominal radiographs or upper GI contrast studies may suggest an underlying HAA when a rim of calcification in the right hypochondrium or a smooth filling defect in the duodenum is demonstrated. Ultrasonography and contrast-enhanced CT scanning will provide the diagnosis in most cases. MRI has been applied to good effect in the diagnosis of HAAs. Color-flow duplex ultrasonography is particularly effective in demonstrating intrahepatic lesions.

Unless severe comorbidities disqualify the patient, all extrahepatic aneurysms greater than 2 cm in diameter should be treated. Pseudoaneurysms, most of which are intrahepatic and can be successfully embolized, are treated when greater than 1 cm.

Extrahepatic aneurysms warrant surgical treatment, except in high-risk patients and in saccular aneurysms. Common HAAs (i.e., those proximal to a patent gastroduodenal artery) may be ligated and excised.

As a rule, extrahepatic aneurysms involving the hepatic artery propria will need vascular reconstruction. Ligation and bypass is necessary for aneurysms of the true hepatic artery beyond the gastroduodenal artery.

Successful percutaneous embolization was first reported in 1977, and several reports have been published that support the use of this technique. An advantage of selective arterial embolization is its precision in limiting hepatic devascularization. It is of particular value in cases of posttraumatic pseudoaneurysms, and because of its lower morbidity, represents an attractive option in high-risk patients.

Splenic Artery Aneurysms

These are the most common visceral artery aneurysms and also most likely to develop pseudoaneurysms.

Symptoms and signs. Most are asymptomatic, usually being discovered incidentally. Chronic vague epigastric and left hypochondrial pain may be reported. The development of acute left upper quadrant pain indicates that rupture may have occurred, especially when signs of hypovolemia are present.

Investigations. The presence of a splenic artery aneurysm (SAA) may be suspected with the appearance of calcification in a corresponding area on a KUB radiograph. CT scanning is valuable in demonstrating size and location of these aneurysms. Angiography confirms the diagnosis, delineates the location and number of these aneurysms, and assists in determining whether an endovascular or open surgical approach should be selected.

Treatment

There is a general consensus that women anticipating pregnancy should have surgical treatment, and patients with symptomatic aneurysms should be promptly treated. Although widely recommended, the indications for treating aneurysms that are larger than 2 cm are less definite.

The recommended procedure for proximally situated aneurysms is exclusion of the lesion with proximal and distal ligation of the splenic artery. Occasionally, opening the aneurysm to oversew feeding vessels from within the lesion may be necessary.

Successful laparoscopic ligation has been reported. Percutaneous embolization with Gianturco coils and gelfoam sponges has been reported with favorable results.

Renal Artery Aneurysms

The incidence of renal arterial aneurysms (RAAs) is estimated to be between 0.09 and 0.7 percent of the population. The incidence rises to 2.5 percent among patients evaluated for hypertension, and is 9.2 percent among patients with fibromuscular disease (FMD) involving the renal artery. Complications are uncommon but can include renovascular hypertension; renal infarction from embolization, dissection, or thrombosis; and arteriovenous fistula formation.

Renal artery aneurysms are slightly more common in women than men and more frequently affect the right than the left renal artery.

The true risk of rupture for renal arterial aneurysms has been overestimated. A disproportionate number of ruptures have occurred in pregnancy.

Management options include observation, transcatheter occlusion, or surgical intervention. Indications for intervention include aneurysm size greater than 2.5 cm, renovascular hypertension with lateralizing serum renin level, symptomatic aneurysms, documented expansion, renal embolization, and young women anticipating pregnancy.

Embolization is particularly useful in patients with saccular aneurysms; small, bleeding aneurysms in patients with arteritis; and in high-risk patients. Transcatheter embolization is also the treatment of choice for intraparenchymal lesions.

Aneurysmectomy and arteriorrhaphy with or without patch angioplasty is the simplest method of aneurysm resection with reconstitution of the renal artery. It is most easily applied to saccular aneurysms with a narrow neck on the patent artery. Ligation and bypass are appropriately applied to fusiform aneurysms. Opening of the aneurysm with oversewing of feeding vessels from within the sac is optimal to preclude progressive enlargement of a ligated aneurysm.

ACUTE ARTERIAL OCCLUSION

One of the most common vascular emergencies is acute lower extremity ischemia; however, sudden-onset acute occlusion of any major vessel (e.g., mesenteric, renal, or upper extremity) presents with severe symptoms, which reflect ischemia in the organ supplied by those vessels. Arteries that undergo slow progressive occlusion permit the development of collaterals such that patients may be asymptomatic or lack the severe symptoms associated with acute ischemia. In the absence of collaterals, however, acute ischemia can result in nonreversible changes within the target organ within h. Consequently, expeditious relief of the obstruction is mandatory, and revascularization of ischemic tissue, resulting in swelling and edema within the target tissues, and washout of lactic acid, myoglobin, and potassium. The vascular surgeon must know how to manage both the local and systemic effects of this postrevascularization syndrome.

Arterial Embolism

Cardiac Sources

The heart is the most common source of distal emboli. In fact, 70 percent of distal emboli are cardiac in origin (atrial fibrillation, ventricular aneurysm, mural thrombus over an area of infection, and endocarditis).

Lower Extremity Acute Ischemia

Clinical manifestations. Acute lower extremity ischemia manifests with the "five Ps": pain, pallor, paresthesias, paralysis, and pulselessness, to which some add a sixth "P"—poikilothermia or "perishing cold." Pain, however, is what causes a patient to present to the emergency room. The most common location for an embolus to lodge in the leg is at the common femoral bifurcation. Typically a patient will complain of foot and calf pain. In addition to absent pulses, there is a variable diminution of sensation, which varies from a mild reduction in sensation compared to the contralateral side to being completely insensate.

Absent bilateral femoral pulses in a patient with bilateral lower extremity ischemia is most likely because of saddle embolus to the aortic bifurcation. A palpable femoral pulse and absent popliteal and distal pulses may either be because of distal common femoral embolus (the pulse being palpable above the level of occlusion) or embolus to the superficial femoral or popliteal arteries. Typically, emboli lodge at bifurcations where there are sudden changes in arterial diameter. A popliteal trifurcation embolus will present with calf ischemia and absent pedal pulses, possibly with a popliteal pulse present. The finding of palpable contralateral pulses in the absence of ipsilateral pulses in the ischemic leg is suggestive of an embolus.

Medical therapy. In the absence of any significant contraindication, the patient with an ischemic lower extremity should be immediately anticoagulated.

Surgery. The groin is opened through a vertical incision, exposing the common femoral artery and its bifurcation. Frequently, the location of the embolus at the femoral bifurcation is readily apparent by the presence of a palpable proximal femoral pulse, which disappears distally. The artery is clamped and opened transversely over the bifurcation. Thrombus is extracted by passing a Fogarty balloon embolectomy catheter. Good back-bleeding and antegrade bleeding suggest that the entire clot has been removed. Completion angiography is advisable. The artery is then closed and the patient fully anticoagulated.

When an embolus lodges in the popliteal artery, in most cases it can be extracted via a femoral incision using the techniques previously described. A femoral approach is preferred because the larger arterial size results in a lessened likelihood of arterial compromise when the artery is closed. The disadvantage is that the embolectomy catheter cannot be specifically directed into each of the infrapopliteal arteries. This can be achieved from the groin using fluoroscopic imaging and an over-the-wire thrombectomy catheter, which can be specifically directed into each of the infrapopliteal vessels. Otherwise, a separate incision exposing the popliteal bifurcation may be necessary to ensure completeness of thrombectomy.

In the postoperative period it is important to seek the source of the embolus using echocardiography and CT scanning of the descending thoracic and abdominal aorta.

A more complex situation arises when a patient has preexisting peripheral vascular disease and in situ thrombosis on top of atheroma; frequently embolectomy catheters will not pass through these occlusions. There are essentially two options: surgical bypass or catheter-based lytic therapy. Angiography is necessary in both situations to determine the extent of the occlusion and to search for inflow and distal outflow vessels to which a bypass graft could be attached. Although the surgeon's preference tends to predominate in the approach to the ischemic limb, both approaches have been demonstrated to be fairly equivalent in terms of limb salvage. Criteria for selecting the appropriate approach are based on the presence or absence of good target vessels and availability of a suitable bypass conduit. If there are good distal vessels—usually inflow vessels are adequate or can be made adequate—and a good saphenous vein is available, surgical bypass is recommended, as it is fast and reliable. In the absence of a good distal target, absent saphenous vein, or in a patient at high risk for surgery, lysis is recommended.

Complications of reperfusion of the ischemic limb. Reperfusion of the ischemic limb is variable in its physiologic effects, which directly relates to the severity and extent of the ischemia. Patients with a saddle embolus of the aortic bifurcation and severely ischemic limbs may sustain the full-blown "reperfusion syndrome." At the other end of the spectrum, patients with minimal muscle ischemia who are rapidly reperfused may have essentially no effects. However, many of these patients have severe underlying cardiac disease and poorly tolerate even short ischemic periods. Complications occurring after revascularization of the lower extremity and causes of recurrent thrombosis are listed. Therapy is directed toward forced alkaline diuresis by adding bicarbonate to the intravenous fluid. Alkalinization increases the solubility of myoglobin in the urine, preventing it from crystallizing in the tubules, which is what promotes acute renal failure.

Compartment syndrome. Compartment syndrome occurs after prolonged ischemia followed by reperfusion. The capillaries leak fluid into the interstitial space in the muscles, which are enclosed within a nondistensible fascial envelope. When the pressure inside the compartment exceeds the capillary perfusion pressure, nutrient flow ceases and progressive ischemia occurs, even in the presence of peripheral pulses. The most commonly affected compartment is the anterior compartment in the leg. Numbness in the web space between the first and second toes is diagnostic because of compression of the deep peroneal nerve. When skin changes occur over the compartment, this indicates advanced ischemia. Compartment pressure is measured by inserting an arterial line into the compartment and recording the pressure. Although controversial, pressures greater than 30 mmHg or below 30 mmHg diastolic are frequently cited. Treatment is by fasciotomy. In the leg, medial and lateral incisions are used via the medial incision. Long openings are then made in the fascia of the superficial and deep posterior compartments. Through the lateral incision, the anterior and peroneal compartments are opened.

Acute Aortic Occlusion

Acute aortic occlusion is a rare vascular catastrophe. It may result from an aortic saddle embolus, in situ thrombosis of a previously atherosclerotic abdominal aorta, sudden thrombosis of small abdominal aortic aneurysms, distal aortic dissection, or other etiologies that embolize to the aortic bifurcation. The diagnosis can easily go unrecognized and has a published mortality rate of 75 percent with conservative treatment. Additionally, the condition often presents with leg paralysis that occasionally leads clinicians to perform an extensive neurologic workup, even if patients have absent femoral pulses, which can lead to delays in diagnosis and operative therapy.

In all patients, an acute onset of bilateral lower extremity ischemia or a sudden exacerbation of preexisting chronic ischemia is the presenting syndrome.

Acute aortic occlusion is a different entity than chronic obstruction, in which a well-developed collateral circulation may minimize symptoms. When an embolus is large enough to occlude the aorta, the source is usually cardiac (i.e., mural thrombus over an infarct, a left ventricular aneurysm, or rheumatic heart disease).

Presenting symptoms. Symptoms include sudden onset of bilateral limb pain, pallor, paralysis, paresthesia, and the absence of palpable pulses. Mottling of the lower extremities, often to the level of the umbilicus, may also be present.

Physical examination. If the physical examination shows the absence of both femoral pulses, the diagnosis of acute aortic occlusion is established. The cause of the occlusion will significantly alter patient management, and thus a detailed history is important. Severe coronary artery disease, known arrhythmias, or ventricular aneurysms suggest a saddle embolus, whereas known aortoiliac disease or a previously diagnosed aortic aneurysm suggests an in situ thrombosis.

Investigations. Patients with suspected in situ abdominal aortic thrombosis with clinically unclear renal or mesenteric arterial involvement should have preoperative angiography. For all other patients, it is recommended that intraoperative angiography with a C-arm be used in the operating room, because it saves time and provides important information should it be needed.

Operative considerations. Because patient prognosis is time-dependent, early recognition, institution of supportive care, and prompt diagnosis (if possible) are essential elements of management. The treatment of acute aortic occlusion is surgical. The cause of occlusion is important because transfemoral embolectomy is likely to restore perfusion in patients with saddle embolus, but is usually unhelpful in patients with in situ thrombosis. When the diagnosis is made, the patient should be heparinized immediately to prevent proximal and distal propagation of the thrombotic process. Bilateral transfemoral embolectomy is the first procedure of choice. If flow is re-established, the groin wounds are closed and postoperative anticoagulation is initiated. If flow cannot be re-established, more extensive surgery, such as aortoiliac bypass or axillobifemoral bypass, should be performed. The choice to perform axillobifemoral bypass versus aortobifemoral bypass is guided by the clinical condition of the patient.

Postoperative management. Postoperative management requires correction of any embolic diathesis. Transthoracic or transesophageal echocardiography should be obtained. A CT scan of the abdomen should be done if not performed preoperatively to rule out the presence of an abdominal aortic aneurysm. If an aneurysm is present and the patient is a reasonable candidate, the aneurysm may be ligated electively. If the patient is known to have an aneurysm that appears to have occluded, then replacement with a prosthetic graft is the procedure of choice. Long-term anticoagulation is necessary for all patients.

AORTOILIAC OCCLUSIVE DISEASE

The distal abdominal aorta and the iliac arteries are common sites of involvement with atherosclerosis. Aortoiliac occlusive disease occurs in a relatively younger group of patients (aged in their mid-50s), compared with patients with femoropopliteal disease. It alone is rarely limb-threatening. Symptoms typically consist of bilateral thigh or buttock claudication and fatigue. Men report diminished penile tumescence, and there may later be complete failure of erectile function. These symptoms constitute Leriche syndrome. Rest pain is unusual with isolated aortoiliac disease. Femoral pulses are usually diminished or absent. There are usually no stigmata of ischemia unless distal disease co-exists. Others may present with "trash foot," representing microembolization into the distal vascular bed.

Noninvasive tests such as pulse volume recordings of the lower extremity with estimation or the thigh-brachial pressure index may be suggestive of aortoiliac disease. Definitive diagnosis, however, can only be established by arteriography.

Preferred Approach to Therapeutic Alternatives

Medical Treatment

There is no effective medical therapy for the management of aortoiliac disease. Patients should have good medical management for atherosclerosis and risk factor modification as described above.

Open Surgical Treatment or Endovascular Therapy

The decision to pursue an open rather than an endovascular approach is made based on the extent of the occlusive disease. The Trans-Atlantic Intersocietal Commission (TASC) has classified the distribution and extent of atherosclerosis and has suggested a therapeutic approach based on this classification. TASC type A lesions are best treated with a catheter-based approach. TASC type D lesions should have open bypass. TASC types B and C remain controversial. However, this is a rapidly evolving field and it is likely that aortoiliac disease will be increasingly treated with a catheter-based approach.

Indications for surgery. Indications for surgery include disabling claudication (severely limiting work or lifestyle), rest pain, limb-threatening ischemia, and microembolization of the toes in which no other source is identified.

Surgical options. Surgical options consist of aortobifemoral bypass grafting, extra-anatomic bypass grafting, and aortoiliac endarterectomy. The procedure selected is determined by several factors, including anatomic distribution of the disease, clinical condition of the patient, and personal preference of the surgeon. Aortobifemoral bypass grafting is an excellent procedure for good risk patients. It reliably relieves symptoms, has an excellent long-term patency of 60–75 percent at 10 years, and can be completed with a tolerable mortality of 2–3 percent.

Procedure. Both femoral arteries are initially exposed to ensure that they are adequate for the distal anastomoses. The abdomen is then opened at the midline. A collagen-impregnated, knitted Dacron graft is then sewn in either end-to-end or end-to-side fashion using 3-0 polypropylene suture.

The limbs of the graft are then tunneled through the retroperitoneum to the groin, where an end-to-side anastomosis is fashioned between the graft and the bifurcation of the common femoral artery using 5-0 polypropylene suture.

Extra-anatomic (axillofemoral) bypass grafting from the axillary artery is an option for those patients with intercurrent medical problems that prohibit a laparotomy.

Postoperative management. All aortic patients are observed in the ICU overnight. Distal pulses are monitored hourly. Loss of a pulse that had been present postoperatively is suggestive of graft occlusion and warrants angiography to assess for re-exploration if the graft has failed.

The patient gets out of bed and into a chair on the second postoperative day and ambulates on the third day. Most patients may be discharged from the hospital 5–7 days postoperatively.

Percutaneous Transluminal Dilatation

Angioplasty is most useful in the treatment of isolated iliac stenoses of less than 4 cm in length. When used for stenoses rather than occlusion, a 2-year patency of 86 percent can be achieved. The complication rate is approximately 2 percent, consisting of distal embolization, medial dissection, and acute thrombosis.

Femoropopliteal Occlusive Disease

One of the most common sites for occlusive disease is in the distal superficial femoral artery (SFA) as it passes deep through the adductor canal. It may be that the entrapment by the adductor hiatus prevents the compensatory dilation that occurs in atherosclerotic vessels. Stenoses, which develop here, progress to occlusion of the distal third of the superficial femoral artery. Although often originating in this location, the SFA is frequently the site of diffuse disease with posterior plaque, which spirals along the artery. When distal SFA occlusion develops slowly it may be totally asymptomatic, and collaterals from the proximal SFA or the profunda femoris artery (PFA) bypass the occlusion and reconstitute the popliteal artery. Symptom development is a function of the extent of occlusion, adequacy of collaterals, and also the activity level of the patients.

Clinical Manifestations

Presenting symptoms of femoropopliteal occlusive disease are broadly classified into two types: limb-threatening and non–limb-threatening ischemia. Claudication (calf pain with exercise) is non–limb-threatening. Rest pain, ulceration, and gangrene are limb-threatening and demand intervention.

In greater than 70 percent of claudicants, the disease is stable, particularly with risk factor modification. It does not lead to progressive occlusion, and in most cases is not limb-threatening. This is extremely important for both the patient and physician to understand. Progression is more likely to occur in patients with diabetes and those who continue to smoke or fail to modify their atherosclerotic risk factors.

In contrast, rest pain is constant, usually occurring in the forefoot across the metatarsophalangeal joint. It is worse at night and requires foot dependency to improve symptoms. Patients may report that they either sleep in a chair or hang the foot off the side of the bed.

Ischemic ulceration most commonly involves the toes and often will progress to gangrene.

Differential Diagnosis

Night cramps often wake patients from sleep with painful calf muscle spasms and are not associated with arterial disease. However, foot ulceration, arterial ulcers that occur on the toes or lateral side of the foot, and venous ulcers, which are quite common and occur above the medial malleolus, usually in an area with the skin changes of lipodermatosclerosis, are associated with arterial disease.

Physical Examination

Diminished popliteal and distal pulses indicate SFA occlusive disease.

Investigations

Segmental pressure measurement and pulse volume recordings (PVRs) will demonstrate the level at which the pressure fall occurs and assist in localizing the affected segment. A pressure drop of greater than 30 mmHg between two adjacent segments is suggestive of significant occlusive disease at that level. Exercise testing with measurement of the ABI after exercise will help identify those patients who, despite significant occlusive disease, have palpable pedal pulses by showing an abrupt fall in ABI after exercise.

Angiography continues to be the best and most reliable test for imaging the entire lower extremity vasculature. Although magnetic resonance angiography (MRA) and computed tomographic angiography (CTA) continue to improve, it has not yet replaced DSA for lower-extremity angiography as anticipated. Lower-extremity duplex arterial mapping is increasing in popularity, but there remain only a few select centers that routinely use this technique for preoperative planning.

Age and comorbidities. Evaluation of the risk benefit ratio is particularly important in the claudicant. A femoral-popliteal bypass in the 50-year-old patient who has to walk as part of their employment is warranted. In contrast, the same operation in an 80-year-old patient is usually not indicated.

Extent of disease. Generally, localized disease (i.e., stenoses and short segment occlusions) is more amenable to a catheter-based approach.

Medical Therapy

Cilostazol has been demonstrated to be effective when compared with both placebo and pentoxifylline in improving walking distance. Likewise, for patients with non–limb-threatening ischemia, an exercise program should be initiated.

Open Surgical Procedures

Endarterectomy. Endarterectomy has a limited, albeit important role in lower extremity occlusive disease. It is most frequently used when there is disease of the common femoral artery or involving the profunda femoris artery. In this procedure, the surgeon opens the diseased segment longitudinally and develops a cleavage plane within the media that is developed proximally and distally.

Bypass grafting. Bypass grafting remains the primary intervention for lower-extremity occlusive disease. The type of bypass and the type of conduit are important variables. Those patients with occlusive disease limited to the SFA, with reconstitution of at least 4 cm (ideally 10 cm) of normal popliteal artery above the knee joint, and with at least one continuous vessel to the foot are treated with an above-knee femoral-to-popliteal bypass graft. In this location (i.e., not crossing the knee joint) the differential in patency between prosthetic (ePTFE) and vein graft is relatively small, therefore either conduit can be used.

Complications. Fifteen percent of vein grafts will develop intrinsic stenoses within the first 18 months following implantation. Consequently all patients with a vein graft should enter a duplex surveillance protocol. Scanning should be performed in the postoperative period at 3, 6, 12, and 18 months. Stenoses greater than 50 percent should be repaired, usually with patch angioplasty.

Wound infection. Because the most common inflow vessel for distal bypass is the common femoral artery, groin infection occurs in 7 percent of cases.

Alternate Bypass Techniques

In diabetic patients the SFA may be spared, and it is appropriate to shorten the bypass graft by performing popliteal-to-tibial grafts. In patients in whom both greater saphenous veins (GSVs) have been harvested, alternate vein sources include the short saphenous veins and upper extremity cephalic and basilic veins.

Endovascular Procedures

Endovascular procedures are undergoing rapid change. Presently, endovascular procedures in the infrainguinal area have a limited role and are confined to short segment stenoses or occlusions. Longer lesions, although treatable, have limited durability because of neointimal hyperplasia.

Mesenteric Artery Occlusive Disease

Blood flow to the intestine is supplied by three vessels: the celiac artery (CA), the superior mesenteric artery (SMA), and the internal mammary artery (IMA). These are the arteries to the foregut (stomach to second part of duodenum), midgut (second part of duodenum to right two thirds of transverse colon), and hind gut (distal third of the transverse colon to the rectum), respectively. Anastomoses exist between the celiac and superior mesenteric arteries via the pancreaticoduodenal arcade, and between the SMA and IMA via the marginal artery of Drummond and the Riolan arc; however, these collateral pathways are inconsistent and cannot be relied on to suffice in either acute or chronic occlusion of the visceral arteries.

Occlusive disease of the mesenteric arteries usually occurs in individuals who are medically debilitated with generalized atherosclerosis. The disease process may evolve in a chronic fashion, as in the case of progressive luminal plaque narrowing because of atherosclerotic progression. On the other hand, mesenteric ischemia can occur suddenly, as in the case of thromboembolism. Despite recent progress in perioperative management and better understanding in pathophysiology, mesenteric ischemia is one of the most lethal vascular disorders, with mortality rates ranging from 50–75 percent. Delay in diagnosis and treatment are the main contributing factors to the high mortality rate. Early recognition and prompt treatment prior to the onset of irreversible intestinal ischemia are essential to improve the outcome.

Types of Mesenteric Artery Occlusive Disease

There are four major types of visceral ischemia involving the mesenteric arteries: (1) acute embolic mesenteric ischemia, (2) acute thrombotic mesenteric ischemia, (3) chronic mesenteric ischemia, and (4) nonocclusive mesenteric ischemia. Despite the variability of these syndromes, a common anatomic pathology is involved in these processes. The SMA is the most commonly involved vessel in acute mesenteric ischemia. Acute thrombotic mesenteric ischemia frequently occurs in patients with underlying mesenteric atherosclerosis, which usually involves the origin of the mesenteric arteries while sparing the collateral branches. The development of collateral vessels is more likely when the occlusive process is a gradual, rather than a sudden, ischemic event. In acute embolic mesenteric ischemia, the emboli typically originate from a cardiac source, and frequently occur in patients with atrial fibrillation or following myocardial infarction. Nonocclusive mesenteric ischemia is characterized by a low-flow state in otherwise normal mesenteric arteries. In contrast, chronic mesenteric ischemia is a functional consequence of a long-standing atherosclerotic process that typically involves at least two of the three main mesenteric vessels, the CA, the SMA, and the IMA.

Several less common syndromes of visceral ischemia involving the mesenteric arteries can also cause serious debilitation. Chronic mesenteric ischemic symptoms can occur because of extrinsic compression of the celiac artery by the diaphragm, which is termed the median arcuate ligament syndrome. Acute visceral ischemia may occur following an aortic operation, because of ligation of the IMA in the absence of adequate collateral vessels. Furthermore, acute visceral ischemia may develop in aortic dissection, which involves the mesenteric arteries. Finally, other unusual causes of ischemia include mesenteric arteritis, radiation arteritis, and cholesterol emboli.

Clinical Presentation

Severe abdominal pain, out of proportion to the findings on exam is the classic presentation in patients with acute mesenteric ischemia. Sudden onset of abdominal cramps with bowel emptying may occur, perhaps with bloody diarrhea. Diffuse abdominal tenderness, rebound, and rigidity are ominous signs and usually herald bowel infarction.

Symptoms of thrombotic mesenteric ischemia may initially be more insidious than those of embolic mesenteric ischemia. Approximately 70 percent of patients with chronic mesenteric ischemia have a history of abdominal angina. In these patients, the chronicity of mesenteric atherosclerosis is important, as it permits collateral vessel formation. The precipitating factor leading to chronic mesenteric occlusion is often an unrelated illness that results in dehydration, such as diarrhea or vomiting, which may further confuse the actual diagnosis. If the diagnosis is not recognized promptly, symptoms may worsen that can lead to progressive abdominal distention, oliguria, increasing fluid requirements, and severe metabolic acidosis.

Abdominal pain is only present in approximately 70 percent of patients with nonocclusive mesenteric ischemia. When present, pain is usually severe, but may vary in location, character, and intensity. In the absence of abdominal pain, progressive abdominal distention with acidosis may be an early sign of ischemia and impending bowel infarction.

Diagnostic Studies

Laboratory evaluation is neither sensitive nor specific in the diagnosis of mesenteric ischemia. Complete blood count (CBC) may reveal hemoconcentration and leukocytosis. Metabolic acidosis develops as a result of anaerobic metabolism. Elevated serum amylase and lactate levels are nonspecific findings. Hyperkalemia and azotemia may occur in the late stages of ischemia. Plain abdominal radiographs may provide helpful information to exclude other abdominal pathologies such as bowel perforation, obstruction, or volvulus, which may exhibit symptoms mimicking intestinal ischemia. Radiographic appearance of an adynamic ileus with a gasless abdomen is the most common finding in patients with acute mesenteric ischemia. Embolic sources should be sought as described under acute ischemia.

The definitive diagnosis of mesenteric thrombosis is made by biplanar mesenteric arteriography, which should be performed promptly in any patient with suspected mesenteric occlusion. It typically shows occlusion or near-occlusion of the CA and SMA at or near their origins from the aorta. In most cases, the IMA has been previously occluded secondary to diffuse infrarenal aortic atherosclerosis. The differentiation of the four different types of mesenteric arterial occlusion may be suggested with a biplanar mesenteric arteriogram. Mesenteric emboli typically lodge in the SMA at the origin of the middle colic artery, creating a "meniscus sign" with an abrupt cutoff of a normal proximal SMA several centimeters from its origin on the aorta. Mesenteric thrombosis, in contrast, occurs at the most proximal SMA, which tapers off at 1–2 cm from its origin. In the case of chronic mesenteric occlusion, the appearance of collateral circulation is usually present. Nonocclusive mesenteric ischemia produces an arteriographic image of segmental mesenteric vasospasm with a relatively normal-appearing main SMA trunk.

Mesenteric arteriography also can play a therapeutic role. Once the diagnosis of nonocclusive mesenteric ischemia is made on the arteriogram, an infusion catheter can be placed at the SMA orifice, and vasodilating agents such as papaverine can be administered intraarterially. The papaverine infusion may be continued postoperatively to treat persistent vasospasm, a common occurrence following mesenteric reperfusion. Transcatheter thrombolytic therapy has little role in the management of thrombotic mesenteric occlusion. Although thrombolytic agents may transiently recannulate the occluded vessels, the underlying occlusive lesions require definitive treatment. Furthermore, thrombolytic therapy typically requires a prolonged period of time to restore perfusion, and the intestinal viability may be difficult to assess.

Treatment

Initial management of patients with acute mesenteric ischemia includes fluid resuscitation and systemic anticoagulation with heparin to prevent further thrombus propagation. Significant metabolic acidosis should be corrected with sodium bicarbonate. The operative management of acute mesenteric ischemia is dictated by the cause of the occlusion. It is helpful to obtain a preoperative mesenteric arteriogram to confirm the diagnosis and to plan appropriate treatment options. However, the diagnosis of mesenteric ischemia frequently cannot be established prior to surgical exploration, and therefore patients in a moribund condition with acute abdominal symptoms should undergo immediate surgical exploration, avoiding the delay required to perform an arteriogram.

Acute embolic mesenteric ischemia. The primary goal of surgical treatment in embolic mesenteric ischemia is to restore arterial perfusion with removal of the embolus from the vessel. The abdomen is explored through a midline incision, which often reveals variable intestinal ischemia from the midjejunum to the ascending or transverse colon. The SMA is approached at the root of the small bowel mesentery and a transverse arteriotomy is made to extract the embolus, using standard balloon embolectomy catheters. Following the restoration of SMA flow, an assessment of intestinal viability must be made, and nonviable bowel must be resected. A second-look procedure should be considered in many patients, and is performed 24–48 h following embolectomy.

Acute thrombotic mesenteric ischemia. In embolic mesenteric ischemia, the SMA itself is normal, and thromboembolectomy will usually suffice to restore mesenteric circulation. However, thrombotic mesenteric ischemia usually involves a severely atherosclerotic vessel, typically the proximal CA and SMA. Therefore, these patients require a reconstructive procedure to the distal SMA. The saphenous vein is the graft material of choice, and prosthetic materials should be avoided in patients with nonviable bowel, because of the risk of bacterial contamination if resection of necrotic intestine is performed. The bypass graft may originate from the aorta (either above the celiac or below the renals or iliac artery).

Chronic mesenteric ischemia. The therapeutic goal in patients with chronic mesenteric ischemia is to revascularize mesenteric circulation and prevent the development of bowel infarction. Mesenteric occlusive disease can be treated successfully by either transaortic endarterectomy or mesenteric artery bypass. Transaortic endarterectomy is indicated for ostial lesions of patent CA and SMA. For occlusive lesions located 1–2 cm distal to the mesenteric origin, mesenteric artery bypass should be performed. Multiple mesenteric arteries are typically involved in chronic mesenteric ischemia, and both the CA and SMA should be revascularized whenever possible; a collateral called the arc of

Riolan may fill the distal SMA from the IMA. In general, bypass grafting may be performed either antegrade from the supraceliac aorta or retrograde from either the infrarenal aorta or iliac artery. Both autogenous saphenous vein grafts and prosthetic grafts have been used with satisfactory and equivalent success. An antegrade bypass also can be performed using a small-caliber bifurcated graft from the supraceliac aorta to both the CA and SMA, which yields an excellent long-term result.

Nonocclusive mesenteric ischemia. The treatment of nonocclusive mesenteric ischemia is primarily pharmacologic, with selective mesenteric arterial catheterization followed by infusion of vasodilatory agents such as tolazoline or papaverine. Once the diagnosis is made via mesenteric arteriography, intraarterial papaverine is given at a dose of 30–60 mg/h.

Celiac Artery Compression Syndrome

Abdominal pain because of narrowing of the origin of the CA may occur as a result of extrinsic compression or impingement by the median arcuate ligament. This condition is known as celiac artery compression syndrome or median arcuate ligament syndrome. CA compression syndrome has been implicated in some variants of chronic mesenteric ischemia. However, significant compression of the CA can be observed frequently on a lateral aortogram in the complete absence of symptoms. A decision to intervene is therefore based on both an appropriate symptom complex and the finding of CA compression in the absence of other findings to explain the symptoms. The patient should be cautioned that relief of the celiac compression cannot be guaranteed to relieve the symptoms. Most patients are young females between 20 and 40 years of age. Abdominal symptoms are nonspecific, but the pain is localized in the upper abdomen and may be precipitated by meals. The treatment goal is to release the ligamentous structure that compresses the proximal CA and to correct any persistent stricture by bypass grafting.

Renal Artery Occlusive Disease

Obstructive lesions of the renal artery can produce hypertension, resulting in a condition known as renovascular hypertension, which is the most common form of hypertension amenable to therapeutic intervention. Renovascular hypertension is believed to affect 5–10 percent of all hypertensive patients in the United States. Patients with renovascular hypertension are at an increased risk for irreversible renal dysfunction if inappropriate pharmacologic therapies are used to control the blood pressure (e.g., ACE inhibitors). In the rare event that a critically ischemic kidney cannot be revascularized, nephrectomy may also be effective in improving hypertension and preserving contralateral renal function.

Causes of Renal Artery Stenosis

Nearly 70 percent of all renal artery occlusive lesions are caused by atherosclerosis, typically occur near the renal artery ostia, and are usually less than 1 cm in length.

Patients with this disease are usually older adult males that have other atherosclerotic disease such as ischemic heart disease and peripheral vascular disease; however, a growing number of patients develop restenosis of previously placed stents.

The second most common cause of renal artery stenosis is fibromuscular dysplasia. Fibromuscular dysplasia of the renal artery represents a heterogeneous group of lesions that produce specific pathologic lesions in various regions of the vessel wall, including the intima, media, or adventitia. The most common variety consists of medial fibroplasia, in which thickened fibromuscular ridges alternate with attenuated media, producing the classic angiographic "string of beads" appearance. It occurs most commonly in young women, who are often multiparous.

Other less common causes of renal artery stenosis include renal artery aneurysm (compressing the adjacent normal renal artery), arteriovenous malformations, neurofibromatosis, renal artery dissections, renal artery trauma, Takayasu disease, and renal artery thrombosis.

Diagnostic Studies

Nearly all diagnostic studies for renovascular hypertension evaluate either the anatomic stenosis or renal parenchymal dysfunction attributed to the stenosis. Functional tests have been largely replaced by direct imaging.

Renal duplex scanning is a noninvasive test assessing renal artery stenosis both by visualization of the vessel and by measurement of the effect of stenosis on blood flow velocity and waveforms. The presence of a severe renal artery stenosis correlates with peak systolic velocities of greater than 180 cm/s and a ratio of these velocities to those in the aorta of greater than 3.5. However, many renal artery ultrasounds are difficult to perform or interpret because of obesity or increased bowel gas pattern. Additionally, renal ultrasonography does not differentiate among renal artery stenoses exceeding 60 percent cross-sectional stenosis. Because this test is highly dependent on the operator's expertise, its role as an effective screening test remains limited. Conventional renal artery angiography is critical to the evaluation of patients with possible renovascular hypertension. A flush aortogram is performed first so that any accessory renal arteries can be detected and the origins of all the renal arteries are adequately displayed. The presence of collateral vessels circumventing a renal artery stenosis strongly supports the hemodynamic importance of the stenosis. A pressure gradient of 10 mmHg or greater is necessary for collateral vessel development, which is also associated with activation of the renin-angiotensin cascade. MRA, particularly with gadolinium contrast enhancement, has become a useful diagnostic tool for renal artery occlusive disease, because of its ability to provide high-resolution images. CT angiography is also being increasingly used.

Treatment

Medical therapy. The development of a new generation of antihypertensive medications including β blockers, calcium channel blockers, and ACE inhibitors has greatly enhanced the ability to control high blood pressure in many patients with renovascular hypertension. Refractory hypertension, particularly that because of bilateral disease or unilateral renal artery stenosis with contralateral parenchymal disease, may respond to the addition of diuretic medications.

If the renal function remains stable and the blood pressure is satisfactorily controlled by medications, it is appropriate to maintain medical therapy for renovascular hypertension. However, a reduction in systemic pressure by drug therapy frequently reduces renal perfusion, which may lead to progressive renal failure. Because renal artery occlusive disease frequently progresses with concomitant loss of renal mass and function, a definitive therapy to restore normal renal blood flow may provide a greater long-term benefit than antihypertensive medical therapy.

Transluminal balloon angioplasty and stenting. Percutaneous transluminal angioplasty of the renal artery is being performed with increasing frequency. A guidewire is inserted into the renal artery from a femoral artery approach and then passed across the stenosis. An angioplasty balloon catheter is next inserted over the guidewire and positioned across the renal artery stenosis. Inflation of the balloon creates a controlled disruption of the vessel wall, thereby eliminating the intraluminal stenosis.

Percutaneous balloon angioplasty has a high success and low recurrence rate as a treatment for fibromuscular dysplasia, particularly of the medial fibroplastic type. More than two-thirds of patients with fibromuscular dysplasia are cured following balloon angioplasty and maintain diastolic pressure below 90 mmHg without antihypertensive medication. Most of the remainder of patients have significant improvement in their renovascular hypertension, although they may require antihypertensive medication.

Renal artery atherosclerotic lesions are typically an extension of aortic disease and are limited to the renal artery ostium where it joins the aorta. Balloon angioplasty in this setting is usually ineffective in achieving satisfactory dilatation because of recoil. Intravascular stents placed during balloon angioplasty are now widely used to support renal angioplasty as primary stenting has become common. Current data suggest that stenting may prove useful in patients with ostial disease, those who develop restenosis after percutaneous balloon angioplasty, or those with complications resulting from percutaneous transluminal renal angioplasty (PTRA), such as dissection. Primary renal artery stenting in patients with atherosclerotic ostial renal artery stenosis has a high technical success rate, with restenosis rates ranging from 10–20 percent at 4 years.

Surgical revascularization. The proper selection of an operative approach relates to the extent of the renal artery occlusive disease, the degree of concomitant aortic atherosclerotic disease, and the preference of the surgeon performing the procedure.

Transaortic renal artery endarterectomy is appropriate for atherosclerotic lesions, but is not applicable in fibrodysplastic disease of the renal artery. The procedure may be accomplished through a transaortic exposure in which the aorta is clamped and opened at the level of the renal arteries via a transverse aortotomy.

Renal artery bypass is the most common approach to correct renal artery stenoses and occlusions. The choice of the type of renal reconstruction depends on the status of the abdominal aorta. An aortorenal bypass is the procedure of choice when the aorta is relatively spared from atherosclerotic change and clamping will not produce injury or distal embolization.

In the event that the aorta is so heavily calcified that it poses a daunting technical challenge to perform an aortorenal grafting procedure, an alternative donor vessel source can be considered. Saphenous vein bypass from the hepatic artery to the right renal artery or splenic artery bypass to the left renal artery are the most appropriate alternatives. Both procedures avoid the embolic and hemodynamic consequences of aortic clamping. Splenorenal grafts are performed by transecting the splenic artery and constructing an anastomosis of one end of the splenic artery to one end or side of the left renal artery, and collateral flow from the short gastric vessels obviates the need for splenectomy. Alternatively, the gastroduodenal artery itself, which communicates between the celiac artery and superior mesenteric artery, can be divided distally and anastomosed to the right renal artery if it is long enough. Reconstructions based on the visceral arteries should only be performed if significant mesenteric artery occlusive disease has been excluded on angiography. Occasionally concurrent aortic disease mandates synchronous aortic reconstruction. Kidney autotransplantation may be a useful treatment modality when dealing with distal renal artery occlusive disease.

Nephrectomy is appropriate in patients with severe renovascular hypertension when the involved kidney is the source of renin production but is so severely damaged from chronic ischemia (< 6 cm in length) that the prospects for retrieval of renal function are poor.

Carotid Artery Occlusive Disease

An occlusive lesion at the origin of the internal carotid artery remains the most common cause of cerebrovascular accidents, which is the third most common cause of death and accounts for 160,000 deaths annually in the United States. Management of cerebrovascular accidents consumes $45 billion annually and is responsible for more than 1 million hospital admissions each year in the United States.

Nomenclature of Cerebrovascular Ischemia

Focal cerebral ischemic disease, or stroke, is defined as a loss of cerebral function lasting more than 24 h that is because of ischemic vascular etiology.

A transient ischemic attack (TIA) is defined in the same manner as is stroke, but lasts less than 24 h. In fact most TIAs resolve within min rather than h. When the frequency of TIAs is greater than two or three per day, it is referred to as crescendo TIA. When the ischemic focal neurologic symptoms last longer than 24 h, but resolve within 3 weeks, the term reversible ischemic neurologic deficit (RIND) is applied. Neurologic deficits lasting longer than 3 weeks are considered completed strokes.

Pathogenesis of Stroke and Transient Ischemic Attacks

Hemispheric symptoms are frequently caused by emboli from the carotid circulation. Vertebrobasilar symptoms originate from either flow-limiting or embolic lesions of the aortic arch vessels, the vertebral arteries, or the basilar artery. The predominant causes of stroke and TIA arise from the occlusive lesion of the extracranial carotid artery, and include internal carotid artery thrombosis, flow-related ischemic events, and cerebral embolization.

Carotid artery thrombosis. Thrombosis of the internal carotid artery represents the terminal event of the atherosclerotic progression of the carotid artery bifurcation. The clinical sequelae of carotid thrombosis depend on several factors, including the presence of cerebral collateral vessels provided by the circle of Willis, the chronicity of the thrombosis, and the extent of the thrombosis. Once the internal carotid artery becomes thrombosed, the column of thrombus usually propagates distally to the ophthalmic artery. However, the thrombus may occasionally extend beyond the ophthalmic artery and propagate into the circle of Willis. If the distal propagation of the thrombus stops at the ophthalmic artery and remains stable, the event of total occlusion may be silent if collateral flow is sufficient. If the thrombus progresses beyond the ophthalmic artery into the middle cerebral artery, a hemispheric event varying from a TIA to a profound stroke occurs.

Carotid artery embolization. Nearly one half of all ischemic carotid territory strokes are because of cholesterol or platelet-fibrin emboli that dislodged from atherosclerotic plaques within the internal carotid artery (ICA) and subsequently occluded distal branches of the ICA, including territories supplied by either the middle cerebral artery and/or the anterior cerebral artery. This mechanism accounts for the occurrence of the Hollenhorst plaques, which are platelet-fibrin aggregates or cholesterol crystals obstructing branches of the retinal artery which are frequently observed during an ophthalmologic exam. TIA or stroke as a consequence of a carotid stenosis has been extensively studied, with clear benefit established in the the North American Symptomatic Carotid Endarterectomy Trial (NASCET) for stenoses greater than 75 percent. The Asymptomatic Carotid Atherosclerosis Study (ACAS) demonstrated benefit even in asymptomatic patients for stenoses greater than 60 percent.

Cardiogenic embolization. Cardiogenic embolization is responsible for less than 10 percent of all ischemic carotid territory strokes.

Miscellaneous causes. Miscellaneous causes account for less than 5 percent of ischemic carotid territory strokes, and include migraine, oral contraceptive use, trauma, dissection, giant cell arteritis, Takayasu arteritis, systemic lupus erythematosus, polyarteritis nodosa, amyloid angiopathy, cocaine abuse, fibromuscular dysplasia, and radiation arteritis. Fibromuscular dysplasia (FMD) is the most common nonatherosclerotic disease affecting the ICA. Approximately one quarter of patients with carotid FMD have associated intracranial aneurysms, and up to two thirds of these patients will have bilateral carotid FMD.

Carotid artery aneurysms. As with aneurysms anywhere else in the body, carotid aneurysms may be either true or false. In the past, most true aneurysms have traditionally been classified as part of the atherosclerotic process. However, emerging evidence suggests that aneurysmal disease may be yet another manifestation of abnormalities of matrix metalloproteinase unless it is associated with other distinct pathologies (e.g., arteritis [giant cell or Takayasu] or FMD). False aneurysms may arise as a consequence of iatrogenic injury, blunt trauma, or carotid patch infection because of prior carotid endarterectomy.

Carotid dissection. Acute carotid dissection can complicate atherosclerosis, FMD, cystic medial necrosis, and blunt trauma. Angiographic studies suggest that the most likely mechanism of acute carotid dissection is an intimal tear followed by an acute intimal dissection, which produces luminal occlusion because of secondary thrombosis. This appears as a flame-shaped occlusion 2–3 cm beyond the bifurcation. Autopsy studies typically reveal a sharply demarcated transition between the normal carotid artery and the dissected carotid segment. The ICA is commonly affected, with the dissection plane typically occurring in the outer medial layer. Treatment is with anticoagulation, and in most cases this results in complete resolution within 1–2 months. Recently there has been increasing use of stenting in severely symptomatic patients.

Carotid body tumor. A carotid body tumor typically presents as a palpable and painless mass over the carotid bifurcation region in the neck. Cranial nerve palsy may occur in up to 25 percent of patients, particularly involving the vagus and hypoglossal nerves. The differential diagnosis includes cervical lymphadenopathy, carotid artery aneurysm, brachial cleft cyst, laryngeal carcinoma, and metastatic tumor.

The treatment of choice of carotid body tumors is surgical excision. Because these tumors are highly vascularized, preoperative tumor embolization may be an advantage to minimize operative blood loss when dealing with tumors greater than 3 cm in diameter. An important surgical principle in carotid body tumor resection is to maintain a dissecting plane along the subadventitial space, which will invariably allow complete tumor removal without interrupting the carotid artery integrity.

Diagnosis

The most important tool in the diagnosis of carotid artery disease is a careful history and complete neurologic examination, which should localize the area of cerebral ischemia responsible for the neurologic deficit. The neurologic examination of the patient should be complemented by a complete physical examination to determine the presence of vascular occlusive disease in either the coronary or peripheral arteries, and to define the other risk factors for stroke, such as acute arrhythmia. The diagnosis of carotid bifurcation disease is facilitated by the relatively superficial location of the carotid artery, rendering it accessible to auscultation and palpation. The cervical carotid pulse is usually normal in patients with carotid bifurcation disease, because the common carotid artery is the only palpable vessel in the neck and is rarely diseased. Carotid bifurcation bruits may be heard just anterior to the sternocleidomastoid muscle near the angle of the mandible. Bruits do not become audible until the stenosis is severe enough to reduce the luminal diameter by at least 50 percent. Bruits may be absent in extremely severe lesions because of the extreme reduction of flow across the stenosis.

The utility of noninvasive carotid imaging modalities has provided more accurate information regarding the nature and severity of the carotid artery lesion. Color-flow duplex scanning uses real-time, B-mode ultrasound and color-enhanced pulsed Doppler flow measurements to determine the extent of the carotid stenosis with reliable sensitivity and specificity. Real-time, B-mode imaging permits localization of the disease and determination of the presence or absence of calcification within the plaque. Determination of the extent of stenosis is based largely on velocity criteria. As the stenosis increasingly obliterates the lumen of the vessel, the velocity of blood must increase in the area of the stenosis so that the total volume of flow remains constant within the vessel. Thus, the velocity is correlated with the extent of carotid artery stenosis.

MRI and MRA have been evaluated as a means of imaging the carotid arteries. These are highly sensitive imaging tools for the evaluation of patients with symptomatic cerebrovascular disease. MRI is more sensitive than CT scanning for the detection of an acute stroke. MRI can detect a stroke immediately after the infarction occurs, whereas CT scanning cannot. MRA, which is evolving rapidly, permits evaluation of both the extracranial and intracranial cerebral circulations. The precision of MRA in determining the extent of stenosis, although improving rapidly, remains inferior to that achieved by conventional angiography. Nonetheless, MRA will likely play an increasingly important role in the diagnostic evaluation of patients with cerebrovascular disease.

Carotid angiography has been the traditional diagnostic tool for the evaluation of cerebrovascular disease. However, fewer hospitals now perform routine contrast angiography on all patients prior to surgery. This is partly because of the potential for angiography-related complications, and improved diagnostic accuracy of noninvasive imaging modalities. Angiography remains the only method that allows complete and detailed visualization of both the intracranial and extracranial arterial circulations.

Surgical Treatment

Carotid endarterectomy is indicated for treatment of patients with hemispheric TIAs and stroke associated with carotid bifurcation occlusive disease. Additionally, prophylactic carotid endarterectomy for asymptomatic patients with high-grade stenosis or complex ulcerated plaques is indicated. A brief overview of three important clinical trials, including the European Carotid Surgery Trial (ECST), NASCET, and ACAS is discussed below.

Overview of the European carotid surgery trial and the North American symptomatic carotid endarterectomy trial. The benefit of carotid endarterectomy for patients with symptomatic cerebrovascular disease has recently been established by both the ECST and NASCET trials. These studies randomized nearly 6000 patients in 200 hospitals around the world comparing "best medical therapy" against "best medical therapy" plus carotid endarterectomy. These studies documented a significant reduction in cerebrovascular events following the procedure compared with patients managed only medically. Both trials showed that carotid endarterectomy conferred significant benefit in symptomatic patients with a 70–99 percent stenosis. Although the NASCET trial observed a small but significant benefit in patients with 50–69 percent stenoses, the ECST trial found no evidence of benefit in patients with lesser degrees of disease. The reason for these apparent discrepancies lies in the method for calculating the degree of stenosis. ECST compared the residual luminal diameter against the diameter of the carotid artery at the level of the stenosis (usually the carotid bulb). NASCET compared the residual luminal diameter against the diameter of the ICA at least 1 cm above the stenosis. As a consequence, ECST tends to systematically overestimate stenoses (as compared with NASCET), particularly in those with mild to moderate disease. In reality, a 60 percent NASCET stenosis is approximately equivalent to an 80 percent ECST stenosis.

The ECST and NASCET trials have identified predictive factors that are associated with a significantly higher risk of late stroke in medically treated patients. These factors include male sex, 90–94 percent stenosis, surface irregularity/ulceration, coexistent intracranial disease, no recruitment of intracranial collaterals, hemispheric symptoms, cerebral events within 2 months, multiple cerebral events, contralateral occlusion, multiple concurrent risk factors, and age of more than 75 years.

Overview of the asymptomatic carotid atherosclerosis study. The ACAS trial was a prospective study that randomized 1600 patients with asymptomatic stenosis of 60 percent or greater to either carotid endarterectomy and aspirin or aspirin alone. This study was interrupted because of a significant benefit identified in patients undergoing carotid endarterectomy. At the time of interruption of the study, a relative reduction in stroke rate by 50 percent was observed by patients undergoing carotid endarterectomy. The benefit was much greater in men than in women. This study used stroke as its primary endpoint.

This group has since substantiated unequivocally the effectiveness of carotid endarterectomy in good-risk patients identified to have high-grade stenosis.

These prospective trials firmly established the role of carotid endarterectomy in the prevention of strokes in patients with high-grade carotid artery stenosis, regardless whether the lesion is symptomatic or asymptomatic. All the patients in these clinical trials were carefully selected, and the carotid endarterectomy was performed by surgeons with proven successful outcomes and low complication rates. For patients with carotid occlusive disease to benefit from surgical intervention, the operation must be performed by experienced surgeons with proven low operative morbidity and mortality rates.

Technique of carotid endarterectomy. The carotid bifurcation is usually approached via a longitudinal incision based on the anterior border of the sternocleidomastoid muscle. Dissection continues medial to the jugular vein, and the common carotid bifurcation is mobilized and exposed. The patient is systemically heparinized and the carotid arteries cross-clamped. If the surgeon chooses to shunt the patient, it is inserted at this time. The plaque is endarterectomized, tacking sutures are inserted if required, and the ECA origin is cleared of plaque using the eversion technique. The carotid arteriotomy is closed primarily using a running suture, and if the ICA is small, a patch angioplasty is performed.

Although carotid endarterectomy has been performed for more than four decades, a wide variety of surgical and anesthetic approaches can be used. This operation can be performed under general endotracheal anesthesia, regional cervical block, or local.

Complications of carotid endarterectomy. The most serious complication of carotid endarterectomy is that of perioperative stroke. Stroke can occur during or after carotid endarterectomy secondary to a variety of mechanisms, including inadequate collateral blood flow to the brain during temporary ICA occlusion, embolization during dissection of the carotid artery, or embolism or thrombosis of the reconstruction during the early postoperative period. Embolization after carotid endarterectomy is usually secondary to platelet aggregates forming on the surface of the endarterectomized vessel. In contrast, thrombosis after carotid endarterectomy usually is a result of sudden intimal dissection because of a loose flap or inadequate distal endarterectomy endpoint.

Postoperative cranial nerve dysfunction can occur in up to 35 percent of patients undergoing carotid endarterectomy, which can occur because of cranial nerve damage resulting from nerve division, excessive traction, or perineural dissection. Common cranial nerve injuries include dysfunction of the recurrent laryngeal nerve, causing hoarseness; dysfunction of the hypoglossal nerve, causing deviation of the tongue toward the side of the injury; and superior laryngeal nerve dysfunction, causing easy fatigability of the voice. Less common is injury of the marginal mandibular nerve, which results in drooping of the nasolabial fold ipsilateral to the injury.

Residual or recurrent carotid artery stenosis can be detected in up to 30 percent of patients undergoing careful postoperative surveillance with carotid duplex scanning. However, less than 3 percent of patients experience symptomatic recurrence.

Carotid balloon angioplasty and stenting. Carotid stent trials (Sapphire Trial, Archer Trial) have now demonstrated that carotid angioplasty and stenting is equal to carotid endarterectomy in terms of stroke and death rate in high risk surgical patients. It is likely that there will be a trend toward increasing stenting and reduced numbers of open endarterectomy.

Non Atherosclerotic Vascular Disease

Popliteal artery. There are three distinct nonatherosclerotic disease entities that may result in lower extremity claudication, predominantly occurring in 40–50-year-old men. Adventitial cystic disease, popliteal artery entrapment syndrome, and Buerger disease should be considered in any young patients presenting with intermittent claudication.

Adventitial Cystic Disease

Adventitial cystic disease is a rare arterial condition occurring at an incidence of 0.1 percent, usually in the popliteal artery. This disease affects men in a ratio of approximately 5:1 and appears predominantly in the fourth and fifth decades. Besides claudication as a symptom, this diagnosis should be considered in young patients who have a mass in a nonaxial vessel in proximity to a related joint. These synovial-like, mucin-filled cysts reside in the subadventitial layer of the vessel wall and have a similar macroscopic appearance to ganglion cysts.

Patients presenting at a young age with bilateral lower extremity claudication and minimal risk factors for atheroma formation should be evaluated for adventitial cystic disease, and the other two nonatherosclerotic vascular lesions described here. Because of luminal encroachment and compression, peripheral pulses may be present in the limb when extended, but then can disappear during knee joint flexion. Noninvasive studies may suggest arterial stenosis with elevated velocities. Color-flow duplex scanning followed by T2-weighted MRI now appears to be the best diagnostic choice. Angiography will demonstrate a smooth, well-defined, crescent-shaped filling defect, the classic "scimitar" sign.

The recommended treatments are excision of the cyst with the cystic wall, enucleation, or simple aspiration when the artery is stenotic. Retention of the cystic lining leads to continued secretion of the cystic fluid and recurrent lesions. In 30 percent of patients who have an occluded artery, resection of the affected artery, followed by an interposition graft using autogenous saphenous vein, is recommended.

Popliteal Artery Entrapment Syndrome

Love and colleagues first coined the term popliteal artery entrapment in 1965 to describe a syndrome combining muscular involvement with arterial ischemia occurring behind the knee, with the successful surgical repair having taken place 6 years earlier. This is a rare disorder with an estimated prevalence of 0.16 percent that occurs with a male-to-female ratio of 15:1. Five types of anatomic entrapment have been defined, according to the position of the medial head of the gastrocnemius muscle, abnormal muscle slips or tendinous bands, or the course of the popliteal artery itself. Concomitant popliteal vein impingement occurs in up to 30 percent. Twenty-five percent of cases are bilateral.

The typical patient presents with swelling and claudication of isolated calf muscle groups following vigorous physical activity. Noninvasive studies with ankle-brachial indices should be performed with the knee extended and the foot in a neutral, forced plantar, and dorsiflexed position. A drop in pressure of 50 percent or greater or dampening of the plethysmographic waveforms in plantar or dorsiflexion is a classic finding. The sudden onset of signs and symptoms of acute ischemia with absent distal pulses is consistent with popliteal artery occlusion secondary to entrapment. Although CT and MRI have been employed, angiography remains the most widely used test. Angiography performed with the foot in a neutral position may demonstrate classical medial deviation of the popliteal artery or normal anatomic positioning. Coexisting abnormalities may include stenosis, luminal irregularity, delayed flow, aneurysm, or complete occlusion. Diagnostic accuracy is increased with the use of ankle stress view-active plantar flexion and passive dorsiflexion.

The treatment of popliteal artery entrapment consists of surgical decompression of the impinged artery with possible arterial reconstruction. Division of the anomalous musculotendinous insertion site with or without saphenous vein interposition grafting to bypass the damaged arterial segment has been described to be the procedure of choice. The natural history of entrapment is progressive arterial degeneration leading to complete arterial thrombosis. In such instances, thrombolytic therapy is needed with subsequent release of the functional arterial impairment. Lysis will improve distal runoff and may improve limb-salvage and bypass patency rates.

Buerger Disease (Thromboangiitis Obliterans)

Buerger disease, also known as thromboangiitis obliterans, is a progressive nonatherosclerotic segmental inflammatory disease that most often affects small and medium-sized arteries, veins, and nerves of the upper and lower extremities. The typical age range for occurrence is 20–50 years, and the disorder is more frequently found in males who smoke. The upper extremities may be involved, and a migratory superficial phlebitis may be present in up to 16 percent of patients, thus indicating a systemic inflammatory response. In young adults presenting to the Mayo Clinic (1953–1981) with lower limb ischemia, Buerger disease was diagnosed in 24 percent. Conversely, the diagnosis was made in 9 percent of patients with ischemic finger ulcerations. The cause of thromboangiitis obliterans is unknown; however, use of or exposure to tobacco is essential to both the diagnosis and progression of the disease.

Pathologically, thrombosis occurs in small to medium size arteries and veins with associated dense polymorphonuclear leukocyte aggregation, microabscesses, and multinucleated giant cells. Buerger's disease typically presents in young male smokers, with symptoms beginning prior to age 40. Patients initially present with foot, leg, arm, or hand claudication, which may be mistaken for joint or neuromuscular problems. Progression of the disease leads to calf claudication and eventually ischemic rest pain and ulcerations on the toes, feet, or fingers. Characteristic angiographic findings show disease confinement to the distal circulation, usually infrapopliteal and distal to the brachial artery. The occlusions are segmental and show "skip" lesions with extensive collateralization, the so-called "corkscrew collaterals."

Treatment involve strict smoking cessation. In patients who are able to abstain, disease remission is impressive and amputation avoidance is increased. The role of surgical intervention is minimal in Buerger's disease, as there is often no acceptable target vessel for bypass. Furthermore, autogenous vein conduits are limited secondary to coexisting migratory thrombophlebitis.

Inflammatory Arteritis and Vasculitides

Chronic inflammatory arteritides and vasculitides include a spectrum of disease processes caused by immunologic mechanism. This results in a necrotizing transmural inflammation of the vessel wall associated with antigen-antibody immune complex deposition within the endothelium and pronounced cellular infiltration in the adventitia, thickened intimal fibrosis, and organized thrombus. Most are treated by corticosteroid therapy or chemotherapeutic agents.

Takayasu Arteritis

Takayasu arteritis is an inflammatory disease of the large medial vessels, affecting primarily the aorta, its main branches and the pulmonary artery. This rare autoimmune disease occurs predominantly in women between the ages of 10 and 40 years who are of Asian descent. Vascular inflammation leads to arterial wall thickening, stenosis, and eventually, fibrosis and thrombus formation. The pathologic changes produce stenosis, dilation, aneurysm formation, and/or occlusion.

The clinical course of Takayasu arteritis begins with a "prepulseless" phase in which the patient demonstrates constitutional symptoms. These include fever, anorexia, weight loss, general malaise, arthralgias, and malnutrition. As the inflammation progresses and stenoses develop, more characteristic features of the disease become evident. During the chronic phase, the disease is inactive or "burned out." It is during this latter stage that patients most frequently present with bruits and vascular insufficiency according to the arterial bed involved. Laboratory data may show elevations in erythrocyte sedimentation rate, C-reactive protein, white blood cell count, or conversely, anemia may predominate. Characteristic clinical features during the second phase vary according to the involved vascular bed, and include hypertension reflecting renal artery stenosis, retinopathy, aortic regurgitation, cerebrovascular symptoms, angina and congestive heart failure, abdominal pain or gastrointestinal bleeding, pulmonary hypertension, or extremity claudication.

The standard criterion for diagnosis remains angiography showing narrowing or occlusion of the entire aorta or its primary branches, or focal or segmental changes in large arteries in the upper or lower extremities. Six types of Takayasu arteritis exist and are graded in terms of severity: type I, affecting the aorta and arch vessels; type IIa, affecting the ascending aorta, aortic arch, and branches; type IIb, affecting the ascending aorta, aortic arch and branches, and thoracic descending aorta; type III, affecting the thoracic descending aorta, abdominal aorta, and/or renal arteries; type IV, affecting the abdominal aorta and/or renal arteries; and type V, with combined features of types IIb and IV.

Treatment consists of steroid therapy initially, with cytotoxic agents used in patients who do not achieve remission. Surgical treatment is performed only in advanced stages, and bypass needs to be delayed during active phases of inflammation. There is no role for endarterectomy, and synthetic or autogenous bypass grafts need to be placed onto disease-free segments of vessels. For focal lesions, there have been reports of success with angioplasty.

Giant Cell Arteritis (Temporal Arteritis)

Patients tend to be white women older than the age of 50 years, with a high incidence in Scandinavia and women of Northern European descent. The inflammatory process typically involves the aorta and its extracranial branches, of which the superficial temporal artery is specifically affected.

The clinical syndrome begins with a prodromal phase of constitutional symptoms, including headache (most common), fever, malaise, and myalgias.

The patients may be initially diagnosed with coexisting polymyalgia rheumatica; an HLA-related association may exist between the two diseases. As a result of vascular narrowing and end-organ ischemia, complications may occur such as visual alterations, including blindness and mural weakness, resulting in acute aortic dissection that may be devastating. Ischemic optic neuritis resulting in partial or complete blindness occurs in up to 40 percent of patients and is considered a medical emergency. Cerebral symptoms occur when the disease process extends to the carotid arteries. Jaw claudication and temporal artery tenderness may be experienced. Aortic lesions are usually asymptomatic until later stages and consist of thoracic aneurysms and aortic dissections.

The diagnostic standard criterion is a temporal artery biopsy, which will show the classic histologic findings of multinucleated giant cells with a dense perivascular inflammatory infiltrate. Treatment regimens are centered on corticosteroids, and giant cell arteritis tends to rapidly respond. Remission rates are high, and treatment tends to have a beneficial and preventative effect on the development of subsequent vascular complications.

Behçet Disease

Behçet disease is a rare syndrome characterized by oral and genital ulcerations and ocular inflammation, affecting males in Japan and the Mediterranean. Vascular involvement is seen in 7–38 percent of patients, and is localized to the abdominal aorta, femoral artery, and pulmonary artery. Vascular lesions may also include venous complications such as deep venous thrombosis or superficial thrombophlebitis. Arterial aneurysmal degeneration can occur; however, this is an uncommon, albeit potentially devastating, complication. Multiple true aneurysms and pseudoaneurysms may develop, and rupture of an aortic aneurysm is the major cause of death in patients with Behçet disease. Multiple aneurysms are relatively common, with a reported occurrence of 36 percent in affected Japanese patients. Furthermore, pseudoaneurysm formation after surgical bypass is common at anastomotic suture lines because of the vascular wall fragility and medial destruction. Systemic therapy with corticosteroids and immunosuppressive agents may diminish symptoms related to the inflammatory process; however, they have no effect on the rate of disease progression and arterial degeneration.

Polyarteritis Nodosa

Polyarteritis nodosa (PAN) is another systemic inflammatory disease process, which is characterized by a necrotizing inflammation of medium-sized or small arteries that spares the smallest blood vessels (i.e., arterioles and capillaries). This disease predominantly affects men over women by a 2:1 ratio. PAN develops subacutely, with constitutional symptoms that last for weeks to months. Intermittent, low-grade fevers, malaise, weight loss, and myalgias are common presenting symptoms. As medium-sized vessels lie within the deep dermis, cutaneous manifestations occur in the form of livedo reticularis, nodules, ulcerations, and digital ischemia. Skin biopsies of these lesions may be sufficient for diagnosis. Inflammation may be seen histologically, with pleomorphic cellular infiltrates and segmental transmural necrosis leading to aneurysm formation.

Neuritis from nerve infarction occurs in 60 percent of patients, and gastrointestinal complications in up to 50 percent. Additionally, renal involvement is found in 40 percent, and manifests as microaneurysms within the kidney or segmental infarctions. Cardiac disease is a rare finding except at autopsy, where thickened, diseased coronary arteries may be seen, and patchy myocardial necrosis. Patients may succumb to renal failure, intestinal hemorrhage, or perforation. End-organ ischemia from vascular occlusion or aneurysm rupture can be disastrous complications with high mortality rates. The mainstay of treatment is steroid and cytotoxic agent therapy. Up to 50 percent of patients with active PAN will experience remission with high dosing.

Raynaud Syndrome

Raynaud syndrome is a heterogeneous symptom array associated with peripheral vasospasm, more commonly occurring in the upper extremities. The characteristically intermittent vasospasm classically follows exposure to various stimuli, including cold temperatures, tobacco, or emotional stress. Formerly, a distinction was made between Raynaud "disease" and Raynaud "phenomenon" for describing a benign disease occurring in isolation or a more severe disease secondary to another underlying disorder, respectively. However, many patients develop collagen vascular disorders at some point after the onset of vasospastic symptoms; progression to a connective tissue disorder ranges from 11–65 percent in reported series. Therefore, the term Raynaud's syndrome is now used to encompass both the primary and secondary conditions. Characteristic color changes occur in response to the arteriolar vasospasm, ranging from intense pallor to cyanosis to redness as the vasospasm occurs. The digital vessels then relax, eventually leading to reactive hyperemia. The majority of patients are young women younger than 40 years of age. Up to 70–90 percent of reported patients are women, although many patients with only mild symptoms may never present for treatment. Certain occupational groups, such as those that use vibrating tools, may be more predisposed to Raynaud syndrome or digital ischemia. The exact pathophysiologic mechanism behind the development of such severe vasospasm remains elusive, and much attention has focused on increased levels of α_2-adrenergic receptors and their hypersensitivity in patients with Raynaud syndrome, and abnormalities in the thermoregulatory response, which is governed by the sympathetic nervous system.

The diagnosis of severe vasospasm may be made using noninvasive measurements in the vascular laboratory. Angiography is usually reserved for those who have digital ulceration and an embolic or obstructive cause is believed to be present and potentially surgically correctable. Different changes in digital blood pressure will occur in patients with Raynaud syndrome. Normal individuals will show only a slight decrease in digital blood pressure in response to external cold stimuli, whereas those with Raynaud syndrome will show a similar curve until a critical temperature is reached. It is at this point that arterial closure acutely occurs.

There is no cure for Raynaud syndrome, thus all treatments mainly palliate symptoms and decrease the severity and perhaps frequency of attacks. Conservative measures predominate, including the wearing of gloves, use of electric or chemically activated hand warmers, avoiding occupational exposure to vibratory tools, abstinence from tobacco, or relocating to a warmer, dryer climate. The majority (90 percent) of patients will respond to avoidance of cold and other stimuli. The remaining 10 percent of patients with more persistent or severe syndromes can be treated with a variety of vasodilatory drugs, albeit with only a 30–60 percent response rate. Calcium-channel blocking agents such as diltiazem and nifedipine are the drugs of choice. The selective serotonin reuptake inhibitor fluoxetine has been shown to reduce the frequency and duration of vasospastic episodes. Intravenous infusions of prostaglandins have been reserved for nonresponders with severe symptoms.

Surgical therapy is limited to débridement of digital ulcerations and amputation of gangrenous digits, which are rare complications. Upper extremity sympathectomy may provide relief in 60–70 percent of patients; however, the results are short-lived with a gradual recurrence of symptoms in 60 percent within 10 years.

Fibromuscular Dysplasia

FMD is a vasculopathy of uncertain etiology that is characterized by segmental arterial involvement. Histologically, fibrous tissue proliferation, smooth muscle cell hyperplasia, and elastic fiber destruction alternate with mural thinning. The characteristic beaded appearance of FMD is because of areas of medial thinning alternating with areas of stenosis. The most commonly affected are medium-sized arteries, including the internal carotid, renal, vertebral, subclavian, mesenteric, and iliac arteries. The internal carotid artery is the second most common site of involvement after the renal arteries. FMD occurs most frequently in women (90 percent) and is recognized at approximately 55 years of age. Only 10 percent of patients with FMD will have complications attributable to the disease. Pathologically, FMD is a heterogenous group of four distinct types of lesions which are subgrouped based on the predominant site of involvement within the vessel wall. Of the four types (medial fibroplasia, intimal fibroplasia, medial hyperplasia, and perimedial dysplasia), medial fibroplasia is the most common pathologic type, affecting the ICA and the renal artery, and occurring in 85 percent of reported cases.

The two main clinical syndromes associated with FMD are transient ischemic attacks from disease in the ICA, and hypertension from renal artery involvement. Symptoms produced by FMD are generally secondary to associated arterial stenosis, and are clinically indistinguishable from those caused by atherosclerotic disease. Often, asymptomatic disease is found incidentally on conventional angiographic studies being performed for other reasons. Within the ICA, FMD lesions tend to be located higher in the extracranial segment than with atherosclerotic lesions, and may not be readily demonstrated by duplex scan.

Clinically, symptoms are because of encroachment on the vessel lumen and a reduction in flow. Additionally, thrombi may form in areas of mural dilatation from a stagnation of flow, leading to distal embolization. Surgical treatment has been favored for symptomatic patients with angiographically proven disease. Owing to the distal location of FMD lesions in the extracranial carotid artery, resection and repair is not usually feasible. Instead, graduated luminal dilatation under direct vision has been used successfully in patients, with antiplatelet therapy continued postoperatively. Percutaneous transluminal angioplasty has been used effectively in patients with FMD-induced hypertension. Several series have documented a high technical success rate, with recurrence rates of 8–23 percent at more than 1 year. However, the therapeutic effect of blood pressure control may continue to be observed despite restenosis. Surgical reconstruction of the renal arteries for FMD has good long-term results and is recommended for recurrent lesions after angioplasty. Open balloon angioplasty of the ICA has been described, which allows for precise fluoroscopic guidance, rather than blind dilatation with calibrated metal probes, and back-bleeding after dilatation to eliminate cerebral embolization. Distal neuroprotective devices may allow this procedure to be performed completely percutaneously, by lessening the threat of cerebral emboli.

UPPER EXTREMITY ARTERIAL DISEASE

Upper extremity arterial disease is much less common than disease in the lower extremity. Indeed most arterial problems in the arms are related to the establishment of arteriovenous access grafts. Although atherosclerosis remains the most common cause of naturally occurring upper extremity vascular disease, there is a much higher incidence of nonatherosclerotic arterial disease in the upper extremity than in the leg. The details of these nonatherosclerotic vascular disorders are described in more detail in that section.

Symptoms

The most common location for atherosclerosis affecting the upper limb is at the origin of the subclavian artery, most commonly the left subclavian artery. Frequently there are no symptoms, because of rich collaterals and reversed flow in the ipsilateral vertebral artery. Symptoms when they do occur manifest as arm pain, described as aching and weakness in the extremity, made worse with exercise of the arm and relieved by rest. Subclavian steal syndrome occurs when posterior circulation symptoms (dizziness, drop attacks, and diplopia) occur during arm exercise in patients with proximal subclavian artery occlusion. This syndrome is relatively rare. Another unusual manifestation of subclavian artery occlusion is coronary-subclavian steal syndrome. This occurs in the setting of proximal (usually left) subclavian artery occlusion in a patient with a prior left internal mammary artery (LIMA) to left anterior descending artery (LAD) graft. Arm exercise may lead to reversed flow in the LIMA and lead to development of chest pain from myocardial ischemia. Because of the collaterals, the limb is threatened only rarely; however, distal embolization can occur from atherosclerotic stenoses or from an axillosubclavian aneurysm, both of which can complicate thoracic outlet syndrome. Embolization usually manifests as small areas of digital gangrene.

Examination

This begins with pulse examination: axillary, brachial, radial, and ulnar. Both the infraclavicular and supraclavicular fossae should be palpated and auscultated for aneurysms and bruits. The blood pressure should be recorded for both brachial arteries. A difference of greater than 20 mmHg is likely to be significant and suggestive of proximal occlusive disease.

Investigations

The subclavian artery is inaccessible for examination and duplex scanning. However, the finding of a pressure difference between the arms and reversed flow in the ipsilateral vertebral artery by duplex scanning is highly suggestive of proximal subclavian stenosis. If this is not associated with symptoms, then further investigation may not be necessary. However, in a symptomatic patient or in a patient in whom an IMA to LAD bypass has been performed, further investigation is warranted. Spiral CT and MRA can be used, but the definitive procedure remains arch angiography. The angiographer should specifically look for reversed flow in the ipsilateral vertebral artery, which leads to late filling of the distal subclavian artery. This is an important observation to determine treatment options and select a distal site for bypass grafting.

Treatment

Intervention is indicated only for patients who are symptomatic. In patients with symptoms suggestive of subclavian steal syndrome and concurrent carotid stenoses, the carotid stenosis is usually treated first. If the carotid lesion is at the origin of the carotid required for carotid subclavian bypass, then synchronous retrograde stenting of the common carotid artery (CCA) origin prior to creating the bypass can be performed.

Both endovascular and open treatment options are available for subclavian disease. We prefer angioplasty and stenting for stenoses and reserve carotid subclavian bypass for total occlusion or for stenoses that have been actively embolizing or where there is intraluminal thrombus on angiography. The open procedure most commonly performed is carotid to subclavian bypass. This is performed through a supraclavicular incision, exposing the proximal CCA. The subclavian is exposed by dividing the scalenus anterior muscle. A short 8-mm Dacron graft is tunneled posterior to the jugular vein between the two arteries and should restore a palpable pulse to the extremity. Transposition of the subclavian artery into the common carotid is another option, made easier if the subclavian is high and tortuous. Although subclavian endarterectomy has been described, these authors believe this is fraught with hazard and should be abandoned. Other revascularization options employed when there is concurrent occlusive disease involving the other supraortic trunks include subclavian to subclavian bypass, axillosubclavian bypass, and in patients with disease involving all the supra-aortic vessels, direct revascularization from the aorta may be necessary.

When arm ischemia occurs because of more distal axillary or brachial artery disease, the physician must verify that the patient does not have atherosclerotic disease. In most cases bypass with reversed saphenous vein is the treatment of choice.

Subclavian stenting can be performed by either a transfemoral or retrograde brachial approach. Primary stenting is most commonly performed to minimize the risk of embolization down the limb or up the vertebral artery.

Subclavian Artery Aneurysms

Subclavian artery aneurysms are uncommon and difficult to treat. They are typically atherosclerotic in etiology and located at the origin of the subclavian artery. Clinical manifestations include pain from arm ischemia secondary to thrombosis or embolization. Additionally, right-sided aneurysms can present with hoarseness because of stretching of the recurrent laryngeal nerve.

An aberrant right subclavian artery, arising from the aortic arch distal to the left subclavian artery, is particularly predisposed to undergoing aneurysmal degeneration, often referred to as a Kommerell diverticulum. Aneurysms of an aberrant right subclavian artery also can present with dysphagia because of compression of the esophagus.

The left subclavian artery and an aberrant right subclavian artery surgically are in very inaccessible locations. An aneurysm of the left subclavian artery is best approached through a left posterolateral thoracotomy. This permits both proximal subclavian or aortic control. The aneurysm is opened, and a 10-mm interposition Dacron graft can be inserted. Care is required when clamping the aorta because of the presence of the left recurrent laryngeal nerve hooking around the aorta medial to the left subclavian artery. On the right side, proximal control is gained via a median sternotomy. Depending on the extent of the aneurysm, distal control can be achieved via either a supraclavicular or infraclavicular incision.

Because of the difficulty in approaching these aneurysms, there has been increasing interest in the use of endovascular grafts to repair these aneurysms. Endografts can be delivered via either a femoral approach or via a retrograde brachial approach. Aneurysms with an adequate proximal and distal neck (>1 cm) are suitable for endografting. Ideally the vertebral artery should be spared; however, if the contralateral vertebral is normal, the ipsilateral vertebral can be sacrificed.

An alternate approach to a proximal subclavian artery aneurysm is ligation with embolization of the vertebral stump and carotid subclavian bypass to maintain antegrade perfusion to the arm and retrograde perfusion to the vertebral artery.

Suggested Readings

Brewster DC, Cronenwett JL, Hallett JW et al. Joint Council of the American Association for Vascular Surgery and Society for Vascular Surgery. Guidelines for the treatment of abdominal aortic aneurysms. Report of a subcommittee of the Joint Council of the American Association for Vascular Surgery and Society for Vascular Surgery. J Vasc Surg 37:1106, 2003.

Chaikof EL, Blankensteijn JD, Harris PL, et al; Ad Hoc Committee for Standardized Reporting Practices in Vascular Surgery of The Society for Vascular Surgery/American Association for Vascular Surgery. Reporting standards for endovascular aortic aneurysm repair. J Vasc Surg 35:1048, 2002.

Salam, T. A., Lumsden, A. B., Martin, L. G., et al. Nonoperative management of visceral aneurysms and pseudoaneurysms. Am. J. Surg 164:215, 1992.

Reilly LM, Sauer L, Weinstein ES, et al. Infrarenal aortic occlusion. Does it threaten renal perfusion or function? J Vasc Surg 11:216, 1990.

Chaikof EL, Smith RB III, Salam AA, et al. Ischemic nephropathy and concomitant aortic disease: a ten-year experience. J Vasc Surg 19:135, 1994.

Barnett HJ, Warlow CP. Carotid endarterectomy and the measurement of stenosis. Stroke 24:1281, 1993.

Barnett HJM, Taylor DW, Eliasziw M, et al. The benefit of carotid endarterectomy in patients with symptomatic moderate or severe stenosis. N Engl J Med 339:1415, 1998.

Love J. Popliteal artery entrapment syndrome. Am J Surg 109:620, 1965.

Hollier LH, Stanson AW, Gloviczki P, et al. Arteriomegaly: classification and morbid implications of diffuse aneurismal disease. Surgery 93:700, 1983.

Weiss VJ, Lumsden AB. Minimally invasive vascular surgery: review of current modalities. World J Surg 23:406, 1999.

Yadav JS, Wholey MH, Kuntz RE, Fayad P, Katzen BT, Mishkel GJ, Bajwa TK, Whitlow P, Strickman NE, Jaff MR, Popma JJ, Snead DB, Cutlip DE, Firth BG, Ouriel K; Stenting and Angioplasty with Protection in Patients at High Risk for Endarterectomy Investigators. Protected carotid artery stenting versus endarterectomy in high risk patients. N Engl J Med 351:1493, 2004.

23 | Venous and Lymphatic Disease

Gregory L. Moneta

VENOUS STRUCTURE/PHYSIOLOGY/ANATOMY

Venous blood flow is dependent on multiple factors such as gravity, venous valves, the cardiac and respiratory cycles, blood volume, and the calf muscle pump. Alterations in the balance of these factors may result in venous pathology.

In the supine patient, normal lower extremity venous flow is phasic, decreasing with inspiration and increasing with expiration. When the patient is upright muscular contractions of the calf, and the one-way venous valves, are required to promote venous return. Flow also can be increased by leg elevation or compression and decreased by sudden elevation of intraabdominal pressure (Valsalva maneuver).

Veins are thin-walled, highly distensible, and collapsible. Unidirectional blood flow is achieved with multiple venous valves. The number of valves is greatest below the knee and decrease in number in the more proximal veins.

Lower extremity veins are divided into superficial, deep, and perforating veins. The superficial venous system lies above the uppermost fascial layer of the leg and thigh and consists of the greater saphenous vein (GSV) and lesser saphenous vein (LSV) and their tributaries. The GSV courses medially and enters the femoral vein approximately 4 cm inferior and lateral to the pubic tubercle. The LSV courses cephalad in the posterior calf. The termination of the LSV is variable. It most often joins the popliteal vein in the popliteal fossa but may enter the deep venous system as high as the mid-posterior thigh.

In the lower leg, paired veins parallel the course of the arteries and join to form the popliteal vein. The popliteal vein continues through the adductor hiatus to become the femoral vein. In the proximal thigh, the femoral vein joins with the deep femoral vein to form the common femoral vein. The common femoral vein becomes the external iliac vein at the inguinal ligament. Perforator veins traverse the deep fascia to connect the superficial and deep venous systems. Venous sinuses are thin-walled, large veins located within the substance of the soleus and gastrocnemius muscles. A large amount of blood can be stored in the venous sinuses. With each contraction of the calf muscle bed, blood is pumped out through the venous channels into the main conduit veins to return to the heart.

There are also deep and superficial veins in the upper extremity. Deep veins follow the named arteries. Superficial veins of the upper extremity are the cephalic and basilic veins and their tributaries. The cephalic vein courses over the ventral surface of the forearm and terminates in the axillary vein. The basilic vein runs medially and joins the deep brachial veins to become the axillary vein.

The axillary vein becomes the subclavian vein at the lateral border of the first rib. At the medial border of the scalenus anterior muscle, the subclavian vein joins with the internal jugular vein to become the brachiocephalic vein. The left and right brachiocephalic veins join to become the superior vena cava.

Clinical Evaluation

Evaluation of the venous system begins with a detailed history and physical examination. Risk factors for venous disease are identified and include increased age, history of prior venous thromboembolism, malignancy, trauma, obesity, pregnancy, and hypercoagulable states, and the postoperative state. Signs suggestive of superficial venous disease are varicose and telangectatic veins, distended subdermal venules near the ankle (corona phlebectatica) and hyperpigmentation of the distal calf and ankle region. Deep veins cannot be directly assessed clinically.

Chronic venous insufficiency (CVI) may lead to characteristic changes in the skin and subcutaneous tissues in the affected limb. CVI results from incompetence of venous valves, venous obstruction, or both. Most CVI involves venous reflux. Severe CVI often reflects a combination of reflux and obstruction. A typical leg affected by CVI is edematous, indurated and pigmented with eczema and dermatitis.

Fibrosis occurs from impaired nutrition, chronic inflammation, and fat necrosis (lipodermatosclerosis). Hemosiderin deposition causes the characteristic pigmentation of chronic venous disease. Ulceration can develop with long-standing venous hypertension. Most commonly venous ulcers are approximately 3 cm proximal to the medial malleolus.

VENOUS THROMBOEMBOLISM

Epidemiology

Deep venous thrombosis (DVT) and pulmonary embolism (PE) are important preventable sources of morbidity and mortality. Venous thromboembolism (VTE) results in approximately 250,000 deaths annually. DVT also causes long-term disability. The 20-year cumulative incidence rate is 26.8 percent and 3.7 percent for the development of venous stasis changes and venous ulcers, respectively, after an episode of DVT.

Risk Factors

Stasis of blood flow, endothelial damage, and hypercoagulability contribute to VTE. Hypercoagulability appears most important in cases of spontaneous DVT. Stasis and endothelial damage play a greater role in DVT following surgical procedures and trauma. Table 23-1 lists specific risk factors for VTE.

TABLE 23-1 Risk Factors for Venous Thromboembolism

History of venous thromboembolism
Age
Major surgery
Malignancy
Obesity
Trauma
Varicose veins/superficial thrombophlebitis
Cardiac disease
Hormones
Prolonged immobilization/paralysis
Pregnancy
Venous catheterization
Hypercoagulable states (most prevalent; resistance to activated protein C)

Over 90 percent of patients hospitalized for VTE have more than one risk factor. The number of risk factors increases with age and the risk of DVT increases dramatically with multiple risk factors.

The risk for VTE in surgical patients is multifactorial. Surgical patients may have a period of activated coagulation, transient depression of fibrinolysis, be immobilized, or have a malignancy. Spinal cord injury (odds ratio 8.59) and femur or tibia fracture (odds ratio 4.82) are among the strongest risk factors for VTE.

Diagnosis

Clinical Evaluation

Venous thrombosis is thought to begin in the calf in an area of relative stasis, such as a soleal sinus vein or downstream to a venous valve. Proximal DVT without tibial vein thrombosis is unusual. Early in the course of a DVT, there may be no clinical findings. Even extensive DVT may be asymptomatic. History and physical examination are unreliable for the diagnosis of DVT. Objective studies are required to confirm or exclude a diagnosis of DVT. DVT has been found with venogram or duplex ultrasound in 50 percent or less of patients where it was clinically suspected. Clinical symptoms are usually worse with DVT that involves the proximal deep veins. Massive DVT can cause a condition called phlegmasia alba dolens. This condition is characterized by pain, pitting edema, and blanching. There is no associated cyanosis. When the thrombosis extends to the collateral veins, massive fluid sequestration and more significant edema ensues, resulting in phlegmasia cerulea dolens. Phlegmasia cerulea dolens is preceded by phlegmasia alba dolens in 50–60 percent of patients. Phlegmasia cerulea dolens is extremely painful, with severe edema, and cyanosis, and may be associated with arterial insufficiency, compartment syndrome and venous gangrene. Venous gangrene may require major amputation.

Duplex Ultrasound

DUS for detection of DVT has a sensitivity and specificity greater than 95 percent in symptomatic patients. DVT can be diagnosed by any of the following DUS findings: lack of spontaneous flow, inability to compress the vein, absence of color filling of the lumen, loss of respiratory flow variation, and venous distention. The primary method of detecting DVT with ultrasound is demonstration of lack of compressibility of the vein with probe pressure on B-mode imaging. Normally, the vein walls coapt with pressure. Lack of coaptation indicates thrombus. Several studies comparing B-mode ultrasound to venography for the detection of femoropopliteal DVT in patients clinically suspected to have DVT report sensitivities greater than 91 percent and specificities greater than 97 percent. DUS ability to assess isolated calf vein DVT varies, with sensitivities reported from 50–93 percent and specificities approaching 100 percent.

Venography

Venography is the most definitive test for the diagnosis of DVT. A small catheter is placed in the dorsum of the foot and contrast injected. A positive study is failure to fill the deep systems with a passage of the contrast medium into the superficial system, or demonstration of discrete filling defects. A normal study virtually excludes the presence of DVT. Venography is, however, no longer routinely used for diagnosis of DVT having been supplanted by duplex ultrasound.

Venous Thromboembolism (VTE) Prophylaxis

The goal of prophylaxis is to prevent the mortality and morbidity of VTE. Without prophylaxis, patients undergoing surgery for intraabdominal malignancy have a 25 percent incidence of DVT, whereas orthopedic patients undergoing hip fracture surgery have a 40–50 percent incidence of DVT. Patients at highest risk for DVT are older adults and undergoing major surgery or those with previous VTE, malignancy, or paralysis.

Prophylaxis involves use of one or more pharmacologic or mechanical modalities. Methods of VTE prophylaxis include low-dose heparin (LDH), low-molecular–weight heparin (LMWH), elastic stockings (ES), intermittent pneumatic compression (IPC), and warfarin. Aspirin alone is not adequate for DVT prophylaxis.

LMWH appears to be more effective than LDH for DVT prophylaxis with a similar risk of major bleeding. There is a 30 percent risk reduction of DVT in patients given LMWH verses those given LDH. LMWH for VTE prophylaxis is contraindicated in patients with intracranial bleeding, spinal hematoma, ongoing and uncontrolled hemorrhage, or coagulopathy. Recommendations for VTE prophylaxis from the American College of Chest Physicians (ACCP) Table 23-2 summarizes the ACCP consensus statement.

Prophylactic insertion of IVC filters has been suggested for VTE prophylaxis in high-risk trauma patients and in patients with malignancy and contraindications to LMWH. A 5-year study of prophylactic IVC filter placement in 132 trauma patients at high risk of PE reported a 0 percent incidence of symptomatic PE in patients with a correctly positioned IVC filter. IVC patency was 97.1 percent at 3 years.

The ACCP recommends IVC filters be placed only if a proximal DVT is present and anticoagulation contraindicated. IVC filter insertion is not recommended for primary prophylaxis. Retrievable IVC filters have been developed for use in patients with a temporarily increased risk of PE. Some of these devices may be removed up to 3 months postinsertion as long as there are no significant emboli contained by the filter. The device can be left in place if it traps a significant embolus.

Treatment Venous Thromboembolism

The theoretic goals of VTE treatment are to prevent mortality and morbidity associated with PE and to prevent the postphlebitic syndrome. However, the only proven benefit of anticoagulation treatment of DVT is to prevent death from PE. Treatment may include antithrombotics (heparin and warfarin), thrombolytics, vena cava interruption, and surgical thrombectomy.

Heparin

Intravenous unfractionated heparin (UFH) has traditionally been the initial treatment for VTE. UFH binds to antithrombin and potentiates antithrombin's inhibition of thrombin and activated factor X (Xa). UFH also catalyzes the inhibition of thrombin by heparin cofactor II.

TABLE 23-2 Recommendations for Venous Thromboembolism Prophylaxis

Indication	Prophylaxis methods
Low-risk general surgery (minor surgery, age < 40, no risk factors)	Early ambulation
Moderate-risk general surgery (minor surgery with risk factors; major surgery, age > 40, no risk factors)	LDH, LMWH, ES, or IPC
High-risk general surgery (minor surgery with risk factors, age > 60; major surgery, age > 40 or additional risk factors)	LDH, LMWH, or IPC
Very high-risk general surgery (multiple risk factors present)	LDH or LMWH combined with ES or IPC
Elective hip replacement	LMWH (started 12 h before surgery) or warfarin (started preoperatively or immediately after surgery with international normalized ratio [INR] target 2.5)
Elective knee replacement	LMWH or warfarin (INR = 2.5)
Hip fracture surgery	LMWH or warfarin (INR = 2.5)
Neurosurgery	IPC with or without ES and LMWH or LDH if feasible
Trauma	ES and/or IPC, LMWH if feasible
Acute spinal cord injury	LMWH with continuation of LMWH or conversion to warfarin (INR = 2.5) in the rehabilitation phase

ES = elastic compression stockings; IPC = intermittent pneumatic compression; LDH = low-dose heparin; LMWH = low molecular weight heparin.

Unfractionated heparin therapy begins with a bolus intravenous (IV) injection followed by a continuous infusion. The half-life is approximately 90 min. The level of anticoagulation should be monitored every 6 h with activated partial thromboplastin time (aPTT) determinations until aPTT levels reach a steady state. Thereafter, aPTT can be obtained daily. aPTT levels must be kept at or above 1.5 times control levels. Weight-based UFH dosages are more effective than standard fixed boluses in rapidly achieving therapeutic levels. Weight-based dosing of UFH is initiated with a bolus of 80 IU/kg IV, and a maintenance continuous infusion is started at 18 IU/kg per hour IV.

Oral anticoagulation with warfarin is started after 1 day of UFH infusion. UFH and warfarin are then administered concurrently for approximately 4 to 5 days. The daily dose of warfarin is adjusted to reach an international normalized ratio (INR) of 2–3. UFH is stopped 2 days after the patient's INR reaches 2–3 on warfarin therapy.

Hemorrhage is the primary complication of UFH therapy. The rate of major hemorrhage is 1 percent in medical patients and 8 percent in surgical patients. Anticoagulation with UFH can be reversed with protamine sulfate. Protamine is administered slowly. The infusion is terminated if side effects occur. Side effects of protamine include hypotension, pulmonary edema, and anaphylaxis. One milligram of protamine will reverse 100 units of UFH. Heparin has other complications. Heparin-induced thrombocytopenia (HIT) results from antibodies against platelet factor 4. It occurs in 1–5 percent of patients being

TABLE 23-3 Recommendations for Long-Term Anticoagulation

Indication	Duration
First VTE event with reversible risk factor (transient immobilization, estrogen use, surgery, trauma)	3–6 months
First idiopathic VTE event	≥ 6 months

treated with heparin. The major form of HIT can lead to disastrous venous or arterial thrombotic complications. Because of HIT, platelet counts should be checked after 3 days of heparin therapy. Heparin should be stopped with a drop in platelet count to < 100,000/μL. Another complication of prolonged high-dose heparin therapy is osteopenia.

Warfarin

Warfarin is the only currently available oral anticoagulant. It acts by inhibiting synthesis of vitamin K–dependent procoagulants (II, VII, IX, X) and anticoagulants (proteins C and S). Warfarin takes several days to achieve its full effect because residual normal coagulation factors have to be cleared. Therefore heparin should be continued for 2 days after achieving a therapeutic INR. The anticoagulation response to warfarin is variable. Warfarin has a half-life of 40 h. It must be withheld 2–3 days prior to any procedure with significant bleeding risk. The recommended INR for VTE therapy in most cases is between 2 and 3.

The major complication of warfarin is hemorrhage. The risk of hemorrhage is related to the magnitude of INR prolongation. Bleeding complications are treated with fresh-frozen plasma or with intravenous vitamin K.

A unique complication of warfarin is skin necrosis. It usually occurs in the first days of therapy and is associated with protein C or S deficiency or malignancy. When individuals with protein C or S deficiency are exposed to warfarin, the sudden decline in proteins C and S leads to thrombus formation in venules with extensive skin and subcutaneous fat necrosis.

Warfarin is not recommended in pregnant patients. It has been associated with spontaneous abortion and birth defects. Pregnant patients with VTE should be treated with heparin and monitored for the development of osteopenia.

Warfarin therapy reduces VTE recurrence after an acute event. The duration of oral anticoagulation for VTE is dependent on the patient's risk factors for VTE. Patients with an initial VTE with identified reversible risk factors such as transient immobilization or estrogen use should be treated for at least 3 months. Patients without identifiable risk factors are at a higher risk of recurrence and should be treated for at least 6 months. Patients with recurrent VTE or irreversible risk factors such as cancer or a hypercoagulable state should be treated for 12 months or longer. Table 23-3 summarizes current ACCP recommendations for duration of warfarin therapy.

Low-Molecular–Weight-Heparins

LMWHs differ from UFH in several ways. LMWHs, like UFH, bind to antithrombin via a specific pentasaccharide sequence. However, unlike UFH, LMWHs lack additional saccharide units to bind to and inactivate thrombin (factor IIa). In comparison to UFH, LMWHs have increased bioavailability, a longer half-life, and more predictable elimination rates.

The anticoagulant response of LMWH is predictable when given in weight-based subcutaneous doses. There is no need for laboratory monitoring of aPTT. LMWHs are eliminated through the kidneys and must be used with caution in patients with creatinine clearance less than 30 mL/min. When required, activity of LMWHs is performed by monitoring anti-Xa levels. Patients who should be monitored include children < 50 kg, obese patients > 120 kg receiving weight-adjusted doses, pregnant patients, and those with renal failure. LMWHs differ in their anti-Xa and anti-IIa activities. The treatment regimen recommended for one LMWH cannot be extrapolated for use with another one. LMWHs are only partially reversed with protamine sulfate.

LMWHs are at least as effective as, and perhaps safer than, UFH. HIT is seen in only 2–3 percent of patients receiving LMWHs but platelet counts should still be ascertained weekly in patients receiving LMWHs.

A major benefit of LMWHs is the ability to treat selected patients with VTE as outpatients. In a randomized study comparing intravenous UFH and the LMWH nadroparin-Ca, there was no significant difference in recurrent thromboembolism or major bleeding complications. There was a 67 percent reduction in mean days in the hospital for the LMWH group.

Pentasaccharides

Fondaparinux is a commercially available, chemically synthesized agent that contains the five-polysaccharide chain that binds and activates antithrombin. It does not affect thrombin (factor IIa). It is administered as a fixed subcutaneous dose and is at least as effective as the LMWH enoxaparin for the prevention of VTE after elective hip and knee replacement surgery. It is specific to antithrombin, does not bind to platelets, and minimizes the risk of HIT.

Hirudin

Hirudin is a class of direct thrombin inhibitors first derived from leeches. The commercially available hirudin, lepirudin, is manufactured by recombinant deoxyribonucleic acid (DNA) technology. Hirudins complex with thrombin and inhibit conversion of fibrinogen to fibrin and thrombin-induced platelet aggregation independent of antithrombin. Hirudins do not bind platelet factor 4. They can be used in patients who develop HIT as a complication of heparin therapy. Lepirudin is administered intravenously with a loading dose of 0.4 mg/kg followed by a continuous infusion of 0.15 mg/kg per h. The aPTT is used to monitor the effects of hirudins. The dose must be adjusted in patients with renal failure. There is no reversal agent. Plasma exchange can reverse the anticoagulant effect of hirudin.

Argatroban

Argatroban is a synthetic direct thrombin inhibitor that reversibly binds to thrombin. It is approved as an anticoagulant for prophylaxis or treatment of thrombosis in patients with heparin-induced thrombocytopenia and for patients with, or at risk for, heparin-induced thrombocytopenia undergoing percutaneous coronary intervention. Argatroban does not require the presence of antithrombin. Argatroban has a half-life of 39–51 min and reaches a steady state with intravenous infusion in 1–3 h. Argatroban can be monitored by the aPTT. There is no reversal agent.

Thrombolytic Agents

Thrombolytic therapy may reverse the hemodynamic consequences of PE and be lifesaving. In clinical practice few patients with PE (< 10 percent) are candidates for thrombolytic therapy. A major complication of systemic thrombolytic therapy is bleeding. Thrombolytic therapy is absolutely contraindicated in patients with active internal bleeding, a recent (< 2 months) cerebrovascular accident, and intracranial pathology. Relative major contraindications include major trauma, uncontrolled hypertension, active gastrointestinal pathology, recent (< 10 days) major surgery, and ocular pathology.

Thrombolytic agents currently available for clinical use are streptokinase, and recombinant tissue plasminogen activator (rtPA). Both activate plasminogen to plasmin, leading to fibrin degradation and thrombolysis. Plasmin also limits thrombus formation by degrading coagulation factors V, VIII, XII, and prekallikrein.

Streptokinase is antigenic and can cause allergic reactions. It can be inactivated by circulating antibodies and requires plasminogen as a cofactor. For PE, streptokinase is given as a 250,000-IU IV loading dose followed by 100,000 IU/h IV for 24 h. Readministration of streptokinase is not recommended between 5 days and 1–2 years of initial use or after recent streptococcal infection because of the presence of neutralizing antibodies.

TPA is found in all human tissues. A recombinant form, rTPA, is available for commercial use. It is more specific than streptokinase for fibrin-bound plasminogen, but is not superior for dissolution of thrombi or for reducing bleeding complications. rTPA to treat PE is given as a 100-mg infusion over 2 h.

There is no clear benefit for thrombolytic therapy in the large majority of patients with DVT. Thrombolytic therapy can be used in patients with massive iliofemoral DVT in an attempt to improve acute symptoms and to decrease the incidence of postthrombotic syndrome. Systemic administration of thrombolytic agents for DVT is not effective as the majority of the thrombus is not exposed to the circulating agent. In an effort to increase efficacy, catheter-directed thrombolytic techniques have been developed for the treatment of symptomatic DVT. In catheter-directed therapy, the lytic agent is administered directly into the thrombus through a catheter.

Catheter-directed thrombolytic therapy in patients with acute (>10 days) iliofemoral DVT has a reasonable chance of clearing the thrombosis. Long-term benefit in preventing the postthrombotic syndrome is unknown. Currently, the ACCP recommends that thrombolytic therapy be considered in patients with hemodynamically unstable PE or massive iliofemoral thrombosis with low bleeding potential.

Vena Caval Filters

Vena cava filters are placed percutaneously through the femoral or internal jugular vein under fluoroscopic or ultrasound guidance. Complications associated with IVC filter placement include insertion site thrombosis, filter migration, erosion of the filter into the IVC wall, and IVC obstruction. The rate of fatal complications is less than 0.12 percent.

Accepted indications for IVC filter placement in a patient with DVT or PE are contraindications to anticoagulation and failure of anticoagulation in a patient who has had a PE or is at high risk of PE. IVC filter placement does not prolong early or late survival in patients with proximal DVT, but does decrease the rate of PE. An increased rate of recurrent DVT has been observed in patients with IVC filters.

Surgical Treatment

Surgical therapy for DVT is generally reserved for patients with phlegmasia cerulea dolens or impending venous gangrene. A fasciotomy of the calf compartments is first performed. For iliofemoral DVT, a longitudinal venotomy is made in the common femoral vein (CFV) and a embolectomy catheter passed through the thrombus into the IVC and pulled back several times until no further thrombus is extracted. Distal thrombus in the leg is removed by application of a tight rubber elastic wrap beginning from the foot and extending to the thigh. If the thrombus in the femoral vein is old and cannot be extracted, the vein is ligated. For a thrombus that extends into the IVC, the IVC is exposed transperitoneally and the IVC is controlled below the renal veins. The IVC is opened and the thrombus is removed by massage. A completion venogram is performed to determine if any residual thrombus or stenosis is present. If a residual iliac vein stenosis is present, angioplasty and stenting can be performed. In most cases, an arteriovenous fistula is created by anastomosing the GSV end-to-side to the superficial femoral artery. Heparin is administered postoperatively and warfarin anticoagulation is maintained for at least 6 months. Complications of iliofemoral thrombectomy include PE in up to 20 percent and death in less than 1 percent of patients. Patients should wear compression stockings for at least 1-year post thrombectomy.

Emergency pulmonary embolectomy for acute PE is rarely indicated. Patients with preterminal massive PE who have failed thrombolysis or have contraindications to thrombolytics may be candidates for this procedure. Mortality rates range between 20 and 40 percent.

Percutaneous techniques for removal of PE involve mechanical thrombus fragmentation or embolectomy with suction devices. Mechanical clot fragmentation is followed by catheter-directed thrombolysis. Results of catheter-based fragmentation are documented in small case series only. Transvenous catheter pulmonary suction embolectomy has been performed for acute massive PE with a reported 76 percent successful extraction rate and a 30-day survival rate of 70 percent.

OTHER FORMS OF VENOUS THROMBOSIS

Superficial Venous Thrombophlebitis

Superficial venous thrombophlebitis (SVT) most commonly occurs in lower extremity varicose veins but can occur in normal superficial veins. This condition arises frequently in veins with indwelling catheters. Upper extremity SVT occurs in up to 38 percent of patients with peripherally inserted central catheters. When SVT recurs at variable sites in normal superficial veins, termed thrombophlebitis migrans, it may signify a hidden malignancy.

Clinical signs of SVT include erythema, warmth, and tenderness along the distribution of the affected vein. There is often a palpable cord. Patients with suppurative SVT may have fever and leukocytosis. DUS should be performed to confirm the diagnosis and to determine if any associated DVT is present. DVT is present in 5–40 percent of patients with SVT. A follow-up DUS should be performed in 5–7 days in patients who have SVT in the proximal GSV. They are at risk for the extension of thrombus into the femoral vein. Ten to

20 percent of patients with SVT in the proximal GSV will progress to deep venous involvement within 1 week.

Treatment of SVT is dependent on the location of the thrombus and severity of symptoms. In patients with GSV SVT >1 cm from the saphenofemoral junction or SVT in varicose veins, treatment consists of compression, warm packs, and administration of antiinflammatory medications. If GSV SVT extends proximally to within 1 cm of the saphenofemoral junction, anticoagulation for 6 weeks or GSV ligation are equally effective in preventing thrombus extension into the deep system. In patients with suppurative SVT, antibiotics and removal of any existing indwelling catheters is mandatory. Excision of the vein may be necessary.

Axillary-Subclavian Vein Thrombosis

Axillary-subclavian vein thromboses (ASVT) are classified into two forms. In primary ASVT, no clear cause for the thrombosis is readily identifiable at initial evaluation. A minority of patients have performed repetitive motions with their upper extremities resulting in damage to the subclavian vein, usually where it passes between the head of the clavicle and the first rib. This condition is known as venous thoracic outlet syndrome. Secondary ASVT is more common and is usually associated with an indwelling catheter or hypercoagulable state.

A patient with ASVT may be asymptomatic or present with upper extremity swelling and tenderness. DUS can confirm the diagnosis. Anticoagulation prevents PE and decrease symptoms. Patients presenting with acute symptomatic primary ASVT may be candidates for thrombolytic therapy. A venogram is performed through a catheter placed in the basilic vein to document the extent of the thrombus. A catheter is placed within the thrombus and a lytic agent infused. Heparin is also administered. After completion of thrombolytic therapy, a follow-up venogram is performed to identify any correctable anatomic abnormalities. Following thrombolytic therapy balloon angioplasty for residual venous narrowing and first rib resection for decompression of the thoracic outlet may be performed.

Mesenteric Venous Thrombosis

Five to 15 percent percent of acute mesenteric ischemia is as a result of mesenteric venous thrombosis (MVT). Mortality rates are as high as 50 percent. Usually the presentation is nonspecific abdominal pain, perhaps followed with diarrhea and nausea and vomiting. Peritoneal signs are present in less than 50 percent. MVT is more common in patients with a hypercoagulable state and malignancy.

In patients with MVT, plain abdominal radiographs usually demonstrate a nonspecific bowel gas pattern and are nondiagnostic. Contrast-enhanced abdominal CT scanning is the diagnostic study of choice in patients with suspected MVT.

Patients with MVT and no peritoneal findings require fluid resuscitation and anticoagulation evaluation for a hyper-coaguable disorder, and close follow up. Urgent laparotomy is indicated in patients with peritoneal findings. Findings at laparotomy are edema and cyanosis of the mesentery and bowel wall and thrombus in the mesenteric veins. The arterial supply of the bowel is usually intact. Nonviable bowel is resected, and primary anastomoses can be performed. If viability of any remaining bowel is in question, a second-look operation is performed within 24 to 48 h. Most patients with MVT are maintained on life-long anticoagulation.

VARICOSE VEINS

Varicose veins are present in 10 percent of the population. Varicose veins include dilated and tortuous veins, telangiectasias, and fine reticular varicosities. Risk factors are obesity, female sex, inactivity, and family history. Varicose veins can be classified as primary or secondary. Primary varicose veins result from intrinsic abnormalities of the venous wall. Secondary varicose veins are associated with venous insufficiency.

Patients with varicose veins may complain of aching, heaviness, and early leg fatigue. Symptoms worsen with prolonged standing and are relieved by leg elevation. Mild edema is often present. More severe signs include thrombophlebitis, hyperpigmentation, lipodermatosclerosis, ulceration, and bleeding.

Elastic compression stockings are effective treatment for many patients with varicose veins. Usually 20–30-mmHg stockings are sufficient.

Additional interventions are indicated in patients with symptoms unrelieved with compression therapy or who have signs of lipodermatosclerosis. Cosmetic concerns also can lead to intervention.

Varicose veins may be managed by injection sclerotherapy or surgical excision or a combination of both techniques. Injection sclerotherapy can be successful in varicose veins less than 3 mm in diameter and in telangiectatic vessels. Sclerosing agents include hypertonic saline, sodium tetradecyl sulfate, and polidocanol. An elastic bandage is worn continuously for 3–5 days postsclerotherapy. Complications of sclerotherapy include allergic reaction, pigmentation, thrombophlebitis, DVT, and possible skin necrosis.

Larger varicose veins are best treated by surgical excision. Standard treatment of residual varicosities is removal by the "stab/avulsion" technique. Two-millimeter incisions are made directly over branch varicosities. The varicosity is dissected proximally and distally as far as possible and is then avulsed with no attempt at ligation. Bleeding is controlled with manual pressure.

In patients with symptomatic GSV reflux, the GSV can be treated with open surgical or catheter based techniques. Surgical excision consists of GSV stripping from the groin to just below the knee. Complications associated with GSV stripping include ecchymosis, lymphocele, infection, and transient numbness in the saphenous nerve distribution. Stripping of the GSV is preferred by most surgeons over simple ligation of the GSV in the groin.

CHRONIC VENOUS INSUFFICIENCY

Chronic venous insufficiency (CVI) affects an estimated 600,000 patients in the United States. Patients complain of leg fatigue, discomfort, and heaviness. Signs of CVI may include varicose veins, pigmentation, lipodermatosclerosis, and venous ulceration. Severe CVI can be present without varicose veins. The most severe form of CVI is venous ulceration. Sixty five percent of chronic leg ulcer patients have severe pain, 81 percent have decreased mobility, and 100 percent experienced a negative impact of their disease on their work capacity. Venous leg ulcers result in an estimated 2 million lost workdays per year.

CVI results from venous reflux, venous obstruction, calf muscle pump dysfunction, or a combination of these factors. Venous reflux is the most important factor in the majority of patients with CVI. Primary valvular incompetence is diagnosed when there is no known underlying etiology of valvular dysfunction.

Secondary valvular reflux is diagnosed when an identifiable etiology is present. The most frequent secondary etiology is DVT.

Evaluation of CVI

Clinical Evaluation

The Trendelenburg test can help determine whether incompetent valves are present, and in the superficial, deep, or perforator veins. With the patient supine, the leg is elevated 45 degrees to empty the veins, and the GSV is occluded with a tourniquet. The patient stands and the superficial veins are observed for filling. When compression on the GSV is released the superficial veins are observed for increased filling. No clinically evident venous reflux is indicated by gradual filling of the veins. A positive result is the sudden filling of veins with standing or release of GSV compression. The perforator veins are thought to be normal with competent valves if the first component of the test is negative. If this part of the test is positive, there are incompetent valves in deep and perforator veins. The GSV valves are competent if the second component of the test is negative, and the GSV valves are incompetent if the second component of the test is positive. The Trendelenburg test is subjective. It has been largely supplanted by more objective noninvasive vascular laboratory tests.

Diagnostic Studies

Early diagnostic studies to evaluate CVI required invasive measurements of venous pressures after exercise. Currently noninvasive studies are preferred.

Plethysmography

Plethysmography methods are based on the measurement of volume changes in the leg. In photoplethysmography (PPG) a light-emitting diode is placed just above the medial malleolus and the patient performs a series of tip-toe maneuvers. PPG measures venous recovery time (VRT), the time required for venous volume in the skin to return to baseline after exercise. In limbs with CVI, VRT is shortened compared to a normal limb. VRT does not localize the site of reflux.

Air plethysmography (APG) also can be used to assess reflux and overall venous function. An air-filled plastic pressure bladder is placed on the calf to detect volume changes in the leg during a standard set of maneuvers. Based on measurements during these maneuvers, venous filling index (a measure of reflux), ejection fraction (a measure of calf muscles function), and residual volume fraction (a measure of overall venous function) are calculated. Theoretically, patients with an increased venous filling index and normal ejection fraction (indicating the presence of reflux with normal calf pump function) would benefit from antireflux surgery, whereas patients with a normal venous filling index and a diminished ejection fraction would not.

Venous Duplex Ultrasound

Duplex ultrasound can be used to evaluate reflux in individual venous segments of the leg. The patient is standing and the leg to be examined is non–weight bearing. Pneumatic pressure cuffs are placed around the thigh, calf, and forefoot. The ultrasound scan head is positioned just proximal to the pneumatic cuff over the venous segment to be examined. The cuff is then inflated to a standard pressure for 3 s and then rapidly deflated and reflux assessed. Reflux for greater than 0.5 s is abnormal. Typically, the common femoral, femoral, popliteal, and posterior tibial, and the greater and lesser saphenous veins, are evaluated.

Nonoperative Treatment of Chronic Venous Insufficiency

Compression Therapy

Prior to the initiation of therapy for CVI a definitive diagnosis of CVI must be made. Patients must be educated about their chronic disease and the need to comply with treatment. Compression therapy is the mainstay of CVI management. Compression can be achieved with elastic compression stockings, paste gauze boots (Unna boot), multilayer elastic wraps/dressings, or pneumatic compression devices. The exact mechanism by which compression therapy can improve CVI remains uncertain. Compression therapy is most commonly achieved with gradient elastic compression stockings. Elastic compression stockings are available in various compositions, strengths, and lengths, and can be customized.

The benefits of elastic compression stocking therapy have been well documented. In a retrospective review of 113 venous ulcer patients, the use of below-knee, 30–40-mm Hg elastic compression stockings, resulted in 93 percent healing. Complete ulcer healing occurred in 99 of 102 (97 percent) patients compliant with stocking use versus 6 of 11 patients (55 percent) who were noncompliant ($p < 0.0001$). The mean time to ulcer healing was 5 months. Ulcer recurrence was less in patients compliant with compression therapy; 29 percent at 5 years for compliant patients and 100 percent at 3 years for noncompliant patients.

Elastic compression therapy can improve quality of life in patients with CVI. In a recent study, 112 patients with CVI documented by DUS and treated with compression stockings were administered a questionnaire to quantify the symptoms of swelling, pain, skin discoloration, cosmesis, activity tolerance, depression, and sleep alterations. Symptom severity scores improved at 1 month after initiation of treatment. Further improvements were noted at 16 months.

The Unna boot is another method of compression consisting of a three-layer dressing. It requires application by trained personnel. A rolled gauze bandage impregnated with calamine, zinc oxide, glycerin, sorbitol, gelatin, and magnesium aluminum silicate is first applied with graded compression from the forefoot to just below the knee. The next layer consists of a 4-inch wide continuous gauze dressing followed by an outer layer of elastic wrap applied with graded compression. The Unna boot is changed weekly or sooner if there is significant drainage.

Other forms of compressive dressings for CVI include multilayered dressings and various legging orthosises. The efficacy of multilayered dressings is dependent on the wrapping technique of health care personnel. A commercially available legging orthosis consisting of multiple adjustable loop-and-hook closure compression bands provides compression similar to the Unna boot and can be applied daily by the patient.

Skin Substitutes

Bioengineered skin ranges in composition from acellular skin substitutes to partial-living skin substitutes. They may serve as delivery vehicles for various growth factors and cytokines important in wound healing.

Apligraf is a bilayered living skin construct that closely approximates human skin. Apligraf is between 0.5 and 1.0 mm thick and is supplied as a disk of living tissue.

A prospective randomized study comparing multilayer compression therapy alone to treatment with Apligraf in addition to multilayered compression therapy has been performed in treatment of venous ulcers. More patients treated with Apligraf had ulcer healing at 6 months (63 vs. 49 percent, $p = 0.02$). The median time to complete ulcer closure was shorter in patients treated with Apligraf (61 days vs. 181 days, $p = 0.003$). The ulcers that showed the greatest benefit were large (>1000 mm^2) or were long-standing (>6 months).

Surgical Therapy of Chronic Venous Insufficiency

Perforator Vein Ligation

Perforator vein incompetence may contribute to development of venous ulcers. The classic technique described by Linton had a high incidence of wound complications and has largely been abandoned. A minimally invasive technique termed subfascial endoscopic perforator vein surgery (SEPS) is now available.

DUS is performed preoperatively to document deep venous competence and to identify perforating veins. An Esmarque bandage and a thigh tourniquet are used to exsanguinate the limb. The knee is flexed, and two small incisions are made in the proximal medial leg away from areas of maximal induration at the ankle. Laparoscopic trocars are then positioned, and the subfascial dissection is performed with a combination of blunt and sharp dissection. Carbon dioxide is then used to insufflate the subfascial space. The thigh tourniquet is inflated to prevent air embolism. Perforators are identified, clipped and divided. After completion of the procedure, the leg is wrapped in a compression bandage for 5 days.

In a report from a large North American registry of 146 patients undergoing SEPS, healing was achieved in 88 percent of ulcers (75 of 85) at 1 year. Adjunctive procedures, primarily superficial vein stripping, were performed in 72 percent of patients. Ulcer recurrence was predicted to be 16 percent at 1 year and 28 percent at 2 years by life table analysis. The efficacy of the technique has not been confirmed in a randomized trial.

Venous Reconstruction

In the absence of significant deep venous valvular incompetence, saphenous vein stripping and perforator vein ligation can be effective in the treatment of CVI. However, in patients with a combination of superficial and deep venous valvular incompetence, the addition of deep venous valvular reconstruction may improve ulcer healing. Many techniques of deep venous valve correction have been reported. These techniques consist of repair of existing valves, transplant of venous segments from the arm, and transposition of an incompetent vein onto an adjacent competent vein.

Successful long-term outcomes of 60–80 percent have been reported for venous valve reconstructions by internal suture repair. However, in patients who initially had ulceration, 40–50 percent still have persistence or recurrence of ulcers. Valve transplantation involves replacement of a segment of incompetent femoral vein or popliteal vein with a segment of axillary or brachial vein with competent valves. Early results are similar to those of venous valve reconstruction. However, the transplanted segments tend to develop incompetence, and long-term outcomes are poorer than those of venous valve reconstructions. The outcomes for venous transposition are similar to those of valve transplantation.

Lymphedema

Pathophysiology

Lymphedema is swelling that results from a reduction in lymphatic transport. Primary lymphedema is subdivided into congenital, praecox, and tarda. Congenital lymphedema is typically present at birth. It can involve a single extremity, multiple limbs, the genitalia, or the face. Lymphedema praecox accounts for 94 percent of cases of primary lymphedema. The onset of swelling is during the childhood or teenage years and involves the foot and calf; 90 percent of patients are female. Lymphedema tarda, accounts for less than 10 percent of cases of primary lymphedema. The onset of edema is later in life than in lymphedema praecox.

Secondary lymphedema is far more common than primary lymphedema. Secondary lymphedema develops as a result of acquired lymphatic obstruction or disruption. Globally, filariasis, is the most common cause of secondary lymphedema. Lymphedema of the arm following axillary node dissection is the most common cause of secondary lymphedema in the United States. Other causes of secondary lymphedema include radiation therapy, trauma, or malignancy.

Diagnosis

Clinical Findings

In most patients the diagnosis of lymphedema is made by history and physical exam alone. There are complaints of heaviness and fatigue in the affected extremity. Limb size increases during the day and decreases over night. The limb never completely normalizes. Swelling involves the dorsum of the foot. The toes have a squared-off appearance. In advanced cases, hyperkeratosis of the skin develops. Recurrent cellulitis is a common complication. Repeated infection results in further lymphatic damage.

Distinguishing lymphedema from other causes of leg swelling can be difficult. Venous insufficiency is often confused with lymphedema. However, patients with advanced venous insufficiency typically have lipodermatosclerosis in the gaiter region, skin ulceration, and greater resolution of swelling with leg elevation.

Imaging Studies

Duplex Ultrasound

It is often difficult to distinguish lymphedema from venous insufficiency. Duplex ultrasound of the venous system can determine if venous reflux is present. Additional studies include:

Lymphoscintigraphy

A radiolabeled sulfur colloid is injected into the subdermal, interdigital region of the affected limb. Lymphatic transport is monitored with a gamma camera. Major lymphatics and nodes can be visualized.

Radiologic Lymphology

Radiologic lymphology visualizes lymphatics with colored dye injected into the hand or foot. The lymphatic channels and nodes are then visualized with traditional roentgenograms.

Management

There is no cure for lymphedema. Goals of treatment are to minimize swelling and to prevent infections. Controlling the chronic limb swelling can improve discomfort, heaviness, and tightness, and potentially reduce the progression of disease.

Bed Rest and Leg Elevation

Elevation is often the first recommended intervention. However, elevation throughout the day can interfere with quality of life. Elevation is an adjunct to lymphedema therapy, but is not the mainstay of treatment.

Compression Garments

Graded compression stockings reduce swelling in the involved extremity. Compression stockings are associated with long-term maintenance of reduced limb circumference. They may also protect the tissues against chronically elevated intrinsic pressures, which lead to thickening of the skin and subcutaneous tissue.

The degree of compression required for controlling lymphedema ranges from 20–60 mmHg and varies among patients. Stockings can be custom-made or prefabricated. The stockings should be worn during waking h and replaced approximately every 6 months.

Sequential External Pneumatic Compression

Intermittent pneumatic compression for 4–6 h per day reduces edema and provides adjunct to compression stockings. Compression stockings are necessary to maintain the volume reduction when the patient is no longer supine.

Lymphatic Massage

Manual lymphatic drainage is a form of massage. In combination with compression stockings, manual lymphatic drainage is associated with a long-term reduction in edema and fewer infections per patient per year.

Antibiotic Therapy

Patients with lymphedema are at increased risk of cellulitis in the affected extremity. Staphylococcus or β-hemolytic Streptococcus are the most common organisms causing soft tissue infection. Aggressive antibiotic therapy is recommended at the earliest signs or symptoms of cellulitis. The drug of choice is penicillin, usually 500 mg orally 3–4 times per day. Patients with a history of lymphedema and recurrent cellulitis should be given a prescription for antibiotics that can be kept at home and initiated at the first sign of infection.

Surgery

Surgical treatment involves either excision of extra tissue or anastomoses of a lymphatic vessel to another lymphatic or vein. With excisional procedures, part or all of the edematous tissue is removed. Microsurgical procedures involve the creation of a lymphaticolymphatic or lymphaticovenous anastomosis, theoretically improving lymphatic drainage. Operative therapy for lymphedema is not well accepted. Operative intervention can further obliterate lymphatic channels, worsening edema.

Summary

Lymphedema is a chronic condition caused by ineffective lymphatic transport that results in edema and skin damage. Lymphedema is not curable but can be controlled with a combination of elastic compression stockings, limb elevation, pneumatic compression, and massage.

Suggested Readings

Mohr DN, Silverstein MD, Heit JA, et al: The venous stasis syndrome after deep venous thrombosis or pulmonary embolism: a population-based study. Mayo Clin Proc 75:1249, 2000.

Lensing AW, Prandoni P, Brandjes D, et al: Detection of deep-vein thrombosis by real-time B-mode ultrasonography. N Engl J Med 320:342, 1989.

Geerts WH, Heit JA, Clagett GP, et al: Prevention of venous thromboembolism. Chest 119:132S, 2001.

Raschke RA, Reilly BM, Guidry JR, et al: The weight-based heparin dosing nomogram compared with a standard care nomogram. A randomized controlled trial. Ann Intern Med 119:874, 1993.

Ridker P, Goldhaber S, Danielson E, et al: Long-term, low-intensity warfarin therapy for the prevention of recurrent venous thromboembolism. N Engl J Med 348:1425, 2003.

Merli G, Spiro TE, Olsson CG, et al: Subcutaneous enoxaparin once or twice daily compared with intravenous unfractionated heparin for treatment of venous thromboembolic disease. Ann Intern Med 134:191, 2001.

Dwerryhouse S, Davies B, Harradine K, et al: Stripping the long saphenous vein reduces the rate of reoperation for recurrent varicose veins: Five-year results of a randomized trial. J Vasc Surg 29:589, 1999.

Mayberry JC, Moneta GL, Taylor LM Jr., et al: Fifteen-year results of ambulatory compression therapy for chronic venous ulcers. Surgery 109:575, 1991.

Gloviczki P, Bergan JJ, Rhodes JM, et al: Mid-term results of endoscopic perforator vein interruption for chronic venous insufficiency: Lessons learned from the North American subfascial endoscopic perforator surgery registry. The North American Study Group. J Vasc Surg 29:489, 1999.

Masuda EM, Kistner RL: Long-term results of venous valve reconstruction: A four- to twenty-one-year follow-up. J Vasc Surg 19:391, 1994.

24 | Esophagus and Diaphragmatic Hernia

Jeffrey H. Peters and Tom R. DeMeester

SURGICAL ANATOMY

The esophagus is a muscular tube that starts as the continuation of the pharynx and ends as the cardia of the stomach.

Manometrically, the length of the esophagus between the lower border of the cricopharyngeus and upper border of the lower sphincter varies according to the height of the individual. The musculature of the esophagus can be divided into an outer longitudinal and an inner circular layer. The upper 2–6 cm of the cervical esophagus contain only striated muscle fibers. From there on, smooth muscle fibers gradually become more abundant. When a surgical myotomy is indicated for a cricopharyngeal disorder, the myotomy incision needs to extend over this distance. Below this distance smooth muscle fibers gradually become more abundant. Most clinically significant esophageal motility disorders involve only the smooth muscle in the lower two thirds of the esophagus and the function of the cervical esophagus is normal.

The lymphatics of the esophagus located in the submucosa of the esophagus are so dense and interconnected that they constitute a single plexus. There are more lymph vessels than blood capillaries in the submucosa. Lymph flow in the submucosal plexus runs in a longitudinal direction, and on injection of a contrast medium, the longitudinal spread is seen to be about 6 times that of the transverse spread. In the upper two-thirds of the esophagus the lymphatic flow is mostly cephalad, and in the lower third caudad. In the thoracic portion of the esophagus, the submucosal lymph plexus extends over a long distance in a longitudinal direction before penetrating the muscle layer to enter lymph vessels in the adventitia. As a consequence of this nonsegmental lymph drainage, a primary tumor can extend for a considerable length superiorly or inferiorly in the submucosal plexus. Consequently, free tumor cells can follow the submucosal lymphatic plexus in either direction for a long distance before they pass through the muscularis and on into the regional lymph nodes. The cervical esophagus has a more direct segmental lymph drainage into the regional nodes, and as a result, lesions in this portion of the esophagus have less submucosal extension and a more regionalized lymphatic spread.

The efferent lymphatics from the cervical esophagus drain into the paratracheal and deep cervical lymph nodes, and those from the upper thoracic esophagus empty mainly into the paratracheal lymph nodes. Efferent lymphatics from the lower thoracic esophagus drain into the subcarinal nodes and nodes in the inferior pulmonary ligaments. The superior gastric nodes receive lymph not only from the abdominal portion of the esophagus, but also from the adjacent lower thoracic segment.

PHYSIOLOGY

Swallowing Mechanism

The act of alimentation requires the passage of food and drink from the mouth into the stomach. One-third of this distance consists of the mouth and hypopharynx, and two thirds is made up by the esophagus. To comprehend the mechanics of alimentation, it is useful to visualize the gullet as a mechanical model in which the tongue and pharynx function as a piston pump with three valves, and the body of the esophagus and cardia function as a worm-drive pump with a single valve. The three valves in the pharyngeal cylinder are the soft palate, the epiglottis, and the cricopharyngeus. The valve of the esophageal pump is the lesser esophageal sphincter (LES). Failure of the valves or the pumps leads to abnormalities in swallowing—that is, difficulty in food propulsion from mouth to stomach—or regurgitation of gastric contents into the esophagus or pharynx.

Food is taken into the mouth in a variety of bite sizes, where it is broken up, mixed with saliva, and lubricated. Once initiated, swallowing is entirely a reflex act. When food is ready for swallowing, the tongue, acting like a piston, moves the bolus into the posterior oropharynx and forces it into the hypopharynx. Concomitantly with the posterior movement of the tongue, the soft palate is elevated, thereby closing the passage between the oropharynx and nasopharynx. This partitioning prevents pressure generated in the oropharynx from being dissipated through the nose. When the soft palate is paralyzed, for example, after a cerebrovascular accident, food is commonly regurgitated into the nasopharynx. During swallowing, the hyoid bone moves upward and anteriorly, elevating the larynx and opening the retrolaryngeal space, bringing the epiglottis under the tongue. The backward tilt of the epiglottis covers the opening of the larynx to prevent aspiration. The entire pharyngeal part of swallowing occurs within 1.5 s.

During swallowing, the pressure in the hypopharynx rises abruptly, to at least 60 mmHg, because of the backward movement of the tongue and contraction of the posterior pharyngeal constrictors. A sizable pressure difference develops between the hypopharyngeal pressure and the less-than-atmospheric mid-esophageal or intrathoracic pressure. This pressure gradient speeds the movement of food from the hypopharynx into the esophagus when the cricopharyngeus or upper esophageal sphincter relaxes. The bolus is both propelled by peristaltic contraction of the posterior pharyngeal constrictors and sucked into the thoracic esophagus. Critical to receiving the bolus is the compliance of the cervical esophagus; when compliance is lost because of muscle pathology, dysphagia can result. The upper esophageal sphincter closes within 0.5 s of the initiation of the swallow, with the immediate closing pressure reaching approximately twice the resting level of 30 mmHg. The postrelaxation contraction continues down the esophagus as a peristaltic wave. The high closing pressure and the initiation of the peristaltic wave prevents reflux of the bolus from the esophagus back into the pharynx. After the peristaltic wave has passed farther down the esophagus, the pressure in the upper esophageal sphincter returns to its resting level.

The pharyngeal phase of swallowing can be started at will, or it can be reflexively elicited by the stimulation of areas in the mouth and pharynx, among them the anterior and posterior tonsillar pillars or the posterior lateral walls of the hypopharynx. The afferent sensory nerves of the pharynx are the glossopharyngeal nerves and the superior laryngeal branches of the vagus nerves.

Once aroused by stimuli entering via these nerves, the swallowing center in the medulla coordinates the complete act of swallowing by discharging impulses through cranial nerves V, VII, X, XI, and XII, and the motor neurons of C1–C3. Discharges through these nerves occur in a rather specific pattern and last for approximately 0.5 s. Little is known about the organization of the swallowing center, except that it can trigger swallowing after a variety of different inputs, but the response is always a rigidly ordered pattern of outflow. Following a cerebrovascular accident, this coordinated outflow may be altered, causing mild to severe abnormalities of swallowing. In more severe injury, swallowing can be grossly disrupted, leading to repetitive aspiration.

The striated muscles of the cricopharyngeus and the upper third of the esophagus are activated by efferent motor fibers distributed through the vagus nerve and its recurrent laryngeal branches. The integrity of innervation is required for the cricopharyngeus to relax in coordination with the pharyngeal contraction, and resume its resting tone once a bolus has entered the upper esophagus. Operative damage to the innervation can interfere with laryngeal, cricopharyngeal, and upper esophageal function, and predispose the patient to aspiration.

The pharyngeal phase of swallowing initiates the esophageal phase. The body of the esophagus functions as a worm-drive propulsive pump because of the helical arrangement of its circular muscles, and is responsible for transferring a bolus of food into the stomach. The esophageal phase of swallowing represents esophageal work done during alimentation, in that food is moved into the stomach from a negative-pressure environment of –6 mmHg intrathoracic pressure, to a positive-pressure environment of 6 mmHg intraabdominal pressure, or over a gradient of 12 mmHg. Effective and coordinated smooth muscle function in the lower third of the esophagus is therefore important in pumping the food across this gradient.

The peristaltic wave generates an occlusive pressure varying from 30–120 mmHg. The wave rises to a peak in 1 s, lasts at the peak for about 0.5 s, and then subsides in about 1.5 s. The whole course of the rise and fall of occlusive pressure may occupy one point in the esophagus for 3–5 s. The peak of a primary peristaltic contraction initiated by a swallow (primary peristalsis) moves down the esophagus at 2–4 cm/s and reaches the distal esophagus about 9 s after swallowing starts. Consecutive swallows produce similar primary peristaltic waves, but when the act of swallowing is rapidly repeated, the esophagus remains relaxed and the peristaltic wave occurs only after the last movement of the pharynx. Progress of the wave in the esophagus is caused by sequential activation of its muscles, initiated by efferent vagal nerve fibers arising in the swallowing center.

Continuity of the esophageal muscle is not necessary for sequential activation if the nerves are intact. If the muscles, but not the nerves, are cut across, the pressure wave begins distally below the cut as it dies out at the proximal end above the cut. This allows a sleeve resection of the esophagus to be done without destroying its normal function. Afferent impulses from receptors within the esophageal wall are not essential for progress of the coordinated wave. Afferent nerves, however, do go to the swallowing center from the esophagus, because if the esophagus is distended at any point, a contractual wave begins with a forceful closure of the upper esophageal sphincter and sweeps down the esophagus. This secondary contraction occurs without any movements of the mouth or pharynx. Secondary peristalsis can occur as an independent local reflex to clear the esophagus of ingested material left behind after the passage of the primary wave. Current studies suggest that secondary peristalsis is not as common as once thought. Despite the powerful occlusive pressure, the propulsive force of the esophagus is relatively feeble. If a subject attempts to swallow a bolus attached by a string to a counterweight, the maximum weight that can be overcome is 5–10 g. Orderly contractions of the muscular wall and anchoring of the esophagus at its inferior end are necessary for efficient aboral propulsion to occur. Loss of the inferior anchor, as occurs with a large hiatal hernia, can lead to inefficient propulsion.

The LES provides a pressure barrier between the esophagus and stomach and acts as the valve on the worm-drive pump of the esophageal body. Although an anatomically distinct LES has been difficult to identify, microdissection studies show that in humans, the sphincter-like function is related to the architecture of the muscle fibers at the junction of the esophageal tube with the gastric pouch. The sphincter actively remains closed to prevent reflux of gastric contents into the esophagus and opens by a relaxation that coincides with a pharyngeal swallow. The LES pressure returns to its resting level after the peristaltic wave has passed through the esophagus. Consequently, reflux of gastric juice that may occur through the open valve during a swallow is cleared back into the stomach.

If the pharyngeal swallow does not initiate a peristaltic contraction, then the coincident relaxation of the LES is unguarded and reflux of gastric juice can occur. This may be an explanation for the observation of spontaneous lower esophageal relaxation, thought by some to be a causative factor in gastroesophageal reflux disease. The power of the worm-drive pump of the esophageal body is insufficient to force open a valve that does not relax. In dogs, a bilateral cervical parasympathetic blockade abolishes the relaxation of the LES that occurs with pharyngeal swallowing or distention of the esophagus. Consequently, vagal function appears to be important in coordinating the relaxation of the LES with esophageal contraction. The antireflux mechanism in human beings is composed of three components: a mechanically effective LES, efficient esophageal clearance, and an adequately functioning gastric reservoir. A defect of any one of these three components can lead to increased esophageal exposure to gastric juice and the development of mucosal injury.

Physiologic Reflux

On 24-h esophageal pH monitoring, healthy individuals have occasional episodes of gastroesophageal reflux. This physiologic reflux is more common when awake and in the upright position than during sleep in the supine position. When reflux of gastric juice occurs, normal subjects rapidly clear the acid gastric juice from the esophagus regardless of their position. There are several explanations for the observation that physiologic reflux in normal subjects is more common when they are awake and in the upright position than during sleep in the supine position. First, reflux episodes occur in healthy volunteers primarily during transient losses of the gastroesophageal barrier, which may be because of a relaxation of the LES or intragastric pressure overcoming sphincter pressure. Gastric juice can also reflux when a swallow-induced relaxation of the LES is not protected by an oncoming peristaltic wave. The average frequency of these "unguarded moments" or of transient losses of the gastroesophageal barrier is far less while asleep and in the supine position than while awake and in the upright position. Consequently, there are fewer opportunities for reflux to occur in the supine position. Second, in the upright position there is a 12-mmHg pressure gradient between the resting, positive intraabdominal pressure measured in the stomach and the most negative intrathoracic pressure measured in the esophagus at midthoracic level. This gradient favors the flow of gastric juice up into the thoracic esophagus when upright. The gradient diminishes in the supine position. Third, the LES pressure in normal subjects is significantly higher in the supine position than in the upright position. This is because of the apposition of the hydrostatic pressure of the abdomen to the abdominal portion of the sphincter when supine. In the upright position, the abdominal pressure surrounding the sphincter is negative compared with atmospheric pressure, and as expected, the abdominal pressure gradually increases the more caudally it is measured. This pressure gradient tends to move the gastric contents toward the cardia and encourages the occurrence of reflux into the esophagus when the individual is upright. By contrast, in the supine position the gastroesophageal pressure gradient diminishes, and the abdominal hydrostatic pressure under the diaphragm increases, causing an increase in sphincter pressure and a more competent cardia.

ASSESSMENT OF ESOPHAGEAL FUNCTION

A thorough understanding of the patient's underlying anatomic and functional deficits prior to making therapeutic decisions is fundamental to the successful treatment of esophageal disease. The diagnostic tests as presently employed may be divided into five broad groups: (1) tests to detect structural abnormalities of the esophagus; (2) tests to detect functional abnormalities of the esophagus; (3) tests to detect increased esophageal exposure to gastric juice; (4) tests to provoke esophageal symptoms; and (5) tests of duodenogastric function as they relate to esophageal disease.

Tests to Detect Structural Abnormalities

Radiographic Evaluation

The first diagnostic test in patients with suspected esophageal disease should be a barium swallow including a full assessment of the stomach and duodenum. Esophageal motility is optimally assessed by observing several individual swallows of barium traversing the entire length of the organ, with the patient in the horizontal position. Hiatal hernias are best demonstrated with the patient prone because the increased intraabdominal pressure produced in this position promotes displacement of the esophagogastric junction above the diaphragm. To detect lower esophageal narrowing, such as rings and strictures, fully distended views of the esophagogastric region are crucial. The density of the barium used to study the esophagus can potentially affect the accuracy of the examination. Esophageal disorders shown clearly by a full-column technique include circumferential carcinomas, peptic strictures, large esophageal ulcers, and hiatal hernias. A small hiatal hernia is usually not associated with significant symptoms or illness, and its presence is an irrelevant finding unless the hiatal hernia is large, the hiatal opening is narrow and interrupts the flow of barium into the stomach, or the hernia is of the paraesophageal variety. Lesions extrinsic but adjacent to the esophagus can be reliably detected by the full-column technique if they contact the distended esophageal wall. Conversely, a number of important disorders may go undetected if this is the sole technique used to examine the esophagus. These include small esophageal neoplasms, mild esophagitis, and esophageal varices. Thus, the full-column technique should be supplemented with mucosal relief or double-contrast films to enhance detection of these smaller or more subtle lesions.

Motion-recording techniques greatly aid in evaluating functional disorders of the pharyngeal and esophageal phases of swallowing. Cine- and videoradiography are more useful to evaluate function than to detect structural abnormalities.

The radiographic assessment of the esophagus is not complete unless the entire stomach and duodenum have been examined. A gastric or duodenal ulcer, partially obstructing gastric neoplasm, or scarred duodenum and pylorus may contribute significantly to symptoms otherwise attributable to an esophageal abnormality.

When a patient's complaints include dysphagia and no obstructing lesion is seen on the barium swallow, it is useful to have the patient swallow a barium-impregnated marshmallow, a barium-soaked piece of bread, or a hamburger mixed with barium. This test may bring out a functional disturbance in esophageal transport that can be missed when liquid barium is used.

Endoscopic Evaluation

In any patient complaining of dysphagia, esophagoscopy is indicated, even in the face of a normal radiographic study. A barium study obtained prior to esophagoscopy is helpful to the endoscopist by directing attention to locations of subtle change, and alerting the examiner to such potential danger spots as a cervical vertebral osteophyte, esophageal diverticulum, a deeply penetrating ulcer, or a carcinoma. Regardless of the radiologist's interpretation of an abnormal finding, each structural abnormality of the esophagus should be confirmed visually.

The flexible fiberoptic esophagoscope is the instrument of choice because of its technical ease, patient acceptance, and the ability to simultaneously assess the stomach and duodenum. When gastroesophageal reflux disease is the suspected diagnosis, particular attention should be paid to detecting the presence of esophagitis and Barrett columnar-lined esophagus. When endoscopic esophagitis is seen, severity and the length of esophagus involved are recorded. Grade I esophagitis is defined as small, circular, nonconfluent erosions. Grade II esophagitis is defined by the presence of linear erosions lined with granulation tissue that bleeds easily when touched. Grade III esophagitis represents a more advanced stage, in which the linear or circular erosions coalesce into circumferential loss of the epithelium, or the appearance of islands of epithelium which on endoscopy appears as a "cobblestone" esophagus. Grade IV esophagitis is the presence of a stricture. Its severity can be assessed by the ease of passing a 36F endoscope. When a stricture is observed, the severity of the esophagitis above it should be recorded. The absence of esophagitis above a stricture suggests a chemical-induced injury or a neoplasm as a cause. The latter should always be considered and is ruled out only by evaluation of a tissue biopsy of adequate size.

Barrett esophagus (BE) is a condition in which the tubular esophagus is lined with columnar epithelium, as opposed to the normal squamous epithelium. Histologically it is identified by the presence of globlet cells, the marker of intestinal metaplasia. It is suspected at endoscopy when there is difficulty in visualizing the squamocolumnar junction at its normal location, and by the appearance of a redder, more luxuriant mucosa than is normally seen in the lower esophagus. Its presence is confirmed by biopsy. Multiple biopsies should be taken in a cephalad direction to determine the level at which the junction of Barrett epithelium with normal squamous mucosa occurs. BE is susceptible to ulceration, bleeding, stricture formation, and most important, malignant degeneration. The earliest sign of the latter is severe dysplasia or intramucosal adenocarcinoma. These dysplastic changes can have a patchy distribution, so a minimum of four biopsy samples spaced 2 cm apart should be taken from the Barrett-lined portion of the esophagus. Changes seen in one biopsy are significant. Nishimaki has determined that 85 percent of tumors occur in an area of specialized columnar epithelium near the squamocolumnar junction in and within 2 cm of the squamocolumnar junction in virtually all patients. Particular attention should be focused in this area in patients suspected of harboring a carcinoma.

Abnormalities of the geometry of the gastroesophageal junction can be visualized by retroflexion of the endoscope. Hill has graded the appearance of the gastroesophageal junction from I–IV according to the deterioration of the normal valve architecture. The appearance of the valve correlates with the presence of increased esophageal acid exposure, occurring predominantly in patients with grade III and IV valves.

A hiatal hernia is endoscopically confirmed by finding a pouch lined with gastric rugal folds lying 2 cm or more above the margins of the diaphragmatic crura, identified by having the patient sniff. A prominent sliding hiatal hernia frequently is associated with increased esophageal exposure to gastric juice. When a paraesophageal hernia is observed, particular attention is taken to exclude a gastric ulcer or gastritis within the pouch. The intragastric retroflex or J maneuver is important in evaluating the full circumference of the mucosal lining of the herniated stomach.

When an esophageal diverticulum is seen, it should be carefully explored with the flexible endoscope to exclude ulceration or neoplasia. When a submucosal mass is identified, biopsies are usually not performed. Normally a submucosal leiomyoma or reduplication cyst can be easily dissected away from the intact mucosa, but if a biopsy sample is taken, the mucosa may become fixed to the underlying abnormality. This complicates the surgical dissection by increasing the risk of mucosal perforation.

Tests to Detect Functional Abnormalities

In many patients with symptoms of an esophageal disorder, standard radiographic and endoscopic evaluation fails to demonstrate a structural abnormality. In these situations, esophageal function tests are necessary to identify a functional disorder.

Stationary Manometry

Esophageal manometry is a widely used technique to examine the motor function of the esophagus and its sphincters. Manometry is indicated whenever a motor abnormality of the esophagus is suspected on the basis of complaints of dysphagia, odynophagia, or noncardiac chest pain, and the barium swallow or endoscopy does not show a clear structural abnormality. Esophageal manometry is particularly necessary to confirm the diagnosis of specific primary esophageal motility disorders (i.e., achalasia, diffuse esophageal spasm, nutcracker esophagus, and hypertensive LES). It also identifies nonspecific esophageal motility abnormalities and motility disorders secondary to systemic

TABLE 24-1 Normal Manometric Values of the Distal Esophageal Sphincter, n = 50

| | | Percentile | |
	Median	2.5	97.5
Pressure (mmHg)	13	5.8	27.7
Overall length (cm)	3.6	2.1	5.6
Abdominal length (cm)	2	0.9	4.7
	Mean	Mean −2 SD	Mean +2 SD
Pressure (mmHg)	13.8 ± 4.6	4.6	23.0
Overall length (cm)	3.7 ± 0.8	2.1	5.3
Abdominal length (cm)	2.2 ± 0.8	0.6	3.8

Source: Reproduced with permission from DeMeester TR, Stein HJ: Gastroesophageal reflux disease, in Moody FG, Carey LC, et al (eds): *Surgical Treatment of Digestive Disease.* Chicago: Year Book Medical, 1990, p 89.

disease such as scleroderma, dermatomyositis, polymyositis, or mixed connective tissue disease. In patients with symptomatic gastroesophageal reflux disease, manometry of the esophageal body can identify a mechanically defective LES, and evaluate the adequacy of esophageal peristalsis and contraction amplitude. Manometry has become an essential tool in the preoperative evaluation of patients prior to antireflux surgery, allowing selection of the appropriate procedure based on the patient's underlying esophageal function.

Table 24-1 shows the values for parameters of the LES in 50 normal volunteers without subjective or objective evidence of a foregut disorder. A mechanically defective sphincter is identified by having one or more of the following characteristics: an average LES pressure of less than 6 mmHg, an average length exposed to the positive-pressure environment in the abdomen of 1 cm or less, and/or an average overall sphincter length of 2 cm or less. Compared with the normal volunteers, these values are below the 2.5 percentile for sphincter pressure and overall length and for abdominal length. It has been shown that the resistance of the sphincter to reflux of gastric juice is determined by the integrated effects of radial pressures extended over the entire length, resulting in three-dimensional computerized imaging of sphincter pressures. Calculating the volume of this image reflects the sphincter's resistance and is called the sphincter pressure vector volume (SPVV).

Patients with gastroesophageal reflux disease and an SPVV below the fifth percentile of normal, or a deficiency of one, two, or all three mechanical components of an LES on standard manometry, have a mechanical defect of their antireflux barrier that a surgical antireflux procedure is designed to correct.

To assess the relaxation and postrelaxation contraction of the LES, a pressure transducer is positioned within the high-pressure zone, with the distal transducer located in the stomach and the proximal transducer within the esophageal body. Ten wet swallows (5 mL water each) are performed. The normal pressure of the LES should drop to the level of gastric pressure during each wet swallow.

The function of the esophageal body is assessed with the five pressure transducers located in the esophagus. The standard procedure is to locate the most proximal pressure transducer 1 cm below the well-defined cricopharyngeal sphincter, allowing a pressure response throughout the whole esophagus to be obtained on one swallow. The relationship of the esophageal contractions following a swallow is classified as peristaltic or simultaneous.

The relaxation of the upper esophageal sphincter is studied by straddling pressure transducers across the sphincter so that one is in the pharynx, one in the sphincter and another in the upper esophagus.

Video- and Cineradiography

High-speed video recording of radiographic studies allows re-evaluation by reviewing the studies at various speeds. This technique is more useful than manometry in the evaluation of the pharyngeal phase of swallowing. Observations suggesting oropharyngeal or cricopharyngeal dysfunction include misdirection of barium into the trachea or nasopharynx, prominence of the cricopharyngeal muscle, a Zenker diverticulum, a narrow pharyngoesophageal segment, and stasis of the contrast medium in the valleculae or hypopharyngeal recesses. These findings are usually not specific, but rather common manifestations of neuromuscular disorders affecting the pharyngoesophageal area. Studies using liquid barium, barium-impregnated solids, or radiopaque pills, aid the evaluation of normal and abnormal motility in the esophageal body. Loss of the normal stripping wave or segmentation of the barium column with the patient in the recumbent position correlates with abnormal motility of the esophageal body. In addition, structural abnormalities such as small diverticula, webs, and minimal extrinsic impressions of the esophagus may be recognized only with motion-recording techniques. The simultaneous computerized capture of videofluoroscopic images and manonometric tracings is now available, and is referred to as manofluorography. Manofluorographic studies allow precise correlation of the anatomic events, such as opening of the upper esophageal sphincter, with manometric observations, such as sphincter relaxation. Manofluorography, although not widely available, is presently the best means available to evaluate complex functional abnormalities.

Tests to Detect Increased Exposure to Gastric Juice

24-H Ambulatory pH Monitoring

The most direct method of measuring increased esophageal exposure to gastric juice is by an indwelling pH electrode, or more recently via a radiotelemetric pH monitoring capsule that can be clipped to the esophageal mucosa. The latter consists of an antimony pH electrode fitted inside a small capsule-shaped device accompanied by a battery and electronics that allow 48-h monitoring and transmission of the pH data via transcutaneous radio telemetry to a waist-mounted data logger. The device can be introduced either transorally or transnasally, and clipped to the esophageal mucosa using a suction fastening techniques. It passes spontaneously within 3–7 days. Prolonged monitoring of esophageal pH is performed by placing the pH probe or telemetry capsule 5 cm above the manometrically measured upper border of the distal sphincter for 24 h. It measures the actual time the esophageal mucosa is exposed to gastric juice, measures the ability of the esophagus to clear refluxed acid, and correlates esophageal acid exposure with the patient's symptoms. A 24–48-h period is necessary so that measurements can be made over one or two complete circadian cycles. This allows measuring the effect of physiologic activity, such as eating or sleeping, on the reflux of gastric juice into the esophagus.

TABLE 24-2 Normal Values for Esophageal Exposure to pH < 4 (n = 50)

Component	Mean	SD	95%
Total time	1.51	1.36	4.45
Upright time	2.34	2.34	8.42
Supine time	0.63	1.0	3.45
No. of episodes	19.00	12.76	46.90
No. > 5 min	0.84	1.18	3.45
Longest episode	6.74	7.85	19.80

SD = Standard deviation.
Source: Reproduced with permission from DeMeester TR, Stein HJ: Gastro-esophageal reflux disease, in Moody FG, Carey LC, et al (eds): *Surgical Treatment of Digestive Disease.* Chicago: Year Book Medical, 1990, p 68.

The 24-h esophageal pH monitoring should not be considered a test for reflux, but rather a measurement of the esophageal exposure to gastric juice. The measurement is expressed by the time the esophageal pH was below a given threshold during the 24-h period. This single assessment, although concise, does not reflect how the exposure has occurred; that is, did it occur in a few long episodes or several short episodes? Consequently, two other assessments are necessary: the frequency of the reflux episodes and their duration.

The units used to express esophageal exposure to gastric juice are (1) cumulative time the esophageal pH is below pH 4, expressed as the percentage of the total, upright, and supine monitored time; (2) frequency of reflux episodes below pH 4, expressed as number of episodes per 24 h; and (3) duration of the episodes, expressed as the number of episodes greater than 5 min per 24 h, and the time in min of the longest episode recorded. Table 24-2 shows the normal values for these components of the 24-h record from 50 normal asymptomatic subjects. The upper limits of normal were established at the ninety-fifth percentile.

To combine the result of the six components into one expression of the overall esophageal acid exposure below a pH threshold, a pH score was calculated by using the standard deviation of the mean of each of the six components measured in the 50 normal subjects as a weighting factor. The upper limits of normal for the composite score for pH threshold less than 4 is 14.7.

Twenty-four hour esophageal pH monitoring has a sensitivity and specificity of 96 percent. (Sensitivity is the ability to detect a disease when known to be present; specificity is the ability to exclude the disease when known to be absent.) This gave a predictive value of a positive and a negative test of 96 percent, and an overall accuracy of 96 percent. Based on extensive clinical experience, 24-h esophageal pH monitoring has emerged as the standard criterion for the diagnosis of gastroesophageal reflux disease.

24-Hour Ambulatory Bile Monitoring

The potentially injurious components that reflux into the esophagus include gastric secretions, such as acid and pepsin, and biliary and pancreatic secretions that regurgitate from the duodenum into the stomach. The presence of duodenal contents within the esophagus can now be determined via an indwelling spectrophotometric probe capable of detecting bilirubin. Bilirubin serves as a marker for the presence of duodenal juice. Ambulatory bilirubin monitoring can be used to identify patients who are at risk for esophageal mucosal injury, and are thus candidates for surgical antireflux treatment.

GASTROESOPHAGEAL REFLUX DISEASE

Gastroesophageal reflux disease (GERD) is a common disease that accounts for approximately 75 percent of esophageal pathology. Despite its high prevalence, it can be one of the most challenging diagnostic and therapeutic problems in benign esophageal disease. A contributing factor to this is the lack of a universally accepted definition of the disease.

The simplest approach is to define the disease by its symptoms. However, symptoms thought to be indicative of GERD, such as heartburn or acid regurgitation, are very common in the general population, and many individuals consider them to be normal and do not seek medical attention. Even when excessive, these symptoms are not specific for GERD, and can be caused by other diseases such as achalasia, diffuse spasm, esophageal carcinoma, pyloric stenosis, cholelithiasis, gastritis, gastric or duodenal ulcer, and coronary artery disease. In addition, patients with GERD can present with atypical symptoms, such as nausea, vomiting, postprandial fullness, chest pain, choking, chronic cough, wheezing, and hoarseness. Furthermore, bronchiolitis, recurrent pneumonia, idiopathic pulmonary fibrosis, and asthma can be primarily because of GERD. To confuse the issue more, GERD can coexist with cardiac and pulmonary disease. Thus using clinical symptoms to define GERD lacks sensitivity and specificity.

An alternative definition for GERD is the presence of endoscopic esophagitis. Using this criterion for diagnosis assumes that all patients who have esophagitis have excessive regurgitation of gastric juice into their esophagus. This is true in 90 percent of patients, but in 10 percent the esophagitis has other causes, the most common being unrecognized chemical injury from prescribed drug ingestion. In addition, the definition leaves undiagnosed those patients who have symptoms of gastroesophageal reflux but do not have endoscopic esophagitis. A third approach to defining GERD is to measure the basic pathophysiologic abnormality of the disease; that is, increased exposure of the esophagus to gastric juice. In the past this was inferred by the presence of a hiatal hernia, later by endoscopic esophagitis, and more recently by a hypotensive LES pressure. The development of miniaturized pH electrodes and data recorders allowed measurement of esophageal exposure to gastric juice by calculating the percentage of time the pH was less than 4 over a 24-h period. This provided an opportunity to objectively identify the presence of the disease.

The Human Antireflux Mechanism and the Pathophysiology of Gastroesophageal Reflux

The human antireflux mechanism consists of a pump, the esophageal body, and a barrier, the LES. The common denominator for virtually all episodes of gastroesophageal reflux in both patients and normal subjects is the loss of the barrier to reflux. This is usually secondary to low or reduced LES resistance. The loss of this resistance may be either permanent or transient. A structurally defective barrier results in a permanent loss of LES resistance, and permits unhampered reflux of gastric contents into the esophagus throughout the circadian cycle. Transient loss of the barrier may occur secondary to gastric abnormalities, including gastric distention with air or food, increased intragastric or intraabdominal pressure, and delayed gastric emptying. These transient losses of sphincter resistance occur in the early stages of GERD, and are likely the mechanism for both physiologic and pathophysiologic postprandial reflux. Thus, GERD may begin with abnormalities of the stomach or over eating.

Data have shown that transient loss of sphincter resistance is because of gastric distention. This results in shortening of the LES, upright reflux, and inflammatory changes at the gastroesophageal junction secondary to unfolding of esophageal squamous mucosa into the gastric environment with shortening. Over time, persistent inflammation results in the permanent loss of LES function.

Several studies support the biomechanical effects of a distended stomach in the pathogenesis of GERD, and provide a mechanical explanation for why patients with a structurally normal LES may have increased esophageal acid exposure. In vivo baboon studies have shown that as gastric volume or distention increases, sphincter length decreases. Furthermore, as the sphincter length decreases, its resting pressure, as measured by a perfused catheter, also decreases. The decrease usually occurs suddenly when an inefficient length of sphincter is reached usually between 1 and 2 cm.

The mechanism by which gastric distention contributes to shortening of sphincter length so that its resistance drops and reflux occurs provides a mechanical explanation for "transient relaxations" of the LES without invoking a neuromuscular reflex. Rather than a "spontaneous" muscular relaxation, there is a mechanical shortening of the sphincter length as a consequence of gastric distention, to the point where it becomes incompetent. After gastric venting, sphincter length is restored and competence returns until distention again shortens the sphincter and encourages further venting and reflux. This sequence results in the common complaints of repetitive belching and bloating heard from patients with GERD. Gastric distention may initially occur because of overeating, stress aerophagia, or delayed gastric emptying, secondary to fatty diet or a systemic disorder. The distention is augmented by an increased swallowing frequency that occurs in patients as they repetitively swallow their saliva in an effort to neutralize the acid refluxed into their esophagus.

The consequence of fundic distention, with the LES being "taken up" into the stretched fundus, is that the squamous epithelium of the sphincter is exposed to gastric juice and mucosal injury. This initial step in the pathogenesis of GERD explains why mild esophagitis is usually limited to the very distal esophagus. Erosions in the terminal squamous epithelium caused by this mechanism may also explain the complaint of epigastric pain so often registered by patients with early disease. It may also be the stimulus to increase the swallowing of saliva to bathe the erosions to alleviate the discomfort induced by exposure to gastric acid. With increased swallowing come aerophagia, gastric distention, bloating, and repetitive belching. During this process there is repeated exposure of the squamous epithelium to gastric juice, because of the sphincter being "taken up" into the stretched fundus, which may cause erosion, ulceration, fibrosis (ring formation), and cardiac metaplasia of the terminal squamous mucosa.

In summary, GERD starts in the stomach. It is caused by gastric distention because of overeating or ingestion of fried foods, typical of the Western diet, which delays gastric emptying. Gastric distention causes unfolding of the sphincter as it is taken up by the distended fundus and exposure of the terminal squamous epithelium within the sphincter to noxious gastric juice. Signs of injury to the exposed squamous epithelium are erosions, ulceration, fibrosis, and columnar metaplasia, with an inflammatory infiltrate or foveolar hyperplasia.

Intestinal metaplasia within the sphincter may result, as in Barrett metaplasia of the esophageal body. This process results in the loss of muscle function, and the sphincter becomes mechanically defective, allowing free reflux with progressively higher degrees of mucosal injury.

The first component of the human antireflux mechanism is a functional LES. The most common cause of a structurally defective LES is inadequate sphincter pressure, secondary to inflammatory injury. The reduced pressure is most likely because of an abnormality of myogenic function. This is supported by two observations. First, the location of the LES, in either the abdomen or the chest, is not a major factor in the genesis of the sphincter pressure, because it can still be measured when the chest and abdomen are surgically opened and the distal esophagus is held free in the surgeon's hand. Second, Biancani and coworkers have shown that the distal esophageal sphincter's muscle response to stretch is reduced in patients with an incompetent cardia. This suggests that sphincter pressure depends on the length and tension properties of the sphincter's smooth muscle. Surgical fundoplication has been shown to improve the mechanical efficiency of the sphincter by restoring normal length-tension characteristics.

Although an inadequate pressure is the most common cause of a structurally defective sphincter, the efficiency of a sphincter with normal pressure can be nullified by an inadequate abdominal length or an abnormally short overall resting length. An adequate abdominal length is important in preventing reflux caused by increases in intraabdominal pressure, and an adequate overall length is important in providing the resistance to reflux caused by gastric distention independent of intraabdominal pressure. Therefore, patients with a low sphincter pressure or those with a normal pressure but a short abdominal length are unable to protect against reflux caused by fluctuations of intraabdominal pressure that occur with daily activities or changes in body position. Patients with a low sphincter pressure or those with a normal pressure but short overall length are unable to protect against reflux related to gastric distention caused by outlet obstruction, aerophagia, gluttony, delayed gastric emptying associated with a fatty diet, or various gastropathies. Persons who have a short overall length on a resting motility study are at a disadvantage in protecting against excessive gastric distention secondary to eating, and suffer postprandial reflux. This is because with normal dilatation of the stomach, sphincter length becomes shorter, and if already shortened in the resting state, there is little tolerance for further shortening before incompetence occurs.

The second component of the human antireflux mechanism is an effective esophageal pump that clears the esophagus after physiologic reflux episodes. Ineffective esophageal clearance can result in an abnormal esophageal exposure to gastric juice in individuals who have a normal LES and gastric function, but fail to clear physiologic reflux episodes. This situation is relatively rare, and ineffectual clearance is more apt to be seen in association with a structurally defective sphincter, which augments the esophageal exposure to gastric juice by prolonging the duration of each reflux episode.

Four factors important in esophageal clearance are gravity, esophageal motor activity, salivation, and anchoring of the distal esophagus in the abdomen. The loss of any one can augment esophageal exposure to gastric juice by contributing to ineffective clearance. This explains why in the absence of peristalsis, reflux episodes are prolonged in the supine position. The bulk of refluxed gastric juice is cleared from the esophagus by a primary peristaltic wave initiated by a pharyngeal swallow. Secondary peristaltic waves are initiated by either distention of the lower esophagus or a drop in the intraesophageal pH. Ambulatory motility studies indicate that secondary waves are less common and play less of a role in clearance than previously thought.

Salivation contributes to esophageal clearance by neutralizing the minute amount of acid that is left following a peristaltic wave. Return of esophageal pH to normal takes significantly longer if salivary flow is reduced, such as after radiotherapy, and is shorter if saliva is stimulated by sucking lozenges.

A hiatal hernia can also contribute to an esophageal propulsion defect because of loss of anchorage of the esophagus in the abdomen. This results in a reduction in the efficiency of acid clearance.

The third component of the human antireflux mechanism is the gastric reservoir. Abnormalities of the gastric reservoir that increase esophageal exposure to gastric juice include gastric distention, increased intragastric pressure, persistent gastric reservoir, and increased gastric acid secretion. The effects of gastric distention on reflux are discussed above. Increased intragastric pressure may be the result of outlet obstruction because of a scarred pylorus or duodenum, or the result of a vagotomy; it can also be found in the diabetic patient with gastroparesis. The latter two conditions are secondary to abnormalities of the normal adaptive relaxation of the stomach. The increase in intragastric pressure because of alteration in the pressure-volume relationship in these abnormalities can overcome the sphincter resistance and results in reflux.

A persistent gastric reservoir results from delayed gastric emptying and increases the exposure of the esophagus to gastric juice by accentuating physiologic reflux. It is caused by myogenic abnormalities such as gastric atony in advanced diabetes, diffuse neuromuscular disorders, anticholinergic medications, and postviral infections. Nonmyogenic causes are vagotomy, antropyloric dysfunction, and duodenal dysmotility. Delayed gastric emptying can result in increased exposure of the gastric mucosa to bile and pancreatic juice refluxed from the duodenum into the stomach, with the development of gastritis.

Gastric hypersecretion can increase esophageal exposure to gastric acid juice by the physiologic reflux of concentrated gastric acid. Barlow has shown that 28 percent of patients with increased esophageal exposure to gastric juice measured by 24-h pH monitoring have gastric hypersecretion. A mechanically defective sphincter seems to be more important than gastric hypersecretion in the development of complications of reflux disease. In this respect, GERD differs from duodenal ulcer disease, as the latter is specifically related to gastric hypersecretion.

Complications of Gastroesophageal Reflux

The complications of gastroesophageal reflux result from the damage inflicted by gastric juice on the esophageal mucosa or respiratory epithelium, and changes caused by their subsequent repair and fibrosis. Complications because of repetitive reflux are esophagitis, stricture, and Barrett esophagus; repetitive aspiration may lead to progressive pulmonary fibrosis. The severity of the complications is directly related to the prevalence of a structurally defective sphincter (Table 24-3). The observation that a structurally defective sphincter occurs in 42 percent of patients without complications (most of whom have one or two components failed) suggests that disease may be confined to the sphincter

TABLE 24-3 Complications of Gastroesophageal Reflux Disease: 150 Consecutive Cases with Proven Gastroesophageal Reflux Disease (24-H Esophageal pH Monitoring Endoscopy, and Motility)

Complication	No.	Structurally normal sphincter	Structurally defective sphincter
None	59	58%	42%
Erosive esophagitis	47	23%	77%[a]
Stricture	19	11%	89%
Barrett esophagus	25	0%	100%
Total	150		

[a]Grade more severe with defective cardia.
Source: Reproduced with permission from DeMeester TR, Stein HJ: Gastroesophageal reflux disease, in Moody FG, Carey LC, et al (eds): *Surgical Treatment of Digestive Disease.* Chicago: Year Book Medical, 1990, p 81.

because of compensation by a vigorously contracting esophageal body. Eventually all three components of the sphincter fail, allowing unrestricted reflux of gastric juice into the esophagus and overwhelming its normal clearance mechanisms. This leads to esophageal mucosal injury with progressive deterioration of esophageal contractility, as is commonly seen in patients with strictures and BE. The loss of esophageal clearance increases the potential for regurgitation into the pharynx with aspiration.

The potential injurious components that reflux into the esophagus include gastric secretions such as acid and pepsin, and biliary and pancreatic secretions that regurgitate from the duodenum into the stomach. There is a considerable body of experimental evidence to indicate that maximal epithelial injury occurs during exposure to bile salts combined with acid and pepsin. These studies have shown that acid alone does minimal damage to the esophageal mucosa, but the combination of acid and pepsin is highly deleterious. Similarly, the reflux of duodenal juice alone does little damage to the mucosa, although the combination of duodenal juice and gastric acid is particularly noxious (Table 24-4).

Experimental animal studies have shown that the reflux of duodenal contents into the esophagus enhances inflammation, increases the prevalence of BE, and results in the development of esophageal adenocarcinoma. The component of duodenal juice thought to be most damaging is bile acids. In order for bile acids to injure mucosal cells, it is necessary that they be both soluble and un-ionized, so that the un-ionized nonpolar form may enter mucosal cells. Before the entry of bile into the gastrointestinal (GI) tract, 98 percent of bile acids are conjugated with either taurine or glycine in a ratio of about 3:1. Conjugation increases the solubility and ionization of bile acids by lowering their pKa. At the normal duodenal pH of approximately 7, over 90 percent of bile salts are in solution and completely ionized. At pH ranges from 2–7, there is a mixture of the ionized salt and the lipophilic, nonionized acid. Acidification of bile to below pH 2

TABLE 24-4 Relation of the Type of Reflux to Injury

	No injury	Esophagitis	Uncomplicated Barrett	Complicated Barrett
Gastric reflux	15 (54%)	13 (38%)	8 (32%)	1 (8%)
Gastroduodenal reflux	13 (38%)	21 (62%)	17 (68%)	12 (92%)

results in an irreversible bile acid precipitation. Consequently, under normal physiologic conditions, bile acids precipitate and are of minimal consequence when an acid gastric environment exists. On the other hand, in a more alkaline gastric environment, such as occurs with excessive duodenogastric reflux and after acid suppression therapy or vagotomy and partial or total gastrectomy, bile salts remain in solution, are partially dissociated, and when refluxed into the esophagus can cause severe mucosal injury by crossing the cell membrane and damaging the mitochondria.

The fact that the combination of refluxed gastric and duodenal juice is more noxious to the esophageal mucosa than gastric juice alone may explain the repeated observation that 25 percent of patients with reflux esophagitis develop recurrent and progressive mucosal damage, often despite medical therapy. A potential reason is that acid suppression therapy is unable to consistently maintain the pH of refluxed gastric and duodenal juice above the range of 6. Lapses into pH ranges from 2–6 encourage the formation of undissociated, nonpolarized, soluble bile acids, which are capable of penetrating the cell wall and injuring mucosal cells. To assure that bile acids remain completely ionized in their polarized form, and thus unable to penetrate the cell, requires that the pH of the refluxed material be maintained above 7, 24 h a day, 7 days a week, for the patient's lifetime. In practice this would not only be impractical but likely impossible, unless very high doses of medications were used. The use of lesser doses would allow esophageal mucosal damage to occur while the patient was relatively asymptomatic. Antireflux operative procedures re-establish the barrier between stomach and esophagus, protecting the esophagus from damage in patients with mixed gastroesophageal reflux. If reflux of gastric juice is allowed to persist and sustained or repetitive esophageal injury occurs, two sequelae can result. First, a luminal stricture can develop from submucosal and eventually intramural fibrosis. Second, the tubular esophagus may become replaced with columnar epithelium. The columnar epithelium is resistant to acid and is associated with the alleviation of the complaint of heartburn. This columnar epithelium often becomes intestinalized, identified histologically by the presence of goblet cells. This specialized intestinal metaplasia is currently required for the diagnosis of BE. Endoscopically, BE can be quiescent or associated with complications of esophagitis, stricture, Barrett ulceration, and dysplasia. The complications associated with BE may be because of the continuous irritation from refluxed duodenogastric juice. This continued injury is pH dependent and may be modified by medical therapy. The incidence of metaplastic Barrett epithelium becoming dysplastic and progressing to adenocarcinoma is approximately 0.5–1 percent per year.

An esophageal stricture can be associated with severe esophagitis or Barrett's esophagus. In the latter situation, it occurs at the site of maximal inflammatory injury (i.e., the columnar-squamous epithelial interface). As the columnar epithelium advances into the area of inflammation, the inflammation extends higher into the proximal esophagus, and the site of the stricture moves progressively up the esophagus. Patients who have a stricture in the absence of Barrett esophagus should have the presence of gastroesophageal reflux documented before the presence of the stricture is ascribed to reflux esophagitis. In patients with normal acid exposure, the stricture may be because of cancer or a drug-induced chemical injury, the latter resulting from the lodgment of a capsule or tablet in the distal esophagus. In such patients, dilation usually corrects the problem of dysphagia. Heartburn, which may have occurred only because of the chemical injury, need not be treated. It is also possible for drug-induced injuries to occur in patients who have underlying esophagitis and a distal esophageal stricture secondary to gastroesophageal reflux. In this situation, a long string-like stricture progressively develops as a result of repetitive caustic injury from capsule or tablet lodgment on top of an initial reflux stricture. These strictures are often resistant to dilation.

When the refluxed gastric juice is of sufficient quantity, it can reach the pharynx, with the potential for pharyngeal tracheal aspiration, causing symptoms of repetitive cough, choking, hoarseness, and recurrent pneumonia. This is often an unrecognized complication of GERD, because either the pulmonary or the GI symptoms may predominate in the clinical situation and focus the physician's attention on one to the exclusion of the other. Three factors are important in these patients. First, it may take up to 7 days for the recovery of the respiratory epithelium secondary to the aspiration of gastric contents, and a chronic cough that is not related to a reflux episode may develop between episodes of aspiration. Second, the presence of an esophageal motility disorder is observed in 75 percent of patients with reflux-induced aspiration, and is believed to promote the aboral movement of the refluxate toward the pharynx. Third, if the pH in the cervical esophagus in patients with increased esophageal acid exposure is below 4 for less than 1 percent of the time, there is a high probability that the respiratory symptoms have been caused by aspiration. Increasingly, benign pulmonary pathology is recognized as being secondary to GERD, including asthma, idiopathic pulmonary fibrosis, and bronchiectases.

Symptomatic Assessment of Gastroesophageal Reflux Disease

Gastroesophageal reflux disease is a functional disorder often accompanied by non–reflux-related GI and respiratory symptoms that will not improve or may be worsened by antireflux surgery. Symptoms consistent with irritable bowel syndrome, such as alternating diarrhea and constipation, bloating, and crampy abdominal pain, should be sought and detailed separately from GERD symptoms. Likewise, symptoms suggestive of gastric pathology including nausea, early satiety, epigastric abdominal pain, anorexia, and weight loss are important. It has become increasingly recognized that oral symptoms such as mouth and tongue burning and sore throat rarely improve with antireflux surgery.

The patient's perception of what each symptom means should be explored in an effort to avoid their misinterpretation. Of equal importance is the classification of symptoms as primary or secondary, for prioritization of therapy and to allow an estimate of the probability of relief of each of the particular symptoms. The response to acid-suppressing medications predicts success and symptom relief after surgery. In contrast to the widely held belief that failure of medical therapy is an indication for surgery, a good response to proton pump inhibitors is desirable, as it predicts that the symptoms are actually because of reflux of gastric contents.

GERD-related symptoms can be classified into "typical" symptoms of heartburn, regurgitation and dysphagia, and "atypical" symptoms of cough, hoarseness, asthma, aspiration, and chest pain. Because there are fewer mechanisms for their generation, typical symptoms are more likely to be secondary to increased esophageal acid exposure than are atypical symptoms. The relationship of atypical symptoms such as cough, hoarseness, wheezing, or sore throat to heartburn and/or regurgitation should be established. Other, more common factors that may contribute to respiratory symptoms also should be investigated. The patient must be made aware of the relatively diminished likelihood of success of surgery when atypical symptoms are the primary symptoms. Of note is the comparatively longer duration required for the respiratory symptoms to improve after surgery.

Medical Therapy

GERD is such a common condition that most patients with mild symptoms carry out self-medication. When first seen with symptoms of heartburn without obvious complications, patients can reasonably be placed on 8–12 weeks of simple antacids before extensive investigations are carried out. In many situations, this successfully terminates the attacks. Patients should be advised to elevate the head of the bed; avoid tight clothing; eat small, frequent meals; avoid eating their nighttime meal shortly before retiring; lose weight; and avoid alcohol, coffee, chocolate, and peppermint, which may aggravate the symptoms.

In patients with persistent symptoms, the mainstay of medical therapy is acid suppression. High-dosage regimens of hydrogen potassium proton pump inhibitors can reduce gastric acidity by as much as 80–90 percent. This usually heals mild esophagitis. In severe esophagitis, healing may occur in only half of the patients. In patients who reflux a combination of gastric and duodenal juice, acid-suppression therapy may give relief of symptoms, although still allowing mixed reflux to occur. This can allow persistent mucosal damage in an asymptomatic patient. Unfortunately, within 6 months of discontinuation of any form of medical therapy for GERD, 80 percent of patients have a recurrence of symptoms.

Once initiated, most patients with GERD will require lifelong treatment with proton pump inhibitors, both to relieve symptoms and control any coexistent esophagitis. Although control of symptoms has historically served as the endpoint of therapy, the wisdom of this approach has recently been questioned, particularly in patients with BE. Evidence suggesting that reflux control may prevent the development of adenocarcinoma and lead to regression of dysplastic and nondysplastic Barrett segments has led many to consider control of reflux, and not symptom control, a better therapeutic endpoint. However, complete control of reflux can be difficult, as has been highlighted by studies of acid breakthrough while on proton pump inhibitor (PPI) therapy.

Suggested Therapeutic Approach

The traditional stepwise approach to the therapy of GERD should be re-examined in view of a more complete understanding of the pathophysiology of gastroesophageal reflux, and the rising incidence of BE. The approach should be to identify risk factors for persistent and progressive disease early in the course of the disease, and encourage surgical treatment when these factors are present. The following approach is suggested.

Patients presenting for the first time with symptoms suggestive of gastroesophageal reflux may be given initial therapy with PPI. In view of the availability of these as over-the-counter medications, many patients will have already self-medicated their symptoms. Failure of PPIs blockers to control the symptoms, or immediate return of symptoms after stopping treatment, suggests either that the diagnosis is incorrect or that the patient has relatively severe disease. Endoscopic examination at this stage of the patient's evaluation provides the opportunity for assessing the severity of mucosal damage and the presence of BE. Both of these findings on initial endoscopy are associated with a high probability that medical control of the disease will be difficult. A measurement of the degree and pattern of esophageal exposure to gastric and duodenal juice, via 24-h pH and bilirubin monitoring, should be obtained at this point. The status of the LES and the function of the esophageal body should also be measured. These studies identify features such as the following, which are predictive of a poor response to medical therapy, frequent relapses, and the development of complications: supine reflux, poor esophageal contractility, erosive esophagitis (or a columnar-lined esophagus at initial presentation), bile in the refluxate, and a structurally defective sphincter. Patients who have these risk factors should be given the option of surgery as a primary therapy, with the expectation of long-term control of symptoms and complications.

Surgical Therapy

Preoperative Evaluation

Before proceeding with an antireflux operation, several factors should be evaluated. First, the propulsive force of the body of the esophagus should be evaluated by esophageal manometry to determine if it has sufficient power to propel a bolus of food through a newly reconstructed valve. Patients with normal peristaltic contractions do well with a 360-degree Nissen fundoplication. When peristalsis is absent or severely disordered, or the amplitude of the contraction is below 20 mm Hg throughout the lower esophagus, a two-thirds partial fundoplication may be the procedure of choice.

Second, anatomic shortening of the esophagus can compromise the ability to do an adequate repair without tension, and lead to an increased incidence of breakdown or thoracic displacement of the repair. Esophageal shortening is identified on a barium swallow roentgenogram by a sliding hiatal hernia that will not reduce in the upright position, or that measures larger than 5 cm between the diaphragmatic crura and gastroesophageal junction on endoscopy. When esophageal shortening is present, a gastroplasty should be performed. In patients who have a global absence of contractility, and have dysphagia or a history of several failed previous antireflux procedures, esophageal resection should be considered as an alternative.

Third, the surgeon should specifically query the patient for complaints of nausea, vomiting, and loss of appetite. In such patients, these symptoms may persist after an antireflux procedure, and patients should be given this information before the operation. In these patients, 24-h bilirubin monitoring and gastric emptying studies can be performed to detect and quantify duodenogastric abnormalities.

Principles of Surgical Therapy

The primary goal of antireflux surgery is to safely restore the structure of the sphincter or to prevent its shortening with gastric distention, although preserving the patient's ability to swallow normally, to belch to relieve gaseous distention, and to vomit when necessary. Regardless of the choice of the procedure, this goal can be achieved if attention is paid to five principles in reconstructing the cardia. First, the operation should restore the pressure of the distal esophageal sphincter to a normal level and its length to at least 3 cm. The fundoplication augments sphincter characteristics in patients in whom they are reduced prior to surgery and prevents unfolding of a normal sphincter in response to gastric distention.

Second, the operation should place an adequate length of the distal esophageal sphincter in the positive-pressure environment of the abdomen by a method that ensures its response to changes in intraabdominal pressure. The permanent restoration of 1.5–2 cm of abdominal esophagus in a patient whose sphincter pressure has been augmented to normal levels will maintain the competency of the cardia over various challenges of intraabdominal pressure.

Third, the operation should allow the reconstructed cardia to relax on deglutition. In normal swallowing, a vagally mediated relaxation of the distal esophageal sphincter and the gastric fundus occurs. The relaxation lasts for approximately 10 s and is followed by a rapid recovery to the former tonicity. To ensure relaxation of the sphincter, three factors are important: (1) only the fundus of the stomach should be used to buttress the sphincter, because it is known to relax in concert with the sphincter; (2) the gastric wrap should be properly placed around the sphincter and not incorporate a portion of the stomach or be placed around the stomach itself, because the body of the stomach does not relax with swallowing; and (3) damage to the vagal nerves during dissection of the thoracic esophagus should be avoided because it may result in failure of the sphincter to relax.

Fourth, the fundoplication should not increase the resistance of the relaxed sphincter to a level that exceeds the peristaltic power of the body of the esophagus. The resistance of the relaxed sphincter depends on the degree, length, and diameter of the gastric fundoplication, and on the variation in intraabdominal pressure. A 360-degree gastric fundoplication should be no longer than 2 cm and constructed easily over a 60F bougie. This will ensure that the relaxed sphincter will have an adequate diameter with minimal resistance. This is not necessary when constructing a partial wrap.

Fifth, the operation should ensure that the fundoplication can be placed in the abdomen without undue tension, and maintained there by approximating the crura of the diaphragm above the repair. Leaving the fundoplication in the thorax converts a sliding hernia into a paraesophageal hernia, with all the complications associated with that condition. Maintaining the repair in the abdomen under tension predisposes to an increased incidence of recurrence. This is likely to occur in patients who have a stricture or BE, and is because of shortening of the esophagus from the inflammatory process. This problem can be resolved by lengthening the esophagus with a Collis gastroplasty.

Procedure Selection

A laparoscopic approach is used in patients with normal esophageal contractility and length. Patients with questionable esophageal length may be best approached transthoracically, in which full esophageal mobilization serves as a lengthening procedure. Those with a failed esophagus characterized by absent esophageal contractions and/or absent peristalsis such as those with scleroderma are best treated either medically or with a partial fundoplication to avoid the increased outflow resistance associated with a complete fundoplication. If the esophagus is short after it is mobilized from diaphragm to aortic arch, a Collis gastroplasty is done to provide additional length and avoid placing the repair under tension. In the majority of patients who have good esophageal contractility and normal esophageal length, the laparoscopic Nissen fundoplication is the procedure of choice for a primary antireflux repair.

Primary Antireflux Repairs

Nissen Fundoplication

The most common antireflux procedure is the Nissen fundoplication. The procedure can be performed through an abdominal or a chest incision, and through a laparoscope. Rudolph Nissen described the procedure as a 360-degree fundoplication around the lower esophagus for a distance of 4–5 cm. Although this provided good control of reflux, it was associated with a number of side effects that have encouraged modifications of the procedure as originally described. These include using only the gastric fundus to envelop the esophagus in a fashion analogous to a Witzel jejunostomy, sizing the fundoplication with a 60F bougie, and limiting the length of the fundoplication to 1–2 cm. The essential elements necessary for the performance of a transabdominal fundoplication are common to both the laparoscopic and open procedures and include the following:

1. Crural dissection, identification, and preservation of both vagi, and the anterior hepatic branch
2. Circumferential dissection of the esophagus
3. Crural closure
4. Fundic mobilization by division of short gastric vessels
5. Creation of a short, loose fundoplication by placing the posterior fundic wall posterior, and the anterior fundus anterior, to the esophagus, meeting at the right lateral position.

The laparoscopic approach. Laparoscopic fundoplication has become commonplace and has replaced the open abdominal Nissen fundoplication as the procedure of choice.

Transthoracic Nissen fundoplication. The indications for performing an antireflux procedure by a transthoracic approach are as follows:

1. A patient who has had a previous hiatal hernia repair. In this situation, a peripheral circumferential incision in the diaphragm is made to provide simultaneous exposure of the upper abdomen. This allows safe dissection of the previous repair from both the abdominal and thoracic sides of the diaphragm.
2. A patient who has a short esophagus. This is usually associated with a stricture or BE. In this situation, the thoracic approach is preferred to allow maximum mobilization of the esophagus, and to perform a Collis gastroplasty to place the repair without tension below the diaphragm.
3. A patient with a sliding hiatal hernia that does not reduce below the diaphragm during a roentgenographic barium study in the upright position. This can indicate esophageal shortening, and again, a thoracic approach is preferred for maximum mobilization of the esophagus, and if necessary, the performance of a Collis gastroplasty.
4. A patient who has associated pulmonary pathology. In this situation, the nature of the pulmonary pathology can be evaluated and the proper pulmonary surgery, in addition to the antireflux repair, can be performed.

5. An obese patient. In this situation, the abdominal repair is difficult because of poor exposure, particularly in men, in whom the intraabdominal fat is more abundant.

Outcome After Fundoplication

Nearly all published reports of laparoscopic fundoplication show that this procedure relieves the typical symptoms of gastroesophageal reflux—heartburn, regurgitation, and dysphagia—in greater than 90 percent of patients. The incidence of persistent postoperative dysphagia has decreased to the 3–5 percent range with increasing experience and attention to the technical details in constructing the fundoplication. Resting LES characteristics and esophageal acid exposure return to normal in nearly all patients. Morbidity after laparoscopic fundoplication is similar to that after open fundoplication, averaging 10–15 percent. Unrecognized perforation of the esophagus or stomach is the most life-threatening complication. Perforations occur most often during hiatal and circumferential dissection of the esophagus, and their incidence is also related to the surgeon's experience. Intraoperative recognition and repair are the keys to preventing a life-threatening complication.

BARRETT'S ESOPHAGUS

The condition whereby the tubular esophagus is lined with columnar epithelium rather than squamous epithelium was first described by Norman Barrett in 1950. He incorrectly believed it to be congenital in origin. It is now realized that it is an acquired abnormality, occurs in 7–15 percent of patients with GERD, and represents the end stage of the natural history of this disease. It is also thought to be distinctly different from the congenital condition in which islands of gastric fundic epithelium are found in the upper half of the esophagus.

The definition of BE has evolved considerably over the past decade. Traditionally, BE was identified by the presence of columnar mucosa extending at least 3 cm into the esophagus. It is now recognized that the specialized intestinal type epithelium found in the Barrett mucosa is the only tissue predisposed to malignant degeneration. Consequently, the diagnosis of BE is presently made given any length of endoscopically identifiable columnar mucosa that proves on biopsy to show intestinal metaplasia. Although long segments of columnar mucosa without intestinal metaplasia do occur, they are less uncommon today than they were previously.

The hallmark of intestinal metaplasia is the presence of intestinal goblet cells. There is a high prevalence of biopsy-demonstrated intestinal metaplasia at the cardia, on the gastric side of the squamocolumnar junction, in the absence of endoscopic evidence of a columnar-lined esophagus. Evidence is accumulating that these patches of what appears to be Barrett in the cardia have a similar malignant potential as the longer segments, and may be the precursors for carcinoma of the cardia.

The long-term relief of symptoms remains the primary reason for performing antireflux surgery in patients with BE. Healing of esophageal mucosal injury and the prevention of disease progression are important secondary goals. In this regard, patients with BE are no different than the broader population of patients with gastroesophageal reflux. They should be considered for antireflux surgery when patient data suggest severe disease or predict the need for long-term medical management. Most patients with BE are symptomatic. Although

TABLE 24-5 Symptomatic Outcome of Surgical Therapy for Barrett Esophagus

Author	Year	No. of patients	% Excellent to good response	Mean follow-up, years
Starnes	1984	8	75	2
Williamson	1990	37	92	3
DeMeester	1990	35	77	3
McDonald	1996	113	82.2	6.5
Ortiz	1996	32	90.6	5

it has been argued that some patients with BE may not have symptoms, careful history taking will reveal the presence of symptoms in most, if not all, patients.

The typical complications in BE include ulceration in the columnar-lined segment, stricture formation, and a dysplasia-cancer sequence. Barrett's ulceration is unlike the erosive ulceration of reflux esophagitis in that it more closely resembles peptic ulceration in the stomach or duodenum, and has the same propensity to bleed, penetrate, or perforate. The strictures found in BE occur at the squamocolumnar junction, and are typically higher than peptic strictures in the absence of BE. Ulceration and stricture in association with BE were commonly reported prior to 1975, but with the advent of potent acid suppression medication they have become less common. In contrast, the complication of adenocarcinoma developing in Barrett mucosa has become more common. Adenocarcinoma developing in Barrett mucosa was considered a rare tumor prior to 1975. Today it occurs in approximately one in every 100 patient-years of follow-up, which represents a risk 40 times that of the general population. Most if not all cases of adenocarcinoma of the esophagus arise in Barrett epithelium.

Few studies have focused on the alleviation of symptoms after antireflux surgery in patients with BE (Table 24-5). Those that are available document excellent to good results in 72–95 percent of patients at 5 years following surgery.

Farrell and associates also reported symptomatic outcome of laparoscopic Nissen fundoplication in 50 patients with both long- and short-segment BE. Mean scores for heartburn, regurgitation, and dysphagia all improved dramatically post-Nissen. Importantly, there was no significant decrement in symptom scores when 1-year results were compared to those at 2–5 years postoperatively. They did find a higher prevalence of "anatomic" failures requiring re-operation in patients with BE when compared to non-Barrett patients with GERD. Others have reported similar results. Taken together these studies document the ability of antireflux surgery to provide long-term symptomatic relief in patients with BE.

Three relevant questions arise concerning the fate, over time, of the metaplastic tissue found in BE: (1) Does antireflux surgery cause regression of Barrett epithelium? (2) Does it prevent progression? and (3) Can the development of Barrett metaplasia be prevented by early antireflux surgery in patients with reflux disease?

The common belief that Barrett epithelium cannot be reversed is likely false. DeMeester and associates reported that after antireflux surgery, loss of intestinal metaplasia (IM) in patients with visible BE was rare, but occurred in 73 percent of patients with inapparent IM of the cardia. This suggests that the metaplastic process may indeed be reversible if reflux is eliminated early in its process, that cardiac mucosa is dynamic, and that as opposed to IM extending several centimeters into the esophagus, IM of the cardia is more likely to regress following antireflux surgery.

Recent evidence suggests that the development of BE may even be preventable. Although a very difficult hypothesis to study, Oberg and coworkers followed a cohort of 69 patients with short-segment, nonintestinalized, columnar-lined esophagus (CLE) over a median of 5 years of surveillance endoscopy. Forty-nine of the patients were maintained on PPI therapy and 20 had antireflux surgery. Patients with antireflux surgery were 10 times less likely to develop IM in these CLE segments over a follow-up span of nearly 15 years than those on medical therapy. This rather remarkable observation supports the two-step hypothesis of the development of BE (cardiac metaplasia followed by intestinal metaplasia), and suggests that the second step can be prevented if reflux disease is recognized and treated early and aggressively.

There is a growing body of evidence to attest to the ability of fundoplication to protect against dysplasia and invasive malignancy. Three studies suggest that an effective antireflux procedure can impact the natural history of BE in this regard. Two prospective randomized studies found less adenocarcinoma in the surgically treated groups. Parrilla and associates reported that although the development of dysplasia and adenocarcinoma was no different overall, the subgroup of surgical patients with normal postoperative pH studies developed significantly less dysplasia and had no adenocarcinoma. Spechler identified one adenocarcinoma 11–13 years after antireflux surgery, compared to four following medical treatment. Most of these authors concluded that there is a critical need for future trials exploring the role of antireflux surgery in protecting against the development of dysplasia in patients with BE.

Atypical Reflux Symptoms

Chronic respiratory symptoms, such as chronic cough, recurrent pneumonias, episodes of nocturnal choking, waking up with gastric contents in the mouth, or soilage of the bed pillow, may also indicate the need for surgical therapy. Patients suffering from repetitive pulmonary aspiration secondary to gastroesophageal reflux often shows signs of pleural thickening, bronchiectasis, and chronic interstitial pulmonary fibrosis on their chest radiograph. If 24-h pH monitoring confirms the presence of increased esophageal acid exposure, and manometry shows normal esophageal body motility, an antireflux procedure can be done with an expected good result. However, these patients usually have a nonspecific motor abnormality of the esophageal body, which tends to propel the refluxed material toward the pharynx. In some of these patients, the motor abnormality will disappear after a surgical antireflux procedure. In others, the motor disorder will persist and contribute to postoperative aspiration of swallowed saliva and food. Consequently, the results of an antireflux procedure in patients with a motor disorder of the esophageal body are variable.

Chest pain may be an atypical symptom of gastroesophageal reflux, and is often confused with coronary artery disease. Fifty percent of patients in whom a cardiac cause of the chest pain has been excluded will have increased esophageal acid exposure as a cause of the episode of pain. An antireflux procedure provides relief of the chest pain more consistently than medical therapy.

Dysphagia, regurgitation, or chest pain on eating in a patient with normal endoscopy and esophageal function studies can be an indication for an antireflux procedure. These symptoms are usually related to the presence of a large paraesophageal hernia, intrathoracic stomach, or a small hiatal hernia with a narrow diaphragmatic hiatus. A Schatzki ring may be present with the latter. All these conditions are easily identified with an upper GI radiographic barium examination done by a knowledgeable radiologist. These patients may have no heartburn, because the LES is usually normal and reflux of gastric acid into the esophagus does not occur. The surgical repair of the hernia usually includes an antireflux procedure because of the potential of destroying the competency of the cardia during the surgical dissection.

MOTILITY DISORDERS OF THE PHARYNX AND ESOPHAGUS

Clinical Manifestations

Difficulty in swallowing (dysphagia) is the primary symptom of esophageal motor disorders. Its perception by the patient is a balance between the severity of the underlying abnormality causing the dysphagia, and the adjustment made by the patient in altering eating habits. Consequently, any complaint of dysphagia must include an assessment of the patient's dietary history. It must be known whether the patient experiences pain, chokes, or vomits with eating; whether the patient requires liquids with the meal, is the last to finish, or is forced to interrupt a social meal; and whether he or she has been admitted to the hospital for food impaction. These assessments, plus an evaluation of the patient's nutritional status, help to determine how severe the dysphagia is and evaluate the indications for surgical therapy.

A surgical myotomy is designed to improve the symptoms of dysphagia caused by a motility disorder. The results can profoundly improve the patient's ability to ingest food, but rarely return the function of the foregut to normal. The principle of the procedure is to destroy esophageal contractility to correct a defect in esophageal motility, resulting in improvement but never a return to normal function. To use a surgical myotomy to treat the problem of dysphagia, the surgeon needs to know the precise functional abnormality causing the symptom. This usually entails a complete esophageal motility evaluation. A clear understanding of the physiologic mechanism of swallowing, and identification of the motility abnormality giving rise to the dysphagia, are essential for determining if surgery is indicated and the extent of the myotomy to be performed. Endoscopy is necessary only to exclude the presence of tumor or inflammatory changes as the cause of dysphagia.

Motility Disorders of the Pharyngoesophageal Segment

Disorders of the pharyngoesophageal phase of swallowing result from a discoordination of the neuromuscular events involved in chewing, initiation of swallowing, and propulsion of the material from the oropharynx into the cervical esophagus. They can be categorized into one or a combination of the following abnormalities: (1) inadequate oropharyngeal bolus transport; (2) inability to pressurize the pharynx; (3) inability to elevate the larynx; (4) discoordination of pharyngeal contraction and cricopharyngeal relaxation; and

(5) decreased compliance of the pharyngoesophageal segment secondary to muscle pathology. The latter results in incomplete anatomic relaxation of the cricopharyngeus and cervical esophagus.

Pharyngoesophageal swallowing disorders are usually because of acquired disease involving the central and peripheral nervous system. This includes cerebrovascular accidents, brain stem tumors, poliomyelitis, multiple sclerosis, Parkinson disease, pseudobulbar palsy, peripheral neuropathy, and operative damage to the cranial nerves involved in swallowing. Muscular diseases such as radiation-induced myopathy, dermatomyositis, myotonic dystrophy, and myasthenia gravis are less common causes. Rarely, extrinsic compression by thyromegaly, cervical lymphadenopathy, or hyperostosis of the cervical spine can cause pharyngoesophageal dysphagia.

Zenker Diverticulum

In the past, the most common recognized sign of pharyngoesophageal dysfunction was the presence of a Zenker diverticulum, originally described by Ludlow in 1769. The eponym resulted from Zenker classic clinicopathologic descriptions of 34 cases published in 1878. Pharyngoesophageal diverticula have been reported to occur in 0.1 percent of 20,000 routine barium examinations, and classically occur in older adult, white males. Zenker diverticula tend to enlarge progressively with time because of the decreased compliance of the skeletal portion of the cervical esophagus that occurs with aging.

Presenting symptoms include dysphagia associated with the spontaneous regurgitation of undigested, bland material, often interrupting eating or drinking. The symptom of dysphagia is due initially to the loss of muscle compliance in the pharyngoesophageal segment, later augmented by the presence of an enlarging diverticulum. On occasion, the dysphagia can be severe enough to cause debilitation and significant weight loss. Chronic aspiration and repetitive respiratory infection are common associated complaints. Once suspected, the diagnosis is established by a barium swallow. Endoscopy is usually difficult in the presence of a cricopharyngeal diverticulum, and potentially dangerous, owing to obstruction of the true esophageal lumen by the diverticulum and the attendant risk of diverticular perforation.

Pharyngocricoesophageal Myotomy

The myotomy can be performed under local or general anesthesia through an incision along the anterior border of the left sternocleidomastoid muscle. The pharynx and cervical esophagus are exposed by retracting the sternocleidomastoid muscle and carotid sheath laterally, and the thyroid, trachea, and larynx medially. When a pharyngoesophageal diverticulum is present, localization of the pharyngoesophageal segment is easy. The diverticulum is carefully freed from the overlying areolar tissue to expose its neck, just below the inferior pharyngeal constrictor and above the cricopharyngeus muscle. It can be difficult to identify the cricopharyngeus muscle in the absence of a diverticulum. A benefit of local anesthesia is that the patient can swallow and demonstrate an area of persistent narrowing at the pharyngoesophageal junction. Furthermore, before closing the incision, gelatin can be fed to the patient to ascertain whether the symptoms have been relieved, and to inspect the opening of the previously narrowed pharyngoesophageal segment. Under general anesthesia, and in the absence of a diverticulum, the placement of a nasogastric tube to the level of the manometrically determined cricopharyngeal sphincter helps in localization of the structures. The myotomy is extended cephalad by dividing 1 to 2 cm of inferior constrictor muscle of the pharynx, and caudad by dividing the cricopharyngeal muscle and the cervical esophagus for a length of 4–5 cm. The cervical wound is closed only when all oozing of blood has ceased, because a hematoma after this procedure is common, and is often associated with temporary dysphagia while the hematoma absorbs. Oral alimentation is started the day after surgery. The patient is usually discharged on the first or second postoperative day.

If a diverticulum is present and is large enough to persist after a myotomy it may be sutured in the inverted position to the prevertebral fascia using a permanent suture (i.e., diverticulopexy). If the diverticulum is excessively large so that it would be redundant if suspended, or if its walls are thickened, a diverticulectomy should be performed.

Endoscopic stapled diverticulotomy recently has been described. The procedure uses a Weerda diverticuloscope with two retractable valves passed into the hypopharynx. The lips of the diverticuloscope are positioned so that one lip lies in the esophageal lumen and the other in the diverticular lumen. The valves of the diverticuloscope are retracted appropriately so as to visualize the septum interposed between the diverticulum and the esophagus. An endoscopic linear stapler is introduced into the diverticuloscope and positioned against the common septum with the anvil in the diverticulum and the cartridge in the esophageal lumen. Firing of the stapler divides the common septum between the posterior esophageal and the diverticular wall over a length of 30 mm, placing three rows of staples on each side. More than one stapler application may be needed, depending on the size of the diverticulum. The patient is allowed to resume liquid feeds either on the same day or the day after, and is usually discharged the day after surgery. Complications are rare and may include perforation at the apex of the diverticulum, and can be repaired with minimally invasive techniques.

Postoperative complications include fistula formation, abscess, hematoma, recurrent nerve paralysis, difficulties in phonation, and Horner's syndrome. The incidence of the first two can be reduced by performing a diverticulopexy. Recurrence of a Zenker diverticulum occurs late, and is more common after diverticulectomy without myotomy, presumably because of persistence of the underlying loss of compliance of the cervical esophagus when a myotomy is not performed.

Motility Disorders of the Esophageal Body and Lower Esophageal Sphincter

Disorders of the esophageal phase of swallowing result from abnormalities in the propulsive pump action of the esophageal body or the relaxation of the LES. These disorders result from either primary esophageal abnormalities, or from generalized neural, muscular, or collagen vascular disease (Table 24-6). The use of standard esophageal manometry techniques has allowed specific primary esophageal motility disorders to be identified out of a pool of nonspecific motility abnormalities. These include achalasia, diffuse esophageal spasm, the so-called nutcracker esophagus, the hypertensive LES, and ineffectiveesophageal motility. Table 24-7 shows the manometric characteristics of these disorders.

TABLE 24-6 Esophageal Motility Disorders

Primary esophageal motility disorders
Achalasia, "vigorous" achalasia
Diffuse and segmental esophageal spasm
Nutcracker esophagus
Hypertensive lower esophageal sphincter
Nonspecific esophageal motility disorders

Secondary esophageal motility disorders
Collagen vascular diseases: progressive systemic sclerosis, polymyositis and dermatomyositis, mixed connective tissue disease, systemic lupus erythematosus, etc.
Chronic idiopathic intestinal pseudo-obstruction
Neuromuscular diseases
Endocrine and metastatic disorders

Achalasia

The best known and best understood primary motility disorder of the esophagus is achalasia, with an incidence of six per 100,000 population per year. Although complete absence of peristalsis in the esophageal body has been proposed as the major abnormality, present evidence indicates achalasia is a primary disorder of the LES. The observation that esophageal peristalsis can return in patients with classic achalasia following dilation or myotomy provides support that achalasia is a primary disease of the LES.

The pathogenesis of achalasia is presumed to be a neurogenic degeneration, which is either idiopathic or because of inflammation. In experimental animals, the disease has been reproduced by destruction of the nucleus ambiguus and the dorsal motor nucleus of the vagus nerve. In patients with the disease, degenerative changes have been shown in the vagus nerve and in the ganglia in the Auerbach plexus of the esophagus itself. This degeneration results in hypertension of the LES, a failure of the sphincter to relax on deglutition, elevation of intraluminal esophageal pressure, esophageal dilatation, and a subsequent loss of progressive peristalsis in the body of the esophagus. The esophageal dilatation results from the combination of a nonrelaxing sphincter, which causes a functional retention of ingested material in the esophagus, and elevation of intraluminal pressure from repetitive pharyngeal air swallowing. With time, the functional disorder results in anatomic alterations seen on radiographic studies, such as a dilated esophagus with a tapering, beak-like narrowing of the distal end. There is usually an air-fluid level in the esophagus from the retained food and saliva, the height of which reflects the degree of resistance imposed by the nonrelaxing sphincter. As the disease progresses, the esophagus becomes massively dilated and tortuous.

Diffuse and Segmental Esophageal Spasm

Diffuse esophageal spasm is characterized by substernal chest pain and/or dysphagia. Diffuse esophageal spasm differs from classic achalasia in that it is primarily a disease of the esophageal body, produces a lesser degree of dysphagia, causes more chest pain, and has less effect on the patient's general condition. True symptomatic diffuse esophageal spasm is a rare condition, occurring about 5 times less frequently than achalasia.

TABLE 24-7 Manometric Characteristics of the Primary Esophageal Motility Disorders

Achalasia
Incomplete lower esophageal sphincter (LES) relaxation (< 75% relaxation)
Aperistalsis in the esophageal body
Elevated LES pressure ≤ 26 mm Hg
Increased intraesophageal baseline pressures relative to gastric baseline

Diffuse Esophageal Spasm (DES)
Simultaneous (nonperistaltic contractions) (> 20% of wet swallows)
Repetitive and multi-peaked contractions
Spontaneous contractions
Intermittent normal peristalsis
Contractions may be of increased amplitude and duration

Nutcracker Esophagus
Mean peristaltic amplitude (10 wet swallows) in distal esophagus ≥ 180 mm Hg
Increased mean duration of contractions (> 7.0 s)
Normal peristaltic sequence

Hypertensive Lower Esophageal Sphincter
Elevated LES pressure (≥ 26 mm Hg)
Normal LES relaxation
Normal peristalsis in the esophageal body

Ineffective Esophageal Motility Disorders
Decreased or absent amplitude of esophageal peristalsis (< 30 mm Hg)
Increased number of nontransmitted contractions

Source: Reproduced with permission from DeMeester TR, Stein HJ, Fuchs KH: Physiologic diagnostic studies, in Zuidema GD, Orringer MB (eds): *Shackelford's Surgery of the Alimentary Tract,* 3rd ed, Vol. I. Philadelphia: WB Saunders, 1991, p 115.

The causation and neuromuscular pathophysiology of diffuse esophageal spasm are unclear. The basic motor abnormality is rapid wave progression down the esophagus secondary to an abnormality in the latency gradient. Hypertrophy of the muscular layer of the esophageal wall and degeneration of the esophageal branches of the vagus nerve have been observed in this disease, although these are not constant findings. Manometric abnormalities in diffuse esophageal spasm may be present over the total length of the esophageal body, but usually are confined to the distal two-thirds. In segmental esophageal spasm, the manometric abnormalities are confined to a short segment of the esophagus.

The classic manometric findings in these patients are characterized by the frequent occurrence of simultaneous waveforms and multipeaked esophageal contractions, which may be of abnormally high amplitude or long duration. Key to the diagnosis of diffuse esophageal spasm is that there remain some peristaltic waveforms in excess of those seen in achalasia. A criterion of 20 percent or more simultaneous waveforms out of 10 wet swallows has been used to diagnose diffuse esophageal spasm. However, this figure is arbitrary and often debated.

The LES in patients with diffuse esophageal spasm usually shows a normal resting pressure and relaxation on deglutition. In patients with advanced disease, the radiographic appearance of tertiary contractions appears helical, and has been termed corkscrew esophagus or pseudodiverticulosis. Patients with segmental or diffuse esophageal spasm can compartmentalize the esophagus and develop an epiphrenic or midesophageal diverticulum.

Diverticula of the Esophageal Body

Radiographic abnormalities such as segmental spasm, corkscrewing, compartmentalization, and diverticulum are the anatomic results of disordered motility function. Of these, the most persistent and easiest to demonstrate is an esophageal diverticulum. Diverticula occur most commonly with nonspecific motility disorders, but can occur with all of the primary motility disorders. In the latter situation, the motility disorder is usually diagnosed before the development of the diverticulum. When present, a diverticulum may temporarily alleviate the symptom of dysphagia by becoming a receptacle for ingested food, and substitute the symptoms of postprandial pain and the regurgitation of undigested food. If a motility abnormality of the esophageal body or LES cannot be identified, a traction or congenital cause for the diverticulum should be considered. Because development in radiology preceded development in motility monitoring, diverticula of the esophagus were considered historically to be a primary abnormality, the cause, rather than the consequence, of motility disorders. Consequently, earlier texts focused on them as specific entities based on their location.

Epiphrenic diverticula arise from the terminal third of the thoracic esophagus and are usually found adjacent to the diaphragm. They have been associated with distal esophageal muscular hypertrophy, esophageal motility abnormalities, and increased luminal pressure. They are "pulsion" diverticula, and have been associated with diffuse spasm, achalasia, or nonspecific motor abnormalities in the body of the esophagus.

Whether the diverticulum should be surgically resected or suspended depends on its size and proximity to the vertebral body. When diverticula are associated with esophageal motility disorders, esophageal myotomy from the distal extent of the diverticulum to the stomach is indicated; otherwise, one can expect a high incidence of suture line rupture because of the same intraluminal pressure that initially gave rise to the diverticulum. If the diverticulum is suspended to the prevertebral fascia of the thoracic vertebra, a myotomy is begun at the neck of the diverticulum and extended across the LES. If the diverticulum is excised by dividing the neck, the muscle is closed over the excision site and a myotomy is performed on the opposite esophageal wall, starting at the level of diverticulum. When a large diverticulum is associated with a hiatal hernia, the diverticulum is excised, a myotomy is performed if there is an associated esophageal motility abnormality, and the hernia is repaired because of the high incidence of postoperative reflux when it is omitted.

Midesophageal or traction diverticula were first described in the nineteenth century. At that time they were frequently noted in patients who had mediastinal lymph node involvement with tuberculosis. It was theorized that adhesions form between the inflamed mediastinal nodes and the esophagus. By contraction, the adhesions exerted traction on the esophageal wall and led to a localized diverticulum. This theory was based on the findings of early dissections, in which adhesions between diverticula and lymph nodes were commonly found. It is now believed that some diverticula in the midesophagus may also be caused by motility abnormalities.

Most midesophageal diverticula are asymptomatic and incidentally discovered during investigation for nonesophageal complaints. In such patients, the radiologic abnormality may be ignored. Patients with symptoms of dysphagia, regurgitation, chest pain, or aspiration, in whom a diverticulum is discovered, should be thoroughly investigated for an esophageal motor abnormality and treated appropriately. Occasionally, a patient will present with a bronchoesophageal fistula manifested by a chronic cough on ingestion of meals. The diverticulum in such patients is most likely to have an inflammatory etiology.

The indication for surgical intervention is the degree of symptomatic disability. Usually midesophageal diverticula can be suspended because of their proximity to the spine. If motor abnormality is documented, a myotomy should be performed similarly to that described for an epiphrenic diverticulum.

Operations

Long esophageal myotomy for motor disorders of the esophageal body. A long esophageal myotomy is indicated for dysphagia caused by any motor disorder characterized by segmental or generalized simultaneous waveforms in a patient whose symptoms are not relieved by medical therapy. Such disorders include diffuse and segmental esophageal spasm, vigorous achalasia, and nonspecific motility disorders associated with a mid- or epiphrenic esophageal diverticulum. However, the decision to operate must be made by a balanced evaluation of the patient's symptoms, diet, lifestyle adjustments, and nutritional status, with the most important factor being the possibility of improving the patient's swallowing disability. The symptom of chest pain alone is not an indication for a surgical procedure.

Twenty-four-h ambulatory motility monitoring has greatly aided in the identification of patients with symptoms of dysphagia and chest pain who might benefit from a surgical myotomy. Ambulatory motility studies have shown that when the prevalence of "effective contractions" (i.e., peristaltic waveforms consisting of contractions with an amplitude above 30 mm Hg) drops below 50 percent during meals, the patient is likely to experience dysphagia. This would suggest that relief from the symptom could be expected with an improvement of esophageal contraction amplitude or amelioration of nonperistaltic waveforms. Prokinetic agents may increase esophageal contraction amplitude, but do not alter the prevalence of simultaneous waveforms. Patients in whom the efficacy of esophageal propulsion is severely compromised because of a high prevalence of simultaneous waveforms usually receive little benefit from medical therapy. In these patients, a surgical myotomy of the esophageal body can improve the patients' dysphagia, provided the loss of contraction amplitude in the remaining peristaltic waveforms, caused by the myotomy, has less effect on swallowing function than the presence of the excessive simultaneous contractions. This situation is reached when the prevalence of effective waveforms during meals drops below 30 percent, i.e., 70 percent of esophageal waveforms are ineffective.

In patients selected for surgery, preoperative manometry is essential to determine the proximal extent of the esophageal myotomy. Most surgeons extend the myotomy distally across the LES to reduce outflow resistance. Consequently, some form of antireflux protection is needed to avoid gastroesophageal reflux if there has been extensive dissection of the cardia. In this situation, most authors prefer a partial, rather than a full, fundoplication, in order not to add back-resistance that will further interfere with the ability of the myotomized esophagus to empty. If the symptoms of reflux are present preoperatively, 24-hour pH monitoring is required to confirm its presence.

The procedure may be performed either open or via thoracoscopy. The open technique is performed through a left thoracotomy in the sixth intercostal space. An incision is made in the posterior mediastinal pleura over the esophagus, and the left lateral wall of the esophagus is exposed. The esophagus is not circumferentially dissected unless necessary. A 2-cm incision is made into the abdomen through the parietal peritoneum at the midportion of the left crus. A tongue of gastric fundus is pulled into the chest. This exposes the gastroesophageal junction and its associated fat pad. The latter is excised to give a clear view of the junction. A myotomy is performed through all muscle layers, extending distally over the stomach 1–2 cm below the gastroesophageal junction, and proximally on the esophagus over the distance of the manometric abnormality. The muscle layer is dissected from the mucosa laterally for a distance of 1 cm. Care is taken to divide all minute muscle bands, particularly in the area of the junction. The gastric fundic tongue is sutured to the margins of the myotomy over a distance of 3–4 cm and replaced into the abdomen. This maintains separation of the muscle and acts as a partial fundoplication to prevent reflux.

If an epiphrenic diverticulum is present, it is excised by dividing the neck and closing the muscle. The myotomy is then performed on the opposite esophageal wall. If a midesophageal diverticulum is present, the myotomy is made so that it includes the muscle around the neck, and the diverticulum is inverted and suspended by attaching it to the paravertebral fascia of the thoracic vertebra.

The results of myotomy for motor disorders of the esophageal body have improved in parallel with the improved preoperative diagnosis afforded by manometry. Previous published series report between 40 and 92 percent improvement of symptoms, but interpretation is difficult because of the small number of patients involved and the varying criteria for diagnosis of the primary motor abnormality. When myotomy is accurately done, 93 percent of the patients have effective palliation of dysphagia after a mean follow-up of 5 years, and 89 percent would have the procedure again if it was necessary. Most patients gain or maintain rather than lose weight after the operation. Postoperative motility studies show that the myotomy reduces the amplitude of esophageal contractions to near zero and eliminates simultaneous peristaltic waves. If the benefit of obliterating the simultaneous waves exceeds the adverse effect on bolus propulsion caused by the loss of peristaltic waveforms, the patient's dysphagia is likely to be improved by the procedure. If not, the patient is likely to continue to complain of dysphagia and to have little improvement as a result of the operation. Preoperative motility studies are thus crucial in deciding which patients are most likely to benefit from a long esophageal myotomy.

Myotomy of the lower esophageal sphincter. Second only to reflux disease, achalasia is the most common functional disorder of the esophagus to require surgical intervention. The goal of treatment is to relieve the functional outflow obstruction secondary to the loss of relaxation and compliance of the LES. This requires disrupting the LES muscle. When performed adequately (i.e., reducing sphincter pressure to < 10 mm Hg), and done early in the course of disease, LES myotomy results in symptomatic improvement with the occasional return of esophageal peristalsis. Reduction in LES resistance can be accomplished intraluminally by hydrostatic balloon dilation, which ruptures the sphincter muscle, or by a surgical myotomy that cuts the sphincter. The difference between these two methods appears to be the greater likelihood of reducing sphincter pressure to less than 10 mm Hg by surgical myotomy as compared with hydrostatic balloon dilation. However, patients whose sphincter pressure has been reduced by hydrostatic balloon dilation to less than 10 mm Hg have an outcome similar to those after surgical myotomy. In performing a surgical myotomy of the LES, there are four important principles: (1) minimal dissection of the cardia, (2) adequate distal myotomy to reduce outflow resistance, (3) prevention of postoperative reflux, and (4) preventing rehealing of the myotomy site. In the past, the drawback of a surgical myotomy was the need for an open procedure. With the advent of limited-access technology, the myotomy can now be performed laparoscopically.

The therapeutic decisions regarding the treatment of patients with achalasia center around three issues. The first issue is the question of whether newly diagnosed patients should be treated with pneumatic dilation or a surgical myotomy. Long-term follow-up studies have shown that pneumatic dilation achieves adequate relief of dysphagia and pharyngeal regurgitation in 50–60 percent of patients. Close follow-up is required, and if dilation fails, myotomy is indicated. For those patients who have a dilated and tortuous esophagus or an associated hiatal hernia, balloon dilation is dangerous and surgery is the better option. Whether it is better to treat a newly diagnosed esophageal achalasia patient by forceful dilation or by operative cardiomyotomy remains undecided. The outcome of the one controlled randomized study (38 patients) comparing the two modes of therapy suggests that surgical myotomy as a primary treatment gives better long-term results. There are several large retrospective series that report the outcome obtained with the two modes of treatment (Table 24-8). Despite objections regarding variations in surgical and dilation techniques and the number of physicians performing the procedures, these collective data would appear to support operative myotomy as the initial treatment of choice, when performed by a surgeon of average skill and experience.

TABLE 24-8 Series with >100 Patients Giving Follow-Up Results of Myotomy of Balloon Dilation for Achalasia

Author	Year	No. of patients	Follow-up years	Good-to-excellent response
Surgical myotomy				
Black et al	1976	108	4	65%
Menzies Gow	1978	102	8	98%
Okike et al	1979	456	1–17	85%
Ellis et al	1984	113	3.5	91%
Csendes et al	1988	100	6.8	92%
Balloon dilation				
Sanderson et al	1970	408	. . .	81%
Vantrappen et al	1979	403	7.8	76%
Okike et al	1979	431	1–18	65%

Source: Reproduced with permission from DeMeester TR, Stein HJ: Surgery for esophageal motor disorders, in Castell DO (ed): *The Esophagus.* Boston: Little, Brown, 1992, p 424.

The second issue is the question of whether a surgical myotomy should be performed through the abdomen or the chest. Myotomy of the LES can be accomplished via either an abdominal or thoracic approach. Recent data suggest that a transabdominal approach is preferable, particularly when done using minimally invasive techniques.

The third issue—and one that has been long debated—is the question of whether an antireflux procedure should be added to a surgical myotomy. A recent preoperative randomized study supports the need for antireflux protection. Further support for an antireflux procedure is the fact that the development of a reflux-induced stricture after an esophageal myotomy is a serious problem, and usually necessitates esophagectomy for relief of symptoms. If an antireflux procedure is used as an adjunct to esophageal myotomy, a complete 360-degree fundoplication should be avoided. Rather, a 270-degree partial fundoplication or a Dor hemifundoplication should be used to avoid the long-term esophageal dysfunction secondary to the outflow obstruction afforded by the fundoplication itself.

Laparoscopic esophageal myotomy. The laparoscopic approach is similar to the Nissen fundoplication in terms of the trocar placement and exposure. The procedure begins by division of the short gastric vessels in preparation for fundoplication. Exposure of the gastroesophageal junction (GEJ) via removal of the gastroesophageal fat pad follows. The anterior vagus nerve is swept right laterally along with the fat pad. Once completed, the GEJ and the left lateral 4–5 cm of esophagus should be bared of any overlying tissue. A left lateral esophageal myotomy is performed. It is generally easiest to begin the myotomy 1–2 cm above the GEJ. Either scissors or a hook-type electrocautery can be used to initiate the incision in the longitudinal and circular muscle. Distally, the myotomy is carried across the GEJ and onto the proximal stomach along the greater curvature for approximately 3 cm. After completion, the muscle edges are separated bluntly from the esophageal mucosa for approximately 50 percent of the esophageal circumference. An antireflux procedure follows completion of the myotomy. A left lateral partial fundoplication that augments the angle of His (Dor) or a posterior lateral partial fundoplication (Toupet) can be performed. The Dor type fundoplication is slightly easier to perform, and does not require disruption of the normal posterior gastroesophageal attachments (a theoretical advantage in preventing postoperative reflux).

Outcome assessment of the therapy for achalasia. Critical analysis of the results of therapy for motor disorders of the esophagus requires objective measurement. The use of symptoms alone as an endpoint to evaluate therapy for achalasia may be misleading. The propensity for patients to unconsciously modify their diet to avoid difficulty swallowing is underestimated, making an assessment of results based on symptoms unreliable. Insufficient reduction in outflow resistance may allow progressive esophageal digitation to develop slowly, giving the impression of improvement because the volume of food able to be ingested with comfort increases. A variety of objective measurements may be used to assess success, including LES pressure, esophageal baseline pressure, and scintigraphic or time barium swallow assessment of esophageal emptying time. Esophageal baseline pressure is usually negative when compared to gastric pressure. Given that the goal of therapy is to eliminate the outflow resistance of a nonrelaxing sphincter, measurement of improvements in esophageal baseline pressure and transit time may be better indicators of success, but are rarely reported.

TABLE 24-9 Reasons for Failure of Esophageal Myotomy

Reason	Author, procedure (n)		
	Ellis, myotomy only (n = 81)	Goulbourne, myotomy only (n = 65)	Malthaner, myotomy + antireflux (n = 22)
Reflux	4%	5%	18%
Inadequate myotomy	2%	...	9%
Megaesophagus	2%	...	...
Poor emptying	4%	3%	...
Persistent chest pain	1%	...	...

Source: Data from Malthaner RA, Tood TR, Miller L, Pearson FG: Long-term results in surgically managed esophageal achalasia. *Ann Thorac Surg* 58:1343, 1994; Ellis FH Jr.: Oesophagomyotomy for achalasia: A 22-year experience. *Br J Surg* 80:882, 1993; and Goulbourne IA, Walbaum PR: Long-term results of Heller's operation for achalasia. *J Royal Coll Surg* 30, 1985.

Bonavina and colleagues reported good to excellent results with trans-abdominal myotomy and Dor fundoplication in 94 percent of patients after a mean follow-up of 5.4 years. No operative mortality occurred in either of these series, attesting to the safety of the procedure. Malthaner and Pearson reported the long-term clinical results in 35 patients with achalasia, having a minimum follow-up of 10 years (Table 24-9). Twenty-two of these patients underwent primary esophageal myotomy and Belsey hemi-fundoplication at the Toronto General Hospital. Excellent to good results were noted in 95 percent of patients at 1 year, declining to 68, 69, and 67 percent at 10, 15, and 20 years, respectively. Two patients underwent early reoperation for an incomplete myotomy, and three underwent an esophagectomy for progressive disease. They concluded that there was a deterioration of the initially good results after surgical myotomy and hiatal repair for achalasia, which is because of late complications of gastroesophageal reflux.

Ellis reported his lifetime experience with transthoracic short esophageal myotomy without an antireflux procedure. One hundred seventy-nine patients were analyzed at a mean follow-up of 9 years, ranging from 6 months to 20 years. Overall 89 percent of patients were improved at the 9-year mark. He also observed that the level of improvement deteriorated with time, with excellent results (patients continuing to be symptom free) decreasing from 54 percent at 10 years to 32 percent at 20 years. Both studies document nearly identical results 10–15 years following the procedure, and both report deterioration over time, probably because of progression of the underlying disease. The addition of an antireflux procedure if the operation is performed transthoracically has no significant effect on the outcome.

The outcome of laparoscopic myotomy and hemifundoplication has been well documented. Two reports of over 100 patients have documented relief of dysphagia in 93 percent of patients. Richter and coworkers reviewed published reports to date, including 254 patients with an average success rate of 93 percent at 2.5 years. Conversion to an open procedure occurs in 0–5 percent of patients. Complications are uncommon, occurring in less than 5 percent of patients. Intraoperative complications consist largely of mucosal perforation, and have been more likely to occur after botulinum toxin injection.

CARCINOMA OF THE ESOPHAGUS

Squamous carcinoma accounts for the majority of esophageal carcinomas worldwide. Its incidence is highly variable, ranging from approximately 20 per 100,000 in the United States and Britain, to 160 per 100,000 in certain parts of South Africa and the Honan Province of China, and even 540 per 100,000 in the Guriev district of Kazakhstan. The environmental factors responsible for these localized high-incidence areas have not been conclusively identified, although additives to local foodstuffs (nitroso compounds in pickled vegetables and smoked meats) and mineral deficiencies (zinc and molybdenum) have been suggested. In Western societies, smoking and alcohol consumption are strongly linked with squamous carcinoma. Other definite associations link squamous carcinoma with long-standing achalasia, lye strictures, tylosis (an autosomal dominant disorder characterized by hyperkeratosis of the palms and soles), and human papillomavirus.

Adenocarcinoma of the esophagus, once an unusual malignancy, is diagnosed with increasing frequency, and now accounts for over 50 percent of esophageal cancer in most Western countries. The shift in the epidemiology of esophageal cancer from predominantly squamous carcinoma seen in association with smoking and alcohol, to adenocarcinoma in the setting of BE, is one of the most dramatic changes that have occurred in the history of human neoplasia. Although esophageal carcinoma is a relatively uncommon malignancy, its prevalence is exploding, largely secondary to the well-established association between gastroesophageal reflux, BE, and esophageal adenocarcinoma. Once a nearly uniformly lethal disease, survival is improving with advances in surveillance, improvements in staging, and surgical techniques, and possibly neoadjuvant therapy have made clinically relevant improvements in the everyday care of patients.

Furthermore, the clinical picture of esophageal adenocarcinoma is changing. It now occurs not only considerably more frequently, but in younger patients, and is often detected at an earlier stage. These facts support rethinking the traditional approach to patients with the disease. The historical focus on palliation of dysphagia in an older adult patient with comorbidities should change when dealing with a young patient with dependent children and a productive life ahead. The potential for cure becomes of paramount importance.

Microscopically, adenocarcinoma almost always originates in metaplastic Barrett mucosa, and resembles gastric cancer. Rarely it arises in the submucosal glands, and forms intramural growths that resemble the mucoepidermal and adenoid cystic carcinomas of the salivary glands.

The most important etiologic factor in the development of primary adenocarcinoma of the esophagus is a metaplastic columnar-lined or BE, which occurs as a complication in approximately 10–15 percent of patients with GERD. When studied prospectively, the incidence of adenocarcinoma in a patient with BE is one in 100–200 patient-years of follow up (i.e., for every 100 patients with BE followed for 1 year, one will develop adenocarcinoma). Although this risk appears to be small, it is at least 30–40 times that expected for a similar population without BE. This risk is similar to the risk for developing lung cancer in a person with a 20-pack-per-year history of smoking. Endoscopic surveillance for patients with BE is recommended for two reasons: (1) at present there is no reliable evidence that medical therapy removes the risk of neoplastic transformation, and (2) malignancy in BE is curable if detected at an early stage.

Clinical Manifestations

Esophageal cancer generally presents with dysphagia, although increasing numbers of relatively asymptomatic patients are now identified on surveillance endoscopy, and/or present with nonspecific upper GI symptoms and undergo upper endoscopy. Extension of the primary tumor into the tracheobronchial tree can cause stridor, and if a tracheoesophageal fistula develops, coughing, choking, and aspiration pneumonia result. Rarely, severe bleeding from erosion into the aorta or pulmonary vessels occurs. Either vocal cord may be invaded, causing paralysis, but most commonly, paralysis is caused by invasion of the left recurrent laryngeal nerve by the primary tumor or lymph node metastasis. Systemic organ metastases are usually manifested by jaundice or bone pain. The situation is different in high-incidence areas in which screening is practiced. In these communities, the most prominent early symptom is pain on swallowing rough or dry food.

Dysphagia usually presents late in the natural history of the disease, because the lack of a serosal layer on the esophagus allows the smooth muscle to dilate with ease. As a result, the dysphagia becomes severe enough for the patient to seek medical advice only when more than 60 percent of the esophageal circumference is infiltrated with cancer. Consequently, the disease is usually advanced if symptoms herald its presence. Tracheoesophageal fistula may be present in some patients on their first visit to the hospital, and more than 40 percent will have evidence of distant metastases. With tumors of the cardia, anorexia and weight loss usually precede the onset of dysphagia. The physical signs of esophageal tumors are those associated with the presence of distant metastases.

Staging of Esophageal Carcinoma

At the initial encounter with a patient diagnosed as having carcinoma of the esophagus, a decision must be made regarding whether he or she is a candidate for curative surgical therapy, palliative surgical therapy, or nonsurgical palliation. Making this decision is difficult, because evaluating the pretreatment disease stage of esophageal carcinoma is imprecise because of the difficulty of measuring the depth of tumor penetration of the esophageal wall and the inaccessibility of the organ's widespread lymphatic drainage.

The introduction of endoscopic ultrasound has made it possible to identify patients who are potentially curable prior to surgical therapy. Using an endoscope, the depth of the wall penetration by the tumor and the presence of five or more lymph node metastases can be determined with 80 percent accuracy. A curative resection should be encouraged if endoscopic ultrasound indicates that the tumor has not invaded adjacent organs, and/or fewer than five enlarged lymph nodes are imaged. Thoracoscopic and laparoscopic staging of esophageal cancer have been recommended; preliminary results indicate that using these techniques, correct staging of esophageal carcinomas approaches 90 percent. If these results are confirmed and the cost is not prohibitive, then thoracoscopic and laparoscopic staging are likely to become valuable tools to determine the extent of disease prior to therapy. At the present time, despite the modern techniques of computed tomography, magnetic resonance imaging, endoscopic ultrasound, and laparoscopic and thoracoscopic technology, pretreatment staging still remains imprecise. This underscores the need for an intraoperative assessment of the potential for cure in each individual patient.

Experience with esophageal resections in patients with early disease has identified characteristics of esophageal cancer that are associated with improved survival. A number of studies suggest that only metastasis to lymph nodes and tumor penetration of the esophageal wall have a significant and independent influence on prognosis. The beneficial effects of the absence of one factor persists, even when the other is present. Factors known to be important in the survival of patients with advanced disease, such as cell type, degree of cellular differentiation, or location of tumor in the esophagus, have no effect on survival of patients who have undergone resection for early disease. Studies also showed that patients having five or fewer lymph node metastases have a better outcome.

Clinical Approach to Carcinoma of the Esophagus and Cardia

The selection of a curative versus a palliative operation for cancer of the esophagus is based on the location of the tumor, the patient's age and health, the extent of the disease, and intraoperative staging.

Tumor Location

The selection of surgical therapy for patients with carcinoma of the esophagus depends not only on the anatomic stage of the disease and an assessment of the swallowing capacity of the patient, but also on the location of the primary tumor.

It is estimated that 8 percent of the primary malignant tumors of the esophagus occur in the cervical portion. They are almost always squamous cell lesions, with a rare adenocarcinoma arising from a congenital inlet patch of columnar lining. These tumors, particularly those in the postcricoid area, represent a separate pathologic entity for a number of reasons: (1) they are more common in females and appear to be a unique entity in this regard; and (2) the efferent lymphatics from the cervical esophagus drain completely differently from those of the thoracic esophagus. The latter drain directly into the paratracheal and deep cervical or internal jugular lymph nodes with minimal flow in a longitudinal direction. Except in advanced disease, it is unusual for intrathoracic lymph nodes to be involved.

Low cervical lesions that reach the level of the thoracic inlet are usually unresectable because of early invasion of the great vessels and trachea. The length of the esophagus below the cricopharyngeus is insufficient to allow intubation or construction of a proximal anastomosis for a bypass procedure. Consequently, palliation of these tumors is difficult, and patients afflicted with disease at this site have a poor prognosis. Upper airway obstruction or the development of tracheoesophageal fistulas in such tumors may require surgical intervention for palliation. If possible, these tumors should be resected after a preoperative course of chemoradiotherapy has reduced their size.

Tumors that arise within the middle or upper third of the thoracic esophagus lie too close to the trachea and aorta to allow an en bloc resection without removal of these vital structures. Consequently, in this location only tumors that have not penetrated through the esophageal wall and have not metastasized to the regional lymph nodes are potentially curable. The resection for a tumor at this level is done similarly whether for palliation or cure, and long-term survival is a chance phenomenon. This does not mean that when resecting such tumors, efforts to remove the adjacent lymph nodes should be abandoned. To do so may inadvertently leave unrecognized metastatic disease behind and compromise the patient's overall survival, because of recurrent local disease and compression of the trachea. It is recommended that a course of preoperative chemoradiotherapy should be given before resection to shrink the size of the tumor. It is recommended that the radiotherapy be limited to 3.5 Gy to allow for tissue healing after surgery.

Tumors of the lower esophagus and cardia are usually adenocarcinomas. However, squamous cell carcinoma of the lower esophagus does occur. Both types of tumor are amenable to en bloc resection. Unless preoperative and intra-operative staging clearly demonstrates an incurable lesion, an en bloc resection in continuity with a lymph node dissection should be performed. Because of the propensity of GI tumors to spread for long distances submucosally, long lengths of grossly normal GI tract should be resected. The longitudinal lymph flow in the esophagus can result in skip areas, with small foci of tumor above the primary lesion, which underscores the importance of a wide resection of esophageal tumors. Wong has shown that local recurrence at the anastomosis can be prevented by obtaining a 10-cm margin of normal esophagus above the tumor. Anatomic studies have also shown that there is no submucosal lymphatic barrier between the esophagus and the stomach at the cardia.

Cardiopulmonary Reserve

Patients undergoing esophageal resection should have sufficient cardiopulmonary reserve to tolerate the proposed procedure. The respiratory function is best assessed with the forced expiratory volume in 1 second (FEV-1), which ideally should be 2 L or more. Any patient with an FEV-1 of less than 1.25 L is compromised for surgery. Clinical evaluation and electrocardiogram are not sufficient indicators of cardiac reserve. Echocardiography and dipyridamole thallium imaging provide accurate information on wall motion, ejection fraction, and myocardial blood flow. A defect on thallium imaging may require further evaluation with preoperative coronary angiography. A resting ejection fraction of less than 40 percent, particularly if there is no increase with exercise, is an ominous sign.

Clinical Stage

Clinical factors that indicate an advanced stage of carcinoma and exclude surgery with curative intent are recurrent nerve paralysis, Horner syndrome, persistent spinal pain, paralysis of the diaphragm, fistula formation, and malignant pleural effusion. Factors that make surgical cure unlikely include a tumor greater than 8 cm in length, abnormal axis of the esophagus on a barium radiogram, multiple enlarged lymph nodes on computed tomography (CT), a weight loss more than 20 percent, and loss of appetite. In patients in whom these findings are not present, staging depends primarily on the degree of wall penetration and lymph node metastasis seen with endoscopic ultrasound.

Surgical Treatment

A patient's nutritional status before surgery has a profound effect on the outcome of an esophageal resection. Low serum protein levels have a deleterious effect on the cardiovascular system, and a poor nutritional status affects the host resistance to infection and the rate of anastomotic and wound healing. A serum albumin level of less than 3.4 g/dL on admission indicates poor caloric intake and an increased risk of surgical complications, including anastomotic breakdown. A feeding jejunostomy tube provides the most reliable and safest method for nutritional support in patients who cannot consume an oral diet and have a functionally normal small bowel. In severely malnourished patients, the jejunostomy is performed as a separate procedure to allow for preoperative nutritional support. In these patients the abdomen is entered through a small supraumbilical midline incision. Otherwise, the jejunostomy tube is placed at the time of esophageal resection, and feeding is begun on the third postoperative day.

Control of the local and regional disease forms the basis for the classic en bloc resection. Nodal recurrence in the field of the resection following en bloc resection is only 1 percent. Six to 10 percent of patients will develop nodes lying along the recurrent laryngeal nerve chains, which are not routinely removed. Performing a more extended mediastinal dissection combined with a radical neck dissection has been advocated by some authors. The increased morbidity and the possibility of permanent hoarseness associated with this approach have discouraged its widespread application. It has been reported that the finding of metastatic disease involving the celiac nodes precludes survival beyond 2 years. By contrast, other authors have reported prolonged survival in patients with celiac axis involvement.

Cervical and Upper Thoracic Esophageal Cancer

It was hoped that the prognosis for patients with cervical esophageal cancer might be better than for those with carcinoma of the thoracic esophagus, but this has not proved to be the case. Early experience with resection of the cervical esophagus resulted in a high mortality rate, and reconstruction by neck flaps often required multiple operations. Because of these complexities and the generally disappointing results, radiotherapy frequently was elected. Immediate mortality decreased, but control of the tumor was not satisfactory.

The difference between the two forms of therapy is the manner in which the disease recurs. Tumors treated with radiation therapy initially tend to recur locally and systemically, and cause unmanageable local disease with eventual erosion into neck vessels and trachea, causing hemorrhage and dyspnea. Patients who undergo surgical therapy have few local recurrences of the tumor, provided total excision is possible, but they succumb to metastatic disease. Collin has reported a local failure rate of 80 percent after definitive radiation therapy, and 20 percent of these patients required palliative surgery to control the disease locally. Improvements in the techniques of immediate esophageal reconstruction have reduced the complications of the surgical treatment of this disease and encouraged a more aggressive surgical approach. The data reported by Collin suggest that an initial aggressive surgical resection yields longer survival than radiation therapy. Positive surgical margins, tracheal invasion that cannot be removed, and vocal cord paralysis correlate with a significantly shorter survival following surgery. Palliation was better achieved in patients who underwent esophagectomy with immediate gastric pull-up than in those who underwent primary radiation therapy or chemotherapy.

Lesions that are not fixed to the spine, do not invade the vessels or trachea, and do not have fixed cervical lymph node metastases should be resected. If lymph node metastases are present or the tumor comes in close proximity to the cricopharyngeus muscle, a course of preoperative chemo- and radiotherapy should be given before surgical resection. This usually consists of two to three cycles of chemotherapy and no more than 3.5 Gy of radiation therapy.

Neoadjuvant therapy is given in an attempt to salvage the larynx, because the larynx is often invaded by microscopic tumors, and in the past, a total laryngectomy in combination with esophagectomy was usually necessary. A simultaneous en bloc dissection of the superior mediastinum and cervical lymph nodes is done, sparing the jugular veins on both sides.

Tumors in the upper thoracic esophagus are removed via a right posterolateral thoracotomy with a corresponding lymphadenectomy. The continuity of the GI tract is re-established by pulling the stomach up through the esophageal bed. If removing the larynx is necessary, a permanent tracheostomy stoma is constructed in the lower flap of the cervical incision. The division of the trachea in some patients may preclude the possibility of a permanent cervical standard tracheostomy, because the remaining tracheal stump distal to the tumor will not reach the suprasternal notch. Removal of the medial head of the clavicles and the manubrium down to the sternal angle of Louis provides excellent exposure and allows the construction of a mediastinal tracheostomy. A bipedicle skin flap over the pectoralis muscle can be advanced upward, or a single-pedicle musculocutaneous flap including the pectoralis muscle and its overlying skin can be rotated to cover the defect. A circular incision in the flap can be used as a port through which the tracheal remnant is brought out to the skin.

Tumors of the Thoracic Esophagus and Cardia

For tumors that arise below the carina, the preference is either an en bloc resection for cure or a transhiatal removal for palliation. A curative procedure is performed according to the principles of an en bloc resection in continuity with the regional lymph nodes. It is attempted in a patient whose preresection physical condition and tumor characteristics have the potential for long-term survival. The en bloc resection is done through three incisions in the following order: (1) right posterolateral thoracotomy, en bloc dissection of the distal esophagus, mobilization of the esophagus above the aortic arch, closure of the thoracotomy, repositioning of the patient in the recumbent position; (2) upper midline abdominal incision, en bloc dissection of the stomach and associated lymph nodes; and (3) left neck incision and proximal division of the esophagus. The specimen is removed transhiatally and the stomach is tubed, preserving the antrum. GI continuity is re-established with a cervical esophagogastric anastomosis. A standard left thoracotomy with intrathoracic anastomosis for lower lesions or an Ivor Lewis combined approach for higher lesions is not advocated because of (1) the proven need to resect long lengths of the esophagus to eradicate submucosal spread, (2) the higher morbidity associated with a thoracic anastomotic leak, and (3) the high incidence of esophagitis secondary to reflux following an intrathoracic anastomosis.

En Bloc Esophagogastrectomy versus Transhiatal Resection for Carcinoma of the Lower Esophagus and Cardia

Many strategies for treatment of esophageal carcinoma limit the role of surgery to removing the primary tumor, with the hope that adjuvant therapy will increase cure rates by destroying systemic disease. This approach emphasizes the concept of biological determinism (i.e., that the outcome of treatment in esophageal cancer is determined at the time of diagnosis, and that surgical therapy aimed at removing more than the primary tumor is not helpful). Lymph node metastases are considered simply markers of systemic disease; the systematic removal of involved nodes is not considered beneficial. The belief that removal of the primary tumor by transhiatal esophagogastrectomy results in the same survival rates as a more extensive en bloc resection is based on the same kind of reasoning.

In the transhiatal procedure there is no specific attempt made to remove lymph node–bearing tissue in the posterior mediastinum. By contrast, the en bloc esophagectomy removes the tumor covered on all surfaces with a layer of normal tissue. A long length of foregut above and below the lesion is resected to incorporate submucosal spread of the tumor. Appropriate cervical mediastinal and abdominal lymph node dissections are included using an en bloc technique to remove potentially involved regional nodes.

Hagen and colleagues recently reviewed 100 consecutive patients who underwent en bloc esophagectomy for esophageal adenocarcinoma. No patient received pre- or postoperative chemotherapy or radiation therapy. The aim of the study was to relate the extent of disease to prognostic features, timing and mode of recurrence, and survival following en bloc resection. The median follow-up of surviving patients was 40 months, with 24 patients surviving 5 years or more. Overall actuarial survival at 5 years was 52 percent. Fifty-five of the tumors were transmural and 63 patients had lymph node involvement. Metastases to celiac ($n = 16$) or other distant node sites ($n = 26$) were not associated with decreased survival. Remarkably, local recurrence was seen in only one patient. Latent nodal recurrence outside the surgical field occurred in nine, and systemic metastases in 31. The authors concluded that long-term survival from adenocarcinoma of the esophagus can be achieved in over half of the patients who undergo en bloc resection. One-third of patients with lymph node involvement survived 5 years, and the authors concluded that local control is excellent following en bloc resection.

Controversy persists over the extent of resection necessary for cure of esophageal adenocarcinoma. Several retrospective studies have shown a benefit to the more extensive node dissection accomplished with a transthoracic en bloc esophagectomy as compared to the transhiatal esophagectomy. These studies have been criticized as suffering from selection bias and for inaccuracy in preoperative staging. Performance of a more complete node dissection also results in the potential for stage migration. Hulscher has reported a prospective randomized control trial that compared transthoracic en bloc to transhiatal esophagectomy. The results were inconclusive but showed a trend toward better survival with the en bloc resection. This trial eliminated many of the criticisms of the retrospective studies but included patients with various stages of disease. This may have obscured the benefits of systematic node dissection by the unequal distribution of patients with early stage disease who did not need a formal lymphadenectomy, and those with advanced disease with extensive lymph node metastases who were not curable by surgery alone. An alternative approach to compare transthoracic en bloc to transhiatal resection has been done by Johansson using a retrospective case control study between nonrandomized patients having similar size transmural (T3) tumors with lymph node metastases (N1). The aim of the study was to determine whether patients with locally advanced (T3N1) esophageal cancer benefit from the performance of a transthoracic en bloc resection. This approach removes the influence of inaccurate preoperative staging and minimizes the influence of postoperative stage migration on survival because all patients had N1 disease. Further, all patients had 20 or more lymph nodes in the surgical specimen which allowed confirmation that the extent of lymph node disease in both groups was comparable. These conditions focused the question regarding which procedure was associated with a better survival. The results, show that a transthoracic en bloc resection confers a survival benefit over a transhiatal resection in patients with transmural (T3) esophageal carcinomas when eight or fewer lymph nodes are involved (N1). The most likely explanation for the improved survival following transthoracic en bloc resection is a more complete removal of local-regional disease, which is unrecognized disease that is removed with an en bloc lymph node dissection but left behind with a transhiatal lymph node dissection. Consequently, transthoracic en bloc resection results in better control of local-regional disease. Indeed, in clinical trials neoadjuvant radiochemotherapy has been added to transhiatal esophagectomy in an effort to control local-regional disease without great success. A more prudent approach would be to use a transthoracic en bloc dissection to control local-regional disease and focus postoperative adjuvant therapy on eliminating systemic disease.

These studies showed that for early cancers of the lower esophagus and cardia, en bloc esophagogastrectomy results in significantly better survival rates than transhiatal esophagogastrectomy. This finding cannot be explained by a bias in the stage of disease resected, a difference in operative mortality, or death from nontumor causes. Rather, it appears to be because of the type of operation performed. Ideally, the question regarding which procedure is the best should be resolved by a prospective randomized study of similiarly staged patients.

Extent of Resection to Cure Disease Confined to the Mucosa

The development of surveillance programs for the detection of early squamous cell carcinoma in endemic areas and for early adenocarcinoma in patients with BE has given rise to controversy over how to manage tumors confined to the mucosa. Some authors have endoscopically resected squamous carcinomas after using endoscopic ultrasound to determine that the depth of the tumor was limited to the mucosa. Surprisingly, large areas of squamous mucosa can be resected without perforation or bleeding, leaving the smooth surface of the muscularis mucosae intact. Re-epithelialization of the large artificially induced ulcer is usually complete in 3 weeks. In order not to miss a squamous cancer that has invaded deeper than expected, it is important to examine the deep margins of the resected specimen carefully, and to perform periodic endoscopic follow-up examinations with vital staining techniques. This technique is not appropriate for multiple and widespread or circumferential squamous lesions because of the risk of developing a stricture during the healing process. In this situation, those acquainted with endoscopic resection would advocate an esophagectomy.

Several studies have shown that intraepithelial carcinoma (i.e., carcinoma in situ or high-grade dysplasia), and intramucosal tumors (i.e., invasive cancer limited by the muscular mucosae), are quite different in their biologic behavior from submucosal tumors. This disfunction is independent of histology (squamous or adenocarcinoma) and histologic grade. Vessel invasion and lymph node metastasis do not occur in severe dysplasia, are uncommon in the intramucosal tumors, but are the rule in submucosal tumors. Consequently, the 5-year survival for intramucosal tumors is significantly better than for submucosal tumors. These findings indicate that both severe dysplasia and intramucosal cancers represent early malignant lesions of the esophagus. A critical issue to be resolved is whether an intramucosal tumor can be correctly discriminated from a submucosal tumor before surgery. The results of using endoscopic ultrasound for determining the depth of tumors confined to the esophageal wall are of questionable accuracy. The resolution of present-day endoscopic ultrasonographic systems is not sufficient to predictably differentiate the fine detail of tumor infiltration when it is limited to the esophageal wall. Currently there is no dependable way, before surgery, of determining whether a tumor extends beyond the muscularis mucosae.

Another complicating factor is that up to 5 percent of patients with intramucosal tumors have lymph node metastases, although the number of involved nodes per patient is usually no more than one. Akiyama and others have reported that even though the number of involved nodes may be small, they can spread to distant nodal regions, including cervical and abdominal nodes.

We have recently used the presence or absence of an endoscopically visible lesion in patients with biopsy-proven high-grade dysplasia (HGD) or intramucosal carcinoma as a predictor of tumor depth and nodal metastases. The data indicate that a positive biopsy in the absence of an endoscopically visible lesion almost always corresponds to an intramucosal tumor without nodal metastases. Of patients with HGD, 43 percent proved to harbor occult adenocarcinoma at resection. Importantly, when there was no visible lesion on endoscopy, 88 percent of the tumors were intramucosal and 12 percent submucosal. Only one of 10 patients with no visible lesion had lymph node involvement, either histologically or immunohistochemically. In contrast, patients with endoscopically visible tumors had a high prevalence of tumors that penetrated beyond the mucosa (75 percent), and 56 percent had positive nodes.

Patients with HGD and intramucosal carcinoma are best treated by a total esophagectomy, removing all Barrett tissue and any potential associated adenocarcinoma. Options include transhiatal esophagectomy, or more recently, vagal-sparing esophagectomy. The vagal-sparing approach is suitable only given confidence of the absence of regional nodal disease. Reconstruction is accomplished with either the stomach (transhiatal) or colon (vagal sparing) with the anastomosis in the neck. The mortality associated with this procedure should be less than 5 percent, particularly in centers experienced in esophageal surgery. Functional recovery is excellent, particularly in the vagal-sparing group.

As the understanding of the pathology of esophageal cancer improves and experience with its resection increases, evidence is accumulating that the best chance for cure of patients with an intramural tumor in the distal esophagus or cardia is an en bloc esophagectomy and proximal gastrectomy, with GI continuity re-established with a either gastric or colon interposition. For patients with a tumor in the upper or cervical esophagus, the best chance for cure is an en bloc esophagectomy and a cervical lymph node dissection with GI continuity re-established with a gastric pull-up. Table 24-10 presents a summary of the extent of resection for tumors extending various depths into the esophageal wall.

Alternative Therapies

Radiation Therapy

Primary treatment with radiation therapy does not produce results comparable with those obtained with surgery. Currently, the use of radiotherapy is restricted to patients who are not candidates for surgery. Palliation of dysphagia is short

TABLE 24-10 Recommended Surgical Therapy for Esophageal Carcinoma

Lesion	Resection
1. Confined areas of high-grade dysplasia (intraepidermal cancer)	Endoscopic mucosal resection (at present only applicable to squamous carcinoma).
2. Widespread or circumferential area of high-grade dysplasia (intraepidermal cancer)	Transhiatal or vagal sparing esophagectomy.
3. Tumor invading through the basement membrane but not through the muscularis mucosae (intramucosal tumors)	Transhiatal or vagal sparing esophagectomy.
4. Tumor deeper than the muscularis mucosae but not through the esophageal wall (intramural tumors)	En bloc esophagectomy with appropriate systematic lymphadenectomy of the cervical, upper mediastinal (above the tracheal bifurcation), lower mediastinal (below the tracheal bifurcation) and abdominal nodes. (For upper and middle third cancers, mediastinal dissection must include the node along the left recurrent laryngeal nerve. For lower third esophageal and cardia cancers, omit cervical and upper mediastinal node dissection, but include the proximal stomach in the resection. For upper third esophageal cancers, omit abdominal lymph node dissection.) Reconstruction with gastric pull-up for middle and upper third tumors, and with colon interposition for lower third and cardia tumors that involve a segmental portion of the stomach.
5. Tumor extending through the muscularis propria (transmural tumors)	Same as for intramural tumors.

term, generally lasting only 2–3 months. Furthermore, the length and course of treatment are difficult to justify in patients with a limited life expectancy. Consequently there is a reluctance to treat patients with advanced disease.

Adjuvant Chemotherapy

The proposal to use adjuvant chemotherapy in the treatment of esophageal cancer began when it became evident that most patients develop postoperative systemic metastasis without local recurrence. This observation led to the hypothesis that undetected systemic micrometastasis had been present at the time of diagnosis, and if effective systemic therapy was added to local regional therapy, survival should improve.

Recently this hypothesis has been supported by the observation of epithelial tumor cells in the bone marrow in 37 percent of patients with esophageal cancer who were resected for cure. These patients had a greater prevalence of relapse at 9 months after surgery compared to those patients without such cells. Such studies emphasize that hematogenous dissemination of viable malignant cells occurs early in the disease, and that systemic chemotherapy may be helpful if the cells are sensitive to the agent. On the other hand, systemic chemotherapy may be a hindrance, because of its immunosuppressive properties, if the cells are resistant. Unfortunately, current technology is not able to test tumor cell sensitivity to chemotherapeutic drugs. This requires that the choice of drugs be made solely on the basis of their clinical effectiveness against grossly similar tumors.

The decision to use preoperative rather than postoperative chemotherapy was based on the ineffectiveness of chemotherapeutic agents when used after surgery, and animal studies suggesting that agents given before surgery were more effective. The claim that patients who receive chemotherapy before resection are less likely to develop resistance to the drugs is unsupported by hard evidence. The claim that drug delivery is enhanced because blood flow is more robust before patients undergo surgical dissection is similarly flawed, because of the fact that if enough blood reaches the operative site to heal the wound or anastomosis, then the flow should be sufficient to deliver chemotherapeutic drugs. There are, however, data supporting the claim that preoperative chemotherapy in patients with esophageal carcinoma can, if effective, facilitate surgical resection by reducing the size of the tumor. This is particularly beneficial in the case of squamous cell tumors above the level of the carina. Reducing the size of the tumor may provide a safer margin between the tumor and the trachea, and allow an anastomosis to a tumor-free cervical esophagus just below the cricopharyngeus. Involved margin at this level usually requires a laryngectomy to prevent subsequent local recurrence.

Preoperative chemotherapy. Three randomized prospective studies with squamous cell carcinoma have shown no survival benefit with preoperative chemotherapy over surgery alone (Table 24-11). This includes a recent U.S. trial reported by Kelson. The possibility that preoperative neoadjuvant 5-fluorouracil (5-FU)/platinum-based chemotherapy may indeed provide a small benefit was recently raised by a medical research council trial in the United Kingdom. This trial is one of the few to include enough patients (800) to detect small differences. Two-thirds had adenocarcinoma and distal third tumors. The trial had a 10 percent absolute survival benefit at 2 years for the neoadjuvant chemotherapy group.

With the exception of the potential to improve resectability of tumors located above the carina, the benefits cited by those in favor of preoperative chemotherapy are questionable. Preoperative chemotherapy alone potentially can downstage the tumor, particularly squamous cell carcinoma. It can also potentially eliminate or delay the appearance of metastasis. There is little evidence, however, that it can prolong survival of patients with resectable carcinoma of the esophagus. Most failures are because of distant metastatic disease, underscoring the need for improved systemic therapy. Postoperative septic and respiratory complications may be more common in patients receiving chemotherapy.

Preoperative combination chem- and radiotherapy. Preoperative chemoradiotherapy using cisplatin and 5-FU in combination with radiotherapy has been reported by several investigators to be beneficial in both adenomatous and squamous cell carcinoma of the esophagus. There has been six randomized prospective studies: four with squamous cell carcinoma, one with both

TABLE 24-11 Esophageal Carcinoma: Randomized Preoperative Chemotherapy Versus Surgery Alone

Author	Year	No. preop chemotherapy/no. surgery alone	Cell type	Regimen	Complete response to chemotherapy	Survival chemotherapy vs. surgery alone
Roth	1988	19/20	Squamous	P, V, B	6%	NS
Nygaard	1992	50/41	Squamous	P, B	...	NS
Schlag	1992	21/24	Squamous	P, 5-FU	5%	NS
Low	1997	74/73	Squamous	P, 5-FU	...	NS
Kelson	1998	233/234	Squamous and adenomatous	P, 5-FU	2.5%	NS

B = bleomycin; 5-FU = 5-fluorouracil; NS = not significant; P = cisplatin; V = vindesine.

squamous and adenocarcinoma, and one with only adenocarcinoma (Table 24-12). Only one showed any survival benefit with preoperative chemoradiotherapy over surgery alone. Most authors report substantial morbidity and mortality to the treatment. However, many have been encouraged by the observation that some patients who had a complete response had remained free of recurrence at 3 years.

Caution must be exercised in trying to isolate the effects of chemotherapy, because the addition of preoperative radiation therapy to chemotherapy elevates the complete response rate and inflates the benefit of chemotherapy. With chemoradiation the complete response rates for adenocarcinoma range from 17–24 percent (Table 24-13). When radiation is removed, the complete response falls to 0–5 percent, which suggests that the effects of chemotherapy are negligible. If radiotherapy is the factor responsible for the improved response rate, surgery alone could do the job as well, because numerous studies in the past have shown that the combination of surgery and radiation does not provide any survival advantages.

The better question is whether a patient with carcinoma of the esophagus should go through three cycles of chemotherapy on the 5 percent chance that they may get a complete response in the primary tumor, and in the face of the paucity of evidence that such a response controls systemic disease. Studies have shown that the rates of infection, anastomotic breakdown, incidence of acute respiratory distress syndrome, and long-term use of a respirator were greater in patients receiving adjuvant therapy as compared with surgery alone.

Current data support giving chemoradiotherapy as a matter of routine in a limited number of clinical settings, including: (1) preoperatively to reduce tumor size in a young person with surgically incurable squamous cell carcinoma above the carina, and (2) chemotherapy as salvage therapy for patients who have not had previous chemotherapy and develop recurrent systemic disease after surgical resection. Adjuvant therapy in patients not in those categories should be limited to the setting of a controlled clinical trial. At present, the strongest predictors of outcome of patients with esophageal cancer are the anatomic extent of the tumor at diagnosis and the completeness of tumor removal by surgical resection. After incomplete resection of an esophageal cancer, the 5-year survival rates are 0–5 percent. In contrast, after complete resection, independent of stage of disease, 5-year survival ranges from 15–40 percent, according to selection criteria and stage distribution. The importance of early recognition and adequate surgical resection cannot be overemphasized.

BENIGN TUMORS AND CYSTS

Benign tumors and cysts of the esophagus are relatively uncommon. From the perspectives of both the clinician and the pathologist, benign tumors may be divided into those that are within the muscular wall and those that are within the lumen of the esophagus.

Intramural lesions are either solid tumors or cysts, and the vast majority are leiomyomas. They are made up of varying portions of smooth muscle and fibrous tissue. Fibromas, myomas, fibromyomas, and lipomyomas are closely related and occur rarely. Other histologic types of solid intramural tumors have been described, such as lipomas, neurofibromas, hemangiomas, osteochondromas, granular cell myoblastomas, and glomus tumors, but they are medical curiosities.

TABLE 24-12 Esophageal Carcinoma: Randomized Preoperative Chemo- or Radiotherapy Versus Surgery Alone

Author	Year	No. preop chemo-radiotherapy/ No. surgery alone	Cell type	Regimen	Survival chemo-radiotherapy vs. surgery alone
Nygaard	1992	47/41	Squamous	P, B, 35 Gy	NS
LePrise	1994	41/45	Squamous	P, 5-FU, 20 Gy	NS
Apinop	1994	35/34	Squamous	P, 5-FU, 40 Gy	NS
Urba	1995	50/50	Squamous and adenomatous	P, 5-FU, V, 45 Gy	NS
Walsh	1996	48/54	Adenomatous	P, 5-FU, 40 Gy	$p = 0.01$
Bosset	1997	143/139	Squamous	P, 18.5 Gy	NS

B = bleomycin; 5-FU = 5-fluorouracil; NS = not significant; P = cisplatin; V = vindesine.

621

TABLE 24-13 Results of Neoadjuvant Therapy in Adenocarcinoma of the Esophagus

Institution	Year	No. of patients	Regimen	Complete pathologic response	Survival
M. D. Anderson	1990	35	P, E, 5-FU	3%	42% at 3 y
SLMC	1992	18	P, 5-FU, RT	17%	40% at 3 y
Vanderbilt	1993	39	P, E, 5-FU, RT	19%	47% at 4 y
Michigan	1993	21	P, VBL, 5-FU, RT	24%	34% at 5 y
MGH	1994	16	P, 5-FU	0%	42% at 4 y
MGH	1994	22	E, A, P	5%	58% at 2 y

A = doxorubicin; E = etoposide; 5-FU = 5-fluorouracil; MGH = Massachusetts General Hospital; P = cisplatin; RT = radiation therapy; SLMC = St. Louis University Medical Center; VBL = vinblastine.

Source: Reproduced with permission from Wright CD, Mathisen DJ, Wain JC, et al: Evolution of treatment strategies for adenocarcinoma of the esophagus and gastroesophageal junction. *Ann Thorac Surg* 58:1574, 1994.

Intraluminal lesions are polypoid or pedunculated growths that usually originate in the submucosa, develop mainly into the lumen, and are covered with normal stratified squamous epithelium. The majority of these tumors are composed of fibrous tissue of varying degrees of compactness with a rich vascular supply. Some are loose and myxoid (e.g., myxoma and myxofibroma), some are more collagenous (e.g., fibroma), and some contain adipose tissue (e.g., fibrolipoma). These different types of tumor are frequently collectively designated as fibrovascular polyps, or simply as polyps. Pedunculated intraluminal tumors should be removed. If the lesion is not too large, endoscopic removal with a snare is feasible.

Leiomyoma

Leiomyomas constitute more than 50 percent of benign esophageal tumors. The average age at presentation is 38, which is in sharp contrast to that seen with esophageal carcinoma. Leiomyomas are twice as common in males. Because they originate in smooth muscle, 90 percent are located in the lower two thirds of the esophagus. They are usually solitary, but multiple tumors have been found on occasion. They vary greatly in size and shape. Tumors as small as 1 cm in diameter and as large as 10 lb have been removed.

Typically, leiomyomas are oval. During their growth, they remain intramural, having the bulk of their mass protruding toward the outer wall of the esophagus. The overlying mucosa is freely movable and normal in appearance. Neither their size nor location correlates with the degree of symptoms. Dysphagia and pain are the most common complaints, the two symptoms occurring more frequently together than separately. Bleeding directly related to the tumor is rare, and when hematemesis or melena occurs in a patient with an esophageal leiomyoma, other causes should be investigated.

A barium swallow is the most useful method to demonstrate a leiomyoma of the esophagus. In profile the tumor appears as a smooth, semilunar, or crescent-shaped filling defect that moves with swallowing, is sharply demarcated, and is covered and surrounded by normal mucosa. Esophagoscopy should be performed to exclude the reported observation of a coexistence with carcinoma. The freely movable mass, which bulges into the lumen, should not be biopsied because of an increased chance of mucosal perforation at the time of surgical enucleation.

Despite their slow growth and limited potential for malignant degeneration, leiomyomas should be removed unless there are specific contraindications. The majority can be removed by simple enucleation. If during removal the mucosa is inadvertently entered, the defect can be repaired primarily. After tumor removal, the outer esophageal wall should be reconstructed by closure of the muscle layer. The location of the lesion and the extent of surgery required will dictate the approach. Lesions of the proximal and middle esophagus require a right thoracotomy, whereas distal esophageal lesions require a left thoracotomy. Videothoracoscopic approaches have been reported. The mortality rate associated with enucleation is less than 2 percent, and success in relieving the dysphagia is near 100 percent. Large lesions or those involving the gastroesophageal junction may require esophageal resection.

ESOPHAGEAL PERFORATION

Perforation of the esophagus constitutes a true emergency. It most commonly occurs following diagnostic or therapeutic procedures. Spontaneous perforation, referred to as Boerhaave syndrome, accounts for only 15 percent of cases of esophageal perforation, foreign bodies for 14 percent, and trauma for 10 percent. Pain is a striking and consistent symptom and strongly suggests that an esophageal rupture has occurred, particularly if located in the cervical area following instrumentation of the esophagus, or substernally in a patient with a history of resisting vomiting. If subcutaneous emphysema is present, the diagnosis is almost certain.

Spontaneous rupture of the esophagus is associated with a high mortality rate because of the delay in recognition and treatment. Although there usually is a history of resisting vomiting, in a small number of patients the injury occurs silently, without any antecedent history. When the chest radiogram of a patient with an esophageal perforation shows air or an effusion in the pleural space, the condition is often misdiagnosed as a pneumothorax or pancreatitis. An elevated serum amylase caused by the extrusion of saliva through the perforation may fix the diagnosis of pancreatitis in the mind of an unwary physician. If the chest radiogram is normal, a mistaken diagnosis of myocardial infarction or dissecting aneurysm is often made.

Spontaneous rupture usually occurs into the left pleural cavity or just above the gastroesophageal junction. Fifty percent of patients have concomitant gastroesophageal reflux disease, suggesting that minimal resistance to the transmission of abdominal pressure into the thoracic esophagus is a factor in the pathophysiology of the lesion. During vomiting, high peaks of intragastric pressure can be recorded, frequently exceeding 200 mmHg, but because extragastric pressure remains almost equal to intragastric pressure, stretching of the gastric wall is minimal. The amount of pressure transmitted to the esophagus varies considerably, depending on the position of the gastroesophageal junction. When it is in the abdomen and exposed to intraabdominal pressure, the pressure transmitted to the esophagus is much less than when it is exposed to the negative thoracic pressure. In the latter situation, the pressure in the lower esophagus will frequently equal intragastric pressure if the glottis remains closed. Cadaver studies have shown that when this pressure exceeds 150 mmHg, rupture of the esophagus is apt to occur. When a hiatal hernia is present and the sphincter remains exposed to abdominal pressure, the lesion produced is usually a Mallory-Weiss mucosal tear, and bleeding rather than perforation is the problem. This is because of the stretching of the supradiaphragmatic portion of the gastric wall. In this situation, the hernia sac represents an extension of the abdominal cavity, and the gastroesophageal junction remains exposed to abdominal pressure.

Diagnosis

Abnormalities on the chest radiogram can be variable and should not be depended on to make the diagnosis. This is because the abnormalities are dependent on three factors: (1) the time interval between the perforation and the radiographic examination, (2) the site of perforation, and (3) the integrity of the mediastinal pleura. Mediastinal emphysema, a strong indicator of perforation, takes at least 1 hour to be demonstrated, and is present in only 40 percent of patients. Mediastinal widening secondary to edema may not occur for several h. The site of perforation also can influence the radiographic findings. In cervical perforation, cervical emphysema is common and mediastinal emphysema rare; the converse is true for thoracic perforations. Frequently, air will be visible in the erector spinae muscles on a neck radiogram before it can be palpated or seen on a chest radiogram. The integrity of the mediastinal pleura influences the radiographic abnormality in that rupture of the pleura results in a pneumothorax, a finding that is seen in 77 percent of patients. In two-thirds of patients the perforation is on the left side, in one fifth it is on the right side, and in one tenth it is bilateral. If pleural integrity is maintained, mediastinal emphysema (rather than a pneumothorax) appears rapidly. A pleural effusion secondary to inflammation of the mediastinum occurs late. In 9 percent of patients the chest radiogram is normal.

The diagnosis is confirmed with a contrast esophagogram, which will demonstrate extravasation in 90 percent of patients. The use of a water-soluble medium such as Gastrografin is preferred. Of concern is that there is a 10 percent false-negative rate. This may be because of obtaining the radiographic study with the patient in the upright position. When the patient is upright, the passage of water-soluble contrast material can be too rapid to demonstrate a small perforation. The studies should be done with the patient in the right lateral decubitus position. In this position the contrast material fills the entire length of the esophagus, allowing the actual site of perforation and its interconnecting cavities to be visualized in almost all patients.

Management

The key to optimum management is early diagnosis. The most favorable outcome is obtained following primary closure of the perforation within 24 h, resulting in 80–90 percent survival. The most common location for the injury is the left lateral wall of the esophagus, just above the gastroesophageal junction. To get adequate exposure of the injury, a dissection similar to that described for esophageal myotomy is performed. A flap of stomach is pulled up and the soiled fat pad at the gastroesophageal junction is removed. The edges of the injury are trimmed and closed using a modified Gambee stitch. The closure is reinforced by the use of a pleural patch or construction of a Nissen fundoplication.

Mortality associated with immediate closure varies between 8 and 20 percent. After 24 h survival, decreases to less than 50 percent, and is not influenced by the type of operative therapy (i.e., drainage alone or drainage plus closure of the perforation). If the time delay prior to closing a perforation approaches 24 h and the tissues are inflamed, division of the cardia and resection of the diseased portion of the esophagus are recommended. The remainder of the esophagus is mobilized, and as much normal esophagus as possible is saved and brought out as an end cervical esophagostomy. In some situations the retained esophagus may be so long that it loops down into the chest. The contaminated mediastinum is drained and a feeding jejunostomy tube is inserted. The recovery from sepsis is often immediate, dramatic, and reflected by a marked improvement in the patient's condition over a 24-h period. On recovery from the sepsis, the patient is discharged and returns on a subsequent date for reconstruction with a substernal colon interposition. Failure to apply this aggressive therapy can result in a mortality rate in excess of 50 percent in patients in whom the diagnosis has been delayed.

Nonoperative management of esophageal perforation has been advocated in select situations. The choice of conservative therapy requires skillful judgment and necessitates careful radiographic examination of the esophagus. This course of management usually follows an injury occurring during dilation of esophageal strictures or pneumatic dilations of achalasia. Conservative management should not be used in patients who have free perforations into the pleural space. Cameron proposed three criteria for the nonoperative management of esophageal perforation: (1) the barium swallow must show the perforation to be contained within the mediastinum and drain well back into the esophagus, (2) symptoms should be mild, and (3) there should be minimal evidence of clinical sepsis. If these conditions are met, it is reasonable to treat the patient with hyperalimentation, antibiotics, and cimetidine to decrease acid secretion and diminish pepsin activity. Oral intake is resumed in 7–14 days, dependent on subsequent radiographic examinations.

CAUSTIC INJURY

Accidental caustic lesions occur mainly in children, and in general, rather small quantities of caustics are taken. In adults or teenagers, the swallowing of caustic liquids is usually deliberate, during suicide attempts, and greater quantities are swallowed. Alkalies are more frequently swallowed accidentally than acids, because strong acids cause an immediate burning pain in the mouth.

Pathology

The swallowing of caustic substances causes both an acute and a chronic injury. During the acute phase, care focuses on controlling the immediate tissue injury and the potential for perforation. During the chronic phase, the focus is on treatment of strictures and disturbances in pharyngeal swallowing. In the acute phase the degree and extent of the lesion are dependent on several factors: the nature of the caustic substance, its concentration, the quantity swallowed, and the time the substance is in contact with the tissues. Acids and alkalies affect tissue in different ways. Alkalies dissolve tissue, and therefore penetrate more deeply, although acids cause a coagulative necrosis that limits their penetration. Animal experiments have shown that there is a correlation between the depth of the lesion and the concentration of sodium hydroxide (NaOH) solution. When a solution of 3.8 percent comes into contact with the esophagus for 10 s, it causes necrosis of the mucosa and the submucosa, but spares the muscular layer. A concentration of 22.5 percent penetrates the whole esophageal wall and into the periesophageal tissues. Cleansing products can contain up to 90 percent NaOH. The strength of esophageal contractions varies according to the level of the esophagus, being weakest at the striated muscle–smooth muscle interface. Consequently, clearance from this area may be somewhat slower, allowing caustic substances to remain in contact with the mucosa longer. This explains why the esophagus is preferentially and more severely affected at this level than in the lower portions.

The lesions caused by lye injury occur in three phases. First is the acute necrotic phase, lasting 1 to 4 days after injury. During this period, coagulation of intracellular proteins results in cell necrosis, and the living tissue surrounding the area of necrosis develops an intense inflammatory reaction. Second is the ulceration and granulation phase, starting 3–5 days after injury. During this period the superficial necrotic tissue sloughs, leaving an ulcerated, acutely inflamed base, and granulation tissue fills the defect left by the sloughed mucosa. This phase lasts 10–12 days, and it is during this period that the esophagus is the weakest. Third is the phase of cicatrization and scarring, which begins the third week following injury. During this period the previously formed connective tissue begins to contract, resulting in narrowing of the esophagus. Adhesions between granulating areas occurs, resulting in pockets and bands. It is during this period that efforts must be made to reduce stricture formation.

TABLE 24-14 Endoscopic Grading of Corrosive Esophageal and Gastric Burns

First degree: Mucosal hyperemia and edema

Second degree: Limited hemorrhage, exudate ulceration, and pseudomembrane formation

Third degree: Sloughing of mucosa, deep ulcers, massive hemorrhage, complete obstruction of lumen by edema, charring, and perforation

Clinical Manifestations

The clinical picture of an esophageal burn is determined by the degree and extent of the lesion. In the initial phase, complaints consist of pain in the mouth and substernal region, hypersalivation, pain on swallowing, and dysphagia. The presence of fever is strongly correlated with the presence of an esophageal lesion. Bleeding can occur, and frequently the patient vomits. These initial complaints disappear during the quiescent period of ulceration and granulation. During the cicatrization and scarring phase, the complaint of dysphagia reappears and is because of fibrosis and retraction, resulting in narrowing of the esophagus. Of the patients who develop strictures, 60 percent do so within 1 month, and 80 percent within 2 months. If dysphagia does not develop within 8 months, it is unlikely that a stricture will occur. Serious systemic reactions such as hypovolemia and acidosis resulting in renal damage can occur in cases in which the burns have been caused by strong acids. Respiratory complications such as laryngospasm, laryngedema, and occasionally pulmonary edema can occur, especially when strong acids are aspirated.

Inspection of the oral cavity and pharynx can indicate that caustic substances were swallowed, but does not reveal that the esophagus has been burned. Conversely, esophageal burns can be present without apparent oral injuries. Because of this poor correlation, early esophagoscopy is advocated to establish the presence of an esophageal injury. To lessen the chance of perforation, the scope should not be introduced beyond the proximal esophageal lesion. Table 24-14 lists criteria by which the degree of injury can be graded. Even if the esophagoscopy is normal, strictures may appear later. Radiographic examination is not a reliable means to identify the presence of early esophageal injury, but is important in later follow-up to identify strictures. Table 24-15 shows the most common locations of caustic injuries.

Treatment

Treatment of a caustic lesion of the esophagus is directed toward management of both the immediate and late consequences of the injury. The immediate

TABLE 24-15 Location of Caustic Injury (n = 62)

Pharynx	10%
Esophagus	70%
Upper	15%
Middle	65%
Lower	2%
Whole	18%
Stomach	20%
Antral	91%
Whole	9%
Both stomach and esophagus	14%

treatment consists of limiting the burn by administering neutralizing agents. To be effective, this must be done within the first hour. Lye or other alkali can be neutralized with half-strength vinegar, lemon juice, or orange juice. Acid can be neutralized with milk, egg white, or antacids. Sodium bicarbonate is not used because it generates CO_2, which might increase the danger of perforation. Emetics are contraindicated, because vomiting renews the contact of the caustic substance with the esophagus and can contribute to perforation if too forceful. Hypovolemia is corrected and broad-spectrum antibiotics are administered to lessen the inflammatory reaction and prevent infectious complications. If necessary a feeding jejunostomy tube is inserted to provide nutrition. Oral feeding can be started when the dysphagia of the initial phase has regressed.

In the past, surgeons waited until the appearance of a stricture before starting treatment. Currently, dilations are started the first day after the injury, with the aim of preserving the esophageal lumen by removing the adhesions that occurred in the injured segments. However, this approach is controversial in that dilations can traumatize the esophagus, causing bleeding and perforation, and there are data indicating that excessive dilations cause increased fibrosis secondary to the added trauma. The use of steroids to limit fibrosis has been shown to be effective in animals, but their effectiveness in human beings is debatable.

Extensive necrosis of the esophagus frequently leads to perforation, and is best managed by resection. When there is extensive gastric involvement, the esophagus is nearly always necrotic or severely burned, and total gastrectomy and near-total esophagectomy are necessary. The presence of air in the esophageal wall is a sign of muscle necrosis and impending perforation and is a strong indication for esophagectomy.

Some authors have advocated the use of an intraluminal esophageal stent in patients who are operated on and found to have no evidence of extensive esophagogastric necrosis. In these patients, a biopsy of the posterior gastric wall should be performed to exclude occult injury. If histologically there is a question of viability, a second-look operation should be done within 36 h. If a stent is inserted it should be kept in position for 21 days, and removed after a satisfactory barium esophagogram. Esophagoscopy should be done and if strictures are present, dilations initiated.

Once the acute phase has passed, attention is turned to the prevention and management of strictures. The length of time the surgeon should persist with dilation before consideration of esophageal resection is problematic. An adequate lumen should be re-established within 6 months to 1 year, with progressively longer intervals between dilations. If during the course of treatment an adequate lumen cannot be established or maintained (i.e., smaller bougies must be used), operative intervention should be considered. Surgical intervention is indicated when there is (1) complete stenosis in which all attempts from above and below have failed to establish a lumen, (2) marked irregularity and pocketing on barium swallow, (3) the development of a severe periesophageal reaction or mediastinitis with dilatation, (4) a fistula, (5) the inability to dilate or maintain the lumen above a 40F bougie, or (6) a patient who is unwilling or unable to undergo prolonged periods of dilation.

DIAPHRAGMATIC HERNIAS

With the advent of clinical radiology, it became evident that a diaphragmatic hernia was a relatively common abnormality and was not always accompanied by symptoms. Three types of esophageal hiatal hernia were identified: (1) the sliding hernia, type I, characterized by an upward dislocation of the cardia in the posterior mediastinum; (2) the rolling or paraesophageal hernia, type II, characterized by an upward dislocation of the gastric fundus alongside a normally positioned cardia; and (3) the combined sliding-rolling or mixed hernia, type III, characterized by an upward dislocation of both the cardia and the gastric fundus. The end stage of type I and type II hernias occurs when the whole stomach migrates up into the chest by rotating 180 degrees around its longitudinal axis, with the cardia and pylorus as fixed points. In this situation the abnormality is usually referred to as an intrathoracic stomach.

Clinical Manifestations

The clinical presentation of a paraesophageal hiatal hernia differs from that of a sliding hernia. There is usually a higher prevalence of symptoms of dysphagia and postprandial fullness with paraesophageal hernias, but the typical symptoms of heartburn and regurgitation present in sliding hiatal hernias can also occur. Both are caused by gastroesophageal reflux secondary to an underlying mechanical deficiency of the cardia. The symptoms of dysphagia and postprandial fullness in patients with a paraesophageal hernia are explained by the compression of the adjacent esophagus by a distended cardia, or twisting of the gastroesophageal junction by the torsion of the stomach that occurs as it becomes progressively displaced in the chest.

Approximately one-third of patients with a paraesophageal hernia are found to be anemic, which is because of recurrent bleeding from ulceration of the gastric mucosa in the herniated portion of the stomach. Respiratory complications are frequently associated with a paraesophageal hernia, and consist of dyspnea from mechanical compression and recurrent pneumonia from aspiration. With time the stomach migrates into the chest and can cause intermittent obstruction because of the rotation that has occurred. In contrast, many patients with paraesophageal hiatal hernia are asymptomatic or complain of minor symptoms. However, the presence of a paraesophageal hernia can be life-threatening in that the hernia can lead to sudden catastrophic events, such as excessive bleeding or volvulus with acute gastric obstruction or infarction. With mild dilatation of the stomach, the gastric blood supply can be markedly reduced, causing gastric ischemia, ulceration, perforation, and sepsis. The probability of incarceration is not well known, although recent analysis using mathematical modeling suggests the risk is small.

The symptoms of sliding hiatal hernias are usually because of functional abnormalities associated with gastroesophageal reflux and include heartburn, regurgitation, and dysphagia. These patients have a mechanically defective LES, giving rise to the reflux of gastric juice into the esophagus and the symptoms of heartburn and regurgitation. The symptom of dysphagia occurs from the presence of mucosal edema, Schatzki ring, stricture, or the inability to organize peristaltic activity in the body of the esophagus as a consequence of the disease.

Diagnosis

A radiogram of the chest with the patient in the upright position can diagnose a hiatal hernia if it shows an air-fluid level behind the cardiac shadow. This is usually caused by a paraesophageal hernia or an intrathoracic stomach. The accuracy of the upper GI barium study in detecting a paraesophageal hiatal hernia is greater than for a sliding hernia, because the latter can often spontaneously reduce. The paraesophageal hiatal hernia is a permanent herniation of the stomach into the thoracic cavity, so a barium swallow provides the diagnosis in virtually every case. Attention should be focused on the position of the gastroesophageal junction, when seen, to differentiate it from a type II hernia. Fiberoptic esophagoscopy is useful in the diagnosis and classification of a hiatal hernia because the scope can be retroflexed. In this position, a sliding hiatal hernia can be identified by noting a gastric pouch lined with rugal folds extending above the impression caused by the crura of the diaphragm, or measuring at least 2 cm between the crura, identified by having the patient sniff, and the squamocolumnar junction on withdrawal of the scope. A paraesophageal hernia is identified on retroversion of the scope by noting a separate orifice adjacent to the gastroesophageal junction into that which gastric rugal folds ascend. A sliding-rolling or mixed hernia can be identified by noting a gastric pouch lined with rugal folds above the diaphragm, with the gastroesophageal junction entering about midway up the side of the pouch.

Treatment

The treatment of paraesophageal hiatal hernia is largely surgical. Controversial aspects include (1) indications for repair, (2) surgical approach, and (3) role of fundoplication.

Indications

The presence of a paraesophageal hiatus hernia has traditionally been considered an indication for surgical repair. This recommendation is largely based on two clinical observations. First, retrospective studies have shown a significant incidence of catastrophic, life-threatening complications of bleeding, infarction, and perforation in patients being followed with known paraesophageal herniation. Second, emergency repair carries a high mortality. In the classic report of Skinner and Belsey, 6 of 21 patients with a paraesophageal hernia, treated medically because of minimal symptoms, died from the complications of strangulation, perforation, exsanguinating hemorrhage, or acute dilatation of the herniated intrathoracic stomach. These catastrophes occurred for the most part without warning. Others have reported similar findings.

Recent studies suggest that catastrophic complications may be somewhat less common. Allen and colleagues followed 23 patients for a median of 78 months with only four patients progressively worsening. There was a single mortality secondary to aspiration that occurred during a barium swallow examination to investigate progressive symptoms. Although emergency repairs had a median hospital stay of 48 days compared to a stay of 9 days in those having elective repair, there were only three cases of gastric strangulation in 735 patient-years of follow-up.

If surgery is delayed and repair is done on an emergency basis, operative mortality is high, compared to less than 1 percent for an elective repair. With this in mind, patients with a paraesophageal hernia are generally counseled to have elective repair of their hernia, particularly if they are symptomatic. Watchful waiting of asymptomatic paraesophageal hernias may be an acceptable option.

Surgical Approach

The surgical approach to repair of a paraesophageal hiatal hernia may be either transabdominal (laparoscopic or open) or transthoracic. Each has its advantages and disadvantages. A transthoracic approach facilitates complete esophageal mobilization and removal of the hernia sac. Thoracotomy also allows for the occasional gastroplasty, which may be required for esophageal lengthening to achieve a tension-free repair.

The transabdominal approach facilitates reduction of the volvulus that is often associated with paraesophageal hernias. Although some degree of esophageal mobilization can be accomplished transhiatally, complete mobilization to the aortic arch is difficult or impossible without risk of injury to the vagal nerves.

Several authors have reported the successful repair of paraesophageal hernias using a laparoscopic approach. Laparoscopic repair of a pure type II, or mixed type III paraesophageal hernia is an order of magnitude more difficult than a standard laparoscopic Nissen fundoplication. Most would recommend that these procedures are best avoided until the surgeon has accumulated considerable experience with laparoscopic antireflux surgery. There are several reasons for this. First, the vertical and horizontal volvulus of the stomach often associated with paraesophageal hernias makes identification of the anatomy, in particular the location of the esophagus, difficult. Second, dissection of a large paraesophageal hernia sac usually results in significant bleeding, obscuring the operative field. Finally, redundant tissue present at the gastroesophageal junction following dissection of the sac frustrates the creation of a fundoplication, which these authors believe should accompany the repair of all paraesophageal hernias. Mindful of these difficulties, and given appropriate experience, patients with paraesophageal hernia may be approached laparoscopically, with expectation of success in the majority.

Results

Most outcome studies report relief of symptoms following surgical repair of paraesophageal hernias in over 90 percent of patients. The current literature suggests that laparoscopic repair of a paraesophageal hiatal hernia can be successful. Most authors report symptomatic improvement in 80–90 percent of patients, and less than 10–15 percent prevalence of recurrent hernia. However, the problem of recurrent hernia following laparoscopic repair of any hiatal hernia is becoming increasingly appreciated. Recurrent hernia is now the most common cause of anatomic failure following laparoscopic Nissen fundoplication done for GERD. The problem of recurrent hernia following repair of large type III hiatal hernias has received less attention. Outcome following repair of these hernias is usually based on symptomatic assessment alone. Although recurrence rates of 6–13 percent have been reported, they have largely been based on the need for reoperation or investigations that are performed on a selective basis. Recent reports have shown some degree of anatomic recurrence in up to 45 percent of patients who underwent laparoscopic repair of their hernia.

The principles of laparoscopic repair of a large intrathoracic hernia are analogous to those for an open procedure, namely reduction of the hernia, excision of the peritoneal sac, crural repair, and fundoplication. However, there are several factors that make the laparoscopic repair of these large hernias complex. First, the hiatal opening in a patient with a large hernia is wide, with the right and left muscular crura often separated by 4 cm or more. This can make closure problematic because of the tension required to bring the crura together. Second, the right crus may be devoid of stout tissue and sutures may pull through it easily. Finally, redundant tissue present at the gastroesophageal junction following dissection of the sac retards the creation of the fundoplication.

The use of prosthetic mesh as an adjunct to repair has been advocated for both open and laparoscopic repair of large hiatal hernias. Whether its use is beneficial or not remains controversial, but most prefer to avoid prosthetic material if possible. In contrast to groin hernias, the esophageal hiatus is a dynamic area with constant movement of the diaphragm, esophagus, stomach, and pericardium. Erosion of prosthetic material placed in this area into the GI tract will occur, the only question is how often. The short-term follow-up of most studies is insufficient to provide insight into this problem.

Suggested Readings

General

Balaji B, Peters JH: Minimally invasive surgery for esophageal motor disorders. Surg Clin North Am 82:763, 2002.

Bremner CG, DeMeester TR, Bremner RM: Esophageal Motility Testing Made Easy. St. Louis, MI: Quality Medical Publishing, 2001.

Castel DW, Richter J (eds): The Esophagus. Boston: Little, Brown & Co., 1999.

Demeester SR (ed): Barrett's esophagus. Problems in General Surgery, 18:2. Hagerstown, MD: Lippincott Williams & Wilkins, 2001.

DeMeester TR, Barlow AP: Surgery and current management for cancer of the esophagus and cardia: Part I. Curr Probl Surg 25:477, 1988.

DeMeester TR, Barlow AP: Surgery and current management for cancer of the esophagus and cardia: Part II. Curr Probl Surg 25:535, 1988.

DeMeester TR, Peters JH, Bremner CG, et al: Biology of gastroesophageal reflux disease; pathophysiology relating to medical and surgical treatment. Annu Rev Med 50:469, 1999.

DeMeester SR, Peters JH, DeMeester TR: Barrett's esophagus. Curr Probl Surg 38:549, 2001.

Hunter JG, Pellagrini CA: Surgery of the esophagus. Surg Clin North Am 77:959, 1997.

McFadyen BV, Arregui ME, Eubanks S, et al: Laparoscopic Surgery of the Abdomen. New York: Springer, 2003.

Stein HJ, DeMeester TR, Hinder RA: Outpatient physiologic testing and surgical management of functional foregut disorders. Curr Probl Surg 24:418, 1992.

Zuidema GD, Orringer MB (eds): Shackelford's Surgery of the Alimentary Tract, 3rd ed, Vol. I. Philadelphia: WB Saunders, 1991.

Surgical Anatomy

Daffner RH, Halber MD, Postlethwait RW, et al: CT of the esophagus. II. Carcinoma. AJR 133:1051, 1979.

Gray SW, Rowe JS Jr., Skandalakis JE: Surgical anatomy of the gastroesophageal junction. Am Surg 45:575, 1979.

Liebermann-Meffert DMI, Meier R, Siewert JR: Vascular anatomy of the gastric tube used for esophageal reconstruction. Ann Thorac Surg 54:1110, 1992.

Liebermann-Meffert D, Siewert JR: Arterial anatomy of the esophagus; a review of the literature with brief comments on clinical aspects. Gullet 2:3, 1992.

Liebermann-Meffert D: The pharyngoesophageal segment; anatomy and innervation. Dis Esophagus 8:242, 1995.

Liebermann-Meffert DMI, Walbrun B, Hiebert CA, et al: Recurrent and superior laryngeal nerves; a new look with implications for the esophageal surgeon. Ann Thorac Surg 67:217, 1999.

Physiology

Barlow AP, DeMeester TR, et al: The significance of the gastric secretory state in gastroesophageal reflux disease. Arch Surg 124:937, 1989.

Biancani P, Zabinski MP, Behar J: Pressure, tension, and force of closure of the human LES and esophagus. J Clin Invest 56:476, 1975.

Bonavina L, Evander A, et al: Length of the distal esophageal sphincter and competency of the cardia. Am J Surg 151:25, 1986.

Davenport HW: Physiology of the Digestive Tract, 5th ed. Chicago: Year Book Medical, 1982, p 52.

DeMeester TR, Lafontaine E, et al: The relationship of a hiatal hernia to the function of the body of the esophagus and the gastroesophageal junction. J Thorac Cardiovasc Surg 82:547, 1981.

DeMeester TR, Stein HJ, Fuchs KH: Physiologic diagnostic studies, in Zuidema GD, Orringer MB (eds): Shackelford's Surgery of the Alimentary Tract, 3rd ed, Vol. I. Philadelphia: WB Saunders, 1991, p 94.

DeMeester TR: What is the role of intraoperative manometry? Ann Thorac Surg 30:1, 1980.

Helm JF, Dodds WJ, et al: Acid neutralizing capacity of human saliva. Gastroenterology 83:69, 1982.

Helm JF, Dodds WJ, et al: Effect of esophageal emptying and saliva on clearance of acid from the esophagus. N Engl J Med 310:284, 1984.

Helm JF, Dodds WJ, Hogan WJ: Salivary responses to esophageal acid in normal subjects and patients with reflux esophagitis. Gastroenterology 93:1393, 1982.

Helm JF, Riedel DR, et al: Determinants of esophageal acid clearance in normal subjects. Gastroenterology 85:607, 1983.

Joelsson BE, DeMeester TR, et al: The role of the esophageal body in the antireflux mechanism. Surgery 92:417, 1982.

Johnson LF, DeMeester TR: Evaluation of elevation of the head of the bed, bethanechol, and antacid foam tablets on gastroesophageal reflux. Dig Dis Sci 26:673, 1981.

Kahrilas PJ, Dodds WJ, Hogan WJ: Effect of peristaltic dysfunction on esophageal volume clearance. Gastroenterology 94:73, 1988.

Kaye MD, Showalter JP: Pyloric incompetence in patients with symptomatic gastro-esophageal reflux. J Lab Clin Med 83:198, 1974.

Liebermann-Meffert D, Allgower M, et al: Muscular equivalent of the esophageal sphincter. Gastroenterology 76:31, 1979.

McCallum RW, Berkowitz DM, Lerner E: Gastric emptying in patients with gastro-esophageal reflux. Gastroenterology 80:285, 1981.

Mittal RK, Lange RC, McCallum RW: Identification and mechanism of delayed esophageal acid clearance in subjects with hiatus hernia. Gastroenterology 92:130, 1987.

Price LM, El-Sharkawy TY, Mui HY, Diamant NE: Effects of bilateral cervical vagotomy on balloon-induced lower esophageal sphincter relaxation in the dog. Gastroenterology 77:324, 1979.

Rao SSC, Madipalli RS, Mujica VR, Patel RS, Zimmerman B: Effects of age and gender on esophageal biomechanical properties and sensation. Am J Gastroenterol 98:1688, 2003.

Zaninotto G, DeMeester TR, Schwizer W, et al: The lower esophageal sphincter in health and disease. Am J Surg 155:104, 1988.

Assessment of Esophageal Function

Adamek RJ, Wegener M, et al: Long-term esophageal manometry in healthy subjects: Evaluation of normal values and influence of age. Dig Dis Sci 39:2069, 1994.

Akberg O, Wahlgren L: Dysfunction of pharyngeal swallowing: A cineradiographic investigation in 854 dysphagial patients. Acta Radiol Diagn 26:389, 1985.

American Gastroenterological Association Patient Care Committee: Clinical esophageal pH recording: A technical review for practice guideline development. Gastroenterology 110, 1982.

Barish CF, Castell DO, Richter JE: Graded esophageal balloon distention: A new provocative test for non-cardiac chest pain. Dig Dis Sci 31:1292, 1986.

Battle WS, Nyhus LM, Bombeck CT: Gastroesophageal reflux: Diagnosis and treatment. Ann Surg 177:560, 1973.

Bechi P: Fiberoptic measurement of "alkaline" gastro-esophageal reflux: Technical aspects and clinical indications. Dis Esophagus 131, 1994.

Bechi P, Pucciani F, et al: Long-term ambulatory enterogastric reflux monitoring. Validation of a new fiberoptic technique. Dig Dis Sci 38:1297, 1991.

Behar J, Biancani P, Sheahan DG: Evaluation of esophageal tests in the diagnosis of reflux esophagitis. Gastroenterology 71:9, 1976.

Benjamin SM, Richter JE, et al: Prospective manometric evaluation with pharmacologic provocation of patients with suspected esophageal motility dysfunction. Gastroenterology 84:893, 1983.

Bennett JR, Atkinson M: Oesophageal acid-perfusion in the diagnosis of precordial pain. Lancet 2:1150, 1966.

Bernstein IM, Baker CA: A clinical test for esophagitis. Gastroenterology 34:760, 1958.

Castell DO, Richter JE, Dalton CB (eds): Esophageal Motility Testing. New York: Elsevier, 1987.

DeMeester TR, Johnson LF, et al: Patterns of gastroesophageal reflux in health and disease. Ann Surg 184:459, 1976.

DeMeester TR, Stein HJ, Fuchs KH: Physiologic diagnostic studies, in Zuidema GD, Orringer MB (eds): Shackelford's Surgery of the Alimentary Tract, 3rd ed, Vol. I. Philadelphia: Saunders, 1991, p 94.

DeMeester TR, Wang CI, et al: Technique, indications and clinical use of 24-hour esophageal pH monitoring. J Thorac Cardiovasc Surg 79:656, 1980.

DeMoraes-Filho JPP, Bettarello A: Lack of specificity of the acid perfusion test in duodenal ulcer patients. Am J Dig Dis 19:785, 1974.

Dent J: A new technique for continuous sphincter pressure measurement. Gastroenterology 71:263, 1976.

Dhiman RK, Saraswat VA, Naik SR: Ambulatory esophageal pH monitoring; technique interpretations and clinical indications. Dig Dis Sci 47:241, 2002.

Dodds WJ: Current concepts of esophageal motor function: Clinical implications for radiology. AJR 128:549, 1977.

Donner MW: Swallowing mechanism and neuromuscular disorders. Semin Roentgenol 9:273, 1974.

Emde C, Armstrong F, et al: Reproducibility of long-term ambulatory esophageal combined pH/manometry. Gastroenterology 100:1630, 1991.

Emde C, Garner A, Blum A: Technical aspects of intraluminal pH-metry in man: Current status and recommendations. Gut 23:1177, 1987.

Fein M, Fuchs K-H, et al: Fiberoptic technique for 24-hour bile reflux monitoring. Standards and normal values for gastric monitoring. Dig Dis Sci 41:216, 1996.

Fisher RS, Malmud LS, et al: Gastroesophageal (GE) scintiscanning to detect and quantitate GE reflux. Gastroenterology 70:301, 1976.

Fuchs KH, DeMeester TR, Albertucci M: Specificity and sensitivity of objective diagnosis of gastroesophageal reflux disease. Surgery 102:575, 1987.

Fuchs KH, DeMeester TR, et al: Concomitant duodenogastric and gastroesophageal reflux: The role of twenty-four-hour gastric pH monitoring, in Siewert JR, Holscher AH (eds): Diseases of the Esophagus. New York: Springer-Verlag, 1988, p 1073.

Glade MJ: Continuous ambulatory esophageal pH monitoring in the evaluation of patients with gastroesophageal reflux. JAMA 274:662, 1995.

Iascone C, DeMeester TR, et al: Barrett's esophagus: Functional assessment, proposed pathogenesis and surgical therapy. Arch Surg 118:543, 1983.

Johnson LF, DeMeester TR: Development of 24-hour intraesophageal pH monitoring composite scoring. J Clin Gastroenterol 8:52, 1986.

Johnson LF, DeMeester TR, Haggitt RC: Endoscopic signs for gastroesophageal reflux objectively evaluated. Gastrointest Endosc 22:151, 1976.

Johnson LF, DeMeester TR: Twenty-four-hour pH monitoring of the distal esophagus: A quantitative measure of gastroesophageal reflux. Am J Gastroenterol 62:325, 1974.

Kauer WKH, Burdiles P, Ireland A, et al: Does duodenal juice reflux into the esophagus in patients with complicated GERD? Evaluation of a fiberoptic sensor for bilirubin. Am J Surg 169:98, 1995.

Kramer P, Hollander W: Comparison of experimental esophageal pain with clinical pain of angina pectoris and esophageal disease. Gastroenterology 29:719, 1955.

Landon RL, Ouyang A, et al: Provocation of esophageal chest pain by ergonovine or edrophonium. Gastroenterology 81:10, 1981.

Mittal RK, Stewart WR, Schirmer BD: Effect of a catheter in the pharynx on the frequency of transient LES relaxations. Gastroenterology 103:1236, 1992.

Pandolfino JE, Richter JE, Ours T, et al: Ambulatory esophageal pH monitoring using a wireless system. Am J Gastroenterol 98:740, 2003.

Reid BJ, Weinstein WM, et al: Endoscopic biopsy can detect high-grade dysplasia or early adenocarcinoma in Barrett's esophagus without grossly recognizable neoplastic lesions. Gastroenterology 94:81, 1988.

Richter JE, Hackshaw BT, Wu WC: Edrophonium: A useful provocative test for esophageal chest pain. Ann Intern Med 103:14, 1985.

Russell COH, Hill LD, et al: Radionuclide transit: A sensitive screening test for esophageal dysfunction. Gastroenterology 80:887, 1981.

Schwesinger WH: Endoscopic diagnosis and treatment of mucosal lesions of the esophagus. Surg Clin North Am 69:1185, 1989.

Schwizer W, Hinder RA, DeMeester TR: Does delayed gastric emptying contribute to gastroesophageal reflux disease? Am J Surg 157:74, 1989.

Seaman WB: Roentgenology of pharyngeal disorders, in Margulis AR, Burhenne JH (eds): Alimentary Tract Roentgenology, 2nd ed, Vol. I. St Louis, MO: Mosby, 1973, p 305.

Shoenut JP, Yaffe CS: Ambulatory esophageal pH testing. Referral patterns, indications, and treatment in a Canadian teaching hospital. Dig Dis Sci 41:1102, 1996.

Smout AJPM: Ambulatory manometry of the oesophagus: The method and the message. Gullet 1:155, 1991.

Stein HJ, DeMeester TR, et al: Three-dimensional imaging of the LES in gastroesophageal reflux disease. Ann Surg 214:374, 1991.

Stein HJ, DeMeester TR, Peters JH, et al: Technique, indications, and clinical use of ambulatory 24-hour gastric pH monitoring in a surgical practice. Surgery 116:758, 1994.

Tolin RD, Malmud LS, et al: Esophageal scintigraphy to quantitate esophageal transit (quantitation of esophageal transit). Gastroenterology 76:1402, 1979.

Tutuian R, Vela MF, Balaji NS, et al: Esophageal function testing with combined multichannel intraluminal impedance and manometry; multicenter study in healthy volunteers. Clin Gastroenterol Hepatol 1:174, 2003.

Welch RW, Lickmann K, et al: Manometry of the normal upper esophageal sphincter and its alteration in laryngectomy. J Clin Invest 63:1036, 1979.

Wickremesinghe PC, Bayrit PQ, et al: Quantitative evaluation of bile diversion surgery utilizing 99mTc HIDA scintigraphy. Gastroenterology 84:354, 1983.

Winans CS: Manometric asymmetry of the lower esophageal high pressure zone. Dig Dis Sci 22:348, 1977.

Gastroesophageal Reflux Disease

Allison PR: Hiatus hernia: A 20 year retrospective survey. Ann Surg 178:273, 1973.

Allison PR: Peptic ulcer of the esophagus. J Thorac Surg 15:308, 1946.

Allison PR: Reflux esophagitis, sliding hiatus hernia and the anatomy of repair. Surg Gynecol Obstet 92:419, 1951.

Altorki NK, Sunagawa M, et al: High-grade dysplasia in the columnar-lined esophagus. Am J Surg 161:97, 1991.

Barlow AP, DeMeester TR, et al: The significance of the gastric secretory state in gastroesophageal reflux disease. Arch Surg 124:937, 1989.

Bonavina L, DeMeester TR, et al: Drug-induced esophageal strictures. Ann Surg 206:173, 1987.

Bremner RM, DeMeester TR, Crookes PF, et al: The effect of symptoms and nonspecific motility abnormalities on surgical therapy for gastroesophageal reflux disease. J Thorac Cardiovasc Surg 107:1244, 1994.

Cadiot G, Bruhat A, et al: Multivariate analysis of pathophysiological factors in reflux oesophagitis. Gut 40:167, 1997.

Castell DO. Nocturnal acid breakthrough in perspective: Let's not throw out the baby with the bathwater. Am J Gastroenterol 98:517, 2003.

Chandrasoma P: Norman Barrett: So close, yet 50 years from the truth. J Gastrointest Surg 3:7, 1999.

Chen MF, Wang CS: A prospective study of the effect of cholecystectomy on duodenogastric reflux in humans using 24-hour gastric hydrogen monitoring. Surg Gynecol Obstet 175:52, 1992.

Clark GWB, Ireland AP, Peters JH, et al: Short segments of Barrett's esophagus: A prevalent complication of gastroesophageal reflux disease with malignant potential. J Gastrointest Surg 1:113, 1997.

DeMeester SR, Campos GMR, DeMeester TR, et al: The impact of an antireflux procedure on intestinal metaplasia of the cardia. Ann Surg 228:547; 1998.

DeMeester TR, Bonavina L, Albertucci M: Nissen fundoplication for gastroesophageal reflux disease: Evaluation of primary repair in 100 consecutive patients. Ann Surg 204:9, 1986.

DeMeester TR, Bonavina L, et al: Chronic respiratory symptoms and occult gastro-esophageal reflux. Ann Surg 211:337, 1990.

DeMeester SR, DeMeester TR: Columnar mucosa and intestinal metaplasia of the esophagus: Fifty years of controversy. Ann Surg 231:303, 2000.

DeMeester TR: Management of benign esophageal strictures, in Stipa S, Belsey RHR, Moraldi A (eds): Medical and Surgical Problems of the Esophagus. New York: Academic Press, 1981, p 173.

DeMeester TR, Fuchs KH, et al: Experimental and clinical results with proximal end-to-end duodenojejunostomy for pathologic duodenogastric reflux. Ann Surg 206:414, 1987.

DeMeester TR, Johansson KE, et al: Indications, surgical technique, and long-term functional results of colon interposition or bypass. Ann Surg 208:460, 1988.

Desai KM, Klingensmith ME, Winslow ER, Frisella P, Soper NJ: Symptomatic outcomes of laparoscopic antireflux surgery in patients eligible for endoluminal therapies. Surg Endosc 16:1669, 2002.

Donahue PE, Samelson S, et al: The floppy Nissen fundoplication: Effective long-term control of pathologic reflux. Arch Surg 120:663, 1985.

Farrell TM, Smith CD, Metreveli RE, et al: Fundoplication provides effective and durable symptom relief in patients with Barrett's esophagus. Am J Surg 178:18, 1999.

Fass R: Epidemiology and pathophysiology of symptomatic gastroesophageal reflux disease. Am J Gastroenterol 98(Suppl):S2, 2003.

Fein M, Ireland AP, Ritter MP, et al: Duodenogastric reflux potentiates the injurious effects of gastroesophageal reflux. J Gastrointest Surg 1:27, 1997.

Fiorucci S, Santucci L, et al: Gastric acidity and gastroesophageal reflux patterns in patients with esophagitis. Gastroenterology 103:855, 1992.

Fletcher J, Wirz A, Young J, et al: Unbuffered highly acidic gastric juice exists at the gastroesophageal junction after a meal. Gastroenterology 121:775, 2001.

Freston JW: Long-term acid control and proton pump inhibitors: Interactions and safety issues in perspective. Am J Gastroenterol 92:51S, 1997.

Fuchs KH, DeMeester TR, et al: Computerized identification of pathologic duodeno-gastric reflux using 24-hour gastric pH monitoring. Ann Surg 213:13, 1991.

Gerson LB, Shetler K, Triadafilopoulos G: Prevalence of Barrett's esophagus in asymptomatic individuals. Gastroenterology 123:461, 2002.

Gillen P, Keeling P, et al: Implication of duodenogastric reflux in the pathogenesis of Barrett's oesophagus. Br J Surg 75:540, 1988.

Gotley DC, Ball DE, Owen RW, et al: Evaluation and surgical correction of esophagitis after partial gastrectomy. Surgery 111:29, 1992.

Graham DY: The changing epidemiology of GERD: Geography and Helicobacter pylori. Am J Gastroenterol 98:1462, 2003.

Gurski RR, Peters JH, Hagen JA, et al: Barrett's esophagus can and does regress following antireflux surgery: A study of prevalence and predictive features. J Am Coll Surg 196:706, 2003.

Henderson RD, Henderson RF, Marryatt GV: Surgical management of 100 consecutive esophageal strictures. J Thorac Cardiovasc Surg 99:1, 1990.

Hill LD, Kozarek RA, et al: The gastroesophageal flap valve. In vitro and in vivo observations. Gastrointest Endosc 44:541, 1996.

Hinder RA, et al: Relationship of a satisfactory outcome to normalization of delayed gastric emptying after Nissen fundoplication. Ann Surg 210:458, 1989.

Hinder RA, Filipi CJ: The technique of laparoscopic Nissen fundoplication. Surg Laparosc Endosc 2:265, 1992.

Hirota WK, Loughney TM, Lazas DJ, et al: Specialized intestinal metaplasia, dysplasia and cancer of the esophagus and esophagogastric junction: Prevalence and clinical data. Gastroenterology 116:277, 1999.

Hofstetter WA, Peters JH, DeMeester TR, et al: Long term outcome of antireflux surgery in patients with Barrett's esophagus. Ann Surg 234:532, 2001.

Ireland AP, Clark GWB, et al: Barrett's esophagus: The significance of p53 in clinical practice. Ann Surg 225:17, 1997.

Isolauri J, Luostarinen M, et al: Long-term comparison of antireflux surgery versus conservative therapy for reflux esophagitis. Ann Surg 225:295, 1997.

Iwakiri K, Kobayashi M, et al: Relationship between postprandial esophageal acid exposure and meal volume and fat content. Dig Dis Sci 41:926, 1996.

Jacob P, Kahrilas PJ, Herzon G: Proximal esophageal pH-metry in patients with "reflux laryngitis." Gastroenterology 100:305, 1991.

Jamieson JR, Hinder RA, et al: Analysis of 32 patients with Schatzki's ring. Am J Surg 158:563, 1989.

Johnson WE, Hagen JA, DeMeester TR, et al: Outcome of respiratory symptoms after antireflux surgery on patients with gastroesophageal reflux disease. Arch Surg 131:489, 1996.

Kahrilas PJ: Diagnosis of symptomatic gastroesophageal reflux disease. Am J Gastroenterol 98(Suppl):S15, 2003.

Kahrilas PJ, Dodds WP, Hogan WJ: Effect of peristaltic dysfunction on esophageal volume clearance. Gastroenterology 94:73, 1988.

Kahrilas PJ: Radiofrequency therapy of the lower esophageal sphincter for treatment of GERD. Gastrointest Endosc 57:723; 2003.

Kauer WKH, Peters JH, DeMeester TR, et al. Mixed reflux of gastric juice is more harmful to the esophagus than gastric juice alone. The need for surgical therapy reemphasized. Ann Surg 222:525, 1995.

Kaul BK, DeMeester TR, et al: The cause of dysphagia in uncomplicated sliding hiatal hernia and its relief by hiatal herniorrhaphy: A roentgenographic, manometric, and clinical study. Ann Surg 211:406, 1990.

Khaitan L, Ray WA, Holzman MD, et al: Health care utilization after medical and surgical therapy for gastroesophageal reflux disease. Arch Surg 138:1356, 2003.

Labenz J, Tillenburg B, et al. Helicobacter pylori augments the pH-increasing effect of omeprazole in patients with duodenal ulcer. Gastroenterology 110:725, 1996.

Liebermann-Meffert D: Rudolf Nissen: Reminiscences 100 years after his birth. Dis Esophagus 9:237, 1996.

Lin KM, Ueda RK, et al: Etiology and importance of alkaline esophageal reflux. Am J Surg 162:553, 1991.

Lind JF, et al: Motility of the gastric fundus. Am J Physiol 201:197, 1961.

Little AG, et al: Duodenogastric reflux and reflux esophagitis. Surgery 96:447, 1984.

Little AG, Ferguson MK, Skinner DB: Reoperation for failed antireflux operations. J Thorac Cardiovasc Surg 91:511, 1986.

Liu JY, Finlayson SRG, Laycock WS, Rothstein RI, et al: Determining the appropriate threshold for referral to surgery for gastroesophageal reflux disease. Surgery 133:5, 2003.

Lundell L, Miettinen P, Myrvold HE, et al: Long-term management of gastro-oesophageal reflux disease with omeprazole or open antireflux surgery: Results of a prospective randomized trial. Eur J Gastroenterol Hepatol 12:879, 2000.

Marshall RE, Anggiansah A, Owen WJ: Bile in the esophagus: Clinical relevance and ambulatory detection. Br J Surg 84:21, 1997.

Narayani RI, Burton MP, Young GS: Utility of esophageal biopsy in the diagnosis of non-erosive reflux disease. Dis Esophagus 16:187, 2003.

Nehra D, Watt P, Pye JK, et al: Automated oesophageal reflux sampler: A new device used to monitor bile acid reflux in patients with gastro-oesophageal reflux disease. J Med Engr Tech 21:1, 1997.

Nissen R: Eine einfache Operation zur Beeinflussung der Refluxoesophagitis. Schweiz Med Wochenschr 86:590, 1956.

Nissen R: Gastropexy and fundoplication in surgical treatment of hiatus hernia. Am J Dig Dis 6:954, 1961.

Notivol R, Coffin B, et al: Gastric tone determines the sensitivity of the stomach to distention. Gastroenterology 108:330, 1995.

Oberg S, Johansson H, Wenner J, et al: Endoscopic surveillance of columnar lined esophagus: Frequency of intestinal metaplasia detection and impact of antireflux surgery. Ann Surg 234:619, 2001.

Oleynikov D, Oelschlager B: New alternatives in the management of gastroesophageal reflux disease. Am J Surg 186:106, 2003.

Orlando RC: The pathogenesis of gastroesophageal reflux disease: The relationship between epithelial defense, dysmotility, and acid exposure. Am J Gastroenterol 92:3S, 1997.

Orringer MB, Skinner DB, Belsey RHR: Long-term results of the Mark IV operation for hiatal hernia and analyses of recurrences and their treatment. J Thorac Cardiovasc Surg 63:25, 1972.

O'Sullivan GC, DeMeester TR, et al: Twenty-four-hour pH monitoring of esophageal function: Its use in evaluation in symptomatic patients after truncal vagotomy and gastric resection or drainage. Arch Surg 116:581, 1981.

Ouatu-Lascar R, Triadafilopoulos G: Complete elimination of reflux symptoms does not guarantee normalization of intraesophageal acid reflux in patients with Barrett's esophagus. Am J Gastroenterol 93:711, 1998.

Parrilla P, Martinez de Haro LF, Ortiz A, et al: Long term results of a randomized prospective study comparing medical and surgical treatment in Barrett's esophagus. Ann Surg 237:291, 2003.

Patti MG, Debas HT, et al: Esophageal manometry and 24-hour pH monitoring in the diagnosis of pulmonary aspiration secondary to gastroesophageal reflux. Am J Surg 163:401, 1992.

Patti MG, Diener E, Tamburini A, et al: Role of esophageal function tests in diagnosis of gastroesophageal reflux disease. Dig Dis Sci 46:597, 2001.

Pearson FG, Cooper JD, et al: Gastroplasty and fundoplication for complex reflux problems. Ann Surg 206:473, 1987.

Pelligrini CA, DeMeester TR, et al: Gastroesophageal reflux and pulmonary aspiration: Incidence, functional abnormality, and results of surgical therapy. Surgery 86:110, 1979.

Peters JH, DeMeester TR: Indications, principles of procedure selection, and technique of laparoscopic Nissen fundoplication. Semin Laparoscopy 2:27, 1995.

Peters JH, Heimbucher J, Incarbone R, et al: Clinical and physiologic comparison of laparoscopic and open Nissen fundoplication. J Am Coll Surg 180:385, 1995.

Provenzale D, Kemp JA, et al: A guide for surveillance of patients with Barrett's esophagus. Am J Gastroenterol 89, 1994.

Richardson JD, Larson GM, Polk HC: Intrathoracic fundoplication for shortened esophagus: Treacherous solution to a challenging position. Am J Surg 143:29, 1982.

Richter JE: Long-term management of gastroesophageal reflux disease and its complications. Am J Gastroenterol 92:30S, 1997.

Romagnuolo J, Meier MA, Sadowski DC: Medical or surgical therapy for erosive reflux esophagitis: Cost utility analysis using a Markov model. Ann Surg 236:191, 2002.

Ropert A, Des Varannes SB, et al: Simultaneous assessment of liquid emptying and proximal gastric tone in humans. Gastroenterology 105:667, 1993.

Salama FD, Lamont G: Long-term results of the Belsey Mark IV antireflux operation in relation to the severity of esophagitis. J Thorac Cardiovasc Surg 100:17, 1990.

Schwizer W, Hinder RA, DeMeester TR: Does delayed gastric emptying contribute to gastroesophageal reflux disease? Am J Surg 157:74, 1989.

Shaker R, Castell DO, Schoenfeld PS, et al: Nighttime heartburn is an under-appreciated clinical problem that impacts sleep and daytime function: The results of a Gallup survey conducted on behalf of the American Gastroenterologic Association. Am J Gastroenterol 98:1487, 2003.

Siewert JR, Isolauri J, Feussuer M: Reoperation following failed fundoplication. World J Surg 13:791, 1989.

Sontag SJ, O'Connell S, Khandelwal S, et al: Asthmatics with gastroesophageal reflux: Long term results of a randomized trial of medical and surgical antireflux therapies. Am J Gastroenterol 98:987, 2003.

Sontag SJ: The medical management of reflux esophagitis: Role of antacids and acid inhibition. Gastroenterol Clin North Am 19:683, 1990.

Spechler SJ, Department of Veterans Affairs Gastroesophageal Reflux Disease Study Group: Comparison of medical and surgical therapy for complicated gastroesophageal reflux disease in veterans. N Engl J Med 326:786, 1992.

Spechler SJ, Lee E, Ahmen D: Long term outcome of medical and surgical therapies for gastroesophageal reflux disease: Follow-up of a randomized controlled trial. JAMA 285:2331, 2001.

Stein HJ, Barlow AP, et al: Complications of gastroesophageal reflux disease: Role of the LES, esophageal acid and acid/alkaline exposure, and duodenogastric reflux. Ann Surg 216:35, 1992.

Stein HJ, Bremner RM, et al: Effect of Nissen fundoplication on esophageal motor function. Arch Surg 127:788, 1992.

Stein HJ, et al: Clinical use of 24-hour gastric pH monitoring vs. O-diisopropyl iminodiacetic acid (DISIDA) scanning in the diagnosis of pathologic duodenogastric reflux. Arch Surg 125:966, 1990.

Stein HJ, Smyrk TC, et al: Clinical value of endoscopy and histology in the diagnosis of duodenogastric reflux disease. Surgery 112:796, 1992.

Stirling MC, Orringer MB: Surgical treatment after the failed antireflux operation. J Thorac Cardiovasc Surg 92:667, 1986.

Vaezi MF, Hicks DM, Abelson TI, et al: Laryngeal signs and symptoms and gastroesophageal reflux disease (GERD): A critical assessment of cause and effect association. Clin Gastroenterol Hepatol 1:333, 2003.

Van Den Boom G, Go PMMYH, et al: Cost effectiveness of medical versus surgical treatment in patients with severe or refractory gastroesophageal reflux disease in the Netherlands. Scand J Gastroenterol 31:1, 1996.

Watson DI, Baigrie RJ, Jamieson GG: A learning curve for laparoscopic fundoplication. Definable, avoidable, or a waste of time? Ann Surg 224:198, 1996.

Wattchow DA, Jamieson GG, et al: Distribution of peptide-containing nerve fibers in the gastric musculature of patients undergoing surgery for gastroesophageal reflux. Ann Surg 290:153, 1992.

Welch NT, Yasui A, et al: Effect of duodenal switch procedure on gastric acid production, intragastric pH, gastric emptying, and gastrointestinal hormones. Am J Surg 163:37, 1992.

Weston AP, Krmpotich P, et al: Short segment Barrett's esophagus: Clinical and histological features, associated endoscopic findings, and association with gastric intestinal metaplasia. Am J Gastroenterol 91:981, 1996.

Wetscher GJ, Hinder RA, et al: Reflux esophagitis in humans is mediated by oxygen-derived free radicals. Am J Surg 170:552, 1995.

Williamson WA, Ellis FH Jr., et al: Effect of antireflux operation on Barrett's mucosa. Ann Thorac Surg 49:537, 1990.

Wright TA: High-grade dysplasia in Barrett's oesophagus. Br J Surg 84:760, 1997.

Zaninotto G, DeMeester TR, et al: Esophageal function in patients with reflux-induced strictures and its relevance to surgical treatment. Ann Thorac Surg 47:362, 1989.

Motility Disorders of the Pharynx and Esophagus

Achem SR, Crittenden J, et al: Long-term clinical and manometric follow-up of patients with nonspecific esophageal motor disorders. Am J Gastroenterol 87:825, 1992.

American Gastroenterologic Society: AGA technical review on treatment of patients with dysphagia caused by benign disorders of the distal esophagus. Gastroenterology 117:233, 1999.

Andreollo NA, Earlam RJ: Heller's myotomy for achalasia: Is an added antireflux procedure necessary? Br J Surg 74:765, 1987.

Anselmino M, Perdikis G, et al: Heller myotomy is superior to dilatation for the treatment of early achalasia. Arch Surg 132:233, 1997.

Bianco A, Cagossi M, et al: Appearance of esophageal peristalsis in treated idiopathic achalasia. Dig Dis Sci 90:978, 1986.

Bonavina L, Khan NA, DeMeester TR: Pharyngoesophageal dysfunctions: The role of cricopharyngeal myotomy. Arch Surg 120:541, 1985.

Bonavina L, Nosadinia A, et al: Primary treatment of esophageal achalasia: Long-term results of myotomy and Dor fundoplication. Arch Surg 127:222, 1992.

Browning TH, et al: Diagnosis of chest pain of esophageal origin. Dig Dis Sci 35:289, 1990.

Cassella RR, Brown AL Jr., et al: Achalasia of the esophagus: Pathologic and etiologic considerations. Ann Surg 160:474, 1964.

Chakkaphak S, Chakkaphak K, et al: Disorders of esophageal motility. Surg Gynecol Obstet 172:325, 1991.

Chen LQ, Chughtau T, Sideris L, et al: Long term effects of myotomy and partial fundoplication for esophageal achalasia. Dis Esophagus 15:171, 2002.

Code CF, Schlegel JF, et al: Hypertensive gastroesophageal sphincter. Mayo Clin Proc 35:391, 1960.

Cook IJ, Blumbergs P, et al: Structural abnormalities of the cricopharyngeus muscle in patients with pharyngeal (Zenker's) diverticulum. J Gastroenterol Hepatol 7:556, 1992.

Cook IJ, Gabb M, et al: Pharyngeal (Zenker's) diverticulum is a disorder of upper esophageal sphincter opening. Gastroenterology 103:1229, 1992.

Csendes A, Braghetto I, et al: Late results of a prospective randomized study comparing forceful dilatation and oesophagomyotomy in patients with achalasia. Gut 30:299, 1989.

Csendes A, Braghetto I, et al: Late subjective and objective evaluation of the results of esophagomyotomy in 100 patients with achalasia of the esophagus. Surgery 104:469, 1988.

Csendes A, Velasco N, et al: A prospective randomized study comparing forceful dilatation and esophagomyotomy in patients with achalasia of the esophagus. Gastroenterology 80:789, 1981.

Dalton CB, Castell DO, Richter JE: The changing faces of the nutcracker esophagus. Am J Gastroenterol 83:623, 1988.

DeMeester TR, Johansson KE, et al: Indications, surgical technique and long-term functional results of colon interposition or bypass. Ann Surg 208:460, 1988.

DeMeester TR, Lafontaine E, et al: The relationship of a hiatal hernia to the function of the body of the esophagus and the gastroesophageal junction. J Thorac Cardiovasc Surg 82:547, 1981.

DeMeester TR, Stein HJ: Surgery for esophageal motor disorders, in Castell DO (ed): The Esophagus. Boston: Little, Brown, 1992, p 401.

Donner MW: Swallowing mechanism and neuromuscular disorders. Semin Roentgenol 9:273, 1974.

Eckardt V, Aignherr C, Bernhard G: Predictors of outcome in patients with achalasia treated by pneumatic dilation. Gastroenterol 103:1732, 1992.

Eckardt VF, Köhne U, et al: Risk factors for diagnostic delay in achalasia. Dig Dis Sci 42:580, 1997.

Ekberg O, Wahlgren L: Dysfunction of pharyngeal swallowing: A cineradiographic investigation in 854 dysphagial patients. Acta Radiol Diagn 26:389, 1985.

Ellis FH Jr., Crozier RE: Cervical esophageal dysphagia: Indications for and results for cricopharyngeal myotomy. Ann Surg 194:279, 1981.

Ellis FH: Long esophagomyotomy for diffuse esophageal spasm and related disorders: An historical overview. Dis Esophagus 11:210; 1998.

Ellis Jr, FH: Oesophagomyotomy for achalasia: A 22-year experience. Br J Surg 80:882, 1993.

Evander A, Little AG, et al: Diverticula of the mid and lower esophagus. World J Surg 10:820, 1986.

Eypasch EP, Stein HJ, et al: A new technique to define and clarify esophageal motor disorders. Am J Surg 159:144, 1990.

Ferguson MK: Achalasia: Current evaluation and therapy. Ann Thorac Surg 52:336, 1991.

Ferguson MK, Skinner DB (eds): Diseases of the Esophagus: Benign Diseases, Vol. 2. Mount Kisco, NY: Futura Publishing, 1990.

Ferguson TB, Woodbury JD, Roper CL: Giant muscular hypertrophy of the esophagus. Ann Thorac Surg 8:209, 1969.

Foker JE, Ring WE, Varco RL: Technique of jejunal interposition for esophageal replacement. J Thorac Cardiovasc Surg 83:928, 1982.

Gillies M, Nicks R, Skyring A: Clinical, manometric, and pathologic studies in diffuse oesophageal spasm. Br Med J 2:527, 1967.

Goulbourne IA, Walbaum PR: Long-term results of Haller's operation for achalasia. J Royal Coll Surg 30:101, 1985.

Gutschow CA, Hamoir M, Rombaux P, et al: Management of pharyngoesophageal (Zenker's) diverticulum: Which technique? Ann Thorac Surg 74:1677, 2002.

Hirano I, Tatum RP, Shi G, et al: Manometric heterogeneity in patients with idiopathic achalasia. Gastroenterology 120:789, 2001.

Kahrilas PJ, Logemann JA, et al: Pharyngeal clearance during swallowing: A combined manometric and videofluoroscopic study. Gastroenterology 103:128, 1992.

Lafontaine E: Pharyngeal dysphagia, in DeMeester TR, Matthews HR (eds): Benign Esophageal Disease: International Trends in General Thoracic Surgery,Vol. 3. St. Louis: CV Mosby, 1987.

Lam HGT, Dekker W, et al: Acute noncardiac chest pain in a coronary care unit. Gastroenterology 102:453, 1992.

Lang IM, Dantas RO, Cook IJ, et al: Videographic, manometric, and electromyographic analysis of canine upper esophageal sphincter. Am J Physiol 260:G911, 1991.

Lerut J, Elgariani A, et al: Zenker's diverticulum. Surgical experience in a series of 25 patients. Acta Gastroenterol Belg 46:189, 1983.

Lerut T, VanRaemdonck D, et al: Pharyngo-oesophageal diverticulum (Zenker's). Clinical, therapeutic and morphologic aspects. Acta Gastroenterol Belg 53:330, 1990.

Little AG, Correnti FS, et al: Effect of incomplete obstruction on feline esophageal function with a clinical correlation. Surgery 100:430, 1986.

Malthaner RA, Todd TR, Miller L, Pearson FG: Long-term results in surgically managed esophageal achalasia. Ann Thorac Surg 58:1343, 1994.

Mellow MH: Return of esophageal peristalsis in idiopathic achalasia. Gastroenterology 70:1148, 1976.

Meshkinpour H, Haghighat P, et al: Quality of life among patients treated for achalasia. Dig Dis Sci 41:352, 1996.

Migliore M, Payne H, et al: Pathophysiologic basis for operation on Zenker's diverticulum. Ann Thorac Surg 57:1616, 1994.

Moser G, Vacariu-Granser GV, et al: High incidence of esophageal motor disorders in consecutive patients with globus sensation. Gastroenterology 101:1512, 1991.

Moses PL, Ellis LM, Anees MR, et al: Antineural antibodies in idiopathic achalasia and gastro-oesophageal reflux disease. Gut 52:629, 2003.

Nehra D, Lord RV, DeMeester TR, et al: Physiologic basis for the treatment of epiphrenic diverticulum. Ann Surg 235:346, 2002.

Oelschlager BK, Chang L, Pellegrini CA: Improved outcome after extended gastric myotomy for achalasia. Arch Surg 138:490, 2003.

Patti MG, Fisichella PM, Peretta S, et al: Impact of minimally invasive surgery on the treatment of esophageal achalasia: A decade of change. J Am Coll Surg 196:698, 2003.

Pellegrini C, Wetter LA, et al: Thoracoscopic esophagomyotomy: Initial experience with a new approach for the treatment of achalasia. Ann Surg 216:291, 1992.

Peters JH: An antireflux procedure is critical to the long-term outcome of esophageal myotomy for achalasia. J Gastrointest Surg 5:17, 2001.

Peters JH, Kauer WKH, Ireland AP, Bremner CG, DeMeester TR: Esophageal resection with colon interposition for end-stage achalasia. Arch Surg 130:632, 1995.

Ponce J, Garrigues V, Pertejo V, Sala T, et al: Individual prediction of response to pneumatic dilation in patients with achalasia. Dig Dis Sci 41:2135, 1996.

Richter JE: Surgery or pneumatic dilation for achalasia: A head-to-head comparison. Gastroenterology 97:1340, 1989.

Shimi SM, Nathanson LK, Cuschieri A: Thoracoscopic long oesophageal myotomy for nutcracker oesophagus: Initial experience of a new surgical approach. Br J Surg 79:533, 1992.

Shoenut J, Duerksen D: A prospective assessment of gastroesophageal reflux before and after treatment of achalasia patients: Pneumatic dilation versus transthoracic limited myotomy. Am J Gastroenterol 92:1109, 1997.

Sivarao DV, Mashimo HL, Thatte HS, Goyal RK: Lower esophageal sphincter is achalasic in nNos(-/-) and hypotensive in W/W(v) mutant mice. Gastroenterology 121:34, 2001.

Spechler S, Castell DO: Classification of oesophageal motility abnormalities. Gut 49:145, 2001.

Stein HJ, DeMeester TR, Eypasch EP: Ambulatory 24-hour esophageal manometry in the evaluation of esophageal motor disorders and non-cardiac chest pain. Surgery 110:753, 1991.

Stein HJ, Eypasch EP, DeMeester TR: Circadian esophageal motility pattern in patients with classic diffuse esophageal spasm and nutcracker esophagus. Gastroenterology 96:491, 1989.

Streitz JM Jr., Glick ME, Ellis FH Jr.: Selective use of myotomy for treatment of epiphrenic diverticula: Manometric and clinical analysis. Arch Surg 127:585, 1992.

Vaezi MF, Baker ME, Achkar E, et al: Timed barium oesophogram: Better predictor of long term success after pneumatic dilation in achalasia than symptom assessment. Gut 50:765, 2002.

Vantrappen G, Janssens J: To dilate or to operate? That is the question. Gut 24:1013, 1983.

Verne G, Sallustio JE, et al: Anti-myenteric neuronal antibodies in patients with achalasia: A prospective study. Dig Dis Sci 42:307, 1997.

Waters PF, DeMeester TR: Foregut motor disorders and their surgical management. Med Clin North Am 54:1235, 1981.

Williams RB, Grehan MJ, Andre J, Cook IJ: Biomechanics, diagnosis, and treatment outcome in inflammatory myopathy presenting as oropharyngeal dysphagia. Gut 52:471, 2003.

Zhao X, Pasricha PJ: Botulinum toxin for spastic GI disorders: A systematic review. Gastrointest Endosc 57:219, 2003.

Carcinoma of the Esophagus

Akiyama H: Surgery for carcinoma of the esophagus. Curr Probl Surg 17:53, 1980.

Akiyama H, Tsurumaru M: Radical lymph node dissection for cancer of the thoracic esophagus. Ann Surg 220:364, 1994.

Akiyama H, Tsurumaru M, et al: Principles of surgical treatment for carcinoma of the esophagus: Analysis of lymph node involvement. Ann Surg 194:438, 1981.

Altorki N, Skinner D: Should en-bloc esophagectomy be the standard of care for esophageal carcinoma? Ann Surg 234:581, 2001.

Badwe RA, Sharma V, Bhansali MS, et al: The quality of swallowing for patients with operable esophageal carcinoma: A randomized trial comparing surgery with radiotherapy. Cancer 85:763, 1999.

Baker JW Jr., Schechter GL: Management of paraesophageal cancer by blunt resection without thoracotomy and reconstruction with stomach. Ann Surg 203:491, 1986.

Blazeby JM, Williams MH, et al: Quality of life measurement in patients with esophageal cancer. Gut 37:505, 1995.

Bolton JS, Ochsner JL, et al: Surgical management of esophageal cancer. A decade of change. Ann Surg 219:475, 1994.

Borrie J: Sarcoma of esophagus: Surgical treatment. J Thorac Surg 37:413, 1959.

Cameron AJ, Ott BJ, Payne WS: The incidence of adenocarcinoma in columnar-lined (Barrett's) esophagus. N Engl J Med 313:857, 1985.

Clark GWB, Ireland AD, et al: Carcinoembryonic antigen measurements in the management of esophageal cancer. An indicator of subclinical recurrence. Am J Surg 170:597, 1995.

Clark GWB, Peters JH, Hagen JA, et al: Nodal metastases and recurrence patterns after en-bloc esophagectomy for adenocarcinoma. Ann Thorac Surg 58:646, 1994.

Clark GWB, Smyrk TC, et al: Is Barrett's metaplasia the source of adenocarcinomas of the cardia? Arch Surg 129:609, 1994.

Collin CF, Spiro RH: Carcinoma of the cervical esophagus: Changing therapeutic trends. Am J Surg 148:460, 1984.

Corley DA, Kerlikowske K, Verma R, et al: Protective association of aspirin/NSAIDs and esophageal cancer: A systematic review and meta-analysis. Gastroenterology 124:47, 2003.

Dallal HJ, Smith GD, Grieve DC, et al: A randomized trial of thermal ablative therapy versus expandable metal stents in the palliative treatment of patients with esophageal carcinoma. Gastrointest Endosc 54:549, 2001.

DeMeester TR, Attwood SEA, et al: Surgical therapy in Barrett's esophagus. Ann Surg 212:528, 1990.

DeMeester TR, Barlow AP: Surgery and current management for cancer of the esophagus and cardia: Part II. Curr Probl Surg 25:535, 1988.

DeMeester TR: Esophageal carcinoma: Current controversies. Semin Surg Oncol 13:217, 1997.

DeMeester TR, Skinner DB: Polypoid sarcomas of the esophagus. Ann Thorac Surg 20:405, 1975.

DeMeester TR, Zaninotto G, Johansson KE: Selective therapeutic approach to cancer of the lower esophagus and cardia. J Thorac Cardiovasc Surg 95:42, 1988.

Duhaylongsod FG, Wolfe WG: Barrett's esophagus and adenocarcinoma of the esophagus and gastroesophageal junction. J Thorac Cardiovasc Surg 102:36, 1991.

Ell C, May A, Gossner L, et al: Endoscopic mucosal resection of early cancer and high grade dysplasia in Barrett's esophagus. Gastroenterology 118:670, 2001.

Ellis FH, Heatley GJ, Krosna MJ, Williamson WA, Balogh K: Esophagogastrectomy for carcinoma of the esophagus and cardia: A comparison of findings and results after standard resection in three consecutive 8 year time intervals, using improved staging criteria. J Thorac Cardiovasc Surg 113:836, 1997.

Frenken M: Best palliation in esophageal cancer; surgery, stenting, radiation or what? Dis Esophagus 14:120, 2001.

Fujita H, Kakegawa T, et al: Mortality and morbidity rates, postoperative course, quality of life, and prognosis after extended radical lymphadenectomy for esophageal cancer. Ann Surg 222:654, 1995.

Gomes MN, Kroll S, Spear SL: Mediastinal tracheostomy. Ann Thorac Surg 43:539, 1987.

Goodner JT: Treatment and survival in cancer of the cervical esophagus. Am J Surg 20:405, 1975.

Guernsey JM, Knudsen DF: Abdominal exploration in the evaluation of patients with carcinoma of the thoracic esophagus. J Thorac Cardiovasc Surg 59:62, 1970.

Hagen JA, DeMeester TR, Peters JH, et al: Curative resection for esophageal adenocarcinoma analysis of 100 en bloc esophagectomies. Ann Surg 234:520, 2001.

Heatley RV, Lewis MH, Williams RHP: Preoperative intravenous feeding: A controlled trial. Postgrad Med J 55:541, 1979.

Heimlich HJ: Carcinoma of the cervical esophagus. J Thorac Cardiovasc Surg 59:309, 1970.

Heitmiller RF, Sharma RR: Comparison of prevalence and resection rates in patients with esophageal squamous cell carcinoma and adenocarcinoma. J Thorac Cardiovasc Surg 112:130, 1996.

Hofstetter W, Swisher SG, Correa AM: Treatment outcomes of resected esophageal cancer. Ann Surg 236:376, 2002.

Hulscher JBF, Van Sandick JW, DeBoer AGEM, et al: Extended transthoracic resection compared with limited transhiatal resection for adenocarcinoma of the esophagus. N Engl J Med 347:1662, 2002.

Iijima K, Henrey E, Moriya A, et al: Dietary nitrate generates potentially mutagenic concentrations of nitric oxide at the gastroesophageal junction. Gastroenterology 122:1248, 2002.

Ikeda M, Natsugoe S, Ueno S, et al: Significant host and tumor related factors for predicting prognosis in patients with esophageal carcinoma. Ann Surg 238:197, 2003.

Jankowski JA, Wight NA, Meltzer SJ, et al: Molecular evolution of the metaplasia-dysplasia-adenocarcinoma sequence in the esophagus. Am J Pathol 154:965, 1999.

Johansson J, DeMeester TR, Hoger JA, et al: En bloc is superior to transhiatal esophagectomy for T3 N1 adenocarcinoma of the distal esophagus and GE junction. Arch Surg 139:627, 2004.

Kaklamanos IG, Walker GR, Ferry K, et al: Neoadjuvant treatment for resectable cancer of the esophagus and the gastroesophageal junction: A meta-analysis of randomized clinical trials. Ann Surg Oncol 10:754, 2003.

Krasna MJ, Reed CE, Nedzwiecki D, et al: CALGB 9380: A prospective trial of the feasibility of thoracoscopy/laparoscopy in staging esophageal cancer. Ann Thorac Surg 71:1073, 2001.

Kirby JD: Quality of life after esophagectomy: The patients' perspective. Dis Esophagus 12:168, 1999.

Kron IL, Joob AW, et al: Blunt esophagectomy and gastric interposition for tumors of the cervical esophagus and hypopharynx. Am Surg 52:140, 1986.

Lagergren J, Bergstrom R, Lindgren A, et al: Symptomatic gastroesophageal reflux as a risk factor for esophageal adenocarcinoma. N Engl J Med 340:825, 1999.

Lavin P, Hajdu SI, Foote FW Jr.: Gastric and extragastric leiomyoblastomas. Cancer 29:305, 1972.

Law SYK, Fok M, Wong J: Pattern of recurrence after oesophageal resection for cancer: Clinical implications. Br J Surg 83:107, 1996.

Law SYK, Fok M, et al: A comparison of outcomes after resection for squamous cell carcinomas and adenocarcinomas of the esophagus and cardia. Surg Gynecol Obstet 175:107, 1992.

Law S, Kwong DLW, Kwok KF, et al: Improvement in treatment results and long term survival of patients with esophageal cancer: Impact of chemoradiation and change in treatment strategy. Ann Surg 238:339, 2003.

Lerut T, Coosemans W, et al: Surgical treatment of Barrett's carcinoma. Correlations between morphologic findings and prognosis. J Thorac Cardiovasc Surg 107:1059, 1994.

Lerut T, De Leyn P, et al: Surgical strategies in esophageal carcinoma with emphasis on radical lymphadenectomy. Ann Surg 216:583, 1992.

Leuketich JD, Alvelo-Rivera M, Buenaventura PO, et al: Minimally invasive esophagectomy: Outcomes in 222 patients. Ann Surg 238:486, 2003.

Levine DS, Reid BJ: Endoscopic diagnosis of esophageal neoplasms. Gastrointest Clin North Am 2:395, 1992.

Lewis I: The surgical treatment of carcinoma of the esophagus with special reference to a new operation for the growths of the middle third. Br J Surg 34:18, 1946.

Logan A: The surgical treatment of carcinoma of the esophagus and cardia. J Thorac Cardiovasc Surg 46:150, 1963.

Lund O, Hasenkam JM, et al: Time related changes in characteristics of prognostic significance of carcinomas of the esophagus and cardia. Br J Surg 76:1301, 1989.

Maerz LL, Deveney CW, et al: Role of computed tomographic scans in the staging of esophageal and proximal gastric malignancies. Am J Surg 165:558, 1993.

McCort JJ: Esophageal carcinosarcoma and pseudosarcoma. Radiology 102:519, 1972.

Medical Research Council Oesophageal Working Party: Surgical resection with or without preoperative chemotherapy in oesophageal cancer: A randomized controlled trial. Lancet 359:1727, 2002.

Moore TC, Battersby JS, et al: Carcinosarcoma of the esophagus. J Thorac Cardiovasc Surg 45:281, 1963.

Murray GF, Wilcox BR, Starek P: The assessment of operability of esophageal carcinoma. Ann Thorac Surg 23:393, 1977.

Naunheim KS, Petruska PJ, et al: Preoperative chemotherapy and radiotherapy for esophageal carcinoma. J Thorac Cardiovasc Surg 103:887, 1992.

Nicks R: Colonic replacement of the esophagus. Br J Surg 54:124, 1967.

Nigro JJ, Hagen JA, DeMeester TR, et al: Occult esophageal adenocarcinoma: Extent of disease and implications for effective therapy. Ann Surg 230:433, 1999.

Orringer MB, Marshall B, Iannettoni MD: Transhiatal esophagectomy: Clinical experience and refinements. Ann Surg 230:392, 1999.

Orringer MB: Transhiatal esophagectomy without thoracotomy for carcinoma of the thoracic esophagus. Ann Surg 200:282, 1984.

Orringer MB, Skinner DB: Unusual presentations of primary and secondary esophageal malignancies. Ann Thorac Surg 11:305, 1971.

Pacifico RJ, Wang KK, Wongkeesong LM, et al: Combined endoscopic mucosal resection and photodynamic therapy versus esophagectomy for management of early adenocarcinoma of the esophagus. Clin Gastroenterol Hepatol 1:252, 2003.

Pera M, Cameron AJ, et al: Increasing incidence of adenocarcinoma of the esophagus and esophagogastric junction. Gastroenterology 104:510, 1993.

Pera M, Trastek VF, et al: Barrett's esophagus with high-grade dysplasia: An indication for esophagectomy? Ann Thorac Surg 54:199, 1992.

Pera M, Trastek VF, et al: Influence of pancreatic and biliary reflux on the development of esophageal carcinoma. Ann Thorac Surg 55:1386, 1993.

Peters JH, Clark GWB, et al: Outcome of adenocarcinoma arising in Barrett's esophagus in endoscopically surveyed and non-surveyed patients. J Thorac Cardiovasc Surg 108:813, 1994.

Peters JH, Hoeft SF, et al: Selection of patients for curative or palliative resection of esophageal cancer based on preoperative endoscopic ultrasound. Arch Surg 129:534, 1994.

Peters JH: Surgical treatment of esophageal adenocarcinoma: Concepts in evolution. J Gastrointest Surg 6:518, 2002.

Piccone VA, Ahmed N, et al: Esophagogastrectomy for carcinoma of the middle third of the esophagus. Ann Thorac Surg 28:369, 1979.

Pouliquen X, Levard H, et al: 5-Fluorouracil and cisplatin therapy after palliative surgical resection of squamous cell carcinoma of the esophagus. Ann Surg 223:127, 1996.

Rasanen JV, Sihvo EIT, Knuuti J, et al: Prospective analysis of accuracy of proton emission tomography, computed tomography and endoscopic ultrasonography in staging of adenocarcinoma of the esophagus and esophagogastric junction. Ann Surg Oncol 10:954, 2003.

Ravitch M: A Century of Surgery. Philadelphia: Lippincott, 1981, p 56.

Reed CE: Comparison of different treatments for unresectable esophageal cancer. World J Surg 19:828, 1995.

Reid BJ, Weinstein WM, et al: Endoscopic biopsy can detect high-grade dysplasia or early adenocarcinoma in Barrett's esophagus without grossly recognizable neoplastic lesions. Gastroenterology 94:81, 1988.

Ribeiro U Jr., Posner MC, et al: Risk factors for squamous cell carcinoma of the oesophagus. Br J Surg 83:1174, 1996.

Rice TW, Boyce GA, et al: Esophageal ultrasound and the preoperative staging of carcinoma of the esophagus. J Thorac Cardiovasc Surg 101:536, 1991.

Robertson CS, Mayberry JF, Nicholson JA: Value of endoscopic surveillance in the detection of neoplastic changes in Barrett's esophagus. Br J Surg 75:760, 1988.

Rösch T, Lorenz R, et al: Endosonographic diagnosis of submucosal upper gastrointestinal tract tumors. Scand J Gastroenterol 27:1, 1992.

Rosenberg JC, Budev H, et al: Analysis of adenocarcinoma in Barrett's esophagus utilizing a staging system. Cancer 55:1353, 1985.

Rosenberg JC, Franklin R, Steiger Z: Squamous cell carcinoma of the thoracic esophagus: An interdisciplinary approach. Curr Probl Cancer 5:1, 1981.

Saidi F, Abbassi A, et al: Endothoracic endoesophageal pull-through operation: A new approach to cancers of the esophagus and proximal stomach. J Thorac Cardiovasc Surg 102:43, 1991.

Sarr MG, Hamilton SR, et al: Barrett's esophagus: Its prevalence and association with adenocarcinoma in patients with symptoms of gastroesophageal reflux. Am J Surg 149:187, 1985.

Schottenfeld D: Epidemiology of cancer of the esophagus. Semin Oncol 11:92, 1984.

Silver CE: Surgical management of neoplasms of the larynx, hypopharynx and cervical esophagus. Curr Probl Surg 14:2, 1977.

Skinner DB, Dowlatshahi KD, DeMeester TR: Potentially curable carcinoma of the esophagus. Cancer 50:2571, 1982.

Skinner DB, Ferguson MK, Little AG: Selection of operation for esophageal cancer based on staging. Ann Surg 204:391, 1986.

Smith R, Gowing WFC: Carcinoma of the esophagus with histological appearances simulating a carcinosarcoma. Br J Surg 40:487, 1953.

Sonnenberg A, Fennerty MB: Medical decision analysis of chemoprevention against esophageal adenocarcinoma. Gastroenterology 124:1758, 2003.

Spechler SJ: Endoscopic surveillance for patients with Barrett's esophagus: Does the cancer risk justify the practice? Ann Intern Med 106:902, 1987.

Stout AP, Humphreys GH, Rottenberg LA: A case of carcinosarcoma of the esophagus. AJR Radium Ther Nucl Med 61:461, 1949.

Streitz JM Jr., Ellis FH Jr., et al: Adenocarcinoma in Barrett's esophagus. Ann Surg 213:122, 1991.

Talbert JL, Cantrell JR: Clinical and pathologic characteristics of carcinosarcoma of the esophagus. J Thorac Cardiovasc Surg 45:1, 1963.

Thomas PA: Physiologic sufficiency of regenerated lung lymphatics. Ann Surg 192:162, 1980.

Turnbull AD, Rosen P, et al: Primary malignant tumors of the esophagus other than typical epidermoid carcinoma. Ann Thorac Surg 15:463, 1973.

Urschel JD, Ashiku S, Thurer R, et al: Salvage or planned esophagectomy after chemoradiation for locally advanced esophageal cancer: A review. Dis Esophagus 16:60, 2003.

Vigneswaran WT, Trastek VK, et al: Extended esophagectomy in the management of carcinoma of the upper thoracic esophagus. J Thorac Cardiovasc Surg 107:901, 1994.

Walsh TN, Noonan N, et al: A comparison of multimodal therapy and surgery for esophageal adenocarcinoma. N Engl J Med 335:462, 1996.

Watson WP, Pool L: Cancer of the cervical esophagus. Surgery 23:893, 1948.

Benign Tumors and Cysts

Bardini R, Segalin A, et al: Videothoracoscopic enucleation of esophageal leiomyoma. Am Thorac Surg 54:576, 1992.

Bonavina L, Segalin A, et al: Surgical therapy of esophageal leiomyoma. J Am Coll Surg 181:257, 1995.

Esophageal Perforation

Brewer LA III, Carter R, et al: Options in the management of perforations of the esophagus. Am J Surg 152:62, 1986.

Bufkin BL, Miller JI Jr., Mansour KA: Esophageal perforation. Emphasis on management. Ann Thorac Surg 61:1447, 1996.

Chang C-H, Lin PJ, et al: One-stage operation for treatment after delayed diagnosis of thoracic esophageal perforation. Ann Thorac Surg 53:617, 1992.

Engum SA, Grosfeld JL, et al: Improved survival in children with esophageal perforation. Arch Surg 131:604, 1996.

Gouge TH, Depan HJ, Spencer FC: Experience with the Grillo pleural wrap procedure in 18 patients with perforation of the thoracic esophagus. Ann Surg 209:612, 1989.

Jones WG II, Ginsberg RJ: Esophageal perforation: A continuing challenge. Ann Thorac Surg 53:534, 1992.

Pate JW, Walker WA, et al: Spontaneous rupture of the esophagus: A 30-year experience. Ann Thorac Surg 47:689, 1989.

Reeder LB, DeFilippi VJ, Ferguson MK: Current results of therapy for esophageal perforation. Am J Surg 169:615, 1995.

Salo JA, Isolauri JO, et al: Management of delayed esophageal perforation with mediastinal sepsis. Esophagectomy or primary repair? J Thorac Cardiovasc Surg 106:1088, 1993.

Sawyer R, Phillips C, Vakil N: Short- and long-term outcome of esophageal perforation. Gastrointest Endosc 41:130, 1995.

Segalin A, Bonavina L, et al: Endoscopic management of inveterate esophageal perforations and leaks. Surg Endosc 10:928, 1996.

Weiman DS, Walker WA, et al: Noniatrogenic esophageal trauma. Ann Thorac Surg 59:845, 1995.

Whyte RI, Iannettoni MD, Orringer MB: Intrathoracic esophageal perforation. The merit of primary repair. J Thorac Cardiovasc Surg 109:140, 1995.

Caustic Injury

Anderson KD, Rouse TM, Randolph JG: A controlled trial of corticosteroids in children with corrosive injury of the esophagus. N Engl J Med 323:637, 1990.

Ferguson MK, Migliore M, et al: Early evaluation and therapy for caustic esophageal injury. Am J Surg 157:116, 1989.

Jeng L-BB, Chen H-Y, et al: Upper gastrointestinal tract ablation for patients with extensive injury after ingestion of strong acid. Arch Surg 129:1086, 1994.

Lahoti D, Broor SL, et al: Corrosive esophageal strictures. Predictors of response to endoscopic dilation. Gastrointest Endosc 41:196, 1995.

Popovici Z: About reconstruction of the pharynx with colon in extensive corrosive strictures. Kurume Med J 36:41, 1989.

Sugawa C, Lucas CE: Caustic injury of the upper gastrointestinal tract in adults: A clinical and endoscopic study. Surgery 106:802, 1989.

Wu M-H, Lai W-W: Esophageal reconstruction for esophageal strictures or resection after corrosive injury. Ann Thorac Surg 53:798, 1992.

Wu M-H, Lai W-W: Surgical management of extensive corrosive injuries of the alimentary tract. Surg Gynecol Obstet 177:12, 1993.

Zargar SA, Kochhar R, et al: The role of fiberoptic endoscopy in the management of corrosive ingestion and modified endoscopic classification of burns. Gastrointest Endosc 37:165, 1991.

Diaphragmatic Hernias

Bombeck TC, Dillard DH, Nyhus LM: Muscular anatomy of the gastroesophageal junction and role of the phrenoesophageal ligament. Ann Surg 164:643, 1966.

Bonavina L, Evander A, et al: Length of the distal esophageal sphincter and competency of the cardia. Am J Surg 151:25, 1986.

Casbella F, Sinanan M, et al: Systematic use of gastric fundoplication in laparoscopic repair of paraesophageal hernias. Am J Surg 171:485, 1996.

Dalgaard JB: Volvulus of the stomach. Acta Chir Scand 103:131, 1952.

DeMeester TR, Bonavina L: Paraesophageal hiatal hernia, in Nyhus LM, Condon RE (eds): Hernia, 3rd ed. Philadelphia: Lippincott, 1989, p 684.

DeMeester TR, Lafontaine E, et al: The relationship of a hiatal hernia to the function of the body of the esophagus and the gastroesophageal junction. J Thorac Cardiovasc Surg 82:547, 1981.

Eliska O: Phreno-oesophageal membrane and its role in the development of hiatal hernia. Acta Anat 86:137, 1973.

Fuller CB, Hagen JA, et al: The role of fundoplication in the treatment of type II paraesophageal hernia. J Thorac Cardiovasc Surg 111:655, 1996.

Hashemi M, Peters JH, DeMeester TR, et al: Laparoscopic repair of large type III hiatal hernia: Objective follow-up reveals high recurrence rate. J Am Coll Surg 190:539, 2000.

Kahrilas PJ, Wu S, et al: Attenuation of esophageal shortening during peristalsis with hiatus hernia. Gastroenterology 109:1818, 1995.

Kleitsch WP: Embryology of congenital diaphragmatic hernia. I. Esophageal hiatus hernia. Arch Surg 76:868, 1958.

Menguy R: Surgical management of large paraesophageal hernia with complete intrathoracic stomach. World J Surg 12:415, 1988.

Myers GA, Harms BA, et al: Management of paraesophageal hernia with a selective approach to antireflux surgery. Am J Surg 170:375, 1995.

Patti MG, Goldberg HI, et al: Hiatal hernia size affects LES function, esophageal acid exposure, and the degree of mucosal injury. Am J Surg 171:182, 1996.

Pierre AF, Luketich JD, Fernando HC, et al: Results of laparoscopic repair of giant paraesophageal hernias: 200 Consecutive patients. Ann Thorac Surg 74:1909, 2002.

Postlethwait RW: Surgery of the Esophagus. New York: Appleton-Century Crofts, 1979, p 195.

Skinner DB, Belsey RHR: Surgical management of esophageal reflux and hiatus hernia: Long-term results with 1030 patients. J Thorac Cardiovasc Surg 53:33, 1967.

Stylopoulos N, Gazelle GS, Ratner DW. Paraesophageal hernias: Operation or observation. Ann Surg 236:492. 2002.

Walther B, DeMeester TR, et al: The effect of paraesophageal hernia on sphincter function and its implication on surgical therapy. Am J Surg 147:111, 1984.

Miscellaneous Esophageal Lesions

Burdick JS, Venu RP, Hogan WJ: Cutting the defiant lower esophageal ring. Gastrointest Endosc 39:616, 1993.

Burt M, Diehl W, et al: Malignant esophagorespiratory fistula: Management options and survival. Ann Thorac Surg 52:1222, 1991.

Chen MYM, Ott DJ, Donati DL: Correlation of lower esophageal mucosal ring and LES pressure. Dig Dis Sci 39:766, 1994.

D'Haens G, Rutgeerts P, et al: The natural history of esophageal Crohn's disease. Three patterns of evolution. Gastrointest Endosc 40:296, 1994.

Eckhardt VF, Kanzler G, Willems D: Single dilation of symptomatic Schatzki rings. A prospective evaluation of its effectiveness. Dig Dis Sci 37:577, 1992.

Klein HA, Wald A, et al: Comparative studies of esophageal function in systemic sclerosis. Gastroenterology 102:1551, 1992.

Mathisen DJ, Grillo HC, et al: Management of acquired nonmalignant tracheoesophageal fistula. Ann Thorac Surg 52:759, 1991.

Poirier NC, Taillefer R, et al: Antireflux operations in patients with scleroderma. Ann Thorac Surg 58:66, 1994.

Soudah HC, Hasler WL, Owyang C: Effect of octreotide on intestinal motility and bacterial overgrowth in scleroderma. N Engl J Med 325:1461, 1991.

Stagias JG, Ciarolla D, Campo S, et al: Vascular compression of the esophagus. A manometric and radiologic study. Dig Dis Sci 39:782, 1994.

Toskes PP: Hope for the treatment of intestinal scleroderma (Letter to the Editor). N Engl J Med 325:1508, 1991.

Wilcox CM, Straub RF: Prospective endoscopic characterization of cytomegalovirus esophagitis in AIDS. Gastrointest Endosc 40:481, 1994.

Techniques of Esophageal Reconstruction

Akiyama H: Esophageal reconstruction. Entire stomach as esophageal substitute. Dis Esophagus 8:7, 1995.

Banki F, Mason RJ, DeMeester SR, et al: Vagal sparing esophagectomy: A more physiologic alternative. Ann Surg 236:324, 2002.

Bonavina L, Anselmino M, et al: Functional evaluation of the intrathoracic stomach as an oesophageal substitute. Br J Surg 79:529, 1992.

Burt M, Scott A, et al: Erythromycin stimulates gastric emptying after esophagectomy with gastric replacement. A randomized clinical trial. J Thorac Cardiovasc Surg 111:649, 1996.

Cheng W, Heitmiller RF, Jones BJ: Subacute ischemia of the colon esophageal interposition. Ann Thorac Surg 57:899, 1994.

Curet-Scott MJ, Ferguson MK, et al: Colon interposition for benign esophageal disease. Surgery 102:568, 1987.

DeMeester TR, Johansson K-E, et al: Indications, surgical technique, and long-term functional results of colon interposition or bypass. Ann Surg 208:460, 1988.

DeMeester TR, Kauer WKH: Esophageal reconstruction. The colon as an esophageal substitute. Dis Esophagus 8:20, 1995.

Dexter SPL, Martin IG, McMahon MJ: Radical thoracoscopic esophagectomy for cancer. Surg Endosc 10:147, 1996.

Ellis FH Jr., Gibb SP: Esophageal reconstruction for complex benign esophageal disease. J Thorac Cardiovasc Surg 99:192, 1990.

Finley RJ, Lamy A, et al: Gastrointestinal function following esophagectomy for malignancy. Am J Surg 169:471, 1995.

Fok M, Cheng SWK, Wong J: Pyloroplasty versus no drainage in gastric replacement of the esophagus. Am J Surg 162:447, 1991.

Gossot D, Cattan P, Fritsch S: Can the morbidity of esophagectomy be reduced by the thoracoscopic approach? Surg Endosc 9:1113, 1995.

Heitmiller RF, Jones B: Transient diminished airway protection after transhiatal esophagectomy. Am J Surg 162:442, 1991.

Honkoop P, Siersema PD, et al: Benign anastomotic strictures after transhiatal esophagectomy and cervical esophagogastrostomy. Risk factors and management. J Thorac Cardiovasc Surg 111:1141, 1996.

Liebermann-Meffert DMI, Meier R, Siewert JR: Vascular anatomy of the gastric tube used for esophageal reconstruction. Ann Thorac Surg 54:1110, 1992.

Maier G, Jehle EC, Becker HD: Functional outcome following oesophagectomy for oesophageal cancer. A prospective manometric study. Dis Esophagus 8:64, 1995.

Naunheim KS, Hanosh J, et al: Esophagectomy in the septuagenarian. Ann Thorac Surg 56:880, 1993.

Nishihra T, Oe H, et al: Esophageal reconstruction. Reconstruction of the thoracic esophagus with jejunal pedicled segments for cancer of the thoracic esophagus. Dis Esophagus 8:30, 1995.

Patil NG, Wong J: Surgery in the "new" Hong Kong. Arch Surg 136:1415, 2001.

Peters JH, Kronson J, Bremner CG, DeMeester TR: Arterial anatomic considerations in colon interposition for esophageal replacement. Arch Surg 130:858, 1995.

Stark SP, Romberg MS, et al: Transhiatal versus transthoracic esophagectomy for adenocarcinoma of the distal esophagus and cardia. Am J Surg 172:478, 1996.

Valverde A, Hay JM, Fingerhut A, Elhadad A: Manual versus mechanical esophagogastric anastomosis after resection for carcinoma. A controlled trial. French Associations for Surgical Research. Surgery 120:476, 1996.

Watson T, DeMeester TR, Kauer WKH, Peters JH, Hagen JA: Esophagectomy for end stage benign esophageal disease. J Thorac Cardiovasc Surg 115:1241, 1998.

Wu M-H, Lai W-W: Esophageal reconstruction for esophageal strictures or resection after corrosive injury. Ann Thorac Surg 53:798, 1992.

25 | Stomach

Daniel T. Dempsey

The stomach is a remarkable organ with important digestive, nutritional, and endocrine functions. It stores and facilitates the digestion and absorption of ingested food, and it helps regulate appetite. Treatable diseases of the stomach are common and the stomach is accessible and relatively forgiving. It is thus a favorite therapeutic target. To provide intelligent diagnosis and treatment, the physician and surgeon must understand gastric anatomy, physiology, and pathophysiology. This includes a sound understanding of the mechanical, secretory, and endocrine processes through which the stomach accomplishes its important functions. It also includes a familiarity with the common benign and malignant gastric disorders of clinical significance, especially peptic ulcer and gastric cancer.

Gross Anatomy

The stomach is readily recognizable as the asymmetrical pear-shaped most proximal abdominal organ of the digestive tract. The superior-most part of the stomach is the distensible floppy fundus, bounded superiorly by the diaphragm and laterally by the spleen. The angle of His is where the fundus meets the left side of the gastroesophageal (GE) junction. The inferior extent of the fundus generally is considered to be the horizontal plane of the GE junction, in which the body (corpus) of the stomach begins. The body of the stomach contains most of the parietal (oxyntic) cells. The gastrin secreting antrum comprises the distal 25–30 percent of the stomach.

The stomach is the most richly vascularized portion of the alimentary canal. Most of the gastric blood supply is from the celiac axis via four named arteries. The left and right gastric arteries form an anastomotic arcade along the lesser curvature, and the right and left gastroepiploic arteries form an arcade along the greater gastric curvature. About 15 percent of the time the left gastric artery supplies an aberrant vessel to the left side of the liver which travels in the gastrohepatic ligament (lesser omentum), but rarely is this the only arterial blood supply to this part of the liver. The second largest artery to the stomach is usually the right gastroepiploic artery which arises fairly consistently from the gastroduodenal artery behind the first portion of the duodenum. The left gastroepiploic artery arises from the splenic artery and together with the right gastroepiploic artery forms the rich gastroepiploic arcade along the greater curvature. The right gastric artery usually arises from the hepatic artery near the pylorus and hepatoduodenal ligament, and runs proximally along the distal stomach. In the fundus along the proximal greater curvature, the short gastric arteries and veins arise from the splenic circulation. There may also be vascular branches to the proximal stomach from the phrenic circulation. The veins draining the stomach generally parallel the arteries. The left gastric (coronary vein) and right gastric veins usually drain into the portal vein, although occasionally the coronary vein drains into the splenic vein. The right gastroepiploic vein drains into the superior mesenteric vein near the inferior border of the pancreatic neck, and the left gastroepiploic vein drains into the splenic vein.

Regions of the stomach usually drain lymph to the closest nodal basins. However, within the gastric wall there is a rich anastomotic network of lymphatics which may drain the stomach in a somewhat unpredictable fashion. Thus a tumor arising in the distal stomach could give rise to positive lymph nodes in the splenic hilum. Sentinel node mapping and lymphoscintigraphy are investigational techniques that may evolve as clinically useful methods for staging gastric cancer. Surgeons and pathologists have numbered the primary and secondary lymph node groups to which the stomach drains.

Both the extrinsic and intrinsic innervation of the stomach play an important role in gastric secretory and motor function. The vagus nerves provide the extrinsic parasympathetic innervation to the stomach and acetylcholine is the most important neurotransmitter. Near the gastroesophageal junction the anterior (left) vagus sends a branch (or branches) to the liver in the gastrohepatic ligament and continues along the lesser curvature as the anterior nerve of Laterjet. Similarly, the posterior (right) vagus sends branches to the celiac plexus and continues along the posterior lesser curvature. The nerves of Laterjet send segmental branches to the body of the stomach before they terminate near the angularis incisura as the "crow's foot," sending branches to the antro-pyloric region. In 50 percent of patients there are more than two vagal nerves at the esophageal hiatus. The branch which the posterior vagus sends to the posterior fundus is termed the criminal nerve of Grassi. This branch typically arises above the esophageal hiatus and is easily missed during truncal or highly selective vagotomy. Most (>75 percent) of the axons contained in the vagal trunks are afferent (i.e., carrying stimuli from the viscera to the brain). The extrinsic sympathetic nerve supply to the stomach originates at spinal levels T5–T10 and travels in the splanchnic nerves to the celiac ganglion. Postganglionic sympathetic nerves then travel from the celiac ganglion to the stomach along the blood vessels. Neurons in the myenteric and submucosal plexuses constitute the intrinsic nervous system of the stomach. The extrinsic (parasympathetic and sympathetic) and intrinsic gastric nervous system have various and diverse neurotransmitters including cholinergic, adrenergic, and peptidergic (e.g., substance P, somatostatin).

Histology

There are four distinct layers of the gastric wall: mucosa, submucosa, muscularis propria, and serosa. The epithelium, lamina propria, and muscularis mucosa constitute the "mucosa." The epithelium of the gastric mucosa is columnar glandular. A scanning electron micrograph shows a smooth mucosal carpet punctuated by the openings of the gastric glands. The gastric glands are lined with different types of epithelial cells depending on the location of the stomach (Table 25-1). There are also endocrine cells (such as histamine-secreting enterochromaffin-like [ECL] cells and somatostatin secreting D cells) present in the gastric glands. Progenitor cells at the base of the glands differentiate and replenish sloughed cells on a regular basis. Throughout the stomach, the "carpet" consists primarily of mucous secreting surface epithelial cells which extend down into the gland pits for a variable distance. These cells also secrete bicarbonate and play an important role in protecting the stomach from injury because of acid, pepsin, and/or ingested irritants.

Parietal cells secrete acid and intrinsic factor into the gastric lumen, and bicarbonate into the intercellular space. Chief cells (also called zymogenic cells) secrete pepsinogen which is activated at pH below 2.5. They tend to be

TABLE 25-1 Epithelial Cells of the Stomach

Cell type	Distinctive ultrastructural features	Major functions
Surface-foveolar mucous cells	Apical stippled granules up to 1 μm in diameter	Production of neutral glycoprotein and bicarbonate to form a gel on the gastric luminal surface; neutralization of hydrochloric acid[a];
Mucous neck cell	Heterogeneous granules 1–2 μm in diameter dispersed throughout the cytoplasm	Progenitor cell for all other gastric epithelial cells; glycoprotein production; production of pepsinogens I and II
Oxyntic (parietal) cell	Surface membrane invaginations (canaliculi); tubulovesicle structures; numerous mitochondria;	Production of hydrochloric acid production of intrinsic factor production of bicarbonate
Chief cell	Moderately dense apical granules up to 2 μm in diameter; prominent supranuclear Golgi apparatus; extensive basolateral granular endoplasmic reticulum	Production of pepsinogens I and II, and of lipase
Cardiopyloric mucous cell	Mixture of granules like those in mucous neck and chief cells; extensive basolateral granular endoplasmic reticulum	Production of glycoprotein Production of pepsinogen II
Endocrine cells		

[a]Bicarbonate is probably produced by other gastric epithelial cells in addition to surface-foveolar mucous cells.
Source: Reproduced with permission from Antonioli DA, Madara JL, in Ming SC, Goldman H (eds): *Pathology of the Gastrointestinal Tract.* Baltimore: Williams & Wilkins, 1998, p 13.

clustered toward the base of the gastric glands and have a low columnar shape. In the antrum, the gastric glands are more branched and shallow, parietal cells are rare, and gastrin-secreting G cells and somatostatin-secreting D cells are present. A variety of hormone secreting cells are present in various proportions throughout the gastric mucosal . Histologic analysis suggests that in the normal stomach, 13 percent of the epithelial cells are oxyntic (parietal) cells, 44 percent chief (zymogenic cells), 40 percent mucous cells, and 3 percent endocrine cells.

Deep to the mucosa is the submucosa that is rich in branching blood vessels, lymphatics, collagen, various inflammatory cells, autonomic nerve fibers, and ganglion cells of Meissner autonomic submucosal plexus. The collagen rich submucosa gives strength to gastrointestinal anastomosis. The mucosa and submucosa are folded into the grossly visible gastric rugae which tend to flatten out as the stomach becomes distended.

Below the submucosa is the thick muscularis propria (also referred to as the muscularis externa) which consists of an incomplete inner oblique layer, a complete middle circular layer (continuous with the esophageal circular muscle and the circular muscle of the pylorus), and a complete outer longitudinal layer (continuous with the longitudinal layer of the esophagus and duodenum). Within the muscularis propria is the rich network of autonomic ganglia and nerves which make up Auerbach myenteric plexus. The outer layer of the stomach is the serosa, which is synonymous with the visceral peritoneum.

PHYSIOLOGY

The stomach stores food and facilitates digestion through a variety of secretory and motor functions. Important secretory functions include the production of acid and intrinsic factor from parietal cells, pepsin from chief cells, mucous from mucous secreting epithelial cells, and a variety of gastrointestinal (GI) hormones from gastric endocrine cells. Important motor functions include food storage (receptive relaxation and accommodation), grinding and mixing, controlled emptying of ingested food, and periodic interprandial "housekeeping."

Acid Secretion

The parietal cell is stimulated to secrete acid when one or more of three membrane receptor types is stimulated by acetylcholine (from vagal nerve fibers), gastrin (from mucosal G cells) or histamine (from mucosal ECL cells). The enzyme H/K-ATPase is the proton pump. The normal human stomach contains about a billion parietal cells, and total gastric acid production is proportional to parietal cell mass. The potent acid suppressing proton pump inhibitor drugs irreversibly interfere with the function of the H/K-ATPase molecule. They must be incorporated into the activated enzyme to be effective and thus work best when taken before or during a meal (when the parietal cell is stimulated). When proton pump inhibitor therapy is stopped, acid secretory capability returns as new hydrogen/potassium-adenosine triphosphatase (H/K-ATPase) is synthesized.

Gastrin, acetylcholine and histamine stimulate the parietal cell to secrete hydrochloric acid. Gastrin binds to type B CCK receptors and acetylcholine binds to M_3 muscarinic receptors. Both stimulate phospholipase C via a G-protein linked mechanism leading to increased production of inositol triphosphate (IP3) from membrane bound phospholipids. IP3 stimulates the release of calcium from intracellular stores which leads to activation of protein kinases and activation of H/K-ATPase. Histamine binds to the histamine 2 (H_2) receptor that stimulates adenylate cyclase, also via a G protein linked mechanism. Activation of adenylate cyclase results in an increase in intracellular cyclic AMP that activates protein kinases leading to increased levels of phosphoproteins and activation of the proton pump. Somatostatin from mucosal D cells binds to membrane receptors and inhibits the activation of adenylate cyclase through an inhibitory G protein.

The acid secretory response that occurs after a meal is traditionally described in three phases: cephalic, gastric, and intestinal. The cephalic or vagal phase begins with the thought, sight, smell, and/or taste of food. These stimuli activate several cortical and hypothalamic sites and signals are transmitted to the stomach by the vagal nerves. Acetylcholine is released leading to stimulation of ECL cells and parietal cells. Although the acid secreted per unit time in the cephalic phase is greater than in the other two phases, the duration of the cephalic phase is briefer. Thus the cephalic phase accounts for no more than 30 percent of total acid secretion in response to a meal. Sham feeding (chew and spit) stimulates gastric acid secretion only via the cephalic phase.

When food reaches the stomach, the gastric phase of acid secretion begins. This phase lasts until the stomach is empty, and accounts for about 60 percent of the total acid secretion in response to a meal. The gastric phase of acid secretion has several components. Amino acids and small peptide directly stimulate antral G cells to secrete gastrin which is carried in the bloodstream to the parietal cells and stimulates acid secretion in an endocrine fashion. Additionally, proximal gastric distention stimulates acid secretion via a vagovagal reflex arc, which is abolished by truncal or highly selective vagotomy. Antral distention also stimulates antral gastrin secretion. Acetylcholine also stimulates gastrin release; and gastrin stimulates histamine release from ECL cells.

The intestinal phase of gastric secretion is poorly understood. It is thought to be mediated by a yet to be discovered hormone released from the proximal small bowel mucosa in response to luminal chyme. This phase starts when gastric emptying of ingested food begins, and continues as long as nutrients remain in the proximal small intestine. It accounts for about 10 percent of meal-induced acid secretion.

ECL cells play a pivotal role in the regulation of gastric acid secretion. A large part of the acid stimulatory effects of both acetylcholine and gastrin are mediated by histamine released from mucosal ECL cells. This explains why the histamine 2 receptor antagonists (H_2RAs) are such effective inhibitors of acid secretion, even though histamine is only one of three parietal cell stimulants. The mucosal D cell, which releases somatostatin, is also an important regulator of acid secretion. Somatostatin inhibits histamine release from ECL cells and gastrin release from D cells. The function of D cells is inhibited by H. pylori infection, and this leads to an exaggerated acid secretory response.

Gastric Mucosal Barrier

The stomach's durable resistance to autodigestion by caustic hydrochloric acid and active pepsin is intriguing. Table 25-2 lists some of the important components of gastric barrier function and cytoprotection. When these defenses break down, ulceration occurs. A variety of factors are important in maintaining an intact gastric mucosal layer. The mucous and bicarbonate secreted by surface epithelial cells forms an unstirred mucous gel with a favorable pH gradient. Cell membranes and tight junctions prevent hydrogen ions from gaining access to the interstitial space. Hydrogen ions that do break through are buffered by the alkaline tide created by basolateral bicarbonate secretion from stimulated

TABLE 25-2 Important Components and Mediators of Mucosal Defenses in the Stomach

Components
Mucous barrier
Bicarbonate secretion
Epithelial barrier
Hydrophobic phospholipids
Tight junctions
Restitution
Microcirculation (reactive hyperemia)
Afferent sensory neurons
Mediators
Prostaglandins
Nitric oxide
Epidermal growth factor
Calcitonin gene-related peptide
Hepatocyte growth factor
Histamine

parietal cells. Any sloughed or denuded surface epithelial cells are rapidly replaced by migration of adjacent cells, a process known as restitution. Mucosal blood flow plays a crucial role in maintaining a healthy mucosa, providing nutrients and oxygen for the cellular functions involved in cytoprotection. "Back diffused" hydrogen is buffered and rapidly removed by the rich blood supply. When "barrier breakers" such as bile or aspirin lead to increased back diffusion of hydrogen ions from the lumen into the lamina propria and submucosa, there is a protective increase in mucosal blood flow. If this protective response is blocked, gross ulceration can occur. Important mediators of these protective mechanisms include prostaglandins, nitric oxide, intrinsic nerves, and peptides (e.g., calcitonin gene related peptide, gastrin). Misoprostol is a commercially available prostaglandin E analogue that has been shown to prevent gastric mucosal damage in chronic nonsteroidal antiinflammatory drug (NSAID) users. Some protective reflexes involve afferent sensory neurons, and can be blocked by the application of topical anesthetics to the gastric mucosa, or the experimental destruction of the afferent sensory nerves. In addition to these local defenses, there are important protective factors in swallowed saliva, duodenal secretions, and pancreatic or biliary secretions.

Gastric Hormones

Gastrin (mostly little gastrin, G-17) is produced by antral G cells and is the major hormonal stimulant of the acid secretion during the gastric phase. The biologically active pentapeptide sequence at the C-terminal end of gastrin is identical to that of CCK. Luminal peptides and amino acids are the most potent stimulants of gastrin release, and luminal acid is the most potent inhibitor of gastrin secretion. The latter effect is predominantly mediated in a paracrine fashion by somatostatin released from antral D cells. Gastrin stimulated acid secretion is significantly blocked by H_2 antagonists, suggesting that the principle mediator of gastrin stimulated acid production is histamine from mucosal ECL cells. Important causes of hypergastrinemia include pernicious anemia, acid suppressive medication, gastrinoma, retained antrum following distal gastrectomy and Billroth II, and vagotomy.

Somatostatin (predominantly somatostatin 14) is produced by D cells located throughout the gastric mucosa. The major stimulus for somatostatin release is antral acidification, and acetylcholine from vagal nerve fibers inhibits its release. Somatostatin inhibits acid secretion from parietal cells, and gastrin release from G cells. It also decreases histamine release from ECL cells. The proximity of the D cells to these target cells suggests that the primary effect of somatostatin is mediated in a paracrine fashion, but an endocrine effect is also possible.

Gastrin-releasing peptide (GRP), the mammalian equivalent of bombesin, stimulates both gastrin and somatostatin release by binding to receptors on the G and D cells. There are nerve terminals ending near the mucosa in the gastric body and antrum which are rich in GRP immunoreactivity. When GRP is given peripherally it stimulates acid secretion, but when it is given centrally into the cerebral ventricles of animals, it inhibits acid secretion apparently via a pathway involving the sympathetic nervous system.

Ghrelin, a small peptide produced primarily in the stomach, is a potent secretogogue of pituitary growth hormone and appears to be an orexigenic regulator of appetite. When ghrelin is elevated, appetite is stimulated and when it is suppressed, appetite is suppressed. The gastric bypass operation, a very effective treatment for morbid obesity, is associated with suppression of plasma ghrelin levels (and appetite) in humans. Resection of the primary source of this hormone, the stomach, may partly account for the anorexia and weight loss seen in some patients following gastrectomy.

Gastric Motility/Emptying

Gastric motor function has several purposes. Interprandial motor activity clears the stomach of undigested debris, sloughed cells, and mucus. When feeding begins, the stomach relaxes to accommodate the meal. Regulated motor activity then breaks down the food into small particles, and controls the output into the duodenum. The stomach accomplishes these functions by coordinated smooth muscle relaxation and contraction of the various gastric segments (proximal, distal, pylorus). Smooth muscle myoelectric potentials are translated into muscular activity which is modulated by extrinsic and intrinsic innervation, and hormones. There are a variety neurotransmitters, which are generally grouped as excitatory (augment muscular activity) and inhibitory (decrease muscular activity). Important excitatory neurotransmitters include acetylcholine and the tachykinins substance P and neurokinin A. Important inhibitory neurotransmitters include nitric oxide (NO) and vasoactive intestinal peptide (VIP). Serotonin has been shown to modulate both contraction and relaxation. A variety of other molecules affect motility including GRP, histamine, neuropeptide Y, norepinephrine, and endogenous opioids. Specialized cells in the muscularis propria are also important modulators of gastrointestinal motility. These cells, called interstitial cells of Cajal, are distinguishable histologically from neurons and myocytes, and appear to amplify both cholinergic excitatory and neurergic inhibitory input to the smooth muscle of the stomach and intestine.

When food is ingested, intragastric pressure falls as the proximal stomach relaxes. This proximal relaxation is mediated by two important vagovagal reflexes, receptive relaxation (reduction in proximal gastric tone associated with food swallowing) and gastric accommodation (proximal gastric relaxation when food enters the stomach). Because both of these reflexes are mediated by afferent and efferent vagal fibers, they are significantly altered by truncal and highly selective vagotomy which tend to increase basal intragastric pressure and may increase the rate of liquid emptying. In addition to receptive relaxation and accommodation, proximal gastric tone is decreased by duodenal distention, colonic distention, and ileal perfusion with glucose (the ileal brake).

The distal stomach breaks up solid food and is the main determinant of gastric emptying of solids. Slow waves of myoelectric depolarization sweep down the distal stomach at a rate of about 3 per min. These waves originate from the proximal gastric pacemaker, high on the greater curvature. The pacing cells may be the interstitial cells of Cajal, which have been shown to have a similar function in the small intestine and colon. Most of these myoelectric waves are below the threshold for smooth muscle contraction in the quiescent state, and thus are associated with negligible changes in pressure. Neural and/or hormonal input which increases the plateau phase of the action potential can trigger muscle contraction, resulting in a peristaltic wave associated with the electrical slow wave and of the same frequency (3 per min).

During fasting, distal gastric motor activity is controlled by the migrating motor complex (MMC), the "gastrointestinal housekeeper." The teleologic function of the MMC is to sweep along any undigested food, debris, sloughed cells, and mucous after the fed phase of digestion is complete. The MMC lasts about 100 min (longer at night, shorter during daytime) and is divided into four phases. Neurohormonal control of the MMC is poorly understood, but it appears that different phases are regulated by different mechanisms. For example, vagotomy abolishes phase II of the gastric MMC, but has little influence on phase III. In fact, phase III persists in the autotransplanted stomach, totally devoid of extrinsic neural input. This suggests that phase III is regulated by intrinsic nerves and/or hormones. Indeed, the initiation of phase III of the MMC in the distal stomach corresponds temporally to elevation in serum levels of motilin, a hormone produced in the duodenal mucosa. Resection of the duodenum abolishes distal gastric phase III in dogs. There are clearly motilin receptors on antral smooth muscle and nerves. Other modulators of gastric MMC activity include NO, endogenous opioids, intrinsic cholinergic and adrenergic nerves, duodenal pH (MMC phase III does not occur if the duodenal pH is below 7).

Feeding abolishes the MMC and leads to the fed motor pattern. The fed motor pattern of gastric activity starts within 10 min of food ingestion and persists until all the food has left the stomach. Gastric motility during the fed pattern resembles phase II of the MMC, with irregular but continuous phasic contractions of the distal stomach. Some contractions are prograde and some are retrograde, serving to mix and grind the solid components of the meal. The magnitude of gastric contractions and the duration of the pattern is influenced by the consistency and composition of the meal.

The pylorus functions as a very effective regulator of gastric emptying, preventing large particles and large boluses of liquid from entering the duodenum in which they could overwhelm normal digestive and homeostatic mechanisms. It also is an effective barrier to duodenogastric reflux. Dysfunction, bypass, transection, or resection of the pylorus may lead to uncontrolled gastric emptying of food and the dumping syndrome, or uncontrolled entry of duodenal contents into the stomach, leading to bile reflux gastritis.

Although an oversimplification, liquid emptying has been attributed to the activity of the proximal stomach, and solid emptying to the activity of the distal stomach. Clearly receptive relaxation and gastric accommodation play a role

TABLE 25-3 Promotility Agents That Accelerate Gastric Emptying

Drug	Mechanism
Metoclopramide	Dopamine antagonist
Domperidone	Dopamine antagonist
Erythromycin	Motilin agonist
Bethanecol	Cholinergic agonist
Neostigmine	Cholinergic agonist

in gastric emptying of liquids. Patients with a denervated (e.g., vagotomy), resected, or plicated (e.g., fundoplication) proximal stomach have decreased gastric compliance and may show accelerated gastric emptying of liquids. Normally, the T1/2 of solid gastric emptying is about 2 h. Unlike liquids which display an initial rapid phase followed by a slower linear phase of emptying, solids have an initial lag phase during which very little emptying of solids occurs It is during this phase that much of the grinding and mixing occurs. A linear emptying phase follows during which the smaller particles are metered out to the duodenum. Solid gastric emptying is a function of meal particle size, caloric content and composition (especially fat). When liquids and solids are ingested together, the liquids empty first. Solids are stored in the fundus and delivered to the distal stomach at constant rates for trituration. Liquids are also sequestered in the fundus but they appear to be readily delivered to the distal stomach for early emptying. The larger the solid component of the meal, the slower the liquid emptying. Patients bothered by dumping syndrome are advised to limit the amount of liquid consumed with the solid meal, taking advantage of this effect. A variety of prokinetic agents have been shown to be clinically useful in increasing gastric emptying. Table 25-3 shows the commonly used agents, mechanisms, and side effects.

EVALUATION OF GASTRIC DISEASE

The most common symptoms of gastric disease are pain, weight loss, early satiety, and anorexia. Nausea, vomiting, bloating and anemia are also frequent complaints. Patients with one or more of the alarm symptoms listed in Table 25-4 should undergo expeditious upper endoscopy (esophagogastroduodenoscopy = EGD). EGD is a very safe and accurate outpatient procedure performed under conscious sedation. To rule out cancer with a high degree of accuracy, all patients with gastric ulcer should have multiple biopsies of the base and rim of the lesion, and brush cytology should be considered. Gastritis is biopsied for histology and to rule out Helicobacter. The most serious complications of EGD are rare and include perforation, pulmonary aspiration,

TABLE 25-4 Alarm Symptoms That Indicate the Need
for Esophagogastroduodenoscopy

Weight loss
Recurrent vomiting
Dysphagia
Bleeding
Anemia

and respiratory depression from excessive sedation. Generally EGD is a more sensitive test than double contrast upper GI series, but these modalities should be considered complementary rather than competitive. Some anatomic abnormalities are more easily demonstrable or quantifiable on barium study than EGD (e.g., diverticula, fistula, tortuosity or stricture location, and size of hiatal hernia). Computed tomography (CT) scan or magnetic resonance imaging (MRI) should be part of the routine staging workup for most patients with a malignant gastric tumor. MRI may prove clinically useful as a quantitative test for gastric emptying, and may even hold some promise for the analysis of myoelectric derangements in patients with gastroparesis. Arteriography is rarely necessary or useful in the diagnosis of gastric disease. It may be helpful in the occasional poor risk patient with exsanguinating gastric hemorrhage, or in the patient with hard to diagnose occult gastric bleeding. Extravasation of contrast indicates the bleeding vessel, and embolization or selective infusion of vasopressin may be therapeutic. Occasionally empiric embolization of the suspected but unproven bleeding vessel helps. Arteriovenous malformations have a characteristic angiographic appearance.

Endoscopic ultrasound (EUS) is useful in the evaluation of some gastric lesions. Local/regional staging of gastric tumors is best accomplished with EUS. Enlarged nodes can be sampled with EUS guided endoscopic needle biopsy. Malignant tumors that are confined to the mucosa on EUS may be amenable to endoscopic resection, although locally advanced tumors may merit neoadjuvant treatment. EUS can also be used to assess the response of gastric lymphoma to chemotherapy.

Analysis of gastric acid output requires gastric intubation. This somewhat uncomfortable test may be useful in the evaluation of patients for Zollinger-Ellison syndrome, patients with refractory ulcer or GERD, and patients with recurrent ulcer after operation. Historically gastric analysis was performed most commonly to test for the adequacy of vagotomy in postoperative patients with recurrent or persistent ulcer. However this can also be done by assessing peripheral pancreatic polypeptide levels in response to sham feeding. A 50 percent increase of PP within 30 min of sham feeding suggests vagal integrity. Nuclear medicine tests can be helpful in the evaluation of gastric emptying and duodenogastric reflux. The standard scintigraphic evaluation of gastric emptying involves the ingestion of a test meal with one or two isotopes and scanning of the patient under a gamma camera. A curve for liquid and solid emptying is plotted and the T1/2 calculated. Normal standards exist for each facility. Duodenogastric reflux can be quantitated by the intravenous administration of dimethyl iminodiacedic acid (HIDA), which is concentrated and excreted by the liver into the duodenum. Software allows a semiquantitative assessment of how much of the isotope refluxes into the stomach. Lymphoscintigraphy may evolve as a useful staging test for gastric cancer.

A variety of tests can help determine whether or not the patient has active Helicobacter infection (Table 25-5). The predictive value (positive and negative) of any of the tests used as a screening tool depends on the prevalence of Helicobacter infection in the screened population. A positive test is quite accurate in predicting Helicobacter infection, but a negative test is characteristically unreliable. Thus in the appropriate clinical setting, treatment for Helicobacter should be initiated on the basis of a positive test, but not necessarily withheld if the test is negative. Antroduodenal motility testing and electrogastrography (EGG)

TABLE 25-5 Tests for *Helicobacter pylori*

Test	When to use	Why	Why not
Serologic test	Test of choice when endoscopy is not indicated and is not an option and when the patient has not received antimicrobial therapy for *H. pylori* infection	Noninvasive; sensitivity of >80%, specificity of about 90%	Does not confirm eradication, because serologic "scar" remains for indefinite period after microbiologic cure
Urea breath test	Preferred for confirming cure of *H. pylori* infection, but no sooner than 4 wk after completion of therapy	Simple; sensitivity and specificity of 90 to 99%	False-negatives possible if testing is done too soon after treatment with proton pump inhibitors, antimicrobials, or bismuth compounds; small radiation exposure with ^{14}C method; expensive
Histologic test	To directly ascertain presence of *H. pylori* when endoscopy is being used; also used when determination of neoplastic status of lesion is necessary	Sensitivity of 80–100%, specificity of >95%; hematoxylin-eosin and Diff-Quik stains are simplest; Genta stain has sensitivity of >95% and specificity of 99%	Requires laboratory facilities and experience; when hematoxylin-eosin stain is nondiagnostic, second staining method is required
Rapid urease test	Simplest method when endoscopy is necessary	Simple; rapid (once biopsy specimen has been obtained); sensitivity of 80 to 95%, specificity of 95 to 100%	Invasive; false-negatives possible if testing is done too soon after treatment with proton pump inhibitors, antimicrobials, or bismuth compounds
Culture	After repeated failure of appropriate combination antibiotic therapy; when antimicrobial resistance is suspected or high level of resistance exists in the population	Allows determination of antibiotic susceptibility	Time-consuming; expensive; usually not necessary unless resistance is suspected

Source: Reproduced with permission from Graham DY, et al: *Postgraduate Medicine* 105:113, 1999.

are performed in specialized centers and may be useful in the evaluation of the patient with poorly explained epigastric symptoms. Electrogastrography consists of the transcutaneous recording of gastric myoelectric activity. Antroduodenal motility testing is done with a tube place transnasally or transorally into distal duodenum. There are pressure recording points extending from the stomach to the distal duodenum. The combination of these two tests together with scintigraphy provides a thorough assessment of gastric motility.

PEPTIC ULCER DISEASE

Peptic ulcer remains a common outpatient diagnosis, but the number of physician visits, hospital admissions, and elective operations for peptic ulcer disease have decreased steadily and dramatically over the past three decades. These trends all predated the advent of fiberoptic endoscopy, highly selective vagotomy, and H_2 blockers. The incidence of emergency operation and the death rate for peptic ulcer are fairly stable however. These epidemiologic trends probably represent the net effect of several factors including decreased prevalence of Helicobacter infection, better medical therapy, increase in outpatient management, and NSAID/aspirin use (with and without ulcer prophylaxis).

Pathophysiology

A variety of factors may contribute to the development of peptic ulcer. Although it is now recognized that the large majority of duodenal and gastric ulcers are "caused by" Helicobacter infestation and/or nonsteroidal antiinflammatory drug use, the final common pathway to ulcer formation is acid-peptic injury of the gastroduodenal mucosal barrier. Thus the adage, "no acid, no ulcer," is as true today as it ever was. Acid suppression either with medication or surgery remains a mainstay in healing both duodenal and gastric ulcers and in preventing recurrence. It is generally thought that Helicobacter predisposes to ulceration both by acid hypersecretion and by compromise of mucosal defense mechanisms. NSAIDs are thought to lead to peptic ulcer predominantly by compromise of mucosal defenses. Duodenal ulcer has typically been thought of as a disease of increased acid peptic aggression on the duodenal mucosa, whereas gastric ulcer has been viewed as a disease of weakened mucosal defenses in the face of relatively normal acid peptic aggression. However increased understanding of the pathophysiology of peptic ulcer has blurred this distinction. Clearly weakened mucosal defenses play a role in many duodenal and most gastric ulcers (e.g., duodenal ulcer in Helicobacter negative patient on NSAIDs; or typical type I gastric ulcer with acid hyposecretion); whereas acid peptic aggression may result in a duodenal or gastric ulcer in the setting of normal mucosal defenses (e.g., duodenal ulcer in patient with Zollinger-Ellison syndrome; gastric ulcer in patient with gastric outlet obstruction, antral stasis, and acid hypersecretion).

Elimination of *H. pylori* infection or NSAID use is important for optimal ulcer healing and perhaps even more important in preventing recurrence and/or complications. A variety of other diseases are known to cause peptic ulcer, including Zollinger-Ellison Syndrome (gastrinoma), antral G-cell hyperfunction and/or hyperplasia, systemic mastocytosis, trauma, burns, and major physiological stress. Other "causative agents" are drugs (all NSAIDs, aspirin, cocaine), smoking, alcohol and psychological stress. Probably in the United

States, over 90 percent of serious peptic ulcer complications can be attributed to Helicobacter infection, NSAID use, and cigarette smoking.

The *H. pylori* bacteria are uniquely equipped for survival in the hostile environment of the stomach. It possesses the urease enzyme which converts urea into ammonia and bicarbonate creating an environment around the bacteria which buffers the acid secreted by the stomach. *H. pylori* infection is associated with decreased levels of gastric mucosal somatostatin production, hypergastrinemia and acid hypersecretion. The acid hypersecretion and the antral gastritis are thought to lead to antral epithelial metaplasia in the post-pyloric duodenum. This duodenal metaplasia allows *H. pylori* to colonize the duodenal mucosa and in these patients the risk of developing a duodenal ulcer increases 50-fold. When *H. pylori* colonizes the duodenum, there is a significant decrease in acid-stimulated duodenal bicarbonate release. Likewise, Helicobacter predisposes to gastric ulcer at least in part by weakening mucosal defenses. It is clear from multiple randomized prospective studies that curing *H. pylori* infection dramatically decreases the risk of recurrent ulcer.

As a rule duodenal ulcer patients secrete more acid than patients with gastric ulcer. It has long been recognized that duodenal ulcer patients as a group have a higher mean basal acid output (BAO) and also a higher mean maximal acid output (MAO) than normal controls. However many duodenal ulcer patients have basal and peak acid outputs in the normal range and there is no correlation between acid secretion and the severity of the ulcer disease. Some patients with duodenal ulcer also have increased rates of gastric emptying which delivers an increased acid load per unit of time to the duodenum. Finally the buffering capacity of the duodenum in many patients with duodenal ulcer is compromised because of decreased duodenal bicarbonate secretion.

In patients with gastric ulcer, acid secretion is variable. Generally, four types of gastric ulcer are described. The most common Johnson type I gastric ulcer is typically located near the angularis incisura on the lesser curvature, close to the border between the antrum and the body of the stomach. Usually these patients have normal or decreased acid secretion. Type II gastric ulcer is associated with active or quiescent duodenal ulcer disease, and type III gastric ulcer is prepyloric. Both type II and type III gastric ulcers are associated with normal or increased gastric acid secretion. Type IV gastric ulcer occurs near the gastroesophageal junction and acid secretion is normal or below normal. Patients with Type I or IV gastric ulcer may have weak mucosal defenses which permit an abnormal amount of injurious acid back-diffusion into the mucosa. Duodenogastric reflux may play a role in weakening the gastric mucosal defenses in patients with gastric ulcer. A variety of components in duodenal juice, including bile, lysolecithin, and pancreatic juice, has been shown to cause injury and inflammation in the gastric mucosa. NSAIDs and aspirin have similar effects.

NSAIDs (including aspirin) are inextricably linked to peptic ulcer disease. Patients with rheumatoid arthritis and osteoarthritis who take NSAIDs have a 15–20 percent annual incidence of peptic ulcer, and the prevalence of peptic ulcer in chronic NSAID users is about 25 percent (15 percent gastric and 10 percent duodenal). Complications of peptic ulcer disease (specifically hemorrhage and perforation) are much more common in patients taking NSAIDs. More than half of patients who present with peptic ulcer hemorrhage or perforation report the recent use of nonsteroidal antiinflammatory drugs, including aspirin. Many of these patients remain asymptomatic up until the time they develop these life threatening complications. This problem is put into prospective when one realizes that approximately 20 million patients in the United States take NSAIDs on a regular basis; perhaps as many regularly take aspirin.

Factors which clearly put patients at increased risk for NSAID-induced GI complications include age older than 60, prior GI event, high NSAID dose, concurrent steroid intake, and concurrent anticoagulant intake. Any patient taking NSAIDs or aspirin who has one or more of these risk factors should receive concomitant acid suppressive medication or misoprostol at a therapeutic dose or should be considered for alternative treatment with cyclooxygenas-2 (COX-2) inhibitors.

Epidemiologic studies suggest that smokers are about twice as likely to develop peptic ulcer disease as nonsmokers. Smoking increases gastric acid secretion and duodenogastric reflux. Smoking decreases both gastroduodenal prostaglandin production and pancreaticoduodenal bicarbonate production. These observations may be related, and any or all could explain the observed association between smoking and peptic ulcer disease. Although difficult to measure, both physiological and psychological stress undoubtedly play a role in the development of peptic ulcer in some patients. In 1842, Curling described duodenal ulcer and/or duodenitis in burn patients. Decades later, Cushing described the appearance of acute peptic ulceration in patients with head trauma (Cushing ulcer). Recently, the use of crack cocaine has been linked to juxtapyloric peptic ulcers with a propensity to perforate. Alcohol is commonly mentioned as a risk factor for peptic ulcer disease, but confirmatory data are lacking.

Clinical Manifestations and Diagnosis

Over 90 percent of patients with peptic ulcer complain of abdominal pain. The pain is typically nonradiating, burning in quality and located in the epigastrium. Other signs and symptoms include nausea, bloating, weight loss, positive stool for occult blood, and anemia. In the young patient with dyspepsia and/or epigastric pain, it may be appropriate to initiate empiric therapy for peptic ulcer disease without confirmatory testing. All patients with the above symptoms over 45 should have an upper endoscopy, and all patients regardless of age should have this study if any alarm symptoms (see Table 25-4) are present. A good double contrast upper GI radiograph study may be useful. All gastric ulcers should be adequately biopsied, and any sites of gastritis should be biopsied to rule out Helicobacter, and for histologic evaluation. Additional testing for Helicobacter may be indicated. Although somewhat controversial, it is not unreasonable to test all peptic ulcer patients for Helicobacter. A baseline serum gastrin is appropriate to rule out gastrinoma.

The three complications of peptic ulcer disease, in decreasing order of frequency, are bleeding, perforation, and obstruction now account for the large majority of operations performed for peptic ulcer disease, and essentially all of the deaths (most of which are because of bleeding).

Medical Treatment of Peptic Ulcer

Patients with peptic ulcer should stop smoking, and avoid alcohol and NSAIDs (including aspirin). If Helicobacter infection is documented, it should be treated with one of numerous acceptable regimens (Table 25-6). If initial Helicobacter testing is negative, the ulcer patient may be treated with H_2 receptor blockers or proton pump inhibitors. Sucralfate or misoprostol may also be effective. If ulcer symptoms persist, an empiric trial of anti-Helicobacter therapy is reasonable

TABLE 25-6 Treatment Regimens for *Helicobacter pylori* Infections

Bismuth triple therapy
Bismuth, 2 tablets four times daily
plus
Metronidazole, 250 mg three times daily
plus
Tetracycline, 500 mg four times daily

PPI triple therapy
PPI twice daily
plus
Amoxicillin, 1000 mg two times daily
plus
Clarithromycin, 500 mg two times daily
or
Metronidazole, 500 mg two times daily

Quadruple therapy
PPI twice daily
plus
Bismuth, 2 tablets four times daily
plus
Metronidazole, 250 mg three times daily
plus
Tetracycline, 500 mg four times daily

Note: Treatment for 10–14 days is recommended.
PPI = proton pump inhibitor.

(false negative Helicobacter tests are not uncommon). Generally antisecretory therapy can be stopped after 3 months if the ulcerogenic stimulus (Helicobacter or NSAIDs or aspirin) has been removed. However long-term maintenance therapy for peptic ulcer should be considered in all patients admitted to hospital with an ulcer complication, all high-risk patients on NSAIDs or aspirin (the older adult or debilitated), and all patients with a history of recurrent ulcer or bleeding. Consideration should be given to maintenance therapy in persistent smokers with a history of peptic ulcer. Misoprostol, sucralfate, and acid suppression may be quite comparable in many of these groups, but misoprostol may cause diarrhea and cramps, and cannot be used in women of child-bearing age because of its abortifacient properties.

Surgical Treatment of Peptic Ulcer

Fundamentally, the vast majority of peptic ulcers requiring operation are adequately treated by a variant of one of three basic procedures: highly selective vagotomy; vagotomy and drainage; vagotomy and distal gastrectomy (Table 25-7).

Highly selective vagotomy (HSV), also called parietal cell vagotomy or proximal gastric vagotomy, is safe (mortality risk <0.5 percent) and causes minimal side effects. The operation severs the vagal supply to the proximal two thirds of the stomach, in which essentially all the parietal cells are located. It preserves the vagal innervation to the antrum and pylorus, and the remaining abdominal viscera. HSV decreases total gastric acid secretion by about 65–75 percent, which is quite comparable to truncal vagotomy or acid suppressive medication. Gastric emptying of solids is typically normal in patients

TABLE 25-7 Clinical Results of Surgery for Duodenal Ulcer

	Parietal cell vagotomy	Truncal vagotomy and pyloroplasty	Truncal vagotomy and antrectomy
Operative mortality rate (%)	0	<1	1
Ulcer recurrence rate (%)	5–15	5–15	< 2
Dumping (%)			
Mild	< 5	10	10–15
Severe	0	1	1–2
Diarrhea (%)			
Mild	< 5	25	20
Severe	0	2	1–2

Source: Modified with permission from Mulholland MW, Debas HT: Chronic duodenal and gastric ulcer. *Surg Clin North Am* 67:489, 1987.

after parietal cell vagotomy; liquid emptying may be normal or increased because of decreased compliance associated with loss of receptive relaxation and accommodation. When applied to uncomplicated duodenal ulcer, the recurrent ulcer rate is higher with HSV than with vagotomy and antrectomy. However our increased understanding of the pathophysiologic role of Helicobacter and NSAIDs in the development of recurrent ulcer may mitigate this concern. HSV has not performed particularly well as a treatment for type II (gastric and duodenal) and III (prepyloric) gastric ulcer, perhaps because of hypergastrinemia caused by gastric outlet obstruction and persistent antral stasis.

Truncal vagotomy and pyloroplasty, and truncal vagotomy and gastrojejunostomy are the paradigmatic vagotomy and drainage procedures (TV and D), although total gastric vagotomy (selective vagotomy [SV]) and drainage, and HSV and gastrojejunostomy have also been shown to be effective ulcer operations in selected patients. The advantage of TV and D is that it can be performed safely and quickly by the experienced surgeon. The main disadvantage is the side effect profile (10 percent with significant dumping and/or diarrhea), and a 10 percent recurrent ulcer rate. Whether the incidence of these postoperative problems (heretofore determined in studies predominantly involving patients with intractable uncomplicated duodenal ulcer) will be different in the current era of complicated ulcer, Helicobacter, and NSAIDs is unknown.

Truncal vagotomy denervates the antropyloric mechanism and therefore some sort of procedure is necessary to ablate or bypass the pylorus, otherwise gastric stasis often results. Gastrojejunostomy or pyloroplasty are the classic drainage procedures.

The advantage of vagotomy and antrectomy (V and A) is the extremely low ulcer recurrence rate and the applicability of the operation to many patients with complicated peptic ulcer (e.g., bleeding duodenal and gastric ulcer; obstructing peptic ulcer; nonhealing gastric ulcer; recurrent ulcer). When applied to gastric ulcer, the resection is usually extended far enough proximally to include the ulcer. The disadvantage of V and A is the somewhat higher operative mortality rate when compared with HSV, or V and D. Following antrectomy, gastrointestinal continuity may be re-established either as a Billroth I gastroduodenostomy or a Billroth II loop gastrojejunostomy. Because antrectomy routinely leaves a 60–70 percent gastric remnant, reconstruction as a Roux gastrojejunostomy should be avoided. The Roux operation is an excellent procedure for keeping duodenal contents out of the stomach and esophagus. But

TABLE 25-8 Surgical Options in the Treatment of Duodenal and
Gastric Ulcer Disease

Indication	Duodenal	Gastric
Bleeding	1. Oversew[a] 2. Oversew, V + D 3. V + A	1. Oversew and biopsy[a] 2. Oversew, biopsy, V + D 3. Distal gastrectomy[b]
Perforation	1. Patch[a] 2. Patch, HSV[b] 3. Patch, V + D	1. Biopsy and patch[a] 2. Wedge excision, V + D 3. Distal gastrectomy[b]
Obstruction	1. HSV + GJ 2. V + A	1. Biopsy; HSV + GJ 2. Distal gastrectomy[b]
Intractability/ nonhealing	1. HSV[b] 2. V + D 3. V + A	1. HSV and wedge excision 2. Distal gastrectomy

[a]Unless the patient is in shock or moribund, a definitive procedure should be considered.
[b]Operation of choice in low-risk patient.
GJ = gastrojejunostomy; HSV = highly-selective vagotomy; V + A = vagotomy and antrectomy; V + D = vagotomy and drainage.

in the presence of a large gastric remnant, this reconstruction will predispose to marginal ulceration and/or gastric stasis.

Distal gastrectomy without vagotomy (usually approximately 50 percent gastrectomy to include the ulcer) has traditionally been the procedure of choice for type I gastric ulcer. Reconstruction may be done as a Billroth I (preferable) or II. Truncal vagotomy is added for Type 2 and 3 gastric ulcers, or if the patient is believed to be at increased risk for recurrent ulcer, and should be considered if Billroth II reconstruction is contemplated. Although not routinely used nowadays in the surgical treatment of peptic ulcer, subtotal gastrectomy (75 percent distal gastrectomy) without vagotomy may be an appealing operation for an occasional ulcer patient.

The choice of operation for the individual patient with peptic ulcer disease depends on a variety of factors including (inter alia) the type of ulcer (duodenal, gastric, recurrent or marginal), the indication for operation, and the condition of the patient. Other important considerations are intraabdominal factors (duodenal scarring/inflammation; adhesions; difficult exposure), the virulence of the ulcer diathesis, the surgeon's experience and personal preference, the Helicobacter status, the need for continued NSAID therapy, previous treatment, and the likelihood of future compliance with treatment. Table 25-8 shows the surgical options for managing various aspects of peptic ulcer disease. In general, resective procedures have a lower ulcer recurrence rate, but a higher operative morbidity and mortality (see Table 25-7) when compared to nonresective ulcer operations. We now know that ulcer recurrence is often related to Helicobacter and/or NSAIDs, and usually is managed adequately without reoperation. Thus gastric resection to minimize recurrence in duodenal ulcer disease is often not justified today; resection for gastric ulcer remains the standard because of the risk of cancer.

Bleeding

Patients coming to operation for bleeding peptic ulcer today are more selected toward a poor surgical result then ever before. The surgical options for treating bleeding peptic ulcer are three: suture ligation of the bleeder (and biopsy for gastric ulcer); suture ligation and definitive nonresective ulcer operation (HSV or V and D); and gastric resection (usually including vagotomy and ulcer excision). Indications for operation in bleeding ulcer are: (1) massive hemorrhage unresponsive to endoscopic control, (2) transfusion requirement of greater than 4 to 6 units of blood despite attempts at endoscopic control. Unavailability of therapeutic endoscopist, recurrent hemorrhage after one or more attempts at endoscopic control, unavailability of blood for transfusion, repeat hospitalization for bleeding duodenal ulcer and concurrent indication for surgery such as perforation or obstruction are also indications for operation. Early operation should be considered in patients over 60, those presenting in shock, those requiring more than four units of blood in 24 h or eight units of blood in 48 h, those with rebleeding, and those with ulcers greater than 2 cm in diameter or strategically located as described above.

The two operations most commonly used for bleeding duodenal ulcer are: vagotomy and drainage combined with oversewing of the ulcer, or vagotomy and antrectomy. The trade-off appears to be an increased risk of rebleeding with the vagotomy and drainage procedure versus the increased operative mortality of vagotomy and antrectomy. When the mortality for reoperation for rebleeding is considered, the overall mortality is probably comparable for the two approaches. Patients who are in shock or medically unstable should not have gastric resection.

Bleeding gastric ulcer tends to occur in older and/or medically complicated patients that tend to increase the operative risk. Although this has been used by some as an excuse not to operate early on these patients, experience shows that planned operation in a resuscitated patient results in a better operative mortality than emergent operation in a patient who has rebled and is in shock. Those patients with gastric ulcer bleeding likely to require operation have bled more than six units and have presented in shock. Endoscopically their ulcers tend to be on the lesser curvature with the usual stigmata of recent hemorrhage. Distal gastric resection to include the bleeding ulcer is the operation of choice for bleeding gastric ulcer. Second best is vagotomy and drainage, with oversewing and biopsy of the ulcer. Oversewing of the bleeder followed by long-term acid suppression is a reasonable alternative in extremely high risk patients. The specter of cancer is ever present in the patient with gastric ulcer whether it is bleeding or not.

Perforation

Perforation is the second most common complication of peptic ulcer. As with bleeding peptic ulcer, NSAIDS also have been inextricably linked with perforated peptic ulcer disease especially in the older adult population. Well over 20 percent of patients older than the age of 60 presenting with a perforated ulcer are taking NSAIDS at the time of perforation. Operation is almost always indicated although occasionally nonoperative treatment can be used in the stable patient without peritonitis and in whom radiologic studies document a sealed perforation. The options for surgical treatment of perforated duodenal ulcer are simple patch closure, patch closure and HSV, or patch closure and TV/D. Simple patch closure alone should be done in patients with hemodynamic instability and/or exudative peritonitis signifying a perforation over 24 h old. In all other patients the addition of a definitive ulcer operation (HSV or V and D) should be considered. Numerous studies have reported a negligible mortality with this approach. Early data now suggest that simple closure of perforated duodenal ulcer may achieve satisfactory long term results when *H. pylori* infection (present in 50–75 percent with perforated duodenal ulcer) is eliminated. On the other hand it is sometimes difficult to determine the *H. pylori* status of the patient having emergent operation for perforated ulcer. Furthermore it is doubtful whether many of these patients will comply with the medication regimen required to eradicate Helicobacter. Thus using possible *H. pylori* infection as an excuse not to do a definitive ulcer operation in any patients with perforated duodenal ulcer is irrational. Perforated gastric ulcer carriers a higher mortality rate than perforated duodenal ulcer (10–40 percent). This is generally through to represent the gastric ulcer patients' higher age, increased medical comorbidities, delay in seeking medical attention and large size of gastric ulcers. Perforated gastric ulcers are associated with NSAIDS and tobacco use, and often present without prior symptoms. All perforated gastric ulcers are best treated by gastric resection (to include the ulcer) with or without truncal vagotomy depending on ulcer type. Vagotomy is usually performed for type II and III gastric ulcers. Patch closure with biopsy; or local excision and closure; or biopsy, closure, truncal vagotomy and drainage are alternative operations. All perforated gastric ulcers even those in the pre pyloric position should be biopsied if they are not removed at surgery.

Obstruction

Gastric outlet obstruction is the least common ulcer complication requiring operative treatment. Endoscopic balloon dilation can often transiently improve obstructive symptoms, but many of these patients ultimately fail and come to operation. The most common operations for obstructing peptic ulcer disease are vagotomy and antrectomy, and vagotomy and drainage. HSV and gastrojejunostomy is an appealing operation for obstruction, both because it can be done as a laparoscopic assisted procedure, and because it does not complicate future resection should this be needed. All gastric ulcers associated with obstruction should be adequately biopsied if not resected.

Intractability/Nonhealing

This should indeed be a rare indication for operation nowadays. Arguably, the patient referred for surgical evaluation because of intractable peptic ulcer disease should raise red flags with the surgeon. Acid secretion can be totally blocked and Helicobacter eradicated with modern medication, so why does the patient have a persistent ulcer diathesis? The surgeon should review the differential diagnosis of nonhealing ulcer (Table 25-9) prior to any consideration of operative treatment. Surgical treatment should be considered in patients with nonhealing or intractable peptic ulcer who have multiple recurrences, large ulcers (>2 cm), complications (obstruction, perforation or hemorrhage), or suspected gastric cancer. Operation should be considered most cautiously in the thin or marginally nourished individual.

If operation is necessary for intractability, less is often better. Our preferred operations for this group of patients is HSV. In patients with nonhealing gastric ulcer, wedge resection either with HSV or TV and D should be considered in thin or frail patients, and it patients with inconveniently situated ulcers (biopsy alone is sometimes appropriate). Otherwise distal gastrectomy (to include the ulcer) is recommended. It is unnecessary to add a vagotomy to distal gastrectomy in all patients with Type I gastric ulcer.

TABLE 25-9 Differential Diagnosis of Intractability or Nonhealing Peptic Ulcer Disease

Cancer
  Gastric
  Pancreatic
  Duodenal
Persistent *H. pylori* infection
  Tests may be false-negative
  Consider empiric treatment
Noncompliant patient
  Failure to take prescribed medication
  Surreptitious use of nonsteroidal anti-inflammatory drugs
Motility disorder
Zollinger-Ellison syndrome

Zollinger-Ellison Syndrome

Zollinger-Ellison syndrome (ZES) is caused by the uncontrolled secretion of abnormal amounts of gastrin by a pancreatic or duodenal neuroendocrine tumor, i.e., gastrinoma. The inherited or familial form of gastrinoma (20 percent of cases) is associated with multiple endocrine neoplasia type I (MEN I) which consists of parathyroid, pituitary, and pancreatic (or duodenal) tumors. Patients with MEN I usually have multiple gastrinoma tumors and surgical cure is unusual. Sporadic gastrinomas are more often solitary and amenable to surgical cure. Nowadays about 50 percent of gastrinomas are malignant, with lymph node, liver, or other distant metastases at presentation. Five-year survival in patients presenting with metastatic disease is around 40 percent.

The most common symptoms of ZES are epigastric pain, GERD, and diarrhea. The average age of presentation is 50 years, and over 90 percent of patients with gastrinoma have peptic ulcer. Most ulcers are in the typical location (proximal duodenum), but atypical ulcer location (distal duodenum, jejunum, multiple ulcers) should prompt an evaluation for gastrinoma. Gastrinoma should also be considered in the differential diagnosis of recurrent or refractory peptic ulcer, secretory diarrhea, gastric rugal hypertrophy, esophagitis with stricture, bleeding or perforated ulcer, familial ulcer, and ulcer in the setting of hypercalcemia. Causes of hypergastrinemia can be divided into those associated with hyperacidity and those associated with hypoacidity (Table 25-10). The diagnosis of ZES is confirmed by the secretin stimulation test.

TABLE 25-10 Differential Diagnosis of Hypergastrinemia

With excessive gastric acid formation (ulcerogenic)
  Zollinger-Ellison syndrome
  Gastric outlet obstruction
  Retained gastric antrum (after Billroth II reconstruction)
  G-cell hyperplasia
Without excessive gastric acid formation (nonulcerogenic)
  Pernicious anemia
  Atrophic gastritis
  Renal failure
  Postvagotomy
  Short gut syndrome (after significant intestinal resection)

Eighty percent of primary tumors are found in the gastrinoma triangle and many tumors are small (<1 cm) making preoperative localization difficult. Transabdominal ultrasound is quite specific, but not very sensitive. CT scan will detect most lesions over 2 cm and MRI is comparable. Endoscopic ultrasound is more sensitive than these other noninvasive imaging tests, but it still misses many of the smaller lesions, and may confuse normal lymph nodes for gastrinoma. Currently, the imaging study of choice for gastrinoma is somatostatin receptor scintigraphy (SRS, the octreotide scan). Arteriography with selective visceral arterial infusion of secretin, and simultaneous hepatic venous gastrin sampling, may help localize the tumor as inside or outside the gastrinoma triangle.

All patients with sporadic (nonfamilial) gastrinoma should be considered for surgical resection and possible cure. Thorough exploration by an experienced surgeon is important. The lesion should be found in 90 percent of patients and 60 percent are cured. Acid hypersecretion in patients with gastrinoma can always be managed with high dose proton pump inhibitors. Highly selective vagotomy may make management easier in some patients and should be considered in patients with surgically untreatable or unresectable gastrinoma.

MALIGNANT NEOPLASMS OF THE STOMACH

The three most common primary malignant gastric neoplasms are adenocarcinoma (95 percent), lymphoma (4 percent), and malignant gastrointestinal stromal tumor (GIST) (1 percent).

Adenocarcinoma (Gastric Cancer)

Gastric cancer is more common in patients with atrophic gastritis, pernicious anemia, blood group A, or a family history of gastric cancer. Other commonly accepted risk factors for gastric cancer include diet (nitrates, salt, fat), gastric adenomas, familial polyposis, hereditary nonpolyposis colorectal cancer, smoking, and Menetrier disease. A variety of genetic abnormalities have been described in gastric cancer (Table 25-11).

Premalignant Conditions of the Stomach

Polyps. There are five types of gastric epithelial polyps: inflammatory, hamartomatous, heterotopic, hyperplastic, and adenoma. The first three types have negligible malignant potential. Adenomas can lead to carcinoma, just like in the colon, and they should be removed when diagnosed. Occasionally, hyperplastic polyps can lead to carcinoma (<2 percent). Patients with familial adenomatous polyposis (FAP) have a high prevalence of gastric adenomatous polyps (about 50 percent), and are 10 times more likely to develop adenocarcinoma of the stomach than the general population.

Atrophic gastritis. Chronic atrophic gastritis is by far the most common precursor for gastric cancer, particularly the intestinal subtype. In many patients, it is likely that Helicobacter is involved in the pathogenesis of atrophic gastritis. An individual's risk of gastric cancer is proportional to the extent of intestinal metaplasia of the gastric mucosa, suggesting that intestinal metaplasia is a precursor lesion to gastric cancer. There is evidence that eradication of Helicobacter infection leads to significant regression of intestinal metaplasia and improvement in atrophic gastritis. Thus Helicobacter treatment is a

TABLE 25-11 Genetic Abnormalities in Gastric Cancer

Abnormalities	Gene	Approximate frequency (%)
Deletion/suppression	*p53*	60–70
	FHIT	60
	APC	50
	DCC	50
	E-cadherin	<5
Amplification/overexpression	*COX-2*	70
	HGF/SF	60
	VEGF	50
	c-met	45
	AIB-1	40
	β-catenin	25
	k-sam	20
	ras	10–15
	c-erb B-2	5–7
Microsatellite instability		25–40
DNA aneuploidy		60–75

Source: Reproduced with permission from Koh TJ, Wang TC in *Sleisenger & Fordtran's Gastrointestinal and Liver Diseases,* 7th ed. Philadelphia: Saunders, 2002.

reasonable recommendation for patients with atrophic gastritis and Helicobacter infection.

Gastric remnant cancer. It has long been recognized that stomach cancer can develop in the gastric remnant, usually years following distal gastrectomy for peptic ulcer disease. The risk is controversial, but the phenomenon is real. Most tumors develop more than 10 years following the initial operation, and they usually arise in an area of chronic gastritis, metaplasia, and dysplasia.

Other premalignant states. Up to 10 percent of gastric cancer cases appear "to run in families", even without a clear cut genetic diagnosis such as familial polyposis. First degree relatives of patients with gastric cancer have an increased risk of 2 to 3 fold. Patients with hereditary nonpolyposis colorectal cancer (HNPCC) have a 10 percent risk of developing gastric cancer, predominantly the intestinal subtype. The mucous cell hyperplasia of Menetrier disease is generally considered to carry a 5–10 percent risk of adenocarcinoma, but the glandular hyperplasia associated with gastrinoma is not premalignant.

Pathology of Stomach Cancer

It is generally accepted that gastric dysplasia is the universal precursor to gastric adenocarcinoma. Clearly, patients with severe dysplasia require some sort of ablative treatment, usually gastric resection. Patients with mild dysplasia should be followed carefully with endoscopic biopsy surveillance.

Early gastric cancer is defined as adenocarcinoma limited to mucosa and submucosa of the stomach, regardless of lymph node status. About 10 percent of patients with early gastric cancer will have lymph node metastases. About 70 percent of early gastric cancers are well differentiated, and 30 percent are poorly differentiated. The overall cure rate with adequate gastric resection and lymphadenectomy in early gastric cancer is 95 percent. In some Japanese centers, 50 percent of gastric cancers treated are early gastric cancer. In the United States, less than 20 percent of resected gastric adenocarcinomas are early.

There are four gross forms of gastric cancer: polypoid, fungating, ulcerative, and scirrhous. In the first two, the bulk of the tumor mass is intraluminal. In the latter two gross subtypes, the bulk of the tumor mass is in the wall of the stomach. Scirrhous tumors (linitis plastica) have a particularly poor prognosis, and not uncommonly involve the entire stomach. Although these latter lesions may be technically resectable with total gastrectomy, not uncommonly both the esophageal and duodenal margin of resection will show microscopic evidence of tumor infiltration. Death from recurrent disease within 6 months is the rule. The location of the primary tumor in the stomach is important in planning operation. Several decades ago, the large majority of gastric cancers were in the distal stomach. Recently there is a proximal migration of tumors in the stomach so that currently the distribution is closer to 40 percent for distal, 30 percent for mid, and 30 percent for proximal.

Histology

The most important prognostic indicators in gastric cancer are both histologic: lymph node involvement and depth of tumor invasion. Tumor grade (degree of differentiation: well, moderate, poor) is also important prognostically. The most widespread system for staging of gastric cancer is the TNM staging system based on depth of tumor invasion (T), extent of lymph node metastases (N), and presence of distant metastases (M).

Clinical Manifestations (History and Physical Examination)

Most patients who are diagnosed with gastric cancer in the United States have advanced stage III or IV disease at the time of diagnosis (Table 25-12). The most common symptoms are weight loss and decreased food intake because of anorexia and early satiety. Abdominal pain (usually not severe and often ignored) is also common. Other symptoms include nausea, vomiting and bloating. Acute GI bleeding is somewhat unusual (5 percent), but chronic occult blood loss is common and manifests as iron deficiency anemia and heme positive stool. Dysphagia is common if the tumor involves the cardia of the stomach. Physical examination is usually normal. Other than weight loss, specific physical findings usually indicate incurability. It is important to check for these findings: cervical, supraclavicular (on the left referred to as Virchow node) and axillary lymphadenopathy; metastatic pleural effusion or aspiration pneumonitis; abdominal mass (large primary tumor, liver metastases, or carcinomatosis); palpable umbilical metastasis (Sister Joseph nodule); ascites; "drop metastases" or rectal shelf of Blumer in the pouch of Douglas.

Diagnostic Evaluation

Distinguishing between peptic ulcer and gastric cancer on clinical grounds alone is often impossible. Essentially all patients in whom gastric cancer is on the differential diagnosis should have endoscopy and biopsy. If suspicion for cancer is high and the biopsy is negative, the patient should be re-endoscoped and more aggressively biopsied. Preoperative staging of gastric cancer is best accomplished with abdominal/pelvic CT scan with intravenous and oral

TABLE 25-12 TNM Staging of Gastric Cancer by the
International Union Against Cancer
and American Joint Committee on Cancer

T: Primary tumor

Tis	Carcinoma in situ; Intraepithelial tumor without invasion of lamina propria
T1	Tumor invades lamina propria or submucosa
T2	Tumor invades muscularis propria or subserosa
T3	Tumor penetrates serosa (visceral peritoneum) without invasion of adjacent structures
T4	Tumor invades adjacent structures

N: Regional lymph node

N0	No regional lymph node metastasis
N1	Metastasis in 1 to 6 regional lymph nodes
N2	Metastasis in 7 to 15 lymph nodes
N3	Metastasis in more than 15 regional lymph nodes

M: Distant metastasis

M0	No distant metastasis
M1	Distant metastasis

Stage grouping

Stage	T	N	M
0	Tis	N0	M0
IA	T1	N0	M0
IB	T1	N1	M0
	T2	N0	M0
II	T1	N2	M0
	T2	N1	M0
	T3	N0	M0
IIIA	T2	N2	M0
	T3	N1	M0
	T4	N0	M0
IIIB	T3	N2	M0
IV	T4	N1–3	M0
	T1–3	N3	M0
	Any T	Any N	M1

Source: Reproduced with permission from Greene FL, *AJCC Cancer Staging Manual,* 6th ed. New York: Springer–Verlag, 2002.

contrast. MRI is probably comparable. The best way to stage the tumor locally is endoscopic ultrasound which gives accurate information about the depth of tumor penetration into the gastric wall and can usually show enlarged perigastric and celiac lymph nodes. In some centers, if the tumor is transmural (T3) or involves lymph nodes (enlarged nodes can usually be needled under ultrasound guidance), preoperative (neoadjuvant) cancer therapy is given. EUS is quite accurate in distinguishing early gastric cancer (T1) from more advanced tumors. PET scan should be considered prior to major operation in patients with particularly high risk tumors, or multiple medical comorbidities. The usefulness of staging laparoscopy and/or peritoneal cytology in gastric cancer depends on the individual patient's situation and the treatment philosophy of the cancer team.

Treatment

Surgery is the only curative treatment for gastric cancer. It is also the best palliation, and provides the most accurate staging. The goal of curative surgical treatment is resection of all tumor (i.e., R0 resection). Thus all margins (proximal, distal, radial) should be negative and an adequate lymphadenectomy performed. Generally, the surgeon strives for a grossly negative proximal and distal margin of at least 5 cm, with frozen section confirmation of histologically negative margins. Patients with positive lymph nodes may be cured by adequate operation, and often nodes thought to be grossly positive at operation turn out to be histologically negative. Thus therapeutic nihilism should be avoided, and in the good risk patient an aggressive attempt to resect all tumor should be made.

Extent of Gastrectomy

The standard operation for gastric cancer is radical subtotal gastrectomy. Reconstruction is usually by Billroth II gastrojejunostomy, but if a small gastric remnant is left (<20 percent) a Roux reconstruction is considered. The operative mortality is around 5 percent. Radical subtotal gastrectomy is generally deemed to be an adequate cancer operation in most Western countries, provided that all gross tumor is resected with negative margins. In the absence of involvement by direct extension, the spleen and pancreatic tail are not removed. Total gastrectomy is not performed unless it is necessary to obtain an R0 resection. There have been several large studies comparing subtotal gastrectomy to total gastrectomy for gastric cancer and the survival results in the two groups have been the same. But the complication rate in the total gastrectomy group is higher. Total gastrectomy with jejunal pouch/esophageal anastomosis may be the best operation for patients with proximal gastric adenocarcinoma.

Extent of Lymphadenectomy

The Japanese have labeled all the lymph node stations which potentially drain the stomach. Generally these are grouped into level N1 (e.g., stations 1–6), level N2 (e.g., stations 7–11), and level N3 (e.g., stations 12–16) nodes. The nodal stations defined as level N1, N2, and N3 varies depending on the location of the tumor. In general, N1 nodes are within 3 cm of the tumor, N2 nodes are along the celiac branches and N3 nodes are the most distant from the tumor (portal triad, retropancreatic, mesenteric root, middle colic, para-aortic). The operation described above, by far the most commonly performed procedure in the United States for gastric cancer, is called a D1 resection because it removes the tumor and the N1 nodes. The standard operation for gastric cancer in the Orient is the D2 gastrectomy, which involves a more extensive lymphadenectomy (removal of N1 and N2 nodes). In addition to the tissue removed in a D1 resection, the standard D2 gastrectomy removes the peritoneal layer over the pancreas and anterior mesocolon, along with nodes along the hepatic and splenic arteries, and the crural nodes. Splenectomy and distal pancreatectomy are not routinely performed, because clearly this has been shown to increase the morbidity of the operation. Randomized prospective trials have not confirmed a survival advantage for the more extensive lymphadenectomy, but the morbidity and mortality in the D2 group was higher (Table 25-13). This was mostly attributable to the splenectomy and distal pancreatectomy which are no longer routinely done as part of the D2 gastrectomy. Some experts have argued that the D2 operation is simply a better staging procedure, and that

TABLE 25-13 Randomized Trials Comparing D1 and D2 Gastrectomy for Gastric Cancer

Authors	Number of patients	Type of surgery	Postoperative complications (%)	Postoperative mortality (%)	5-year survival (%)
Bonenkamp et al.	711	D1	25	4	45
		D2	43	10	47
Cuschieri et al.	400	D1	28	6.5	35
		D2	46	13	33

Source: Data from Bonenkamp JJ, Hermans J, Sasako M, van de Velde CJH: Extended lymph node dissection for gastric cancer. *N Engl J Med* 340:908, 1999; and Cuschieri A, Fayers P, Fielding J, et al: Postoperative morbidity and mortality after D1 and D2 resections for gastric cancer: Preliminary results of the MRC randomized controlled surgical trial. *Lancet* 347:995, 1996.

the apparent improved survival with this more extensive dissection is simply an epiphenomenon of improved pathologic staging. All experts would agree that to avoid understaging of gastric cancer, a minimum of 15 nodes should be resected with the gastrectomy specimen.

Chemotherapy and Radiation for Gastric Cancer

Adjuvant treatment with chemotherapy (5 FU and leucovorin) and radiation (4500 cGy) has demonstrated a survival benefit in resected patients with stage II and III adenocarcinoma of the stomach. There is no indication for the routine use of radiation alone in the adjuvant setting, but in certain patients it can be very effective palliation for bleeding or pain. In patients with gross unresectable, metastatic, or recurrent disease, palliative chemotherapy has not been demonstrated to conclusively prolong survival, but an occasional patient has a dramatic response. These patients should be considered for clinical trials. Agents that have shown activity against gastric cancer include 5 FU, cisplatin, Adriamycin, and methotrexate. Neoadjuvant treatment of gastric adenocarcinoma is being evaluated.

Endoscopic Resection

The Japanese have demonstrated that some patients with early gastric cancer can be adequately treated by an endoscopic mucosal resection. Small tumors (<3 cm) confined to the mucosa have an extremely low chance of lymph node metastasis (3 percent) which approaches the operative mortality rate for gastrectomy. If the resected specimen demonstrates no ulceration, no lymphatic invasion, and size less than 3 cm, the risk of lymph node metastases is less than 1 percent. Thus some patients with early gastric cancer might be better treated with the endoscopic technique. Currently this should be limited to patients with tumors less than 2 cm, which on EUS are node-negative and confined to the mucosa.

Prognosis

The 5 year survival for gastric adenocarcinoma has increased from 15–22 percent in the United States over the past 25 years. Survival is dependent on pathologic stage (TNM stage, see Table 25-12) and degree of tumor differentiation.

Screening for Gastric Cancer

In Japan it has clearly been shown that patients participating in gastric cancer screening programs have a significantly decreased risk of dying from gastric cancer. Thus screening is effective in a high risk population. Certainly screening the general population in the United States (a low-risk country) does not make sense, but patients clearly at risk for gastric cancer should probably have periodic endoscopy and biopsy. This includes patients with FAP, HNPCC, gastric adenomas, Menetrier disease, intestinal metaplasia, dysplasia, and remote gastrectomy or gastrojejunostomy.

Gastric Lymphoma

Gastric lymphomas generally account for about 4 percent of gastric malignancies. Over half of patients with non-Hodgkin lymphoma have involvement of the GI tract. The stomach is the most common site of primary GI lymphoma, and over 95 percent are non-Hodgkin type. Most are B-cell type, thought to arise in mucosa associated lymphoid tissue (MALT). In populations with a high incidence of gastric lymphoma, there is a high incidence of Helicobacter infection. And patients with gastric lymphoma usually have Helicobacter. Low-grade MALT lymphomas, essentially a monoclonal proliferation of B cells, presumably arise in a background of chronic gastritis associated with Helicobacter. Remarkably, when the Helicobacter is eradicated and the gastritis improves, the low grade MALT lymphoma often disappears. Thus low-grade MALT lymphoma is not a surgical lesion. Obviously careful follow-up is necessary.

These relatively innocuous "MALTomas" may undergo degeneration to high grade lymphoma, which is the usual variety seen by the surgeon. These patients require aggressive oncologic treatment for cure, and present with many of the same symptoms as gastric cancer patients. However, systemic symptoms such as fever, weight loss, and night sweats occur in about 50 percent of patients with gastric lymphoma. The tumors may bleed and/or obstruct. Lymphadenopathy and/or organomegaly suggest systemic disease. Diagnosis is by endoscopy and biopsy. Much of the tumor may be submucosal and an assiduous attempt at biopsy is necessary. A diligent search for extragastric disease is necessary before the diagnosis of localized primary gastric lymphoma is made. This includes endoscopic ultrasound, CT scan of the chest, abdomen and pelvis, and bone marrow biopsy.

For gastric lymphoma limited to the stomach and regional nodes, radical subtotal gastrectomy may be performed, especially for bulky tumors with bleeding and/or obstruction. Palliative gastrectomy for tumor complications also has a role. Recently, patients have been treated with primary chemotherapy and radiation without operation, and the results have been quite good. Perforation and bleeding especially from thick tumors is a recognized complication of this approach. Certainly, a multidisciplinary team should be involved with the treatment plan for patients with primary gastric lymphoma.

Malignant Gastrointestinal Stromal Tumor

GI stromal tumors arise in mesenchymal tissue from an indistinct (probably multipotential) cell line of origin. There are varying patterns of differentiation including smooth muscle type, formerly called leiomyosarcoma, and epithelioid type. Two-thirds of all gut GISTs occur in the stomach. GISTs are submucosal tumors, which are slow growing. Smaller lesions are usually found incidentally, although they occasionally may ulcerate and cause impressive bleeding. Larger lesions generally produce symptoms of weight loss, abdominal pain, fullness, early satiety, and bleeding. An abdominal mass may be palpable. Spread is by the hematogenous route often to liver and/or lung, although positive lymph nodes are occasionally seen in resected specimens. Diagnosis is by endoscopy and biopsy, although the interpretation of the latter may be problematic. Endoscopic ultrasound may be helpful, but symptomatic tumors and tumors over 2 cm should be removed. Metastatic workup entails CT of chest, abdomen and pelvis (chest radiograph may suffice in lieu of CT of chest). Wedge resection with clear margins is adequate treatment, and prognosis depends on tumor size and mitotic count. Most patients with low grade lesions are cured (80 percent 5-year survival), but most patients with high-grade lesions are not (30 percent 5-year survival). GIST are usually positive for the proto-oncogene, c-kit. Gleevec, a chemotherapeutic agent which blocks the activity of the tyrosine kinase product of c-kit, shows promising activity in patients with this tumor.

Gastric Carcinoid Tumors

Gastric carcinoids comprise about 3 percent of GI carcinoids, and they clearly have malignant potential. Patients with pernicious anemia or atrophic gastritis are at risk for gastric carcinoid tumors, but thus far chronic pharmacologic suppression of acid has not been recognized as a risk factor. The tumors are submucosal and may be quite small. They are often confused with heterotopic pancreas or small leiomyomas. Biopsy may be difficult because of the submucosal location, and EUS can be helpful in defining the size and depth of the lesion. Gastric carcinoids should be resected. Small lesions confined to the mucosa may be removed endoscopically. Larger lesions should be removed by D1 gastrectomy. Survival is excellent for node negative patients (>90 percent 5-year survival); node positive patients have a 50 percent 5-year survival.

BENIGN GASTRIC NEOPLASMS

The most common gastric polyp (about 75 percent in most series) is the hyperplastic or regenerative polyp which frequently occurs in the setting of gastritis and has a low but real malignant potential. Adenomatous polyps may undergo malignant transformation, similar to adenomas in the colon. They constitute about 10–15 percent of gastric polyps. Hamartomatous, inflammatory, and heterotopic polyps have negligible malignant potential. Polyps which are symptomatic, larger than 2 cm, or adenomatous should be removed, usually by endoscopic snare polypectomy. Consideration should also be given to removing hyperplastic polyps, especially if large. Repeat esophagogastroduodenoscopy (EGD) for surveillance should be done following removal of adenomatous polyps, and perhaps after removal of hyperplastic polyps as well.

What used to be called leiomyoma is now termed GI stromal tumor. The typical leiomyoma is submucosal and firm. If ulcerated it has an umbilicated appearance, and it may bleed. Histologically these lesions appear to be of smooth muscle origin. Lesions less than 2 cm are usually asymptomatic and benign. Larger lesions have greater malignant potential, and a greater likelihood to cause symptoms such as bleeding, obstruction, or pain. Asymptomatic lesions less than 2 cm may be observed; larger lesions and symptomatic lesions should be removed by wedge resection (often possible laparoscopically). When these lesions are observed rather than resected, the patient should be made aware of their presence and the small possibility for malignancy.

Lipomas are benign submucosal fatty tumors which are usually asymptomatic, found incidentally on upper GI series or EGD. Endoscopically, they have a characteristic appearance; there is also a characteristic appearance on endoscopic ultrasound. Excision is unnecessary unless the patient is symptomatic.

GASTRIC MOTILITY DISORDERS

Most patients with primary gastroparesis present with nausea and vomiting. Bloating, early satiety, and abdominal pain are common. Eighty percent of patients are women. Some are diabetic. The gastroparesis and vomiting significantly complicates the management of the diabetes; frequently the patient takes parenteral insulin, eats, then vomits, then becomes dangerously hypoglycemic. In patients with gastroparesis, it is important to rule out mechanical gastric outlet obstruction, and small bowel obstruction. Upper GI series may suggest slow gastric emptying and relative atony or it may be normal. EGD may show bezoars but is frequently normal. Gastric emptying scintigraphy shows delayed solid emptying, and often delayed liquid emptying. Gastroparesis can be a manifestation of a variety of problems (Table 25-14). Medical treatment includes promotility agents, antiemetics, and perhaps botulinum injection into the pylorus. If appropriate, the patient with severe diabetic gastroparesis should be evaluated for pancreas transplant prior to any invasive abdominal procedure because some patients improve substantially after pancreas transplant. Gastrostomy (for decompression) and jejunostomy (for feeding and prevention of hypoglycemia) may be effective. Other surgical options include implantation of gastric pacemaker, and gastric resection but the latter should be done infrequently, if at all for primary gastroparesis.

MISCELLANEOUS LESIONS OF THE STOMACH

Menetrier disease (hypertrophic gastropathy) is characterized by epithelial hyperplasia and giant gastric folds, associated with protein losing gastropathy and hypochlorhydria. There are large rugal folds in the proximal stomach, and the antrum is usually spared. Mucosal biopsy shows diffuse hyperplasia of the surface mucous secreting cells. The etiology is unclear, and there may be an increased risk of gastric cancer. Most patients with Menetrier disease are middle aged men who present with epigastric pain, weight loss, diarrhea, and hypoproteinemia. Sometimes the disease regresses spontaneously. Gastric resection may be indicated for bleeding, severe hypoproteinemia, or cancer in some patients with this rare problem.

The parallel red stripes atop the mucosal folds of the distal stomach give this rare entity its sobriquet, watermelon stomach (gastric antral vascular ectasia). Histologically gastric antral vascular ectasia is characterized by dilated mucosal blood vessels in the lamina propria, often containing thrombi. Mucosal fibromuscular hyperplasia and hyalinization are often present. The histologic appearance can resemble portal gastropathy, but the latter usually affects the proximal stomach, whereas watermelon stomach predominantly affects the distal stomach. Patients with gastric antral vascular ectasia are usually older adult women with transfusion requiring chronic GI blood loss. Most have an associated autoimmune connective tissue disorder, and at least 25 percent have chronic liver disease. Antrectomy may be required to control blood loss, but

TABLE 25-14 Etiology of Gastroparesis

Idiopathic
Endocrine or metabolic
  Diabetes mellitus
  Thyroid disease
  Renal insufficiency
After gastric surgery
  After resection
  After vagotomy
Central nervous system disorders
  Brain stem lesions
  Parkinson disease
Peripheral neuromuscular disorders
  Myotonia dystrophica
  Duchenne muscular dystrophy
Connective tissue disorders
  Scleroderma
  Polymyositis/dermatomyositis
Infiltrative disorders
  Lymphoma
  Amyloidosis
Diffuse gastrointestinal motility disorder
  Chronic intestinal pseudo-obstruction
Medication-induced
Electrolyte imbalance
  Potassium, calcium, magnesium
Miscellaneous conditions
  Infections (especially viral)
  Paraneoplastic syndrome
  Ischemic conditions
  Gastric ulcer

Source: Reproduced with permission from Packman HP, Fisher RS: Disorders of gastric emptying in Yamada T (ed): *Textbook of Gastroenterology,* 2003.

in patients with portal hypertension, transvenous intrahepatic portasystemic shunt (TIPS) should be considered first.

Bezoars are concretions of undigestible matter that accumulate in the stomach. Trichobezoars, composed of hair, occur most commonly in young women who swallow their hair. Phytobezoars are composed of vegetable matter and in this country are usually seen in association with gastroparesis or gastric outlet obstruction. Most commonly, bezoars produce obstructive symptoms, but they may cause ulceration and bleeding. Diagnosis is suggested by upper GI series and confirmed by endoscopy. Treatment options include enzyme therapy (papain, cellulase, acetylcysteine), endoscopic disruption and removal, or surgical removal.

Dieulafoy's lesion is a congenital arteriovenous malformation characterized by an unusually large tortuous submucosal artery. If this artery is eroded, impressive bleeding may occur. To the operating surgeon, this appears as a stream of arterial blood emanating from what appears grossly to be a normal gastric mucosa. The lesion typically occurs in middle-age or older adult men. Patients present with upper GI bleeding, which may be intermittent, and endoscopy can miss the lesion if not actively bleeding. Treatment options include endoscopic hemostatic therapy (usually injection), angiographic embolization, or operation. At surgery, the lesion may be oversewn or resected.

Gastric diverticula are usually solitary and may be congenital or acquired. Congenital diverticula are true diverticula and contain a full coat of muscularis propria, whereas acquired diverticula (perhaps caused by pulsion) usually have a negligible outer muscle layer. Most gastric diverticula occur in the posterior cardia or fundus and are asymptomatic. However if they can become inflamed, they may produce pain or bleeding. Perforation is rare. Asymptomatic diverticula do not require treatment, but symptomatic lesions should be removed. This can often be done laparoscopically.

Ingested foreign bodies are usually asymptomatic. Removal of sharp or large objects should be considered. This can usually be done endoscopically, with an overtube technique. Recognized dangers include aspiration of the foreign body during removal, and rupture of drug containing bags in "body packers." Both complications can be fatal. Surgical removal is recommended in body packers, and in patients with large jagged objects.

The Mallory-Weiss lesion is a longitudinal tear in the mucosa of the GE junction. It is presumably caused by forceful vomiting and/or retching, and is commonly seen in alcoholics. It typically presents with impressive upper GI bleeding, often with hematemesis. Endoscopy confirms the diagnosis and may be useful in controlling the bleeding, but 90 percent of patients stop bleeding spontaneously. Other options to control the bleeding include balloon tamponade, angiographic embolization or selective infusion of vasopressin, systemic vasopressin, and operation. Surgical treatment consists of oversewing the bleeding lesion through a long gastrotomy.

Gastric volvulus is a twist of the stomach, which usually occurs in association with a large hiatal hernia. It can also occur in patients with an unusually mobile stomach without hiatal hernia. Typically, the stomach twists along its long axis (organoaxial volvulus), with the greater curvature "flipping up". If the stomach twists around the transverse axis, it is called mesenteroaxial rotation. Usually, volvulus is a chronic condition which can be surprisingly asymptomatic. In these instances, expectant nonoperative management is usually advised, especially in the older adult. The risk of strangulation and infarction has been overestimated in asymptomatic patients. Symptomatic patients should be considered for operation, especially if the symptoms are severe and/or progressive.

GASTROSTOMY

A gastrostomy is performed either for alimentation or for gastric drainage/decompression. Gastrostomy may be done percutaneously, laparoscopically, or via open technique. Currently, percutaneous endoscopic gastrostomy is the most common method used, usually with the Ponsky technique. In this procedure, the insufflated stomach is accessed percutaneously with a thin trocar needle under direct endoscopic vision. A long braided wire is passed through the needle into the stomach, snared endoscopically, and pulled out the mouth where it is attached to the outside end of a special gastrostomy tube. The wire and attached tube are then pulled down the esophagus, into the stomach and out the dilated trocar needle track and is secured. By far the most common open technique is the Stamm gastrostomy, which can be done open or laparoscopically. Complications of gastrostomy include infection, dislodgement, and aspiration pneumonia. Although gastrostomy tubes usually do prevent tense gastric dilatation, they may not adequately drain the stomach, especially when the patient is bedridden.

POSTGASTRECTOMY PROBLEMS

A variety of abnormalities affect some patients after a gastric operation that usually has been performed because of ulcer or tumor. Some of the more common disorders result from disturbance of the normal anatomic and physiologic mechanisms that control gastric motor function, and a discussion of these follows.

Dumping syndrome is a phenomenon caused by the destruction or bypass of the pyloric sphincter. Clinically significant dumping occurs in 5–10 percent of patients after pyloroplasty, pyloromyotomy, or distal gastrectomy, and consists of a constellation of postprandial symptoms ranging in severity from annoying to disabling. The symptoms are thought to be the result of the abrupt delivery of a hyperosmolar load into the small bowel. Rapid fluid influx into the bowel lumen and wall results, along with an incompletely understood neuroendocrine response. There is peripheral and splanchnic vasodilatation. About 15–30 min after a meal, the patient becomes diaphoretic, weak, lightheaded, and tachycardic. These symptoms may be ameliorated by recumbence or saline infusion. Diarrhea often follows. This is referred to as early dumping, and should be distinguished from postprandial (reactive) hypoglycemia, also called "late dumping" which usually occurs later (2–3 h following a meal), and is relieved by the administration of sugar. A variety of hormonal aberrations have been observed in early dumping, including increased vasoactive intestinal peptide (VIP), CCK, neurotensin, PYY, renin/angiotensin/aldosterone and decreased atrial natriuretic peptide. Late dumping is associated with hypoglycemia and hyperinsulinemia.

The medical therapy for the dumping syndrome consists of dietary management and somatostatin analogue (octreotide). Octreotide ameliorates the abnormal hormonal pattern seen in patients with dumping symptoms. It also promotes restoration of a "fasting" motility pattern in the small intestine (i.e., restoration of the MMC). The α-glucosidase inhibitor acarbose may be particularly helpful in ameliorating the symptoms of late dumping. Only a small percentage of patients with dumping symptoms ultimately require operation. The results of remedial operation for dumping are variable and unpredictable. Patients with disabling dumping after loop gastrojejunostomy can be considered for simple takedown of this anastomosis provided that (1) there is some vagal innervation to the antrum and (2) the pyloric channel is open endoscopically. Taking advantage of the disordered motility of the Roux limb, surgeons have used conversion of Billroth I or II to Roux gastrojejunostomy in the management of the dumping syndrome. Although this is probably the procedure of choice in the small group of patients requiring operation for severe dumping following gastric resection, gastric stasis and/or marginal ulceration may result, particularly if a large gastric remnant is left.

Truncal vagotomy is associated with clinically significant diarrhea in 5–10 percent of patients. It occurs soon after operation, tends to improve over time (months and years), and is usually not associated with other symptoms, a fact that helps to distinguish it from dumping. The cause of postvagotomy diarrhea is unclear. Possible mechanisms include intestinal dysmotility and accelerated transit, bile acid malabsorption, rapid gastric emptying, and bacterial overgrowth. Although bacterial overgrowth can be confirmed with the hydrogen breath test, a simpler test is an empirical trial of oral antibiotics. Some patients with postvagotomy diarrhea respond to cholestyramine, although in others codeine or loperamide may be useful. Another theoretical cause of diarrhea following gastric operation is fat malabsorption because of acid inactivation of pancreatic enzymes or poorly coordinated mixing of food and digestive juices. In the rare patient who is debilitated by postvagotomy diarrhea that is unresponsive to medical management, the operation of choice is a 10 cm reversed jejunal interposition placed in continuity 100 cm distal to the ligament of Treitz. Another option is the onlay antiperistaltic distal ileal graft. Both operations can cause obstructive symptoms and/or bacterial overgrowth.

Gastric stasis following operation on the stomach may be because of a problem with gastric motor function or an obstruction. The gastric motility abnormality may have been preexisting and unrecognized by the operating surgeon. Alternatively, it may be secondary to deliberate or unintentional vagotomy or resection of the dominant gastric pacemaker. An obstruction may be mechanical (e.g., anastomotic stricture, efferent limb kink from adhesions or constricting mesocolon, or a proximal small bowel obstruction), or functional (e.g., retrograde peristalsis in a Roux limb). Gastric stasis presents with vomiting (often of undigested food), bloating, epigastric pain, and weight loss. The evaluation of a patient with suspected postoperative gastric stasis includes EGD, upper GI, gastric emptying scan, and gastric motor testing. Once mechanical obstruction has been ruled out, medical treatment is successful in most cases of motor dysfunction following previous gastric surgery. This consists of dietary modification and promotility agents. Intermittent oral antibiotic therapy may be helpful in treating bacterial overgrowth with its attendant symptoms of bloating, flatulence, and diarrhea. Gastroparesis following vagotomy and drainage may be treated with subtotal (75 percent) gastrectomy. Billroth-II anastomosis with Braun enteroenterostomy may be preferable to Roux-en-Y reconstruction. This latter option may be associated with persistent emptying problems which will subsequently require near-total or total gastrectomy, a nutritionally unattractive option. Gastric pacing is promising, but it has not achieved widespread clinical usefulness in the treatment of postoperative gastric atony.

Bile reflux gastritis. Most patients who have undergone ablation or resection of the pylorus have bile in the stomach on endoscopic examination, along with some degree of gross or microscopic gastric inflammation. Therefore attributing postoperative symptoms to bile reflux is problematic, because most asymptomatic patients have bile reflux too. However it is generally accepted that a small subset of patients have bile reflux gastritis, and present with nausea, bilious vomiting, and epigastric pain and quantitative evidence of excess enterogastric reflux. Curiously, symptoms often develop months or years after the index operation. The differential diagnosis includes afferent or efferent loop obstruction, gastric stasis, and small bowel obstruction. Bile reflux may be quantitated with gastric analysis, or more commonly scintigraphy (bile reflux scan). Remedial operation will eliminate the bile from the vomitus and may improve the epigastric pain, but it is quite unusual to render these patients completely asymptomatic, especially if they are narcotic dependent. Bile reflux gastritis after distal gastric resection may be treated by one of the following options: Roux-en-Y gastrojejunostomy; interposition of a 40-cm isoperistaltic jejunal loop between the gastric remnant and the duodenum (Henley loop); Billroth-II gastrojejunostomy with Braun enteroenterostomy. To avoid bile reflux into the stomach the Roux limb should be at least 45 cm long. The Braun enteroenterostomy should be placed a similar distance from the stomach. Primary bile reflux gastritis (i.e. no previous operation) is rare, and may be treated with the duodenal switch operation, essentially an end-to-end Roux-en-Y to the proximal duodenum. The Achilles heel of this operation is, not surprisingly, marginal ulceration. Thus it should be combined with highly selective vagotomy, and perhaps H_2 blockers.

Roux syndrome. A subset of patients who have had distal gastrectomy and Roux-en-Y gastrojejunostomy will have great difficulty with gastric emptying in the absence of mechanical obstruction. These patients present with vomiting, epigastric pain, and weight loss. This clinical scenario has been labeled the Roux syndrome. Endoscopy may show bezoar formation, dilation of the gastric remnant, and/or dilation of the Roux limb. Upper GI confirms these findings and may show delayed gastric emptying. This is better quantitated by a gastric emptying scan which always shows delayed solid emptying, and may show delayed liquid emptying as well.

GI motility testing shows abnormal motility in the Roux limb, with propulsive activity toward rather than away from the stomach. Gastric motility may also be abnormal. The disorder seems to be more common in patients with a generous gastric remnant. Truncal vagotomy has also been implicated. Medical treatment consists of promotility agents. Surgical treatment consists of paring down the gastric remnant. If gastric motility is severely disordered, 95 percent gastrectomy should be done. The Roux limb should be resected if it is dilated and flaccid, and doing so does not put the patient at risk for short bowel problems. Gastrointestinal continuity may be re-established with another Roux, a Billroth II with Braun enteroenterostomy, or an isoperistaltic jejunal interposition between the stomach and the duodenum (Henley loop). Truncal vagotomy should probably not be done. Long term acid suppression may be necessary.

Weight loss is common in patients who have had a vagotomy and/or gastric resection. The degree of weight loss tends to parallel the magnitude of the operation. It may be insignificant in the large person, or devastating in the asthenic female. The surgeon should always reconsider before performing a gastric resection for benign disease in a thin female. The causes of weight loss after gastric surgery generally fall into one of two categories: altered dietary intake or malabsorption. If a stool stain for fecal fat is negative, it is likely that decreased caloric intake is the cause. This is the most common cause of weight loss after gastric surgery and may be because of small stomach syndrome, postoperative gastroparesis, or self-imposed dietary modification because of dumping and/or diarrhea. Specific problems may be treated as outlined above. Consultation with an experienced dietitian may prove invaluable.

Anemia. Iron absorption takes place primarily in the proximal gastrointestinal tract, and is facilitated by an acidic environment. Intrinsic factor, essential for the enteric absorption of vitamin B12, is made by the parietal cells of the stomach. Vitamin B12 bioavailability is also facilitated by an acidic environment. Patients with small gastric pouch, decreased compliance or anastomotic stricture may avoid bulky green vegetables, a rich source of folate. Patients who have had gastric surgery should be monitored for anemia, and for iron, folate, and B12 deficiency. Prophylactic vitamin and iron supplementation may be prudent, with therapeutic supplementation required to correct any documented deficiency. Of course, patients who have had a total gastrectomy will all develop B12 deficiency without parenteral vitamin B12 supplementation.

Bone disease. Gastric surgery not uncommonly disturbs calcium and vitamin D metabolism. Calcium absorption occurs primarily in the duodenum, which is bypassed with gastrojejunostomy. Fat malabsorption may occur because of blind loop syndrome and bacterial overgrowth, or because of inefficient mixing of food and digestive enzymes. This can significantly affect the absorption of vitamin D, a fat-soluble vitamin. Both abnormalities of calcium and vitamin D metabolism can contribute to metabolic bone disease in patients following gastric surgery. The problems usually manifest as pain and/or fractures years after the index operation. Musculoskeletal symptoms should prompt a study of bone density. Dietary supplementation of calcium and vitamin D may be useful in preventing these complications. Routine skeletal monitoring of patients at high risk (e.g., older adult male and female; postmenopausal females) may prove useful in identifying skeletal deterioration that with appropriate treatment may be arrested.

Suggested Readings

Ming S-C, Goldman H (eds): Pathology of the Gastrointestinal Tract (2nd ed). Baltimore: Williams & Wilkins, 1998.

Mercer DW, Liu TH, Castaneda A: Anatomy and physiology of the stomach, in Zuidema GD, Yeo CJ (eds): Shackelford's Surgery of the Alimentary Tract (5th edition), vol II, Saunders, 2002, pp 3–15.

Feldman M: Gastric Secretion, in Feldman M (ed): Sleisenger and Fordtran's Gastrointestinal and Liver Disease, 7th edition, Elsevier, 2002, pp 715–731.

Hasler WL: Physiology of gastric motility and gastric emptying, in Yamada T, et al. (eds): Textbook of Gastroenterology (4th edition). Philadelphia, Lippincott, Williams & Wilkins, 2003, pp 195–219.

Ponsky JL, Dumot JA: Diagnostic evaluation of the stomach and duodenum, in Zuidema GD, Yeo CJ (eds): Shackelford's Surgery of the Alimentary Tract (5th edition), vol II, Saunders, 2002, pp. 34–45.

Peterson WL, Graham DY: Helicobacter Pylori, in Feldman M (ed): Sleisenger and Fordtran's Gastrointestinal and Liver Disease, 7th edition, Elsevier, 2002, pp 732–746.

Harbison SP, Dempsey DT: Peptic Ulcer Disease. Current Problems in Surgery, 2005.

Seymour NE, Andersen DK: Surgery for peptic ulcer disease and postgastrectomy syndromes, in Yamada T, et al, (eds): Textbook of Gastroenterology (4th edition). Philadelphia, Lippincott, Williams & Wilkins, 2003, pp 1441–1454.

Wells SA Jr: Surgery for the Zollinger-Ellison syndrome. N Engl J Med 341:689–690, 1999.

Leung WK, Ng EKW, Sung JJY: Tumors of the stomach. In Yamada T, et al. (eds): Textbook of Gastroenterology (4th edition). Philadelphia, Lippincott, Williams & Wilkins, 2003, pp 1416–1440.

Bonenkamp JJ, Hermans J, Sasako M, van de Velde CJH: Extended lymph node dissection for gastric cancer. N Engl J Med 340:908–914, 1999.

Macdonald JS, Smalley SR, Benedetti J, Hundahl SA, et al: Chemoradiotherapy after surgery compared with surgery alone for adenocarcinoma of the stomach or gastroesophageal junction. N Engl J Med 345(10):725–30, 2001.

Parkman HP, Fisher RS: Disorders of gastric emptying, in Yamada T, et al. (eds): Textbook of Gastroenterology (4th edition). Philadelphia, Lippincott, Williams & Wilkins, 2003, pp 1292–1320.

26 | The Surgical Management of Obesity

Philip R. Schauer and Bruce David Schirmer

THE DISEASE OF OBESITY

Obesity is a serious disease that carries substantial morbidity and mortality. The degrees of obesity are defined by body mass index [BMI = weight (kg)/height $(m)^2$], which correlates body weight with height. Patients are classified as overweight, obese, or severely obese (sometimes referred to as morbidly obese) (Table 26-1). Morbidly obese individuals generally exceed ideal body weight by 100 lb or more, or are 100 percent over ideal body weight, but more uniformly have a BMI of more than 40 kg/m². Superobesity is a term sometimes used to define individuals who have a body weight exceeding a BMI of 50 kg/m² or greater.

Prevalence and Contributing Factors

Morbid obesity is reaching epidemic proportions in the United States. Since 1960, surveys of the prevalence of obesity have been conducted every decade by the National Center for Health Statistics. Twenty-five percent of adult Americans were overweight in 1980 compared to 34 percent in 1990. This trend has even increased in the past decade. In 1990, conservative estimates put the number of Americans with a BMI between 35 and 40 kg/m² at 4 million, with an additional 4 million having a BMI exceeding 40 kg/m². Current estimates put that patient population at over 20 million. Despite the expenditure of over $30 billion annually on weight loss products, the prevalence of obesity is increasing. Obesity is most common in minorities, low-income groups, and women.

The increase in obesity is multifactorial. Genetics play an important role in the development of obesity. Although children of parents of normal weight have a 10 percent chance of becoming obese, the children of two obese parents have an 80–90 percent chance of developing obesity by adulthood. The weight of adopted children correlates strongly with the weight of their birth parents. Furthermore, concordance rates for obesity in monozygotic twins are doubled compared to others.

Diet and culture are important factors as well; these environmental factors contribute significantly to the epidemic of obesity in the United States because the rapid increase in obesity during the past two decades cannot be explained by any genetic etiology.

Clinical Presentation

The morbidly obese patient often presents with chronic weight-related problems, detailed below. The morbidly obese almost uniformly endure discrimination, prejudice, ridicule, and inappropriately disrespectful treatment from the public. Consequently, the stigma of morbid obesity has a major impact on social function and emotional well-being.

Significant comorbidities, defined as medical problems associated with or caused by obesity, are numerous. The most prevalent and acknowledged of

TABLE 26-1 Assessing Disease Risk Using Body Mass Index and Waist Size

Category	BMI	Men (< 40 in.) women (< 35 in.)	Men (> 40 in.) women (> 35 in.)
Underweight	< 18.5	−	−
Normal	18.5–24.9	−	−
Overweight	25.0–29.9	+	+
Obesity	^{3}30		
Class I	30.0–34.9	+	++
Class II	35.0–39.9	++	++
Class III (extreme obesity)	^{3}40	+++	

these include degenerative joint disease, low back pain, hypertension, obstructive sleep apnea, gastroesophageal reflux disease (GERD), cholelithiasis, type 2 diabetes, hyperlipidemia, hypercholesterolemia, asthma, hypoventilation syndrome of obesity, fatal cardiac arrhythmias, right sided heart failure, migraine headaches, pseudotumor cerebri, venous stasis ulcers, deep venous thrombosis, fungal skin rashes, skin abscesses, stress urinary incontinence, infertility, dysmenorrhea, depression, abdominal wall hernias, and an increased incidence of various cancers such as those of the uterus, breast, colon, and prostate.

Prognosis

Obesity has a profound effect on overall health and life expectancy, largely secondary to weight-related comorbidities. Obesity is now considered to be the second leading cause of preventable death behind cigarette smoking. The incidence of morbidity and mortality is directly related to the degree of obesity. In a study with 12-year follow-up, mortality rates for those weighing 50 percent over average weight were doubled. A study carried out by the Veterans Administration demonstrated a 12-fold increase in mortality among morbidly obese men aged 25–34 years, and a 6-fold increase among morbidly obese men aged 35–44 years.

Medical Management

Treatment of morbid obesity should begin with simple lifestyle changes, including moderation of diet and initiation of regular exercise such as walking. The treatment of associated comorbidities should be addressed expeditiously. However, because the only effective treatment for morbid obesity is bariatric surgery, these are the initial steps to be taken in preparation for the more definitive, albeit invasive, treatment.

Pharmacotherapy is a second tier therapy usually used in heavier patients (BMI > 27) or when lifestyle changes alone have failed. Sibutramine and orlistat are the only current Food and Drug Administration (FDA)–approved drugs for weight loss treatment. Orlistat is a potent and selective inhibitor of gastric and pancreatic lipases that reduces lipid intestinal absorption, although sibutramine is a noradrenaline and 5-hydroxytryptamine reuptake inhibitor that works as an appetite suppressant. Despite their different mechanisms of action, they effectively produce weight loss of 6–10 percent of initial body weight at 1 year, but much of this weight is regained once the drug is stopped.

OVERVIEW OF BARIATRIC SURGERY

The goal of bariatric surgery is to improve health in morbidly obese patients by achieving long-term, durable weight loss. It involves reducing caloric intake and/or absorption of calories from food, and may modify eating behavior by promoting slow ingestion of small boluses of food.

Restrictive operations restrict the amount of food intake by reducing the quantity of food that can be consumed at one time, which results in a reduction in caloric intake. Malabsorptive procedures limit the absorption of nutrients and calories from ingested food by bypassing the duodenum and predetermined lengths of small intestine.

The operations currently in use for the management of morbid obesity involve gastric restriction with or without intestinal malabsorption. Purely gastric restrictive procedures include vertical banded gastroplasty (VBG) and laparoscopic adjustable gastric banding (LAGB). Primarily malabsorptive procedures include biliopancreatic diversion (BPD), and biliopancreatic diversion with duodenal switch (BPD-DS). Roux-en-Y gastric bypass (RYGB) has features of primary restriction with some malabsorption. The advent of laparoscopic techniques allowed surgeons to offer minimally invasive approaches to these bariatric procedures.

Indications

Patients that have a BMI of 35 kg/m^2 or more with comorbidity, or those with a BMI of 40 kg/m$_2$ or greater regardless of comorbidity, are eligible for bariatric surgery. Candidates should have attempted weight loss in the past by medically supervised diet regimens, exercise, or medications, but this is not mandatory. They must be motivated to comply with postoperative dietary and exercise regimens and follow up. Traditionally, surgeons have offered bariatric surgery to patients aged 18–60 years. However, bariatric surgery is now offered to carefully selected older adults at some institutions with no reported increase in morbidity or mortality. Adolescent patients with morbid obesity may be considered for bariatric surgery under selected circumstances. A summary of appropriate indications for bariatric surgery and approved bariatric operations was recently published after a consensus conference held by the American Association for Bariatric Surgery (ASBS).

Contraindications

Patients who are unable to undergo general anesthesia because of cardiac, pulmonary, or hepatic disease, or those who are unwilling or unable to comply with postoperative lifestyle changes, diet, supplementation, or follow up should not undergo these procedures. Patients with ongoing substance abuse, unstable psychiatric illness, or inadequate ability to understand the consequences of surgery are also considered to be poor surgical candidates.

Preparation for Surgery

Comorbidities are identified during the medical and surgical history taking and physical examination of the patient. Preoperative testing should be performed and additional studies should be considered, depending on the patient's comorbidities. A preoperative electrocardiogram should be obtained for all patients. Patients with cardiovascular disease should have preoperative evaluation by a cardiologist. Echocardiography, stress testing, and cardiac catheterization may be indicated.

Symptoms of loud snoring or daytime sleepiness in a morbidly obese patient should prompt a work-up for obstructive sleep apnea. The diagnosis is established by polysomnography at a sleep center. Patients with significant sleep apnea are treated with nasal continuous positive airway pressure. Obesity hypoventilation syndrome is characterized by hypoxemia (partial pressure of arterial oxygen [$Pao_2 < 55$ mmHg]) and hypercarbia (partial pressure of carbon dioxide [$Paco_2 > 47$ mmHg]), with severe pulmonary hypertension and polycythemia. These patients require preoperative evaluation by a pulmonologist, and consideration of intensive care monitoring postoperatively. They also are possibly at increase risk for venous thromboembolic complications.

Patients with severe gastroesophageal reflux should undergo upper endoscopy with possible biopsy to rule out esophagitis or Barrett esophagus. Because of the high incidence of gallstones in the obese population, many surgeons advocate routine preoperative sonography, and cholecystectomy when stones are present.

Nutritional evaluation and education is invaluable in the preoperative period. The dietitian may help determine whether the patient is able to understand the necessary changes in postoperative eating habits and food choices.

The objective of psychologic screening for obesity surgery is to determine whether a patient has realistic expectations about the results of the procedure, and a fundamental understanding of the impact that it will have on his or her life. It may also help to identify patients suffering from depression, history of abusive relationships, or psychotic disorders that were previously unrecognized and that may require intervention.

Assessment of Results

Weight loss has traditionally been used as the main outcome measure in bariatric surgery. Although an easily measured objective parameter, weight alone is insufficient as a single outcome goal in bariatric surgery outcomes.

The National Institute of Health (NIH) Conference recommended statistical reporting of surgical results, including quality of life, to provide a clearer assessment of outcomes. It underlines the fact weight loss should be considered the main postoperative outcome, but improvement of medical conditions associated with obesity is also desirable. The Bariatric Analysis and Reporting Outcome System (BAROS) has been developed to standardize and compare outcomes of bariatric surgical series.

Follow-up

A bariatric electronic database is very useful for outcomes reporting and further analyses. All bariatric surgeons should record such data so as to be aware of their outcomes.

The ASBS recommends visits during the immediate postoperative period, and then at variable intervals for life, with additional visits as needed, depending on the patient's condition. A typical schedule for visits is 1–2 weeks, 4–6 weeks, 3 months, 6 months, 1 year, then annually after surgery. Patients are encouraged to comply with lifelong follow-up, exercise, and vitamin supplementation after undergoing bariatric surgery. Follow-up includes assessment of weight loss trends and regular monitoring of metabolic and nutritional parameters.

Efficacy

Past randomized controlled trials have established the superiority of surgical weight loss procedures over nonsurgical approaches in achieving durable weight loss. The Swedish Obese Subjects (SOS) matched pair cohort study compared surgery with nonsurgical treatment. Weight loss at 2 years was 28 ± 15 kg among the operated patients and 0.5 ± 8.9 kg among the obese controls. At 8 years weight loss remained significantly different. There was also a reduction in the incidence of diabetes and hypertension at 2 years, which remained for diabetes at 8 years. The SOS trial also provides evidence for improvement in quality of life.

Gastric bypass produces weight loss of 68 percent to 62 percent of excess weight at one to three years postoperatively. Long-term (5 to 14 years) excess weight loss has been 49–62 percent. Laparoscopic and open approaches to RYGB appear to result in similar weight loss. Studies reporting gastric banding results collectively demonstrate a 40–60 percent mean estimated weight loss (EWL) at 3–5 years. Patients with malabsorption procedures had up to 78 percent EWL at 18 years.

BARIATRIC SURGICAL PROCEDURES

Vertical Banded Gastroplasty

The VBG is listed and described here as much for historic reasons as for practical applicability today. It represents the procedure least commonly done in the United States over the past several years. Its abandonment has been largely because of the poor overall long-term weight loss observed in many studies.

The VBG is purely restrictive in nature. A proximal gastric pouch empties through a calibrated stoma, which is reinforced by a strip of mesh or a Silastic ring.

Technique

Mason first described the VBG in 1982. A 32F Ewald tube is passed orally into the stomach and positioned against the lesser curvature. A circular stapler is positioned against it and used to create a 2.5-cm window through the stomach 8–9 cm below the angle of His. A line of four rows of 90-mm staples leads from the circular opening to the angle of His to create a pouch 50 mL in size or smaller. Using a linear stapler to divide this tissue prevents staple line breakdown. A 7×1.5 cm. strip of polypropylene mesh is placed around the lesser curvature channel and is sewn to itself to create a 5.0–5.5-cm collar. The laparoscopic technique follows the same steps.

Another technique involves use of a linear cutting stapler to excise a wedge of fundus, thereby creating a 20-mL pouch without the use of a circular stapler. A polypropylene mesh or polytetrafluoroethylene band is sutured around the distal end of the gastroplasty.

Efficacy

VBG achieves acceptable short- to medium-term weight loss. In a series of 305 patients followed for a minimum of 2 years, a mean excess weight loss of 61 percent was reported. Studies have shown excess weight loss of 63 percent after 7 years.

A significant number of patients have required reoperation following VBG. In a study from Spain, 25 percent of patients required reoperation for complications related to the technique. A prospective study of 71 patients who underwent VBG with a 99 percent 10-year follow up reported that only 26 percent had maintained a loss of at least 50 percent of their excess weight, and 17 percent had a bariatric reoperation. In a study of 60 patients followed for a median of 9.6 years, only 40 percent maintained their original weight loss, although 60 percent regained a significant amount of weight and 31 percent returned to preoperative weight. Patients who regain weight were found to change eating patterns to adopt a diet high in high-calorie soft and liquid foods.

Complications

The overall operative morbidity rate with VBG is under 10 percent and the mortality rate is 0–0.38 percent. Late complications include stomal stenosis, which may occur in 15–20 percent, and staple line dehiscence, which occurs in up to 48 percent if the linear staple line is not a divided one. In a series from MacLean and associates, 30 percent of all patients required reoperations for this problem. Reflux esophagitis may occur in 16–38 percent of patients, and some patients may require conversion to Roux-en-Y gastric bypass for severe symptoms. Intractable vomiting one or more times a week was seen in as many as 30–50 percent of patients.

Advantages and Disadvantages

Weight loss following VBG can significantly improve comorbidities. VBG is associated with minimal long-term metabolic or nutritional deficiencies. It is technically easier to perform than RYGB, and requires less operative time. These relative advantages of VBG, however, are more than overshadowed by the disadvantages of poor long-term weight loss and the high incidence of long-term complications listed above.

Laparoscopic Adjustable Gastric Banding

Technique

The patient is placed in reverse Trendelenburg position. Six laparoscopic ports are placed. A 5-mm liver retractor is used to elevate the left hepatic lobe. A 15-mL gastric calibration balloon is used to identify the location for the initial dissection. A retrogastric tunnel is created starting at the base of the right diaphragmatic crus, using the pars flaccida technique. The silicone band is passed through the tunnel so that it encircles the cardia of the stomach about 1 cm below the gastroesophageal junction. The tail of the silicone band is passed through the buckle of the band and locked into place. A calibration tube is reinserted to determine the stoma diameter. Interrupted sutures are placed to imbricate the anterior stomach over the band in all but the buckle area. The end of the silicone tube is brought out through the abdominal wall and connected to the access port. The port, which will subsequently be used for injection or withdrawal of saline postoperatively for band volume adjustment, is secured to the anterior rectus sheath.

Postoperative Care

Patients are given clear liquids a few h after the procedure. A Gastrografin swallow is obtained on the first postoperative day to confirm band position and patency. Patients can generally be discharged 1–2 days after surgery with a liquid diet for 4 weeks.

Band adjustment may be performed with fluoroscopic guidance initially at 8–12 weeks. Patients are assessed monthly for weight loss and tolerance of oral intake. Band adjustments are made accordingly and as needed every 4–8 weeks during the first year, with the band progressively tightened as needed to provide slow but steady weight loss of 1–2 kg per week.

Efficacy

Suter et al observed mean excess weight loss after LAGB at 1 and 2 years was 55 and 56 percent, respectively. O'Brien and associates reported a series of over 700 patients undergoing LAGB and observed steady progression of weight loss, with 52 ± 19 percent EWL at 24 months ($n = 333$), 52 ± 24 percent EWL at 48 months ($n = 108$), 54 ± 24 percent EWL at 60 months ($n = 30$). Major improvements occurred in diabetes, asthma, GERD, dyslipidemia, sleep apnea, and depression. Quality of life showed highly significant improvement.

Data on 1893 patients who underwent LAGB were reported by the Italian Collaborative Study Group for the Lap-Band System. Weight loss was evaluated at 24, 36, 48, 60, and 72 months, with a BMI of 34.8, 34.1, 32.7, 34.8, and 32 kg/m^2, respectively.

Complications

During LAGB, intraoperative complications include splenic injury, esophageal or gastric injury (0–1 percent), conversion to an open procedure (1–2 percent), and bleeding (0–1 percent). Early postoperative complications include bleeding (0.5 percent), wound infection (0–1 percent), and food intolerance (0–11 percent). Late complications include slippage of the band (7.3–21 percent), band erosion (1.9–7.5 percent), tubing-related problems (4.2 percent), leakage of the reservoir, persistent vomiting (13 percent), pouch dilatation (5.2 percent) and gastroesophageal reflux.

In O'Brien's report, there were no deaths perioperatively or during follow up in 700 patients. Postoperative complications occurred in 1.2 percent of patients. Reoperation was needed for prolapse (slippage) in 12.5 percent, erosion of the band into the stomach in 2.8 percent, and for tubing breaks in 3.6 percent of patients. Among the patients requiring reoperation, 12 (1.7 percent) had the device removed.

The Italian Cooperative Group reported a postoperative mortality of 0.53 percent, a conversion to open rate of 3.1 percent, and a postoperative complication rate of 10.2 percent. Complications included tube port failure 4.1 percent, gastric pouch dilation (4.9 percent), and gastric erosion (1.1 percent).

Advantages and Disadvantages

LAGB is a relatively simple procedure that takes less operative time than the more complex procedures such as laparoscopic RYGB or laparoscopic BPD. The mortality rate is very low (0.06 percent), as are conversion rates (0–4 percent). No staple lines or anastomoses are required. Recovery is rapid and hospital stay is short. Performance as an outpatient has been reported. The adjustable nature of the laparoscopic band allows the degree of restriction to be optimized.

Disadvantages include the potential for port site complications and the need for frequent postoperative visits for band adjustment. Some patients

(5–10 percent) experience band slipping or gastric prolapse, which usually requires reoperation. Other potential problems include band erosion, GERD, alterations in esophageal motility, and esophageal dilatation.

Open Roux-en-Y Gastric Bypass

Technique

The peritoneum between the angle of His and the tip of the superior pole of the spleen is opened. The gastrohepatic ligament is opened, and the mesentery between the first and second branches of the left gastric artery is divided. Blunt dissection is carried out between the opening in the gastrohepatic omentum and the angle of His. An appropriate size (28F–36F) red rubber tube or Mallekot catheter is placed behind the stomach, and the open end of the tube is then brought through the opening in the mesentery and used to guide a linear stapler across the stomach. The stomach is completely divided using the linear stapler, creating the proximal gastric pouch.

The ligament of Treitz is identified and a point 15–45 cm distally is identified. The jejunum is divided with a linear stapling device. The mesentery is divided between clamps to mobilize the Roux limb, and a side-to-side jejuno-jejunostomy is created with a linear stapler to create a 50–75-cm Roux limb for a standard gastric bypass, or a 150-cm limb for a long-limb modification in the superobese. The enterotomy is closed as is the mesenteric defect.

The Roux limb is most commonly brought through the transverse mesocolon and behind the stomach, but may also be brought anterior to the colon or anterior to the stomach. A gastrojejunal anastomosis is created between the gastric pouch and the proximal end of the Roux limb, using either a linear stapler, circular stapler or a hand-sewn technique. The integrity of the anastomosis is tested by injecting methylene blue or air under pressure (to distend the pouch). All mesenteric defects are closed.

Postoperative Care

Early ambulation postoperatively is important to help prevent deep venous thrombosis. Pain control must be adequate to allow coughing and use of incentive spirometry. Although controversial, we obtain a Gastrografin swallow on postoperative day 1 to document pouch size, proximal and distal anastomotic patency, lack of obstruction, and reconfirm the absence of leakage (although clinical criteria outweigh the results of such testing for determining reoperation for suspected leak). Liquids are started after this study, if all appears well. Patients are generally discharged 2–4 days after surgery.

Efficacy

RYGB results in weight loss that is slightly superior to that of purely restrictive operations. Five-year weight loss results have ranged from 48–74 percent excess weight loss. One series of 608 patients followed over 14 years with less than 3 percent of patients lost to follow up has demonstrated a 49 percent excess weight loss.

RYGB has been demonstrated not only to prevent the progression of non–insulin-dependent diabetes mellitus, but also to reduce the mortality from diabetes mellitus, primarily because of a reduction in the number of deaths from cardiovascular disease. Durable control of diabetes mellitus is achieved following RYGB, along with amelioration or resolution of other comorbidities such as hypertension, sleep apnea, GERD, and cardiopulmonary failure. Other obesity-related medical illnesses that have shown improvement or resolution following RYGB include hyperlipidemia, hypertension, asthma, osteoarthritis, angina, venous stasis, and obesity-hypoventilation syndrome.

Complications

Early complications include anastomotic leak with peritonitis (1.2 percent), acute distal gastric dilatation, Roux limb obstruction, severe wound infection (4.4 percent), and minor wound infection or seroma (11.4 percent). Late complications include stomal stenosis (15 percent), marginal ulcer (13 percent), intestinal obstruction (2 percent), internal hernia (1 percent), staple line disruption (0 to 1 percent), incisional hernia (16.9 percent), cholecystitis (10 percent). Mortality in the best of series is as low as 0.4 percent, and more commonly at 1–2 percent in general practice. Metabolic complications include deficiencies of vitamin B12 (26–40 percent), iron (20–49 percent), and anemia (18–35 percent).

A few postoperative complications are specific to RYGB, including distal gastric distention and internal hernia. Distal gastric distention, usually because of obstruction at or distal to the enteroenterostomy, is an emergency requiring percutaneous or operative decompression of the distal stomach. Internal hernias, at times difficult to diagnose, may present with vague periumbilical pain, nausea, and vomiting. A radiographic upper gastrointestinal study or computed tomography (CT) scan may be helpful in diagnosis, but may not be diagnostic. Operative exploration and repair is indicated if this diagnosis is being entertained.

Advantages and Disadvantages

The RYGB is more effective than VBG in terms of weight loss, as is detailed above. This is true even if diet preferences are selected for preoperatively. Overall resolution of comorbidities, especially those of diabetes, GERD, and perhaps hyperlipidemias appear better after RYGB than after any of the restrictive operations. RYGB has become the most popular bariatric operation in the United States, because of its overall effectiveness and relatively low need for reoperation.

Dumping syndrome occurs in a variable number of patients following gastric bypass. Patients may experience bloating, nausea, diarrhea, and abdominal pain after ingesting sweets or milk products. Vasomotor symptoms such as palpitations, diaphoresis, and lightheadedness also may occur. Dumping syndrome may provide a beneficial effect in promoting weight loss by causing patients to avoid sweets.

Laparoscopic Roux-en-Y Gastric Bypass

Technique

Laparoscopic RYGB was first described by Wittgrove, Clark, and Tremblay in 1994. After pneumoperitoneum is established, five or six access ports are inserted. A vertically oriented proximal gastric pouch measuring 15–30 mL is created from the proximal lesser curvature portion of the stomach using sequential applications of a linear endoscopic stapler.

The ligament of Treitz is identified, and the jejunum is divided 20–50 cm distally with a linear stapler. More distal division is needed if an antecolic route of the Roux limb is planned. A 75–150-cm Roux limb (once again based on patient's preoperative weight) is constructed and a side-to-side jejunojejunostomy is created with linear endoscopic staplers. Some groups use an elongated Roux limb of 150–250 cm for superobesity.

The gastrojejunal anastomosis may be stapled or hand-sewn. Several stapling techniques have been described. For a circular stapled anastomosis with transoral passage of the anvil, upper endoscopy is performed and a looped wire is used to pass the anvil of a circular stapler into and through the wall of the pouch. An incision is made near the end of the Roux limb to admit the circular stapler, which is mated with the anvil to create the stapled anastomosis.

To create a circular stapled anastomosis with transgastric anvil insertion, a gastrotomy is created on the anterior stomach and the anvil is introduced into the stomach. The tip is brought through the gastric wall; the pouch is then created using sequential firings of the linear stapler.

For a linear-stapled anastomosis, a posterior layer of sutures is placed to approximate the Roux limb to the pouch. A 45-mm linear stapler is used to create the gastrojejunostomy. Closure of the stapler defect is performed with two layers of sutures.

The gastrojejunal anastomosis may also be completely hand-sewn in two layers using absorbable suture.

Insufflation of the gastric pouch with air by endoscopy or orogastric tube or with methylene blue is performed to test the integrity of the anastomosis. Port sites larger than 5 mm are closed at the fascial level.

Postoperative Care

Some surgeons place a Jackson-Pratt or Blake drain at the anastomosis, which is left in place for a varying length of time, depending on surgeon preference. Nasogastric tubes are not used routinely. Early postoperative mobilization is emphasized. Parameters used for open RYGB are similarly used for LRYGB.

Efficacy

Mean excess weight loss after LRYGB ranges from 69–82 percent with follow-up of 24 months or less. Wittgrove and associates demonstrated a mean excess weight loss of 73 percent with follow up of 60 months. Schauer and associates showed the mean excess weight loss was 83 and 77 percent at 24 and 30 months, respectively. Most comorbidities were improved or eradicated, including diabetes mellitus, hypertension, sleep apnea, and GERD. Quality of life was improved significantly.

Complications

Postoperative complications observed after LRYGB include pulmonary embolism (0–1.5 percent), anastomotic leak (1.5–5.8 percent), bleeding (0–3.3 percent), and pulmonary complications (0–5.8 percent). Stenosis of the gastrojejunostomy is observed in 1.6–6.3 percent. Other complications include internal hernia (2.5–5 percent), gallstones (1.4 percent), marginal ulcer (1.4 percent), and staple-line failure (1 percent). Conversion to an open procedure occurs in 3–9 percent. The mortality rate is 0–1.5 percent.

Advantages and Disadvantages

LRYGB offers the advantages over open RYGB of better cosmesis, less postoperative pain, and attenuation of the postoperative stress response. Patients recover rapidly and have a shorter hospital stay. There is an improvement in postoperative pulmonary function with the laparoscopic procedure. The principal advantage of the laparoscopic approach has been in reducing perioperative morbidity, in particular the marked reduction in wound-related complications, including incisional hernias.

LRYGB, although safe and feasible, is a technically challenging, advanced laparoscopic procedure with a steep learning curve. This approach may be more difficult in superobese patients, those with large livers, and those who have a preponderance of fat in the abdominal area.

Biliopancreatic Diversion

Indications

BPD is primarily indicated for the superobese, for those who have failed restrictive bariatric procedures, or for those patients wishing to have less restriction on their ability to eat after surgery but willing to accept the consequences of increased bowel frequency and diarrhea.

Contraindications

Patients with anemia, hypocalcemia, and osteoporosis, and those who are not motivated to comply with stringent postoperative supplementation regimens may not be appropriate for this procedure. Patients whose social situation and geographic location suggest they may be noncompliant with follow up also are not good candidates. The laparoscopic approach may be especially challenging in patients who have undergone multiple previous abdominal surgeries, previous weight loss surgery, patients with an enlarged fatty liver, and in those with a large amount of intraabdominal fat.

Technique

The BPD was developed by Nicola Scopinaro of Italy. The procedure combines mild to moderate gastric restriction with an intestinal malabsorptive procedure.

A subtotal distal gastrectomy is performed, leaving a proximal 200-mL gastric pouch for the superobese patient, or up to a 400-mL pouch for the others. The terminal ileum is measured, and the intestine divided 250 cm proximal to the ileocecal valve. The distal end of this divided bowel is anastomosed to the gastric pouch with a 2–3-cm stoma. An enteroenterostomy is created 50–100 cm proximal to the ileocecal valve to incorporate the distal end of the biliopancreatic limb into the alimentary stream. A concomitant cholecystectomy is performed.

Biliopancreatic Diversion with Duodenal Switch

A modification of this technique is called the biliopancreatic diversion with BPD-DS. This involves performing a greater curvature sleeve gastrectomy, with maintenance of the continuity of the antrum, pylorus, and first portion of the duodenum. The distal bowel division and connections are the same, except the anastomosis to the stomach is instead performed to the distal stump of the retained first portion of the duodenum. This may be an end to side or end to end anastomosis, and is often performed using a circular stapler.

The BPD-DS allows for a lower marginal ulcer rate (0–1 percent) and a lower incidence of dumping syndrome. For the laparoscopic approach, six to eight laparoscopic ports are inserted. A sleeve gastrectomy is performed to create a gastric reservoir of 150–200 mL. As in the open procedure, the ileum is divided 250 cm proximal to the ileocecal valve and is anastomosed to the first portion of the duodenum. An enteroenterostomy is created laparoscopically, leaving a 100 cm common channel.

Postoperative Care

The patient must be on lifelong vitamin, calcium, and iron supplementation, and must comply with lifelong follow up because of the risk of malnutrition. Fat soluble vitamin supplementation is indicated, and this must often be done using the parenteral route. Careful follow-up is necessary to be on alert for the potential for protein-calorie malnutrition, which is important to recognize and treat aggressively with parenteral nutrition or even, if persistent, revision and lengthening of the common channel.

Efficacy

Weight loss results with BPD are excellent and durable. At 8 years, patients weighing up to 120 percent of ideal body weight, and those weighing more than 120 percent of ideal body weight maintained 72 and 77 percent mean excess weight loss, respectively. A group of 40 patients had a mean excess weight loss of 70 percent for a 15-year period.

The results of laparoscopic BPD-DS in 40 patients were reported. Median preoperative BMI was 60 kg/m². There was one conversion to an open procedure (2.5 percent). Median length of stay was 4 days. Mean excess weight loss at 6 and 9 months was 46 ± 2 percent and 58 ± 3 percent, respectively, with a median follow up of 6 months.

Complications

The incidence of postoperative complications, including nutritional ones, is substantial following BPD. The most common morbidities include anemia (30 percent), protein-calorie malnutrition (20 percent), dumping syndrome, and marginal ulceration (10 percent). The duodenal switch modification is associated with a lower ulceration rate (1 percent) and a lower incidence of dumping syndrome. Other complications include vitamin B12 deficiency, hypocalcemia, fat-soluble vitamin deficiencies, osteoporosis, night blindness, and prolongation of prothrombin time. The postoperative mortality rate ranges from 0.4–2.5 percent.

From Scopinaro's series, early surgical complications included wound infection and dehiscence (1.2 percent). Late complications included incisional hernia (8.7 percent), intestinal obstruction (1.2 percent), protein malnutrition (7 percent), iron deficiency anemia (< 5 percent), stomal ulcer (2.8 percent), and acute biliopancreatic limb obstruction. Bone demineralization was seen in 25 percent preoperatively; at 1–2 years, it was observed in 29 percent. At 3–5 years, it was present in 53 percent, and in 14 percent at 6–10 years.

In a laparoscopic series from Ren and colleagues, there was one death (2.5 percent). The major morbidity rate was 15 percent, including anastomotic leak (2.5 percent), venous thrombosis (2.5 percent), staple-line hemorrhage (10 percent), and subphrenic abscess (2.5 percent).

Advantages and Disadvantages

Even if patients consume a great quantity of food, the malabsorptive component of the BPD allows for excellent results in terms of weight loss. This operation may be more effective than RYGB or LAGB in the patients with BMI greater than 70 kg/m²), or in those who have failed to maintain weight loss following those operations. Patients are not as restricted in terms of types of food that they may eat. Of the BPD or BPD-DS options, the BPD is generally felt to be technically easier to perform, as the duodenoileostomy anastomosis is challenging. On the other hand, the BPD-DS does offer a lower incidence of dumping and marginal ulcer postoperatively. The laparoscopic versions of the BPD or BPD-DS procedures have the same advantages as the open approach versions.

The disadvantages of BPD include the fact it is technically more complex than any restrictive procedure. Protein malnutrition with anemia, hypoalbuminemia, edema, and alopecia are among the serious adverse sequelae of this operation. Severe iron and fat-soluble vitamin deficiencies may occur, leading to anemia, osteoporosis and night-blindness. Treatment requires prolonged supplementation, often parenteral. Routine replacement of fat-soluble vitamins is needed for patients following BPD or BPD-DS. Patients typically have four to six foul-smelling stools per day and may also experience bloating and heartburn.

Protein calorie malnutrition is a potentially life-threatening complication, which occurs in 3–20 percent of patients. It requires total parenteral nutrition to correct its acute phase, then improved diet intake and modification. If recurrent hypoalbuminemia persists, the common channel must be lengthened at reoperation.

The laparoscopic approaches to the BPD or BPD-DS are both especially challenging procedures technically, and are generally felt to be the most technically difficult laparoscopic bariatric operations to perform.

SPECIAL ISSUES RELATING TO THE BARIATRIC PATIENT

Bariatric Procedures in the Adolescent Patient

Bariatric surgery in morbidly obese adolescents is controversial. An estimated 25 percent of children in the United States are obese, a number that has doubled over a 30-year period. Although very little information has been published on the subject of obesity surgery in adolescents, review of the available literature shows that bariatric surgery in adolescents is safe and is associated with significant weight loss, correction of obesity-related comorbidities, and improved self-image and socialization.

Surgery may be indicated in this population because of the dismal failure of conservative methods of weight control. All patients should meet NIH criteria for bariatric surgery. Issues of preoperative consent and compliance with follow up suggest that patients who do undergo such procedures must have a more intensive multidiscipline team approach to preparation for and follow up after surgery.

The reports in the literature report small numbers of patients at any institution. Sugerman and associates described 33 adolescents who underwent gastroplasty ($n = 3$) or RYGB ($n = 30$). There were two late sudden deaths (2 and 6 years postoperatively), unrelated to the bariatric procedure. Significant weight loss was maintained in the majority of patients for up to 14 years after surgery. Most of comorbidities resolved at 1 year. Self-image was greatly enhanced, resulting in successful marriages and educational achievements. Capella and colleagues reported 19 adolescent patients undergoing banded RYGB who experienced an 80 percent excess weight loss at 5.5-year follow-up. Abu-Abeid reported 11 patients who underwent LAGB. Their mean BMI dropped from 46.6 down to 32.1 kg/m^2, with marked improvement in medical conditions.

Bariatric Surgery in Older Adult Patients

Information about the association between body weight and mortality at higher ages is sparse. Indices of visceral obesity may be better indicators of risk than BMI in these age groups. Not only actual weight, but also weight development over the last decades of life may predict outcome. Little is known about the benefits of diets or drugs that induce weight loss in this age group. Osteoarthritis and static respiratory complications seem to improve with weight loss, even at higher ages. Recent studies suggest that bariatric surgery, previously considered contraindicated in obese patients above age 60, can be safely performed even in patients above age 70, with the same benefits as those seen in younger patients.

Some surgeons have considered age 50 years or older as a relative contraindication to bariatric surgery. Gonzales et al demonstrated safety and efficacy in a group of patients aged 50 years or older undergoing RYGB. Macgregor and Rand reported that patients aged 55 years and older undergoing gastric restrictive surgery had an average loss of 57 percent excess body weight and 20–48 percent reduction of comorbidities. Nehoda and colleagues reported patients over age 50 who underwent LAGB experienced the same clinical outcome as younger patients.

The Female Patient: Pregnancy and Gynecologic Issues in the Bariatric Surgery Patient

Pregnancy in morbidly obese women carries increased risks, and should be managed as a high-risk pregnancy. The incidence of gestational diabetes and hypertension is increased, and macrosomia is common. Following the pregnancy is difficult because of limitations of the physical examinations. More costly, more frequent ultrasound examinations are needed. There is a 2–3-fold increase in the rate of cesarean sections, with more complications. However, fetal morbidity does not appear to be changed when maternal weight gain is limited.

Bariatric surgery reduces both a woman's weight and the incidence of obesity-related comorbidities, and appears to confer decreased risk to pregnancy. Dixon and associates suggest that morbidly obese women have higher obstetric risks and poorer neonatal outcomes. However, weight loss reduced obstetric risk. They noticed decreased maternal weight gain during pregnancy for women who underwent LAGB. No difference in birth weights was noted for women before and after LAGB. Obstetric complications were minimal, and there were no premature or low birth weight infants.

Wittgrove's group evaluated the rate of complications in patients becoming pregnant following RYGB or LRYGB. They found a lower risk of gestational diabetes, macrosomia, and cesarean section in postsurgical patients than in those who were obese and had not had bariatric surgery. Another study showed medical complications that were frequent during pregnancy whereas individuals were severely obese (hypertension 26.7 percent, preeclampsia 12.8 percent, diabetes 7.0 percent, and deep vein thrombosis 7.0 percent) did not occur after weight loss and weight stabilization. Because surgical patients after RYGB have had an operation that restricts food intake, some dietary precautions should be taken when they become pregnant. They are at risk for developing severe iron deficiency anemia because of poor absorption of iron.

The incidence of infertility is increased in morbidly obese women. Obesity-induced hormonal disorders contribute to biologic imbalance, and thus favor the development of dysfunctional ovulation. An abnormal menstrual history is common. In one study, infertility problems were present preoperatively in 29.3 percent of female patients. Bariatric surgery results in normalization of many gynecologic and obstetric risks and problems from obesity. Menstrual irregularities decreased from 40.4–4.6 percent after bariatric surgery in one report.

The polycystic ovary syndrome results from a systemic hormonal dysfunction. Women with polycystic ovaries are frequently obese and have a higher risk of infertility, anovulation, hyperandrogenism, dyslipidemia, insulin resistance, and abnormal menses. Improvement of these problems may occur after surgically induced weight loss.

Obesity has a major impact on stress urinary incontinence. Women suffering from obesity manifest increased intraabdominal pressures, which adversely stress the pelvic floor and may contribute to the development of urinary incontinence. Additionally, obesity may affect the neuromuscular function of the genitourinary tract, thereby also contributing to incontinence. Dwyer and colleagues reported on incontinent women who underwent urodynamic assessment: 63 percent were diagnosed as having genuine stress incontinence and 27 percent as having detrusor instability. Obesity was significantly more common in women with genuine stress incontinence and detrusor instability than in the normal population. Weight reduction after bariatric surgery improves urinary incontinence in obese women. In one study, the incidence decreased from 61.2–11.6 percent.

Gallbladder Disease in the Bariatric Surgery Patient

Rapid weight loss after diets or bariatric surgery is known to be associated with increased gallstone formation. After RYGB, this incidence has been quantified as being as high as 38–53 percent of patients who preoperatively did not have stones. The incidence of cholecystectomy in such at-risk patients after RYGB is described as being from 10–27 percent within 3 years after surgery. Most bariatric surgeons recommend simultaneous cholecystectomy when stones are known to be present at the time of the bariatric operation. This is especially true for open procedures and malabsorptive procedures.

Routine cholecystectomy concomitant with a LRYGB remains controversial. The safety of combining laparoscopic cholecystectomy and LRYGB has been established, but performing both in one procedure may increase the length of hospital stay and adds 30–60 min to the operative time. If cholecystectomy is not performed, excellent data exist that the prophylactic use of oral ursodiol after RYGB is indicated. It has been shown that ursodiol, if taken in doses of 300 mg twice daily for the first 6 months postoperatively, decreases the incidence of postoperative gallstones formation to 2 percent.

Choledocholithiasis after RYGB or BPD becomes a difficult clinical problem because of a loss of endoscopic access to the duodenum. Anchoring the remnant stomach to the anterior abdominal wall, preferably with a radiologic marker, may provide a safe point for percutaneous access for endoscopic retrograde cholangiopancreatography, especially if known gallstones are left in situ.

Diabetes in the Bariatric Surgery Patient

Paralleling the rise in incidence of morbid obesity is the incidence of type II diabetes, often as a component of the metabolic syndrome (syndrome X) comprising central obesity, glucose intolerance, dyslipidemia, and hypertension.

Several recently published outcome studies demonstrate the value of bariatric operations in improving diabetes in the morbidly obese. LAGB resulted in complete resolution or definite improvement of diabetes in 97 percent of patients. In a study by Schauer and associates, 21 percent of 1160 patients undergoing laparoscopic LRYGB demonstrated impaired fasting glucose or type II diabetes mellitus. After surgery, fasting plasma glucose and glycosylated hemoglobin concentrations returned to normal levels (83 percent) or were markedly improved (17 percent) in all patients. A significant reduction in the use of oral antidiabetic agents (80 percent) and insulin (79 percent) was also observed. Patients with the shortest duration (<5 years), the mildest form of diabetes (diet-controlled), and the greatest weight loss after surgery, were most likely to achieve complete resolution of diabetes.

Plastic Surgery Following Weight Loss

Most patients who lose massive amounts of weight are troubled by hanging skin and rolls of skin and fat. Although smaller in size, their clothes fit poorly. Skin macerates under an abdominal pannus, hanging inner thighs, and ptotic breasts. Body aroma is unpleasant. Heavy flaps of skin burden the back and inhibit vigorous exercise. Intimate relations may be untenable. Plastic surgery can substantially improve or correct the skin changes resulting from weight loss.

Body contouring surgery advanced considerably during the 1990s, and these procedures have been modified for this new post–bariatric surgery population. The massive weight loss patient has a deflated shape that is related to genetically defined fat deposition patterns. The most susceptible regions are the anterior neck, upper arms, breasts, lower back, flanks, abdomen, mons pubis, and thighs. Problematic areas for women include the subcutaneous abdomen and hips and thighs; in men, they are the flanks, abdomen, and breasts. The deformity reflects the initial BMI and its change. Because the etiology of the skin laxity is not understood, there is no medical therapy. The widest possible areas of skin are excised and closed. Operative planning is based on the deformity and patient priorities. Most have excess tissue of the lower torso and thighs removed through a circumferential abdominoplasty and lower body lift. Starting prone and then turning supine, the operation removes a wide swath of skin and fat along the bikini line. A panniculectomy that corrects the overhanging pannus is included. The circumferential abdominoplasty removes the redundant skin of the lower abdomen, flattens the abdomen, and incorporates the lower body lift. A medial high transverse thighplasty usually accompanies the lower body lift in massive weight loss patients. Unwanted skin redundancy distal to the mid-thighs requires long vertical medial excision of skin.

Mid-back and epigastric rolls and sagging breasts are corrected with an upper body lift. The upper body lift is a reverse abdominoplasty, removal of mid-torso excess skin, and reshaping of the breasts. For highly selected individuals, and with a well organized team, a single-stage total body lift, which includes a circumferential abdominoplasty, lower body lift, medial thighplasty, an upper body lift, and breast reshaping, can be performed safely in under 8 h.

The opportunity that these large numbers of massive weight loss patients provide for plastic surgery innovation, treatment, and professional satisfaction is extraordinary. Patients are uniformly pleased with their improvements. Research in adipocyte physiology, skin biomechanics, and alternative surgical technique should lead to improved care.

Acknowledgment

The authors would like to thank the following for their contributions to this chapter: Dennis Hurwitz, M. D., Clinical Professor of Plastic Surgery, University of Pittsburgh, Paul Thoidiyl, M. D., Fellow in Laparoscopic and Bariatric Surgery, University of Pittsburgh, and Tomasz Rogula, M. D. Fellow in Laparoscopic and Bariatric Surgery University of Pittsburgh.

Suggested Readings

Scopinaro N, Adami GF, Marinari GM, et al: Biliopancreatic diversion. World J Surg 22:936, 1998.

Schauer PR, Ikramuddin S, Gourash W, et al: Outcomes after laparoscopic Roux-en-Y gastric bypass for morbid obesity. Ann Surg 232:515, 2000.

Nguyen NT, et al: Laparoscopic versus open gastric bypass: A randomized study of outcomes, quality of life, and costs. Ann Surg 234:279, 2001; discussion 289.

Balsiger BM, Poggio JL, Mai J, et al: Ten and more years after vertical banded gastroplasty as primary operation for morbid obesity. J Gastrointest Surg 4:598, 2000.

O'Brien PE, et al: The laparoscopic adjustable gastric band (Lap-Band): A prospective study of medium-term effects on weight, health and quality of life. Obes Surg 12:652, 2002.

Angrisani L, et al: Lap Band adjustable gastric banding system: The Italian experience with 1863 patients operated on 6 years. Surg Endosc 17:409, 2003.

Ren CJ, Patterson E, Gagner M: Early results of laparoscopic biliopancreatic diversion with duodenal switch: A case series of 40 consecutive patients. Obes Surg 10:514, 2000; discussion 524.

Schauer PR, et al: Effect of laparoscopic Roux-en Y gastric bypass on type 2 diabetes mellitus. Ann Surg 238:467, 2003; discussion 84.

Buchwald H, Avidor Y, Braunwald E, et al. Bariatric Surgery. A systematic review and meta-analysis. JAMA 2004; 292:1724–37.

Buchwald H. Bariatric Surgery for Morbid Obesity: Health Implications for Patients, Health Professionals, and Third-Party Payers. J Am Coll Surg 2005; 200:593–604.

27 | Small Intestine

*Edward E. Whang, Stanley W. Ashley,
and Michael J. Zinner*

GROSS ANATOMY

The small intestine is a tubular structure that consists of three segments lying in series: the duodenum, the jejunum, and the ileum. The duodenum, the most proximal segment, lies in the retroperitoneum immediately adjacent to the head and inferior border of the body of the pancreas. The duodenum is demarcated from the jejunum by the ligament of Treitz. The jejunum and ileum lie within the peritoneal cavity and are tethered to the retroperitoneum by a broad-based mesentery. No distinct anatomic landmark demarcates the jejunum from the ileum; the proximal 40 percent of the jejunoileal segment is arbitrarily defined as the jejunum and the distal 60 percent as the ileum.

The small intestine contains mucosal folds known as plicae circulares or valvulae conniventes that are visible on gross inspection. These folds are also visible radiographically and help to distinguish between small intestine and colon (which does not contain them) on abdominal radiographs. Gross examination of the small-intestinal mucosa also reveals aggregates of lymphoid follicles. Those follicles are most prominent in the ileum, in which they are designated Peyer patches.

Most of the duodenum derives its arterial blood from branches of both the celiac and the superior mesenteric arteries. The distal duodenum, the jejunum, and the ileum derive their arterial blood from the superior mesenteric artery. Their venous drainage occurs via the superior mesenteric vein. Lymph drainage occurs through lymphatic vessels coursing parallel to corresponding arteries. This lymph drains through mesenteric lymph nodes to the cisterna chyli, then through the thoracic duct, and ultimately into the left subclavian vein. The parasympathetic and sympathetic innervation of the small intestine is derived from the vagus and splanchnic nerves, respectively.

HISTOLOGY

The wall of the small intestine consists of four distinct layers: mucosa, submucosa, muscularis propria, and serosa.

The mucosa is the innermost layer, which itself consists of three layers: epithelium, lamina propria, and muscularis mucosae. The epithelium is exposed to the intestinal lumen and is the surface through which absorption from and secretion into the lumen occurs. The lamina propria is located immediately external to the epithelium and consists of connective tissue and a heterogeneous population of cells. It is demarcated from the more external submucosa by the muscularis mucosae, a thin sheet of smooth-muscle cells.

The mucosa is organized into villi and crypts (crypts of Lieberkühn). Villi are finger-like projections of epithelium and underlying lamina propria that contain blood and lymphatic vessels (lacteals) that extend into the intestinal lumen. Epithelial cellular proliferation is confined to the crypts. All epithelial cells in each crypt are derived from yet uncharacterized multipotent stem cells located at or near the crypt's base. Their descendants undergo differentiation along one of four pathways that ultimately yield enterocyte and goblet, enteroendocrine, and Paneth cells.

Enterocytes are the predominant absorptive cell of the intestinal epithelium. Their apical (lumen-facing) cell membrane contains microvilli and specialized digestive enzymes and transporter mechanisms. Goblet cells produce mucin believed to play a role in mucosal defense against pathogens. Enteroendocrine cells are characterized by secretory granules containing regulatory agents. Paneth cells are located at the base of the crypt and contain secretory granules containing growth factors, digestive enzymes, and antimicrobial peptides. Additionally, the intestinal epithelium contains M cells and intraepithelial lymphocytes, both components of the immune system.

The submucosa consists of dense connective tissue and a heterogeneous population of cells, including leukocytes and fibroblasts. The submucosa also contains an extensive network of vascular and lymphatic vessels, nerve fibers, and ganglion cells of the submucosal (Meissner) plexus.

The muscularis propria consists of an outer, longitudinally oriented layer and an inner, circularly oriented layer of smooth-muscle fibers. Located at the interface between these two layers are ganglion cells of the myenteric (Auerbach) plexus.

The serosa consists of a single layer of mesothelial cells and is a component of the visceral peritoneum.

DEVELOPMENT

The gut tube is formed from the endoderm during the fourth week of gestation. The gut tube initially communicates with the yolk sac; however, the communication between these two structures narrows by the sixth week to form the vitelline duct. Incomplete obliteration of the vitelline duct results in the spectrum of defects associated with Meckel diverticula.

At approximately the fifth week of gestation, the bowel begins to lengthen to an extent greater than that which can be accommodated by the developing abdominal cavity, resulting in the extracoelomic herniation of the developing bowel. The bowel is retracted back into the abdominal cavity during the tenth week of gestation. Coincident with extrusion and retraction, the bowel undergoes a 270-degree counterclockwise rotation relative to the posterior abdominal wall. Errors in this process can result in intestinal malrotation.

During the sixth week of gestation, the lumen of the developing bowel becomes obliterated as bowel epithelial proliferation accelerates. Vacuoles form within the bowel substance during the subsequent weeks and coalesce to form the intestinal lumen by the ninth week of gestation. Errors in this recanalization may account for defects such as intestinal webs and stenoses.

PHYSIOLOGY

Digestion and Absorption

Eight to 9 L of fluid enter the small intestine daily. Most of this volume consists of salivary, gastric, biliary, pancreatic, and intestinal secretions. Under normal conditions, the small intestine absorbs more than 80 percent of this fluid, leaving approximately 1.5 L that enters the colon.

Carbohydrate Digestion and Absorption

Pancreatic amylase is the major enzyme of starch digestion, although salivary amylase initiates the process. The terminal products of amylase-mediated starch digestion are oligosaccharides, maltotriose, maltose, and α-limit dextrins. These products, and the major disaccharides in the diet (sucrose and lactose) undergo hydrolytic cleavage into their constituent monosaccharides, primarily glucose, galactose, and fructose, which are absorbed through specific transmembrane carriers.

Protein Digestion and Absorption

Protein digestion begins in the stomach with the action of pepsins. Digestion continues in the duodenum with the actions of a variety of pancreatic peptidases. The final products of intraluminal protein digestion consist of amino acids and peptides that are two to six amino acids in length. Additional digestion occurs through the actions of peptidases that exist in the enterocyte brush border and cytoplasm. Epithelial absorption occurs for both single amino acids and di- or tripeptides via specific membrane-bound transporters. Absorbed amino acids and peptides then enter the portal venous circulation. Of all amino acids, glutamine appears to be a unique, major source of energy for enterocytes.

Fat Digestion and Absorption

Ingested fat, primarily in the form of triglycerides, is converted into an emulsion by the mechanical actions of mastication and antral peristalsis. Although lipolysis of triglycerides to form fatty acids and monoglycerides is initiated in the stomach by gastric lipase, its principal site is the proximal intestine, in which pancreatic lipase is the catalyst.

Bile acids form mixed micelles with the products of lipolysis to aid in their solubilization in water. Most lipids are absorbed in the proximal jejunum, whereas bile salts are absorbed in the distal ileum. Within the enterocytes, triglycerides are resynthesized and incorporated into chylomicrons that are secreted into the intestinal lymphatics and ultimately enter the thoracic duct.

The steps described above are required for the digestion and absorption of triglycerides containing long-chain fatty acids. However, triglycerides containing short- and medium-chain fatty acids are more hydrophilic and are directly absorbed and enter the portal venous circulation rather than the lymphatics.

Vitamin Absorption

Vitamin B12 (cobalamin) malabsorption can result from a variety of surgical manipulations. The vitamin is initially bound by saliva-derived R protein. In the duodenum, R protein is hydrolyzed by pancreatic enzymes, allowing free cobalamin to bind to gastric parietal cell-derived intrinsic factor. The cobalamin-intrinsic factor complex is able to escape hydrolysis by pancreatic enzymes, allowing it to reach the terminal ileum, which expresses specific receptors for intrinsic factor, facilitating cobalamin absorption. Because each of these steps is necessary for cobalamin assimilation, gastric resection, gastric bypass, and ileal resection can each result in vitamin B12 insufficiency.

Barrier and Immune Function

Factors contributing to epithelial defense include immunoglobulin A (IgA), mucins, and the relative impermeability of the brush border membrane and tight junctions to macromolecules and bacteria.

The intestinal component of the immune system is known as the gut-associated lymphoid tissue (GALT). The GALT is conceptually divided into inductive and effector sites. Inductive sites include Peyer's patches, mesenteric lymph nodes, and smaller, isolated lymphoid follicles scattered throughout the small intestine. At inductive sites, naïve lymphocytes become primed following antigen exposure, then exit through the draining lymphatics to enter the mesenteric lymph nodes where they undergo differentiation. These lymphocytes then migrate into the systemic circulation via the thoracic duct, and ultimately accumulate in the intestinal mucosa at effector sites.

Effector lymphocytes are distributed into distinct compartments. T cell subsets are located in the epithelium and lamina propria where they play regulatory and cytotoxic roles. Plasma cells, located in the lamina propria secrete IgA, which is transported through the intestinal epithelial cells into the lumen, in which it exists in the form of a dimer complexed with a secretory component. This configuration renders IgA resistant to proteolysis by digestive enzymes. IgA is believed both to help prevent the entry of microbes through the epithelium and to promote excretion of antigens or microbes that have already penetrated into the laminal propria.

Motility

Contractions of the muscularis propria are responsible for small-intestinal peristalsis. Contractions of the muscularis mucosae contribute to mucosal or villus motility, but not to peristalsis.

The regulatory mechanisms driving small-intestinal motility consist of both pacemakers intrinsic to the small intestine and external neurohumoral modulatory signals. The interstitial cells of Cajal are pleomorphic mesenchymal cells located within the muscularis propria of the intestine that generate the electrical slow wave (basic electrical rhythm or pacesetter potential) that plays a pacemaker role in setting the fundamental rhythmicity of small-intestinal contractions. In general, the sympathetic motor supply is inhibitory to the enteric motor system; therefore, increased sympathetic input into the intestine leads to decreased intestinal smooth-muscle activity. The parasympathetic motor supply is more complex, with projections to both inhibitory and excitatory enteric motor system motor neurons.

Endocrine Function

More than 30 peptide hormone genes have been identified as being expressed in the gastrointestinal tract.

Table 27-1 summarizes examples of regulatory peptides produced by enteroendocrine cells of the small-intestinal epithelium and their most commonly ascribed functions. Some of these peptides, or their analogues, are used in routine clinical practice. For example, therapeutic applications of octreotide, a long-acting analogue of somatostatin, include the amelioration of symptoms associated with neuroendocrine tumors (e.g., carcinoid syndrome), postgastrectomy dumping syndrome, enterocutaneous fistulas, and the initial treatment of acute hemorrhage caused by esophageal varices. The gastrin secretory response to secretin administration forms the basis for the standard test used to establish the diagnosis of Zollinger-Ellison syndrome. Cholecystokinin is used in evaluations of gallbladder ejection fraction, a parameter that may have utility in patients who have symptoms of biliary colic but are not found to have gallstones.

TABLE 27-1 Representative Regulatory Peptides Produced in the Small Intestine

Hormone	Source[a]	Actions
Somatostatin	D cell	Inhibits gastrointestinal secretion, motility, and splanchnic perfusion
Secretin	S cell	Stimulates exocrine pancreatic secretion; stimulates intestinal secretion
Cholecystokinin	I cell	Stimulates pancreatic exocrine secretion; simulates gallbladder emptying; inhibits sphincter of Oddi contraction
Motilin	M cell	Stimulates intestinal motility
Peptide YY	L cell	Inhibits intestinal motility and secretion
Glucagon-like peptide 2	L cell	Stimulates intestinal epithelial proliferation
Neurotensin	N cell	Stimulates pancreatic and biliary secretion; inhibits small bowel motility; stimulates intestinal mucosal growth

[a]This table indicates which enteroendocrine cell types located in the intestinal epithelium produce these peptides. These peptides are also widely expressed in nonintestinal tissues.

Of the peptides listed in Table 27-1, glucagon-like peptide 2 (GLP-2) is the most recently characterized. This product of the proglucagon gene has potent trophic activity that is specific for the intestinal epithelium. It is currently under clinical evaluation as an intestinotrophic agent in patients suffering from the short bowel syndrome.

SMALL-BOWEL OBSTRUCTION

Epidemiology

Mechanical small-bowel obstruction is the most frequently encountered surgical disorder of the small intestine. Intraabdominal adhesions related to prior abdominal surgery is the etiologic factor in up to 75 percent of cases of small-bowel obstruction. Other common etiologies include hernias and Crohn disease. Although congenital abnormalities capable of causing small-bowel obstruction usually become evident during childhood, they sometimes are diagnosed for the first time in adult patients. For example, intestinal malrotation and mid-gut volvulus should be considered when considering the differential diagnosis of adult patients with acute or chronic symptoms of small-bowel obstruction, especially those without a history of prior abdominal surgery. A rare etiology of obstruction is the superior mesenteric artery syndrome, characterized by compression of the third portion of the duodenum by the superior mesenteric artery as it crosses over this portion of the duodenum. This condition should be considered in young asthenic individuals who have chronic symptoms suggestive of proximal small-bowel obstruction.

Pathophysiology

The obstructing lesion can be conceptualized according to its anatomic relationship to the intestinal wall as (1) intraluminal (e.g., foreign bodies,

TABLE 27-2 Small-Bowel Obstruction: Common Etiologies

Adhesions
Neoplasms
Primary small-bowel neoplasms
Secondary small-bowel cancer (e.g., melanoma-derived metastasis)
Local invasion by intraabdominal malignancy
Carcinomatosis
Hernias
External
Internal
Crohn disease
Volvulus
Intussusception
Radiation-induced stricture
Postischemic stricture
Foreign body
Gallstone ileus
Diverticulitis
Meckel diverticulum
Hematoma
Congenital abnormalities (e.g., webs, duplications, and malrotation)

gallstones, or meconium), (2) intramural (e.g., tumors, Crohn disease-associated inflammatory strictures, or hematomas), or (3) extrinsic (e.g., adhesions, hernias, or carcinomatosis).

With onset of obstruction, gas and fluid accumulate within the intestinal lumen proximal to the site of obstruction. With ongoing gas and fluid accumulation, the bowel distends and intraluminal and intramural pressures rise. If the intramural pressure becomes high enough, microvascular perfusion to the intestine is impaired, leading to intestinal ischemia, and, ultimately, necrosis. This condition is termed strangulating bowel obstruction.

With partial small-bowel obstruction, only a portion of the intestinal lumen is occluded, allowing passage of some gas and fluid. The progression of pathophysiologic events described above tends to occur more slowly than with complete small-bowel obstruction, and development of strangulation is less likely. In contrast, progression to strangulation occurs especially rapidly with closed loop obstruction in which a segment of intestine is obstructed both proximally and distally (e.g., with volvulus).

Clinical Presentation

The symptoms of small-bowel obstruction are colicky abdominal pain, nausea, vomiting, and obstipation. Continued passage of flatus and/or stool beyond 6–12 h after onset of symptoms is characteristic of partial rather than complete obstruction. The signs of small-bowel obstruction include abdominal distention and hyperactive bowel sounds. Laboratory findings reflect intravascular volume depletion and consist of hemoconcentration and electrolyte abnormalities. Mild leukocytosis is common.

Features of strangulated obstruction include tachycardia, localized abdominal tenderness, fever, marked leukocytosis, and acidosis. It is important to note that these parameters lack sufficient predictive value to allow for differentiation between simple and strangulated obstruction prior to the onset of irreversible intestinal ischemia.

Diagnosis

The diagnostic evaluation should focus on the following goals: distinguishing mechanical obstruction from ileus; determining the etiology of the obstruction; discriminating partial from complete obstruction; and discriminating simple from strangulating obstruction.

Important elements to obtain on history include prior abdominal operations (suggesting the presence of adhesions) and the presence of abdominal disorders (e.g., intraabdominal cancer or inflammatory bowel disease) that may provide insights into the etiology of obstruction. On examination, a meticulous search for hernias (particularly in the inguinal and femoral regions) should be conducted. The stool should be checked for gross or occult blood, the presence of which is suggestive of intestinal strangulation.

The diagnosis of small-bowel obstruction is usually confirmed with radiographic examination. The abdominal series consists of a radiograph of the abdomen with the patient in a supine position, a radiograph of the abdomen with the patient in an upright position, and a radiograph of the chest with the patient in an upright position. The finding most specific for small-bowel obstruction is the triad of dilated small-bowel loops (>3 cm in diameter), air–fluid levels seen on upright films, and a paucity of air in the colon. False-negative findings on radiographs can result when the site of obstruction is located in the proximal small bowel and when the bowel lumen is filled with fluid but no gas, thereby preventing visualization of air–fluid levels or bowel distention.

Computed tomographic (CT) scan findings of small-bowel obstruction include a discrete transition zone with dilation of bowel proximally, decompression of bowel distally, intraluminal contrast that does not pass beyond the transition zone, and a colon containing little gas or fluid. Strangulation is suggested by thickening of the bowel wall, pneumatosis intestinalis (air in the bowel wall), portal venous gas, mesenteric haziness, and poor uptake of intravenous contrast into the wall of the affected bowel. CT scanning also offers a global evaluation of the abdomen and may therefore reveal the etiology of obstruction.

A limitation of CT scanning is its low sensitivity in the detection of low-grade or partial small-bowel obstruction. In such cases, contrast examinations of the small bowel, either small-bowel series (small-bowel follow-through) or enteroclysis, can be helpful. For standard small-bowel series, contrast is swallowed or instilled into the stomach through a nasogastric tube. Abdominal radiographs are then taken serially as the contrast travels distally in the intestine. Although barium can be used, water-soluble contrast agents, such as Gastrografin, should be used if the possibility of intestinal perforation exists. For enteroclysis, 200–250 mL of barium followed by 1–2 L of a solution of methylcellulose in water is instilled into the proximal jejunum via a long nasoenteric catheter. Enteroclysis is rarely performed in the acute setting, but offers greater sensitivity than small-bowel series in the detection of lesions that may be causing partial small-bowel obstruction.

Therapy

Small-bowel obstruction is usually associated with a marked depletion of intra-vascular volume caused by decreased oral intake, vomiting, and sequestration of fluid in bowel lumen and wall. Therefore, fluid resuscitation is integral to treatment. An indwelling bladder catheter is placed to monitor urine output. Central venous or pulmonary artery catheter monitoring may be necessary, particularly in patients with underlying cardiac disease. Broad-spectrum antibiotics are commonly administered because of concerns that bacterial translocation may occur in the setting of small-bowel obstruction. The stomach should be continuously evacuated of air and fluid, using a nasogastric (NG) tube, to decrease nausea, distention, and the risk of vomiting and aspiration.

The standard therapy for small-bowel obstruction is expeditious surgery, with the exception of specific situations described below. The operative procedure performed varies according to the etiology of the obstruction. For example, adhesions are lysed, tumors are resected, and hernias are reduced and repaired. Regardless of the etiology, the affected intestine should be examined, and nonviable bowel resected. Criteria suggesting viability are normal color, peristalsis, and marginal arterial pulsations. Usually visual inspection alone is adequate in judging viability. In borderline cases, a Doppler probe may be used to check for pulsatile flow to the bowel, and arterial perfusion can be verified by visualizing intravenously administered fluorescein dye in the bowel wall under ultraviolet illumination. In general, if the patient is hemodynamically stable, short lengths of bowel of questionable viability should be resected and primary anastomosis of the remaining intestine performed. However, if the viability of a large proportion of the intestine is in question, a concerted effort to preserve intestinal tissue should be made. In such situations, the bowel of uncertain viability should be left intact and the patient reexplored in 24–48 h in a "second-look" operation. At that time, definitive resection of nonviable bowel is completed.

Exceptions to the recommendation for expeditious surgery for intestinal obstruction include partial small-bowel obstruction, obstruction occurring in the early postoperative period, intestinal obstruction as a consequence of Crohn disease, and carcinoma-tosis.

Progression to strangulation is less likely to occur with partial small-bowel obstruction, and an attempt at nonoperative resolution is warranted. However, most patients with partial small obstruction whose symptoms do not improve within 48 h after initiation of nonoperative therapy should undergo surgery. Patients undergoing nonoperative therapy should be closely monitored for signs suggestive of peritonitis, the development of which would mandate urgent surgery.

Obstruction that occurs in the early postoperative period is usually partial and only rarely is associated with strangulation. Therefore, a period of extended nonoperative therapy consisting of bowel rest, hydration, and total parenteral nutrition (TPN) administration is usually warranted. However, if complete obstruction is demonstrated or if signs suggestive of peritonitis are detected, expeditious reoperation should be undertaken without delay.

Intestinal obstruction in patients with Crohn disease often responds to medical therapy and is discussed in more detail later under "Crohn Disease." Twenty-five to 33 percent of patients with a history of cancer who present with small-bowel obstruction have adhesions as the etiology of their obstruction and therefore should not be denied appropriate therapy. Even in cases in which the obstruction is related to recurrent malignancy, palliative resection or bypass can be considered. Patients with obvious carcinomatosis pose a difficult challenge, given their limited prognosis. Management must be tailored to an individual patient's prognosis and desires.

Outcomes

The perioperative mortality rate associated with surgery for nonstrangulating small-bowel obstruction is less than 5 percent, with most deaths occurring in older adult patients with significant comorbidities. Mortality rates associated with surgery for strangulating obstruction range from 8–25 percent.

ILEUS AND OTHER DISORDERS OF INTESTINAL MOTILITY

Epidemiology

Ileus and intestinal pseudo-obstruction designate clinical syndromes caused by impaired intestinal motility and are characterized by symptoms and signs of intestinal obstruction in the absence of a lesion-causing mechanical obstruction.

Ileus is temporary and generally reversible if the inciting factor can be corrected. In contrast, chronic intestinal pseudo-obstruction comprises a spectrum of specific disorders associated with irreversible intestinal dysmotility.

Pathophysiology

The most frequently encountered factors cauing ileus are abdominal operations, infection and inflammation, electrolyte abnormalities, and drugs.

Among the proposed mechanisms responsible for postoperative ileus are surgical stress-induced sympathetic reflexes, inflammatory response-mediator release, and anesthetic/analgesic effects, each of which can inhibit intestinal motility.

Chronic intestinal pseudo-obstruction can be caused by a large number of specific abnormalities affecting intestinal smooth muscle, the myenteric plexus, or the extraintestinal nervous system. Both sporadic and familial forms of visceral myopathies and neuropathies exist. Systemic disorders involving the smooth muscle such as progressive systemic sclerosis and progressive muscular dystrophy, and neurologic diseases such as Parkinson disease also can be complicated by chronic intestinal pseudo-obstruction. Additionally, viral infections, such as those associated with cytomegalovirus and Epstein-Barr virus can cause intestinal pseudo-obstruction.

Clinical Presentation

The clinical presentation of ileus resembles that of small-bowel obstruction. Inability to tolerate liquids and solids by mouth, nausea, and lack of flatus or bowel movements are the most common symptoms. Vomiting and abdominal distention may occur. Bowel sounds are characteristically diminished or absent, in contrast to the hyperactive bowel sounds that usually accompany mechanical small-bowel obstruction. The clinical manifestations of chronic intestinal pseudo-obstruction include variable degrees of nausea, vomiting, abdominal pain, and distention.

Diagnosis

Routine postoperative ileus should be expected and requires no diagnostic evaluation. If ileus persists beyond 3–5 days postoperatively or occurs in the absence of abdominal surgery, diagnostic evaluation to detect specific underlying factors capable of inciting ileus and to rule out the presence of mechanical obstruction is warranted.

Patient medication lists should be reviewed for the presence of drugs known to be associated with impaired intestinal motility. Measurement of serum electrolytes may demonstrate hypokalemia, hypocalcemia, hypomagnesemia, hypermagnesemia, or other electrolyte abnormalities commonly associated with ileus. Abdominal radiographs are often obtained, but the distinction between ileus and mechanical obstruction may be difficult based on this test alone. In the postoperative setting, CT scanning is the test of choice because it can demonstrate the presence of an intraabdominal abscess or other evidence of peritoneal sepsis that may be causing ileus and can exclude the presence of complete mechanical obstruction.

The diagnosis of chronic pseudo-obstruction is suggested by clinical features and confirmed by radiographic and manometric studies. Diagnostic laparotomy or laparoscopy with full-thickness biopsy of the small intestine may be required to establish the specific underlying cause.

Therapy

The management of ileus consists of limiting oral intake and correcting the underlying inciting factor. If vomiting or abdominal distention are prominent, the stomach should be decompressed using a nasogastric tube. Fluid and electrolytes should be administered intravenously until ileus resolves. If the duration of ileus is prolonged, TPN may be required.

The therapy of patients with chronic intestinal pseudo-obstruction focuses on palliation of symptoms and fluid, electrolyte, and nutritional management. Surgery should be avoided if at all possible. Prokinetic agents, such as metoclopramide and erythromycin, are associated with poor efficacy. Cisapride has been associated with palliation of symptoms; however, because of cardiac toxicity and reported deaths, this agent is restricted to compassionate use.

CROHN DISEASE

Epidemiology

Crohn disease is a chronic, idiopathic inflammatory disease with a propensity to affect the distal ileum, although any part of the alimentary tract can be involved. The median age at which patients are diagnosed with Crohn disease is approximately 30 years; however, age of diagnosis can range from early childhood through the entire life span. Both genetic and environmental factors appear to influence the risk for developing Crohn disease. The relative risk among first-degree relatives of patients with Crohn disease is 14–15 times higher than that of the general population.

Pathophysiology

Crohn disease is characterized by sustained inflammation. Various hypotheses on the roles of environmental factors, including infectious agents, and derangements in immune regulation have been proposed. Specific genetic defects associated with Crohn disease in human patients are beginning to be defined. For example, the presence of a locus on chromosome 16 (the so-called IBD1 locus) has been linked to Crohn disease. The IBD1 locus has been identified as the NOD2 gene. Persons with allelic variants on both chromosomes have a 40-fold relative risk of Crohn disease when compared to those without variant NOD2 genes.

Pathology

The earliest lesion characteristic of Crohn disease is the aphthous ulcer. These superficial ulcers are up to 3 mm in diameter and are surrounded by a halo of erythema. In the small intestine, aphthous ulcers typically arise over lymphoid aggregates. Granulomas are highly characteristic of Crohn disease and are reported to be present in up to 70 percent of intestinal specimens obtained during surgical resection. These granulomas are noncaseating and can be found in both areas of active disease and apparently normal intestine, in any layer of the bowel wall, and in mesenteric lymph nodes.

As disease progresses, aphthae coalesce into larger, stellate-shaped ulcers. Linear or serpiginous ulcers may form when multiple ulcers fuse in a direction parallel to the longitudinal axis of the intestine. With transverse coalescence of ulcers, a cobblestone appearance of the mucosa may arise.

With advanced disease, inflammation can be transmural. Serosal involvement results in adhesion of the inflamed bowel to other loops of bowel or other adjacent organs. Transmural inflammation also can result in fibrosis, with stricture formation, intraabdominal abscesses, fistulas, and, rarely, free perforation. Inflammation in Crohn disease can affect discontinuous portions of intestine: so-called "skip lesions" that are separated by intervening normal-appearing intestine.

A feature of Crohn disease that is grossly evident and helpful in identifying affected segments of intestine during surgery is the presence of fat wrapping (encroachment of mesenteric fat onto the serosal surface of the bowel).

Clinical Presentation

The most common symptoms of Crohn disease are abdominal pain, diarrhea, and weight loss. However, the clinical features are highly variable among individual patients and depend on which segment(s) of the gastrointestinal tract is (are) predominantly affected, the intensity of inflammation, and the presence or absence of specific complications. The onset of symptoms is insidious, and once present, their severity follows a waxing and waning course. Constitutional symptoms, particularly weight loss and fever, or growth retardation in children, may also be prominent and are occasionally the sole presenting features of Crohn disease.

The distal ileum is the single most frequently affected site, being diseased at some time in 75 percent of patients with Crohn disease. The small bowel alone is affected in 15–30 percent of patients, both the ileum and colon are affected in 40–60 percent of patients, and the colon alone is affected in 25–30 percent of patients. Isolated perineal and anorectal disease occurs in 5–10 percent of affected patients.

An estimated 25 percent of all patients with Crohn disease will have an extraintestinal manifestation of their disease. One-fourth of those affected will have more than one manifestation. Table 27-3 lists the most common extraintestinal manifestations.

TABLE 27-3 Extraintestinal Manifestations of Crohn Disease

Dermatologic
  Erythema nodosum
  Pyoderma gangrenosum

Rheumatologic
  Peripheral arthritis
  Ankylosing spondylitis
  Sacroiliitis

Ocular
  Conjunctivitis
  Uveitis/iritis
  Episcleritis

Hepatobiliary
  Hepatic steatosis
  Cholelithiasis
  Primary sclerosing cholangitis
  Pericholangitis

Urologic
  Nephrolithiasis
  Ureteral obstruction

Miscellaneous
  Thromboembolic disease
  Vasculitis
  Osteoporosis
  Endocarditis, myocarditis, pleuropericarditis
  Interstitial lung disease
  Amyloidosis
  Pancreatitis

Diagnosis

Clinical situations in which the diagnosis of Crohn disease should be considered include the presence of acute or chronic abdominal pain, especially when localized to the right lower quadrant, chronic diarrhea, evidence of intestinal inflammation on radiography or endoscopy, the discovery of a bowel stricture or fistula arising from the bowel, and evidence of inflammation or granulomas on intestinal histology. Disorders associated with clinical presentations that resemble those of Crohn disease include ulcerative colitis, functional bowel disorders such as irritable bowel syndrome, mesenteric ischemia, collagen vascular diseases, carcinoma and lymphoma, diverticular disease, and infectious enteritides. Infectious enteritides are most frequently diagnosed in immunocompromised patients but also can occur in patients with normal immune function. Acute ileitis caused by Campylobacter and Yersinia species can be difficult to distinguish from that caused by an acute presentation of Crohn disease. Typhoid enteritis caused by Salmonella typhosa can lead to overt intestinal bleeding and perforation, most often affecting the terminal ileum. The distal ileum and cecum are the most common sites of intestinal involvement by infection caused by *Mycobacterium tuberculosis*. This condition can result in intestinal inflammation, strictures, and fistula formation, similar to those seen in Crohn disease. Cytomegalovirus (CMV) can cause intestinal ulcers, bleeding, and perforation.

The diagnosis is based on a complete assessment of the clinical presentation with confirmatory findings derived from radiographic, endoscopic, and, in most cases, pathologic tests. Contrast examinations of the small bowel and colon may reveal strictures or networks of ulcers and fissures leading to the typical "cobblestone appearance" of the mucosa. CT scanning may reveal intraabdominal abscesses and is useful in acute presentations to rule out the presence of other intraabdominal disorders. Colonoscopy is used to visualize and biopsy disease in the colon; occasionally the distal ileum can be reached as well. Esophagogastroduodenoscopy (EGD) is done for disease of the proximal alimentary tract.

Therapy

Because no curative therapies are available for Crohn disease, the goal of treatment is to palliate symptoms. Medical therapy is used to induce and maintain disease remission. Surgery is reserved for specific indications described below. Additionally, nutritional support in the form of aggressive enteral regimens or, if necessary, parenteral nutrition, is used to manage the malnutrition that is common in patient's with Crohn disease.

Medical Therapy

Pharmacologic agents used to treat Crohn disease include antibiotics, aminosalicylates, corticosteroids, and immunomodulators. Antibiotics have an adjunctive role in the treatment of infectious complications associated with Crohn disease. They are also used to treat patients with perianal disease, enterocutaneous fistulas, and active colonic disease.

Infliximab is a chimeric monoclonal anti–tumor-necrosis-factor antibody that has recently been shown to promote remission and closure of enterocutaneous fistulas. Infliximab is generally well tolerated but should not be used in patients with ongoing septis.

Surgical Therapy

Seventy to 80 percent of patients with Crohn disease will ultimately require surgical therapy for their disease. Surgery is generally reserved for patients whose disease is unresponsive to aggressive medical therapy or who develop complications of their disease.

One third of patients with Crohn disease will require surgery for intestinal obstruction. Growth retardation constitutes an indication for surgery in 30 percent of children with Crohn disease. Less-common complications that require surgical intervention are acute gastrointestinal hemorrhage and cancer.

During surgery, thorough examination of the entire intestine should be performed. The presence of active disease is suggested by thickening of the bowel wall, narrowing of the lumen, serosal inflammation and coverage by creeping fat, and thickening of the mesentery. Skip lesions are present in approximately 20 percent of cases and should be sought. The length of uninvolved small intestine should be noted.

Segmental intestinal resection of grossly evident disease followed by primary anastomosis is the usual procedure of choice. Microscopic evidence of Crohn disease at the resection margins does not compromise a safe anastomosis, and frozen-section analysis of resection margins is unnecessary.

An alternative to segmental resection for obstructing lesions is stricturoplasty. This technique allows for preservation of intestinal surface area and is especially well-suited to patients with extensive disease and fibrotic strictures who may have undergone previous resection and are at risk for developing short-bowel syndrome. In this technique, the bowel is opened longitudinally to expose the lumen. Depending on the length of the stricture, the reconstruction can be fashioned in a manner similar to the Heinecke-Mikulicz pyloroplasty (for strictures less than 12 cm in length) or the Finney pyloroplasty (for longer strictures as much as 25 cm in length). Stricturoplasty is associated with recurrence rates that are no different from those associated with segmental resection. Stricturoplasty is contraindicated in patients with intraabdominal abscesses or intestinal fistulas.

An uncommon, but not rare, scenario is the intraoperative discovery of inflammation limited to the terminal ileum during operations performed for presumed appendicitis. This scenario can result from an acute presentation of Crohn disease or from acute ileitis caused by bacteria such as Yersinia or Campylobacter. Both conditions should be treated medically; ileal resection is not generally indicated. However, the appendix, even if normal appearing, should be removed (unless the cecum is inflamed, increasing the potential morbidity of this procedure) to eliminate appendicitis from the differential diagnosis of abdominal pain in these patients, particularly those with Crohn disease who may be destined to have recurring symptoms.

Since the 1990s, laparoscopic surgical techniques have been applied to patients with Crohn disease. However, it is important to remember that the inflammatory changes associated with Crohn disease, such as thickened and foreshortened mesentery, obliterated tissue planes, and friable tissues with engorged vasculature, potentially make laparoscopic surgery difficult and dangerous.

Outcomes

Overall complication rates following surgery for Crohn disease range from 15–30 percent. Wound infections, postoperative intraabdominal abscesses, and anastomotic leaks account for most of these complications.

Most patients whose disease is resected eventually develop recurrence. If recurrence is defined endoscopically, 70 percent recur within 1 year of a bowel resection and 85 percent by 3 years. Clinical recurrence, defined as the return of symptoms confirmed as being caused by Crohn disease, affects 60 percent of patients by 5 years and 94 percent by 15 years after intestinal resection. Reoperation becomes necessary in approximately one-third of patients by 5 years after the initial operation.

INTESTINAL FISTULAS

Epidemiology

A fistula is defined as an abnormal communication between two epithelialized surfaces. The communication occurs between two parts of the gastrointestinal tract or adjacent organs in an internal fistula (e.g., enterocolonic fistula or colovesicular fistula). An external fistula (e.g., enterocutaneous fistula or rectovaginal fistula) involves the skin or another external surface epithelium. Enterocutaneous fistulas that drain less than 200 mL of fluid per day are known as low-output fistulas, whereas those that drain more than 500 mL of fluid per day are known as high-output fistulas.

More than 80 percent of enterocutaneous fistulas represent iatrogenic complications that occur as the result of enterotomies or intestinal anastomotic dehiscences. Fistulas that arise spontaneously without antecedent iatrogenic injury are usually manifestations of underlying Crohn disease or cancer.

Pathophysiology

The manifestations of fistulas depend on which structures are involved. Low-resistance enteroenteric fistulas, which allow luminal contents to bypass a significant proportion of the small intestine, may result in clinically significant malabsorption. Enterovesicular fistulas often cause recurrent urinary tract infections. The drainage emanating from enterocutaneous fistulas is irritating to the skin and cause excoriation. The loss of enteric luminal contents, particularly from high-output fistulas originating from the proximal small intestine, results in dehydration, electrolyte abnormalities, and malnutrition.

Clinical Presentation

Iatrogenic enterocutaneous fistulas usually become clinically evident between the fifth and tenth postoperative days. Fever, leukocytosis, prolonged ileus, abdominal tenderness, and wound infection are the initial signs. The diagnosis becomes obvious when drainage of enteric material through the abdominal wound or through existing drains occurs. These fistulas are often associated with intraabdominal abscesses.

Diagnosis

CT scanning is the most useful initial test. Intraabdominal abscesses should be sought and drained percutaneously. If the anatomy of the fistula is not clear on CT scanning, a small-bowel series or enteroclysis examination can be obtained to demonstrate the fistula's site of origin in the bowel. Occasionally, contrast administered into the intestine does not demonstrate the fistula tract. A fistulogram, in which contrast is injected under pressure through a catheter placed percutaneously into the fistula tract, may offer greater sensitivity in localizing the fistula origin.

Therapy

The treatment of enterocutaneous fistulas should proceed through an orderly sequence of steps. Step 1: Stabilization. Fluid and electrolyte resuscitation is begun. Nutrition is provided, usually through the parenteral route initially. Sepsis is controlled with antibiotics and drainage of abscesses. The skin is protected from the fistula effluent with ostomy appliances or fistula drains. Step 2: Investigation. The anatomy of the fistula is defined using the studies described above. Step 3: Rehabilitation. Probability of spontaneous closure is maximized. Nutrition and time are the key components of this phase. Most patients will require TPN; however, a trial of oral or enteral nutrition should be attempted in patients with low-output fistulas originating from the distal intestine. The somatostatin analogue octreotide is a useful adjunct, particularly in patients with high-output fistulas, because its administration reduces the volume of fistula output, thereby facilitating fluid and electrolyte management. Furthermore, octreotide may accelerate the rate at which fistulas close.

If the fistula fails to resolve by 2–3 months, surgery may be required, during which the fistula tract, together with the segment of intestine from which it originates, should be resected. Simple closure of the opening in the intestine from which the fistula originates is associated with high recurrence rates.

Outcomes

Enterocutaneous fistulas are associated with a 10–15 percent mortality rate, mostly related to sepsis or underlying disease. Overall, 50 percent of intestinal fistulas close spontaneously. A useful mnemonic designates factors that inhibit spontaneous closure of intestinal fistulas: FRIEND (foreign body within the fistula tract; radiation enteritis; infection/inflammation at the fistula origin; epithelialization of the fistula tract; neoplasm at the fistula origin; distal obstruction of the intestine). Surgery for fistulas is associated with a greater than 50 percent morbidity rate, including a 10 percent recurrence rate.

SMALL-BOWEL NEOPLASMS

Epidemiology

Adenomas are the most common benign neoplasm of the small intestine. Other benign tumors include fibromas, lipomas, hemangiomas, lymphangiomas, and neurofibromas.

Primary small-bowel cancers are rare, with an estimated incidence of 5300 cases per year in the United States. Among small-bowel cancers, adenocarcinomas comprise 35–50 percent of all cases, carcinoid tumors comprise 20–40 percent, and lymphomas comprise approximately 10–15 percent. Gastrointestinal stromal tumors (GISTs) are the most common mesenchymal tumors arising in the small intestine and comprise up to 15 percent of small-bowel malignancies. The small intestine is frequently affected by metastases from or local invasion by cancers originating at other sites. Melanoma, in particular, is associated with a propensity for metastasis to the small intestine.

Reported risk factors for developing small-intestinal adenocarcinoma include consumption of red meat, ingestion of smoked or cured foods, Crohn disease, celiac sprue, hereditary nonpolyposis colorectal cancer (HNPCC), familial adenomatous polyposis (FAP), and Peutz-Jeghers syndrome. Patients with FAP have a nearly 100 percent cumulative lifetime risk of developing duodenal adenomas that have the potential to undergo malignant transformation. The risk of duodenal cancer in these patients is more than 100-fold than in the general population.

Pathogenesis

Small-intestinal adenocarcinomas are believed to arise from preexisting adenomas through a sequential accumulation of genetic abnormalities in a model similar to that described for the pathogenesis of colorectal cancer. Adenomas are histologically classified as tubular, villous, and tubulovillous. Tubular adenomas have the least-aggressive features. Villous adenomas have the most-aggressive features and tend to be large, sessile, and located in the second portion of the duodenum. Malignant degeneration has been reported to be present in up to 45 percent of villous adenomas by the time of diagnosis.

A defining feature of GISTs is their expression of the receptor tyrosine kinase KIT (CD117). The majority of GISTs have activating mutations in the c-kit protooncogene, which cause KIT to become constitutively activated, presumably leading to persistence of cellular growth or survival signals. Because the interstitial cells of Cajal normally express KIT, these cells have been implicated as the cell of origin for GISTs.

Clinical Presentation

Most small-intestinal neoplasms are asymptomatic until they become large. Partial small-bowel obstruction, with associated symptoms of crampy abdominal pain and distention, nausea, and vomiting, is the most common mode of presentation. Obstruction can be the result of either luminal narrowing by the tumor itself or intussusception, with the tumor serving as the lead point. Hemorrhage, usually indolent, is the second most common mode of presentation.

Physical examination may reveal an abdominal mass or signs of intestinal obstruction. Fecal occult blood test may be positive. Cachexia or ascites may be present with advanced disease.

Adenocarcinomas, and adenomas (from which most are believed to arise), are most commonly found in the duodenum, except in patients with Crohn disease, in whom most are found in the ileum. Lesions in the periampullary location can cause obstructive jaundice or pancreatitis. Adenocarcinomas located in the duodenum tend to be diagnosed earlier in their progression than those located in the jejunum or ileum, which are rarely diagnosed prior to the onset of locally advanced or metastatic disease.

Carcinoid tumors of the small intestine are also usually diagnosed after the development of metastatic disease. These tumors are associated with a more aggressive behavior than the more common appendiceal carcinoid tumors. Approximately 25–50 percent of patients with carcinoid tumor-derived liver metastases will develop manifestations of the carcinoid syndrome. These manifestations include diarrhea, flushing, hypotension, tachycardia, and fibrosis of the endocardium and valves of the right heart. Candidate tumor-derived mediators of the carcinoid syndrome, such as serotonin, bradykinin, and substance P, undergo nearly complete metabolism during first passage through the liver. As a result, symptoms of carcinoid syndrome are rare in the absence of liver metastases.

Lymphoma may involve the small intestine primarily or as a manifestation of disseminated systemic disease. Primary small-intestinal lymphomas are most commonly located in the ileum, which contains the highest concentration of lymphoid tissue in the intestine. Although partial small-bowel obstruction is the most common mode of presentation, 10 percent of patients with small-intestinal lymphoma present with bowel perforation.

Sixty to 70 percent of GISTs are located in the stomach. The small intestine is the second most common site, containing 25–35 percent of GISTs. There appears to be no regional variation in the prevalence of GISTs within the small intestine. GISTs have a greater propensity to be associated with overt hemorrhage than the other small-intestinal malignancies.

Metastatic tumors involving the small intestine can induce intestinal obstruction and bleeding.

Diagnosis

Because of the absent or nonspecific symptoms associated with most small-intestinal neoplasms, these lesions are rarely diagnosed preoperatively. Laboratory tests are nonspecific, with the exception of elevated serum 5-hydroxyindole acetic acid (5-HIAA) levels in patients with the carcinoid syndrome.

Contrast radiography of the small intestine may demonstrate benign and malignant lesions. Enteroclysis has a sensitivity of greater than 90 percent in the detection of small-bowel tumors and is the test of choice, particularly for tumors located in the distal small bowel. CT scanning has low sensitivity for detecting mucosal or intramural lesions, but can demonstrate large tumors and is useful in the staging of intestinal malignancies. Tumors associated with significant bleeding can be localized with angiography or radioisotope-tagged red blood cell (RBC) scans. Tumors located in the duodenum can be visualized and biopsied on EGD.

Therapy

Benign neoplasms of the small intestine that are symptomatic should be surgically resected or removed endoscopically, if feasible. Duodenal adenomas occurring in the setting of FAP require an especially aggressive approach to management. Patients with FAP should undergo screening EGD starting sometime during their second or third decade of life. Adenomas detected should be removed endoscopically, if possible, followed by surveillance endoscopy at 6 months and yearly thereafter, in the absence of recurrence. If surgery is required, pancreaticoduodenectomy is generally necessary because adenomas in patients with FAP tend to be multiple and sessile, with a predilection for the periampullary region.

The surgical therapy of small-intestinal malignancies usually consists of wide–local resection of the intestine harboring the lesion. For adenocarcinomas, a wide excision of corresponding mesentery is done to achieve regional lymphadenectomy. For most adenocarcinomas of the duodenum, except those in the distal duodenum, pancreaticoduodenectomy is required. In the presence of locally advanced or metastatic disease, palliative intestinal resection or bypass is performed. Chemotherapy has no proven efficacy in the adjuvant or palliative treatment of small-intestinal adenocarcinomas.

The goal of surgical therapy for carcinoids is resection of all visible disease. Localized small-intestinal carcinoid tumors should be treated with segmental intestinal resection and regional lymphadenectomy. In approximately 30 percent of cases, multiple small-intestinal carcinoid tumors are present. Therefore, the entire small intestine should be examined before planning the extent of resection. In the presence of metastatic disease, tumor debulking should be conducted because it can be associated with long-term survival and amelioration of symptoms of the carcinoid syndrome. Response rates of 30–50 percent have been reported to chemotherapy regimens based on agents such as doxorubicin, 5-fluorouracil, and streptozocin. However, none of these regimens is associated with a clearly demonstrable impact on the natural history of disease. Octreotide is the most effective pharmacologic agent for management of symptoms of carcinoid syndrome.

Localized small-intestinal lymphoma should be treated with segmental resection of the involved intestine and adjacent mesentery. If the small intestine is diffusely affected by lymphoma, chemotherapy, rather than surgical resection, should be the primary therapy. The value to adjuvant chemotherapy after resection of localized lymphoma is controversial.

Small-intestinal GISTs should be treated with segmental intestinal resection. If the diagnosis is known prior to resection, wide lymphadenectomy can be avoided because GISTs are rarely associated with lymph node metastases. GISTs are resistant to conventional chemotherapy agents. Imatinib (Gleevec, formerly known as ST1571) is a tyrosine kinase inhibitor with potent activity against tyrosine kinase KIT. Recent clinical trials show that 80 percent of patients with unresectable or metastatic GISTs derive clinical benefit from the administration of imatinib, with 50–60 percent having objective evidence of reduction in tumor volume.

Metastatic cancers affecting the small intestine that are symptomatic should be treated with palliative resection or bypass except in the most advanced cases.

Outcomes

Complete resection of duodenal adenocarcinomas is associated with postoperative 5-year survival rates ranging from 50–60 percent. Complete resection of adenocarcinomas located in the jejunum or ileum is associated with 5-year survival rates of only 5–30 percent. Five-year survival rates of 75–95 percent following resection of localized small-intestinal carcinoid tumors have been reported. In the presence of carcinoid tumor-derived liver metastases, 5-year survival rates of 19–54 percent have been reported. The overall 5-year survival rate for patients diagnosed with intestinal lymphoma ranges from 20–40 percent. For patients with localized lymphoma amenable to surgical resection, the 5-year survival rate is 60 percent.

The 5-year survival rate following surgical resection of GISTs ranges from 35–60 percent. Both tumor size and mitotic index are independently correlated with prognosis.

RADIATION ENTERITIS

Epidemiology

Acute radiation enteritis is a transient condition that occurs in approximately 75 percent of patients undergoing radiation therapy for abdominal and pelvic cancers. Chronic radiation enteritis is inexorable and develops in approximately 5–15 percent of these patients.

Pathophysiology

The principal mechanism of radiation-induced cell death is believed to be apoptosis resulting from free radical-induced breaks in double-stranded deoxyribonucleic acid (DNA). Because radiation has its greatest impact on rapidly proliferating cells, the small-intestinal epithelium is acutely susceptible to radiation-induced injury. The intensity of injury is related to the dose of radiation administered, with most cases occurring in patients who have received at least 4500 cGy. Risk factors for acute radiation enteritis include conditions that may limit splanchnic perfusion such as hypertension, diabetes mellitus, coronary artery disease, and restricted motility of the small intestine caused by adhesions. Injury is potentiated by concomitant administration of chemotherapeutic agents that act as radiation-sensitizers such as doxorubicin, 5-fluorouracil, actinomycin D, and methotrexate.

Chronic radiation enteritis is characterized by a progressive occlusive vasculitis that leads to chronic ischemia and fibrosis that affects all layers of the intestinal wall.

Clinical Presentation

The most common manifestations of acute radiation enteritis are nausea, vomiting, diarrhea, and crampy abdominal pain. Symptoms are generally transient and subside after the discontinuation of radiation therapy. Because the diagnosis is usually obvious, given the clinical context, no specific diagnostic tests are required. However, if patients develop signs suggestive of peritonitis, CT scanning should be performed to rule out the presence of other conditions capable of causing acute abdominal syndromes.

The clinical manifestations of chronic radiation enteritis usually become evident within 2 years of radiation administration, although they can begin as early as several months or as late as decades afterwards. The most common clinical presentation is one of partial small-bowel obstruction with nausea, vomiting, intermittent abdominal distention, crampy abdominal pain, and weight loss being the most common symptoms. The terminal ileum is the most frequently affected segment. Other manifestations of chronic radiation enteritis include complete bowel obstruction, acute or chronic intestinal hemorrhage, and abscess or fistula formation.

Diagnosis

Enteroclysis is the most accurate imaging test for diagnosing chronic radiation enteritis. CT scanning should be obtained to rule out the presence of recurrent cancer because its clinical manifestations may overlap with those of chronic radiation enteritis.

Therapy

Most cases of acute radiation enteritis are self-limited. Supportive therapy, including the administration of antiemetics, is usually sufficient. Patients with diarrhea-induced dehydration may require hospital admission and parenteral fluid administration.

The treatment of chronic radiation enteritis represents a formidable challenge. Surgery for this condition is difficult, is associated with high morbidity rates, and should be avoided in the absence of specific indications such as high-grade obstruction, perforation, hemorrhage, intraabdominal abscesses, and fistulas. The goal of surgery is limited resection of diseased intestine with primary anastomosis between healthy bowel segments. If limited resection is not achievable, an intestinal bypass procedure may be an option, except in cases for which hemorrhage is the surgical indication.

Outcomes

Acute radiation injury to the intestine is self-limited; its severity is not correlated with the probability of chronic radiation enteritis developing. Surgery for chronic radiation enteritis is associated with high morbidity rates and reported mortality rates averaging 10 percent.

MECKEL DIVERTICULUM

Epidemiology

Meckel diverticula are designated true diverticula because their walls contain all of the layers found in normal small intestine. Approximately 60 percent of Meckel diverticula contain heterotopic mucosa, of which more than 60 percent consist of gastric mucosa. A useful mnemonic describing Meckel diverticula is the "rule of twos": 2 percent prevalence, 2:1 female predominance, location 2 feet proximal to the ileocecal valve in adults, and half of those who are symptomatic are younger than 2 years of age.

Pathophysiology

During the eighth week of gestation, the omphalomesenteric (vitelline) duct normally undergoes obliteration. Failure or incomplete vitelline duct obliteration results in a spectrum of abnormalities, the most common of which is Meckel diverticulum. Other abnormalities include omphalomesenteric fistula, enterocysts, and a fibrous band connecting the intestine to the umbilicus. A remnant of the left vitelline artery can persist to form a mesodiverticular band tethering a Meckel diverticulum to the ileal mesentery.

Bleeding associated with Meckel diverticulum is usually the result of ileal mucosal ulceration that occurs adjacent to acid-producing, heterotopic gastric mucosa located within the diverticulum. Intestinal obstruction associated with Meckel diverticulum can result from several mechanisms: (1) volvulus of the intestine around the fibrous band attaching the diverticulum to the umbilicus; (2) entrapment of intestine by a mesodiverticular band; (3) intussusception with the diverticulum acting as a lead point; or (4) stricture secondary to chronic diverticulitis.

Clinical Presentation

Meckel diverticula are asymptomatic unless associated complications arise. Bleeding is the most common presentation in children with Meckel diverticula, representing more than 50 percent of Meckel diverticulum-related complications among patients who are younger than 18 years of age. Intestinal obstruction is the most common presentation in adults with Meckel diverticula. Diverticulitis, present in 20 percent of patients with symptomatic Meckel diverticula, and is associated with a clinical syndrome that is indistinguishable from acute appendicitis.

Diagnosis

In the absence of bleeding, Meckel diverticula rarely are diagnosed prior to the time of surgical intervention. Enteroclysis is associated with an accuracy of 75 percent, but is usually not applicable during acute presentations of complications related to Meckel diverticula. Radionuclide scans (99mTc-pertechnetate) suggest the diagnosis of Meckel diverticulum when uptake occurs in associated ectopic gastric mucosa, or when extravasation occurs during active bleeding. Angiography can localize the site of bleeding during acute hemorrhage related to Meckel diverticula.

Therapy

The surgical treatment of symptomatic Meckel diverticula should consist of diverticulectomy with removal of associated bands connecting the diverticulum to the abdominal wall or intestinal mesentery. If the indication for diverticulectomy is bleeding, segmental resection of ileum that includes both the diverticulum and the adjacent ileal peptic ulcer should be performed. Segmental ileal resection may also be necessary if the diverticulum contains a tumor, or if the base of the diverticulum is inflamed or perforated. The management of incidentally found (asymptomatic) Meckel diverticula remains controversial.

ACQUIRED DIVERTICULA

Epidemiology

Acquired diverticula are designated false diverticula because their walls consist of mucosa and submucosa but lack a complete muscularis. Acquired diverticula in the duodenum tend to be located adjacent to the ampulla; such diverticula are known as periampullary, juxtapapillary, or peri-Vaterian diverticula. Acquired diverticula in the jejunum or ileum are known as jejunoileal diverticula.

The prevalence of duodenal diverticula is reported to range from 5–27 percent. The prevalence of jejunoileal diverticula has been estimated to range from 1–5 percent.

Pathophysiology

The pathogenesis of acquired diverticula is hypothesized to be related to acquired abnormalities of intestinal smooth muscle or dysregulated motility, leading to herniation of mucosa and submucosa through weakened areas of muscularis.

Acquired diverticula can be associated with bacterial overgrowth, leading to vitamin B12 deficiency, megaloblastic anemia, malabsorption, and steatorrhea. Periampullary duodenal diverticula have been described to become distended with intraluminal debris and to compress the common bile duct or pancreatic duct, thus causing obstructive jaundice or pancreatitis, respectively. Jejunoileal diverticula can also cause intestinal obstruction through intussusception or compression of adjacent bowel.

Clinical Presentation

Acquired diverticula are asymptomatic unless associated complications arise. Such complications are estimated to occur in 6–10 percent of patients with acquired diverticula and include intestinal obstruction, diverticulitis, hemorrhage, perforation, and malabsorption. Periampullary duodenal diverticula may be associated with choledocholithiasis, cholangitis, recurrent pancreatitis, and sphincter of Oddi dysfunction.

Diagnosis

Most acquired diverticula are discovered incidentally. On ultrasound and CT scanning, duodenal diverticula may be mistaken for pancreatic pseudocysts and fluid collections, biliary cysts, and periampullary neoplasms. These lesions can be missed on endoscopy and are best diagnosed on upper gastrointestinal radiographs. Enteroclysis is the most sensitive test for detecting jejunoileal diverticula.

Therapy

Asymptomatic acquired diverticula should be left alone. Bacterial overgrowth associated with acquired diverticula is treated with antibiotics. Other complications, such as bleeding and diverticulitis, are treated with segmental intestinal resection for diverticula located in the jejunum or ileum. Bleeding and obstruction related to lateral duodenal diverticula are generally treated with diverticulectomy alone. These procedures can be technically difficult for medial duodenal diverticula that penetrate into the substance of the pancreas.

Complications related to these diverticula should be managed nonoperatively if possible.

MESENTERIC ISCHEMIA

Mesenteric ischemia can present as one of two distinct clinical syndromes: acute mesenteric ischemia and chronic mesenteric ischemia.

Pathophysiology

Four distinct pathophysiologic mechanisms can lead to acute mesenteric ischemia: arterial embolus, arterial thrombosis, vasospasm (also known as nonocclusive mesenteric ischemia, or NOMI), and venous thrombosis. Regardless of the pathophysiologic mechanism, acute mesenteric ischemia can lead to intestinal mucosal sloughing within 3 h of onset and full-thickness intestinal infarction by 6 h.

In contrast, chronic mesenteric ischemia develops insidiously, allowing for development of collateral circulation, and, therefore, rarely leads to intestinal infarction. Chronic mesenteric arterial ischemia results from atherosclerotic lesions in the main splanchnic arteries (celiac, superior mesenteric, and inferior mesenteric arteries). In most patients with symptoms attributable to chronic mesenteric ischemia, at least two of these arteries are either occluded or severely stenosed. A chronic form of mesenteric venous thrombosis can involve the portal or splenic veins and may lead to portal hypertension, with resulting esophagogastric varices, splenomegaly, and hypersplenism.

Clinical Presentation

Abdominal pain for which the severity is out of proportion to the degree of tenderness on examination is the hallmark of acute mesenteric ischemia. Associated symptoms can include nausea, vomiting, and diarrhea. Physical findings are characteristically absent early in the course of ischemia. With the onset of bowel infarction, abdominal distention, peritonitis, and passage of bloody stools occur.

With chronic mesenteric ischemia, postprandial abdominal pain is the most prevalent symptom, producing a characteristic aversion to food ("food-fear") and weight loss. Most patients with chronic mesenteric venous thrombosis are asymptomatic because of the presence of extensive collateral venous drainage routes. However, some patients with chronic mesenteric venous thrombosis present with bleeding from esophagogastric varices.

Diagnosis

It is important to consider and pursue the diagnosis of acute mesenteric ischemia in any patient who has the classic early finding of severe abdominal pain out of proportion to physical findings. Laboratory test abnormalities, such as leukocytosis and acidosis are late findings; no laboratory tests have clinically useful sensitivity for the detection of acute mesenteric ischemia prior to the onset of intestinal infarction.

Patients suspected of having acute mesenteric ischemia and who have physical findings suggestive of peritonitis should undergo emergent laparotomy. In the absence of such findings, diagnostic imaging should be performed.

Although angiography is the most reliable method for diagnosing acute mesenteric arterial occlusion, it is invasive, time-consuming, and costly.

Therefore, most patients suspected of having acute mesenteric ischemia should undergo CT scanning as the initial imaging test. CT scans should be evaluated for (1) disorders other than acute mesenteric ischemia that might account for abdominal pain; (2) evidence of ischemia in the intestine and the mesentery; and (3) evidence of occlusion or stenosis of the mesenteric vasculature. CT scanning is also the test of choice for diagnosing acute mesenteric venous thrombosis.

Angiography should be performed if CT scanning reveals no evidence of mesenteric ischemia or other conditions that could account for acute abdominal pain and a high clinical suspicion for the presence of mesenteric ischemia remains. Additionally, because the CT findings of NOMI are nonspecific, patients at risk and suspected of having NOMI should undergo angiography without delay. The angiographic findings of NOMI include diffuse narrowing of mesenteric vessels in the absence of obstructing lesions and reduced opacification of bowel parenchyma.

The gold standard for the diagnosis of chronic arterial mesenteric ischemia is angiography, although CT angiography with three-dimensional reconstruction is noninvasive and offers good resolution. CT findings suggestive of chronic mesenteric ischemia include the presence of atherosclerotic calcified plaques at or near the origins of proximal splanchnic arteries and obvious focal stenosis of proximal mesenteric vessels with prominent collateral development.

Therapy

For embolus or thrombus-induced acute mesenteric ischemia, the standard treatment is surgical revascularization (embolectomy/thrombectomy/mesenteric bypass). These procedures are not indicated if most of the bowel supplied by the affected artery has already become infarcted, or if the patient is too unstable to undergo additional surgery beyond resection of infarcted intestine. For patients diagnosed with embolus or thrombus-induced acute mesenteric ischemia who do not have signs of peritonitis, thrombolysis, using agents such as streptokinase, urokinase, or recombinant tissue plasminogen activator, is an alternative therapeutic option.

The standard treatment of NOMI is selective infusion of a vasodilator, most commonly papaverine hydrochloride, into the superior mesenteric artery. If signs of peritonitis develop, emergent laparotomy should be performed and infarcted intestine resected.

The standard treatment of acute mesenteric venous thrombosis is anticoagulation. Heparin administration is associated with reductions in mortality and recurrence rates, and should be initiated as soon as the diagnosis is made. As for mesenteric ischemia of arterial origin, signs of peritonitis mandate laparotomy, and infarcted bowel should be resected. Most patients should be maintained on warfarin to achieve chronic anticoagulation for 6–12 months.

The standard therapy for chronic arterial mesenteric ischemia is surgical revascularization using aortomesenteric bypass grafting and mesenteric endarterectomy procedures. An alternative therapy is percutaneous transluminal mesenteric angioplasty alone or with stent insertion. The durability of these procedures in inducing relief of symptoms appears to be less than that associated with surgical revascularization.

Patients with chronic venous mesenteric thrombosis who have an underlying thrombophilia identified should be treated with chronic anticoagulation.

Additional therapy is indicated to control or prevent recurrent bleeding caused by esophagogastric varices. Pharmacologic agents such as propanol and endoscopic therapy are the first-line modalities. Surgical portosystemic shunts are indicated in patients whose bleeding cannot be controlled by conservative measures and who have a suitable vein for portosystemic venous anastomosis.

Outcomes

Recently reported mortality rates among patients with acute arterial mesenteric ischemia range from 59–93 percent. Reported mortality rates among patients with acute mesenteric venous thrombosis range from 20–50 percent.

Reported perioperative mortality rates associated with surgical therapy for chronic mesenteric ischemia range from 0–16 percent, with lower mortality rates predominating in recent series.

MISCELLANEOUS CONDITIONS

Obscure GI Bleeding

Obscure GI bleeding refers to gastrointestinal bleeding for which no source has been identified by routine endoscopic studies (EGD and colonoscopy). The small bowel contains most of the lesions responsible for obscure GI bleeding. Small-intestinal angiodysplasias account for approximately 75 percent of cases in adults; neoplasms account for approximately 10 percent. Meckel's diverticulum is the most common etiology of obscure GI bleeding in children. Other etiologies of obscure GI bleeding include Crohn disease, infectious enteritides, nonsteroidal antiinflammatory drug (NSAID)-induced ulcers and erosions, vasculitis, ischemia, varices, diverticula, and intussusception.

Four endoscopic techniques for visualizing the small intestine are available: push enteroscopy, sonde enteroscopy, intraoperative enteroscopy, and wireless capsule enteroscopy.

Push enteroscopy entails advancing a long endoscope (such as a pediatric or adult colonoscope or a specialized instrument) beyond the ligament of Treitz into the proximal jejunum. This procedure can enable visualization of approximately 60 cm of the proximal jejunum. In addition to diagnosis, push enteroscopy enables cauterization of bleeding sites.

In sonde enteroscopy, a long, thin fiberoptic instrument is propelled through the intestine by peristalsis following inflation of a balloon at the instrument's tip. Visualization is done during instrument withdrawal; approximately 50–75 percent of the small intestinal mucosa can be examined. However, this instrument lacks biopsy or therapeutic capability.

Intraoperative enteroscopy can be done during either laparotomy or laparoscopy. An endoscope (usually a colonoscope), is inserted into the small bowel through peroral intubation or through an enterotomy made in the small bowel or cecum. The endoscope is advanced by successively telescoping short segments of intestine onto the end to the instrument. Identified lesions should be marked with a suture placed on the serosal surface of the bowel; these lesions can be resected after completion of endoscopy.

Wireless capsule enteroscopy relies on a radiotelemetry capsule enteroscope that is small enough to swallow and has no external wires, fiberoptic bundles, or cables. While the capsule is being propelled through the intestine by peristalsis, video images are transmitted using radiotelemetry to an array of detectors attached to the patient's body. These detectors capture the images and permit continuous triangulation of the capsule location in the abdomen, facilitating the localization of lesions detected. The entire system is portable, allowing the patient to be ambulatory during the entire examination. Initial comparative studies indicate that the diagnostic yield of wireless capsule enteroscopy in patients with obscure GI bleeding is as good or better than that of push enteroscopy.

For patients in whom bleeding from an obscure GI source has apparently stopped, push and/or sonde enteroscopy or capsule enteroscopy (if available) is a reasonable initial study. If these examinations do not reveal a potential source of bleeding, then enteroclysis should be performed. If still no diagnosis has been made, a watch-and-wait approach is reasonable, although angiography should be considered if the prior episode of bleeding was severe. Angiography can reveal angiodysplasia and vascular tumors in the small intestine, even in the absence of ongoing bleeding.

For persistent mild bleeding from an obscure GI source, push and/or sonde enteroscopy should be used initially, if available. The role of capsule enteroscopy in this setting remains to be defined. If these examinations are nondiagnostic, then 99mTc-labeled RBC scanning should be performed and, if positive, followed by angiography to localize the source of bleeding. 9mTc-pertechnetate scintigraphy to diagnose Meckel diverticulum should be considered, although its yield in patients older than 40 years of age is extremely low. Patients who remain undiagnosed but who continue to bleed, and those patients with recurrent episodic bleeding significant enough to require blood transfusions, should then undergo exploration with intraoperative enteroscopy.

Patients with persistent severe bleeding from an obscure source should undergo angiography. Push enteroscopy can be attempted, but sonde and capsule enteroscopy are too slow to be applicable in this setting. If these examinations fail to localize the source of bleeding, exploratory laparoscopy or laparotomy with intraoperative enteroscopy is indicated. If bleeding is massive enough to cause hemodynamic derangements, expeditious exploration avoiding the delays inherent with angiography may be necessary.

Small-Bowel Perforation

Iatrogenic injury incurred during gastrointestinal endoscopy is the most common cause of small-bowel perforation. Other etiologies of small-bowel perforation include infections (especially tuberculosis, typhoid, and cytomegalovirus [CMV]), Crohn disease, ischemia, drugs (e.g., potassium- and NSAID-induced ulcers), radiation-induced injury, Meckel and acquired diverticula, neoplasms (especially lymphoma, adenocarcinoma, and melanoma), and foreign bodies.

Perforation of the jejunum and ileum occurs into the peritoneal cavity and usually causes overt symptoms and signs, such as abdominal pain, tenderness, and distention accompanied by fever and tachycardia. Perforations of the duodenum distal to its bulb, because of its retroperitoneal location, tend to be locally contained and can present insidiously. Manifestations of contained duodenal perforation following ERCP can resemble those of ERCP-induced pancreatitis, including hyperamylasemia.

Plain abdominal radiographs may reveal free intraperitoneal air if intraperitoneal perforation has occurred. If perforation is suspected but not clinically obvious, contrast radiography using a water-soluble contrast agent or CT scanning should be performed. CT scanning is the most sensitive test for diagnosing duodenal perforations.

Iatrogenic small-bowel perforation incurred during endoscopy, if immediately recognized, can sometimes be repaired using endoscopic techniques. Ampullary injury incurred during ERCP can usually be managed by biliary stent placement. Additionally, contained select cases of retroperitoneal perforations of the duodenum can be managed nonoperatively, in the absence of progression and sepsis. However, intraperitoneal duodenal perforations require surgical repair with pyloric exclusion and gastrojejunostomy or tube duodenostomy. Jejunal and ileal perforations require surgical repair or segmental resection.

Chylous Ascites

Chylous ascites refers to the accumulation of triglyceride-rich peritoneal fluid with a milky or creamy appearance that is caused by the presence of intestinal lymph in the peritoneal cavity.

The most common etiologies of chylous ascites in Western countries are abdominal malignancies and cirrhosis. In Eastern and developing countries, infectious etiologies, such as tuberculosis and filariasis, account for most cases. Chylous ascites can also develop as a complication of abdominal and thoracic operations and trauma. Other etiologies of chylous ascites include congential lymphatic abnormalities (e.g., primary lymphatic hypoplasia), radiation, pancreatitis, and right-sided heart failure.

Three mechanisms have been postulated to cause chylous ascites: (1) exudation of chyle from dilated lymphatics on the wall of the bowel and in the mesentery caused by obstruction of lymphatic vessels at the base of the mesentery or the cisterna chili (e.g., by malignancies); (2) direct leakage of chyle through a lymphoperitoneal fistula (e.g., those which develop as a result of trauma or surgery); and (3) exudation of chyle through the wall of dilated retroperitoneal lymphatic vessels (e.g., in congenital lymphangiectasia or thoracic duct obstruction).

Patients with chylous ascites develop abdominal distention over a period of weeks to months. Postoperative chylous ascites can present acutely during the first postoperative week. Paracentesis is the most important diagnostic test. Fluid triglyceride concentrations above 110 mg/dL are diagnostic. CT scanning may be useful in identifying pathologic intraabdominal lymph nodes and masses and in identifying extent and localization of fluid. Lymphangiography and lymphoscintigraphy may help to localize lymph leaks and obstruction.

Management of patients with chylous ascites should focus on evaluating and treating the underlying causes, especially for patients with infectious, inflammatory, or hemodynamic etiologies for this condition.

Most patients respond to administration of a high-protein and low-fat diet supplemented with medium-chain triglycerides. This regimen is designed to minimize chyle production and flow. Medium-chain triglycerides are absorbed by the intestinal epithelium and are transported to the liver through the portal vein; they do not contribute to chylomicron formation.

Patients who do not respond to this approach should be fasted and placed on TPN. Octreotide can further decrease lymph flow. Paracentesis is indicated for respiratory difficulties related to abdominal distention. Approximately 30 percent of patients will require surgical therapy for chylous ascites. In general, postoperative and trauma-related cases that fail to respond to initial nonoperative therapy are best managed by surgical repair. Lymphatic leaks are localized and repaired with fine nonabsorbable sutures. If extravasation of chyle is localized to the periphery of the small-bowel mesentery, then a limited small-bowel resection can be performed instead. For patients who are poor surgical candidates and who do not respond to prolonged conservative therapy, peritoneovenous shunting may be an option.

SHORT-BOWEL SYNDROME

Epidemiology

Short-bowel syndrome has been arbitrarily defined as the presence of less than 200 cm of residual small bowel in adult patients. A functional definition, in which insufficient intestinal absorptive capacity results in the clinical manifestations of diarrhea, dehydration, and malnutrition, is more broadly applicable.

In adults, the most common etiologies of short-bowel syndrome are acute mesenteric ischemia, malignancy, and Crohn disease. In pediatric patients, intestinal atresias, volvulus, and necrotizing enterocolitis are the most common etiologies of short-bowel syndrome.

Pathophysiology

Clinically significant malabsorption occurs when greater than 50–80 percent of the small intestine has been resected. Among adult patients who lack a functional colon, lifelong TPN dependence is likely to persist if there is less than 100 cm of residual small intestine. Among adult patients who have an intact and functional colon, lifelong TPN dependence is likely to persist if there is less than 60 cm of residual small intestine. Among infants with short-bowel syndrome, weaning from TPN-dependence has been achieved with as little as 10 cm of residual small intestine.

Residual bowel length is not the only factor predictive of achieving independence from TPN (enteral autonomy), however. First, is the presence or absence of an intact colon because the colon has the capacity to absorb large fluid and electrolyte loads. Additionally, the colon can play an important, albeit small, role in nutrient assimilation by absorbing short-chain fatty acids. Second, an intact ileocecal valve is believed to be associated with decreased malabsorption. The ileocecal valve delays transit of chyme from the small intestine into the colon, thereby prolonging the contact time between nutrients and the small-intestinal absorptive mucosa. Third, a healthy, rather than diseased, residual small intestine is associated with decreased severity of malabsorption. Fourth, resection of jejunum is better tolerated than resection of ileum, because the capacity for bile salt and vitamin B12 absorption is specific to the ileum.

Malabsorption in patients who have undergone massive small-bowel resection is exacerbated by a characteristic hypergastrinemia-associated gastric acid hypersecretion that persists for 1–2 years postoperatively. The increased acid load delivered to the duodenum inhibits absorption by a variety of mechanisms, including the inhibition of digestive enzymes, most of which function optimally under alkaline conditions.

Also during the first 1–2 years following massive small-bowel resection, the remaining intestine undergoes compensatory adaptation. Clinically, the period of adaptation is associated with reductions in volume and frequency of bowel movements, increases in the capacity for enteral nutrient assimilation, and reductions in TPN requirements.

THERAPY

Medical Therapy

For patients having undergone massive small-bowel resection, the initial treatment priorities include management of the primary condition precipitating the intestinal resection and the repletion of fluid and electrolytes lost in the severe diarrhea that characteristically occurs. Most patients will require TPN, at least initially. Enteral nutrition should be gradually introduced, once ileus has resolved. High-dose histamine$_2$ receptor antagonists or proton pump inhibitors should be administered to reduce gastric acid secretion. Antimotility agents, such as loperamide hydrochloride or di-phenoxylate, may be administered to delay small-intestinal transit. Octreotide can be administered to reduce the volume of gastrointestinal secretions.

During the period of adaptation, generally lasting 1–2 years postoperatively, TPN and enteral nutrition are titrated in an attempt to allow for independence from TPN. Patients who remain dependent on TPN face TPN-associated morbidities, including catheter sepsis, venous thrombosis, liver and kidney failure, and osteoporosis. Because of these problems, alternative therapies for short-bowel syndrome are under investigation.

Nontransplant Surgical Therapy

Among patients with stomas, restoration of intestinal continuity should be performed, whenever possible, to capitalize on the absorptive capacity of all residual intestine.

Operations designed to slow intestinal transit include segmental reversal of the small bowel, interposition of a segment of colon between segments of small bowel, construction of small-intestinal valves, and electrical pacing of the small intestine. Intestinal lengthening procedures include the longitudinal intestinal lengthening and tailoring (LILT) procedure, first described by Bianchi, and the more recently described serial transverse enteroplasty procedure (STEP). These operations are associated with unclear efficacy and/or substantial morbidities, and therefore should not be applied routinely.

Intestinal Transplantation

Approximately 100 intestinal transplants are performed in the United States annually, with most of these procedures applied to patients with short-bowel syndrome. The currently accepted indication for intestinal transplantation is the presence of life-threatening complications attributable to intestinal failure and/or long-term TPN therapy. Specific complications for which intestinal transplantation is indicated include impending or overt liver failure, thrombosis of major central veins, frequent episodes of catheter-related sepsis, and frequent episodes of severe dehydration.

Isolated intestinal transplantation is used for patients with intestinal failure who have no significant liver disease or failure of other organs. Combined intestine/liver transplantation is used for patients with both intestinal and liver failure. Nearly 80 percent of survivors have full intestinal graft function with no need for TPN. However, morbidities associated with intestinal transplantation are substantial and include acute and chronic rejection, CMV infection, and posttransplant lymphoproliferative disease.

Outcomes

Approximately 50–70 percent of patients with short-bowel syndrome who initially require TPN are ultimately able to achieve independence from TPN.

Suggested Readings

Brandt LJ, Boley SJ: AGA technical review on intestinal ischemia. Gastroenterol 118:954, 2000.

Buchman AL, Solapio J, Fryer J: AGA technical review on short bowel syndrome and intestinal transplantation. Gastroenterology 124:1111, 2003.

Demetri GD, Mehren M, Blanke C, et al: Efficacy and safety of imatinib mesylate in advanced gastrointestinal stromal tumors. N Engl J Med 347:472, 2002.

Geoghegan J, Pappas TN: Clinical uses of gut peptides. Ann Surg 225:145, 1997.

Judson I: Gastrointestinal stromal tumors (GIST): Biology and treatment. Ann Oncol 13(Suppl 4):287, 2002.

Luckey A, Livingston E, Tache Y: Mechanisms and treatment of postoperative ileus. Arch Surg 138:206, 2003.

Schraut WH: The surgical management of Crohn's disease. Gastroenterol Clin North Am 31:255, 2002.

Tavvakolizadeh A, Whang EE: Understanding and augmenting human intestinal adaptation: A call for more clinical research. JPEN J 26:251, 2002.

Thompson JS, Langnas AN: Surgical approaches to improving intestinal function in the short-bowel syndrome. Arch Surg 134:706, 1999.

Yahchouchy EK, Marano AF, Etienne JC, et al: Meckel's diverticulum. J Am Coll Surg 192:654, 2001.

28 | Colon, Rectum, and Anus

Kelli M. Bullard and David A. Rothenberger

ANATOMY

Anatomic divisions of the large intestine:

1. Colon
2. Rectum
3. Anal canal

Layers of the colon and rectum:

1. Mucosa
2. Submucosa
3. Inner circular muscle – Coalesces distally to create the internal anal sphincter.
4. Outer longitudinal muscle – Separated into three teniae coli in the colon; teniae converge proximally at the appendix and distally at the rectum.
5. Serosa – Covers the intraperitoneal colon and one third of the rectum.

Colorectal and Anorectal Vascular Supply

The arterial supply to the colon is highly variable. In general, the arterial supply to the colon is as follows:

1. Superior mesenteric artery branches
   a. Ileocolic artery (absent in up to 20 percent of people) supplies blood flow to the terminal ileum and proximal ascending colon.
   b. Right colic artery supplies the ascending colon.
   c. Middle colic artery supplies the transverse colon.
2. Inferior mesenteric artery branches
   a. Left colic artery supplies the descending colon.
   b. Sigmoidal branches supply the sigmoid colon.
   c. Superior rectal artery supplies the proximal rectum.
   The terminal branches of each artery form anastomoses with the terminal branches of the adjacent artery and communicate via the marginal artery of Drummond (complete in only 15–20 percent of people).
3. Internal iliac artery branches
   a. Middle rectal artery (variable presence and size).
   b. Internal pudendal artery branch.
      i. Inferior rectal artery supplies the lower rectum and anal canal.

A rich network of collaterals connects the terminal arterioles of each of these arteries, thus making the rectum relatively resistant to ischemia.

Except for the inferior mesenteric vein, the veins of the colon, rectum, and anus parallel their corresponding arteries and bear the same terminology. The inferior mesenteric vein ascends in the retroperitoneal plane over the psoas muscle and continues posterior to the pancreas to join the splenic vein. The venous drainage of the rectum parallels the arterial supply. The superior rectal vein drains into the portal system via the inferior mesenteric vein. The middle rectal vein drains into the internal iliac vein. The inferior rectal vein drains into the internal pudendal vein, and subsequently into the internal iliac vein. A submucosal plexus deep to the columns of Morgagni forms the hemorrhoidal plexus and drains into all three veins.

Colorectal and Anorectal Lymphatic Drainage

The lymphatic drainage of the colon originates in a network of lymphatics in the muscularis mucosa. Lymphatic vessels and lymph nodes follow the regional arteries. Lymphatic channels in the upper and middle rectum drain superiorly into the inferior mesenteric lymph nodes. Lymphatic channels in the lower rectum drain both superiorly into the inferior mesenteric lymph nodes and laterally into the internal iliac lymph nodes. The anal canal has a more complex pattern of lymphatic drainage. Proximal to the dentate line, lymph drains into both the inferior mesenteric lymph nodes and the internal iliac lymph nodes. Distal to the dentate line, lymph primarily drains into the inguinal lymph nodes, but also can drain into the inferior mesenteric lymph nodes and internal iliac lymph nodes.

Colorectal and Anorectal Nerve Supply

The nerves to the colon and rectum parallel the course of the arteries.

1. Sympathetic (inhibitory) arise from T6-T12 and L1-L3.
2. Parasympathetic (stimulatory) innervation to the right and transverse colon is from the vagus nerve; parasympathetic nerves to the left colon arise from sacral nerves S2–S4 to form the nervi erigentes. The external anal sphincter and puborectalis muscles are innervated by the inferior rectal branch of the internal pudendal nerve. The levator ani receives innervation from both the internal pudendal nerve and direct branches of S3–S5. Sensory innervation to the anal canal is provided by the inferior rectal branch of the pudendal nerve. Whereas the rectum is relatively insensate, the anal canal below the dentate line is sensate.

CLINICAL EVALUATION

Endoscopy

1. Anoscopy – The anoscope is useful for examination of the anal canal and can generally allow examination of the distal 6–8 cm of the anus. Anoscopy can be diagnostic or therapeutic (e.g., sclerotherapy or rubber band ligation of hemorrhoids).
2. Proctoscopy – The rigid proctoscope is useful for examination of the rectum and distal sigmoid colon and is occasionally used therapeutically (e.g., polypectomy, electrocoagulation, or detorsion of a sigmoid volvulus).
3. Flexible Sigmoidoscopy and Colonoscopy – Flexible sigmoidoscopy and colonoscopy provide excellent visualization of the colon and rectum. Sigmoidoscopes measure 60 cm in length and may allow visualization as high as the splenic flexure. Partial preparation with enemas is usually adequate for sigmoidoscopy and most patients can tolerate this procedure without sedation.

Colonoscopes measure 100–160 cm in length and are capable of examining the entire colon and terminal ileum. A complete oral bowel preparation usually is necessary for colonoscopy and the duration and discomfort of the procedure usually require conscious sedation. Both sigmoidoscopy and colonoscopy can be used diagnostically and therapeutically.

Imaging

1. Plain radiograph of the abdomen (supine, upright, and diaphragmatic views) are useful for detecting free intraabdominal air, bowel gas patterns suggestive of small or large bowel obstruction, and volvulus.

2. Contrast studies are useful for evaluating obstructive symptoms, delineating fistulous tracts, and diagnosing small perforations or anastomotic leaks. Gastrografin is recommended if perforation or leak is suspected. Double-contrast barium enema is more sensitive for the detection of mass lesions greater than 1 cm in diameter.

3. Computed Tomography – Computed tomography (CT) is commonly employed in the evaluation of patients with abdominal complaints. Its utility is primarily in the detection of extraluminal disease, such as intraabdominal abscesses and pericolic inflammation, and in staging colorectal carcinoma. Extravasation of oral or rectal contrast also may confirm the diagnosis of perforation or anastomotic leak. Nonspecific findings such as bowel wall thickening or mesenteric stranding may suggest inflammatory bowel disease, enteritis/colitis, or ischemia. A standard CT scan is relatively insensitive for the detection of intraluminal lesions.

4. Virtual Colonoscopy (CT colography) – Virtual colonoscopy is a technique that is designed to overcome some of the limitations of traditional CT scanning. This technology uses helical CT and three-dimensional reconstruction to detect intraluminal colonic lesions. Oral bowel preparation, oral and rectal contrast, and colon insufflation are used to maximize sensitivity.

5. Magnetic Resonance Imaging (MRI) – The main use of MRI in colorectal disorders is in evaluation of pelvic lesions. MRI is more sensitive than CT for detecting bony involvement or pelvic sidewall extension of rectal tumors. MRI with an endorectal coil can be helpful in the detection and delineation of complex fistulas in ano.

6. Positron Emission Tomography (PET) – Positron emission tomography is used for imaging tissues with high levels of anaerobic glycolysis, such as malignant tumors. PET has been used as an adjunct to CT in the staging of colorectal cancer and may prove useful in discriminating recurrent cancer from fibrosis.

7. Angiography – Angiography is occasionally used for the detection of brisk bleeding (approximately 0.5–1.0 mL per minute) within the colon or small bowel. If extravasation of contrast is identified, infusion of vasopressin or angiographic embolization can be therapeutic.

8. Endorectal and Endoanal Ultrasound – Endorectal ultrasound is primarily used to evaluate the depth of invasion of neoplastic lesions in the rectum. Ultrasound can reliably differentiate most benign polyps from invasive tumors and can differentiate superficial (T1–T2) from deeper (T3–T4) tumors. This modality also can detect enlarged perirectal lymph nodes. Ultrasound may also prove useful for early detection of local recurrence after surgery.

Endoanal ultrasound is used to evaluate the layers of the anal canal. Internal anal sphincter, external anal sphincter, and puborectalis muscle can be differentiated. Endoanal ultrasound is particularly useful for detecting sphincter defects and for outlining complex anal fistulas.

Physiologic and Pelvic Floor Investigations

Anorectal physiologic testing techniques are useful in the evaluation of patients with incontinence, constipation, rectal prolapse, obstructed defecation, and other disorders of the pelvic floor.

1. Manometry – Anorectal manometry measures pressure in the anal canal. The resting pressure in the anal canal reflects the function of the internal anal sphincter (normal: 40–80 mmHg), whereas the squeeze pressure, defined as the maximum voluntary contraction pressure minus the resting pressure, reflects function of the external anal sphincter (normal: 40–80 mmHg above resting pressure). The high-pressure zone estimates the length of the anal canal (normal: 2.0–4.0 cm).

2. Neurophysiology – Neurophysiologic testing assesses function of the pudendal nerves and recruitment of puborectalis muscle fibers. Pudendal nerve terminal motor latency measures the speed of transmission of a nerve impulse through the distal pudendal nerve fibers (normal: 1.8–2.2 msec); prolonged latency suggests the presence of neuropathy. EMG recruitment assesses the contraction and relaxation of the puborectalis muscle during attempted defecation. Normally, recruitment increases when a patient is instructed to "squeeze," and decreases when a patient is instructed to "push." Inappropriate recruitment is an indication of paradoxical contraction (nonrelaxation of the puborectalis).

3. Rectal Evacuation Studies – Rectal evacuation studies include the balloon expulsion test and video defecography. Balloon expulsion assesses a patient's ability to expel an intrarectal balloon. Video defecography provides a more detailed assessment of defecation.

Evaluation of Common Symptoms

Pain

Abdominal pain. Abdominal pain related to the colon and rectum can result from obstruction, inflammation, perforation, or ischemia. Plain radiographs and judicious use of contrast studies and/or a CT scan can often confirm the diagnosis. Gentle retrograde contrast studies (barium or Gastrografin enema) may be useful in delineating the degree of colonic obstruction. Sigmoidoscopy and/or colonoscopy performed by an experienced endoscopist can assist in the diagnosis of ischemic colitis, infectious colitis, and inflammatory bowel disease. However, if perforation or obstruction is suspected, colonoscopy and/or sigmoidoscopy are generally contraindicated.

Pelvic pain. Pelvic pain can originate from the distal colon and rectum or from adjacent urogenital structures. Tenesmus may result from proctitis or from a rectal or retrorectal mass. Cyclic pain associated with menses suggests a diagnosis of endometriosis. Pelvic inflammatory disease also can produce significant abdominal and pelvic pain. The extension of a peridiverticular abscess or periappendiceal abscess into the pelvis may also cause pain. CT scan and/or MRI may be useful in differentiating these diseases. Proctoscopy (if tolerated) also can be helpful. Occasionally, laparoscopy will yield a diagnosis.

Anorectal pain. Anorectal pain most often is secondary to an anal fissure or perirectal abscess and/or fistula. Physical examination can usually differentiate these conditions. Other, less common causes of anorectal pain include anal canal neoplasms, perianal skin infection, and dermatologic conditions.

Proctalgia fugax results from levator spasm and may present without any other anorectal findings. Physical examination is critical in evaluating patients with anorectal pain. If a patient is too tender to examine in the office, an examination under anesthesia is necessary. MRI may be helpful in select cases in which the etiology of pain is elusive.

Lower Gastrointestinal Bleeding

The first goal in evaluating and treating a patient with gastrointestinal hemorrhage is adequate resuscitation. The principles of ensuring a patent airway, supporting ventilation, and optimizing hemodynamic parameters apply and coagulopathy and/or thrombocytopenia should be corrected. The second goal is to identify the source of hemorrhage. Because the most common source of gastrointestinal hemorrhage is esophageal, gastric, or duodenal, nasogastric aspiration should always be performed; return of bile suggests that the source of bleeding is distal to the ligament of Treitz. If aspiration reveals blood or nonbile secretions, or if symptoms suggest an upper intestinal source, esophagogastroduodenoscopy is performed. Anoscopy and/or limited proctoscopy can identify hemorrhoidal bleeding. A technetium-99 (99mTc)-tagged red blood cell (RBC) scan is extremely sensitive and is able to detect as little as 0.1 mL/h of bleeding; however, localization is imprecise. If the 99mTc-tagged RBC scan is positive, angiography can then be employed to localize bleeding. Infusion of vasopressin or angioembolization may be therapeutic. Alternatively, a catheter can be left in the bleeding vessel to allow localization at the time of laparotomy. If the patient is hemodynamically stable, a rapid bowel preparation (over 4–6 h) can be performed to allow colonoscopy. Colonoscopy may identify the cause of the bleeding, and cautery or injection of epinephrine into the bleeding site may be used to control hemorrhage. Colectomy may be required if bleeding persists despite these interventions. Intraoperative colonoscopy and/or enteroscopy may assist in localizing bleeding. If colectomy is required, a segmental resection is preferred if the bleeding source can be localized. "Blind" subtotal colectomy very rarely may be required in a patient who is hemodynamically unstable with ongoing colonic hemorrhage of an unknown source. In this setting, it is crucial to irrigate the rectum and examine the mucosa by proctoscopy to ensure that the source of bleeding is not distal to the resection margin.

Hematochezia is commonly caused by hemorrhoids or fissure. Sharp, knife-like pain and bright-red rectal bleeding with bowel movements suggest the diagnosis of fissure. Painless, bright-red rectal bleeding with bowel movements is often secondary to a friable internal hemorrhoid that is easily detected by anoscopy. In the absence of a painful, obvious fissure, any patient with rectal bleeding should undergo a careful digital rectal examination, anoscopy, and proctosigmoidoscopy. Failure to diagnose a source in the distal anorectum should prompt colonoscopy.

Diarrhea and Irritable Bowel Syndrome

Diarrhea is a common complaint and is usually a self-limited symptom of infectious gastroenteritis. If diarrhea is chronic or is accompanied by bleeding or abdominal pain, further investigation is warranted. Bloody diarrhea and pain are characteristic of colitis; etiology can be an infection, inflammatory bowel disease, or ischemia. Stool wet-mount and culture can often diagnose infection. Sigmoidoscopy or colonoscopy can be helpful in diagnosing inflammatory bowel disease or ischemia. However, if the patient has abdominal tenderness, particularly with peritoneal signs, or any other evidence of perforation, endoscopy is contraindicated.

Chronic diarrhea may present a more difficult diagnostic dilemma. Chronic ulcerative colitis, Crohn's colitis, infection, malabsorption, and short-gut syndrome can cause chronic diarrhea. Rarely, carcinoid syndrome and islet cell tumors present with this symptom. Large villous lesions may cause secretory diarrhea. Collagenous colitis can cause diarrhea without any obvious mucosal abnormality. Along with stool cultures, tests for malabsorption, and metabolic investigations, colonoscopy with biopsies can be invaluable.

Irritable bowel syndrome is a particularly troubling constellation of symptoms consisting of crampy abdominal pain, bloating, constipation, and urgent diarrhea. Work-up reveals no underlying anatomic or physiologic abnormality. Once other disorders have been excluded, dietary restrictions and avoidance of caffeine, alcohol, and tobacco may help to alleviate symptoms. Antispasmodics and bulking agents may be helpful.

Defecation Disorders, Constipation, and Incontinence

Defecation is a complex, coordinated mechanism involving colonic mass movement, increased intraabdominal and rectal pressure, and relaxation of the pelvic floor. Distention of the rectum causes a reflex relaxation of the internal anal sphincter (the rectoanal inhibitory reflex) that allows the contents to make contact with the anal canal. This "sampling reflex" allows the sensory epithelium to distinguish solid stool from liquid stool and gas. If defecation does not occur, the rectum relaxes and the urge to defecate passes (the accommodation response). Defecation proceeds by coordination of increasing intraabdominal pressure via the Valsalva maneuver, increased rectal contraction, relaxation of the puborectalis muscle, and opening of the anal canal.

The maintenance of fecal continence requires adequate rectal wall compliance, appropriate neurogenic control of the pelvic floor and sphincter mechanism, and functional internal and external sphincter muscles. At rest, the puborectalis muscle creates a "sling" around the distal rectum, forming an acute angle that distributes intraabdominal forces onto the pelvic floor. With defecation, this angle straightens, allowing downward force to be applied along the axis of the rectum and anal canal. The internal and external sphincters are tonically active at rest. The internal sphincter is responsible for most of the resting, involuntary sphincter tone (resting pressure). The external sphincter is responsible for most of the voluntary sphincter tone (squeeze pressure). Branches of the pudendal nerve innervate both the internal and external sphincter. Hemorrhoidal cushions may contribute to continence by mechanically blocking the anal canal.

Constipation and Obstructed Defecation

Constipation has a myriad of causes. Underlying metabolic, pharmacologic, endocrine, psychologic, and neurologic causes often contribute to the problem. A stricture or mass lesion should be excluded by colonoscopy or barium enema. After these causes have been excluded, evaluation focuses on differentiating slow-transit constipation from outlet obstruction. Transit studies, in which radiopaque markers are swallowed and then followed radiographically, are useful for diagnosing slow-transit constipation. Anorectal manometry and electromyography can detect nonrelaxation of the puborectalis, which contributes to outlet obstruction. The absence of an anorectal inhibitory reflex suggests Hirschsprung disease and may prompt a rectal mucosal biopsy.

Defecography can identify rectal prolapse, intussusception, rectocele, or enterocele.

Medical management is the mainstay of therapy for constipation and includes fiber, increased fluid intake, and laxatives. Outlet obstruction from non-relaxation of the puborectalis often responds to biofeedback. Surgery to correct rectocele and rectal prolapse has a variable effect on symptoms of constipation, but can be successful in selected patients. Subtotal colectomy is considered only for patients with severe slow-transit constipation (colonic inertia) refractory to maximal medical interventions.

Incontinence

Incontinence ranges in severity from occasional leakage of gas and liquid stool to daily loss of solid stool. The underlying cause of incontinence often is multifactorial and diarrhea often is contributory. In general, causes of incontinence can be classified as neurogenic or anatomic. Neurogenic causes include diseases of the central nervous system and spinal cord along with pudendal nerve injury. Anatomic causes include congenital abnormalities, procidentia, overflow incontinence secondary to impaction or neoplasm, and trauma. The most common traumatic cause of incontinence is injury to the anal sphincter during vaginal delivery. Other causes include anorectal surgery, impalement, and pelvic fracture.

Therapy depends on the underlying abnormality. Diarrhea should be treated medically. Even in the absence of frank diarrhea, the addition of dietary fiber may improve continence. Some patients may respond to biofeedback. Many patients with a sphincter defect are candidates for an overlapping sphincteroplasty. Innovative technologies such as sacral nerve stimulation or artificial bowel sphincter are proving useful in patients who fail other interventions.

GENERAL SURGICAL CONSIDERATIONS

Resections

The extent of colonic resection is determined by the nature of the primary pathology (malignant or benign), the intent of the resection (curative or palliative), the precise location(s) of the primary pathology, and the condition of the mesentery (thin and soft or thickened and indurated). Curative resection of a colorectal cancer is usually best accomplished by performing a proximal mesenteric vessel ligation and radical mesenteric clearance of the lymphatic drainage basin of the tumor site with concomitant resection of the overlying omentum. Resection of a benign process does not require wide mesenteric resection and the omentum can be preserved if desired.

Emergency Resection

Emergency resection may be required because of obstruction, perforation, or hemorrhage. In this setting, the bowel almost always is unprepared and the patient may be unstable. The surgical principles described above apply and an attempt should be made to resect the involved segment along with its lymphovascular supply. If the resection involves the right colon or proximal transverse colon (right or extended right colectomy), a primary ileocolonic anastomosis can usually be performed safely as long as the remaining bowel appears healthy and the patient is stable. For left-sided tumors, the traditional approach has involved resection of the involved bowel and end colostomy, with or without a mucus fistula. However, there is an increasing body of data to suggest that a primary anastomosis with an on-table lavage, with or without a diverting ileostomy, may be equally safe in this setting. If the proximal colon looks unhealthy (vascular compromise, serosal tears, perforation), a subtotal colectomy can be performed with a small bowel to rectosigmoid anastomosis. Resection and diversion (ileostomy or colostomy) remains safe and appropriate if the bowel looks compromised or if the patient is unstable, malnourished, or immunosuppressed.

Laparoscopic Resection

Many procedures that previously have required laparotomy can now be performed laparoscopically. To date, most studies have demonstrated equivalence between laparoscopic and open resection in terms of extent of resection. However, laparoscopic colon resections are technically demanding and consistently require longer operative time than do open procedures. Return of bowel function and length of hospital stay are highly variable. Long-term outcome has yet to be determined.

Colectomy

A variety of terms are used to describe different types of colectomy. Ileocolic Resection – used to remove disease involving ileum, cecum, and/or appendix. If curable malignancy is suspected, more radical resections (right hemicolectomy) are generally indicated.

Right Colectomy – used to remove lesions or disease in the right colon and is oncologically the most appropriate operation for curative intent resection of proximal colon carcinoma.

Extended Right Colectomy – used for curative intent resection of lesions located at the hepatic flexure or proximal transverse colon.

Transverse Colectomy – may be used to resect lesions in the mid and distal transverse colon (an extended right colectomy may be safer with an equivalent functional result).

Left Colectomy – used to resect lesions confined to the distal transverse colon, splenic flexure, or descending colon.

Extended Left Colectomy – used to resect lesions in the distal transverse colon.

Sigmoid Colectomy – used to resect lesions in the sigmoid colon. In general, the entire sigmoid colon should be resected to the level of the peritoneal reflection and an anastomosis created between the descending colon and upper rectum.

Total and Subtotal Colectomy – may be required for patients with fulminant colitis, attenuated familial adenomatous polyposis, or synchronous colon carcinomas. Total abdominal colectomy refers to resection of the entire colon, including the sigmoid colon, with or without an ileorectal anastomosis. Subtotal colectomy refers to resection of the right, transverse, and left colon with or without an anastomosis between the ileum and sigmoid colon. If an anastomosis is contraindicated, an end-ileostomy is created and the remaining sigmoid or rectum is managed either as a mucus fistula or a Hartmann pouch.

Proctocolectomy

Total Proctocolectomy – removal of the entire colon, rectum, and anus with creation of an ileostomy. Restorative proctocolectomy (total proctocolectomy with ileoanal pouch) refers to removal of the entire colon and rectum, with preservation of the anal sphincters. Bowel continuity is restored by anastomosis of an ileal reservoir to the anal canal.

Anterior Resection – a general term used to describe resection of the rectum from an abdominal approach.

High Anterior Resection – used to describe resection of the distal sigmoid colon and upper rectum; appropriate for benign lesions at the rectosigmoid junction.

Low Anterior Resection – used to remove lesions in the upper and mid rectum. Circular stapling devices have greatly facilitated the conduct and improved the safety of the colon to extraperitoneal rectal anastomosis.

Extended Low Anterior Resection – used to remove lesions located in the distal rectum, but several centimeters above the sphincter. After resection, a coloanal anastomosis can be created. Because the risk of an anastomotic leak and subsequent sepsis is higher when an anastomosis is created in the distal rectum or anal canal, creation of a temporary ileostomy should be considered in this setting. Although an anastomosis may be technically feasible very low in the rectum or anal canal, it is important to note that postoperative function and continence may be poor.

Hartmann's Procedure and Mucus Fistula – refers to a colon or rectal resection without an anastomosis in which a colostomy or ileostomy is created proximally and the distal colon or rectum is left as a closed off blind pouch (Hartmann pouch). A mucus fistula is an option if the distal colon is long enough to reach the abdominal wall. It can be created by opening the defunctioned bowel and suturing it to the skin.

Abdominoperineal Resection – removal of the entire rectum, anal canal, and anus with construction of a permanent colostomy from the descending or sigmoid colon.

Anastomoses

Anastomoses may be created between two segments of bowel in a multitude of ways. The geometry of the anastomosis may be end-to-end, end-to-side, side-to-end, or side-to-side. The anastomotic technique may be handsewn (single or double layer) or stapled. The choice of anastomosis depends on the operative anatomy and surgeon preference.

Ostomies

Depending on the clinical situation, a stoma may be temporary or permanent. It may be end-on or a loop. However, regardless of the indication for a stoma, placement and construction are crucial for function. A stoma should be located within the rectus muscle to minimize the risk of a postoperative parastomal hernia. It also should be placed where the patient can see it and easily manipulate the appliance. The surrounding abdominal soft tissue should be as flat as possible to ensure a tight seal and prevent leakage. Preoperative evaluation by an enterostomal therapy nurse to identify the ideal stoma site and to counsel and educate the patient is invaluable.

Ileostomy

Temporary Ileostomy. A temporary ileostomy often is used to "protect" an anastomosis that is at risk for leakage (low in the rectum, in an irradiated field, in an immunocompromised or malnourished patient, and in some emergency operations). The stoma often is constructed as a loop ileostomy. The advantage of a loop ileostomy is that subsequent closure often can be accomplished without a formal laparotomy.

Permanent Ileostomy. A permanent ileostomy is sometimes required after total proctocolectomy or in patients with obstruction. An end ileostomy is the preferred configuration for a permanent ileostomy because a symmetric protruding nipple can be fashioned more easily than with a loop ileostomy.

Complications of Ileostomy

Anatomic

1. Stoma necrosis
2. Stoma retraction
3. Skin irritation
4. Obstruction: intraabdominally or at the site where the stoma exits the fascia
5. Parastomal hernia (less common than after colostomy)
6. Prolapse (rare)

Functional. Dehydration and fluid/electrolyte abnormalities: The creation of an ileostomy bypasses the fluid-absorbing capability of the colon, and dehydration with fluid and electrolyte abnormalities is not uncommon. Ideally, ileostomy output should be maintained at less than 1500 mL/day to avoid this problem. Bulk agents and antidiarrheal agents are useful.

Colostomy

Most colostomies are created as end colostomies. Because a protruding stoma is considerably easier to pouch, colostomies also should be matured in a Brooke fashion. Closure of a colostomy usually requires laparotomy.

Complications of Colostomy

Anatomic.

1. Colostomy necrosis
2. Colostomy retraction (less problematic with a colostomy than with an ileostomy because the stool is less irritating to the skin than succus entericus)
3. Obstruction (intraabdominal or at the site where the bowel exits the fascia)
4. Parastomal hernia is the most common late complication of a colostomy and requires repair if it is symptomatic. Repair usually requires resiting the stoma to the contralateral side of the abdomen.
5. Prolapse (rare)

Bowel Preparation

The rationale for bowel preparation is that decreasing the bacterial load in the colon and rectum will decrease the incidence of postoperative infection. Mechanical bowel preparation uses cathartics to rid the colon of solid stool the night before surgery. The most commonly used regimens include polyethylene glycol (PEG) solutions or sodium phosphate. Antibiotic prophylaxis also is recommended. A combination of three doses of neomycin (1 g) and erythromycin base (1 g) is most commonly used. Some surgeons substitute metronidazole (500 mg) for erythromycin to avoid gastrointestinal upset. Ciprofloxacin also has been used in this setting. A broad-spectrum parenteral antibiotic(s) should be administered just prior to the skin incision. There is no proven benefit to using antibiotics postoperatively after an uncomplicated colectomy.

INFLAMMATORY BOWEL DISEASE

General Considerations

Epidemiology

Inflammatory bowel disease includes ulcerative colitis, Crohn disease, and indeterminate colitis. Multiple etiologies for inflammatory bowel disease have been proposed, but none are proven. Suggested etiology includes an environmental factor (diet, infection), smoking, alcohol, oral contraceptive use, and/or an autoimmune mechanism. Ten to 30 percent of patients will have a family history of irritable bowel disease (IBD). Regardless of the underlying cause of either ulcerative colitis or Crohn disease, both disorders are characterized by intestinal inflammation and medical therapy is largely based on reducing inflammation.

Pathology and Differential Diagnosis

1. Ulcerative Colitis: Ulcerative colitis is a mucosal process in which the colonic mucosa and submucosa are infiltrated with inflammatory cells. The mucosa may be atrophic and crypt abscesses are common. Endoscopically, the mucosa is frequently friable and may possess multiple inflammatory pseudopolyps. In long-standing ulcerative colitis, the colon may be foreshortened and the mucosa replaced by scar. In quiescent ulcerative colitis, the colonic mucosa may appear normal both endoscopically and microscopically. A key feature of ulcerative colitis is the continuous involvement of the rectum and colon; rectal sparing or skip lesions suggests a diagnosis of Crohn disease. Symptoms are related to the degree of mucosal inflammation and the extent of colitis. Patients typically complain of bloody diarrhea and crampy abdominal pain. Severe abdominal pain and fever raises the concern of fulminant colitis or toxic megacolon. Physical findings are nonspecific and range from minimal abdominal tenderness and distention to frank peritonitis. In the nonemergent setting, the diagnosis is typically made by colonoscopy and mucosal biopsy.
2. Crohn Disease: Crohn disease is a transmural inflammatory process that can affect any part of the gastrointestinal tract. Mucosal ulcerations, an inflammatory cell infiltrate, and noncaseating granulomas are characteristic pathologic findings. Chronic inflammation may ultimately result in fibrosis, strictures, and fistulas in either the colon or small intestine. The endoscopic appearance of Crohn colitis is characterized by deep serpiginous ulcers and a "cobblestone" appearance. Skip lesions and rectal sparing are common. Symptoms of Crohn disease depend on the severity of inflammation and/or fibrosis and the location of inflammation in the gastrointestinal tract. Acute inflammation may produce diarrhea, crampy abdominal pain, and fever. Strictures may produce symptoms of obstruction. Weight loss is common, both because of obstruction and from protein loss. Perianal Crohn disease may present with pain, swelling, and drainage from fistulas or abscesses. Physical findings also are related to the site and severity of disease.
3. Indeterminate Colitis: In 15 percent of patients with colitis from IBD, differentiation of ulcerative colitis from Crohn colitis proves impossible.

Endoscopic and pathologic findings usually include features common to both diseases.
4. Differential Diagnosis: Differential diagnoses include infectious colitides, especially *Campylobacter jejuni*, *Entamoeba histolytica*, *C. difficile*, *Neisseria gonococcus*, Salmonella, and Shigella species.

Extraintestinal Manifestations

1. Hepatic
   A. Fatty infiltration (40–50 percent) – reversible
   B. Cirrhosis (2–5 percent) – irreversible
   C. Primary Sclerosing cholangitis – irreversible
   D. Pericholangitis
   E. Bile duct carcinoma – rare
2. Rheumatologic
   A. Arthritis – reversible
   B. Sacroiliitis – irreversible
   C. Ankylosing spondylitis – irreversible
   D. Erythema nodosum (5–15 percent)
   E. Pyoderma gangrenosum (rare)
3. Ocular (10 percent)
   A. Uveitis
   B. Iritis
   C. Episcleritis
   D. Conjunctivitis

Principles of Nonoperative Management

Medical therapy for inflammatory bowel disease focuses on decreasing inflammation and alleviating symptoms, and many of the agents used are the same for both ulcerative colitis and Crohn disease. In general, mild to moderate flares may be treated in the outpatient setting. More severe signs and symptoms mandate hospitalization. Pancolitis generally requires more aggressive therapy than limited disease. Because ulcerative proctitis and proctosigmoiditis are limited to the distal large intestine, topical therapy with salicylate and/or corticosteroid suppositories and enemas can be extremely effective. Systemic therapy rarely is required in these patients.

Salicylates. Sulfasalazine (Azulfidine), 5-ASA, and related compounds are first-line agents in the medical treatment of mild to moderate inflammatory bowel disease. Multiple preparations are available for administration to different sites in the small intestine and colon (sulfasalazine, mesalamine [Pentasa], Asacol, Rowasa).

Antibiotics. Antibiotics are used to decrease the intraluminal bacterial load in Crohn disease. Metronidazole has been reported to improve Crohn colitis and perianal disease, but the evidence is weak. Fluoroquinolones also may be effective in some cases. In the absence of fulminant colitis or toxic megacolon, antibiotics are not used to treat ulcerative colitis.

Corticosteroids. Corticosteroids (oral or parenteral) are a key component of treatment for an acute exacerbation of either ulcerative colitis or Crohn disease. Seventy-five to 90 percent of patients will improve with the administration of these drugs. Corticosteroid enemas provide effective local therapy for proctitis and proctosigmoiditis and have fewer side effects than systemic corticosteroids. Failure to wean systemic corticosteroids is a relative indication for surgery.

Immunosuppressive Agents

1. Antimetabolites: Azathioprine and 6-mercatopurine (6-MP) interfere with nucleic acid synthesis and thus decrease proliferation of inflammatory cells. These agents are useful for treating ulcerative colitis and Crohn disease in patients who have failed salicylate therapy or who are dependent on or are refractory to corticosteroids. Onset of action of these drugs takes 6–12 weeks, and concomitant use of corticosteroids almost always is required.
2. Cyclosporine: Cyclosporine interferes with T-cell function. Although cyclosporine is not routinely used to treat inflammatory bowel disease, up to 80 percent of patients with an acute flare of ulcerative colitis will improve with its use. However, the majority of these patients will ultimately require colectomy. Cyclosporine also is occasionally used to treat exacerbations of Crohn's disease and approximately two-thirds of patients will note some improvement.
3. Methotrexate: Methotrexate is a folate antagonist. Although the efficacy of this agent is unproven, there are reports that more than 50 percent of patients will improve with administration of this drug.
4. Infliximab: Infliximab (Remicade) is a monoclonal antibody against tumor necrosis factor alpha (TNF-α). Intravenous infusion of this agent decreases inflammation systemically. More than 50 percent of patients with moderate to severe Crohn disease will improve with infliximab therapy. This agent also has been useful in treating patients with perianal Crohn disease. Recurrence is common, however, and many patients require infusions on a bimonthly basis. Infliximab has not been used as extensively for treatment of ulcerative colitis; however, there are reports of efficacy in this setting.

Nutrition. Patients with inflammatory bowel disease are often malnourished. Parenteral nutrition should be strongly considered early in the course of therapy for either Crohn disease or ulcerative colitis. The nutritional status of the patient also should be considered when planning operative intervention and nutritional parameters such as serum albumin, prealbumin, and transferrin should be assessed. In extremely malnourished patients, especially those who also are being treated with corticosteroids, creation of a stoma often is safer than a primary anastomosis.

Ulcerative Colitis

Ulcerative colitis is a dynamic disease characterized by remissions and exacerbations. The clinical spectrum ranges from an inactive or quiescent phase to low-grade active disease to fulminant disease. The onset of ulcerative colitis may be insidious, with minimal bloody stools, or the onset can be abrupt, with severe diarrhea and bleeding, tenesmus, abdominal pain, and fever. The severity of symptoms depends on the degree and extent of inflammation. Although anemia is common, massive hemorrhage is rare. Physical findings often are nonspecific.

Diagnosis of ulcerative colitis almost always is made endoscopically. Because the rectum is invariably involved, proctoscopy may be adequate to establish the diagnosis. A complete evaluation with colonoscopy or barium enema during an acute flare is contraindicated because of the risk of perforation.

Because the inflammation in ulcerative colitis is purely mucosal, strictures are highly uncommon. Any stricture diagnosed in a patient with ulcerative colitis must be presumed to be malignant until proven otherwise.

Indications for Surgery

Emergency surgery is required for patients with life-threatening hemorrhage, toxic megacolon, or fulminant colitis who fail to respond rapidly to medical therapy. Patients with fulminant colitis should be treated with bowel rest, hydration, broad-spectrum antibiotics, and parenteral corticosteroids. Colonoscopy and barium enema are contraindicated and antidiarrheal agents should be avoided. Clinical deterioration or failure to improve within 24 h mandates surgery.

Indications for elective surgery include intractability despite maximal medical therapy, development of major complications from medical therapy, and risk of developing colorectal carcinoma. Risk of malignancy increases with pancolonic disease and the duration of symptoms; the risk is approximately 2 percent after 10 years, 8 percent after 20 years, and 18 percent after 30 years. Unlike sporadic colorectal cancers, carcinoma developing in the context of ulcerative colitis is more likely to arise from areas of flat dysplasia and may be difficult to diagnose at an early stage. For this reason, it is recommended that patients with long-standing ulcerative colitis undergo colonoscopic surveillance with multiple (40–50), random biopsies to identify dysplasia before invasive malignancy develops. Surveillance is recommended annually after 8 years in patients with pancolitis, and annually after 15 years in patients with left-sided colitis. Although low-grade dysplasia was long thought to represent minimal risk, more recent studies show that invasive cancer may be present in up to 20 percent of patients with low-grade dysplasia. For this reason, any patient with dysplasia should be advised to undergo proctocolectomy. Controversy exists over whether prophylactic proctocolectomy should be recommended for patients who have had chronic ulcerative colitis for greater than 10 years in the absence of dysplasia.

Operative Management

Emergent operation. In a patient with fulminant colitis or toxic megacolon, total abdominal colectomy with end ileostomy is recommended. Although the rectum is invariably diseased, most patients improve dramatically after an abdominal colectomy, and this operation avoids a difficult and time-consuming pelvic dissection in a critically ill patient. Rarely, a loop ileostomy and decompressing colostomy may be necessary if the patient is too unstable to withstand colectomy.

Elective operation. Total proctocolectomy with end ileostomy has been the "gold standard" for patients with chronic ulcerative colitis. This operation removes the entire affected intestine, but leaves the patient with a permanent ileostomy. Total proctocolectomy with continent ileostomy (Kock pouch) was developed to improve function and quality of life after total proctocolectomy, but morbidity is significant and restorative proctocolectomy is generally preferred today. Restorative proctocolectomy with ileal pouch–anal anastomosis has become the procedure of choice for most patients who require total proctocolectomy but wish to avoid a permanent ileostomy.

Crohn Disease

Crohn disease is characterized by exacerbations and remissions and may affect any portion of the intestinal tract, from mouth to anus. Diagnosis may be made by colonoscopy or esophagogastroduodenoscopy, or by barium small bowel study or enema, depending on which part of the intestine is most affected. Skip lesions are key in differentiating Crohn colitis from ulcerative colitis, and rectal sparing occurs in approximately 40 percent of patients. The most common site of involvement in Crohn disease is the terminal ileum and cecum, followed by the small bowel, and then by the colon and rectum. Crohn disease may affect the distal rectum and anal canal and may present as complex perianal/perirectal fistulas and/or abscesses.

Indications for Surgery

Because Crohn disease can affect any part of the gastrointestinal tract, the therapeutic rationale is fundamentally different from that of ulcerative colitis. In Crohn disease, it is impossible to remove all of the at-risk intestine; therefore surgical therapy is reserved for complications of the disease.

Crohn disease may present as an acute inflammatory process or as a chronic fibrotic process. During the acute inflammatory phase, patients may present with intestinal inflammation complicated by fistulas and/or intraabdominal abscesses. Maximal medical therapy should be instituted, including antiinflammatory medications, bowel rest, and antibiotics. Parenteral nutrition should be considered if the patient is malnourished. Most intraabdominal abscesses can be drained percutaneously with the use of CT scan guidance. Although the majority of these patients will ultimately require surgery to remove the diseased segment of bowel, these interventions allow the patient's condition to stabilize, nutrition to be optimized, and inflammation to decrease prior to embarking on a surgical resection.

Chronic fibrosis may result in strictures in any part of the gastrointestinal tract. Chronic strictures rarely improve with medical therapy. Optimal timing for surgery should take into account the patient's underlying medical and nutritional status. Strictures may be treated with resection or stricturoplasty. Associated fistulas generally require resection of the segment of bowel with active Crohn disease; the secondary sites of the fistula are often otherwise normal and do not generally require resection after division of the fistula. Simple closure of the secondary fistula site usually suffices.

Ileocolic and Small-Bowel Crohn Disease

The terminal ileum and cecum are involved in Crohn disease in up to 41 percent of patients; the small intestine is involved in up to 35 percent of patients. The most common indications for surgery are internal fistula or abscess (30–38 percent) and obstruction (35–37 percent). Psoas abscess may result from ileocolic Crohn disease. Sepsis should be controlled with percutaneous drainage of abscess(es) and antibiotics, if possible. The extent of resection depends on the amount of involved intestine. Because many patients with Crohn disease will require multiple operations, the length of bowel removed should be minimized. Short segments of inflamed small intestine and right colon, and isolated chronic strictures should be resected. Bowel should be resected to an area with grossly normal margins. In patients with multiple fibrotic strictures that would require extensive small-bowel resection, stricturoplasty is a safe and effective alternative to resection. A primary anastomosis may be safely created if the patient is medically stable, nutritionally replete, and taking few immunosuppressive medications. Creation of a stoma should be strongly considered in any patient who is hemodynamically unstable, septic, malnourished, or receiving high-dose immunosuppressive therapy and in patients with extensive intraabdominal contamination. Risk of recurrence after resection for ileocolic and small-bowel Crohn disease is high. More than 50 percent of patients will experience a recurrence within 10 years and the majority of these will require a second operation.

Crohn Colitis

Crohn disease of the large intestine may present as fulminant colitis or toxic megacolon. In this setting, treatment is identical to treatment of fulminant colitis and toxic megacolon secondary to ulcerative colitis. Other indications for surgery in chronic Crohn colitis are intractability, complications of medical therapy, and risk of or development of malignancy. Unlike ulcerative colitis, Crohn colitis may be segmental and rectal sparing often is observed. A segmental colectomy may be appropriate if the remaining colon and/or rectum appear normal. An isolated colonic stricture also may be treated by segmental colectomy. Crohn colitis (especially pancolitis) carries nearly the same risk for cancer as ulcerative colitis and similar surveillance and treatment are recommended. Ileal pouch–anal reconstruction is not recommended because of the risk for development of Crohn disease within the pouch and the high risk of complications and pouch failure.

Anal and Perianal Crohn Disease

Anal or perianal disease occurs in 35 percent of all patients with Crohn disease. Isolated anal Crohn disease is uncommon, affecting only 3 to 4 percent of patients. Detection of anal Crohn disease, therefore, should prompt evaluation of the remainder of the gastrointestinal tract. The most common perianal lesions in Crohn disease are skin tags. Fissures also are common and tend to occur in unusual locations. Perianal abscess and fistulas are common and can be particularly challenging. Fistulas tend to be complex and often have multiple tracts. Treatment of anal and perianal Crohn disease focuses on alleviation of symptoms. In general, skin tags and hemorrhoids should not be excised unless they are extremely symptomatic because of the risk of creating chronic, nonhealing wounds. Fissures may respond to local or systemic therapy; sphincterotomy is relatively contraindicated because of the risk of creating a chronic, nonhealing wound, and because of the increased risk of incontinence in a patient with diarrhea from underlying colitis or small bowel disease. Examination under anesthesia often is necessary to exclude an underlying abscess or fistula and to assess the rectal mucosa in patients with severe anal pain.

Recurrent abscess(es) or complex anal fistulas should raise the possibility of Crohn disease. Treatment focuses on control of sepsis, delineation of complex anatomy, treatment of underlying mucosal disease, and sphincter preservation. Abscesses often can be drained locally, and mushroom catheters are useful for maintaining drainage. Endoanal ultrasound and pelvic MRI are useful for mapping complex fistulous tracts. Liberal use of setons can control many fistulas and avoid division of the sphincter. Many patients with anal Crohn disease function well with multiple setons left in place for years. Endoanal advancement flaps may be considered for definitive therapy if the rectal mucosa is uninvolved. In 10–15 percent of cases, intractable perianal sepsis requires proctectomy.

Medical treatment of underlying proctitis with salicylate and/or cortico-steroid enemas may be helpful; however, control of sepsis is the primary goal of therapy. Metronidazole also has been used with some success in this setting. Infliximab has shown some efficacy in healing chronic fistulas secondary to Crohn disease. However, it is of paramount importance to drain any and all abscesses before initiating immunosuppressive therapy such as corticosteroids or infliximab.

Indeterminate Colitis

Approximately 15 percent of patients with inflammatory bowel disease mani-fest clinical and pathologic characteristics of both ulcerative colitis and Crohn disease. The indications for surgery are the same as those for ulcerative colitis. In the setting of indeterminate colitis in a patient who prefers a sphincter-sparing operation, a total abdominal colectomy with end ileostomy may be the best initial procedure. Pathologic examination of the entire colon may then allow a more accurate diagnosis. Elective proctectomy with or without reconstruction can be undertaken once the final pathologic diagnosis is known.

DIVERTICULAR DISEASE

Diverticulosis

Diverticulosis refers to the presence of diverticula without inflammation. It is estimated that half of the population older than age 50 years has colonic diverticula. The sigmoid colon is the most common site of diverticulosis. The majority of colonic diverticula are false diverticula in which the mucosa and muscularis mucosa have herniated through the colonic wall. These diverticula occur between the teniae coli, at points where the main blood vessels penetrate the colonic wall (presumably creating an area of relative weakness in the colonic muscle). They are thought to be pulsion diverticula resulting from high intraluminal pressure. Although diverticulosis is common, most cases are asymptomatic and complications occur in the minority of people with this condition.

Inflammatory Complications (Diverticulitis)

Diverticulitis refers to inflammation and infection associated with a diverticu-lum and is estimated to occur in 10–25 percent of people with diverticulosis. Infection results from a perforation (macroscopic or microscopic) of a diver-ticulum, which leads to contamination, inflammation, and infection.

Uncomplicated diverticulitis is characterized by left lower quadrant pain and tenderness. CT findings include pericolic soft-tissue stranding, colonic wall thickening, and/or phlegmon. Some patients with uncomplicated divertic-ulitis will respond to outpatient therapy with broad-spectrum oral antibiotics and a low-residue diet. Patients with more severe pain, tenderness, fever, and leukocytosis should be treated in the hospital with parenteral antibiotics and bowel rest. Most patients improve within 48–72 h. Failure to improve may suggest abscess formation. CT can be extremely useful in this setting and many pericolic abscesses can be drained percutaneously. Deterioration in clinical condition and/or the development of peritonitis are indications for laparotomy.

Most patients with uncomplicated diverticulitis will recover without surgery and 50–70 percent will have no further episodes. However, the risk of com-plications increases with recurrent disease. For this reason, elective sigmoid colectomy often is recommended after the second episode of diverticulitis. Resection may be indicated after the first episode in young patients and in immunosuppressed patients, and often is recommended after the first episode of complicated diverticulitis. In the elective setting, a sigmoid colectomy with a primary anastomosis is the procedure of choice. The resection should always be extended to the rectum distally because the risk of recurrence is high if a segment of sigmoid colon is retained. The proximal extent of the resection should include all thickened or inflamed bowel; however, resection of all diverticula is unnecessary.

Complicated diverticulitis includes diverticulitis with abscess, obstruction, diffuse peritonitis (free perforation), or fistulas between the colon and adjacent structures. The Hinchey staging system often is used to describe the severity of complicated diverticulitis:

Stage I – colonic inflammation with a pericolic abscess

Stage II – colonic inflammation with a retroperitoneal or pelvic abscess

Stage III – purulent peritonitis

Stage IV – fecal peritonitis

Treatment depends on the patient's overall clinical condition and the degree of peritoneal contamination and infection. Small abscesses (< 2 cm diameter) may be treated with parenteral antibiotics. Larger abscesses are best treated with CT-guided percutaneous drainage. The majority of these patients will ultimately require resection, but percutaneous drainage may allow a one-stage, elective procedure. Urgent or emergent laparotomy may be required if an abscess is inaccessible to percutaneous drainage, if the patient's condition deteriorates or fails to improve, or if the patient presents with free intraabdominal air or peritonitis. In almost all cases, an attempt should be made to resect the affected segment of bowel. Patients with small, localized pericolic or pelvic abscesses (Hinchey stages I and II) may be candidates for a sigmoid colectomy with a primary anastomosis (a one-stage operation). In patients with larger abscesses, peritoneal soiling, or peritonitis, sigmoid colectomy with end colostomy and Hartmann pouch is the most commonly used procedure. Success also has been reported after sigmoid colectomy, primary anastomosis, ± on-table lavage, and proximal diversion (loop ileostomy). The presence of inflammation and phlegmon may increase the risk of ureteral damage during mobilization of the sigmoid colon, and preoperative placement of ureteral catheters can be invaluable. In extremely unstable patients, or in the presence of such severe inflammation that resection would harm adjacent organs, proximal diversion and local drainage have been employed. However, this approach is generally avoided because of high morbidity and mortality rates, along with the requirement for multiple operations.

Obstructive symptoms occur in approximately 67 percent of patients with acute diverticulitis, and complete obstruction occurs in 10 percent. Patients with incomplete obstruction often respond to fluid resuscitation, nasogastric suction, and gentle, low-volume water or Gastrografin enemas. Relief of obstruction allows full bowel preparation and elective resection. A high-volume oral bowel preparation is contraindicated in the presence of obstructive symptoms. Obstruction that does not rapidly respond to medical management mandates laparotomy and sigmoid colectomy.

Approximately 5 percent of patients with complicated diverticulitis develop fistulas between the colon and an adjacent organ. Colovesical fistulas are most common, followed by colovaginal and coloenteric fistulas. Two key points in the evaluation of fistulas are to define the anatomy of the fistula and exclude other diagnoses. Contrast enema and/or small bowel studies are useful in defining the course of the fistula. CT scan can identify associated abscesses or masses. The differential diagnosis includes malignancy, Crohn disease, and radiation-induced fistulas. Once the anatomy of the fistula has been defined and other diagnoses excluded, operative management should include resection of the affected segment of the colon (usually with a primary anastomosis) and simple repair of the secondarily involved organ. Suspicion of carcinoma may mandate a wider, en bloc resection.

Because colon carcinoma may have an identical clinical presentation to diverticulitis, all patients must be evaluated for malignancy after resolution of the acute episode. Sigmoidoscopy or colonoscopy is recommended 4–6 weeks after recovery. Inability to exclude malignancy is an indication for resection.

Hemorrhage

Bleeding from a diverticulum results from erosion of the peridiverticular arteriole and may result in massive hemorrhage. Most significant lower gastrointestinal hemorrhage occurs in older adult patients in whom both diverticulosis and angiodysplasia are common. Consequently, the exact bleeding source may be difficult to identify. Fortunately, in 80 percent of patients, bleeding stops spontaneously. Clinical management should focus on resuscitation and localization of the bleeding site as described for lower gastrointestinal hemorrhage. Colonoscopy may occasionally identify a bleeding diverticulum that may then be treated with epinephrine injection or cautery. Angiography may be diagnostic and therapeutic in this setting. In the rare instance in which diverticular hemorrhage persists or recurs, laparotomy and segmental colectomy may be required.

ADENOCARCINOMA AND POLYPS

Epidemiology (Risk Factors)

Colorectal carcinoma is the most common malignancy of the gastrointestinal tract. Risk factors include the following:

1. Aging – Aging is the dominant risk factor for colorectal cancer, with incidence rising steadily after age 50. However, individuals of any age can develop colorectal cancer, so symptoms such as a significant change in bowel habits, rectal bleeding, melena, unexplained anemia, or weight loss require a thorough evaluation.
2. Hereditary Risk Factors – Approximately 80 percent of colorectal cancers occur sporadically, whereas 20 percent arise in patients with a known family history of colorectal cancer. Assays currently exist to detect the most common genetic abnormalities.
3. Environmental and Dietary Factors – A diet high in saturated or polyunsaturated fats increases risk of colorectal cancer, whereas a diet high in oleic acid (olive oil, coconut oil, fish oil) does not increase risk. In contrast, a diet high in vegetable fiber appears to be protective. A correlation between alcohol intake and incidence of colorectal carcinoma also has been suggested. Ingestion of calcium; selenium; vitamins A, C, and E; carotenoids; and plant phenols may decrease the risk of developing colorectal cancer. Obesity and sedentary lifestyle dramatically increase cancer-related mortality in a number of malignancies, including colorectal carcinoma.

4. Inflammatory Bowel Disease – Patients with long-standing colitis from inflammatory bowel disease are at increased risk for the development of colorectal cancer.

5. Other Risk Factors – Cigarette smoking is associated with an increased risk of colonic adenomas, especially after more than 35 years of use. Patients with ureterosigmoidostomy are at increased risk for both adenoma and carcinoma formation. Acromegaly, which is associated with increased levels of circulating human growth hormone and insulin-like growth factor-1, increases risk as well. Pelvic irradiation may increase the risk of developing rectal carcinoma.

Pathogenesis of Colorectal Cancer

Genetic Pathways

Two major pathways for tumor initiation and progression have been described: the loss of heterozygosity (LOH) pathway and the replication error (RER) pathway. The LOH pathway is characterized by chromosomal deletions and tumor aneuploidy. Eighty percent of colorectal carcinomas appear to arise from mutations in the LOH pathway. The remaining 20 percent of colorectal carcinomas are thought to arise from mutations in the RER pathway, which is characterized by errors in mismatch repair during DNA replication.

LOH Pathway

1. APC gene defects – Defects in the APC gene were first described in patients with Familial Adenomatous Polyposis (FAP). By investigating these families, characteristic mutations in the APC gene were identified. They are now known to be present in 80 percent of sporadic colorectal cancers as well. The APC gene is a tumor-suppressor gene. Mutations in both alleles are necessary to initiate polyp formation. In FAP, the site of mutation correlates with the clinical severity of the disease. APC inactivation alone does not result in a carcinoma. Instead, this mutation sets the stage for the accumulation of genetic damage that results in malignancy via mutations accumulated in the loss of heterozygosity (LOH) pathway.

2. K-ras: K-ras is classified as a proto-oncogene because mutation of only one allele will perturb the cell cycle. The K-ras gene product is a G-protein involved in intracellular signal transduction. When active, K-ras binds guanosine triphosphate (GTP); hydrolysis of GTP to guanosine diphosphate (GDP) then inactivates the G-protein. Mutation of K-ras results in an inability to hydrolyze GTP, thus leaving the G-protein permanently in the active form. It is thought that this then leads to uncontrolled cell division.

3. DCC – DCC is a tumor-suppressor gene and loss of both alleles is required for malignant degeneration. The role of the DCC gene product is poorly understood, but it might be involved in cellular differentiation. DCC mutations are present in more than 70 percent of colorectal carcinomas and may negatively impact prognosis.

4. p53 – The p53 protein, a tumor suppressor, appears to be crucial for initiating apoptosis in cells with irreparable genetic damage and has been characterized in a large number of malignancies. Mutations in p53 are present in 75 percent of colorectal cancers.

The Replication Error Repair (RER) Pathway

A number of genes have been identified that appear to be crucial for recognizing and repairing DNA replication errors. These mismatch repair genes include hMSH2, hMLH1, hPMS1, hPMS2, and hMSH6/GTBP. A mutation in one of these genes predisposes a cell to mutations and accumulation of these errors, then leads to genomic instability and ultimately to carcinogenesis.

The RER pathway is associated with microsatellite instability. Microsatellites are regions of the genome in which short base-pair segments are repeated several times. These areas are particularly prone to replication error. Consequently, a mutation in a mismatch repair gene produces variable lengths of these repetitive sequences, a finding that has been described as microsatellite instability (MSI).

Tumors with MSI are more likely to be right sided, possess diploid DNA, and are associated with a better prognosis than tumors that arise from the LOH pathway that are microsatellite stable (MSS).

Polyps

It is now well accepted that the majority of colorectal carcinomas evolve from adenomatous polyps; this sequence of events is the adenoma–carcinoma sequence. Colorectal polyps may be classified as neoplastic (tubular adenoma, villous adenoma, tubulovillous adenomas), hamartomatous (juvenile, Peutz-Jeghers, Cronkite-Canada), inflammatory (pseudopolyp, benign lymphoid polyp), or hyperplastic.

Neoplastic Polyps

Adenomatous polyps are common, occurring in up to 25 percent of the population older than 50 years of age in the United States. By definition, these lesions are dysplastic. The risk of malignant degeneration is related to both the size and type of polyp. Tubular adenomas are associated with malignancy in only 5 percent of cases, whereas villous adenomas may harbor cancer in up to 40 percent. Tubulovillous adenomas are at intermediate risk (22 percent). Invasive carcinomas are rare in polyps smaller than 1 cm; the incidence increases with size. The risk of carcinoma in a polyp larger than 2 cm is 35–50 percent. Although most neoplastic polyps do not evolve to cancer, most colorectal cancers originate as a polyp.

Polyps may be pedunculated or sessile. Most pedunculated polyps are amenable to colonoscopic snare excision. Removal of sessile polyps often is more challenging. Special colonoscopic techniques, including saline lift and piecemeal snare excision, facilitate successful removal of many sessile polyps. For rectal sessile polyps, transanal operative excision is preferred because it produces an intact, single pathology specimen that can be used to determine the need for further therapy. Interpretation of the precise depth of invasion of a cancer arising in a sessile polyp after piecemeal excision often is impossible. The site of sessile polypectomies should be marked by injection of methylene blue or India ink to guide follow-up colonoscopy sessions to ensure that the polyp has been completely removed, and to facilitate identification of the involved bowel segment should operative resection be necessary. Colectomy is reserved for cases in which colonoscopic removal is impossible, such as large, flat lesions or if a focus of invasive cancer is confirmed in the specimen. These patients may be ideal candidates for laparoscopic colectomy.

Complications of polypectomy include perforation and bleeding. A small perforation (microperforation) in a fully prepared, stable patient may be managed with bowel rest, broad-spectrum antibiotics, and close observation. Signs of sepsis, peritonitis, or deterioration in clinical condition are indications for laparotomy. Bleeding may occur immediately after polypectomy or may be delayed. The bleeding will usually stop spontaneously, but colonoscopy may be required to re-snare a bleeding stalk, cauterize the lesion, or inject epinephrine around the bleeding vessel. Occasionally angiography and infusion of vasopressin may be necessary. Rarely, colectomy is required.

Hamartomatous Polyps (Juvenile Polyps)

Hamartomatous polyps (juvenile polyps) are not usually premalignant. These lesions are the characteristic polyps of childhood but may occur at any age. Bleeding is a common symptom and intussusception and/or obstruction may occur. Because the gross appearance of these polyps is identical to adenomatous polyps, these lesions also should be treated by polypectomy.

Familial juvenile polyposis is an autosomal dominant disorder in which patients develop hundreds of polyps in the colon and rectum. Unlike solitary juvenile polyps, these lesions may degenerate into adenomas, and eventually carcinoma. Annual screening should begin between the ages of 10 and 12 years. Treatment is surgical and depends in part on the degree of rectal involvement.

Peutz-Jeghers syndrome is characterized by polyposis of the small intestine, and to a lesser extent, polyposis of the colon and rectum. Characteristic melanin spots often are noted on the buccal mucosa and lips of these patients. The polyps of Peutz-Jeghers syndrome are generally considered to be hamartomas and are not thought to be at significant risk for malignant degeneration. However, carcinoma may occasionally develop. Because the entire length of the gastrointestinal tract may be affected, surgery is reserved for symptoms such as obstruction or bleeding or for patients in whom polyps develop adenomatous features. Screening consists of a baseline colonoscopy and upper endoscopy at age 20 years, followed by annual flexible sigmoidoscopy thereafter.

Cronkite-Canada syndrome is a disorder in which patients develop gastrointestinal polyposis in association with alopecia, cutaneous pigmentation, and atrophy of the fingernails and toenails. Diarrhea is a prominent symptom, and vomiting, malabsorption, and protein-losing enteropathy may occur. Most patients die of this disease despite maximal medical therapy, and surgery is reserved for complications of polyposis such as obstruction.

Cowden syndrome is an autosomal dominant disorder with hamartomas of all three embryonal cell layers. Facial trichilemmomas, breast cancer, thyroid disease, and gastrointestinal polyps are typical of the syndrome. Patients should be screened for cancers. Treatment is otherwise based on symptoms.

Inflammatory Polyps (Pseudopolyps)

Inflammatory polyps occur most commonly in the context of inflammatory bowel disease, but also may occur after amebic colitis, ischemic colitis, and schistosomal colitis. These lesions are not premalignant, but they cannot be distinguished from adenomatous polyps based on gross appearance and therefore should be removed.

Hyperplastic Polyps

Hyperplastic polyps are extremely common in the colon. These polyps are usually small (< 5 mm) and show histologic characteristics of hyperplasia without any dysplasia. They are not considered premalignant, but cannot be distinguished from adenomatous polyps colonoscopically and are therefore often removed. In contrast, large hyperplastic polyps (> 2 cm) may have a slight risk of malignant degeneration. Moreover, large polyps may harbor foci of adenomatous tissue and dysplasia. Hyperplastic polyposis is a rare disorder in which multiple large hyperplastic polyps occur in young adults.

Inherited Colorectal Carcinoma

Familial Adenomatous Polyposis

This rare autosomal dominant condition accounts for only approximately 1 percent of all colorectal adenocarcinomas. The genetic abnormality in FAP is a mutation in the APC gene, located on chromosome 5q. Of patients with FAP, APC mutation testing is positive in 75 percent of cases. Although most patients with FAP will have a known family history of the disease, up to 25 percent present without other affected family members. Clinically, patients develop hundreds to thousands of adenomatous polyps shortly after puberty. The lifetime risk of colorectal cancer in FAP patients approaches 100 percent by age 50 years.

Flexible sigmoidoscopy of first-degree relatives of FAP patients beginning at age 10–15 years has been the traditional mainstay of screening. Today, following genetic counseling, APC gene testing may be used to screen family members, providing an APC mutation has been identified in a family member. If APC testing is positive in a relative of a patient with a known APC mutation, annual flexible sigmoidoscopy beginning at age 10–15 years is done until polyps are identified. If APC testing is negative, the relative can be screened starting at age 50 years per average-risk guidelines.

FAP patients also are at risk for the development of adenomas anywhere in the gastrointestinal tract, particularly in the duodenum. Periampullary carcinoma is a particular concern. Upper endoscopy is therefore recommended for surveillance every 1–3 years beginning at age 25–30 years.

Once the diagnosis of FAP has been made and polyps are developing, treatment is surgical. Four factors affect the choice of operation: age of the patient; presence and severity of symptoms; extent of rectal polyposis; and presence and location of cancer or desmoid tumors. Three operative procedures can be considered: total proctocolectomy with either an end (Brooke) ileostomy or continent (Kock) ileostomy; total abdominal colectomy with ileorectal anastomosis; and restorative proctocolectomy with ileal pouch–anal anastomosis with or without a temporary ileostomy. Most patients elect to have an ileal pouch–anal anastomosis in the absence of a distal rectal cancer, a mesenteric desmoid tumor that prevents the ileum from reaching the anus or poor sphincter function. Total abdominal colectomy with an ileorectal anastomosis is also an option in these patients, but requires vigilant surveillance of the retained rectum for development of rectal cancer. There is increasing data suggesting that the administration of COX-2 inhibitors (celecoxib, sulindac) may slow or prevent the development of polyps.

FAP may be associated with extraintestinal manifestations such as congenital hypertrophy of the retinal pigmented epithelium, desmoid tumors, epidermoid cysts, mandibular osteomas (Gardner syndrome), and central nervous system tumors (Turcot syndrome).

Attenuated FAP

Patients with attenuated FAP present later in life with fewer polyps (usually 10 to 100) dominantly located in the right colon. Colorectal carcinoma develops in more than 50 percent of these patients, but occurs later (average age 50 years). Patients also are at risk for duodenal polyposis. APC mutation testing is positive in approximately 60 percent of patients. If the family mutation is unknown, screening colonoscopy is recommended beginning at age 13–15 years, then every 4 years to age 28 years, and then every 3 years. These patients often are candidates for a total abdominal colectomy with ileorectal anastomosis because the limited polyposis in the rectum can usually be treated by colonoscopic snare excision. Prophylaxis with COX-2 inhibitors also may be appropriate.

Hereditary Nonpolyposis Colon Cancer (Lynch Syndrome)

Hereditary nonpolyposis colon cancer (HNPCC or Lynch syndrome) is more common than FAP, but is still extremely rare (1–3 percent). The genetic defects associated with HNPCC arise from errors in mismatch repair genes. HNPCC is inherited in an autosomal dominant pattern and is characterized by the development of colorectal carcinoma at an early age (average age: 40–45 years). Approximately 70 percent of affected individuals will develop colorectal cancer. Cancers appear in the proximal colon more often than in sporadic colorectal cancer and have a better prognosis regardless of stage. The risk of synchronous or metachronous colorectal carcinoma is 40 percent. HNPCC also may be associated with extracolonic malignancies, including endometrial, ovarian, pancreas, stomach, small bowel, biliary, and urinary tract carcinomas. The diagnosis of HNPCC is made based on family history. The Amsterdam criteria for clinical diagnosis of HNPCC are three affected relatives with histologically verified adenocarcinoma of the large bowel (one must be a first-degree relative of one of the others) in two successive generations of a family with one patient diagnosed before age 50 years. The presence of other HNPCC-related carcinomas should raise the suspicion of this syndrome.

Screening colonoscopy is recommended annually for at-risk patients beginning at either age 20–25 years or 10 years younger than the youngest age at diagnosis in the family, whichever comes first. Because of the high risk of endometrial carcinoma, transvaginal ultrasound or endometrial aspiration biopsy also is recommended annually after age 25–35 years. Because there is a 40 percent risk of developing a second colon cancer, total colectomy with ileorectal anastomosis is recommended once adenomas or a colon carcinoma is diagnosed, or if prophylactic colectomy is decided on. Annual proctoscopy is necessary because the risk of developing rectal cancer remains high. Similarly, prophylactic hysterectomy and bilateral salpingo-oophorectomy should be considered in women who have completed childbearing.

Familial Colorectal Cancer

Nonsyndromic familial colorectal cancer accounts for 10–15 percent of patients with colorectal cancer. The lifetime risk of developing colorectal cancer increases with a family history of the disease. The lifetime risk of colorectal cancer in a patient with no family history of this disease (average-risk population) is approximately 6 percent, but rises to 12 percent if one first-degree relative is affected and to 35 percent if two first-degree relatives are affected. Age of onset also impacts risk and a diagnosis before the age of 50 years is associated with a higher incidence in family members. Screening colonoscopy is recommended every 5 years beginning at age 40 years or beginning 10 years before the age of the earliest diagnosed patient in the pedigree.

Prevention: Screening and Surveillance

Because the majority of colorectal cancers are thought to arise from adenomatous polyps, preventive measures focus on identification and removal of these premalignant lesions. Additionally, many cancers are asymptomatic and screening may detect these tumors at an early and curable stage (Table 28-1). Screening guidelines are meant for asymptomatic patients. Any patient with a gastrointestinal complaint (bleeding, change in bowel habits, pain, etc) requires a complete evaluation, usually by colonoscopy.

1. Fecal Occult Blood Testing (FOBT) – FOBT is used as a screening test for colonic neoplasms in asymptomatic, average-risk individuals. The efficacy of this test is based on serial testing because the majority of colorectal malignancies will bleed intermittently. FOBT has been a nonspecific test for peroxidase contained in hemoglobin; consequently, occult bleeding from any gastrointestinal source will produce a positive result. Nonetheless, the direct evidence that FOBT screening is efficacious and decreases both the incidence and mortality of colorectal cancer is so strong that national guidelines recommend annual FOBT screening for asymptomatic, average-risk Americans older than 50 years of age as one of several accepted strategies. Newer immunohistochemical methods for detecting human globin may prove to be more sensitive and specific. A positive FOBT test should be followed by colonoscopy.
2. Flexible Sigmoidoscopy – Screening by flexible sigmoidoscopy every 5 years may lead to a 60–70 percent reduction in mortality from colorectal cancer, chiefly by identifying high-risk individuals with adenomas. Patients found to have a polyp, cancer, or other lesion on flexible sigmoidoscopy will require colonoscopy. The combination of FOBT plus sigmoidoscopy is more sensitive for detection of polyps and/or cancer than either test alone, therefore the combination of the two tests has been suggested as a reasonable screening strategy. American Cancer Society recommendations for average-risk Americans include the combination of FOBT annually and flexible sigmoidoscopy every 5 years.
3. Colonoscopy – Colonoscopy is currently the most accurate and most complete method for examining the large bowel. This procedure is highly sensitive for detecting even small polyps (<1 cm) and allows biopsy, polypectomy, control of hemorrhage, and dilation of strictures. However, colonoscopy does require mechanical bowel preparation and the discomfort associated with the procedure requires conscious sedation in most patients. Additionally, the risk of complications, although low, is greater than with other screening modalities.
4. Air-Contrast Barium Enema (ACBE) – ACBE also is highly sensitive for detecting polyps greater than 1 cm in diameter (90 percent sensitivity). Accuracy is greatest in the proximal colon but may be compromised in the sigmoid colon if there is significant diverticulosis. For this reason, barium

TABLE 28-1 Advantages and Disadvantages of Screening Modalities for Asymptomatic Individuals

	Advantages	Disadvantages
Fecal occult blood testing	Ease of use and noninvasive	May not detect most polyps
	Low cost	Low specificity
	Good sensitivity with repeat testing	Colonoscopy required for positive result
		Poor compliance with serial testing
Sigmoidoscopy	Examines colon most at risk	Invasive
	Very sensitive for polyp detection in left colon	Uncomfortable
		Slight risk of perforation or bleeding
	Does not require full bowel preparation (enemas only)	May miss proximal lesions
		Colonoscopy required if polyp identified
Colonoscopy	Examines entire colon	Most invasive
	Highly sensitive and specific	Uncomfortable and requires sedation
	Therapeutic	Requires bowel preparation
		Risk of perforation or bleeding
		Costly
Double-contrast barium enema	Examines entire colon	Requires bowel preparation
	Good sensitivity for polyps >1 cm	Less sensitivity for polyps <1 cm
		May miss lesions in the sigmoid colon
		Colonoscopy required for positive result
CT Colonography (virtual colonoscopy)	Examines entire colon	Requires bowel preparation
	Noninvasive	Insensitive for small polyps
	Sensitivity may be as good as colonoscopy	Minimal experience and data
		Colonoscopy required for positive result
		Costly

CT = Computed tomography

enema is often combined with flexible sigmoidoscopy for screening purposes. The major disadvantages of barium enema are the need for mechanical bowel preparation and the requirement for colonoscopy if a lesion is discovered.

5. CT Colonography (Virtual Colonoscopy) – CT colonography makes use of helical CT technology and three-dimensional reconstruction to image the intraluminal colon. Patients require a mechanical bowel preparation. The colon is then insufflated with air, a spiral CT is performed, and both two-dimensional and three-dimensional images are generated. In the hands

of a qualified radiologist, sensitivity appears to be as good as colonoscopy for colorectal cancers and polyps greater than 1 cm in size. Colonoscopy is required if a lesion is identified.

Guidelines for Screening

Current American Cancer Society guidelines advocate screening for the average-risk population (asymptomatic, no family history of colorectal carcinoma, no personal history of polyps or colorectal carcinoma, no familial syndrome) beginning at age 50 years. Recommended procedures include yearly FOBT, flexible sigmoidoscopy every 5 years, FOBT and flexible sigmoidoscopy in combination, air-contrast barium enema every 5 years, or colonoscopy every 10 years. Patients with other risk factors should be screened earlier and more frequently (Table 28-2).

Routes of Spread and Natural History

Carcinoma of the colon and rectum arises in the mucosa. The tumor subsequently invades the bowel wall and eventually adjacent tissues and other viscera. Tumors may become bulky and circumferential, leading to colon obstruction. Local extension (especially in the rectum) may occasionally cause obstruction of other organs such as the ureter.

Regional lymph node involvement is the most common form of spread of colorectal carcinoma and usually precedes distant metastasis or the development of carcinomatosis. The likelihood of nodal metastasis increases with tumor size, poorly differentiated histology, lymphovascular invasion, and depth of invasion. The T stage (depth of invasion) is the single most significant predictor of lymph node spread. Carcinoma in situ (Tis) in which there is no penetration of the muscularis mucosa (basement membrane) also has been called high-grade dysplasia and should carry no risk of lymph node metastasis. Small lesions confined to the bowel wall (T1 and T2) are associated with lymph node metastasis in 5–20 percent of cases, whereas larger tumors that invade through the bowel wall or into adjacent organs (T3 and T4) are likely to have lymph node metastasis in more than 50 percent of cases. The number of lymph nodes with metastases correlates with the presence of distant disease and inversely with survival. Four or more involved lymph nodes predict a poor prognosis. Lymphatic spread usually follows the major venous outflow from the involved segment of the colon or rectum.

The most common site of distant metastasis from colorectal cancer is the liver. These metastases arise from hematogenous spread via the portal venous system. The risk of hepatic metastasis increases with tumor size and grade. However, even small tumors may produce distant metastasis. The lung is also a site of hematogenous spread for colorectal carcinoma. Pulmonary metastases rarely occur in isolation. Carcinomatosis (diffuse peritoneal metastases) occurs by peritoneal seeding and has a dismal prognosis.

Staging and Preoperative Evaluation

Clinical Presentation

Symptoms of colon and rectal cancers are nonspecific and generally develop when the cancer is locally advanced. The classic first symptoms are a change in bowel habits and rectal bleeding. Abdominal pain, bloating, and other signs of obstruction typically occur with larger tumors and suggest more advanced disease. Left-sided tumors are more likely to cause obstruction than are right-sided

TABLE 28-2 Screening Guidelines for Colorectal Cancer

Population	Initial age	Recommended screening test
Average risk	50 years	Annual FOBT *or* Flexible sigmoidoscopy every 5 years *or* Annual FOBT and flexible sigmoidoscopy every 5 years *or* Air contrast barium enema every 5 years *or* Colonoscopy every 10 years
Adenomatous polyps	50 years	Colonoscopy at first detection; then colonoscopy in 3 years If no further polyps, colonoscopy every 5 years If polyps, colonoscopy every 3 years Annual colonoscopy for > 5 adenomas
Colorectal cancer	At diagnosis	Pretreatment colonoscopy; then at 12 months after curative resection; then colonoscopy after 3 years; then colonoscopy every 5 years, if no new lesions
Ulcerative colitis Crohn colitis	At diagnosis; then after 8 years for pancolitis, after 15 years for left-sided colitis	Colonoscopy with multiple biopsies every 1–2 years
FAP	10–12 years	Annual flexible sigmoidoscopy Upper endoscopy every 1–3 years after polyps appear
Attenuated FAP	20 years	Annual flexible sigmoidoscopy Upper endoscopy every 1–3 years after polyps appear
HNPCC	20–25 years	Colonoscopy every 1–2 years Endometrial aspiration biopsy every 1–2 years
Familial colorectal cancer 1st degree relative	40 years or 10 years before the age of the youngest affected relative	Colonoscopy every 5 years Increase frequency if multiple family members are affected, especially before 50 years

FAP = familial adenomatous polyposis
FOBT = fecal occult blood test
HNPCC = hereditary nonpolyposis colorectal cancer

tumors. Rectal tumors may cause bleeding, tenesmus, and pain. Alternatively, patients may be asymptomatic and/or present with unexplained anemia or weight loss.

Staging

Colorectal cancer staging is based on tumor depth and the presence or absence of nodal or distant metastases. Older staging systems, such as the Dukes Classification and its Astler-Coller modification, have been largely replaced by

TABLE 28-3 TNM Staging of Colorectal Carcinoma

Tumor stage (T)	Definition
Tx	Cannot be assessed
T0	No evidence of cancer
Tis	Carcinoma in situ
T1	Tumor invades submucosa
T2	Tumor invades muscularis propria
T3	Tumor invades through muscularis propria into subserosa or into nonperitonealized pericolic or perirectal tissues
T4	Tumor directly invades other organs or tissues or perforates the visceral peritoneum of specimen
Nodal stage (N)	
NX	Regional lymph nodes cannot be assessed
N0	No lymph node metastasis
N1	Metastasis to one to three pericolic or perirectal lymph nodes
N2	Metastasis to four or more pericolic or perirectal lymph nodes
N3	Metastasis to any lymph node along a major named vascular trunk
Distant metastasis (M)	
MX	Presence of distant metastasis cannot be assessed
M0	No distant metastasis
M1	Distant metastasis present

the TNM staging system (Table 28-3). In colon cancer, differentiating stages I, II, and III depends on examination of the resected specimen. In rectal cancer, endorectal ultrasound may predict the stage (ultrasound stage, uTxNx) preoperatively, but the final determination depends on pathology examination of the resected tumor and adjacent lymph nodes (pathologic stage, pTxNx). Disease stage correlates with 5-year survival (Table 28-4). Although nodal involvement is the single most important prognostic factor in colorectal carcinoma, tumor characteristics, such as degree of differentiation, mucinous or signet-ring cell histology, vascular invasion, and DNA aneuploidy, also affect prognosis.

Preoperative Evaluation

Once a colon or rectal carcinoma has been diagnosed, a staging evaluation should be undertaken. The colon must be evaluated for synchronous tumors, usually by colonoscopy. Synchronous disease will be present in up to 5 percent

TABLE 28-4 TNM Staging of Colorectal Carcinoma and 5-Year Survival

Stage	TNM	5-Year Survival
I	T1–2, N0, M0	70–95%
II	T3–4, N0, M0	54–65%
III	Tany, N1-3, M0	39–60%
IV	Tany, Nany, M1	0–16%

of patients. For rectal cancers, digital rectal examination and rigid proctoscopy with biopsy should be done to assess tumor size, location, morphology, histology, and fixation. Endorectal ultrasound can be invaluable in staging rectal cancer and is used to classify the ultrasound T and N stage of rectal cancers. A chest radiograph and abdominal/pelvic CT scan should be obtained to evaluate for distant metastases. CT scan of the chest is only necessary if the chest radiograph is abnormal. Pelvic CT scan, and sometimes MRI, can be invaluable in large rectal tumors and in recurrent disease to determine the extent of local invasion. In patients with obstructive symptoms, a water-soluble contrast study (Gastrografin enema) may be useful for delineating the degree of obstruction. It is important to avoid mechanical bowel preparation (for either colonoscopy or surgery) in a patient who appears to be obstructed. PET scan may be useful in evaluating lesions seen on CT scan, and in patients in whom a risky or highly morbid operation is planned (pelvic exenteration, sacrectomy). Preoperative CEA often is obtained, and may be useful for postoperative follow up.

THERAPY FOR COLONIC CARCINOMA

Principles of Resection

The objective in treatment of carcinoma of the colon is to remove the primary tumor along with its lymphovascular supply. Because the lymphatics of the colon accompany the main arterial supply, the length of bowel resected depends on which vessels are supplying the segment involved with the cancer. Any adjacent organ or tissue, such as the omentum that has been invaded, should be resected en bloc with the tumor. If all of the tumor cannot be removed, a palliative procedure should be considered.

The presence of synchronous cancers or adenomas or a strong family history of colorectal neoplasms suggests that the entire colon is at risk for carcinoma (a field defect) and a subtotal or total colectomy should be considered. Metachronous tumors (a second primary colon cancer) identified during follow-up studies should be treated similarly. If unexpected metastatic disease is encountered at the time of a laparotomy, the primary tumor should be resected, if technically feasible and safe. In the rare instance in which the primary tumor is not resectable, a palliative procedure can be performed and usually involves a proximal stoma or bypass. Hemorrhage in an unresectable tumor can sometimes be controlled with angiographic embolization.

Stage-Specific Therapy

Stage 0 (Tis, N0, M0). Polyps containing carcinoma in situ (high-grade dysplasia) carry no risk of lymph node metastasis. However, the presence of high-grade dysplasia increases the risk of finding an invasive carcinoma within the polyp. For this reason, these polyps should be excised completely and pathologic margins should be free of dysplasia.

Stage I: The malignant polyp (T1, N0, M0). Treatment of a malignant polyp is based on the risk of local recurrence and the risk of lymph node metastasis. The risk of lymph node metastases depends primarily on the depth of invasion. Invasive carcinoma in the head of a pedunculated polyp with no stalk involvement carries a low risk of metastasis (< 1 percent) and may be completely resected endoscopically. However, lymphovascular invasion, poorly differentiated histology, or tumor within 1 mm of the resection margin greatly increases the risk of local recurrence and metastatic spread. Segmental colectomy is then indicated. Invasive carcinoma arising in a sessile polyp extends into the submucosa and is usually best treated with segmental colectomy.

Stages I and II: Localized colon carcinoma (T1–3, N0, M0). The majority of patients with stages I and II colon cancer will be cured with surgical resection. However, up to 46 percent of patients with completely resected stage II disease will ultimately die from colon cancer. For this reason, adjuvant chemotherapy has been suggested for selected patients with stage II disease (young patients, tumors with "high-risk" histologic findings).

Stage III: Lymph Node Metastasis (T any, N1, M0). Patients with lymph node involvement are at significant risk for both local and distant recurrence, and adjuvant chemotherapy has been recommended routinely in these patients. 5-Fluorouracil–based regimens (with levamisole or leucovorin) reduce recurrences and improve survival in this patient population. Newer chemotherapeutic agents such as capecitabine, irinotecan, oxaliplatin, angiogenesis inhibitors, and immunotherapy also show promise.

Stage IV: Distant metastasis (T any, N any, M1). Survival is extremely limited in stage IV colon carcinoma. Of patients with systemic disease, approximately 15 percent will have metastases limited to the liver. Of these, 20 percent are potentially resectable for cure. Survival is improved in these patients (20–40 percent 5-year survival) when compared to patients who do not undergo resection. Hepatic resection of synchronous metastases from colorectal carcinoma may be performed as a combined procedure or in two stages. All patients require adjuvant chemotherapy.

The remainder of patients with stage IV disease cannot be cured surgically and therefore the focus of treatment should be palliation.

Therapy for Rectal Carcinoma

Principles of Resection

The biology of rectal adenocarcinoma is presumed to be identical to the biology of colonic adenocarcinoma, and the operative principles of complete resection of the primary tumor, its lymphatic bed, and any other involved organ apply to surgical resection of rectal carcinoma. However, the anatomy of the pelvis and proximity of other structures (ureters, bladder, prostate, vagina, iliac vessels, and sacrum) make resection more challenging and often require a different approach than for colonic adenocarcinoma. Moreover, it is more difficult to achieve negative radial margins in rectal cancers that extend through the bowel wall because of the anatomic limitations of the pelvis. Therefore, local recurrence is higher than with similar stage colon cancers. However, unlike the intraperitoneal colon, the relative paucity of small bowel and other radiation-sensitive structures in the pelvis makes it easier to treat rectal tumors with radiation. Therapeutic decisions, therefore, are based on the location and depth of the tumor and its relationship to other structures in the pelvis.

Local Therapy

The distal 10 cm of the rectum are accessible transanally. For this reason, several local approaches have been proposed for treating rectal neoplasms. Transanal excision (full thickness or mucosal) is an excellent approach for noncircumferential, benign, villous adenomas of the rectum. Although this technique can be used for selected T1, and possibly some T2, carcinomas, local excision does not allow pathologic examination of the lymph nodes and might therefore understage patients. Local recurrence rates are high without the addition of adjuvant chemoradiation therapy. Transanal endoscopic microsurgery (TEM) makes use of a specially designed proctoscope, magnifying system, and instruments similar to those used in laparoscopy to allow local excision of lesions higher in the rectum (up to 15 cm). Local excision of any rectal neoplasm should be considered an excisional biopsy because final pathologic examination of the specimen may reveal a more deeply invasive carcinoma than suggested by preoperative staging. More radical therapy may be indicated.

Ablative techniques, such as electrocautery or endocavitary radiation, also have been used. The disadvantage of these techniques is that no pathologic specimen is retrieved to confirm the tumor stage. Fulguration is generally reserved for extremely high-risk patients with a limited life span who cannot tolerate more radical surgery.

Radical Resection

Radical resection is preferred to local therapy for most rectal carcinomas. Radical resection involves removal of the involved segment of the rectum along with its lymphovascular supply. A 2-cm, distal mural margin is sought for curative resections.

Total mesorectal excision (TME) is a technique that uses sharp dissection along anatomic planes to ensure complete resection of the rectal mesentery during low and extended low anterior resections. For upper rectal or rectosigmoid resections, a partial mesorectal excision of at least 5 cm distal to the tumor appears adequate. Total mesorectal excision both decreases local recurrence rates and improves long-term survival rates. Moreover, this technique is associated with less blood loss and less risk to the pelvic nerves and presacral plexus than is blunt dissection. The principles of total mesorectal excision should be applied to all radical resections for rectal cancer.

Extensive involvement of other pelvic organs (often in the presence of recurrent cancer) may require a pelvic exenteration. The rectal and perineal portions of this operation are similar to an abdominoperineal resection but en bloc resection of the ureters, bladder, and prostate or uterus and vagina also are performed. A permanent colostomy and an ileal conduit to drain the urinary tract may be necessary. The sacrum also may be resected if necessary (sacrectomy) up to the level of the S2–S3 junction.

Pretreatment staging of rectal carcinoma often relies on endorectal ultrasound to determine the T and N status of a rectal cancer. Ultrasound evaluation can guide choice of therapy in most patients.

Stage 0 (Tis, N0, M0). Villous adenomas harboring carcinoma in situ (high-grade dysplasia) are ideally treated with local excision. A 1-cm margin should be obtained. Rarely, radical resection will be necessary if transanal excision is not technically possible (large circumferential lesions).

Stage I: Localized rectal carcinoma (T1–2, N0, M0). Invasive carcinoma confined to the head of a pedunculated polyp carries a very low risk of metastasis (< 1 percent). Polypectomy with clear margins is appropriate therapy. Although local excision has been used for small, favorable sessile uT1N0 and uT2N0 rectal cancers, local recurrence rates may be as high as 20 and 40 percent, respectively. For this reason, radical resection is strongly recommended in all good-risk patients. Lesions with unfavorable histologic characteristics and those located in the distal third of the rectum, in particular, are prone to recurrence. In high-risk patients and in those patients who refuse radical surgery because of the risk of need for a permanent colostomy, local excision may be adequate, but strong consideration should be given to adjuvant chemoradiation to improve local control.

Stage II: Localized rectal carcinoma (T3–4, N0, M0). Larger rectal tumors are more likely to recur locally. There are two schools of thought, each differing in their approach to control local recurrences. Advocates of total mesorectal resection suggest that optimization of operative technique will obviate the need for any adjuvant chemoradiation to control local recurrence after resection. The opposing school suggests that stages II and III rectal cancers will benefit from chemoradiation. Both preoperative chemoradiation (neoadjuvant therapy) and postoperative chemoradiation (adjuvant therapy) have been recommended. Recent evidence favors neoadjuvant therapy.

Stage III: Lymph node metastasis (T any, N1, M0). Because of the risk of either local or systemic recurrence, adjuvant or neoadjuvant chemoradiation is routinely recommended for patients with rectal cancer and nodal metastases. Both preoperative chemoradiation (neoadjuvant therapy) and postoperative chemoradiation (adjuvant therapy) have been shown to decrease local recurrence and prolong survival in locally advanced rectal cancer.

Stage IV: Distant metastasis (T any, N any, M1). Like stage IV colon carcinoma, survival is limited in patients with distant metastasis from rectal carcinoma. Isolated hepatic metastases are rare, but when present may be resected for cure in selected patients. Most patients will require palliative procedures. Local therapy using cautery, endocavitary radiation, or laser ablation may be adequate to control bleeding or prevent obstruction. Intraluminal stents may be useful in the uppermost rectum, but often cause pain and tenesmus lower in the rectum. Occasionally, a proximal diverting colostomy will be required to alleviate obstruction. A mucus fistula should be created if possible to vent the distal colon.

Follow-Up and Surveillance

Patients who have been treated for one colorectal cancer are at risk for the development of recurrent disease (either locally or systemically) or metachronous disease (a second primary tumor). In theory, metachronous cancers should be preventable by using surveillance colonoscopy to detect and remove polyps before they progress to invasive cancer. For most patients, a colonoscopy should be performed within 12 months after the diagnosis of the original cancer (or sooner if the colon was not examined in its entirety prior to the original resection). If that study is normal, colonoscopy should be repeated every 3–5 years thereafter.

The optimal method of following patients for recurrent cancer remains controversial. The goal of close follow-up observation is to detect resectable recurrence and to improve survival. Re-resection of local recurrence and resection of distant metastasis to liver, lung, or other sites is often technically challenging and highly morbid, with only a limited chance of achieving long-term survival. Thus, only selected patients who would tolerate such an approach should be followed intensively. Because most recurrences occur within 2 years of the original diagnosis, surveillance focuses on this time period. CEA often is followed every 2–3 months for 2 years. CT scans are not routinely employed, but may be useful if CEA is elevated. More intensive surveillance is appropriate in high-risk patients such as those with possible HNPCC syndrome or T3 N+ cancers. Although intensive surveillance improves detection of resectable recurrences, it is important to note that a survival benefit has never been proven.

Treatment of Recurrent Colorectal Carcinoma

Between 20 and 40 percent of patients who have undergone curative intent surgery for colorectal carcinoma will eventually develop recurrent disease. Most recurrences occur within the first 2 years after the initial diagnosis, but preoperative chemoradiation therapy may delay recurrence. Although most of these patients will present with distant metastases, a small proportion will have isolated local recurrence and may be considered for salvage surgery. Recurrence after colon cancer resection usually occurs at the local site within the abdomen or in the liver or lungs. Resection of other involved organs may be necessary. Recurrence of rectal cancer can be considerably more difficult to manage because of the proximity of other pelvic structures. If the patient has not received chemotherapy and radiation, then adjuvant therapy should be administered prior to salvage surgery. Radical resection may require extensive resection of pelvic organs (pelvic exenteration with or without sacrectomy). Pelvic MRI is useful for identifying tumor extension that would prevent successful resection (extension of tumor into the pelvic sidewall, involvement of the iliac vessels or bilateral sacral nerves, and sacral invasion above the S2–S3 junction). Patients also should undergo a thorough preoperative evaluation to identify distant metastases (CT of chest, abdomen, and pelvis, and PET scan) before undergoing such an extensive procedure.

OTHER NEOPLASMS

Rare Colorectal Tumors

Carcinoid Tumors

Carcinoid tumors occur most commonly in the gastrointestinal tract and up to 25 percent of these tumors are found in the rectum. Most small rectal carcinoids are benign, and overall survival is greater than 80 percent. However, the risk of malignancy increases with size, and more than 60 percent of tumors greater than 2 cm in diameter are associated with distant metastases. Rectal carcinoids appear to be less likely to secrete vasoactive substances than carcinoids in other locations, and carcinoid syndrome is uncommon in the absence of hepatic metastases. Small carcinoids can be locally resected, either transanally or using transanal endoscopic microsurgery. Larger tumors or tumors with obvious invasion into the muscularis require more radical surgery. Carcinoid tumors in the proximal colon are less common and are more likely to be malignant. Size also correlates with risk of malignancy, and tumors less than 2 cm in diameter rarely metastasize. However, the majority of carcinoid tumors in the proximal colon present as bulky lesions and up to two-thirds will have metastatic spread at the time of diagnosis. These tumors should usually be treated with radical resection. Because carcinoid tumors are typically slow growing, patients with distant metastases may expect reasonably long survival. Symptoms of carcinoid syndrome often can be alleviated with somatostatin analogues (octreotide) and/or interferon-α. Tumor debulking can offer effective palliation in selected patients.

Carcinoid Carcinomas

Composite carcinoid carcinomas (adenocarcinoids) have histologic features of both carcinoid tumors and adenocarcinomas. The natural history of these tumors more closely parallels that of adenocarcinomas.

Lipomas

Lipomas occur most commonly in the submucosa of the colon and rectum. They are benign lesions, but rarely may cause bleeding, obstruction, or intussusception, especially when greater than 2 cm in diameter. Small asymptomatic lesions do not require resection. Larger lipomas should be resected by colonoscopic techniques or by a colotomy and enucleation or limited colectomy.

Lymphoma

Lymphoma involving the colon and rectum is rare, but accounts for about 10 percent of all gastrointestinal lymphomas. The cecum most often is involved. Symptoms include bleeding and obstruction, and these tumors may be clinically indistinguishable from adenocarcinomas. Bowel resection is the treatment of choice. Adjuvant therapy may be given based on the stage of disease.

Leiomyoma and Leiomyosarcoma

Leiomyomas are benign tumors of the smooth muscle of the bowel wall and occur most commonly in the upper gastrointestinal tract. Most patients are asymptomatic, but large lesions can cause bleeding or obstruction. Because it is difficult to differentiate a benign leiomyoma from a malignant leiomyosarcoma, these lesions should be resected. Recurrence is common after local resection, but most small leiomyomas can be adequately treated with limited resection. Lesions larger than 5 cm should be treated with radical resection because the risk of malignancy is high.

Leiomyosarcoma is rare in the gastrointestinal tract. When this malignancy occurs in the large intestine, the rectum is the most common site. Symptoms include bleeding and obstruction. A radical resection is indicated for these tumors.

Retrorectal Tumors

Tumors occurring in the retrorectal space are rare. The retrorectal space contains multiple embryologic remnants derived from a variety of tissues (neuroectoderm, notochord, and hindgut). Tumors that develop in this space often are heterogeneous.

Congenital lesions are most common (67 percent). The remainder are classified as neurogenic, osseous, inflammatory, or miscellaneous lesions. Malignancy is more common in the pediatric population than in adults, and solid lesions are more likely to be malignant than are cystic lesions. Inflammatory lesions may be solid or cystic (abscess) and usually represent extensions of infection either in the perirectal space or in the abdomen.

Patients may present with pain (lower back, pelvic, or lower extremity), gastrointestinal symptoms, or urinary tract symptoms. Most lesions are palpable on digital rectal examination. Although plain radiograph and CT scans often are used to evaluate these lesions, pelvic MRI is the most sensitive and specific imaging study. Myelogram occasionally is necessary if there is central nervous system involvement. Biopsy is not indicated, especially if the lesion appears to be resectable, because of the risk of infection and/or tumor seeding. Treatment almost always is surgical resection. The approach depends in part on the nature of the lesion and its location. High lesions may be approached via a transabdominal route, whereas low lesions may be resected transsacrally. Intermediate lesions may require a combined abdominal and sacral operation.

Anal Canal and Perianal Tumors

Cancers of the anal canal are uncommon and account for approximately 2 percent of all colorectal malignancies. Neoplasms of the anal canal can be divided into those affecting the anal margin (distal to the dentate line) and those affecting the anal canal (proximal to the dentate line). In many cases, therapy depends on whether the tumor is located in the anal canal or at the anal margin.

Anal Intraepithelial Neoplasia (Bowen Disease)

Bowen disease refers to squamous cell carcinoma in situ of the anus. Pathologically, carcinomas in situ and high-grade squamous intraepithelial dysplasia appear identical, and the term anal intraepithelial neoplasia (AIN) recently has been used to describe these lesions. AIN is a precursor to an invasive squamous cell carcinoma (epidermoid carcinoma) and is associated with infection with the human papilloma virus, especially HPV types 16 and 18. Treatment of AIN is aimed at either resection or ablation. Because of a high recurrence and/or reinfection rate, these patients require extremely close surveillance. High-risk, immunosuppressed patients should be followed with frequent anal Papanicolaou (Pap) smears every 3–6 months. An abnormal Pap smear should be followed by an examination under anesthesia and anal mapping using high-resolution anoscopy, biopsy, and ablation of dysplastic lesions.

Epidermoid Carcinoma

Epidermoid carcinoma of the anus includes squamous cell carcinoma, cloacogenic carcinoma, transitional carcinoma, and basaloid carcinoma. Epidermoid carcinoma is a slow-growing tumor, and usually presents as an anal or perianal mass. Epidermoid carcinoma of the anal margin may be treated in a similar fashion as squamous cell carcinoma of the skin in other locations (wide local excision) because adequate surgical margins can usually be achieved without resecting the anal sphincter. Epidermoid carcinoma occurring in the anal canal or invading the sphincter cannot be excised locally, and first-line therapy relies on chemotherapy and radiation (the Nigro protocol). More than 80 percent of these tumors can be cured by using this regimen. Recurrence usually requires radical resection (abdominoperineal resection).

Verrucous Carcinoma (Buschke-Lowenstein Tumor, Giant Condyloma Acuminata)

Verrucous carcinoma is a locally aggressive form of condyloma acuminata. Although these lesions do not metastasize, they can cause extensive local tissue destruction and may be grossly indistinguishable from epidermoid carcinoma. Wide local excision is the treatment of choice when possible.

Basal Cell Carcinoma

Basal cell carcinoma of the anus is rare and resembles basal cell carcinoma elsewhere on the skin. This is a slow-growing tumor that rarely metastasizes.

Wide local excision is the treatment of choice, but recurrence occurs in up to 30 percent of patients.

Adenocarcinoma

Adenocarcinoma of the anus is extremely rare, and usually represents downward spread of a low rectal adenocarcinoma. Adenocarcinoma may occasionally arise from the anal glands or may develop in a chronic fistula. Radical resection with or without adjuvant chemoradiation is usually required.

Extramammary perianal Paget disease is adenocarcinoma in situ arising from the apocrine glands of the perianal area. These tumors are often associated with a synchronous gastrointestinal adenocarcinoma, so a complete evaluation of the intestinal tract should be performed. Wide local excision is usually adequate treatment for perianal Paget disease.

Melanoma

Anorectal melanoma is extremely rare. Overall 5-year survival is less than 10 percent, and many patients present with systemic metastasis and/or deeply invasive tumors at the time of diagnosis. A few patients with anorectal melanoma, however, present with isolated local or locoregional disease that is potentially resectable for cure. In these patients, wide local excision with a 1–2 cm margin is recommended if technically feasible. Radical resection (APR) may be necessary for circumferential lesions or tumors invading the anal sphincter.

OTHER BENIGN COLORECTAL CONDITIONS

Rectal Prolapse and Solitary Rectal Ulcer Syndrome

Rectal Prolapse

Rectal prolapse refers to a circumferential, full-thickness protrusion of the rectum through the anus and also has been called "first-degree" prolapse, "complete" prolapse, or procidentia. Internal prolapse occurs when the rectal wall intussuscepts but does not protrude (internal intussusception). Mucosal prolapse is a partial-thickness protrusion often associated with hemorrhoidal disease and usually is treated with banding or hemorrhoidectomy.

In adults, this condition is far more common among women, with a female-to-male ratio of 6:1. Prolapse becomes more prevalent with age in women and peaks in the seventh decade of life. In men, prevalence is unrelated to age. Symptoms include tenesmus, a sensation of tissue protruding from the anus that may or may not spontaneously reduce, and a sensation of incomplete evacuation. Mucus discharge and leakage may accompany the protrusion. Patients also present with a myriad of functional complaints, from incontinence and diarrhea to constipation and outlet obstruction.

A thorough preoperative evaluation, including colonic transit studies, anorectal manometry, tests of pudendal nerve terminal motor latency, electromyography, and cinedefecography, may be useful. The colon should be evaluated by colonoscopy or air-contrast barium enema to exclude neoplasms or diverticular disease. Cardiopulmonary condition should be thoroughly evaluated because comorbidities may influence the choice of surgical procedure.

Surgical therapy for rectal prolapse: The primary therapy for rectal prolapse is surgery.

1. Abdominal procedures
   A. Reduction of the perineal hernia and closure of the cul-de-sac (Moschowitz repair)
   B. Fixation of the rectum, either with a prosthetic sling (Ripsten and Wells rectopexy) or by suture rectopexy
   C. Resection of redundant sigmoid colon
   D. Resection combined with rectal fixation (resection rectopexy)
2. Perineal procedures
   A. Tightening the anus with a variety of prosthetic materials
   B. Reefing the rectal mucosa (Delorme procedure)
   C. Resection of the prolapsed bowel from the perineum (perineal rectosigmoidectomy or Altemeier procedure)

Because rectal prolapse occurs most commonly in older adult women, the choice of operation depends in part on the patient's overall medical condition. Abdominal rectopexy (with or without sigmoid resection) offers the most durable repair, with recurrence occurring in fewer than 10 percent of patients. Perineal rectosigmoidectomy avoids an abdominal operation and may be preferable in high-risk patients, but is associated with a higher recurrence rate. Reefing the rectal mucosa is effective for patients with limited prolapse. Anal encirclement procedures generally have been abandoned.

Solitary Rectal Ulcer Syndrome

Solitary rectal ulcer syndrome and colitis cystica profunda commonly are associated with internal intussusception. Patients may complain of pain, bleeding, mucus discharge, or outlet obstruction. In solitary rectal ulcer syndrome, one or more ulcers are present in the distal rectum, usually on the anterior wall. In colitis cystica profunda, nodules or a mass may be found in a similar location. Evaluation should include anorectal manometry, defecography, and either colonoscopy or barium enema to exclude other diagnoses. Biopsy of an ulcer or mass is mandatory to exclude malignancy. Nonoperative therapy (high-fiber diet, defecation training to avoid straining, and laxatives or enemas) is effective in the majority of patients. Surgery (either abdominal or perineal repair of prolapse as described above) is reserved for highly symptomatic patients who have failed all medical interventions.

Volvulus

Volvulus occurs when an air-filled segment of the colon twists about its mesentery. A volvulus may reduce spontaneously, but more commonly produces bowel obstruction, which can progress to strangulation, gangrene, and perforation. Chronic constipation may produce a large, redundant colon (chronic megacolon) that predisposes to volvulus.

1. Sigmoid Volvulus (80 percent) – Sigmoid volvulus produces a characteristic bent inner tube or coffee bean appearance on abdominal radiographs, with the convexity of the loop lying in the right upper quadrant (opposite the site of obstruction). Gastrografin enema shows a narrowing at the site of the volvulus and a pathognomonic bird's beak. Unless there are obvious signs of gangrene or peritonitis, the initial management of sigmoid volvulus is resuscitation followed by endoscopic detorsion. A rectal tube may be inserted to maintain decompression. Although these techniques are successful in reducing sigmoid volvulus in the majority of patients, the risk of recurrence

is high (40 percent). For this reason, an elective sigmoid colectomy should be performed after the patient has been stabilized and undergone an adequate bowel preparation. Clinical evidence of gangrene or perforation mandates immediate surgical exploration without an attempt at endoscopic decompression.

2. Cecal Volvulus (<20 percent) – Cecal volvulus results from nonfixation of the right colon. Rotation occurs around the ileocolic blood vessels and vascular impairment occurs early. Abdominal radiographs show a characteristic kidney-shaped, air-filled structure in the left upper quadrant (opposite the site of obstruction), and a Gastrografin enema confirms obstruction at the level of the volvulus.

   Unlike sigmoid volvulus, cecal volvulus can almost never be detorsed endoscopically. Moreover, because vascular compromise occurs early in the course of cecal volvulus, surgical exploration is necessary when the diagnosis is made. Right hemicolectomy with a primary ileocolic anastomosis can usually be performed safely and prevents recurrence. Simple detorsion or detorsion and cecopexy are associated with a high rate of recurrence.

3. Transverse Colon Volvulus (rare) – Nonfixation of the colon and chronic constipation with megacolon may predispose to transverse colon volvulus. The radiographic appearance resembles sigmoid volvulus, but Gastrografin enema will reveal a more proximal obstruction. Although colonoscopic detorsion is occasionally successful in this setting, most patients require emergent exploration and resection.

Megacolon

Megacolon describes a chronically dilated, elongated, hypertrophied large bowel. Megacolon may be congenital or acquired and usually is related to chronic mechanical or functional obstruction. In general, the degree of megacolon is related to the duration of obstruction. Evaluation must always include examination of the colon and rectum (either endoscopically or radiographically) to exclude a surgically correctable mechanical obstruction.

Congenital megacolon caused by Hirschsprung disease results from the failure of migration of neural crest cells to the distal large intestine. Surgical resection of the aganglionic segment is curative. Although Hirschsprung disease is primarily a disease of infants and children, it occasionally presents later in adulthood, especially if an extremely short segment of the bowel is affected (ultrashort-segment Hirschsprung disease).

Acquired megacolon may result from infection or chronic constipation. Infection with the protozoan Trypanosoma cruzi (Chagas disease) destroys ganglion cells and produces both megacolon and megaesophagus. Chronic constipation from slow transit or secondary to medications (especially anticholinergic medications) or neurologic disorders (paraplegia, poliomyelitis, amyotrophic lateral sclerosis, multiple sclerosis) may produce progressive colonic dilatation. Diverting ileostomy or subtotal colectomy with an ileorectal anastomosis is occasionally necessary in these patients.

Colonic Pseudo-Obstruction (Ogilvie Syndrome)

Colonic pseudo-obstruction (Ogilvie syndrome) is a functional disorder in which the colon becomes massively dilated in the absence of mechanical obstruction. Pseudo-obstruction most commonly occurs in hospitalized patients and is associated with the use of narcotics, bedrest, and comorbid disease.

Pseudo-obstruction is thought to result from autonomic dysfunction and severe adynamic ileus. The diagnosis is made based on the presence of massive dilatation of the colon (usually predominantly the right and transverse colon) in the absence of a mechanical obstruction. Initial treatment consists of cessation of narcotics, anticholinergics, or other medications that may contribute to ileus. Strict bowel rest and intravenous hydration are crucial. Most patients will respond to these measures. In patients who fail to improve, colonoscopic decompression often is effective. Recurrence occurs in up to 40 percent of patients. Intravenous neostigmine (an acetylcholinesterase inhibitor) also is extremely effective in decompressing the dilated colon and is associated with a low rate of recurrence (20 percent). However, neostigmine may produce transient but profound bradycardia and may be inappropriate in patients with cardiopulmonary disease. Because the colonic dilatation is typically greatest in the proximal colon, placement of a rectal tube is rarely effective. It is crucial to exclude mechanical obstruction (usually with a Gastrografin or barium enema) prior to medical or endoscopic treatment.

Ischemic Colitis

Intestinal ischemia occurs most commonly in the colon. Unlike small-bowel ischemia, colonic ischemia is rarely associated with major arterial or venous occlusion. Instead, most colonic ischemia appears to result from low flow and/or small-vessel occlusion. Risk factors include vascular disease, diabetes mellitus, vasculitis, and hypotension. Additionally, ligation of the inferior mesenteric artery during aortic surgery predisposes to colonic ischemia. Occasionally, thrombosis or embolism may cause ischemia. Although the splenic flexure is the most common site of ischemic colitis, any segment of the colon may be affected. The rectum is relatively spared because of its rich collateral circulation.

Signs and symptoms of ischemic colitis reflect the extent of bowel ischemia. In mild cases, patients may have diarrhea (usually bloody) without abdominal pain. With more severe ischemia, intense abdominal pain (often out of proportion to the clinical examination), tenderness, fever, and leukocytosis are present. Peritonitis and/or systemic toxicity are signs of full-thickness necrosis and perforation.

The diagnosis of ischemic colitis often is based on the clinical history and physical examination. Plain films may reveal thumb printing, which results from mucosal edema and submucosal hemorrhage. CT often shows nonspecific colonic wall thickening and pericolic fat stranding. Angiography usually is not helpful because major arterial occlusion is rare. Although sigmoidoscopy may reveal characteristic dark, hemorrhagic mucosa, the risk of precipitating perforation is high. For this reason, sigmoidoscopy is relatively contraindicated in any patient with significant abdominal tenderness. Contrast studies (Gastrografin or barium enema) are similarly contraindicated during the acute phase of ischemic colitis.

Treatment of ischemic colitis depends on clinical severity. Unlike ischemia of the small bowel, the majority of patients with ischemic colitis can be treated medically. Bowel rest and broad-spectrum antibiotics are the mainstay of therapy and 80 percent of patients will recover with this regimen. Hemodynamic parameters should be optimized, especially if hypotension and low flow appear to be the inciting cause. Long-term sequelae include stricture (10–15 percent) and chronic segmental ischemia (15–20 percent). Colonoscopy should be performed after recovery to evaluate strictures and to rule out other diagnoses such as inflammatory bowel disease or malignancy. Failure to improve after 2–3 days of medical management, progression of symptoms, or deterioration in clinical condition is indication for surgery. In this setting, all necrotic bowel should be resected. Primary anastomosis should be avoided. Occasionally, repeated exploration (a second-look operation) may be necessary.

Infectious Colitis

Pseudomembranous Colitis (*Clostridium difficile* Colitis)

C. difficile colitis is extremely common and is the leading cause of nosocomially acquired diarrhea. The spectrum of disease ranges from watery diarrhea to fulminant, life-threatening colitis. Colitis is thought to result from overgrowth of *C. difficile* after depletion of the normal commensal flora of the gut with the use of antibiotics, and almost any antibiotic may cause this disease. Immunosuppression, medical comorbidities, prolonged hospitalization or nursing home residence, and bowel surgery increase the risk. *C. difficile* colitis usually is diagnosed based on the presence of toxins in the stool (toxin A, an enterotoxin, and toxin B, a cytotoxin). The diagnosis also may be made endoscopically by detection of characteristic ulcers, plaques, and pseudomembranes. Management should include immediate cessation of the offending antimicrobial agent. Patients with mild disease (diarrhea but no fever or abdominal pain) may be treated as outpatients with oral metronidazole or oral vancomycin (second-line agent). More severe diarrhea associated with dehydration and/or fever and abdominal pain is best treated with bowel rest, intravenous hydration, and oral metronidazole or vancomycin. Proctosigmoiditis may respond to vancomycin enemas. Recurrent colitis occurs in up to 20 percent of patients and may be treated by a longer course of oral metronidazole or vancomycin (up to 1 month). Reintroduction of normal flora by ingestion of probiotics has been suggested as a possible treatment for recurrent or refractory disease. Fulminant colitis, characterized by septicemia and/or evidence of perforation, requires emergent laparotomy. A total abdominal colectomy with end ileostomy may be lifesaving.

Other Infectious Colitides

1. Bacterial
   A. Common: enterotoxic *E. coli*, *Campylobacter jejuni*, *Yersinia enterocolitica*, *Salmonella typhi*, Shigella, *Neisseria gonorrhoeae*
   B. Less common – Mycobacterium tuberculosis, Mycobacterium bovis, Actinomycosis israelii, Treponema pallidum (syphilis)
2. Parasitic – amebiasis, cryptosporidiosis, giardiasis
3. Fungal (rare) – Candida species, histoplasmosis
4. Viral – HIV, herpes simplex viruses, cytomegalovirus

Most symptoms of infection are nonspecific and consist of diarrhea (with or without bleeding), crampy abdominal pain, and malaise. A thorough history may offer clues to the etiology (other medical conditions, especially immunosuppression; recent travel or exposures; and ingestions). Diagnosis usually is made by identification of a pathogen in the stool, either by microscopy or culture. Serum immunoassays also may be useful (amebiasis, HIV, CMV). Occasionally, endoscopy with biopsy may be required. Treatment is tailored to the infection.

ANORECTAL DISEASES

Hemorrhoids

Hemorrhoids are cushions of submucosal tissue containing venules, arterioles, and smooth-muscle fibers that are located in the anal canal. Three hemorrhoidal cushions are found in the left lateral, right anterior, and right posterior positions and are thought to function as part of the continence mechanism. Because hemorrhoids are a normal part of anorectal anatomy, treatment is only indicated if they become symptomatic.

1. External hemorrhoids are located distal to the dentate line and are covered with anoderm. Thrombosis of an external hemorrhoid may cause significant pain. Treatment of external hemorrhoids and skin tags are only indicated for symptomatic relief.
2. Internal hemorrhoids are located proximal to the dentate line and covered by insensate anorectal mucosa. Internal hemorrhoids may prolapse or bleed, but rarely become painful unless they develop thrombosis and necrosis. Internal hemorrhoids are graded according to the extent of prolapse:
   First-degree hemorrhoids—bulge into the anal canal
   Second-degree hemorrhoids—prolapse through the anus but reduce spontaneously
   Third-degree hemorrhoids—prolapse through the anal canal and require manual reduction
   Fourth-degree hemorrhoids—prolapse but cannot be reduced and are at risk for strangulation
3. Combined internal and external hemorrhoids straddle the dentate line and have characteristics of both internal and external hemorrhoids.
4. Postpartum hemorrhoids result from straining during labor, which results in edema, thrombosis, and/or strangulation.
5. Rectal varices may result from portal hypertension. Despite the anastomoses between the portal venous system (middle and upper hemorrhoidal plexuses) and the systemic venous system (inferior rectal plexuses), hemorrhoidal disease is no more common in patients with portal hypertension than in the normal population. Rectal varices, however, may cause significant hemorrhage. In general, rectal varices are best treated by lowering portal venous pressure. Surgical hemorrhoidectomy should be avoided in these patients because of the risk of massive, difficult-to-control variceal bleeding.

Treatment

Medical Therapy (dietary fiber, stool softeners, increased fluid intake, and avoidance of straining) – appropriate for bleeding first- and second-degree hemorrhoids.

Rubber Band Ligation, sclerotherapy, infrared photocoagulation – appropriate for bleeding first-, second-, and selected third-degree hemorrhoids.

Excision of Thrombosed External Hemorrhoids. Acutely thrombosed external hemorrhoids generally cause intense pain and a palpable perianal mass during the first 24–72 h after thrombosis. The thrombosis can be effectively treated with an elliptical excision performed in the office under local anesthesia. Because the clot is usually loculated, simple incision and drainage is rarely effective. After 72 h, the clot begins to resorb, and the pain resolves spontaneously. Sitz baths and analgesics often are helpful.

Operative hemorrhoidectomy. A number of surgical procedures have been described for elective resection of symptomatic hemorrhoids. All are based on decreasing blood flow to the hemorrhoidal plexuses and excising redundant anoderm and mucosa:

1. Closed Submucosal Hemorrhoidectomy
2. Open Hemorrhoidectomy
3. Whitehead Hemorrhoidectomy
4. Stapled Hemorrhoidectomy

Complications of hemorrhoidectomy

1. Postoperative pain – Pain can be significant following excisional hemorrhoidectomy, and requires analgesia with oral narcotics, nonsteroidal anti-inflammatory drugs, muscle relaxants, topical analgesics, and sitz baths.
2. Urinary retention – Urinary retention occurs in 10–50 percent of patients after hemorrhoidectomy. The risk of urinary retention can be minimized by limiting intraoperative and perioperative intravenous fluids, and by providing adequate analgesia.
3. Fecal impaction – Risk of impaction may be decreased by preoperative enemas or a limited mechanical bowel preparation, liberal use of laxatives postoperatively, and adequate pain control.
4. Bleeding – Massive hemorrhage can occur after hemorrhoidectomy. Bleeding may occur in the immediate postoperative period (often in the recovery room) as a result of inadequate ligation of the vascular pedicle, and mandates an urgent return to the operating room. Bleeding may also occur 7–10 days after hemorrhoidectomy when the necrotic mucosa overlying the vascular pedicle sloughs. Although some of these patients may be safely observed, others will require an exam under anesthesia to ligate the bleeding vessel or to oversew the wounds if no specific site of bleeding is identified.
5. Infection – Infection is uncommon after hemorrhoidectomy; however, necrotizing soft-tissue infection can occur with devastating consequences. Severe pain, fever, and urinary retention may be early signs of serious infection. If this is suspected, an emergent examination under anesthesia, drainage of abscess, and/or débridement of all necrotic tissue are required.
6. Long-term sequelae
   A. incontinence (usually transient)
   B. anal stenosis
   C. ectropion (Whitehead deformity)

Anal Fissure

A fissure in ano is a tear in the anoderm distal to the dentate line. Most anal fissures occur in the posterior midline. Ten to 15 percent occur in the anterior midline. Less than 1 percent of fissures occur off midline.

Symptoms and Findings: Characteristic symptoms include tearing pain with defecation and hematochezia. On physical examination, the fissure can often be seen in the anoderm by gently separating the buttocks. Patients are often too tender to tolerate digital rectal examination, anoscopy, or proctoscopy. An acute fissure is a superficial tear of the distal anoderm and almost always heals with medical management. Chronic fissures develop ulceration and heaped-up edges with the white fibers of the internal anal sphincter visible at the base of the ulcer. There is often an associated external skin tag and/or a hypertrophied anal papilla internally. These fissures are more challenging to treat and may require surgery. A lateral location of a chronic anal fissure may be evidence of an underlying disease such as Crohn disease, human immunodeficiency virus, syphilis, tuberculosis, or leukemia.

Treatment

Therapy focuses on breaking the cycle of pain, spasm, and ischemia:

1. Dietary changes – bulk agents, stool softeners, and warm sitz baths.
2. Topical agents – Lidocaine jelly or other analgesic creams, nitroglycerin ointment, oral and topical diltiazem, and topical nifedipine (effective in most acute fissures, but will heal only approximately 50–60 percent of chronic fissures).
3. Botulinum toxin – Botulinum toxin causes temporary muscle paralysis by preventing acetylcholine release from presynaptic nerve terminals, and has been proposed as an alternative to surgical sphincterotomy for chronic fissure. Although there is limited experience with this approach, results appear to be superior to other medical therapy, and complications such as incontinence are rare.
4. Surgical sphincterotomy – Surgical therapy has been recommended for chronic fissures that have failed medical therapy, and lateral internal sphincterotomy is the procedure of choice for most surgeons. Approximately 30 percent of the internal sphincter fibers are divided. Healing is achieved in more than 95 percent of patients by using this technique and most patients experience immediate pain relief. Recurrence is rare (less than 10 percent), but the risk of minor incontinence ranges from 5–15 percent.

Anorectal Sepsis and Cryptoglandular Abscess

Relevant Anatomy

Infection of an anal gland in the intersphincteric space results in the formation of an abscess that enlarges and spreads along one of several planes in the perianal and perirectal spaces. The anatomy of these spaces influences the location and spread of infection.

1. Perianal space – surrounds the anus and laterally becomes continuous with the fat of the buttocks
2. Intersphincteric space – separates the internal and external anal sphincters.
3. Ischiorectal space (ischiorectal fossa) – located lateral and posterior to the anus and bounded medially by the external sphincter, laterally by the ischium, superiorly by the levator ani, and inferiorly by the transverse septum. The two ischiorectal spaces connect posteriorly above the anococcygeal ligament but below the levator ani muscle, forming the deep postanal space.
4. Supralevator spaces – above the levator ani on either side of the rectum (communicate posteriorly).

Diagnosis

Pain is the most common presenting complaint. A palpable mass often is detected by inspection of the perianal area or by digital rectal examination. Occasionally, patients will present with fever, urinary retention, or life-threatening sepsis. The diagnosis of a perianal or ischiorectal abscess can usually be made with physical exam alone. However, complex or atypical presentations may require imaging studies (CT or MRI) to fully delineate the anatomy of the abscess.

Treatment

Anorectal abscesses should be treated by drainage as soon as the diagnosis is established. If the diagnosis is in question, an examination under anesthesia is often the most expeditious way both to confirm the diagnosis and to treat the problem. Antibiotics are only indicated if there is extensive cellulitis or if the patient is immunocompromised, has diabetes mellitus, or has valvular heart disease. Surgical treatment is based in part on the location of the abscess:

Perianal Abscess – painful swelling at the anal verge. Most can be drained under local anesthesia. Larger, more complicated abscesses may require drainage in the operating room.

Ischiorectal Abscesses – may become extremely large and may involve one or both sides, forming a "horseshoe" abscess. Simple ischiorectal abscesses are drained through an incision in the overlying skin. Horseshoe abscesses require drainage of the deep postanal space and often require counterincisions over one or both ischiorectal spaces.

Intersphincteric Abscess – occur in the intersphincteric space and are notoriously difficult to diagnose. The diagnosis is made based on a high index of suspicion and usually requires an examination under anesthesia. Once identified, an intersphincteric abscess can be drained through a limited, usually posterior, internal sphincterotomy.

Supralevator Abscess – is uncommon and may result from extension of an intersphincteric or ischiorectal abscess upward, or extension of an intraperitoneal abscess downward. It is essential to identify the origin of a supralevator abscess prior to treatment. If the abscess is secondary to an upward extension of an intersphincteric abscess, it should be drained through the rectum. If a supralevator abscess arises from the upward extension of an ischiorectal abscess, it should be drained through the ischiorectal fossa. If the abscess is secondary to intraabdominal disease, the primary process requires treatment and the abscess is drained via the most direct route.

Perianal sepsis in the immunocompromised patient. Because of leukopenia, immunocompromised patients may develop serious perianal infection without any of the cardinal signs of inflammation. Although broad-spectrum antibiotics may cure some of these patients, an exam under anesthesia should not be delayed because of neutropenia. An increase in pain or fever, and/or clinical deterioration mandates an exam under anesthesia. Any indurated area should be incised and drained, biopsied to exclude a leukemic infiltrate, and cultured to aid in the selection of antimicrobial agents.

Necrotizing soft-tissue infection of the perineum. Necrotizing soft-tissue infection of the perineum is a rare, but lethal, condition. Most of these infections are polymicrobial and synergistic. The source of sepsis is commonly an undrained or inadequately drained cryptoglandular abscess or a urogenital infection. Immunocompromised patients and diabetic patients are at increased risk. Surgical débridement of all nonviable tissue is required to treat all necrotizing soft-tissue infections. Multiple operations may be necessary to ensure that all necrotic tissue has been resected. Broad-spectrum antibiotics are frequently employed, but adequate surgical débridement remains the mainstay of therapy. Despite early recognition and adequate surgical therapy, the

mortality of necrotizing perineal soft-tissue infections remains approximately 50 percent.

Fistula in Ano

Drainage of an anorectal abscess results in cure for about 50 percent of patients. The remaining 50 percent develop a persistent fistula in ano. The fistula usually originates in the infected crypt (internal opening) and tracks to the external opening. The course of the fistula often can be predicted by the anatomy of the previous abscess.

Diagnosis

Patients present with persistent drainage from the internal and/or external openings. In general, fistulas with an external opening anteriorly connect to the internal opening by a short, radial tract. Fistulas with an external opening posteriorly track in a curvilinear fashion to the posterior midline (Goodsall rule). However, exceptions to this rule often occur. Fistulas are categorized based on their relationship to the anal sphincter complex and treatment options are based on these classifications. The goal of treatment of fistula in ano is eradication of sepsis without sacrificing continence. Because fistulous tracks encircle variable amounts of the sphincter complex, surgical treatment is dictated by the location of the internal and external openings and the course of the fistula.

1. Intersphincteric fistula – tracks through the distal internal sphincter to an external opening near the anal verge; often treated by fistulotomy (opening the fistulous tract), curettage, and healing by secondary intention.
2. Transsphincteric fistula – results from an ischiorectal abscess and extends through both the internal and external sphincters. "Horseshoe" fistulas usually have an internal opening in the posterior midline and extend anteriorly and laterally to one or both ischiorectal spaces by way of the deep postanal space. Fistulas that include less than 30 percent of the sphincter muscles often can be treated by sphincterotomy. High transsphincteric fistulas, which encircle a greater amount of muscle, are more safely treated by initial placement of a seton.
3. Suprasphincteric fistula – originates in the intersphincteric plane and tracks up and around the entire external sphincter and is usually treated with a seton.
4. Extrasphincteric fistula – originates in the rectal wall and tracks around both sphincters to exit laterally, usually in the ischiorectal fossa. Treatment depends on both the anatomy of the fistula and its etiology. In general, the portion of the fistula outside the sphincter should be opened and drained. A primary tract at the level of the dentate line also may be opened if present. Complex fistulas with multiple tracts may require numerous procedures to control sepsis and facilitate healing. Liberal use of drains and setons is helpful.
5. Complex, nonhealing fistula – Complex and/or nonhealing fistulas may result from Crohn disease, malignancy, radiation proctitis, or unusual infection. Proctoscopy should be performed in all cases of complex and/or nonhealing fistulas to assess the health of the rectal mucosa. Biopsies of the fistula tract should be taken to rule out malignancy.

A seton is a drain placed through a fistula to maintain drainage and/or induce fibrosis. Cutting setons consist of a suture or a rubber band that is placed

through the fistula and intermittently tightened. Tightening the seton results in fibrosis and gradual division of the sphincter, thus eliminating the fistula while maintaining continuity of the sphincter. A noncutting seton is a soft plastic drain (often a vessel loop) placed in the fistula to maintain drainage. The fistula tract may subsequently be laid open with less risk of incontinence because scarring prevents retraction of the sphincter. Alternatively, the seton may be left in place for chronic drainage. Higher fistulas may be treated by an endorectal advancement flap. Fibrin glue also has been used to treat persistent fistulas with variable results.

Rectovaginal Fistula

A rectovaginal fistula is a connection between the vagina and the rectum or anal canal proximal to the dentate line and is classified based on location.

1. Low – rectal opening close to the dentate line and vaginal opening in the fourchette; commonly caused by obstetric injuries or trauma from a foreign body.
2. Middle – vaginal opening between the fourchette and cervix; may result from more severe obstetric injury, but also occur after surgical resection of a mid-rectal neoplasm, radiation injury, or extension of an undrained abscess.
3. High – vaginal opening near the cervix; result from operative or radiation injury, complicated diverticulitis, or Crohn disease.

Diagnosis

Patients describe symptoms varying from the sensation of passing flatus from the vagina to the passage of solid stool from the vagina. Contamination may result in vaginitis. Large fistulas may be obvious on anoscopic and/or vaginal speculum examination, but smaller fistulas may be difficult to locate. Occasionally, a barium enema or vaginogram may identify these fistulas. Endorectal ultrasound also may be useful. With the patient in the prone position, installation of methylene blue into the rectum while a tampon is in the vagina may confirm the presence of a small fistula.

Treatment

The treatment of rectovaginal fistula depends on the size, location, etiology, and condition of surrounding tissues. Because up to 50 percent of fistulas caused by obstetric injury heal spontaneously, it is prudent to wait 3–6 months before embarking on surgical repair in these patients. If the fistula was caused by a cryptoglandular abscess, drainage of the abscess may allow spontaneous closure.

Low and mid-rectovaginal fistulas are usually best treated with an endorectal advancement flap. If a sphincter injury is present, an overlapping sphincteroplasty should be performed concurrently. High rectovaginal, colovaginal, and enterovaginal fistulas are usually best treated via a transabdominal approach. The diseased tissue, which caused the fistula (upper rectum, sigmoid colon, or small bowel), is resected and the hole in the vagina closed. Rectovaginal fistulas caused by Crohn disease, radiation injury, or malignancy almost never heal spontaneously. Because differentiating radiation damage from malignancy can be extremely difficult, all fistulas resulting from radiation should be biopsied to rule out cancer.

Perianal Dermatitis

Pruritus Ani

1. Anatomic causes – prolapsing hemorrhoids, ectropion, fissure, fistula, and neoplasms.
2. Infectious causes – fungus (Candida species, Monilia, and Epidermophyton organisms), parasites (*Enterobius vermicularis* [pinworms], *Pediculus pubis* [a louse], and *Sarcoptes scabiei* [scabies]), bacteria (*Corynebacterium minutissimum* [erythrasma] and *Treponema pallidum* [syphilis]), or viruses (human papilloma virus [*condyloma acuminata*]).
3. Noninfectious/dermatologic causes – seborrhea, psoriasis, contact dermatitis.
4. Systemic diseases – jaundice, diabetes.
5. Idiopathic causes – The majority of pruritus ani is idiopathic and probably related to local hygiene, neurogenic, or psychogenic causes.

Treatment focuses on removal of irritants, improving perianal hygiene, dietary adjustments, and avoiding scratching. Biopsy and/or culture may be required to rule out an infectious or dermatologic cause. Hydrocortisone ointment 0.5–1.0 percent can provide symptomatic relief but should not be used for prolonged periods of time because of dermal atrophy. Skin barriers such as Calmoseptine also can provide relief. Systemic antihistamines or tricyclic antidepressants also have been used with some success.

Nonpruritic Lesions

Leprosy, amebiasis, actinomycosis, and lymphogranuloma venereum produce characteristic perianal lesions. Neoplasms such as Bowen disease, Paget disease, and invasive carcinomas also may appear first in the perianal skin. Biopsy usually can distinguish these diagnoses.

Sexually Transmitted Diseases

1. Bacterial Infections
   A. Proctitis – *N. gonorrhoeae*, *C. trachomatis*, *T. pallidum* (syphilis), *Haemophilus ducreyi* (chancroid), Donovania (*granuloma inguinale*).
   B. Diarrhea – Campylobacter, Shigella, other.
2. Parasitic Infections – *Entamoeba histolytica, Giardia lamblia*
3. Viral Infections
   A. Herpes Simplex Virus – may cause extremely painful proctitis.
   B. Human Papilloma Virus – may cause condyloma acuminata (anogenital warts), anal intraepithelial neoplasia, squamous cell carcinoma. HPV serotypes 16 and 18 appear to predispose to malignancy and often cause flat dysplasia in skin unaffected by warts. HPV types 6 and 11 commonly cause warts, but do not appear to cause malignant degeneration. Treatment of anal condyloma includes topical application of bichloracetic acid or podophyllin (small warts), Imiquimod (Aldara), and surgical excision/fulguration (larger or more extensive warts).

Pilonidal Disease

Pilonidal disease (cyst, infection) consists of a hair-containing sinus or abscess occurring in the intergluteal cleft. These ingrown hairs may then become infected and present acutely as an abscess in the sacrococcygeal region. An acute abscess should be incised and drained as soon as the diagnosis is made. Once an acute episode has resolved, recurrence is common. Definitive surgical treatment may include:

1. Unroofing the tract, curetting the base, and marsupializing the wound
2. Small lateral incision and pit excision
3. Flap closure, Z-plasty, advancement flap, or rotational flap (extensive and/or recurrent pilonidal disease)

Hidradenitis Suppurativa

Hidradenitis suppurativa is an infection of the cutaneous apocrine sweat glands. The infection may mimic complex anal fistula disease, but stops at the anal verge because there are no apocrine glands in the anal canal. Treatment involves incision and drainage of acute abscesses and unroofing and débridement of all chronically inflamed fistulas.

TRAUMA

Penetrating Colorectal Injury

Management of colonic injury depends on the mechanism of injury, the delay between the injury and surgery, the overall condition and stability of the patient, the degree of peritoneal contamination, and the condition of the injured colon. A primary repair may be considered in hemodynamically stable patients with few additional injuries and minimal contamination if the colon appears otherwise healthy. Contraindications to primary repair include shock, injury to more than two other organs, mesenteric vascular damage, and extensive fecal contamination. A delay of greater than 6 h between the injury and the operation is a relative contraindication to primary repair. Injuries caused by high-velocity gunshot wounds or blast injuries are usually treated by fecal diversion after débridement of all nonviable tissue.

Primary repair of the rectum is more difficult than primary repair of the colon and most rectal injuries are associated with significant contamination. The majority of penetrating rectal injuries should be treated with proximal fecal diversion and copious irrigation of the rectum (distal rectal washout). If there is extensive fecal contamination, presacral drains may be useful. Small, clean rectal injuries may be closed primarily without fecal diversion in an otherwise stable patient.

Blunt Colorectal Injury

Blunt trauma can cause colon perforation and shear injury to the mesentery can devascularize the intestine. Management of these injuries should follow the same principles outlined for management of penetrating injuries. Blunt injury to the rectum may result from significant trauma, such as a pelvic crush injury, or may result from local trauma caused by an enema or foreign body. Crush injuries, especially with an associated pelvic fracture, often are associated with significant rectal damage and contamination. These patients require débridement of all nonviable tissue, proximal fecal diversion, and a distal rectal washout, with or without drain placement. Blunt trauma from an enema or foreign body may produce a mucosal hematoma, which requires no surgical treatment if the mucosa is intact. Small mucosal tears may be closed primarily if the bowel is relatively clean and there is little contamination.

Iatrogenic Injury

Intraoperative Injury

The key to managing these injuries is early recognition. The vast majority of iatrogenic colorectal injuries may be closed primarily if there is little contamination and if the patient is otherwise stable. Delayed recognition of colorectal injuries may result in significant peritonitis and life-threatening sepsis. In these cases, fecal diversion almost always is required and the patient may need repeated exploration for drainage of abscesses.

Injury from Barium Enema

Colorectal injury from a barium enema is an extremely rare complication associated with a high rate of morbidity and mortality. Perforation with spillage of barium, especially above the peritoneal reflection, may result in profound peritonitis, sepsis, and a systemic inflammatory response. If the perforation is recognized early, it may be closed primarily and the abdomen irrigated to remove stool and barium. However, if the patient has developed sepsis, fecal diversion (with or without bowel resection) is almost always required.

Colonoscopic Perforation

Colonoscopic perforation occurs in less than 1 percent of patients. Management of colonoscopic perforation depends on the size of the perforation, the duration of time since the injury, and the overall condition of the patient. A large perforation recognized during the procedure requires surgical exploration; most can be repaired primarily. If there is significant contamination, if there has been a delay in diagnosis with resulting peritonitis, or if the patient is hemodynamically unstable, proximal diversion with or without resection is the safest approach. Polypectomy using electrocautery may produce a full-thickness burn, resulting in postpolypectomy syndrome in which a patient develops abdominal pain, fever, and leukocytosis without evidence of diffuse peritonitis. Many of these patients will have a "microperforation" which will resolve with bowel rest, broad-spectrum antibiotics, and close observation. Evidence of peritonitis or any deterioration in clinical condition mandates exploration. Free retroperitoneal or intraperitoneal air may be discovered incidentally after colonoscopy. In a completely asymptomatic patient, this finding is thought to result from barotrauma and dissection of air through tissue planes without a free perforation. Many of these patients can be successfully treated with bowel rest and broad-spectrum antibiotics. Surgical exploration is indicated for any clinical deterioration.

Anal Sphincter Injury and Incontinence

The most common cause of anal sphincter injury is obstetric trauma during vaginal delivery. Sphincter damage also may result from hemorrhoidectomy, sphincterotomy, abscess drainage, or fistulotomy. Patients with incontinence and a suspected sphincter injury can be evaluated with anal manometry, electromyography (EMG), and endoanal ultrasound. Mild incontinence, even in the presence of a sphincter defect, may respond to dietary changes and/or biofeedback. More severe incontinence may require surgical repair.

Surgical Repairs

The most common method of repair of the anal sphincter is a wrap-around sphincteroplasty. In cases in which there has been significant loss of sphincter muscle, or in which prior repairs have failed, more complex techniques, such as gracilis muscle transposition or artificial anal sphincter may be indicated. Sacral nerve stimulation via an implanted pulse generator is a new technique used for neurogenic incontinence when the sphincter is intact.

Foreign Body

Depending on the level of entrapment, a foreign body may cause damage to the rectum, rectosigmoid, or descending colon. Generalized abdominal pain suggests intraperitoneal perforation. Evaluation of the patient includes inspection of the perineum and a careful abdominal examination to detect any evidence of perforation. Plain films of the abdomen are mandatory to detect free intraabdominal air. Foreign bodies lodged low in the rectum often may be removed under conscious sedation with or without a local anesthetic block. Objects impacted higher in the rectum may require regional or general anesthesia for removal. Only rarely will a laparotomy be required to remove the object. After removal of the foreign body, proctoscopy and/or flexible sigmoidoscopy should be performed to evaluate the rectum and sigmoid colon for injury.

THE IMMUNOCOMPROMISED PATIENT (HUMAN IMMUNODEFICIENCY VIRUS OR IMMUNOSUPPRESSION FOR TRANSPLANTATION)

1. Diarrhea
   A. Bacteria – *C. difficile*, Salmonella, Shigella, Campylobacter, Chlamydia, and Mycobacterium species
   B. Fungi – Histoplasmosis, Coccidiosis, Cryptococcus
   C. Protozoa – Toxoplasmosis, Cryptosporidiosis, Isosporiasis
   D. Viruses – CMV, HSV colitis
2. Malignancy
   A. Kaposi sarcoma (most common malignancy in AIDS patients)
   B. Gastrointestinal lymphoma (usually non–Hodgkin lymphoma)
   C. Posttransplant lymphoproliferative disease
   D. Anal squamous cell carcinoma (associated with HPV infection)
3. Perianal disease
   A. Sexually transmitted diseases (more common in HIV disease)
   B. Abscesses and fistulas (may be complex and/or difficult to recognize)
4. Diverticulitis (may be more common in some populations of transplant patients and may have a more virulent course)
5. Graft-versus-host disease (unique to transplant patients)

The Neutropenic Patient

Neutropenic enterocolitis (typhlitis) is a life-threatening problem with a mortality rate of greater than 50 percent. This syndrome is characterized by abdominal pain and distention, fever, diarrhea (often bloody), nausea, and vomiting in a patient with fewer than 1000 neutrophils from any cause (bone marrow transplantation, solid-organ transplantation, or chemotherapy). CT scan of the abdomen often shows a dilated cecum with pericolic stranding. However, a normal-appearing CT scan does not exclude the diagnosis. Some patients will respond to bowel rest, broad-spectrum antibiotics, parenteral nutrition, and granulocyte infusion or colony-stimulating factors. Evidence of perforation, generalized peritonitis, or deterioration in clinical condition are indications for operation.

Suggested Readings

Smith RA, von Eschenbach AC, Wender R, et al: American Cancer Society guidelines for the early detection of cancer: Update of early detection guidelines for prostate, colorectal and endometrial cancers. CA Cancer J Clin 51:38, 2001.

Levin B, Brooks D, Smith R: Emerging technologies in screening for colorectal cancer: CT colography, immunochemical fecal occult blood tests, and stool screening using molecular markers. CA Cancer J Clin 53:44, 2003.

Bonen DK, Cho JH: The genetics of inflammatory bowel disease. Gastroenterology 124:521, 2003.

Wong WD, Wexner SD, Lowry A, et al: The Standards Task Force. The American Society of Colon and Rectal Surgeons. Practice parameters for the treatment of sigmoid diverticulitis. Dis Colon Rectum 43:289, 2000.

Greene FL, Page DL, Fleming, et al: AJCC Cancer Staging Manual, 6th ed. New York: Springer-Verlag, 2002.

Madoff R, Fleshman J: AGA technical review on the diagnosis and care of patients with anal fissure. Gastroenterology 124:235, 2003.

Rothenberger DA, Garcia-Aguilar J: Management of cancer in a polyp, in Saltz L (ed): Colorectal Cancer: Multimodality Management. NJ: Humana Press, 2002, p. 325.

National Comprehensive Cancer Network: Colon cancer clinical practice guidelines in oncology. J NCCN 1:40, 2003.

National Comprehensive Cancer Network: Rectal cancer clinical practice guidelines in oncology. J NCCN 1:54, 2003.

National Comprehensive Cancer Network: Anal canal cancer clinical practice guidelines in oncology. J NCCN 1:64, 2003.

29 | The Appendix

David H. Berger and Bernard M. Jaffe

ANATOMY AND FUNCTION

The appendix first becomes visible in the eighth week of development as a protuberance off the cecum. During development the growth rate of the cecum exceeds that of the appendix, displacing the appendix medially toward the ileocecal valve. The relationship of the base of the appendix to the cecum remains constant, whereas the tip can be found in a retrocecal, pelvic, subcecal, preileal, or right pericolic position. The three taenia coli converge at the junction of the cecum with the appendix. The appendix can vary in length from less than 1 cm to greater than 30 cm; most appendices are 6–9 cm in length.

The appendix is an immunologic organ that participates in the secretion of immunoglobulins, particularly immunoglobulin A (IgA). Although the appendix is an integral component of the gut-associated lymphoid tissue (GALT) system, its function is not essential and appendectomy is not associated with any manifestation of immune compromise. Lymphoid tissue first appears in the appendix approximately 2 weeks after birth. The amount of lymphoid tissue increases throughout puberty, remains steady for the next decade, and then begins a steady decrease with age.

ACUTE APPENDICITIS

Historical Background

The greatest contributor to the treatment of appendicitis is Charles McBurney. In 1889, he published his landmark paper in the New York Medical Journal describing the indications for early laparotomy for the treatment of appendicitis. It is in this paper that he described McBurney's point as the point of "maximum tenderness, when one examines with the fingertips is, in adults, one-half to two inches inside the right anterior spinous process of the ilium on a line drawn to the umbilicus." McBurney subsequently published a paper describing the incision that bears his name in 1894. Semm is widely credited with performing the first successful laparoscopic appendectomy in 1982.

Incidence

The lifetime rate of appendectomy is 12 percent for men and 25 percent for women, with approximately 7 percent of all people undergoing appendectomy for acute appendicitis. Over a 10-year period from 1987 to 1997, the overall appendectomy rate decreased parallel to a decrease in incidental appendectomy. However, the rate of appendectomy for appendicitis has remained constant at 10 per 10,000 patients per year. Appendicitis is most frequently seen in patients in their second through fourth decades of life, with a mean age of 31.3 years and a median age of 22 years. There is a slight male to female predominance (M:F 1.2–1.3:1). Despite increased use of ultrasonography, computed tomography (CT) scanning, and laparoscopy between 1987 and 1997, the rate of misdiagnosis of appendicitis has remained constant (15.3 percent), as has the rate of appendiceal rupture. The percentage of misdiagnosis of appendicitis is significantly higher among women than men (22.2 vs. 9.3 percent). The negative appendectomy rate for women of reproductive age is 23.2 percent, with the highest rates identified in women age 40–49 years. The highest negative appendectomy rate is reported for women older than 80 years of age.

Etiology and Pathogenesis

There is a predictable sequence of events leading to appendiceal rupture. Proximal obstruction of the appendiceal lumen produces a closed-loop obstruction, and continuing secretion by the appendiceal mucosa produces distention. Distention of the appendix stimulates nerve endings of visceral afferent stretch fibers, producing vague, dull, diffuse pain in the mid-abdomen or lower epigastrium. Peristalsis is also stimulated by the sudden distention, so that some cramping may be superimposed on the visceral pain early in the course of appendicitis. Distention continues from continued mucosal secretion and from multiplication of the resident bacteria of the appendix. Distention of this magnitude causes reflex nausea and vomiting, and the diffuse visceral pain becomes more severe. As pressure in the organ increases, venous pressure is exceeded. Capillaries and venules are occluded, but arteriolar inflow continues, resulting in engorgement and vascular congestion. The inflammatory process soon involves the serosa of the appendix and in turn parietal peritoneum in the region, producing the characteristic shift in pain to the right lower quadrant.

The mucosa of the appendix is susceptible to impairment of blood supply, thus its integrity is compromised early in the process, allowing bacterial invasion. As progressive distention encroaches on first the venous return and subsequently the arteriolar inflow, the area with the poorest blood supply suffers most. As distention, bacterial invasion, compromise of vascular supply, and infarction progress, perforation occurs, usually through one of the infarcted areas on the antimesenteric border. Perforation generally occurs just beyond the point of obstruction rather than at the tip. This sequence is not inevitable, however, and some episodes of acute appendicitis apparently subside spontaneously.

Bacteriology

The bacteriology of the normal appendix is similar to that of the normal colon. The bacteria cultured in cases of appendicitis are therefore similar to those seen in other colonic infections such as diverticulitis. The principal organisms seen in the normal appendix, in acute appendicitis, and in perforated appendicitis are Escherichia coli and Bacteroides fragilis. However, a wide variety of both facultative and anaerobic bacteria and mycobacteria may be present (Table 29-1). Appendicitis is a polymicrobial infection, with some series reporting up to 14 different organisms cultured in patients with perforation.

TABLE 29-1 Common Organisms Seen in Patients with Acute Appendicitis

Aerobic and facultative	Anaerobic
Gram-negative bacilli	Gram-negative bacilli
E. coli	*Bacteroides fragilis*
Pseudomonas aeruginosa	*Bacteroides* species
Klebsiella species	*Fusobacterium* species
Gram-positive cocci	Gram-positive cocci
Streptococcus anginosus	*Peptostreptococcus* species
Streptococcus species	Gram-positive bacilli
Enterococcus species	*Clostridium* species

The routine use of intraperitoneal cultures in patients with either perforated or nonperforated appendicitis is questionable. As discussed above, the flora is known and therefore broad-spectrum antibiotics are indicated. By the time culture results are available, the patient often has recovered from the illness. Additionally, the number of organisms cultured and the ability of a specific lab to culture anaerobic organisms vary greatly. Peritoneal culture should be reserved for patients who are immunosuppressed, and for patients who develop an abscess after the treatment of appendicitis. Antibiotic coverage is limited to 24–48 h in cases of nonperforated appendicitis. For perforated appendicitis, 7–10 days is recommended. Intravenous antibiotics are usually given until the white blood cell count is normal and the patient is afebrile for 24 h.

Clinical Manifestations

Symptoms

Abdominal pain is the prime symptom of acute appendicitis. Classically, pain is initially diffusely centered in the lower epigastrium or umbilical area, is moderately severe, and is steady, sometimes with intermittent cramping superimposed. After a period varying from 1–12 h, the pain localizes to the right lower quadrant. This classic pain sequence, although usual, is not invariable. In some patients, the pain of appendicitis begins in the right lower quadrant and remains there. Variations in the anatomic location of the appendix account for many of the variations in the principal locus of the somatic phase of the pain. Anorexia nearly always accompanies appendicitis. It is so constant that the diagnosis should be questioned if the patient is not anorectic. Although vomiting occurs in 75 percent of patients, it is neither prominent nor prolonged.

Most patients give a history of obstipation beginning prior to the onset of abdominal pain, and many feel that defecation would relieve their abdominal pain. However, diarrhea occurs in some patients, particularly children, so that the pattern of bowel function is of little differential diagnostic value.

The sequence of symptom appearance has great differential diagnostic significance. In more than 95 percent of patients with acute appendicitis, anorexia is the first symptom, followed by abdominal pain, which is followed, in turn, by vomiting. If vomiting precedes the onset of pain, the diagnosis of appendicitis should be questioned.

Signs

Physical findings are determined principally by the anatomic position of the inflamed appendix, and by whether the organ has already ruptured when the patient is first examined.

Vital signs are minimally changed by uncomplicated appendicitis. Temperature elevation is rarely more than 1°C (33.8°F) and the pulse rate is normal or slightly elevated. Changes of greater magnitude usually indicate that a complication has occurred or that another diagnosis should be considered.

Patients with appendicitis usually prefer to lie supine, with the thighs, drawn up, because any motion increases pain. The classic right lower quadrant physical signs are present when the inflamed appendix lies in the anterior position. Tenderness is often maximal at or near the McBurney point. Direct rebound tenderness is usually present. Additionally, referred or indirect rebound tenderness is present. This referred tenderness is felt maximally in the right lower quadrant, indicating localized peritoneal irritation. The Rovsing sign—pain in the right lower quadrant when palpatory pressure is exerted in the left lower quadrant—also indicates the site of peritoneal irritation. Cutaneous hyperesthesia in the area supplied by the spinal nerves on the right at T10, T11, and T12 frequently accompanies acute appendicitis. Muscular resistance to palpation of the abdominal wall parallels the severity of the inflammatory process.

Anatomic variations in the position of the inflamed appendix lead to deviations in the usual physical findings. The psoas sign indicates an irritative focus in proximity to that muscle. The test is performed by having patients lay on their left side as the examiner slowly extends the right thigh, thus stretching the iliopsoas muscle. The test is positive if extension produces pain. Similarly, a positive obturator sign of hypogastric pain on stretching the obturator internus indicates irritation in the pelvis. The test is performed by passive internal rotation of the flexed right thigh with the patient supine.

Laboratory Findings

Mild leukocytosis, ranging from 10,000–18,000/mm^3, is usually present in patients with acute, uncomplicated appendicitis and is often accompanied by a moderate polymorphonuclear predominance. However, white blood cell counts are variable. It is unusual for the white blood cell count to be greater than 18,000/mm^3 in uncomplicated appendicitis. White blood cell counts above this level raise the possibility of a perforated appendix. Urinalysis is useful to rule out the urinary tract as the source of infection. Although several white or red blood cells can be present from ureteral or bladder irritation as a result of an inflamed appendix, bacteriuria in a catheterized urine specimen is not seen with acute appendicitis.

Imaging Studies

Plain films of the abdomen, although frequently obtained as part of the general evaluation of a patient with an acute abdomen, are rarely helpful in diagnosing acute appendicitis. However, plain radiographs can be of significant benefit in ruling out other pathology. In patients with acute appendicitis, one often sees an abnormal bowel gas pattern, which is a nonspecific finding. The presence of a fecalith is rarely noted on plain films, but if present, is highly suggestive of the diagnosis.

Graded compression sonography has been suggested as an accurate way to establish the diagnosis of appendicitis. The technique is inexpensive, can be performed rapidly, does not require contrast, and can be used in pregnant patients. Sonographically, the appendix is identified as a blind-ending, nonperistaltic bowel loop originating from the cecum. With maximal compression, the diameter of the appendix is measured in the anteroposterior dimension. A scan is considered positive if a noncompressible appendix 6 mm or greater in the anteroposterior direction is demonstrated. The presence of an appendicolith establishes the diagnosis. The presence of thickening of the appendiceal wall and periappendiceal fluid is highly suggestive. Sonographic demonstration of a normal appendix excludes the diagnosis of acute appendicitis. The study is considered inconclusive if the appendix is not visualized and there is no pericecal fluid or mass. When the diagnosis of acute appendicitis is excluded by sonography, a brief survey of the remainder of the abdominal cavity should be performed to establish an alternative diagnosis. In females of child-bearing age, the pelvic organs must be adequately visualized. The sonographic diagnosis of acute appendicitis has a reported sensitivity of 55–96 percent and a specificity of 85–98 percent.

Some studies have reported that graded compression sonography improved the diagnosis of appendicitis over clinical exam, specifically decreasing the percentage of negative explorations for appendectomies from 37 down to 13 percent. Sonography also decreases the time before operation. Sonography identified appendicitis in 10 percent of patients who were believed to have a low likelihood of the disease on physical examination. The positive and negative predictive values of ultrasonography have been reported as 91 or 92 percent, respectively. However, in a recent prospective multicenter study, routine ultrasonography did not improve the diagnostic accuracy or rates of negative appendectomy or perforation when compared to clinical assessment.

High-resolution, helical, computer tomography also has been used to diagnose appendicitis. On CT scan, the inflamed appendix appears dilated and the wall is thickened. There is usually evidence of inflammation, with "dirty fat," thickened mesoappendix, and even an obvious phlegmon. Fecaliths can be easily visualized, but their presence is not necessarily pathognomonic of appendicitis. An important suggestive abnormality is the arrowhead sign. This is caused by thickening of the cecum, which funnels contrast toward the orifice of the inflamed appendix. CT scanning is also an excellent technique for identifying other inflammatory processes masquerading as appendicitis.

Several CT techniques have been used, including focused and nonfocused CT scans and enhanced and nonenhanced helical CT scanning. Surprisingly, all these techniques have yielded similar rates of diagnostic accuracy, i.e., 92–97 percent sensitivity, 85–94 percent specificity, 90–98 percent accuracy, and 75–95 percent positive and 95–99 percent negative predictive values. A number of studies have documented improvement in diagnostic accuracy with the liberal use of CT scanning in the workup of suspected appendicitis. Computed tomography lowered the rate of negative appendectomies from 19 down to 12 percent in one study, and the incidence of negative appendectomies in women from 24 down to 5 percent in another. The use of this imaging study altered the care of 24 percent of patients studied and provided alternative diagnoses in half of the patients with normal appendices on CT scan.

Problems exist with routine CT scanning for suspected appendicitis. CT scanning is expensive, exposes the patients to significant radiation, and cannot be used during pregnancy. Allergy contraindicates the application of intravenous contrast in some patients, and others cannot tolerate the oral ingestion of luminal dye, particularly in the presence of nausea and vomiting. Finally, not all studies have documented the utility of CT scanning in all patients with right lower quadrant pain.

Studies comparing the effectiveness of ultrasound to helical CT in establishing the diagnosis of appendicitis have demonstrated CT scanning superior. In one study, 600 ultrasounds and 317 CT scans revealed sensitivities of 80 and 97 percent, specificities of 93 and 94 percent, diagnostic accuracies of 89 and 95 percent, positive predictive values of 91 and 92 percent, and negative predictive values of 88 and 98 percent, respectively. In another study, ultrasound positively impacted the management of 19 percent of patients, as compared to 73 percent of patients for CT. Finally, in a third study, patients studied by ultrasonography had a 17 percent negative appendix rate compared to a 2 percent negative appendix rate in patients who underwent helical CT scanning.

One issue that has not been resolved is which patients are candidates for imaging studies. The concept that all patients with right lower quadrant pain should undergo CT scanning has been strongly supported by two reports by

TABLE 29-2 Alvarado Scale for the Diagnosis of Appendicitis

	Manifestations	Value
Symptoms	Migration of pain	1
	Anorexia	1
	Nausea/vomiting	1
Signs	RLQ tenderness	2
	Rebound	1
	Elevated temperature	1
Laboratory values	Leukocytosis	2
	Left shift	1
		Total Points 10

RLQ = right lower quadrant.
Source: From Alvarado, with permission.

Rao and his colleagues at the Massachusetts General Hospital. In one, this group documented a fall in the negative appendectomy rate from 20 down to 7 percent, and a decline in the perforation rate from 22 down to 14 percent, and establishing an alternative diagnosis in 50 percent of patients. In the second study, published in the New England Journal of Medicine, they documented that CT scanning prevented 13 unnecessary appendectomies, saved 50 inpatient hospital days, and lowered the per patient cost by $447. In contrast, several studies failed to prove an advantage of routine CT scanning, documenting that surgeon accuracy approached that of the imaging study and expressing concern that the imaging studies could adversely delay appendectomy in affected patients.

The rational approach is the selective use of CT scanning. This has been documented by several studies in which imaging was performed based on an algorithm or protocol. The likelihood of appendicitis can be ascertained using the Alvarado scale (Table 29-2). This scoring system was designed to improve the diagnosis of appendicitis and was devised by giving relative weight to specific clinical manifestation.

Laparoscopy can serve as both a diagnostic and therapeutic maneuver for patients with acute abdominal pain and suspected acute appendicitis. Laparoscopy is most useful in the evaluation of females with lower abdominal complaints because appendectomy is performed on a normal appendix in as many as 30–40 percent of these patients. Differentiating acute gynecologic pathology from acute appendicitis can be effectively accomplished by using the laparoscope.

Appendiceal Rupture

Immediate appendectomy has long been the recommended treatment of acute appendicitis because of the risk of rupture. The overall rate of perforated appendicitis is 25.8 percent. Children younger than age 5 years and patients older than age 65 years have the highest rate of perforation (45 and 51 percent, respectively). It has been suggested that delays in presentation are responsible for the majority of perforated appendices. There is no accurate way of determining when and if an appendix will rupture prior to resolution of the inflammatory process. Although it has been suggested that observation and antibiotic therapy alone may be an appropriate treatment for acute appendicitis, nonoperative treatment exposes the patient to the increased morbidity and mortality associated with a ruptured appendix.

Appendiceal rupture should be suspected in the presence of fever greater than 39°C (102°F) and a white blood cell count greater than 18,000/mm^3. In the majority of cases, rupture is contained and patients display localized rebound tenderness. Generalized peritonitis will be present if the walling-off process is ineffective in containing the rupture.

In 2–6 percent of cases, an ill-defined mass will be detected on physical examination. This could represent a phlegmon or a periappendiceal abscess. Patients who present with a mass have a longer duration of symptoms, usually at least 5–7 days. The ability to distinguish acute, uncomplicated appendicitis from acute appendicitis with perforation on the basis of clinical findings is often difficult, but it is important to make the distinction because their treatment differs. CT scan may be beneficial in guiding therapy. Phlegmons and small abscesses can be treated conservatively with intravenous antibiotics; well-localized abscesses can be managed with percutaneous drainage; complex abscesses should be considered for surgical drainage. If operative drainage is required, it should be performed by using an extraperitoneal approach, with appendectomy reserved for cases in which the appendix is easily accessible. Interval appendectomy performed at least 6 weeks following the acute event has classically been recommended for all patients treated either nonoperatively or with simple drainage of an abscess.

Differential Diagnosis

The differential diagnosis of acute appendicitis is essentially the diagnosis of the "acute abdomen" (see Chapter 34). This is because clinical manifestations are not specific for a given disease, but are specific for disturbance of a physiologic function or functions. Thus, an essentially identical clinical picture can result from a wide variety of acute processes within or near the peritoneal cavity.

The accuracy of preoperative diagnosis should be approximately 85 percent. If it is consistently less, it is likely that some unnecessary operations are being performed, and a more rigorous preoperative differential diagnosis is in order. A diagnostic accuracy rate consistently greater than 90 percent should also cause concern, because this may mean that some patients with atypical, but bona fide cases of, acute appendicitis are being "observed" when they should have prompt surgical intervention. The Haller group has shown, however, that this is not invariably true. Before the group's study, the perforation rate at the hospital in which the study took place was 26.7 percent, and acute appendicitis was found in 80 percent of the operations. By a policy of intensive in-hospital observation when the diagnosis of appendicitis was unclear, the group raised the rate of acute appendicitis found at operation to 94 percent, although the perforation rate remained unchanged at 27.5 percent.

There are a few conditions in which operation is contraindicated. Other disease processes that are confused with appendicitis are also surgical problems, or, if not, are not made worse by surgical intervention. A common error is to make a preoperative diagnosis of acute appendicitis only to find some other condition (or nothing) at operation; much less frequently, acute appendicitis is found after a preoperative diagnosis of another condition. The most common erroneous preoperative diagnoses—accounting for more than 75 percent—in descending order of frequency are acute mesenteric lymphadenitis, no organic pathologic conditions, acute pelvic inflammatory disease, twisted ovarian cyst or ruptured graafian follicle, and acute gastroenteritis.

The differential diagnosis of acute appendicitis depends on four major factors: the anatomic location of the inflamed appendix; the stage of the process (i.e., simple or ruptured); the patient's age; and the patient's sex.

Acute Appendicitis in the Young

The establishment of a diagnosis of acute appendicitis in young children is more difficult than in the adult. The more rapid progression to rupture and the inability of the underdeveloped greater omentum to contain a rupture lead to significant morbidity rates in children. Children younger than 5 years of age have a negative appendectomy rate of 25 percent and an appendiceal perforation rate of 45 percent. This is compared to a negative appendectomy rate of less than 10 percent and a perforated appendix rate of 20 percent for children 5–12 years of age. The incidence of major complications after appendectomy in children is correlated with appendiceal rupture. The wound infection rate after the treatment of nonperforated appendicitis in children is 2.8 percent as compared to a rate of 11 percent after the treatment of perforated appendicitis. The incidence of intraabdominal abscess is also higher after the treatment of perforated appendicitis as compared to nonperforated cases (6 percent vs. 3 percent). The treatment regimen for perforated appendicitis generally includes immediate appendectomy and irrigation of the peritoneal cavity. Antibiotic coverage is limited to 24–48 h in cases of nonperforated appendicitis. For perforated appendicitis, 7–10 days of antibiotics is recommended. Intravenous antibiotics are usually given until the white blood cell count is normal and the patient is afebrile for 24 h. Laparoscopic appendectomy has been shown to be safe and effective for the treatment of appendicitis in children.

Acute Appendicitis in Older Adults

Although the incidence of appendicitis in older adults is lower than in younger patients, the morbidity and mortality are significantly increased in this patient population. Delays in diagnosis, a more rapid progression to perforation, and comorbid disease are all contributing factors. The diagnosis of appendicitis may be subtler and less typical than in younger individuals, and a high index of suspicion should be maintained. In patients older than age 80 years, perforation rates of 49 percent and mortality rates of 21 percent have been reported.

Acute Appendicitis During Pregnancy

Appendicitis is the most frequently encountered extrauterine disease requiring surgical treatment during pregnancy. The incidence is approximately 1 in 2000 pregnancies. Acute appendicitis can occur at any time during pregnancy, but is more frequent during the first two trimesters. As fetal gestation progresses, the diagnosis of appendicitis becomes more difficult as the appendix is displaced laterally and superiorly. Nausea and vomiting after the first trimester or new-onset nausea and vomiting should raise the consideration of appendicitis. Abdominal pain and tenderness will be present, although rebound and guarding are less frequent because of laxity of the abdominal wall. Elevation of the white blood cell count above the normal pregnancy levels of $15,000–20,000/\mu L$, with a predominance of polymorphonuclear cells, is usually present. When the diagnosis is in doubt, abdominal ultrasound may be beneficial. Laparoscopy may be indicated in equivocal cases, especially early in pregnancy. The performance of any operation during pregnancy carries a risk of premature labor of

10–15 percent. The most significant factor associated with both fetal and maternal death is appendiceal perforation. Fetal mortality increases from 3–5 percent in early appendicitis to 20 percent with perforation. The suspicion of appendicitis during pregnancy should prompt rapid diagnosis and surgical intervention.

Appendicitis in Patients with AIDS or HIV Infection

The incidence of acute appendicitis in HIV-infected patients is reported to be 0.5 percent. This is higher than the 0.1–0.2 percent incidence reported for the general population. The presentation of acute appendicitis in HIV-infected patients is similar to that of noninfected patients. The majority of HIV-infected patients with appendicitis will have fever, periumbilical pain radiating to the right lower quadrant (91 percent), right lower quadrant tenderness (91 percent), and rebound tenderness (74 percent). HIV-infected patients will not manifest an absolute leukocytosis; however, if a baseline leukocyte count is available, nearly all HIV-infected patients with appendicitis will demonstrate a relative leukocytosis.

There appears to be an increased risk of appendiceal rupture in HIV-infected patients. In one large series of HIV-infected patients who underwent appendectomy for presumed appendicitis, 43 percent of patients were found to have perforated appendicitis at laparotomy. The increased risk of appendiceal rupture may be related to the delay in presentation seen in this patient population. The mean duration of symptoms prior to arrival in the emergency room has been reported to be increased in HIV-infected patients, with more than 60 percent of patients reporting the duration of symptoms to be longer than 24 h. A low CD4 count is also associated with an increase in appendiceal rupture.

The differential diagnosis of right lower quadrant pain in HIV-infected patients should include the possibility of an opportunistic infection. These opportunistic infections include cytomegalovirus (CMV), Kaposi sarcoma, tuberculosis, lymphoma, and other causes of infectious colitis. In the HIV-infected patient with classic signs and symptoms of appendicitis, immediate appendectomy is indicated. In those patients with diarrhea as a prominent symptom, colonoscopy may be warranted. In patients with equivocal findings, CT scan is usually helpful. The majority of pathologic findings identified in HIV-infected patients who undergo appendectomy for presumed appendicitis are typical. The negative appendectomy rate is 5–10 percent. However, up to 25 percent of patients will have AIDS-related entities in the operative specimens, including CMV, Kaposi sarcoma, and *Mycobacterium aviumintracellulare*.

In a report of 77 human immunodeficiency virus (HIV)-infected patients from 1988–1995, the 30-day mortality rate for patients undergoing appendectomy was reported to be 9.1 percent. More recent series report 0 percent mortality in this group of patients. Morbidity rates for HIV-infected patients with nonperforated appendicitis are similar to those seen in the general population. Postoperative morbidity rates appear to be higher in HIV-infected patients with perforated appendicitis. Additionally, the length of hospital stay for HIV-infected patients undergoing appendectomy is twice that of the general population.

Treatment

Once the decision to operate for presumed acute appendicitis has been made, the patient should be prepared for the operating room. Adequate hydration should be ensured; electrolyte abnormalities corrected; and preexisting cardiac, pulmonary, and renal conditions should be addressed. Many trials have demonstrated the efficacy of preoperative antibiotics in lowering the infectious complications in appendicitis. For intraabdominal infections of gastrointestinal tract origin of mild to moderate severity, the Surgical Infection Society has recommended single-agent therapy with cefoxitin, cefotetan, or ticarcillin-clavulanic acid. For more severe infections, single-agent therapy with carbapenems or combination therapy with a third-generation cephalosporin, monobactam, or aminoglycoside plus anaerobic coverage with clindamycin or metronidazole is indicated.

Open Appendectomy

Most surgeons employ either a McBurney (oblique) or Rocky-Davis (transverse) right lower quadrant muscle-splitting incision in patients with suspected appendicitis. The incision should be centered over either the point of maximal tenderness or a palpable mass. If an abscess is suspected, a laterally placed incision is imperative to allow retroperitoneal drainage and to avoid generalized contamination of the peritoneal cavity. If the diagnosis is in doubt, a lower midline incision is recommended to allow a more extensive examination of the peritoneal cavity. This is especially relevant in older patients with possible malignancy or diverticulitis.

Several techniques can be used to locate the appendix. Because the cecum is usually visible within the incision, the convergence of the taeniae can be followed to the base of the appendix. A sweeping lateral to medial motion can aid in delivering the appendiceal tip into the operative field. Occasionally, limited mobilization of the cecum is needed to aid in adequate visualization. Once identified, the appendix is mobilized by dividing the mesoappendix, taking care to ligate the appendiceal artery securely.

The appendiceal stump can be managed by simple ligation or by ligation and inversion with either a purse-string or Z stitch. As long as the stump is clearly viable and the base of the cecum not involved with the inflammatory process, the stump can be safely ligated with a nonabsorbable suture. The mucosa is frequently obliterated to avoid the development of mucocele. The peritoneal cavity is irrigated and the wound closed in layers. If perforation or gangrene is found in adults, the skin and subcutaneous tissue should be left open and allowed to heal by secondary intent or closed in 4–5 days as a delayed primary closure. In children, who generally have little subcutaneous fat, primary wound closure has not led to an increased incidence of wound infection. If appendicitis is not found, a methodical search for an alternative diagnosis must be performed.

Laparoscopy

Laparoscopic appendectomy is performed under general anesthesia. A nasogastric tube and a urinary catheter are placed prior to obtaining a pneumoperitoneum. Laparoscopic appendectomy usually requires the use of three ports. Four ports may occasionally be necessary to mobilize a retrocecal appendix. The surgeon usually stands to the patient's left. One assistant is required to operate the camera. One trocar is placed in the umbilicus (10 mm), with a second trocar placed in the suprapubic position. Some surgeons will place this second port in the left lower quadrant. The suprapubic trocar is either 10 or 12 mm, depending on whether a linear stapler will be used. The placement of the third trocar (5 mm) is variable and is usually either in the left lower quadrant, epigastrium, or right upper quadrant. Placement is based on location of the appendix and surgeon preference. Initially, the abdomen is thoroughly explored to exclude other pathology. The appendix is identified by following the anterior taeniae to its base. Dissection at the base of the appendix enables the surgeon to create a window between the mesentery and base of the appendix. The mesentery and base of the appendix are then secured and divided separately. When the mesoappendix is involved with the inflammatory process, it is often best to divide the appendix first with a linear stapler, and then to divide the mesoappendix immediately adjacent to the appendix. The base of the appendix is not inverted. The appendix is removed from the abdominal cavity through a trocar site or within a retrieval bag. The base of the appendix and the mesoappendix should be evaluated for hemostasis. The right lower quadrant should be irrigated. Trocars are removed under direct vision.

The largest meta-analysis comparing open to laparoscopic appendectomy included 47 studies, 39 of which were studies of adult patients. This analysis demonstrated that the duration of surgery and operation costs were higher for laparoscopic appendectomy than for open appendectomy. Wound infections were approximately half as likely after laparoscopic appendectomy than after open appendectomy. However, intraabdominal abscess was three times greater after laparoscopic appendectomy than after open appendectomy. Patient-reported pain on the first postoperative day is significantly less after laparoscopic appendectomy. However, the difference has been calculated to be only 8 on a 100-point visual analogue scale. Hospital length of stay also is statistically significantly less after laparoscopic appendectomy. In most studies this difference is less than 1 day. The more important determinant of length of stay after appendectomy is the pathology at operation; specifically whether a patient has perforated or nonperforated appendicitis. In nearly all studies, laparoscopic appendectomy is associated with a shorter return to normal activity, return to work, and return to sports. Although the majority of studies have been performed in adults, similar data has been obtained in children.

There appears to be little benefit to laparoscopic appendectomy over open appendectomy in thin males between the ages of 15 and 45 years. In these patients, the diagnosis is usually straightforward. Open appendectomy has been associated with outstanding results for several decades. Laparoscopic appendectomy should be considered an option in these patients, based on surgeon and patient preference. Laparoscopic appendectomy may be beneficial in obese patients in whom it may be difficult to gain adequate access through a small right lower quadrant incision. Additionally, there may be a decreased risk of postoperative wound infection after laparoscopic appendectomy in obese patients.

Diagnostic laparoscopy has been advocated as a potential tool to decrease the number of negative appendectomies performed. However, the morbidity associated with laparoscopy and general anesthesia is acceptable only if pathology requiring surgical treatment is present and is amenable to laparoscopic techniques. The question of leaving a normal appendix in situ is a controversial one. Seventeen to 26 percent of normal-appearing appendices at exploration have a pathologic histologic finding. The availability of diagnostic laparoscopy may lower the threshold for exploration, thus impacting the negative appendectomy rate adversely. Fertile women with presumed appendicitis constitute the group of patients most likely to benefit from diagnostic laparoscopy. Up to one third of these patients will not have appendicitis at exploration. Most of these patients without appendicitis will have gynecologic pathology identified.

A meta-analysis demonstrated that in fertile women in whom appendectomy was deemed necessary, diagnostic laparoscopy reduced the number of unnecessary appendectomies. Additionally, the number of women without a final diagnosis was smaller. It appears that leaving a normal-appearing appendix in fertile women with identifiable gynecologic pathology is safe.

In summary, it has not been resolved whether laparoscopic appendectomy is more effective at treating acute appendicitis than the time-proven method of open appendectomy. It does appear that laparoscopic appendectomy is effective in the management of acute appendicitis. Laparoscopic appendectomy should be considered part of the surgical armamentarium available to treat acute appendicitis. The decision regarding how to treat any single patient with appendicitis should be based on surgical skill, patient characteristics, clinical scenario, and patient preference.

Interval Appendectomy

The accepted algorithm for the treatment of appendicitis associated with a palpable or radiographically documented mass (abscess or phlegmon) is conservative therapy with interval appendectomy 6–10 weeks later. This technique has been quite successful and provides much lower morbidity and mortality rates than immediate appendectomy. This treatment is associated with added expense and longer hospitalization. The initial treatment consists of intravenous antibiotics and bowel rest. Although generally effective, there is a 9–15 percent failure rate, with operative intervention required at 3–5 days after presentation. Percutaneous or operative drainage of abscesses is not considered a failure of conservative therapy.

The data support the need for interval appendectomy. In a prospective series, 19 of 48 (40 percent) patients who were successfully treated conservatively needed appendectomy earlier (4.3 weeks) than the 10 weeks planned because of bouts of appendicitis. Overall, the rate of late failure as a consequence of acute disease averages 20 percent. An additional 14 percent of patients either continue to have, or redevelop, right lower quadrant pain. Although the appendix may occasionally be pathologically normal, persistent periappendiceal abscesses and adhesions are found in 80 percent of patients. Additionally, almost 50 percent have histologic evidence of inflammation in the organ itself. Several neoplasms also have been detected in the resected appendix.

The timing of interval appendectomy is controversial. Appendectomy may be required as early as 3 weeks following conservative therapy. Two thirds of the cases of recurrent appendicitis occur within 2 years, and this is the outside limit.

Interval appendectomy is associated with a morbidity rate of 3 percent or less and a hospitalization of 1–3 days in length. The laparoscopic approach has been used recently and has been successful in 68 percent of procedures.

Prognosis

The mortality from appendicitis in the United States has steadily decreased from a rate of 9.9 per 100,000 in 1939, to 0.2 per 100,000 as of 1986. Principal factors in mortality are whether rupture occurs before surgical treatment and the age of the patient. The overall mortality rate for a general anesthetic is 0.06 percent. The overall mortality rate in ruptured acute appendicitis is about 3 percent—a 50-fold increase. The mortality rate of ruptured appendicitis in older adults is approximately 15 percent—a 5-fold increase from the overall rate.

Morbidity rates parallel mortality rates, being significantly increased by rupture of the appendix and to a lesser extent by old age. Complications occur in 3 percent of patients with nonperforated appendicitis and in 47 percent of patients with perforations. Most of the serious early complications are septic and include abscess and wound infection. Wound infection is common, but is nearly always confined to the subcutaneous tissues and promptly responds to wound drainage. Wound infection predisposes the patient to wound dehiscence. The type of incision is relevant; complete dehiscence rarely occurs in a McBurney incision.

The incidence of intraabdominal abscesses secondary to peritoneal contamination from gangrenous or perforated appendicitis has decreased markedly because the introduction of potent antibiotics. The sites of predilection for abscesses are the appendiceal fossa, pouch of Douglas, subhepatic space, and between loops of intestine. The latter are usually multiple. Transrectal drainage is preferred for an abscess that bulges into the rectum.

Fecal fistula is an annoying, but not particularly dangerous, complication of appendectomy that may be caused by sloughing of that portion of the cecum inside a constricting purse-string suture; by the ligature's slipping off an appendiceal stump; or by necrosis from an abscess encroaching on the cecum.

CHRONIC APPENDICITIS

The existence of chronic appendicitis as a clinical entity has been questioned for many years. Recent clinical data document the existence of this uncommon disease. Histologic criteria have been established. The pain lasts longer and is less intense than that of acute appendicitis, but is in the same location. There is a much lower incidence of vomiting, but anorexia and occasionally nausea, pain with motion, and malaise are characteristic. Leukocyte counts are predictably normal and CT scans are generally nondiagnostic.

At operation, surgeons can establish the diagnosis with 94 percent specificity and 78 percent sensitivity. There is an excellent correlation between clinical symptomatology, intraoperative findings, and histologic abnormalities. Laparoscopy can be effectively used in the management of this clinical entity. Appendectomy is curative. Symptoms resolve postoperatively in 82–93 percent of patients. Many of those whose symptoms are not cured or recur are ultimately diagnosed with Crohn disease.

APPENDICEAL PARASITES

A number of intestinal parasites cause appendicitis. Although *Ascaris lumbricoides* is the most common, a wide spectrum of helminths have been implicated, including *Enterobius vermicularis*, *Strongyloides stercoralis*, and *Echinococcus granulosis*. The live parasites occlude the appendiceal lumen, causing obstruction. The presence of parasites in the appendix at operation makes ligation and stapling of the appendix technically difficult. Once appendectomy has been performed and the patient recovered, therapy with helminthicide is necessary to clear the remainder of the gastrointestinal tract.

Amebiasis can also cause appendicitis. Invasion of the mucosa by trophozoites of *Entamoeba histolytica* incites a marked inflammatory process. Appendiceal involvement is a component of more generalized intestinal amebiasis.

Appendectomy must be followed by appropriate antibiotic therapy (metronidazole).

INCIDENTAL APPENDECTOMY

The decisions regarding the efficacy of incidental appendectomy should be based on the epidemiology of appendicitis. The best data were published by the Centers for Disease Control and Prevention (CDC) based on the period from 1979–1984. During this period, there was an average of 250,000 cases of appendicitis in the United States. The highest annual incidence of appendicitis was in patients 9–19 years of age (23.3 per 10,000 population). Males were more likely to develop appendicitis than females. Accordingly, the incidence during teenage years was 27.6 in males and 20.5 in females per 10,000 population per year. Beyond age 19 years, the annual incidence fell. After 45 years of age, the annual incidence was 6 in 10,000 males and 4 in 10,000 females. Using the life table technique, the data identified a lifetime risk of appendicitis of 8.6 percent in men and 6.7 percent in women. Although men were more likely to develop appendicitis, the preoperative diagnosis was correct in 91.2 percent of men and 78.6 percent of women. Similarly, perforation occurred more commonly in men (19.2 vs. 17.8 percent in women). In contrast to the cases of appendicitis, 310,000 incidental appendectomies were performed between 1979 and 1984, 62 percent of the total appendectomies in men and 17.7 percent in women. Based on these data, 36 incidental appendectomies had to be performed to prevent 1 patient from developing appendicitis.

Indications to consider incidental appendectomy include children about to undergo chemotherapy, the disabled who cannot describe symptoms or react normally to abdominal pain, Crohn disease patients in whom the cecum is free of macroscopic disease, and individuals who are about to travel to remote places in which there is no access to medical/surgical care.

TUMORS

Appendiceal malignancies are extremely rare. Primary appendiceal cancer is diagnosed in 0.9–1.4 percent of appendectomy specimens. These tumors are only rarely suspected preoperatively. Additionally, less than 50 percent of cases are diagnosed at operation. Most series report that carcinoid is the most common appendiceal malignancy, representing more than 50 percent of the primary lesions of the appendix. However, a recent review from The National Cancer Institute's (NCI) Surveillance, Epidemiology, and End Results (SEER) program found the age-adjusted incidence of appendiceal malignancies to be 0.12 cases per 1,000,000 people per year, and identified mucinous adenocarcinoma as the most frequent histologic diagnosis with 37 percent of total reported cases. Carcinoid was the second most frequent histologic diagnosis, comprising 33 percent of total cases.

Carcinoid

The appendix is the most common site of gastrointestinal carcinoid, followed by the small bowel and then rectum. Carcinoid syndrome is rarely associated with appendiceal carcinoid unless widespread metastases are present, which occur in 2.9 percent of cases. Symptoms attributable directly to the carcinoid are rare, although the tumor can occasionally obstruct the appendiceal lumen much like a fecalith and result in acute appendicitis.

The majority of carcinoids are located in the tip of the appendix. Malignant potential is related to size, with tumors less than 1 cm rarely resulting in extension outside of the appendix or adjacent to the mass. In one report, 78 percent of appendiceal carcinoids were less than 1 cm, 17 percent were 1–2 cm, and only 5 percent were greater than 2 cm. Treatment rarely requires more than simple appendectomy. For tumors smaller than 1 cm with extension into the mesoappendix, and for all tumors larger than 1.5 cm, a right hemicolectomy should be performed.

Adenocarcinoma

Primary adenocarcinoma of the appendix is a rare neoplasm of three major histologic subtypes: mucinous adenocarcinoma, colonic adenocarcinoma, and adenocarcinoid. The most common mode of presentation for appendiceal carcinoma is that of acute appendicitis. Patients may also present with ascites or a palpable mass, or the neoplasm may be discovered during an operative procedure for an unrelated cause. The recommended treatment for all patients with adenocarcinoma of the appendix is a formal right hemicolectomy. Appendiceal adenocarcinomas have a propensity for early perforation, although they are not clearly associated with a worsened prognosis. Overall 5-year survival is 55 percent and varies with stage and grade. Patients with appendiceal adenocarcinoma are at significant risk for both synchronous and metachronous neoplasms, approximately half of which will originate from the gastrointestinal tract.

Mucocele

An appendiceal mucocele leads to progressive enlargement of the appendix from the intraluminal accumulation of a mucoid substance. Mucoceles are of four histologic types, and the type dictates the course of the disease and prognosis: retention cysts, mucosal hyperplasia, cystadenomas, and cystadenocarcinomas. A mucocele of benign etiology is adequately treated by a simple appendectomy.

Pseudomyxoma Peritonei

Pseudomyxoma peritonei is a rare condition in which diffuse collections of gelatinous fluid are associated with mucinous implants on peritoneal surfaces and omentum. Pseudomyxoma is two to three times more common in females than males. There is controversy in the literature regarding whether pseudomyxoma arises from the appendix or the ovary in female patients. Recent immunocytologic and molecular studies suggest that the appendix is the site of origin for most cases of pseudomyxoma. Pseudomyxoma is invariably caused by neoplastic mucous-secreting cells within the peritoneum. These cells may be difficult to classify as malignant because they may be sparse, widely scattered, and have a low-grade cytologic appearance. Patients with pseudomyxoma usually present with abdominal pain, distention, or a mass. Primary pseudomyxoma usually does not cause abdominal organ dysfunction. However, ureteral obstruction and obstruction of venous return can be seen.

The use of imaging before surgery is advantageous to plan surgery. CT scanning is the preferred imaging modality. At surgery a variable volume of mucinous ascites is found together with tumor deposits involving the right hemidiaphragm, right retrohepatic space, left paracolic gutter, ligament of Treitz, and the ovaries in women. Peritoneal surfaces of the bowel are usually free of tumor. Thorough surgical debulking is the mainstay of treatment. All gross disease should be removed. Appendectomy is routinely performed. Hysterectomy with bilateral salpingo-oophorectomy is performed in women. Ultraradical surgery has not been shown to be of significant benefit. Additionally, adjuvant intraperitoneal chemotherapy (with or without hyperthermia) or systemic postoperative chemotherapy have not been shown to be of benefit. Pseudomyxoma is a disease that progresses slowly and in which recurrences may take years to develop or become symptomatic. In a series from the Mayo Clinic, 76 percent of patients developed recurrences within the abdomen. Lymph node metastasis and distant metastasis are uncommon. Recurrences are treated by additional surgery. Surgery for recurrent disease is usually difficult and associated with an increased incidence of enterotomies, anastomotic leaks, and fistulas. With adequate primary surgery and debulking of recurrences, the median survival of pseudomyxoma is 5.9 years, with 53 percent of patients surviving 5 years.

Lymphoma

Lymphoma of the appendix is uncommon. The gastrointestinal tract is the most frequently involved extranodal site for non-Hodgkin lymphoma. Other types of lymphoma, such as Burkitt, and leukemia, have also been reported. The frequency of primary lymphoma of the appendix is 1–3 percent of gastrointestinal lymphomas. Appendiceal lymphoma usually presents as acute appendicitis and is rarely suspected preoperatively. Findings on CT scan of an appendiceal diameter greater than or equal to 2.5 cm or surrounding soft-tissue thickening should prompt suspicion of an appendiceal lymphoma. The management of appendiceal lymphoma confined to the appendix is appendectomy. Right hemicolectomy is indicated if there is extension of tumor onto the cecum or mesentery. A postoperative staging workup is indicated prior to initiating adjuvant therapy. Adjuvant therapy is not indicated for lymphoma confined to the appendix.

Suggested References

Addiss DG, Shaffer N, Fowler BS, et al: The epidemiology of appendicitis and appendectomy in the United States. Am J Epidemiol 132:910, 1990.

Hale DA, Molloy M, Pearl RH, et al: Appendectomy: A contemporary appraisal. Ann Surg 225:252, 1997.

Flum DR, Morris A, Koepsell T, et al: Has misdiagnosis of appendicitis decreased over time? A population-based analysis. JAMA 286:1748, 2001.

Soffer D, Zait S, Klausner J, et al: Peritoneal cultures and antibiotic treatment in patients with perforated appendicitis. Eur J Surg 167:214, 2001.

Rettenbacher T, Hollerweger A, Gritzmann N, et al: Appendicitis: Should diagnostic imaging be performed if the clinical presentation is highly suggestive of the disease? Gastroenterology 123:992, 2002.

Alvarado A: A practical score for the early diagnosis of acute appendicitis. Ann Emerg Med 15:557, 1986.

Paulson EK, Kalady MF, Pappas TN: Clinical practice. Suspected appendicitis. N Engl J Med 348:236, 2003.

Knight PJ, Vassy LE: Specific diseases mimicking appendicitis in childhood. Arch Surg 116:744, 1981.

Sauerland S, Lefering R, Neugebauer EA: Laparoscopic versus open surgery for suspected appendicitis. Cochrane Database Syst Rev (1):CD001546, 2002.

McCusker ME, Cote TR, Clegg LX, et al: Primary malignant neoplasms of the appendix: A population-based study from the Surveillance, Epidemiology and End Results program, 1973–1998. Cancer 94:3307, 2002.

30 | Liver

Steven A. Curley and Timothy D. Sielaff

LIVER ANATOMY

One of the greatest advances in hepatic surgery is the understanding of the segmental anatomy of the liver. The Couinaud system for liver segmental nomenclature is widely accepted in practice. The liver is divided into longitudinal planes drawn through each hepatic vein to the vena cava, and a transverse plane at the level of the main portal bifurcation. The plane of the middle hepatic vein and the primary bifurcation of the portal vein divide the liver into a right and left lobe. This runs from the inferior vena cava to the tip of the gallbladder fossa (also known as the Cantlie line or the portal fissure). The secondary portal bifurcations on the right and left give rise to four sectors (or sections). On the right side this produces the anterior and posterior sectors, which are split by the plane of the right hepatic vein. The tertiary branches on the right supply four segments, two in each sector. The ascending branch of the left gives off recurrent branches to the medial sector of the left lobe. However, the left lateral sector is supplied by separate branches that supply the two segments (segments II and III,). Segment I, the caudate lobe, receives blood supply from both the left and right portal pedicles; bile ducts from segment I also drain into the right and left hepatic ducts.

Portal Vein

The portal vein is a valveless structure that is formed by the confluence of the superior mesenteric vein and the splenic vein. The portal vein provides approximately 75 percent of the total liver blood supply by volume. In the hepatoduodenal ligament, the portal vein is found most commonly posterior to the bile duct and hepatic artery. The normal pressure in the portal vein is between 3 and 5 mmHg. Because the portal vein and its tributaries are without valves, increases in venous pressure are distributed throughout the splanchnic circulation. In the setting of portal venous hypertension, portosystemic collaterals develop secondary to the increased pressure. The most clinically important portosystemic connections include those fed through the coronary (left gastric) and short gastric veins through the fundus of the stomach and distal esophagus to the azygos vein, resulting in gastroesophageal varices. Recanalization of the round ligament/umbilical vein leads to a caput medusa around the umbilicus. Portal hypertension through the inferior mesenteric veins and hemorrhoidal plexuses can lead to engorged external hemorrhoids.

Hepatic Veins

The majority of the venous drainage of the liver occurs through three hepatic veins. The right hepatic vein drains segments V, VI, VII, and VIII, and enters directly into the vena cava. The middle hepatic vein drains segments IVA, IVB, V, and VIII, and enters into a common orifice with the left hepatic vein that drains segments II and III. A number of small short hepatic veins enter directly into the vena cava from the undersurface of the liver in segment I. Direct venous drainage into the vena cava is through small, short hepatic veins, although large segmental branches may also be present.

Hepatic Artery

From the level of the hepatic plate (the interface of the portal bifurcation with the liver capsule), the hepatic arterial anatomy is part of the portal triad and follows the segmental anatomy. The extrahepatic arterial anatomy can be highly variable. In roughly half of the population, the common hepatic artery arises from the celiac trunk, giving off the gastroduodenal artery followed by a right gastric artery. The proper hepatic artery gives rise to the right and left hepatic arteries. However, there is great variation in hepatic artery anatomy that is important to understand and detect in performing cholecystectomies, portal dissections, and liver resections. Replaced hepatic arteries are lobar vessels that arise from either the superior mesenteric artery (replaced right hepatic artery) or left gastric artery (replaced left hepatic artery). The replaced right hepatic artery travels posterior to the portal vein in close proximity to the posterior aspect of the pancreas and bile duct. A replaced right hepatic artery is felt behind both the bile duct and the portal vein when palpating the portal triad structures through the foramen of Winslow. The left hepatic artery, regardless of its origin, enters the liver at the base of the round ligament. A replaced or accessory left hepatic artery will run in the lesser omentum anterior to the caudate lobe and is typically very easily identified. In contrast to a replaced hepatic artery, an accessory hepatic artery is one that exists in addition to an anatomically typical originating vessel. Accessory right hepatic arteries often supply the posterior sector of the right lobe (segment VI and VII). An accessory left hepatic artery will typically supply the left lateral segment. The cystic artery most commonly arises from the right hepatic artery, but has a variety of common anomalies as well.

Biliary System

The bile duct arises at the cellular level from the hepatocyte membrane which coalesces with adjacent hepatocytes to form canaliculi. Larger collections of canaliculi form small ducts. The bile ducts follow the segmental anatomy of the intrahepatic vasculature as previously described. The confluence of the right and left hepatic ducts may be intrahepatic. The right hepatic duct is found to be largely intrahepatic, although the left hepatic duct is extrahepatic and runs perpendicular to the common hepatic duct to the level of the round ligament, in which it is formed by a confluence of ducts from segment IV and segments II/III. The confluence of the left and right hepatic ducts is cephalad and ventral to the portal vein bifurcation.

The hepatic bile duct confluence gives rise to the common hepatic duct, the duct between the confluence and the cystic duct takeoff. The common bile duct extends from the cystic duct to the ampulla of Vater. A normal common bile duct is less than 10 mm in diameter in the adult. The blood supply to the bile duct arises from the right hepatic artery superiorly and from the gastroduodenal artery inferiorly. A rich anastomosis between the right and left hepatic arteries has been demonstrated with corrosion cast analyses of the hilum, indicating that preservation of these intrahepatic anastomoses will preserve bile duct blood flow, even with extrahepatic ligation of one or the other arterial structures.

Lymphatics

The spaces of Disse and clefts of Mall produce lymph fluid at the cellular level that is collected through sub-Glissonian and periportal lymphatics that ultimately drain into larger lymphatics emptying through the porta hepatis into the cisterna chyli. The anatomy and physiology of lymphatic drainage is important in the development of ascites and in the process of tumor metastasis.

Neural Innervation

Parasympathetic fibers from the hepatic branches of the vagus nerve and both parasympathetic and sympathetic fibers derived from the celiac plexus innervate the liver and gallbladder, the latter traveling along the hepatic arteries. The functions of these nerves is not well understood, but liver transplantation shows that the nerves are not essential for normal liver function. Irritation or stretching of the Glisson capsule or gallbladder cause referred pain to the right shoulder through the third and forth cervical nerves.

INTERPRETATION OF LIVER TESTS

Liver tests are broken down into tests of liver function, parenchymal injury, and biliary obstruction (Table 30-1). The pattern of liver test abnormalities is more important than any individual test result. Deviation from this normal time course should prompt specific evaluation for potentially correctable vascular (portal vein thrombosis) or biliary (obstructive) pathology.

RADIOLOGIC EVALUATION OF THE LIVER

The liver most commonly is evaluated as part of right upper quadrant ultrasound studies for gallbladder disease. However, the indications for directed evaluation of the liver include screening or assessment of malignancy, the study of a newly diagnosed cirrhotic patient, or evaluation for living donor transplantation. A comprehensive understanding of the available tests is critical to patient management.

Ultrasound

Transcutaneous ultrasound is frequently the first radiologic evaluation performed on the liver. Ultrasound is an excellent test for identifying biliary tract stones and intrahepatic biliary ductal dilation. The echo-texture of the liver can suggest cirrhosis or fatty infiltration, and cystic and solid characteristics of tumors can be delineated. Ultrasonography is commonly used in programs that screen high-risk populations for the development of hepatocellular carcinoma (HCC). In studies from the United States and Europe, ultrasonography

TABLE 30-1 Serum Liver Tests

Parenchymal (hepatocytes)	AST, ALT
Canalicular (biliary)	ALP, 5′NT, GGT, bilirubin
Synthetic function and metabolism	INR, factors V and VII, bilirubin, albumin

ALP = alkaline phosphatase; ALT = alanine aminotransferase; AST = aspartate aminotransferase; 5′NT = 5′ nucleotidase; GGT = gamma glutamyl transferase; INR = International Normalized Ratio.

has been shown to be superior to serum α-fetoprotein (AFP) measurement to detect early HCC in patients who suffer from chronic viral hepatitis.

Intraoperative ultrasonography (IOUS) has become the gold standard against which all other diagnostic imaging modalities are compared to detect the number, extent, and association of tumors with intrahepatic blood vessels in both primary and metastatic liver tumors. IOUS can be performed laparoscopically or during laparotomy. Placement of the probe directly on the surface of the liver enhances discrimination and sensitivity. Laparoscopic evaluation and laparoscopic ultrasonography have reduced the rate of unwarranted exploratory laparotomies, and thereby increased the proportion of patients who undergo successful hepatic resection at the time of laparotomy. Like IOUS, laparoscopic ultrasonography detects small metastatic or primary liver tumors not visualized on preoperative computed tomography (CT) scans or magnetic resonance imaging (MRI) studies in up to 15 percent of patients. IOUS also can be used to map the line of resection as it relates to relevant vascular structures, to avoid and anticipate possible sources of bleeding. IOUS is necessary for intraoperative image-guided procedures such as biopsy and radiofrequency ablation (RFA).

Computed Tomography Scan

Modern CT scans are helical and are highly sensitive at spatial discrimination and quantitation of lesions in the liver. Lesions can be characterized as solid or cystic and the enhancement characteristics can be evaluated during the arterial, portal, and delayed phases. The smallest detectable lesion size is approximately 1 cm. Dual- and triple-phase bolus intravenous contrast helical CT is more accurate than standard CT or portal venous phase CT in detecting colorectal liver metastases. However, the overall detection rate compared to intraoperative and pathologic findings is still approximately 85 percent with a false-positive rate of up to 5 percent. For HCC, the helical CT detection rate for small tumors is less than that for detecting hepatic metastases. The detection rate of small HCCs (< 2 cm), 40–60 percent, is based on the difficulty of detecting small tumors in cirrhotic livers, particularly in reference to the problem of distinguishing HCC from macroregenerative nodules. CT remains the preferred method for evaluating the remainder of the abdomen. Among patients with liver metastases, a CT scan is used to evaluate for the presence of peritoneal disease, portal lymphadenopathy, and other remote lesions.

Magnetic Resonance Imaging

MRI technology also is rapidly advancing. MRI is somewhat less sensitive at spatial discrimination of lesions, but provides additional tumor characterization benefits that are not available with CT scanning. MRI scans are slightly less accurate than helical CT in detecting the extent of colorectal liver metastases, but are more sensitive for detecting early HCC and in distinguishing HCC from macroregenerative nodules. Contrast enhancement provides an evaluation of vascular enhancement similar to CT, but MRI allows for better differentiation of cystic lesions and hemangiomas using T2-weighted images. This technique also is useful in magnetic resonance cholangiography MRC). MRC is an excellent study for the evaluation of the intrahepatic biliary tree, and is critical to the operative planning for hilar bile duct malignancies requiring liver resection. Magnetic resonance venography is a very sensitive technique for the noninvasive study of the extrahepatic portal system, and is especially useful in confirming extrahepatic portal vein thrombosis.

Positron Emission Tomography

Positron emission tomography (PET) is a whole-body, multiaxial technology that has been used to detect a variety of cancers including melanoma, breast cancer, and colorectal cancer. 18F-fluorodeoxyglucose (FDG) is injected systemically through an intravenous catheter, and axial tomography is performed of the entire body. It has been called a metabolic imaging method because FDG is taken up by active tissues (e.g., the brain) and cancer. The FDG PET is especially useful in the evaluation of patients with hepatic metastases of colorectal cancer to rule out the presence of extrahepatic disease. Similarly to other diagnostic studies, PET does have a false-negative rate of 7–10 percent, but the false-positive rate appears to be significantly lower than this value. In patients with a history of colorectal cancer, a rising serum carcinoembryonic antigen (CEA) level, and no recurrent or metastatic disease evident on CT or MRI images of the chest, abdomen, and pelvis, PET images demonstrating hypermetabolic areas may provide a clue regarding the site of recurrent disease. PET has been less useful in the evaluation of patients with HCC, as many of these tumors do not have a significantly higher uptake of the radioisotope compared to the surrounding hepatic parenchyma. Until further studies are undertaken, the use of PET scanning should be tied very closely to other forms of axial imaging studies. One method is fusion of PET scans with CT scanning. If there is a failure to correlate a hypermetabolic focus on PET scan with a tumor mass on CT scan, then directed evaluation, including biopsy of the hypermetabolic focus, should be performed prior to proceeding with liver resection.

PERCUTANEOUS BIOPSY

The role of image-guided percutaneous biopsy has become less important as the sensitivity and specificity of radiologic imaging studies had improved. In patients with a clinical picture and radiologic findings that point to a specific type of lesion, percutaneous biopsy is rarely indicated to initiate liver-directed therapy. In patients in whom the diagnosis is not evident based on clinical and radiographic grounds, a percutaneous biopsy can be done safely using either ultrasound or CT guidance. The target lesion should be accessed through a quantity of normal liver tissue sufficient to avoid free rupture of tumor into the peritoneum. This is especially important with HCCs, which are friable and vascular lesions.

LIVER FAILURE

Liver failure can be divided into two general categories: acute and chronic. Acute liver failure is relatively uncommon, with approximately 5000 new cases reported annually in the United States. The pathophysiology is related to an acute, massive loss of hepatocyte functional mass. However, there are usually no long-term sequelae in survivors. In chronic liver failure (long-term liver injury)—whether derived from viral hepatitis, metabolic diseases, ethanol abuse, or toxins—ongoing and progressive hepatocyte necrosis produces a fibrotic response and liver cell regeneration that leads to cirrhosis. Twenty-five thousand people die each year from cirrhosis, making it the eighth leading cause of death from disease in the United States.

Cirrhosis is a histologic term that describes generalized hepatic fibrosis and nodular regeneration of the liver. Despite the wide variety of etiologies of cirrhosis, the histologic end results often are indistinguishable. As described earlier, one of the unique physiologic capabilities of the liver is regeneration. The response of the liver to hepatocyte necrosis is collapse of portal tracks with fibrous replacement and nodular regeneration.

Grossly, cirrhosis can be described as micronodular, macronodular, or mixed. The CT findings of cirrhosis can be subtle, but include right lobe atrophy, ascites, caudate lobe hypertrophy, recanalization of the umbilical vein, enlargement of the portal vein caliber and splenomegaly. Laboratory findings in the unsuspected and compensated cirrhotic patient may be absent or include mild elevations in serum transaminases, borderline thrombocytopenia, or elevations in the INR.

Risks of General Surgical Procedures in Portal Hypertension

The Child classification was originally developed to evaluate the risk of portocaval venous shunt surgery for portal hypertension, but it also has been shown to be useful in predicting the risks of other abdominal operations in cirrhotic patients and was subsequently modified by others (Table 30-2).

A dysregulation of the compensatory blood flow response (e.g., increased hepatic arterial flow in response to decreased portal vein flow) is seen in cirrhosis. A variety of studies have shown that American Society of Anesthesiologists (ASA) score, renal insufficiency, and higher Child scores are adverse prognostic factors that predict an increased probability of complications and mortality after an operation. In elective procedures, attention to preoperative control of ascites, electrolyte abnormalities, and coagulopathy are critical to the success of elective surgery. Prevention of postoperative ascites begins with restriction of sodium-containing intravenous fluids in the operating room. As ascites accumulates, continued fluid restriction, diuretic therapy, bedrest, and intermittent paracentesis may be needed. Chronic peritoneal catheter drainage should be avoided because of the risk of retrograde contamination of the peritoneal cavity. Ascites in this setting is highly morbid, especially if complicated by bacterial infection. Encephalopathy also should be anticipated. Administration of narcotic pain medicines and sedatives should be limited when possible, as the hepatic metabolism of most drugs is compromised.

TABLE 30-2 Revised Child Classification of Clinical Severity of Cirrhosis

	Class		
	A	B	C
Nutritional status	Excellent	Good	Poor
Ascites	None	Minimal, controlled	Moderate to severe
Encephalopathy	None	Minimal, controlled	Moderate to severe
Serum bilirubin (mg/dL)	< 2	2–3	> 3
Serum albumin (g/dL)	> 3.5	2.8–3.5	< 2.8
Prothrombin time (% of control)	> 70	40–70	< 40

Portal Hypertension

Portal hypertension may be classified as presinusoidal, sinusoidal, or postsinusoidal. Sinusoidal causes are the most common in the Western Hemisphere because of alcoholic cirrhosis that results from fibrous replacement in the space of Disse. Chronic liver insufficiency is common. Postsinusoidal portal hypertension often has a vascular etiology and also is associated with some degree of liver dysfunction. In contrast, patients with presinusoidal portal hypertension may have well-preserved hepatic function. Etiologies include schistosomiasis, extrahepatic portal vein thrombosis, and congenital hepatic fibrosis (most commonly seen in children).

Budd-Chiari Syndrome

Budd-Chiari syndrome, which is a rare cause of postsinusoidal liver failure and cirrhosis, can occur as a spectrum of presentations that range from asymptomatic disease to fulminant liver failure. The pathophysiology is related to thrombosis of the three major hepatic veins at the level of the inferior vena cava. The disease is more common in women and is associated with a variety of hypercoagulable states: protein C, S, or antithrombin III deficiency; polycythemia vera; lupus anticoagulant; estrogen exposure; myeloproliferative disorders; and Behçet disease. Patients often will present with jaundice, ascites and hepatomegaly. Transcutaneous Doppler-flow ultrasound will show thrombosed hepatic veins and may demonstrate large collaterals into the retrohepatic inferior vena cava. CT findings include striking caudate lobe hypertrophy and inhomogeneous contrast enhancement. Anticoagulation is the standard immediate therapy. Treatment of acute decompensated Budd-Chiari includes placement of a transjugular intrahepatic portosystemic shunt (TIPS) or a nonselective shunt.

Acute Bleeding

Patients with portal hypertension may require surgical intervention after an episode of acute upper gastrointestinal (GI) bleeding. After intravenous fluid resuscitation and correction of coagulation abnormalities, the single most important diagnostic and potentially therapeutic procedure to be performed in the cirrhotic patient with an upper GI bleed is endoscopy. The differential diagnosis must include sources other than bleeding from esophageal varices, because as many as 20 percent of patients will have bleeding from gastritis or duodenal ulcer disease.

Esophageal varices are the most common cause of massive bleeding in patients with cirrhosis, and result from shunting of blood through the coronary (left gastric) vein into the submucosal plexus of the esophagus. Prevention of the first bleeding event with prophylactic beta-adrenergic blockade is more effective than placebo, and the addition of a systemic vasodilator agent is slightly more efficacious, but at the expense of increased peripheral edema. Sclerotherapy, TIPS, or surgical shunts have not been associated with a reduction in first bleeding risk in Western, alcoholic-cirrhotic patients. Prophylaxis is important because variceal bleeding in cirrhotic patients is a grave prognostic event with 70 percent of patients dying within 1 year.

The most critical treatment for acute hemorrhage in cirrhotic patients is prompt endoscopic intervention and therapy. Acute esophageal variceal bleeding can be managed with endoscopic variceal banding in 85 percent of patients. Administration of intravenous vasopressin or octreotide can decrease splanchnic blood flow, and are useful in reducing bleeding from esophageal varices in the acute phase of management.

Hepatic encephalopathy from absorption of the intestinal blood load, and azotemia from large-volume blood replacement, should be anticipated. It may be necessary to use oral or nasogastric lactulose elixir to promote catharsis. Emergency TIPS is successful in treating acute bleeding and in preventing rebleeding in approximately 80 percent of patients. The procedure has supplanted the surgical shunt at most institutions for the treatment of refractory bleeding.

Surgical shunts are associated with long-term survival rates of more than 70 percent in Child class A and B patients. A nonselective portocaval shunt will have the most immediate and durable effect in the acute setting. In patients who are potential liver transplant candidates, an interposition mesocaval shunt or central splenorenal shunt will avoid portal dissection and not complicate a subsequent liver transplant operation. If the patient has complete portal vein thrombosis, an end-to-side portocaval shunt will be effective and is technically straightforward.

Prevention of Rebleeding

Repeated endoscopic therapy employing sclerotherapy or banding can eradicate varices and prevent rebleeding in up to 80 percent of patients in the first year. Use of beta-adrenergic blockade or octreotide has been demonstrated to significantly reduce rebleeding rates in combination with endoscopic therapy. In the cirrhotic patient with significant hepatic dysfunction, liver transplantation must be considered. The long-term outlook in patients with preserved hepatic function may be significantly different, and these patients are candidates for surgical shunts.

Portosystemic Shunts

Transjugular intrahepatic portosystemic shunt. The TIPS procedure is minimally invasive and creates the equivalent of a nonselective surgical shunt. The indications for TIPS include bleeding refractory to endoscopic and medical management, refractory ascites, Budd-Chiari syndrome, and hepatopulmonary syndromes. The procedure involves the placement of an expandable wire mesh stent between the middle hepatic vein and region of the portal bifurcation using ultrasound and radiographic direction. The stent is expanded to a diameter that reduces the portosystemic gradient to less than 12 mmHg. TIPS is associated with postprocedure encephalopathy rates of approximately 25 percent, and patients with renal insufficiency are at risk for worsened renal function. The long-term problem with TIPS is stenosis of the shunt, which occurs in as many as two thirds of patients.

Surgical shunts. Surgical shunts are best used in patients with relatively well-preserved liver function (Child class A and B) who are not candidates for liver transplantation or who have limited access to the medical surveillance necessary for TIPS monitoring. Patients who may require liver transplant in the future (> 1 year) are also candidates for surgical shunts because surgical shunt patency is superior to that of TIPS.

Surgical shunts can be divided into two general categories: selective and nonselective. Nonselective shunts are associated with a high risk of encephalopathy, especially in patients with marginal liver function. Selective shunts are associated with a lower incidence of encephalopathy, as they maintain hepatopetal flow although lowering portal pressure. Currently, the most useful surgical shunts are the small-diameter portacaval H graft shunt and distal splenorenal shunt (DSRS).

In general, nonselective shunts are appropriate for the management of medically refractory bleeding in the patient with preserved liver function who is not a liver transplant candidate and who has intractable ascites. In patients with complete intrahepatic portal vein thrombosis, an end-to-side portocaval shunt is the easiest to perform and the most effective shunt.

LIVER INFECTIONS

Pyogenic Liver Abscesses

Pyogenic liver abscesses have been well known for over 100 years and were a common cause of morbidity and mortality in patients with untreated appendicitis and pylephlebitis. Currently, the most common etiologies of pyogenic liver abscesses include biliary tract manipulation, diverticular disease, inflammatory bowel disease, and systemic infections such as bacterial endocarditis.

The clinical presentation of patients with pyogenic liver abscesses is rarely subtle. Patients present with right upper quadrant abdominal pain, fever, and occasionally jaundice. In patients with chronic symptomatology, fever and weight loss with progressive fatigue may be seen. Interestingly, as many as one third of patients with pyogenic liver abscesses will not have an identifiable primary source of infection.

Ultrasound examination will demonstrate a cystic mass in the liver, often with multiple complex septations or in homogeneous fluid characteristics. CT findings will include a complex hypodense mass with peripheral enhancement. In patients with a solitary dominant abscess, percutaneous aspiration with evaluation by gram stain and culture is essential to direct further antimicrobial and drainage therapy. The placement of a percutaneous drainage catheter at the time of aspiration is beneficial for patients with a complex abscess or an abscess containing particularly thick fluid. In an immunosuppressed patient who has multiple abscesses, hepatosplenic candidiasis should be considered, and more conventional pyogenic etiologies.

In patients with intraabdominal sources leading to hepatic abscesses, Gram-negative aerobes, Gram-positive aerobes, and anaerobes are the predominant organisms found in liver abscesses. Commonly encountered organisms include *Escherichia coli*, *Klebsiella pneumoniae*, *Enterococcus faecalis* and *faecium*, and anaerobic or facultative anaerobic species such as *Bacteroides fragilis*. In patients with systemic infections from subacute bacterial endocarditis and indwelling catheter infections, Staphylococcus and Streptococcus species are more common. Monomicrobial abscesses are found in approximately 40 percent of patients, an additional 40 percent are polymicrobial, although the remaining cases are culture negative.

Parasitic Liver Abscesses

Hydatid Disease

Cystic hydatid disease is caused by the larval/cyst stage of *Echinococcus granulosus*, in which humans are an intermediate host. Hydatid cysts can be uncomplicated and asymptomatic. However, these lesions may rupture, can become secondarily infected, or may infect other organs. The diagnosis is based on an enzyme-linked immunosorbent assay (ELISA) test for echinococcal antigens, which is positive in over 85 percent of infected patients. Ultrasound and CT scanning will typically demonstrate either simple or complex cysts with a cyst wall of varying thickness. The treatment of hydatid disease involves the use of oral anthelmintics such as albendazole. In patients with anatomically appropriate lesions percutaneous aspiration, instillation of absolute alcohol, and reaspiration (PAIR) is the preferred initial treatment. The efficacy of PAIR in managing hydatid cysts is greater than 75 percent. For patients whose disease is refractory to PAIR, laparoscopic or open complete cyst removal with instillation of a scolicidal agent generally is curative. If surgical cystectomy with removal of the germinal laminated layers is not technically feasible, then formal liver resection can be employed. During aspiration or surgical treatment of hydatid cysts, extreme caution must be taken to avoid rupture of the cyst with release of protoscolices into the peritoneal cavity.

Amebiasis

Entamoeba histolytica enters into humans in a cyst form but transforms into a trophozoite in the colon. It enters into the colonic mucosa and invades the portal venous system, infecting the liver. Although resulting from a colonic infection, a recent history of severe diarrhea is uncommon. Patients typically present with sweating and chills, usually of at least 1 week duration. Fevers can be high and patients typically have right upper quadrant abdominal pain and tenderness. The majority of patients have a positive fluorescent antibody test for *E. histolytica* and mild abnormalities in liver enzymes; hyperbilirubinemia is relatively uncommon.

In patients who live in or who have recently visited an endemic area and who present with right upper quadrant tenderness and hepatomegaly, an ultrasound showing an abscess should be considered diagnostic for the presence of amebiasis. Patients diagnosed with amebic liver abscesses should be treated with metronidazole for at least 1 week. Most patients will respond rapidly with complete defervescence within 3 days. Aspiration of the abscess is rarely necessary and should be avoided, except in patients in whom secondary infection from pyogenic organisms is suspected.

CYSTIC DISEASES OF THE LIVER

Noninfectious cystic lesions in the liver are common throughout all decades of life. The vast majority of hepatic cysts are asymptomatic and are found incidentally. Cysts can be categorized as congenital or neoplastic.

Congenital Cysts

Congenital cysts include simple hepatic cysts, which are the most common benign lesions found in the liver. Simple cysts result from excluded hyperplastic bile duct rests and they are commonly identified on imaging studies as unilocular, homogeneous fluid-filled structures with a thin wall without projections. The epithelium of the cyst secretes clear fluid that does not contain bile, and they rarely are symptomatic unless they are large, in which case patients may complain of pain, epigastric fullness or a mass, or early satiety related to gastric compression. Simple aspiration is not recommended as an initial therapy; however, useful information about symptom resolution often is obtained. PAIR has a success rate as high as 80 percent. In patients with easily accessible lesions and appropriate interventional radiology support, PAIR is an excellent first line of therapy in the management of simple, congenital, hepatic cysts.

The surgical management of simple cysts centers on wide cyst fenestration. These procedures are performed laparoscopically, if technically feasible. The recurrence rate after wide cyst fenestration is usually less than 5 percent. The excised cyst wall is sent for pathologic analysis, and the remaining cyst wall within the liver should be carefully examined for the presence of gross neoplastic changes. Cystic fluid analysis by cytology and tumor markers is not indicated unless there is concern for neoplasia. A symptomatic simple cyst rarely requires complete resection, either as an enucleation or as a formal liver resection.

Polycystic Liver Disease

Polycystic disease occurs as an autosomal dominant disease presenting in adulthood. An autosomal recessive process that is associated with hepatic fibrosis also occurs in rare instances in infancy. A wide spectrum of clinical and anatomic presentations is seen in polycystic liver disease (PCLD). Symptoms of fullness, early satiety, dysphagia, and pain are often chronic and unrelenting, and as with any consideration for liver surgery of benign processes, other contributing factors should be ruled out.

In patients with dominant cysts and associated symptoms, PAIR should be used for the initial approach to manage symptoms. Obliteration of a treated cyst is normally seen in 80 percent of cases; however, careful patient selection is necessary to avoid recurrence. In patients who are not candidates for PAIR or who have failed PAIR, fenestration or resection of the cyst(s) should be undertaken. Formal lobectomy along the border of the majority of the cystic disease may be required and is expected to be associated with a durable correction of symptoms in up to 90 percent of carefully selected patients. In patients with massive hepatomegaly but no dominant anatomic presentation, a transverse hepatectomy (resection of segments III, IVB, V, and VI at the level of the rib cage) has been reported to be associated with excellent improvement of symptoms.

Neoplastic Cysts

Neoplastic cysts are more common in women and in those individuals older than 40 years of age. Neoplastic cysts tend to have papillary excrescences and may have multiple loculations within the cyst. Percutaneous aspiration is rarely indicated, but if performed will typically yield mucinous fluid.

The surgical management of neoplastic cysts further relies on the initial differentiation between biliary cystadenoma and biliary cystadenocarcinoma. Biliary cystadenocarcinoma is uncommon and is associated with marked thickening of the cyst wall and vascular enhancement on axial imaging studies. Biliary cystadenomas can be either enucleated or resected as dictated by the anatomy.

BENIGN SOLID LIVER TUMORS

Benign solid liver tumors are increasingly identified with the more common use of axial imaging studies. Differentiation of benign tumors from malignancies including metastatic lesions is achieved based on the clinical scenario and interpretation of radiologic images.

Hepatic Adenoma

Hepatic adenomas (e.g., liver cell adenoma and hepatocellular adenoma) are the most significant benign liver tumors that surgeons encounter. These lesions occur in reproductive-aged women, and are an order of magnitude more common in women who use oral contraceptive pills (OCPs). Histologically, these lesions are composed of sheets of hepatocytes with no nonparenchymal cells (Kupffer cells) or bile ducts present. Up to 75 percent of adenomas may be symptomatic at the time of presentation, with abdominal pain being the most common presenting symptom. Hepatocellular adenomas are significant in that they can rupture and as many as 25 percent of these lesions are identified after an acute episode of hemorrhage.

Radiographically, it is difficult to distinguish hepatic adenomas from focal nodular hyperplasia (FNH). Both lesions demonstrate rapid contrast enhancement followed by rapid washout of contrast within the tumor on CT scan and MRI. Adenomas may demonstrate increased fat signal on MRI when compared to FNH, and do not have a central scar, which is frequently seen in FNH.

The management of patients with hepatic adenomas is evolving. Cessation of OCPs in patients with lesions less than 4 cm in diameter is prudent. Regression of the lesion is commonly seen and such a regression may obviate or facilitate liver-directed intervention. Surgical intervention is recommended in patients with lesions larger than 4 cm in diameter, in patients whose lesions do not shrink after cessation of OCP use, those who medically cannot stop OCP use, or in patients who plan to become pregnant.

Focal Nodular Hyperplasia

In contrast to hepatic adenomas, focal nodular hyperplasia typically is not associated with symptoms and does not pose any risks of rupture or malignant degeneration. Characteristically, up to two thirds of lesions will demonstrate a central scar. The lesions are often peripherally located and histologically composed of regenerative nodules with hyperplastic bile ducts and connective tissue septae.

FNH is rarely symptomatic. Therefore other etiologies for symptoms should be explored. In patients with symptoms related to FNH, resection is indicated. Because the lesions often are peripheral, minimally invasive (laparoscopic) approaches to resection should be advocated for the experienced surgeon.

Hemangiomas

Hemangiomas, also known as cavernous hemangiomas, are common benign liver lesions generally discovered incidentally on axial imaging studies. Patients with hemangiomas may present with chronic low-intensity right upper quadrant abdominal pain, especially when the lesions are quite large. Ultrasound can be helpful in identifying hemangiomas, but a CT scan or contrast-enhanced MRI are diagnostic. CT and MRI will demonstrate peripheral nodular contrast enhancement followed by gradual centripetal enhancement, and finally washout of contrast in the lesion on further delayed films. On MRI, these lesions will be bright on T2-weighted evaluation. In rare instances, hemangiomas are difficult to differentiate on MRI and are termed atypical hemangiomas. An atypical hemangioma can be further evaluated using 99Tc-labeled red cell study. Angiography is rarely necessary.

As with other benign lesions, when symptoms are present other causes of abdominal pain should always be ruled out. Resection can be recommended if symptoms can be clearly ascribed to a large hemangioma. Hemangiomas can be resected by enucleation or more standard formal liver resection. Enucleation of hemangiomas follows the line of compressed liver tissue, and great care must be taken to ensure control of any biliary radicals that are opened in the process.

Bile Duct Hamartomas

Bile duct hamartomas are the most common liver lesions seen at laparotomy. Hamartomas are peripheral in location, and are firm, smooth, and white in appearance. They are less than 1 cm in size and usually only 1–3 mm in diameter. The lesions can be difficult to differentiate from miliary metastatic lesions, especially those derived from colorectal cancer and bile duct cancers. Biopsy is indicated for grossly equivocal lesions.

MALIGNANT LIVER TUMORS

Hepatocellular cancer (HCC) is one of the most common solid human cancers, with an annual incidence estimated to be approximately 1 million new patients. In addition to being a common site for the development of primary malignancy, the liver is second only to lymph nodes as a common site of metastasis from other solid cancers. It is not uncommon, particularly in patients with colorectal adenocarcinoma, for the liver to be the only site of metastatic disease. Surgical resection of HCC, colorectal cancer hepatic metastases, and carefully selected patients with liver-only metastases from other types of primary tumors can result in significant long-term survival benefit in 20–45 percent of patients.

Indications for Resection

The important role of liver resection as a treatment for colorectal cancer metastases was solidified by the report in 1988 from the Registry of Hepatic Metastases. This retrospective chart review from 24 institutions identified 859 patients who underwent resection of colorectal liver metastases between 1948 and 1985. The 5-year actuarial survival rate in these patients was 33 percent, with a 5-year actuarial disease-free survival rate of 21 percent.

The Registry of Hepatic Metastases report is a retrospective review of patients who underwent operation largely before the availability of adequate preoperative and intraoperative imaging modalities. Furthermore, careful pathologic analysis and an accurate count of the number of lesions were not available in all of the patients. Most of the patients were identified by the development of symptoms, abnormalities in serum liver tests, or an elevated serum tumor marker in the later period of the study. The study included 509 (59 percent) patients with a solitary liver metastasis, indicating that this was a highly selected group of patients. Of the 149 patients who had three or more metastases, a breakdown of survival by number of metastases was not provided, and the actuarial 5-year survival rate for this group was 18 percent.

Recent re-evaluations of the number of metastases that should be considered for resection have demonstrated that there is a potential survival benefit in patients with four or more metastases. A study of 235 patients from Japan who underwent hepatic resection for metastatic colorectal cancer included 53 patients (22.6 percent) who had more than four metastases, including some patients with as many as 10–15 lesions. The actuarial 10-year life expectancy of patients with four or more lesions was 29 percent, which was almost equivalent to the long-term survival of patients who underwent resection of a solitary metastasis. Patients with two or three metastases actually had a slightly worse long-term survival than patients with more than four tumors. A study from the United States of 155 patients who underwent resection of more than four colorectal liver metastases revealed an overall 5-year survival rate of 23 percent. As the number of resected metastases increased above nine, there was a significant reduction in long-term survival probability. On multivariate analysis, only positive resection margins and a large number of metastases were significant prognostic indicators for poor outcome.

The indications for resection of HCC also have been re-evaluated. Studies from the 1980s and early 1990s suggested that the presence of cirrhosis or multiple tumors were harbingers of poor outcome after resection of HCC. However, these studies were performed during a time when operative mortality rates in cirrhotic HCC patients ranged from 6–15 percent, and the need for intraoperative and postoperative blood transfusion was common. Improved outcomes have been demonstrated in more recent studies in which modern hepatic resection techniques were employed. Specifically, perioperative blood transfusion rates fell from 69–87 percent in the earlier time period to 23–39 percent in more recent series. The operative and hospital death rate was reduced from 13.2 percent to under 2 percent, and 5-year survival rates improved from 19–32 percent to 25–49 percent, despite all patients harboring pathologically proven cirrhosis.

Laparoscopic Hepatic Resection

Laparoscopy has a definite role in the diagnosis and staging of patients with gastrointestinal malignancies. A therapeutic role for laparoscopic liver resection has yet to be established. The development of endoscopic vascular staplers and the harmonic scalpel have increased interest in laparoscopic approaches to benign and malignant liver tumors, although minimally invasive liver resection has not advanced as far as laparoscopic colon, adrenal, and spleen resection. The large majority of liver resection cases completed laparoscopically have been left lateral segmentectomies, segmental or partial segmental resections, or wedge resections. Laparoscopic ultrasonography is performed to localize tumors and to mark the surface of the liver with electrocautery to ensure an adequate margin-negative resection. The parenchyma can be transected using endovascular staplers, the harmonic scalpel, or with finger fracture through a hand port using a pneumosleeve.

Repeat Hepatectomy for Recurrent Malignant Tumors

The long-term, disease-free survival rates for patients undergoing surgical resection of primary or metastatic liver tumors is usually below 40 percent in the most optimistic reports, and may be below 20 percent in others. Clearly, the majority of patients develop recurrent malignant disease after hepatic resection. In a subset of these patients, the only site of recurrence will be new tumor deposits in the liver. Yet a further subset of these patients may have undergone significant hepatic regeneration and have tumors in locations amenable to repeat liver resection.

The group of patients most frequently considered for repeat hepatectomy are those with recurrent colorectal metastases. Only 10–15 percent of patients who develop recurrent disease after liver resection for colorectal metastases will be considered as candidates for a second or third resection. The incidence of extrahepatic disease in patients being considered for repeat hepatectomy may be as high as 30 percent; thus they should undergo thorough preoperative evaluation with state-of-the-art helical CT imaging and PET scans. Although technically challenging because of adhesions and altered vascular anatomy related to the previous hepatic resection, repeat hepatectomy can be performed with low morbidity and mortality rates.

Repeat hepatic resection also may be applied in selected patients with HCC. Intrahepatic recurrence as the only site of disease is more common in HCC patients than those with metastatic liver tumors, but the number of patients who are candidates for repeated surgical treatment is less than 10 percent of those who develop recurrent disease. Patients who develop hepatic recurrence of HCC after hepatic resection of their primary tumor may not be candidates for repeat resection because of multifocality, vascular invasion by tumor, or the severity of underlying cirrhosis. In properly selected patients, repeat hepatic resection for HCC can be performed and result in long-term survival rates of up to 30 percent.

Portal Vein Embolization

Direct tumor invasion of a lobar portal vein branch may lead to ipsilateral hepatic lobe atrophy and contralateral lobe hypertrophy. The development of compensatory hypertrophy of a lobe or segments of the liver following tumor occlusion of contralateral portal venous branches led to the concept of planned portal vein embolization (PVE) to initiate hypertrophy in segments of the liver that would remain following a major liver resection.

Indications for Portal Vein Embolization

In patients with normal hepatic parenchyma, preservation of a perfused section of liver comprising 25 percent of the total hepatic volume is usually sufficient to prevent major postoperative complications and hepatic insufficiency. This 25 percent value has been determined somewhat empirically, and there is a paucity of data regarding the exact volume of liver that can be resected safely without postoperative liver failure when the remaining liver parenchyma is completely normal. The functional capacity of liver compromised by cholestasis, acute or chronic inflammation, steatosis, or cirrhosis is variable. A larger future liver remnant is required to avoid posthepatectomy hepatic insufficiency or failure in patients with diseased hepatic parenchyma. Two recent studies suggest that at least 40 percent of the total hepatic volume should remain to minimize postoperative complications in patients who have underlying chronic liver disease or who have received high-dose chemotherapy.

Preoperative Volumetric Determination of the Future Liver Remnant

Rapid-sequence, thin-section, helical CT is used to make direct measurements of total liver volume, volume of the liver to be resected, and volume of the future liver remnant. The total liver volume also can be estimated based on the described association between body surface area (BSA) and the total liver volume, in which total liver volume $= 706.2 \times BSA$ (in m^2) $+ 2.4$. The future liver remnant volume, for example the volume of segments I, II, and III in a patient undergoing an extended right hepatectomy, can be directly measured on a helical CT, and then divided by the total estimated liver volume to calculate the percentage of the future liver remnant. If the future liver remnant is estimated to be too small when also considering the presence or absence of chronic liver disease, PVE may be considered to increase the size of the future liver remnant.

Approach for Portal Vein Embolization

A percutaneous transhepatic approach has become the standard technique for PVE. The principal advantage of this technique is that it allows direct access to the portal venous branches of the lobe and segments to be embolized via an ipsilateral approach. This technique minimizes the risk of thrombosis of the main trunk of the portal vein and vascular injury to the portal venous branches supplying the future liver remnant. The side effects are minor and transient and include pain from the transhepatic access site and low-grade fever.

It is important to embolize not only the main right portal vein, but also the portal venous branches to segment IV if an extended right hepatic lobectomy is planned. Systematic embolization of segment IV branches is imperative for two reasons. First, all segments of the liver-bearing tumor are embolized to minimize the risk of accelerated tumor growth. Accelerated tumor growth has been reported when incomplete right trisectoral embolization has been performed. Second, embolization of segment IV portal vein branches in addition to the main right portal vein may contribute to better hypertrophy of segments I, II, and III prior to the extended right hepatic lobectomy.

Results After Portal Vein Embolization

Preoperative PVE has been used to treat primary liver malignancies, including HCC and cholangiocarcinoma, and metastatic liver tumors, particularly colorectal cancer metastases. Studies that report outcome after PVE indicate that the predicted future liver remnant volume increased from 19–36 percent of total liver volume preembolization to 31–59 percent postembolization. Complications are rare (0–10 percent) and there were no reported deaths after PVE. Not all patients who undergo PVE undergo surgery, because some patients fail to develop adequate hypertrophy, or more commonly will develop intrahepatic or extrahepatic progression of their disease in the interval between PVE and the planned resection.

Almost 250 reported extended liver resections have been performed following PVE. Perioperative mortality rates range from 0–7 percent, with no significantly higher mortality rate in cirrhotic compared to noncirrhotic patients. The reported complication rate of more than 15 percent following extended hepatic resection in patients who first underwent PVE is equivalent or better than most reports describing complication rates following this type of procedure without preoperative PVE. Unfortunately, few of the studies report long-term outcome and survival data.

RADIOFREQUENCY ABLATION

A radiofrequency (RF) needle electrode is advanced into the liver tumor to be treated via either a percutaneous, laparoscopic, or open (laparotomy) route. Using transcutaneous or intraoperative ultrasonography to guide placement, the needle electrode is advanced to the targeted area of the tumor, and then the individual wires or tines of the electrode are deployed into the tissues. Once the tines have been deployed, the needle electrode is attached to a RF generator and dispersive electrodes (return or grounding pads) are placed on the patient, one or two on each thigh. The RF energy is then applied following an established treatment algorithm to create a zone of cellular necrosis. Tumors less than 2.5 cm in their greatest dimension can be ablated with the placement of a needle electrode with an array diameter of 3.5–4.0 cm when the electrode is positioned in the center of the tumor. Tumors larger than 2.5 cm require more than one deployment of the needle electrode. For larger tumors, multiple placements and deployments of the electrode array may be necessary to completely destroy the tumor. To mimic a surgical margin in these unresectable tumors, the needle electrode is used to produce a thermal lesion that incorporates not only the tumor, but also nonmalignant liver parenchyma in a zone 1-cm wide surrounding the tumor. Tumors in proximity to major blood vessels also may require additional probe deployment and duration of RFA, as these structures can act as heat sinks.

Indications for Radiofrequency Ablation of Liver Tumors

RF energy has been used to produce coagulative necrosis in hepatic malignancies in patients who did not meet the criteria for resectability of HCC and metastatic liver tumors, and yet were candidates for a liver-directed procedure based on the presence of disease confined to the liver. The selection of patients to be treated with RFA is based on rational principles and goals. Any local therapy for malignant hepatic tumors, be it surgical resection, RFA, or some other tumor ablative technique, is generally performed with curative intent; however, a significant proportion of patients will subsequently develop hepatic or extrahepatic recurrence from their coexistent micrometastatic disease. Occasionally, patients with tumor types usually associated with disseminated, systemic metastatic disease, such as breast or renal cancer, may be considered for RFA if they have been treated with at least 6 months of effective systemic chemotherapy, and have only liver metastasis. Thus RFA should be performed only in patients with no preoperative or intraoperative evidence of extrahepatic disease, and only for tumor histologies with a reasonable probability of disease metastatic only to the liver. The notable exception to considering RFA in patients with low-volume extrahepatic disease and multiple liver metastases is the subgroup of patients with functional endocrine syndromes from neuroendocrine tumor liver metastases, as some patients can survive years with their disease. The goal of RFA in this group is to perform a safe, palliative, rather than curative, treatment.

RFA can be used to treat patients with a solitary hepatic tumor in a location that precludes a margin-negative hepatic resection, such as a tumor nestled between the inferior vena cava and the entry of the three hepatic veins into the liver. The only area of the liver to avoid when treating a tumor with RFA is the hilar plate in which the portal vein and hepatic arterial branches enter the liver. Although these blood vessels can tolerate the heat associated with the RFA treatment, the large bile ducts coursing with them do not, and biliary fistulae or strictures are likely to occur. Lastly, RFA is ideally suited to treat small HCCs in cirrhotic patients who may not be candidates for resection based on the severity of their liver dysfunction.

When considering patients for a combined approach of liver resection of large tumors and RFA of smaller lesions in the opposite lobe, standard surgical considerations apply. Thus an adequate volume of perfused, functional hepatic parenchyma must remain to avoid postoperative liver failure. The volume of liver that must remain varies from patient to patient, depending on the presence of normal liver versus diseased liver related to chronic hepatitis viral infection, ethanol abuse, or some other cause of chronic hepatic inflammation leading to cirrhosis. RFA does not replace standard hepatic resection in patients with resectable disease. RFA expands the population of patients who may be treated with aggressive liver-directed therapy in attempts to improve survival, quality of life, or palliation. Some patients heretofore not candidates for surgical therapy because of the presence of bilobar liver tumors now can be treated with a combination of liver resection and RFA.

Radiofrequency Ablation of Primary Liver Tumors

One hundred and ten HCC patients were followed for a minimum of 12 months after RFA; the median follow-up period was 19 months. Percutaneous or intraoperative RFA was performed in 76 (69 percent) and 34 patients (31 percent), respectively, and a total of 149 discrete HCC tumor nodules were treated with RFA. Local tumor recurrence at the RFA site developed in four patients (3.6 percent), all with tumors greater than 4.0 cm in diameter; all four subsequently developed recurrent HCC in other areas of the liver. New liver tumors or extrahepatic metastases developed in 50 patients (45.5 percent), but 56 patients (50.9 percent) had no evidence of recurrence. Clearly, a longer follow-up period is required to establish long-term, disease-free, and overall survival rates.

Procedure-related complications were minimal in patients with HCC. There were no treatment-related deaths, but complications developed in 12.7 percent of the HCC patients. The overall complication rate following RFA of HCC was low, which is particularly notable because there were 50 child class A, 31 class B, and 29 class C cirrhotic patients treated.

Radiofrequency Ablation of Metastatic Liver Tumors

Procedure-related complications were infrequent in patients with metastatic liver tumors. A few of the sites (10 percent) of intraoperative RFA expressed bleeding when the needle was withdrawn from the needle electrode track, but in all cases this was minimal (< 5 mL) and controlled easily with electrocauterization of the puncture site at the surface of the liver. Complications following RFA arose in less than 10 percent of the patients.

Local recurrence or persistence of metastatic tumors at the site of the RFA occurred in approximately 7 percent of the patients, and over 80 percent of the local recurrences developed in tumors more than 5 cm in diameter. All regions of recurrence or persistence were at the periphery of the necrotic tissue of the ablated tumors. No recurrence or persistence was noted within the center of the thermal lesions produced by RFA. New occurrences of additional hepatic or extrahepatic metastases were found in 46 percent of patients within 18 months post-RFA. The use of a combination of regional and systemic chemotherapy after RFA of colorectal cancer liver metastases to reduce recurrence and improve survival is currently under study by the authors.

The results of 109 patients with 172 metastatic hepatic lesions who underwent percutaneous RFA were described. The median follow-up period was 3 years (range 5–52 months), and local control was achieved in 121 (70 percent) of the lesions, but local recurrence developed in 51 (30 percent). Of these

51 lesions, 24 had repeat RFA and 11 (45 percent) achieved local control. A significant difference in local recurrence rates was observed when comparing lesions less than 3 cm (16 percent) to those greater than 3 cm (56 percent) in diameter. Median time to local recurrence was 16 months. There were no deaths and only one major complication (colonic perforation) after 162 RFA sessions (0.6 percent), with seven minor complications (4 percent). New metastases developed in 50 percent of the patients at a median time to recurrence of 12 months after RFA. Overall 2- and 3-year survival rates were 67 and 33 percent, respectively, with a median survival of 30 months. Thus percutaneous RFA was associated with a high incomplete treatment (local recurrence) rate because of less accurate resolution with transabdominal ultrasonography, making precise needle electrode placement to ablate the entire tumor and a surrounding rim of hepatic parenchyma more difficult.

Neuroendocrine tumors metastatic to the liver often produce symptoms secondary to excessive hormone production and release. Although only a minority of patients with neuroendocrine liver metastases may be curable by surgical techniques, significant symptomatic relief can be obtained by debulking, which may include resection combined with RFA, or RFA alone. One group reported 18 patients with 115 neuroendocrine tumors (carcinoid, islet cell, or medullary thyroid cancers) treated with RFA. The mean lesion size was 3.2 cm (range 1.3–10.0 cm), and the average number of lesions ablated per patient was six (range 1–14). Fifteen patients (83 percent) with 100 lesions were followed for a mean of 12.1 months (range 3–35 months). Local recurrence in tumors treated with RFA was detected in six lesions (6 percent) in three of these 15 patients (20 percent); three patients died of progressive metastatic disease during follow up. Although the exact number was not indicated, the authors reported that most patients had significant improvement in hormone-related symptoms following RFA.

MICROWAVE COAGULATION THERAPY FOR HEPATIC TUMORS

Background and Principles of Microwave Coagulation Therapy

The generators developed for microwave coagulation therapy (MCT) produce microwaves with a frequency of 2450 MHz and a wavelength of 12 cm. Biologically, microwaves applied to living tissues produce dielectric heat by stimulation of water molecules within the tissue and cells. The rapid agitation of water molecules within cells and tissues with direct application of microwaves produces rapid frictional heating and coagulative necrosis. The microwave generators available for clinical use have an output of 70–90 watts. The microwave-emitting needle (14–22-gauge) is placed directly into the hepatic tumor to be treated, usually using ultrasonographic guidance, then is attached to the microwave generator, the generator is activated, and each area of the tumor is treated for 30 to 60 s at 70–90 watts of power. The rapid generation of heat using MCT produces 10–25-mm zones of coagulative necrosis after only 30–60 s. The lesions can range from spherical to elliptical in shape. The rapid development of coagulative necrosis within the tissue around the MCT needle produces a tissue coagulum that inhibits further dissipation of heat into the tissue. MCT can be performed percutaneously using ultrasound or CT guidance for needle placement, or can be performed laparoscopically or during an open surgical procedure using intraoperative ultrasound guidance to place the MCT needle.

Results of Microwave Coagulation Therapy for Treatment of Malignant Hepatic Tumors

A study of 19 patients with unresectable HCC reported that MCT was performed during laparotomy in 12 patients, laparoscopically in 5 patients, and using a thoracotomy approach in two patients with tumors at the dome of the liver. A solitary HCC tumor was treated in 13 patients, although the remaining six patients had between two and five HCC tumors treated with MCT. MCT was performed to palliate symptoms from a large tumor in 6 of the 19 patients who had additional intrahepatic or extrahepatic metastases. The mean size of the tumors treated with MCT was 21 mm (range 5–90 mm), and the mean duration of operation was 4.7 h (range 1.8–7.0 h). The reproducible and reliable zone of complete coagulative necrosis around the MCT needle electrode is only 10 mm; thus the mean number of electrode insertions to treat the HCC tumors was 46 (range 10–135). The authors report that the follow-up period in these patients ranged from 4–64 months; there were two patients treated with curative intent who were alive 47 and 64 months, respectively, after MCT, with no evidence of recurrent or new metastatic HCC. In the entire group of 19 patients, six patients had died of recurrent HCC or progressive liver failure, 10 were alive without radiographic evidence of recurrent HCC, and three were alive with evidence of new HCC metastases. The authors reported that there was no evidence of local recurrence in 28 of the 31 nodules (90 percent) treated with MCT. However, it is difficult to assess the true local recurrence rate, because most of the patients were treated with hepatic arterial chemoembolization after MCT.

There is a striking paucity of data on local recurrence rates and complications following MCT to treat HCC or other malignant liver tumors. Some authors mention that MCT should not be performed near the hepatic hilum, where major bile ducts and blood vessels are located, or near any major hepatic blood vessels, suggesting that there is experience with vascular and biliary complications related to treatment of tumors in these locations. It is unlikely that MCT will be widely applied to treat patients with unresectable malignant hepatic tumors unless modifications in equipment and treatment algorithms occur to produce larger zones of coagulative necrosis around the MCT needle.

Suggested Readings

Harisinghani MG, Hahn PF: Computed tomography and magnetic resonance imaging evaluation of liver cancer. Gastroenterol Clin North Am 31:759, 2002.

Helton WS, Maves R, Wicks K, et al: Transjugular intrahepatic portasystemic shunt vs. surgical shunt in good-risk cirrhotic patients: A case-control comparison. Arch Surg 136:17, 2001.

Horton KM, Bluemke DA, Hruban RH, et al: CT and MR imaging of benign hepatic and biliary tumors. Radiographics 19:431, 1999.

Bilimoria MM, Lauwers GY, Doherty DA, et al: Underlying liver disease, not tumor factors, predicts long-term survival after resection of hepatocellular carcinoma. Arch Surg 136:528, 2001.

Resection of the liver for colorectal carcinoma metastases: A multi-institutional study of indications for resection. Registry of Hepatic Metastases. Surgery 103:278, 1988.

Minagawa M, Makuuchi M, Torzilli G, et al: Extension of the frontiers of surgical indications in the treatment of liver metastases from colorectal cancer: Long-term results. Ann Surg 231:487, 2000.

Abdalla EK, Barnett CC, Doherty DA, et al: Extended hepatectomy in hepatobiliary malignancies with and without preoperative portal vein embolization. Arch Surg 137:675, 2002.

Curley SA, Izzo F, Ellis LM, et al: Radiofrequency ablation of hepatocellular cancer in 110 patients with cirrhosis. Ann Surg 232:381, 2000.

Sato M, Watanabe Y, Ueda S, et al: Microwave coagulation therapy for hepatocellular carcinoma. Gastroenterology 110:1507, 1996.

Abdalla EK, Vauthey JN, Ellis LM, Ellis V, Pollock R, Broglio KR, Hess K, Curley SA. Recurrence and outcomes following hepatic resection, radiofrequency ablation and combined resection/ablation for colorectal liver metastases. Ann Surg 2004;239: 818–827.

31 | Gallbladder and Extrahepatic Biliary System

Margrét Oddsdóttir and John G. Hunter

ANATOMY

The Gallbladder

The gallbladder is a pear-shaped sac, about 7–10 cm long with an average capacity of 30–50 mL. When obstructed, the gallbladder can distend markedly and contain up to 300 mL. The same peritoneal lining that covers the liver covers the fundus and the inferior surface of the gallbladder. The gallbladder is lined by a single, highly folded, tall columnar epithelium that contains cholesterol and fat globules. The epithelial lining of the gallbladder is supported by a lamina propria. The muscle layer has circular longitudinal and oblique fibers, but without well-developed layers. The perimuscular subserosa contains connective tissue, nerves, vessels, lymphatics, and adipocytes. It is covered by the serosa except where the gallbladder is embedded in the liver. The gallbladder differs histologically from the rest of the gastrointestinal tract in that it lacks a muscularis mucosa and submucosa.

The cystic artery that supplies the gallbladder usually is a branch of the right hepatic artery (>90 percent of the time). The course of the cystic artery may vary, but it nearly always is found within the hepatocystic triangle, the area bound by the cystic duct, common hepatic duct, and the liver margin (triangle of Calot). Venous return is carried either through small veins that enter directly into the liver, or rarely to a large cystic vein that carries blood back to the portal vein. Gallbladder lymphatics drain into nodes at the neck of the gallbladder. Frequently, a visible lymph node overlies the insertion of the cystic artery into the gallbladder wall. The nerves of the gallbladder arise from the vagus and from sympathetic branches that pass through the celiac plexus.

The Bile Ducts

The extrahepatic bile ducts consist of the right and left hepatic ducts, the common hepatic duct, the cystic duct, and the common bile duct or choledochus. The common bile duct enters the second portion of the duodenum through a muscular structure, the sphincter of Oddi.

The left hepatic duct is longer than the right and has a greater propensity for dilatation as a consequence of distal obstruction. The two ducts join to form a common hepatic duct, close to their emergence from the liver. The common hepatic duct is 1–4 cm in length and has a diameter of approximately 4 mm. It lies in front of the portal vein and to the right of the hepatic artery. The common hepatic duct is joined at an acute angle by the cystic duct to form the common bile duct.

Variations of the cystic duct and its point of union with the common hepatic duct are surgically important. The segment of the cystic duct adjacent to the gallbladder neck bears a variable number of mucosal folds called the spiral valves of Heister. The common bile duct is about 7–11 cm in length and 5–10 mm in diameter. The common bile duct runs obliquely downward within

821

the wall of the duodenum for 1–2 cm before opening on a papilla of mucous membrane (ampulla of Vater), about 10 cm distal to the pylorus. The pancreatic duct frequently joins the common bile duct outside the duodenal wall and traverses the duodenal wall as a single duct. The sphincter of Oddi controls the flow of bile, and in some cases pancreatic juice, into the duodenum.

The extrahepatic bile ducts are lined by a columnar mucosa with numerous mucous glands in the common bile duct. A fibroareolar tissue containing scant smooth muscle cells surrounds the mucosa. The arterial supply to the bile ducts is derived from the gastroduodenal and the right hepatic arteries, with major trunks running along the medial and lateral walls of the common duct.

Anomalies

The classic description of the extrahepatic biliary tree and its arteries applies only in about one third of patients. The gallbladder may have abnormal positions, be intrahepatic, be rudimentary, have anomalous forms, or be duplicated. Isolated congenital absence of the gallbladder is rare. Duplication of the gallbladder with two separate cavities and two separate cystic ducts has an incidence of about one in every 4000 persons. A partial or totally intrahepatic gallbladder is associated with an increased incidence of cholelithiasis.

Small ducts (of Luschka) may drain directly from the liver into the body of the gallbladder. If present, but not recognized at the time of a cholecystectomy, a bile leak with the accumulation of bile (biloma) may occur in the abdomen. An accessory right hepatic duct occurs in about 5 percent of patients. Anomalies of the hepatic artery and the cystic artery are quite common, occurring in as many as 50 percent of patients.

PHYSIOLOGY

Bile Formation and Composition

The liver produces bile continuously and excretes it into the bile canaliculi. The normal adult consuming an average diet produces within the liver 500–1000 mL of bile a day. The secretion of bile is responsive to neurogenic, humoral, and chemical stimuli. With an intact sphincter of Oddi, bile flow is directed into the gallbladder.

Bile is mainly composed of water, electrolytes, bile salts, proteins, lipids, and bile pigments. Sodium, potassium, calcium, and chlorine have the same concentration in bile as in plasma or extracellular fluid. The primary bile salts, cholate and chenodeoxycholate, are synthesized in the liver from cholesterol. They are conjugated there with taurine and glycine, and act within the bile as anions (bile acids) that are balanced by sodium. Bile salts are excreted into the bile by the hepatocyte and aid in the digestion and absorption of fats in the intestines. About 95 percent of the bile acid pool is reabsorbed and returned via the portal venous system to the liver, the so-called enterohepatic circulation. Five percent is excreted in the stool, leaving the relatively small amount of bile acids to have maximum effect.

Cholesterol and phospholipids synthesized in the liver are the principal lipids found in bile. The synthesis of phospholipids and cholesterol by the liver is in part regulated by bile acids. The color of the bile is because of the presence of the pigment bilirubin diglucuronide, which is the metabolic product from the breakdown of hemoglobin, and is present in bile in concentrations 100 times greater than in plasma. Once in the intestine, bacteria convert it into urobilino-gen, a small fraction of which is absorbed and secreted into the bile.

Gallbladder Function

The gallbladder, the bile ducts, and the sphincter of Oddi act together to store and regulate the flow of bile. The main function of the gallbladder is to concentrate and store hepatic bile and to deliver bile into the duodenum in response to a meal.

Absorption and Secretion

In the fasting state, approximately 80 percent of the bile secreted by the liver is stored in the gallbladder. It rapidly absorbs sodium, chloride, and water against significant concentration gradients, concentrating the bile as much as tenfold and leading to a marked change in bile composition. The epithelial cells of the gallbladder secrete at least two important products into the gallbladder lumen: glycoproteins and hydrogen ions. The mucosal glands in the infundibulum and the neck of the gallbladder secrete mucus glycoproteins. This mucus makes up the colorless "white bile" seen in hydrops of the gallbladder resulting from cystic duct obstruction. The transport of hydrogen ions by the gallbladder epithelium leads to a decrease in the gallbladder bile pH. The acidification promotes calcium solubility, thereby preventing its precipitation as calcium salts.

Motor Activity

Gallbladder filling is facilitated by tonic contraction of the sphincter of Oddi, which creates a pressure gradient between the bile ducts and the gallbladder. In response to a meal, the gallbladder empties by a coordinated motor response of gallbladder contraction and sphincter of Oddi relaxation. One of the main stimuli to gallbladder emptying is the hormone cholecystokinin (CCK). CCK is released endogenously from the duodenal mucosa in response to a meal. When stimulated by eating, the gallbladder empties 50–70 percent of its contents within 30–40 min. Over the following 60–90 min the gallbladder gradually refills. This is correlated with a reduced CCK level.

Neurohormonal Regulation

The vagus nerve stimulates contraction of the gallbladder, and splanchnic sympathetic stimulation is inhibitory to its motor activity. Antral distention of the stomach causes both gallbladder contraction and relaxation of the sphincter of Oddi.

Hormonal receptors are located on the smooth muscles, vessels, nerves, and epithelium of the gallbladder. CCK is a peptide that comes from epithelial cells of the upper gastrointestinal tract and is found in the highest concentrations in the duodenum. CCK acts directly on smooth muscle receptors of the gallbladder and stimulates gallbladder contraction. It also relaxes the terminal bile duct, the sphincter of Oddi, and the duodenum. VIP inhibits contraction and causes gallbladder relaxation. Somatostatin and its analogues are potent inhibitors of gallbladder contraction.

Sphincter of Oddi

The sphincter of Oddi regulates flow of bile (and pancreatic juice) into the duodenum, prevents the regurgitation of duodenal contents into the biliary tree, and diverts bile into the gallbladder. The sphincter of Oddi is about 4–6 mm in length and has a basal resting pressure of about 13 mmHg above the duodenal pressure. Relaxation occurs with a rise in CCK, allowing increased flow of bile into the duodenum.

DIAGNOSTIC STUDIES

Blood Tests

An elevated white blood cell (WBC) count may indicate or raise suspicion of cholecystitis. If associated with an elevation of conjugated bilirubin, alkaline phosphatase, and aminotransferase, cholangitis should be suspected. Cholestasis, an obstruction to bile flow, is characterized by an elevation of bilirubin and a rise in alkaline phosphatase. Serum aminotransferases may be normal or mildly elevated. In patients with biliary colic, blood tests typically will be normal.

Ultrasonography

An ultrasound is the initial investigation of any patient suspected of disease of the biliary tree. It is dependent on the skills and the experience of the operator and it is dynamic. Adjacent organs can frequently be examined at the same time. Obese patients, patients with ascites, and patients with distended bowel may be difficult to examine satisfactorily with an ultrasound.

An ultrasound will show stones in the gallbladder with sensitivity and specificity of over 90 percent. Stones are acoustically dense and reflect the ultrasound waves back to the ultrasonic transducer. Because stones block the passage of sound waves to the region behind them, they also produce an acoustic shadow. Stones also move with changes in position. Some stones form a layer in the gallbladder; others a sediment or sludge. A thickened gallbladder wall and local tenderness indicate cholecystitis. The patient has acute cholecystitis if a layer of edema is seen within the wall of the gallbladder or between the gallbladder and the liver. When a stone obstructs the neck of the gallbladder, the gallbladder may become very large, but thin walled. A contracted, thick-walled gallbladder indicates chronic cholecystitis.

The extrahepatic bile ducts also are well visualized by ultrasound, except for the retroduodenal portion. Dilation of the ducts in a patient with jaundice establishes an extrahepatic obstruction as a cause for the jaundice. Frequently the site, and sometimes the cause of obstruction, can be determined by ultrasound. Small stones in the common bile duct frequently get lodged at the distal end of it, behind the duodenum, and are therefore difficult to detect. Periampullary tumors can be difficult to diagnose on ultrasound, but beyond the retroduodenal portion, the level of obstruction and the cause may be visualized quite well. Ultrasound can be helpful in evaluating tumor invasion and flow in the portal vein, an important guideline for resectability of periampullary tumors.

Oral Cholecystography

Oral Cholecystography involves oral administration of a radiopaque compound that is absorbed, excreted by the liver, and passed into the gallbladder. Stones are noted on a film as filling defects in a visualized, opacified gallbladder. Oral cholecystography is of no value in patients with intestinal malabsorption, vomiting, obstructive jaundice, and hepatic failure.

Biliary Radionuclide Scanning (HIDA Scan)

Biliary scintigraphy provides a noninvasive evaluation of the liver, gallbladder, bile ducts, and duodenum with both anatomic and functional information. 99m-Technetium-labeled derivatives of dimethyl iminodiacetic acid (HIDA) are injected intravenously, cleared by the Kupffer cells in the liver, and excreted in the bile. Uptake by the liver is detected within 10 min, and the gallbladder, the bile ducts, and the duodenum are visualized within 60 min in fasting subjects. The primary use of biliary scintigraphy is in the diagnosis of acute cholecystitis, which appears as a nonvisualized gallbladder, with prompt filling of the common bile duct and duodenum. Filling of the gallbladder and common bile duct with delayed or absent filling of the duodenum indicates an obstruction at the ampulla. Biliary leaks as a complication of surgery of the gallbladder or the biliary tree can be confirmed and frequently localized by biliary scintigraphy.

Computed Tomography

Abdominal computed tomography (CT) scans are inferior to ultrasonography in diagnosing gallstones. CT scan is the test of choice in evaluating the patient with suspected malignancy of the gallbladder, the extrahepatic biliary system, or nearby organs, in particular the head of the pancreas. Use of CT scan is an integral part of the differential diagnosis of obstructive jaundice. Spiral CT scanning provides additional staging information, including vascular involvement in patients with periampullary tumors.

Percutaneous Transhepatic Cholangiography

An intrahepatic bile duct is accessed percutaneously with a small needle under fluoroscopic guidance. Once the position in a bile duct has been confirmed, a guidewire is passed and subsequently a catheter passed over the wire. Through the catheter, a cholangiogram can be performed and therapeutic interventions done, such as biliary drain insertions and stent placements. Percutaneous transhepatic cholangiography is particularly useful in patients with bile duct strictures and tumors, as it defines the anatomy of the biliary tree proximal to the affected segment.

Magnetic Resonance Imaging

Using magnetic resonance imaging (MRI) with newer techniques and contrast materials, accurate anatomic images can be obtained of the bile ducts and the pancreatic duct. It has a sensitivity and specificity of 95 and 89 percent, respectively, at detecting choledocholithiasis. If available, MRI with magnetic resonance cholangiopancreatography (MRCP) offers a single noninvasive test for the diagnosis of biliary tract and pancreatic disease.

Endoscopic Retrograde Cholangiography and Endoscopic Ultrasound

Using a side-viewing endoscope, the common bile duct can be cannulated and a cholangiogram performed using fluoroscopy. Endoscopic retrograde cholangiography (ERC) provides direct visualization of the ampullary region and direct access to the distal common bile duct, with the possibility of therapeutic intervention. The test rarely is needed for uncomplicated gallstone disease. Once the endoscopic cholangiogram has shown ductal stones, sphincterotomy and stone extraction can be performed, and the common bile duct cleared of stones. In the hands of experts, the success rate of common bile duct cannulation and cholangiography is more than 90 percent. Complications of diagnostic ERC include pancreatitis and cholangitis, and occur in up to 5 percent of patients.

An endoscopic ultrasound requires a special endoscope with an ultrasound transducer at its tip. It offers noninvasive imaging of the bile ducts and adjacent structures. It is of particular value in the evaluation of tumors and their resectability. The ultrasound endoscope has a biopsy channel, allowing needle biopsies of a tumor under ultrasonic guidance.

GALLSTONE DISEASE

Prevalence and Incidence

Gallstone disease is one of the most common problems affecting the digestive tract. Autopsy reports have shown a prevalence of gallstones from 11–36 percent. Obesity, pregnancy, dietary factors, Crohn disease, terminal ileal resection, gastric surgery, hereditary spherocytosis, sickle cell disease, and thalassemia all are associated with an increased risk of developing gallstones. Women are three times more likely to develop gallstones than men, and first-degree relatives of patients with gallstones have a 2-fold greater prevalence.

Natural History

Most patients will remain asymptomatic from their gallstones throughout life. For unknown reasons some patients progress to a symptomatic stage, with biliary colic caused by a stone obstructing the cystic duct. Symptomatic gallstone disease may progress to complications related to the gallstones. Rarely, complication of gallstones is the presenting picture.

Gallstones in patients without biliary symptoms are commonly diagnosed incidentally. Approximately 3 percent of asymptomatic individuals develop biliary colic each year. Once symptomatic, patients tend to have recurring bouts of biliary colic. Complicated gallstone disease develops in 3–5 percent of symptomatic patients per year. Over a 20-year period, about two-thirds of asymptomatic patients with gallstones remain symptom free.

Since few patients develop complications without previous biliary symptoms, prophylactic cholecystectomy in asymptomatic persons with gallstones rarely is indicated. For older adult patients with diabetes, for individuals who will be isolated from medical care for extended periods of time, and in populations with increased risk of gallbladder cancer, a prophylactic cholecystectomy may be advisable. Porcelain gallbladder, a rare premalignant condition in which the wall of the gallbladder becomes calcified, is an absolute indication for cholecystectomy.

Gallstone Formation

Gallstones form as a result of solids settling out of solution. Gallstones are classified by their cholesterol content as either cholesterol stones or pigment stones. Pigment stones can be further classified as either black or brown. In Western countries, about 80 percent of gallstones are cholesterol stones and about 15–20 percent are black pigment stones. Brown pigment stones account for only a small percentage. Both types of pigment stones are more common in Asia.

Cholesterol Stones

Pure cholesterol stones are uncommon and account for less than 10 percent of all stones. They usually occur as single large stones with smooth surfaces. Most other cholesterol stones contain variable amounts of bile pigments and calcium, but are always more than 70 percent cholesterol by weight. These stones are usually multiple, of variable size, and may be hard and faceted or irregular, mulberry-shaped and soft. Colors range from whitish yellow and green to black. Most cholesterol stones are radiolucent. Whether pure or of mixed nature, the common primary event in the formation of cholesterol stones is supersaturation of bile with cholesterol.

Pigment Stones

Pigment stones contain less than 20 percent cholesterol and are dark because of the presence of calcium bilirubinate. Otherwise, black and brown pigment stones have little in common and should be considered as separate entities.

Black pigment stones are usually small, brittle, black, and sometimes spiculated. They are formed by supersaturation of calcium bilirubinate, carbonate, and phosphate, most often secondary to hemolytic disorders such as hereditary spherocytosis and sickle cell disease, and in those with cirrhosis. Like cholesterol stones, they almost always form in the gallbladder. When altered conditions lead to increased levels of deconjugated bilirubin in bile, precipitation with calcium occurs. In Asian countries such as Japan, black stones account for a much higher percentage of gallstones than in the Western hemisphere.

Brown stones are usually less than 1 cm in diameter, brownish-yellow, soft, and often mushy. They may form either in the gallbladder or in the bile ducts, usually secondary to bacterial infection caused by bile stasis. Precipitated calcium bilirubinate and bacterial cell bodies compose the major part of the stone. Brown stones are typically found in the biliary tree of Asian populations and are associated with stasis secondary to parasite infection. In Western populations, brown stones occur as primary bile duct stones in patients with biliary strictures or other common bile duct stones that cause stasis and bacterial contamination.

Symptomatic Gallstones

Chronic Cholecystitis

About two thirds of patients with gallstone disease present with chronic cholecystitis characterized by recurrent attacks of pain, often inaccurately labeled biliary colic. The pain develops when a stone obstructs the cystic duct, resulting in a progressive increase of tension in the gallbladder wall. The pathologic changes, vary from an apparently normal gallbladder with minor chronic inflammation in the mucosa, to a shrunken, nonfunctioning gallbladder with gross transmural fibrosis and adhesions to nearby structures.

Clinical presentation. The chief symptom associated with symptomatic gallstones is pain. The pain is constant and increases in severity over the first half hour or so and typically lasts 1–5 h. It is located in the epigastrium or right upper quadrant and frequently radiates to the right upper back or between the scapulae. The pain is severe and comes on abruptly, typically during the night or after a fatty meal. It often is associated with nausea and sometimes vomiting. The pain is episodic. The patient suffers discrete attacks of pain, between which they feel well. Physical examination may reveal mild right upper quadrant tenderness during an episode of pain. If the patient is pain free, the physical exam usually is unremarkable. Laboratory values, such as white blood cell count and liver function tests, usually are normal in patients with uncomplicated gallstones.

Atypical presentation of gallstone disease is common. In patients with atypical presentation, other conditions with upper abdominal pain should be sought out, even in the presence of gallstones. When the pain lasts more than 24 h, an impacted stone in the cystic duct or acute cholecystitis (see below) should be suspected. An impacted stone will result in what is called hydrops of the gallbladder. The bile gets absorbed, but the gallbladder epithelium continues to secrete mucus and the gallbladder becomes distended with mucinous material. Early cholecystectomy generally is indicated to avoid complications.

Diagnosis. An abdominal ultrasound is the standard diagnostic test for gallstones. Sometimes only sludge in the gallbladder is demonstrated on ultrasonography. If the patient has recurrent attacks of typical biliary pain and sludge is detected on two or more occasions, cholecystectomy is warranted. In addition to sludge and stones, cholesterolosis and adenomyomatosis of the gallbladder may cause typical biliary symptoms and may be detected on ultrasonography. In symptomatic patients, cholecystectomy is the treatment of choice for patients with these conditions.

Management. Patients with symptomatic gallstones should be advised to have elective laparoscopic cholecystectomy. While waiting for surgery, or if surgery has to be postponed, the patient should be advised to avoid dietary fats and large meals. Diabetic patients with symptomatic gallstones should have a cholecystectomy promptly, as they are more prone to develop acute cholecystitis that often is severe. Pregnant women with symptomatic gallstones who cannot be managed expectantly with diet modifications can safely undergo laparoscopic cholecystectomy during the second trimester. Laparoscopic cholecystectomy is safe and effective in children and in older adults. Cholecystectomy, open or laparoscopic, for patients with symptomatic gallstones offers excellent long-term results. About 90 percent of patients with typical biliary symptoms and stones are rendered symptom free after cholecystectomy. For patients with atypical symptoms or dyspepsia (flatulence, belching, bloating, and dietary fat intolerance) the results are not as favorable.

Acute Cholecystitis

Pathogenesis. Acute cholecystitis is secondary to gallstones in 90–95 percent of cases. Acute acalculous cholecystitis is a condition that typically occurs in patients with other acute systemic diseases (see acalculous cholecystitis section, below). In less than 1 percent of acute cholecystitis, the cause is a tumor obstructing the cystic duct. Obstruction of the cystic duct by a gallstone is the initiating event that leads to gallbladder distention, inflammation, and edema of the gallbladder wall. Initially, acute cholecystitis is an inflammatory process. Secondary bacterial contamination is documented in over one half of patients undergoing early cholecystectomy for acute uncomplicated cholecystitis. In acute cholecystitis the gallbladder wall becomes grossly thickened and reddish with subserosal hemorrhages. Pericholecystic fluid often is present.

The mucosa may show hyperemia and patchy necrosis. In severe cases, about 5–10 percent, the inflammatory process progresses and leads to ischemia and necrosis of the gallbladder wall. More frequently, the gallstone is dislodged and the inflammation resolves.

When the gallbladder remains obstructed and secondary bacterial infection supervenes, an acute gangrenous cholecystitis develops and an abscess or empyema forms within the gallbladder. Rarely, perforation of ischemic areas occurs. The perforation usually is contained in the subhepatic space by the omentum and adjacent organs.

Clinical manifestations. About 80 percent of patients with acute cholecystitis give a history compatible with chronic cholecystitis. Acute cholecystitis begins as an attack of biliary colic, but in contrast to biliary colic, the pain does not subside; it is unremitting and may persist for several days. The patient often is febrile, complains of anorexia, nausea, and vomiting, and is reluctant to move, as the inflammatory process affects the parietal peritoneum. On physical exam, focal tenderness and guarding are usually present in the right upper quadrant. A mass, the gallbladder and adherent omentum, is occasionally palpable; however, guarding may prevent this. A Murphy's sign, an inspiratory arrest with deep palpation in the right subcostal area, is characteristic of acute cholecystitis.

A mild to moderate leukocytosis (12,000–15,000 cells/mm^3) usually is present. However, some patients may have a normal WBC. Serum liver chemistries usually are normal, but a mild elevation of serum bilirubin, less than 4 mg/mL, may be present along with mild elevation of alkaline phosphatase, transaminases, and amylase. Severe jaundice is suggestive of common bile duct stones or obstruction of the bile ducts by severe pericholecystic inflammation secondary to impaction of a stone in the infundibulum of the gallbladder that mechanically obstructs the bile duct (Mirizzi syndrome). In older adult patients and in those with diabetes mellitus, acute cholecystitis may have a subtle presentation resulting in a delay in diagnosis. The incidence of complications is higher in these patients, who also have approximately tenfold the mortality rate compared to that of younger and healthier patients.

Diagnosis. Ultrasonography is the most useful radiologic test for diagnosing acute cholecystitis. It has a sensitivity and specificity of 95 percent. It will show the thickening of the gallbladder wall and the pericholecystic fluid. Focal tenderness over the gallbladder when compressed by the sonographic probe (sonographic Murphy sign) also is suggestive of acute cholecystitis. Biliary radionuclide scanning (HIDA scan) may be of help in the atypical case. A normal HIDA scan excludes acute cholecystitis. CT scan is frequently performed on patients with acute abdominal pain. It demonstrates thickening of the gallbladder wall, pericholecystic fluid, and the presence of gallstones and air in the gallbladder wall, but is less sensitive than ultrasonography.

Treatment. Patients who present with acute cholecystitis will need intravenous fluids, antibiotics, and analgesia. The antibiotics should cover Gram-negative aerobes and anaerobes. Although the inflammation in acute cholecystitis may be sterile in some patients, more than one half will have positive cultures from the gallbladder bile.

Cholecystectomy is the definitive treatment for acute cholecystitis. Early cholecystectomy performed within 2–3 days of the illness is preferred over interval or delayed cholecystectomy that is performed 6–10 weeks after initial medical treatment and recuperation. Early cholecystectomy offers the patient a definitive solution in one hospital admission, quicker recovery times, and an earlier return to work.

Laparoscopic cholecystectomy is the procedure of choice for acute cholecystitis. The conversion rate to an open cholecystectomy is higher (10–15 percent) in the setting of acute cholecystitis than with chronic cholecystitis. The procedure is more tedious and takes longer than in the elective setting.

When patients present late, after 3–4 days of illness, or are for some reason unfit for surgery, they are treated with antibiotics with laparoscopic cholecystectomy scheduled for approximately 2 months later. Approximately 20 percent of patients will fail to respond to initial medical therapy and require an intervention. For those unfit for surgery, a percutaneous cholecystostomy or an open cholecystostomy under local analgesia can be performed. Failure to improve after cholecystostomy usually is because of gangrene of the gallbladder or perforation. For these patients, surgery is unavoidable. For those who respond after cholecystostomy, the tube can be removed once cholangiography through it shows a patent ductus cysticus. Laparoscopic cholecystectomy may then be scheduled in the near future.

Choledocholithiasis

Common bile duct stones may be small or large, single or multiple, and are found in 6–12 percent of patients with stones in the gallbladder. The incidence increases with age. About 20–25 percent of patients older than the age of 60 with symptomatic gallstones have stones in the common bile duct and in the gallbladder. The vast majority of ductal stones in Western countries are formed within the gallbladder and migrate down the cystic duct to the common bile duct. These are classified as secondary common bile duct stones, in contrast to the primary stones that form in the bile ducts.

Clinical manifestations. Choledochal stones may be silent and often are discovered incidentally. They may cause obstruction, complete or incomplete, or they may manifest with cholangitis or gallstone pancreatitis. The pain caused by a stone in the bile duct is similar to that of biliary colic. Nausea and vomiting are common. Physical exam may be normal, but mild epigastric or right upper quadrant tenderness and mild icterus are common. The symptoms may also be intermittent, such as pain and transient jaundice caused by a stone that temporarily impacts the ampulla but subsequently moves away, acting as a ball valve. A small stone may pass through the ampulla spontaneously with resolution of symptoms. Finally the stones may become completely impacted, causing severe progressive jaundice. Elevation of serum bilirubin, alkaline phosphatase, and transaminases are commonly seen in patients with bile duct stones. However, in about one third of patients with common bile duct stones, the liver chemistries are normal.

Commonly the first test, ultrasonography is useful for documenting stones in the gallbladder, and determining the size of the common bile duct. As stones in the bile ducts tend to move down to the distal part of the common duct, bowel gas can preclude their demonstration on ultrasonography. A dilated common bile duct (> 8 mm in diameter) on ultrasonography in a patient with gallstones, jaundice, and biliary pain is highly suggestive of common bile duct stones. Magnetic resonance cholangiography (MRC) provides excellent anatomic detail and has a sensitivity and specificity of 95 and 89 percent, respectively, at detecting choledocholithiasis. Endoscopic cholangiography is the gold standard for diagnosing common bile duct stones. It has the distinct advantage of providing a therapeutic option at the time of diagnosis. In experienced hands, cannulation of the ampulla of Vater and diagnostic cholangiography are achieved in over 90 percent of cases, with associated morbidity of less than 5 percent (mainly cholangitis and pancreatitis). Percutaneous transhepatic cholangiography (PTC) rarely is needed in patients with secondary common bile duct stones, but frequently is performed for both diagnostic and therapeutic reasons in patients with primary bile duct stones.

Treatment. For patients with symptomatic gallstones and suspected common bile duct stones, either preoperative endoscopic cholangiography or an intraoperative cholangiogram will document the bile duct stones. If an endoscopic cholangiogram reveals stones, sphincterotomy and ductal clearance of the stones is appropriate, followed by a laparoscopic cholecystectomy. An intraoperative cholangiogram at the time of cholecystectomy also will document the presence or absence of bile duct stones. Laparoscopic common bile duct exploration via the cystic duct or with formal choledochotomy allows the stones to be retrieved in the same setting (see following section). If the expertise and/or the instruments for laparoscopic common bile duct exploration are not available, a drain should be left adjacent to the cystic duct and the patient scheduled for endoscopic sphincterotomy the following day. An open common bile duct exploration is an option if the endoscopic method has already been tried or is for some reason not feasible. If a choledochotomy is performed, a τ tube is left in place. Stones impacted in the ampulla may be difficult for both endoscopic ductal clearance and common bile duct exploration (open or laparoscopic). In these cases the common bile duct usually is quite dilated (about 2 cm in diameter). A choledochoduodenostomy or a Roux-en-Y choledochojejunostomy may be the best option for these circumstances.

Retained or recurrent stones following cholecystectomy are best treated endoscopically. If a common bile duct exploration was performed and a τ tube left in place, a τ-tube cholangiogram is obtained prior to its removal. Retained stones can be retrieved either endoscopically or via the τ-tube tract once it has matured (2–4 weeks). Under fluoroscopic guidance the stones are retrieved with baskets or balloons. Recurrent stones may be multiple and large. A generous endoscopic sphincterotomy will allow stone retrieval and spontaneous passage of retained and recurrent stones.

Cholangitis

Cholangitis is one of the two main complications of choledochal stones, the other being gallstone pancreatitis. Acute cholangitis is an ascending bacterial infection in association with partial or complete obstruction of the bile ducts. Hepatic bile is sterile, and bile in the bile ducts is kept sterile by continuous bile flow and by the presence of antibacterial substances in bile such as immunoglobulin. The combination of both significant bacterial contamination and biliary obstruction is required for its development. Gallstones are the most common cause of obstruction in cholangitis. The most common organisms cultured from bile in patients with cholangitis include *Escherichia coli*, *Klebsiella pneumoniae*, *Streptococcus faecalis*, and *Bacteroides fragilis*.

Clinical presentation. Cholangitis may present as anything from a mild, intermittent, and self-limited disease to a fulminant, potentially life-threatening septicemia. The most common presentation is fever, epigastric or right upper quadrant pain, and jaundice. These classic symptoms, well known as Charcot triad, are present in about two thirds of patients. The illness may progress rapidly with septicemia and disorientation, known as Reynolds pentad (e.g., fever, jaundice, right upper quadrant pain, septic shock, and mental status changes). However, the presentation may be atypical, with little if any fever, jaundice, or pain. This occurs most commonly in older adults, who may have unremarkable symptoms until they collapse with septicemia. On abdominal examination, the findings are indistinguishable from those of acute cholecystitis.

Diagnosis and management. Leukocytosis, hyperbilirubinemia, and elevation of alkaline phosphatase and transaminases are common, and when present, support the clinical diagnosis of cholangitis. Ultrasonography is helpful if the patient has not been diagnosed previously with gallstones, as it will document the presence of gallbladder stones and demonstrate dilated ducts. The definitive diagnostic test is ERC. In cases in which ERC is not available, PTC is indicated. Both ERC and PTC will show the level and the reason for the obstruction, allow culture of the bile, possibly allow the removal of stones if present, and drainage of the bile ducts with drainage catheters or stents. CT scanning and MRI will show pancreatic and periampullary masses, if present, in addition to the ductal dilatation.

The initial treatment of patients with cholangitis includes intravenous antibiotics and fluid resuscitation. Most patients will respond to these measures. However, the obstructed bile duct must be drained as soon as the patient has been stabilized. About 15 percent of patients will not respond to antibiotics and fluid resuscitation, and an emergency biliary decompression may be required. Biliary decompression may be accomplished endoscopically, via the percutaneous transhepatic route, or surgically. Patients with choledocholithiasis or periampullary malignancies are best approached endoscopically, with sphincterotomy and stone removal, or by placement of an endoscopic biliary stent. In patients in whom the obstruction is more proximal or perihilar, percutaneous transhepatic drainage is used. Where neither ERC nor PTC is possible, an emergent operation and decompression of the common bile duct with a τ tube may be necessary and life-saving. Definitive operative therapy should be deferred until the cholangitis has been treated and the proper diagnosis established. Patients with indwelling stents and cholangitis usually require repeated imaging and exchange of the stent over a guidewire.

Acute cholangitis is associated with an overall mortality rate of approximately 5 percent.

Biliary Pancreatitis

Gallstones in the common bile duct are associated with acute pancreatitis. Obstruction of the pancreatic duct by an impacted stone or temporary obstruction by a stone passing through the ampulla may lead to pancreatitis. An ultrasonogram of the biliary tree in patients with pancreatitis is essential. If gallstones are present and the pancreatitis is severe, an ERC with sphincterotomy and stone extraction may abort the episode of pancreatitis. Once the pancreatitis has subsided, the gallbladder should be removed during the same admission. When gallstones are present and the pancreatitis is mild and self-limited, the stone has probably passed. For these patients a cholecystectomy and an intraoperative cholangiogram or a preoperative ERC is indicated.

Cholangiohepatitis

Cholangiohepatitis, also known as recurrent pyogenic cholangitis, is endemic to the Orient. It also has been encountered in the Chinese population in the United States and in Europe and Australia. Cholangiohepatitis is caused by bacterial contamination (commonly *E. coli*, Klebsiella species, Bacteroides species, or Enterococcus faecalis) of the biliary tree, and often is associated with biliary parasites such as *Clonorchis sinensis, Opisthorchis viverrini*, and *Ascaris lumbricoides*. Bacterial enzymes cause deconjugation of bilirubin, which precipitates as bile sludge. The sludge and dead bacterial cell bodies form brown pigment stones. These stones are formed throughout the biliary tree and cause partial obstruction that contributes to the repeated bouts of cholangitis

The patient usually presents with pain in the right upper quadrant and epigastrium, fever, and jaundice. Recurrence of symptoms is one of the most characteristic features of the disease. An ultrasound will detect stones in the biliary tree, pneumobilia from infection because of gas-forming organisms, liver abscesses, and occasionally strictures. MRCP and PTC are the mainstays of biliary imaging for cholangiohepatitis. The long-term goal of therapy is to extract stones and debris and relieve strictures. It may take several procedures and require a Roux-en-Y hepaticojejunostomy to establish biliary-enteric continuity.

OPERATIVE INTERVENTIONS FOR GALLSTONE DISEASE

Cholecystostomy

A cholecystostomy decompresses and drains the distended, inflamed, hydropic, or purulent gallbladder. Ultrasound guided percutaneous drainage with a pigtail catheter is the procedure of choice. By passing the catheter through the liver, the risk of bile leak around the catheter is minimized. The catheter can be removed when the inflammation has resolved and the patient's condition improved.

Cholecystectomy

Cholecystectomy is the most common major abdominal procedure performed in Western countries. Open cholecystectomy is a safe and effective treatment for both acute and chronic cholecystitis. In 1987, laparoscopic cholecystectomy was introduced. Today laparoscopic cholecystectomy is the treatment of choice for symptomatic gallstones.

Symptomatic gallstones are the main indication for cholecystectomy. Absolute contraindications for the procedure are uncontrolled coagulopathy and end-stage liver disease. When important anatomic structures cannot be clearly identified or when no progress is made over a set period of time, a conversion to an open procedure usually is indicated. In the elective setting, conversion to an open procedure is needed in about 5 percent of patients. Emergent procedures may require more skill on the part of the surgeon, and be needed in patients with complicated gallstone disease; the incidence of conversion is 10–30 percent. Serious complications are rare. The mortality rate for laparoscopic cholecystectomy is about 0.1 percent. Wound infection and cardiopulmonary complication rates are considerably lower following laparoscopic cholecystectomy than are those for an open procedure, in which injury to the bile ducts is slightly more frequent.

Patients undergoing cholecystectomy should have a complete blood count (CBC) and liver function tests preoperatively. Prophylaxis against deep venous thrombosis with either low-molecular-weight heparin or compression stockings is indicated.

Laparoscopic Cholecystectomy

The patient is placed supine on the operating table with the surgeon standing at the patient's left side. The pneumoperitoneum is created with carbon dioxide gas, either with an open technique or by closed needle technique. Once an adequate pneumoperitoneum is established, a 10-mm trocar is inserted through the supraumbilical incision. The laparoscope with the attached video camera is passed through the umbilical port and the abdomen inspected. Three additional ports are placed under direct vision.

Through the lateral-most port a grasper is used to grasp the gallbladder fundus. The dissection starts at the junction of the gallbladder and the cystic duct. A helpful anatomic landmark is the cystic artery lymph node. The peritoneum, fat, and loose areolar tissue around the gallbladder and the cystic duct-gallbladder junction is dissected off toward the bile duct. The next step is the identification of the cystic artery, which usually runs parallel to and somewhat behind the cystic duct. A wide cystic duct may be too big for clips, requiring the placement of a pretied loop ligature to close. The cystic artery is then clipped and divided. Finally, the gallbladder is dissected out of the gallbladder fossa, using either a hook or scissors with electrocautery. The gallbladder is removed through the umbilical incision. If the gallbladder is acutely inflamed or gangrenous, or if the gallbladder is perforated, it is placed in a retrieval bag before it is removed from the abdomen. A closed suction drain can be placed through one of the 5-mm ports and left underneath the right liver lobe close to the gallbladder fossa.

Open Cholecystectomy

Open cholecystectomy has become an uncommon procedure, usually performed either as a conversion from laparoscopic cholecystectomy or as a second procedure in patients who require laparotomy for another reason. After the cystic artery and cystic duct have been identified, the gallbladder is dissected free from the liver bed, starting at the fundus. The dissection is carried proximally toward the cystic artery and the cystic duct, which are then ligated and divided.

Intraoperative Cholangiogram or Ultrasound

The bile ducts are visualized under fluoroscopy by injecting contrast through a catheter placed in the cystic duct. Routine intraoperative cholangiography will detect stones in approximately 7 percent of patients, and outlining the anatomy and detecting injury. A selective intraoperative cholangiogram can be performed when the patient has a history of abnormal liver function tests, pancreatitis, jaundice, a large duct and small stones, a dilated duct on preoperative ultrasonography, and if preoperative endoscopic cholangiography for the above reasons was unsuccessful. Laparoscopic ultrasonography is as accurate as intraoperative cholangiography in detecting common bile duct stones and it is less invasive; however, it requires more skill to perform and interpret.

Choledochal Exploration

Common bile duct stones that are detected intraoperatively on intraoperative cholangiography or ultrasonography may be managed with laparoscopic choledochal exploration as a part of the laparoscopic cholecystectomy procedure. Patients with common bile duct stones detected preoperatively, but endoscopic clearance was either not available or unsuccessful, should also have their ductal stones managed during the cholecystectomy.

If the stones in the duct are small, they may sometimes be flushed into the duodenum with saline irrigation via the cholangiography catheter after the sphincter of Oddi has been relaxed with glucagon. By managing common bile duct stones at the time of the cholecystectomy, the patients can have all of their gallstone disease treated with one invasive procedure. It does, however, depend on the available surgical expertise.

Choledochal Drainage Procedures

Rarely, when the stones cannot be cleared and/or when the duct is very dilated (larger than 1.5 cm in diameter), a choledochal drainage procedure is performed.

Transduodenal Sphincterotomy

In the majority of cases, endoscopic sphincterotomy has replaced open transduodenal sphincterotomy. If an open procedure for common bile duct stones is being done in which the stones are impacted, recurrent, or multiple, the transduodenal approach may be feasible. The duodenum is incised transversely. The sphincter then is incised at the 11 o'clock position to avoid injury to the pancreatic duct. The impacted stones are removed as are large stones from the duct.

OTHER BENIGN DISEASES AND LESIONS

Acalculous Cholecystitis

Acute inflammation of the gallbladder can occur without gallstones. Acalculous cholecystitis typically develops in critically ill patients in the intensive care unit. The cause is unknown, but gallbladder distention with bile stasis and ischemia have been implicated as causative factors.

The symptoms and signs depend on the condition of the patient, but in the alert patient they are similar to acute calculous cholecystitis. In the sedated or unconscious patient the clinical features often are masked, but fever and elevated white blood cell count, and elevation of alkaline phosphatase and bilirubin are indications for further investigation.

Ultrasonography is usually the diagnostic test of choice. Abdominal CT scan is as sensitive as ultrasonography and additionally allows imaging of the abdominal cavity and chest. A HIDA scan will not visualize the gallbladder. Acalculous cholecystitis requires urgent intervention. Percutaneous ultrasound- or CT-guided cholecystostomy is the treatment of choice for these patients, as they usually are unfit for surgery. About 90 percent of patients will improve with the percutaneous cholecystostomy. However, if they do not improve, other steps, such as open cholecystostomy or cholecystectomy, may be required.

Biliary Cysts

Choledochal cysts are congenital cystic dilatations of the extrahepatic and/or intrahepatic biliary tree. They are rare—the incidence is between 1:100,000 and 1:150,000. Choledochal cysts affect females three to eight times more often than males. Although frequently diagnosed in infancy or childhood, as many as one half of the patients have reached adulthood when diagnosed. The cause is unknown. Choledochal cysts are classified into five types. The cysts are lined with cuboidal epithelium and can vary in size from 2 cm in diameter to giant cysts.

Adults commonly present with jaundice or cholangitis. Less than one half of patients present with the classic clinical triad of abdominal pain, jaundice, and a mass. Ultrasonography or CT scanning will confirm the diagnosis, but endoscopic, transhepatic, or MRC is required to assess the biliary anatomy and to plan the appropriate surgical treatment. For types I, II, and IV, excision of the extrahepatic biliary tree, including cholecystectomy, with a Roux-en-Y hepaticojejunostomy are ideal. In type IV, additional segmental resection of the liver may be appropriate, particularly if intrahepatic stones, strictures, or abscesses are present, or if the dilatations are confined to one lobe. The risk of cholangiocarcinoma developing in choledochal cysts is as high as 15 percent in adults, and supports complete excision when they are diagnosed. For type III, sphincterotomy is recommended.

Sclerosing Cholangitis

Sclerosing cholangitis is an uncommon disease characterized by inflammatory strictures involving the intrahepatic and extrahepatic biliary tree. It is a progressive disease that eventually results in secondary biliary cirrhosis. Sometimes, biliary strictures are clearly secondary to bile duct stones, acute cholangitis, previous biliary surgery, or toxic agents, and are termed secondary sclerosing cholangitis. However, primary sclerosing cholangitis is a disease entity of its own, with no known attributing cause. It is associated with ulcerative colitis in about two thirds of patients. Other diseases associated with sclerosing cholangitis include Riedel thyroiditis and retroperitoneal fibrosis. Patients with sclerosing cholangitis are at risk for developing cholangiocarcinoma. Eventually 10–20 percent of the patients will develop cancer.

The mean age of presentation is 30–45 years and men are affected twice as commonly as women. The usual presentation is intermittent jaundice, fatigue, weight loss, pruritus, and abdominal pain. In several patients with ulcerative colitis, abnormal liver function tests found on routine testing lead to the diagnosis. The clinical course in sclerosing cholangitis is highly variable, but cyclic remissions and exacerbations are typical. However, some patients remain asymptomatic for years, although others progress rapidly with the obliterative inflammatory changes leading to secondary biliary cirrhosis and liver failure. The median survival for patients with primary sclerosing cholangitis from the time of diagnosis ranges from 10 to 12 years, and most die from hepatic failure.

The clinical presentation and elevation of alkaline phosphatase and bilirubin may suggest the diagnosis, but ERC, revealing multiple dilatations and strictures (beading) of both the intra- and extrahepatic biliary tree confirms it. The hepatic duct bifurcation is often the most severely affected segment. Sclerosing cholangitis is followed by ERC and liver biopsies to provide appropriate management.

There is no known effective medical therapy for primary sclerosing cholangitis and no known curative treatment. Corticosteroids, immunosuppressants, ursodeoxycholic acid, and antibiotics have been disappointing. Biliary strictures can be dilated and stented either endoscopically or percutaneously. Surgical management with resection of the extrahepatic biliary tree and hepaticojejunostomy has produced reasonable results in patients with extrahepatic and bifurcation strictures. In patients with sclerosing cholangitis and advanced liver disease, liver transplantation is the only option. It offers excellent results with overall 5-year survival as high as 85 percent. Primary sclerosing cholangitis recurs in 10–20 percent of patients and may require retransplantation.

Stenosis of the Sphincter of Oddi

A benign stenosis of the outlet of the common bile duct usually is associated with inflammation, fibrosis, or muscular hypertrophy. Episodic pain of the biliary type with abnormal liver function tests is a common presentation. However, recurrent jaundice or pancreatitis also may play a role. A dilated common bile duct that is difficult to cannulate with delayed emptying of the contrast are useful diagnostic features. If the diagnosis is well established, endoscopic or operative sphincterotomy will yield good results.

Bile Duct Strictures

Benign bile duct strictures can have numerous causes. However, the vast majority are caused by operative injury, most commonly by laparoscopic cholecystectomy (see below). Other causes include fibrosis because of chronic pancreatitis, common bile duct stones, acute cholangitis, biliary obstruction because of cholecystolithiasis (Mirizzi syndrome), sclerosing cholangitis, cholangiohepatitis, and strictures of a biliary-enteric anastomosis. Bile duct strictures that go unrecognized or are improperly managed may lead to recurrent cholangitis, secondary biliary cirrhosis, and portal hypertension.

Patients with bile duct strictures most commonly present with episodes of cholangitis. An ultrasound or a CT scan will show dilated bile ducts proximal to the stricture, and provide some information about the level of the stenosis. MRC will also provide good anatomic information about the location and the degree of dilatation. In patients with intrahepatic ductal dilatation, a percutaneous transhepatic cholangiogram will outline the proximal biliary tree, define the stricture and its location, and allow decompression of the biliary tree with transhepatic catheters or stents. An endoscopic cholangiogram will outline the distal bile duct. Percutaneous or endoscopic dilatation and/or stent placement give good results in more than one half of patients. Surgery with Roux-en-Y choledochojejunostomy or hepaticojejunostomy is the standard of care with good or excellent results in 80–90 percent of patients. Choledochoduodenostomy may be a choice for strictures in the distal-most part of the common bile duct.

INJURY TO THE BILIARY TRACT

The Gallbladder

Injuries to the gallbladder are uncommon. Penetrating injuries usually are caused by gunshot wounds or stab wounds, and rarely by a needle biopsy procedure of the liver. The treatment of choice is cholecystectomy and the prognosis is directly related to the type and incidence of associated injury.

The Extrahepatic Bile Ducts

Penetrating trauma to the extrahepatic bile ducts is rare and usually is associated with trauma to other viscera. The great majority of injuries of the extrahepatic biliary duct system are iatrogenic, occurring in the course of laparoscopic or open cholecystectomies. The exact incidence of bile duct injury during cholecystectomy is unknown, but data suggest that during open cholecystectomy the incidence is relatively low (about 0.1–0.2 percent). However, the incidence during laparoscopic cholecystectomy, as derived from state and national databases, estimates the rate of major injury to be about 0.55 percent, and the incidence of minor injuries and bile leaks to be about 0.3 percent, a total of 0.85 percent.

Factors associated with bile duct injury include acute or chronic inflammation, obesity, anatomic variations, and bleeding. Surgical technique with inadequate exposure and failure to identify structures before ligating or dividing them are the most common cause of significant biliary injury. The bile ducts may be narrow and can be mistaken for the cystic duct. The cystic duct may run along side the common bile duct before joining it, leading the surgeon to the wrong place. Additionally, the cystic duct may enter the right hepatic duct, and the right hepatic duct may run aberrantly, coursing through the triangle of Calot and entering the common hepatic duct. Intraoperative technical factors implicated in biliary injuries include excessive cephalad retraction of the gallbladder, the use of an end-viewing laparoscope instead of an angled one, careless use of electrocautery, dissection deep into the liver parenchyma and poor clip placement.

The routine use of intraoperative cholangiography to prevent bile duct injury is controversial. If a bile duct injury is suspected during cholecystectomy, a cholangiogram must be obtained to identify the anatomic features.

Diagnosis

Only about 25 percent of major bile duct injuries (common bile duct or hepatic duct) are recognized at the time of operation. Most commonly, intraoperative bile leakage, recognition of the correct anatomy, and an abnormal cholangiogram lead to the diagnosis of a bile duct injury. Within the first postoperative month more than half of patients with injury have presented. The remainder present months or years later. Bile leak, most commonly from the cystic duct stump, a transected aberrant right hepatic duct, or a lateral injury to the main bile duct usually presents with pain, fever, and a mild elevation of liver function tests. A CT scan or an ultrasound will show either a collection (biloma) in the gallbladder area or free fluid (bile) in the peritoneum. Bilious drainage through operatively placed drains or through the wounds is abnormal. An active leak and the site of the bile leak can be confirmed noninvasively with a HIDA scan. CT scan and ultrasound also are important in the initial evaluation of the jaundiced patient, as they can demonstrate the dilated part of the biliary tree proximal to the stenosis or obstruction, and may identify the level of the extrahepatic bile duct obstruction. In the jaundiced patient with dilated intrahepatic ducts, a percutaneous cholangiogram will outline the anatomy and the proximal extent of the injury and allow decompression of the biliary tree with catheter or stent placements. An endoscopic cholangiogram demonstrates the anatomy distal to the injury and may allow the placement of stents across a stricture to relieve an obstruction. MRI cholangiography, if available, provides an excellent, noninvasive delineation of the biliary anatomy both proximal and distal to the injury.

Management

Initial proper treatment of bile duct injury diagnosed during the cholecystectomy can avoid the development of a bile duct stricture. If a major injury is discovered and an experienced biliary surgeon is not available, an external drain and, if necessary, transhepatic biliary catheters, are placed and the patient is transferred to a referral center.

Transected bile ducts smaller than 3 mm or those draining a single hepatic segment can safely be ligated. If the injured duct is 4 mm or larger, it is likely to drain multiple segments or an entire lobe, and thus needs to be reimplanted. Lateral injury to the common bile duct or the common hepatic duct, recognized at the time of surgery, is best managed with a τ-tube placement. If the injury is a small incision in the duct, the τ tube may be placed through it as if it were a formal choledochotomy. In more extensive lateral injuries the τ tube should be placed through a separate choledochotomy and the injury closed over the τ tube end to minimize the risk of subsequent stricture formation.

Major bile duct injuries such as transection of the common hepatic or common bile duct are best managed at the time of injury. In many of these major injuries the bile duct has not only been transected, but a variable length of the duct removed. This injury usually requires a biliary enteric anastomosis with a jejunal loop. Transhepatic biliary catheters are placed through the anastomosis to stent it and to provide access to the biliary tract for drainage and imaging. Although rare, when the injury is to the distal common bile duct, a choledochoduodenostomy can be performed. If there is no or minimal loss of ductal length, a duct-to-duct repair may be done over a τ tube that is placed through a separate incision. Cystic duct leaks usually can be managed with percutaneous drainage of intraabdominal fluid collections followed by an endoscopic biliary stenting.

Major injuries diagnosed postoperatively require transhepatic biliary catheter placement for biliary decompression and percutaneous drainage of intraabdominal bile collections, if any. When the acute inflammation has resolved 6–8 weeks later, operative repair is performed.

Patients with bile duct stricture from an injury or as a sequela of previous repair usually present with either progressive elevation of liver function tests or cholangitis. The initial management usually includes transhepatic biliary drainage catheter placement for decompression and for defining the anatomy and the location and the extent of the damage. An anastomosis is performed between the duct proximal to the injury and a Roux loop of jejunum. Self-expanding metal or plastic stents, placed either percutaneously or endoscopically across the stricture, can provide temporary drainage, and in the high-risk patient, permanent drainage of the biliary tree.

Outcome

Good results can be expected in 70 to 90 percent of patients with bile duct injuries. The best results are obtained when the injury is recognized during the cholecystectomy and repaired by an experienced biliary tract surgeon. The operative mortality rate is about 5–8 percent. Restenosis of a biliary enteric anastomosis occurs in about 10 percent of patients, and may manifest up to 20 years after the initial procedure. Approximately two thirds of recurrent strictures become symptomatic within 2 years after repair. The more proximal strictures are associated with a lower success rate than are distal ones. Patients with deteriorating liver function are candidates for liver transplants.

TUMORS

Carcinoma of the Gallbladder

Cancer of the gallbladder is a rare malignancy that occurs predominantly in older adults. It is an aggressive tumor, with poor prognosis except when incidentally diagnosed at an early stage after cholecystectomy for cholelithiasis. The overall reported 5-year survival rate is about 5 percent.

Incidence

Gallbladder cancer is the fifth most common gastrointestinal malignancy in Western countries. However, it accounts for only 2–4 percent of all malignant gastrointestinal tumors. It is two to three times more common in females than males, and the peak incidence is in the seventh decade of life. Approximately 1 percent of patients undergoing cholecystectomy for gallstone disease are found incidentally to have gallbladder cancer. The incidence of gallbladder cancer is particularly high in native populations of the United States, Mexico, and Chile. The annual incidence in Native American females with gallstones approaches 75 per 100,000, compared with the overall incidence of gallbladder cancer of 2.5 cases per 100,000 residents in the United States.

Etiology

Approximately 90 percent of patients with carcinoma of the gallbladder have gallstones. However, the 20-year risk of developing cancer for patients with gallstones is less than 0.5 percent for the overall population and 1.5 percent for high-risk groups. Polypoid lesions of the gallbladder are associated with increased risk of cancer, particularly in polyps larger than 10 mm. The calcified "porcelain" gallbladder is associated with more than a 20 percent incidence of gallbladder carcinoma. These gallbladders should be removed, even if the patients are asymptomatic.

Pathology

Between 80 and 90 percent of the tumors are adenocarcinomas. The histologic subtypes of gallbladder adenocarcinomas include papillary, nodular, and tubular. Cancer of the gallbladder spreads through the lymphatics, with venous drainage, and with direct invasion into the liver parenchyma. Lymphatic flow from the gallbladder drains first to the cystic duct node (Calot), then the pericholedochal and hilar nodes. The gallbladder veins drain directly into the adjacent liver, usually segments IV and V, although tumor invasion is common. When diagnosed, about 25 percent of gallbladder cancers are localized to the gallbladder wall, 35 percent have regional nodal involvement and/or extension into adjacent liver, and approximately 40 percent have distant metastasis.

Clinical Manifestations and Diagnosis

Signs and symptoms of carcinoma of the gallbladder are generally indistinguishable from those associated with cholecystitis and cholelithiasis. These include abdominal discomfort, right upper quadrant pain, nausea, and vomiting. Jaundice, weight loss, anorexia, ascites, and abdominal mass are less common presenting symptoms. More than one-half of gallbladder cancers are not diagnosed before surgery. Ultrasonography often reveals a thickened, irregular gallbladder wall or a mass replacing the gallbladder. Ultrasonography may visualize tumor invasion of the liver, lymphadenopathy, and a dilated biliary tree. The sensitivity of ultrasonography in detecting gallbladder cancer ranges from 70–100 percent. CT scan may demonstrate a gallbladder mass or an invasion into adjacent organs. Additionally, a spiral CT scan demonstrates the vascular anatomy. MRCP has evolved into a single noninvasive imaging method that allows complete assessment of biliary, vascular, nodal, hepatic, and adjacent organ involvement. If diagnostic studies suggest that the tumor is unresectable, a CT scan or ultrasound-guided biopsy of the tumor can be obtained.

Treatment

Surgery remains the only curative option for gallbladder cancer and for cholangiocarcinoma. However, palliative procedures for patients with unresectable cancer and jaundice or duodenal obstruction remain the most frequently performed surgery for gallbladder cancers. Today, patients with obstructive jaundice can frequently be managed with either endoscopic or percutaneously placed biliary stents. There are no proven effective options for adjuvant radiation or chemotherapy for patients with gallbladder cancer.

Patients without evidence of distant metastasis warrant exploration for tissue diagnosis, pathologic staging, and possible curative resection.

Tumors limited to the muscular layer of the gallbladder (T1), usually are identified incidentally, after cholecystectomy for gallstone disease. There is near-universal agreement that simple cholecystectomy is an adequate treatment for T1 lesions and results in a near 100 percent overall 5-year survival rate. When the tumor invades the perimuscular connective tissue without extension beyond the serosa or into the liver (T2 tumors), an extended cholecystectomy should be performed. That includes resection of liver segments IVB and V, and lymphadenectomy of the cystic duct, and pericholedochal, portal, right celiac, and posterior pancreatoduodenal lymph nodes. One half of patients with T2 tumors are found to have nodal disease on pathologic examination. For tumors that grow beyond the serosa or invade the liver or other organs (T3 and T4 tumors), there is a high likelihood of intraperitoneal and distant spread. If no peritoneal or nodal involvement is found, complete tumor excision with an extended right hepatectomy (segments IV, V, VI, VII, and VIII) must be performed for adequate tumor clearance. An aggressive approach in patients who will tolerate surgery has resulted in an increased survival for T3 and T4 lesions.

Prognosis

Most patients with gallbladder cancer have unresectable disease at the time of diagnosis. The 5-year survival rate of all patients with gallbladder cancer is less than 5 percent, with a median survival of 6 months. Patients with T1 disease treated with cholecystectomy have an excellent prognosis (85–100 percent 5-year survival rate). The 5-year survival rate for T2 lesions treated with an extended cholecystectomy and lymphadenectomy compared with simple cholecystectomy is over 70 percent versus 25–40 percent, respectively. The median survival for patients with distant metastasis at the time of presentation is only 1–3 months.

Recurrence after resection of gallbladder cancer occurs most commonly in the liver or the celiac or retropancreatic nodes. The prognosis for recurrent disease is very poor. Death occurs most commonly secondary to biliary sepsis or liver failure.

Bile Duct Carcinoma

Cholangiocarcinoma is a rare tumor arising from the biliary epithelium and may occur anywhere along the biliary tree. About two-thirds are located at the hepatic duct bifurcation. Surgical resection offers the only chance for cure, however, many patients have advanced disease at the time of diagnosis. Therefore palliative procedures aimed to provide biliary drainage to prevent liver failure and cholangitis are often the only therapeutic possibilities. Most patients with unresectable disease die within a year of diagnosis.

Incidence

The autopsy incidence of bile duct carcinoma is about 0.3 percent. The overall incidence of cholangiocarcinoma in the United States is about 1.0 per 100,000 people per year.

Etiology

Risk factors associated with cholangiocarcinoma include primary sclerosing cholangitis, choledochal cysts, ulcerative colitis, hepatolithiasis, biliary-enteric anastomosis, and biliary tract infections with Clonorchis or in chronic typhoid carriers.

Pathology

Over 95 percent of bile duct cancers are adenocarcinomas. Morphologically they are divided into nodular (the most common type), scirrhous, diffusely infiltrating, or papillary. Anatomically they are divided into distal, proximal, or perihilar tumors. Intrahepatic cholangiocarcinomas occur, but they are treated like hepatocellular carcinoma, with hepatectomy when possible. About two thirds of cholangiocarcinomas are located in the perihilar location. Perihilar cholangiocarcinomas, also referred to as Klatskin tumors, are further classified based on anatomic location by the Bismuth-Corlette classification.

Clinical Manifestations and Diagnosis

Painless jaundice is the most common presentation. Pruritus, mild right upper quadrant pain, anorexia, fatigue, and weight loss also may be present.

The initial tests are usually ultrasound or CT scan. A perihilar tumor causes dilatation of the intrahepatic biliary tree, but normal or collapsed gallbladder and extrahepatic bile ducts distal to the tumor. Distal bile duct cancer leads to dilatation of the extra- and the intrahepatic bile ducts and the gallbladder. Ultrasound can establish the level of obstruction and rule out the presence of bile duct stones as the cause of the obstructive jaundice. The biliary anatomy is defined by cholangiography. PTC defines the proximal extent of the tumor, which is the most important factor in determining resectability. ERC is used, particularly in the evaluation of distal bile duct tumors. MRI, a single noninvasive test, has the potential of evaluating the biliary anatomy, lymph nodes, and vascular involvement, and the tumor growth itself.

Tissue diagnosis may be difficult to obtain nonoperatively except in advanced cases. Patients with potentially resectable disease should therefore be offered surgical exploration based on radiographic findings and clinical suspicion.

Treatment

Surgical excision is the only potentially curative treatment for cholangiocarcinoma. Patients should undergo surgical exploration if they have no signs of metastasis or locally unresectable disease. However, more than one half of the patients who are explored are found to have peritoneal implants, nodal or hepatic metastasis, or locally advanced disease that precludes resection. For these patients surgical bypass for biliary decompression and cholecystectomy to prevent the occurrence of acute cholecystitis should be performed.

For unresectable perihilar cholangiocarcinoma, Roux-en-Y cholangiojejunostomy to either segment II or III bile ducts or to the right hepatic duct can be performed.

For curative resection, the location and local extension of the tumor dictates the extent of the resection. Perihilar tumors involving the bifurcation or proximal common hepatic duct (Bismuth-Corlette type I or II) with no signs of vascular involvement are candidates for local tumor excision with portal lymphadenectomy, cholecystectomy, common bile duct excision, and bilateral Roux-en-Y hepatico jejunostomies. If the tumor involves the right or left hepatic duct (Bismuth-Corlette type IIIa or IIIb), right or left hepatic lobectomy, respectively, should also be performed. Distal bile duct tumors more often are resectable. They are treated with pylorus-preserving pancreatoduodenectomy (Whipple procedure). For patients with distal bile duct cancer found to be unresectable on surgical exploration, Roux-en-Y hepaticojejunostomy, cholecystectomy, and gastrojejunostomy to prevent gastric outlet obstruction should be performed.

Nonoperative biliary decompression is performed for patients with unresectable disease on diagnostic evaluation. Percutaneous placement of expandable metal stents or drainage catheters is usually the appropriate approach for proximal tumors. However, for distal bile duct tumors, endoscopic placement is often the preferred approach. There is no proven role for adjuvant chemotherapy in the treatment of cholangiocarcinoma. Adjuvant radiation therapy also has not been shown to increase either quality of life or survival in resected patients.

Prognosis

Most patients with perihilar cholangiocarcinoma present with advanced, unresectable disease. Patients with unresectable disease have a median survival between 5 and 8 months. The most common causes of death are hepatic failure and cholangitis. The overall 5-year survival rate for patients with resectable perihilar cholangiocarcinoma is between 10 and 30 percent, but for patients with negative margins it may be as high as 40 percent. The operative mortality for perihilar cholangiocarcinoma is 6–8 percent. The overall 5-year survival rate for patients with distal cholangiocarcinoma is 30–50 percent, and the median survival is 32–38 months.

Selected Readings

Scott-Conner CEH, Dawson DL: Operative Anatomy. Philadelphia: JB Lippincott Company, 1993, p 388.

Liu TH, Consorti ET, Kawashima A, et al: Patient evaluation and management with selective use of magnetic resonance cholangiography and endoscopic retrograde cholangiopancreatography before laparoscopic cholecystectomy. Ann Surg 234:33, 2001.

Strasberg SM: The pathogenesis of cholesterol gallstones a review. J Gastrointest Surg 2:109, 1998.

Stewart L, Oesterle AL, Erdan I, et al: Pathogenesis of pigment gallstones in Western societies: The central role of bacteria. J Gastrointest Surg 6:891, 2002.

Ko C, Lee S: Epidemiology and natural history of common bile duct stones and prediction of disease. Gastrointest Endosc 56:S165, 2002.

Khaitan L, Apelgren K, Hunter J, et al: A report on the Society of American Gastrointestinal Endoscopic Surgeons (SAGES) Outcomes Initiative: What have we learned and what is its potential? Surg Endosc 17:365, 2003.

Lipsett PA, Pitt HA: Surgical treatment of choledochal cysts. J Hepatobiliary Pancreat Surg 10:352, 2003.

Strasberg SM: Avoidance of biliary injury during laparoscopic cholecystectomy. J Hepato-Biliary-Pancreat Surg 9:543, 2002.

Grobmyer SR, Lieberman MD, Daly JM: Gallbladder cancer in the twentieth century: Single institution's experience. World J Surg 28:47, 2004.

Mulholland MW, Yahanda A, Yeo CJ: Multidisciplinary management of perihilar bile duct cancer. J Am Coll Surg 193:440, 2001.

32 | Pancreas

William E. Fisher, Dana K. Andersen, Richard H. Bell, Jr., Ashok K. Saluja, and F. Charles Brunicardi

ANATOMY AND PHYSIOLOGY

Situated deep in the center of the abdomen, the pancreas is surrounded by numerous important structures and major blood vessels. Surgeons typically describe the location of pathology within the pancreas in relation to four regions: the head, neck, body, and tail. The neck of the pancreas lies directly over the portal vein. At the inferior border of the neck of the pancreas, the superior mesenteric vein joins the splenic vein and then continues toward the porta hepatis as the portal vein. The common bile duct runs in a deep groove on the posterior aspect of the pancreatic head until it passes through the pancreatic parenchyma to join the main pancreatic duct at the ampulla of Vater. The body and tail of the pancreas lie just anterior to the splenic artery and vein.

Pancreatic Duct Anatomy

An understanding of embryology is required to appreciate the common variations in pancreatic duct anatomy. The pancreas is formed by the fusion of a ventral and dorsal bud. The duct from the smaller ventral bud, which arises from the hepatic diverticulum, connects directly to the common bile duct. The duct from the larger dorsal bud, which arises from the duodenum, drains directly into the duodenum. The duct of the ventral anlage becomes the duct of Wirsung, and the duct from the dorsal anlage becomes the duct of Santorini. With gut rotation, the ventral anlage rotates to the right and around the posterior side of the duodenum to fuse with the dorsal bud. The ventral anlage becomes the inferior portion of the pancreatic head and the uncinate process, although the dorsal anlage becomes the body and tail of the pancreas. The ducts from each anlage usually fuse together in the pancreatic head such that most of the pancreas drains through the duct of Wirsung, or main pancreatic duct, into the common channel formed from the bile duct and pancreatic duct. The length of the common channel is variable. In about one third of patients the two ducts remain distinct to the end of the papilla, the two ducts merge at the end of the papilla in another one third, and in the remaining one-third a true common channel is present for a distance of several millimeters. Commonly, the duct from the dorsal anlage, the duct of Santorini, persists as the lesser pancreatic duct, and sometimes drains directly into the duodenum through the lesser papilla just proximal to the major papilla. In approximately 30 percent of patients, the duct of Santorini ends as a blind accessory duct and does not empty into the duodenum. In 10 percent of patients, the ducts of Wirsung and Santorini fail to fuse. This results in the majority of the pancreas draining through the duct of Santorini and the lesser papilla, although the inferior portion of the pancreatic head and uncinate process drains through the duct of Wirsung and major papilla. This normal anatomic variant, which occurs in one out of 10 patients, is referred to as pancreas divisum. In a minority of these patients, the minor papilla can be inadequate to handle the flow of pancreatic juices from the majority of the gland. This relative outflow obstruction can

845

result in pancreatitis and is sometimes treated by sphincteroplasty of the minor papilla.

Vascular and Lymphatic Anatomy

The blood supply to the pancreas comes from multiple branches from the celiac and superior mesenteric arteries. The common hepatic artery gives rise to the gastroduodenal artery before continuing toward the porta hepatis as the proper hepatic artery. The gastroduodenal artery becomes the superior pancreaticoduodenal artery as it passes behind the first portion of the duodenum and branches into the anterior and posterior superior pancreaticoduodenal arteries. As the superior mesenteric artery passes behind the neck of the pancreas, it gives off the inferior pancreaticoduodenal artery at the inferior margin of the neck of the pancreas. This vessel quickly divides into the anterior and posterior inferior pancreaticoduodenal arteries. The superior and inferior pancreaticoduodenal arteries join together within the parenchyma of the anterior and posterior sides of the head of the pancreas along the medial aspect of the C-loop of the duodenum to form arcades that give off numerous branches to the duodenum and head of the pancreas. Therefore it is impossible to resect the head of the pancreas without devascularizing the duodenum, unless a rim of pancreas containing the pancreaticoduodenal arcade is preserved. Variations in the arterial anatomy occur in one out of five patients. The right hepatic artery, common hepatic artery, or gastroduodenal arteries can arise from the superior mesenteric artery. In 15–20 percent of patients, the right hepatic artery will arise from the superior mesenteric artery and travel upwards toward the liver along the posterior aspect of the head of the pancreas (referred to as a "replaced right hepatic artery"). During the Whipple procedure, it is important to look for this variation so the hepatic artery is recognized and injury is avoided. The body and tail of the pancreas are supplied by multiple branches of the splenic artery. The splenic artery arises from the celiac trunk and travels along the posterior-superior border of the body and tail of the pancreas toward the spleen. The inferior pancreatic artery arises from the superior mesenteric artery and runs to the left along the inferior border of the body and tail of the pancreas, parallel to the splenic artery. Three vessels run perpendicular to the long axis of the pancreatic body and tail and connect the splenic artery and inferior pancreatic artery. They are, from medial to lateral, the dorsal, great, and caudal pancreatic arteries. These arteries form arcades within the body and tail of the pancreas, and account for the rich blood supply of the organ. The venous drainage of the pancreas follows a pattern similar to that of the arterial supply. The lymphatic drainage from the pancreas is diffuse and widespread and this contributes to the fact that pancreatic cancer often presents with positive lymph nodes and a high incidence of local recurrence after resection.

Neuroanatomy

The pancreas is innervated by the sympathetic and parasympathetic nervous systems. The parasympathetic system stimulates endocrine and exocrine secretion and the sympathetic system inhibits secretion. The pancreas also has a rich supply of afferent sensory fibers, which are responsible for the intense pain associated with advanced pancreatic cancer, and acute and chronic pancreatitis. These somatic fibers travel superiorly to the celiac ganglia. Interruption of these somatic fibers can stop transmission of pain sensation.

HISTOLOGY AND PHYSIOLOGY

The exocrine pancreas accounts for about 85 percent of the pancreatic mass; 10 percent of the gland is accounted for by extracellular matrix, and 4 percent by blood vessels and the major ducts, whereas only 2 percent of the gland is comprised of endocrine tissue. The endocrine and exocrine pancreas are sometimes thought of as functionally separate, but these different components of the organ are coordinated to allow an elegant regulatory feedback system for digestive enzyme and hormone secretion.

Exocrine Pancreas

The pancreas secretes approximately 500–800 mL per day of colorless, odorless, alkaline, isosmotic pancreatic juice. Pancreatic juice is a combination of acinar cell and duct cell secretions. The acinar cells secrete amylase, proteases and lipases, enzymes responsible for the digestion of all three food types: carbohydrate, protein, and fat. The acinar cells are pyramid-shaped, with their apices facing the lumen of the acinus. Near the apex of each cell are numerous enzyme-containing zymogen granules which fuse with the apical cell membrane.

Amylase is the only pancreatic enzyme secreted in its active form, and it hydrolyzes starch and glycogen to glucose, maltose, maltotriose, and dextrins. These simple sugars are transported across the brush border of the intestinal epithelial cells by active transport mechanisms. The proteolytic enzymes are secreted as proenzymes that require activation. Trypsinogen is converted to its active form, trypsin, by another enzyme, enterokinase, which is produced by the duodenal mucosal cells. Trypsin in turn activates the other proteolytic enzymes. Chymotrypsinogen is activated to form chymotrypsin. Elastase, carboxypeptidase A and B, and phospholipase also are activated by trypsin. Trypsin, chymotrypsin, and elastase cleave bonds between amino acids within a target peptide chain, and carboxypeptidase A and B cleave amino acids at the end of peptide chains. Individual amino acids and small dipeptides are then actively transported into the intestinal epithelial cells. Pancreatic lipase hydrolyzes triglycerides to 2-monoglyceride and fatty acid. Pancreatic lipase is secreted in an active form. Colipase also is secreted by the pancreas and binds to lipase, changing its molecular configuration and increasing its activity. Phospholipase A2 is secreted by the pancreas as a proenzyme which becomes activated by trypsin. Phospholipase A2 hydrolyzes phospholipids, and as with all lipases, requires bile salts for its action. Carboxylic ester hydrolase and cholesterol esterase hydrolyze neutral lipid substrates like esters of cholesterol, fat-soluble vitamins, and triglycerides. The hydrolyzed fat is then packaged into micelles for transport into the intestinal epithelial cells, in which the fatty acids are reassembled and packaged inside chylomicrons for transport through the lymphatic system into the bloodstream. The centroacinar and intercalated duct cells secrete the water and electrolytes present in the pancreatic juice.

Endocrine Pancreas

There are nearly one million islets of Langerhans in the normal adult pancreas. They vary greatly in size from 40–900 μm. Most islets contain 3000–4000 cells of four major types: alpha cells which secrete glucagon, beta cells which secrete insulin, delta cells which secrete somatostatin, and pancreatic polypeptide (PP) cells, which secrete pancreatic polypeptide.

There are two phases of insulin secretion. In the first phase, stored insulin is released. This phase lasts about 5 min after a glucose challenge. The second phase of insulin secretion is a longer, sustained release because of ongoing production of new insulin. Insulin's function is to inhibit endogenous (hepatic) glucose production and to facilitate glucose transport into cells, thus lowering plasma glucose levels. Insulin also inhibits glycogenolysis, fatty acid breakdown and ketone formation, and stimulates protein synthesis. If the remaining portion of the pancreas is healthy, about 80 percent of the pancreas can be resected without the patient becoming diabetic. In patients with chronic pancreatitis, or other conditions in which much of the gland is diseased, resection of a smaller fraction of the pancreas can result in diabetes.

Glucagon promotes hepatic glycogenolysis and gluconeogenesis and counteracts the effects of insulin through its hyperglycemic action. Somatostatin inhibits endocrine and exocrine secretion and affects neurotransmission, gastrointestinal and biliary motility, intestinal absorption, vascular tone and cell proliferation. Pancreatic polypeptide is known to inhibit bile secretion, gallbladder contraction, and secretion by the exocrine pancreas. A number of studies suggest that PPs most important role is in glucose regulation through its regulation of hepatic insulin receptor gene expression. Deficiencies in PP secretion because of proximal pancreatectomy or severe chronic pancreatitis, are associated with diminished hepatic insulin sensitivity because of reduced hepatic insulin receptors.

In addition to the four main peptides secreted by the pancreas, there are a number of other peptide products of the islet cells, including amylin and pancreastatin, and neuropeptides such as VIP, galanin, and serotonin. Amylin or islet amyloid polypeptide (IAPP) is stored along with insulin in secretory granules. The function of IAPP seems to be the modulation or counterregulation of insulin secretion and function. Pancreastatin is a recently discovered pancreatic islet peptide product that inhibits insulin, and possibly somatostatin release, and augments glucagon release. In addition to this effect on the endocrine pancreas, pancreastatin inhibits pancreatic exocrine secretion.

ACUTE PANCREATITIS

Definition and Incidence

Acute pancreatitis is an inflammatory disease of the pancreas that is associated with little or no fibrosis of the gland. It can be initiated by several factors including gallstones, alcohol, trauma, and infections, and in some cases it is hereditary. Very often patients with acute pancreatitis develop additional complications such as sepsis, shock, and respiratory and renal failure, resulting in considerable morbidity and mortality.

The etiology of acute pancreatitis is a complex subject because many different factors have been implicated in the causation of this disease, and sometimes there are no identifiable causes. Two factors, biliary tract stone disease and alcoholism, account for 80–90 percent of the cases. The remaining 10–20 percent is accounted for either by idiopathic disease or by a variety of miscellaneous causes including trauma, surgery, drugs, heredity, infection and toxins. A tumor should be considered in a nonalcoholic patient with acute pancreatitis who has no demonstrable biliary tract disease. Approximately 1–2 percent of patients with acute pancreatitis have pancreatic carcinoma, and an episode of acute pancreatitis can be the first clinical manifestation of a periampullary tumor. Acute pancreatitis can be associated with a number of surgical procedures, most commonly those performed on or close to the pancreas, such as pancreatic biopsy, biliary duct exploration, distal gastrectomy, and splenectomy. Endoscopic retrograde cholangiopancreatography results in pancreatitis in 2–10 percent of patients, because of direct injury and/or intraductal hypertension.

Certain drugs are known to be capable of causing acute pancreatitis. These include the thiazide diuretics, furosemide, estrogens, azathioprine, L-asparaginase, 6-mercaptopurine, methyldopa, the sulfonamides, tetracycline, pentamidine, procainamide, nitrofurantoin, dideoxyinosine, valproic acid, and acetylcholines-terase inhibitors. Patients with types I and V hyperlipoproteinemia often experience attacks of abdominal pain that are thought to indicate episodes of acute pancreatitis. These episodes are frequently associated with marked hypertriglyceridemia and lactescent serum, and can be prevented by dietary modifications that restrict serum triglycerides. Hypercalcemic states arising from hyperparathyroidism can result in both acute and chronic pancreatitis; the mechanism most likely involves hypersecretion and the formation of calcified stones intraductally. Finally, no apparent cause can be ascribed to some episodes of acute pancreatitis, and these constitute the group referred to as "idiopathic pancreatitis." Some of these patients are eventually found to have gallstone-related pancreatitis, which calls for caution in labeling any episode "idiopathic."

Pathophysiology

Pancreatitis begins with the activation of digestive zymogens inside acinar cells which cause acinar cell injury. Recent studies suggest that the ultimate severity of the resulting pancreatitis may be determined by the events that occur subsequent to acinar cell injury. These include inflammatory cell recruitment and activation, and generation and release of cytokines and other chemical mediators of inflammation.

Diagnosis

The clinical diagnosis of pancreatitis is one of exclusion. The other upper abdominal conditions that can be confused with acute pancreatitis include perforated peptic ulcer, a gangrenous small bowel obstruction, and acute cholecystitis. Because these conditions often have a fatal outcome without surgery, urgent intervention is indicated in the small number of cases in which doubt persists.

All episodes of acute pancreatitis begin with severe pain, generally following a substantial meal. The pain is usually epigastric, but can occur anywhere in the abdomen or lower chest. It has been described as "knifing" or "boring through" to the back, and may be relieved by the patient leaning forward. It precedes the onset of nausea and vomiting, with retching often continuing after the stomach has emptied. Vomiting does not relieve the pain, which is more intense in necrotizing than in edematous pancreatitis. An episode of acute pancreatic inflammation in a patient with known chronic pancreatitis has the same findings.

On examination the patient may show tachycardia, tachypnea, hypotension, and hyperthermia. The temperature is usually only mildly elevated in uncomplicated pancreatitis. Voluntary and involuntary guarding can be seen over the epigastric region. The bowel sounds are decreased or absent. There are usually no palpable masses. The abdomen may be distended with intraperitoneal fluid. There may be pleural effusion, particularly on the left side.

With increasing severity of disease, the intravascular fluid loss may become life-threatening as a result of sequestration of edematous fluid in the retroperitoneum. Hemoconcentration then results in an elevated hematocrit. However, there also may be bleeding into the retroperitoneum or the peritoneal cavity. In some patients (approximately 1 percent), the blood from necrotizing pancreatitis may dissect through the soft tissues and manifest as a blueish discoloration around the umbilicus (Cullen sign) or in the flanks (Grey Turner sign). The severe fluid loss may lead to prerenal azotemia with elevated blood urea nitrogen and creatinine levels. There also may be hyperglycemia, hypoalbuminemia, and hypocalcemia sufficient in some cases to produce tetany.

Serum Markers

Because pancreatic acinar cells synthesize, store, and secrete a large number of digestive enzymes (e.g., amylase, lipase, trypsinogen, and elastase), the levels of these enzymes are elevated in the serum of most pancreatitis patients. Because of the ease of measurement, serum amylase levels are measured most often. Serum amylase concentration increases almost immediately with the onset of disease and peaks within several h. It remains elevated for 3–5 days before returning to normal. There is no significant correlation between the magnitude of serum amylase elevation and severity of pancreatitis; in fact, a milder form of acute pancreatitis is often associated with higher levels of serum amylase as compared with that in a more severe form of the disease.

It is important to note that hyperamylasemia also can occur as a result of conditions not involving pancreatitis. For example, hyperamylasemia can occur in a patient with small bowel obstruction, perforated duodenal ulcer, or other intraabdominal inflammatory conditions. In contrast, a patient with acute pancreatitis may have a normal serum amylase level.

Other pancreatic enzymes also have been evaluated to improve the diagnostic accuracy of serum measurements. Specificity of these markers ranges from 77–96 percent, the highest being for lipase. Measurements of many digestive enzymes also have methodologic limitations and cannot be easily adapted for quantitation in emergency labs. Because serum levels of lipase remain elevated for a longer time than total or pancreatic amylase, it is the serum indicator of highest probability of the disease.

Abdominal ultrasound examination is the best way to confirm the presence of gallstones in suspected biliary pancreatitis. It also can detect extrapancreatic ductal dilations and reveal pancreatic edema, swelling, and peripancreatic fluid collections. However, in about 20 percent of patients, the ultrasound examination does not provide satisfactory results because of the presence of bowel gas, which may obscure sonographic imaging of the pancreas. A computed tomographic (CT) scan of the pancreas more commonly is used to diagnose pancreatitis. CT scanning is used to distinguish milder (nonnecrotic) forms of the disease from more severe necrotizing or infected pancreatitis, in patients whose clinical presentation raises the suspicion of advanced disease.

Assessment of Severity

An early discrimination between mild edematous and severe necrotizing forms of the disease is of the utmost importance to provide optimal care to the patient. In 1974, Ranson identified a series of prognostic signs for early identification of patients with severe pancreatitis. Out of these 11 objective parameters, 5

TABLE 32-1 Ranson's Prognostic Signs of Pancreatitis

Criteria for acute pancreatitis not due to gallstones

At admission	*During the initial 48 h*
Age > 55 y	Hematocrit fall >10 points
WBC > 16,000/mm^3	BUN elevation > 5 mg/dL
Blood glucose > 200 mg/dL	Serum calcium < 8 mg/dL
Serum LDH > 350 IU/L	Arterial Po$_2$ < 60 mm Hg
Serum AST > 250 U/dL	Base deficit > 4 mEq/L
	Estimated fluid sequestration >6 L

Criteria for acute gallstone pancreatitis

At admission	*During the initial 48 h*
Age > 70 y	Hematocrit fall >10 points
WBC > 18,000/mm^3	BUN elevation > 2 mg/dL
Blood glucose > 220 mg/dL	Serum calcium < 8 mg/dL
Serum LDH > 400 IU/L	Base deficit > 5 mEq/L
Serum AST > 250 U/dL	Estimated fluid sequestration > 4 L

AST = aspartate transaminase; BUN = blood urea nitrogen; LDH = lactate dehydrogenase; Po$_2$ = partial pressure of oxygen; WBC = white blood cell count.
Source: Reproduced with permission from Ranson JHC: Etiological and prognostic factors in human acute pancreatitis: A review. *Am J Gastroenterol* 77:633, 1982.

are measured at the time of admission, whereas the remaining 6 are measured within 48 h of admission (Table 32-1). Morbidity and mortality of the disease are directly related to the number of signs present. If the number of positive Ranson signs is less than 2, the mortality is generally zero; with 3–5 positive signs, mortality is increased to 10–20 percent. The mortality rate increases to more than 50 percent when there are more than seven positive Ranson signs. It is important to realize that Ranson prognostic signs are best used within the initial 48 h of hospitalization and have not been validated for later time intervals.

Several recent research studies have suggested additional markers that may have prognostic value, including acute phase proteins such as C-reactive protein (CRP), α2-macroglobulin, PMN-elastase, α1-antitrypsin, and phospholipase A2. While CRP measurement is commonly available many of the others are not. Therefore, at this time CRP seems to be the marker of choice in clinical settings.

Computed Tomography Scan

CT scanning with bolus intravenous contrast has become the standard criterion for detecting and assessing the severity of pancreatitis. While clinically mild pancreatitis usually is associated with interstitial edema, severe pancreatitis is associated with necrosis. In interstitial pancreatitis, the microcirculation of the pancreas remains intact, and the gland shows uniform enhancement on intravenous, contrast-enhanced CT scan. In necrotizing pancreatitis, however, the microcirculation is disrupted; therefore the enhancement of the gland on contrast-enhanced CT scan is considerably decreased. The presence of air bubbles on a CT scan is an indication of infected necrosis or pancreatic abscess.

Currently, intravenous (bolus), contrast-enhanced CT scanning is routinely performed on patients who are suspected of harboring severe pancreatitis, regardless of their Ranson or APACHE scores.

Treatment

The severity of acute pancreatitis covers a broad spectrum of illness, ranging from the mild and self-limiting to the life-threatening necrotizing variety. Regardless of severity, hospitalization of the patient with suspected acute pancreatitis for observation and diagnostic study is usually mandatory. On confirmation of the diagnosis, patients with moderate to severe disease should be transferred to the intensive care unit for observation and maximal support. The most important initial treatment is conservative intensive care with the goals of oral food and fluid restriction, replacement of fluids and electrolytes parenterally as assessed by central venous pressure and urinary excretion, and control of pain. In severe acute pancreatitis, or when signs of infection are present, most experts recommend broad-spectrum antibiotics (e.g., imipenem) and careful surveillance for complications of the disease.

Mild Pancreatitis

The current principles of treatment are physiologic monitoring, metabolic support, and maintenance of fluid balance, which can become dangerously disturbed even in mild acute pancreatitis because of fluid sequestration, vomiting, and sudoresis. Because hypovolemia can result in pancreatic and other visceral ischemia, fluid balance should be assessed at least every 8 h initially.

Cautious resumption of oral feeding consisting of small and slowly increasing meals is permissible after the abdominal pain and tenderness have subsided, serum amylase has returned to normal, and the patient experiences hunger. This usually occurs within a week of the onset of an attack of mild acute pancreatitis. A low-fat, low-protein diet is advocated as the initial form of nutrition following an attack of acute pancreatitis.

Severe Pancreatitis

Pancreatitis can be classified as severe based on predictors such as APACHE-II scores and Ranson signs, and any evidence that the condition is severe mandates care of the patient in the intensive care unit. Such evidence may take various forms, such as the onset of encephalopathy, a hematocrit over 50, urine output less than 50 mL/h, hypotension, fever, or peritonitis. Older adult patients with three or more Ranson criteria also should be monitored carefully despite the absence of severe pain.

Patients may develop adult respiratory distress syndrome (ARDS), and many patients who die during the early stages of severe acute pancreatitis have this complication. The presence of ARDS usually requires assisted ventilation with positive end-expiratory pressure. The value of peritoneal lavage in removing enzyme-rich ascites remains unclear. It has been advocated in patients with deteriorating respiratory function and/or shock that is refractory to maximal management, but its effectiveness in reducing the mortality risk of severe acute pancreatitis remains unproven.

Acute pancreatitis may be accompanied by cardiovascular events such as cardiac arrhythmia, myocardial infarction, cardiogenic shock, and congestive heart failure. The conventional modalities of treatment apply in these cases in addition to the support described above.

Infections

Infection is a serious complication of acute pancreatitis and is the most common cause of death. It is caused most often by translocated enteric bacteria, and is seen commonly in necrotizing rather than interstitial pancreatitis. If there is an indication of infection (e.g., retroperitoneal air on CT scan), then a CT- or ultrasound-guided fine-needle aspiration should be performed for Gram stain and culture of the fluid or tissue, and the indicated antibiotic therapy initiated. However, antibiotics alone may not be effective in infected necrosis, which has a mortality of nearly 50 percent unless débrided surgically. The long-held opinion that antibiotic prophylaxis in necrotizing pancreatitis is of little use has been altered by recent studies showing a beneficial prophylactic effect with antibiotics such as metronidazole, imipenem, and third-generation cephalosporins. Because Candida species are common inhabitants of the upper gastrointestinal tract, Candida sepsis and secondary fungal infection of pancreatic necrosis is a risk in severe disease. The role of empiric therapy with fluconazole in cases of severe acute pancreatitis is currently being investigated in large-scale clinical trials.

Sterile Necrosis

Patients with sterile necrosis have a far better prognosis than those with infected necrosis, with a reported mortality of near zero in the absence of systemic complications. However, others report mortality rates as high as 38 percent in patients with a single systemic complication.

Treatment of sterile necrotic pancreatitis falls into three degrees of aggressiveness. At one end of the scale is the patient with no systemic complications and no concerns about secondary infections, who can be managed with the supportive care described previously and be cautiously brought back to refeeding. The area of sterile necrosis may evolve into a chronic pseudocyst, or may resolve. An intermediate course is demonstrated by the patient who develops systemic complications, and in whom a secondary infection is suspected. A CT-guided, fine-needle aspiration then confirms or disproves infection, and in the latter instance the patient can be managed medically. The last and most serious condition is that of the patient who appears to be very ill, has high APACHE-II and Ranson scores, and shows evidence of systemic toxicity including shock. Patients in this category have a poor chance of survival without aggressive débridement, and a decision may be made to proceed with exploration simply because of a relentless course of deterioration despite maximal medical therapy. It must be emphasized that current opinion is against débridement in sterile necrosis unless it is accompanied by life-threatening systemic complications.

Pancreatic Abscess

A pancreatic abscess occurs 2–6 weeks after the initial attack, in contrast to infected necrosis, which occurs in the first few h or days. The mechanism of delayed infection is not clear, but the treatment consists of external drainage, whether established by surgical or by percutaneous catheter-based methods.

Nutritional Support

The guiding principle of resting the pancreas dictates that patients with acute pancreatitis not be fed orally until their clinical condition improves. This generally occurs in 3–7 days in patients with mild pancreatitis, but the situation in patients with severe pancreatitis is more complicated, requiring nutritional support for several weeks. This can be provided by total parenteral nutrition (TPN) or by enteral nutrition through a jejunal tube. There is some debate regarding the preferred route, because TPN is known to result in early atrophy of the gut mucosa, a condition that favors transmigration of luminal bacteria, and intrajejunal feeding still stimulates pancreatic exocrine secretion through the release of enteric hormones. Recent animal studies and preliminary clinical trials on humans suggest that on balance, jejunal feeding may be superior to TPN.

Treatment of Biliary Pancreatitis

Gallstones are the most common cause of acute pancreatitis worldwide. Most patients pass the offending gallstone(s) during the early h of acute pancreatitis, but have additional stones capable of inducing future episodes. This raises the question of the timing of surgical or endoscopic clearance of gallstones. The issue of when to intervene is controversial. When choledocholithiasis is suspected, clearance of stones by endoscopic retrograde cholangiography is indicated. Most surgeons favor cholecystectomy during the same hospitalization as the acute episode of pancreatitis but surgery is delayed until the pancreatitis is resolved. Routine endoscopic retrograde cholangiopancreatography (ERCP) for examination of the bile duct is discouraged in cases of biliary pancreatitis, as the probability of finding residual stones is low, and the risk of ERCP-induced pancreatitis is significant.

CHRONIC PANCREATITIS

Etiology

Worldwide, alcohol consumption and abuse is associated with chronic pancreatitis in up to 70 percent of cases. Other major causes worldwide include tropical (nutritional) and idiopathic disease, and hereditary causes.

Alcohol

There is a linear relationship between exposure to alcohol and the development of chronic pancreatitis. The risk of disease is present in patients with even a low or occasional exposure to alcohol (1–20 g/day), so there is no threshold level of alcohol exposure below which there is no risk of developing chronic pancreatitis. Furthermore, although the risk of disease is dose related, and highest in heavy (150 g/day) drinkers, fewer than 15 percent of confirmed alcohol abusers suffer from chronic pancreatitis. However, the duration of alcohol consumption is definitely associated with the development of pancreatic disease. The onset of disease typically occurs between ages 35–40, after 16–20 years of heavy alcohol consumption. Recurrent episodes of acute pancreatitis are typically followed by chronic symptoms after 4 or 5 years. It remains to be determined whether alcohol sensitizes the pancreas of susceptible individuals to another cause of acute inflammation, or whether genetic or other factors predispose to direct alcohol-related injury.

Hereditary pancreatitis. Typically, patients first present in childhood or adolescence with abdominal pain, and are found to have chronic calcific pancreatitis on imaging studies. Progressive pancreatic dysfunction is common, and many patients present with symptoms because of pancreatic duct obstruction. The risk of subsequent carcinoma formation is increased, reaching a prevalence in some series of 40 percent, but the age of onset for carcinoma is typically over 50 years. The disorder is characterized by an autosomal dominant pattern of inheritance, with 80 percent penetrance and variable expression. The incidence is equal in both sexes. Whitcomb and colleagues, and separately Le-Bodic and associates, performed gene linkage analysis and identified a linkage for hereditary pancreatitis to chromosome 7q35. Subsequently, the region was sequenced, and revealed eight trypsinogen genes. Mutational analysis revealed a missense mutation resulting in an Arg to His substitution at position 117 of the cationic trypsinogen gene, or PRSS1, one of the primary sites for proteolysis of trypsin. This mutation prevents trypsin from being inactivated by itself or other proteases, and results in persistent and uncontrolled proteolytic activity and autodestruction within the pancreas. The position 117 mutation of PRSS1 and an additional mutation, now known collectively as the R122H and N291 mutations of PRSS1, account for about two-thirds of cases of hereditary pancreatitis. Recently, Schneider and Whitcomb described a probable mutation in the anionic trypsinogen gene which may also be present in some cases. Thus, hereditary pancreatitis results from one or more mutational defects, which incapacitate an autoprotective process that normally prevents proteolysis within the pancreas.

Similarly, PSTI, also known as SPINK1, has been found to have a role in hereditary pancreatitis. SPINK1 specifically inhibits trypsin action by competitively blocking the active site of the enzyme. Witt and colleagues investigated 96 unrelated children with chronic pancreatitis in Germany and found a variety of SPINK1 mutations in 23 percent of the patients. Several studies have now confirmed an association of SPINK1 mutations with familial and idiopathic forms of chronic pancreatitis, and tropical pancreatitis. SPINK1 mutations are common in the general population as well, and the frequency of these mutations varies in different cohorts of idiopathic chronic pancreatitis, from 6.4 percent in France to 25.8 percent in the United States. It is likely that many of the "idiopathic" forms of chronic pancreatitis, and some patients with the more common forms of the disease, will be found to have a genetic linkage or predisposition.

Autoimmune pancreatitis. A variant of chronic pancreatitis is a nonobstructive, diffusely infiltrative disease associated with fibrosis, a mononuclear cell (lymphocyte, plasma cell, or eosinophil) infiltrate, and an increased titer of one or more autoantibodies. Compressive stenosis of the intrapancreatic portion of the common bile duct is frequently seen, along with symptoms of obstructive jaundice. Increased levels of serum β-globulin or immunoglobulin G also are present. Steroid therapy is uniformly successful in ameliorating the disease, including any associated bile duct compression. The differential diagnosis includes lymphoma, plasmacytoma ("pseudotumor" of the pancreas), and diffuse infiltrative carcinoma. Although the diagnosis is confirmed on pancreatic biopsy, presumptive treatment with steroids usually is undertaken, especially when clinical and laboratory findings support the diagnosis. Failure to obtain a cytologic specimen may lead to an unnecessary resectional procedure, and an untreated inflammatory component may cause sclerosis of the extrahepatic or intrahepatic bile ducts, with eventual liver failure.

Pancreas divisum represents a special case of obstructive pancreatitis. It is the most common congenital anomaly involving the pancreas and occurs in up to 10 percent of children. It is thought to predispose the pancreas to recurrent acute pancreatitis and chronic pancreatitis, because of functional obstruction of a diminutive duct of Santorini which fails to communicate with the Wirsung duct. However, the classic picture of obstructive pancreatopathy with a dilated dorsal duct is unusual in pancreas divisum, so a decompressive operation or a lesser papilla sphincteroplasty is frequently not feasible or unsuccessful. Endoscopic stenting through the lesser papilla may result in temporary relief of symptoms, and this response would increase the possibility that a permanent surgical or endoscopic intervention will be successful. Although some authors emphasize the pathologic implications of pancreas divisum, others express skepticism that it represents a true risk to pancreatic secretory capacity or contributes to the development of chronic pancreatitis.

Idiopathic pancreatitis. When a definable cause for chronic pancreatitis is lacking, the term "idiopathic" is used to categorize the illness. Not surprisingly, as diagnostic methods and clinical awareness of disease improve, fewer patients fall into the idiopathic category. Classically, the idiopathic group includes young adults and adolescents who lack a family history of pancreatitis, but who may represent individuals with spontaneous gene mutations encoding for regulatory proteins in the pancreas. Additionally, the idiopathic group has included a large number of older patients for whom no obvious cause of recurrent or chronic pancreatitis can be found. However, because the prevalence of biliary calculi increases steadily with age, it is not surprising that as methods to detect biliary stone disease and microlithiasis have improved, a larger proportion of older adult "idiopathic" pancreatitis patients are found to have biliary tract disease.

Radiology

Radiologic imaging of chronic pancreatitis assists in four areas: (1) diagnosis, (2) the evaluation of severity of disease, (3) detection of complications, and (4) assistance in determining treatment options. With the advent of cross-sectional imaging techniques such as CT and magnetic resonance imaging (MRI), the contour, content, ductal pattern, calcifications, calculi, and cystic disease of the pancreas are all readily discernible. Endoscopic ultrasound (EUS) is now frequently employed as a preliminary step in the evaluation of patients with pancreatic disease, and magnetic resonance cholangiopancreatography (MRCP) is increasingly being used to select patients who are candidates for the most invasive imaging method, ERCP. The staging of disease is important in the care of patients, and a combination of imaging methods is usually employed.

Presentation, Natural History, and Complications

Presenting Signs and Symptoms

Pain is the most common symptom of chronic pancreatitis. It is usually midepigastric in location, but may localize or involve either the left or right upper quadrant of the abdomen. Occasionally it is perceived in the lower mid-abdomen, but is frequently described as penetrating through to the back. The pain is typically steady and boring, but not colicky. It persists for h or days, and may be chronic with exacerbations caused by eating or drinking alcohol. Chronic alcoholics also describe a steady, constant pain that is temporarily relieved by alcohol, followed by a more severe recurrence h later.

Patients with chronic pancreatic pain typically flex their abdomen and either sit or lie with their hips flexed, or lie on their side in a fetal position. Unlike ureteral stone pain or biliary colic, the pain causes the patient to be still. Nausea or vomiting may accompany the pain, but anorexia is the most common associated symptom.

Malabsorption and Weight Loss

When pancreatic exocrine capacity falls below 10 percent of normal, diarrhea and steatorrhea develop. Patients describe a bulky, foul-smelling, loose (but not watery) stool that may be pale in color and float on the surface of toilet water. Frequently, patients will describe a greasy or oily appearance to the stool, or may describe an "oil slick" on the water's surface. In severe steatorrhea, an orange, oily stool often is reported. As exocrine deficiency increases, symptoms of steatorrhea often are accompanied by weight loss. Patients may describe a good appetite despite weight loss, or diminished food intake because of abdominal pain.

In severe symptomatic chronic pancreatitis, anorexia or nausea may occur with or separate from abdominal pain. The combination of decreased food intake and malabsorption of nutrients usually results in chronic weight loss. As a result, many patients with severe chronic pancreatitis are below ideal body weight.

Pancreatogenic Diabetes

The islets comprise only 2 percent of the mass of the pancreas, but they are preferentially conserved when pancreatic inflammation occurs. In chronic pancreatitis, acinar tissue loss and replacement by fibrosis is greater than the degree of loss of islet tissue, although islets are typically smaller than normal, and may be isolated from their surrounding vascular network by the fibrosis. With progressive destruction of the gland, endocrine insufficiency commonly occurs. Frank diabetes is seen initially in about 20 percent of patients with chronic pancreatitis, and impaired glucose metabolism can be detected in up to 70 percent of patients.

Pancreatogenic diabetes is more common after surgical resection for chronic pancreatitis. Distal pancreatectomy and Whipple procedures have a higher incidence of diabetes than do drainage procedures, and the severity of diabetes is frequently worse after partial pancreatectomy.

The etiology and pathophysiology of pancreatogenic or type III diabetes is distinct from that of either insulin-dependent (type I) or non–insulin-independent (type II) diabetes. In pancreatogenic diabetes, because of the loss of functioning pancreatic tissue by disease or surgical removal, there is a global deficiency of all three glucoregulatory islet cell hormones: insulin, glucagon, and PP. Additionally, there is a paradoxical combination of enhanced peripheral sensitivity to insulin, and decreased hepatic sensitivity to insulin. As a result, insulin therapy is frequently difficult; patients are hyperglycemic when insulin replacement is insufficient (because of unsuppressed hepatic glucose production) or hypoglycemic when insulin replacement is barely excessive (because of enhanced peripheral insulin sensitivity and a deficiency of pancreatic glucagon secretion to counteract the hypoglycemia).

This form of diabetes is referred to as "brittle" diabetes, and requires special attention.

Laboratory Studies

Indirect tests of pancreatic exocrine function are based on the measurement of metabolites of compounds which are altered ("digested") by pancreatic exocrine products, and which can be quantified by serum or urine measurements. A commonly used indirect test is the bentiromide test, in which nitroblue tetrazolium-paraaminobenzoic acid (NBT-PABA) is ingested by the subject, and the urinary excretion of the proteolytic metabolite paraaminobenzoic acid (PABA) is measured. Free PABA is absorbed from the small intestine and excreted by the kidney in a linear correlation with the degree of chymotrypsin degradation of NBT-PABA. Although the sensitivity of the test is as high as 100 percent in patients with severe chronic pancreatitis, it identifies only 40–50 percent of patients with mild disease. Furthermore, reduced PABA excretion is found in patients with a variety of other gastrointestinal, hepatic, and renal diseases. Therefore the test is of value not for the diagnosis of chronic pancreatitis, but for determining the extent of exocrine pancreatic insufficiency in patients with known disease.

The quantification of stool fat also has been used as a measure of pancreatic lipase secretion, either through the direct measurement of total fecal fat levels while the subject consumes a diet of known fat content, or by the measurement of exhaled $4CO_2$ after ingestion of [4C]-triolein or [4C]-olein. This so-called triolein breath test avoids the necessity of stool collections and analysis, but has a high false-negative rate.

Prognosis and Natural History

The prognosis for patients with chronic pancreatitis is dependent on the etiology of disease, the development of complications, and on the age and socioeconomic status of the patient. Several studies have demonstrated that although symptoms of pain decrease over time in about half of the patients, this decline also is accompanied by a progression of exocrine and endocrine insufficiency. In general, the likelihood of eventual pain relief is dependent on the stage of disease at diagnosis, and the persistence of alcohol use in patients with alcoholic chronic pancreatitis. Miyake and colleagues found that pain relief was achieved in 60 percent of alcoholic patients who successfully discontinued drinking, but in only 26 percent who did not.

In addition to progressive endocrine and exocrine dysfunction, and the risk of the specific complications outlined below, the other significant long-term risk for the patient with chronic pancreatitis is the development of pancreatic carcinoma. There is a progressive, cumulative increased risk of carcinoma development in patients with chronic pancreatitis, which continues throughout the subsequent lifetime of the patient. The incidence of carcinoma in patients with chronic pancreatitis ranges from 1.5–2.7 percent, which is at least tenfold greater than that of patients of similar age seen in a hospital setting. In patients with advanced chronic pancreatitis referred for surgical therapy, the risk of indolent carcinoma can be over 10 percent. The development of carcinoma in the setting of chronic pancreatitis is no doubt related to the dysregulation of cellular proliferation and tissue repair processes in the setting of chronic inflammation, as is seen throughout the alimentary tract and elsewhere. In the setting of chronic pancreatitis, carcinoma development can be especially cryptic, and the diagnosis of early stage tumors is particularly difficult. Awareness of this risk justifies close surveillance for cancer in patients with chronic pancreatitis. Periodic measurement of tumor markers such as CA19-9, and periodic imaging of the pancreas with CT scan and EUS are necessary to detect the development of carcinoma in the patient with chronic pancreatitis.

Complications

Pseudocyst. A chronic collection of pancreatic fluid surrounded by a nonepithelialized wall of granulation tissue and fibrosis is referred to as a pseudocyst. Pseudocysts occur in up to 10 percent of patients with acute pancreatitis, and in 20–38 percent of patients with chronic pancreatitis, and thus they comprise the most common complication of chronic pancreatitis.

Acute pseudocysts may resolve spontaneously in up to 50 percent of cases, over a course of 6 weeks or longer. Pseudocysts larger than 6 cm resolve less frequently than smaller ones, but may regress over a period of weeks to months. Pseudocysts are multiple in 17 percent of patients, or may be multilobulated. Pseudocysts may become secondarily infected, in which case they become abscesses. They can compress or obstruct adjacent organs or structures, leading to superior mesenteric-portal vein thrombosis or splenic vein thrombosis. They can erode into visceral arteries and cause intracystic hemorrhage or pseudoaneurysms. They also can perforate and cause peritonitis or intraperitoneal bleeding.

Pseudocysts usually cause symptoms of pain, fullness, or early satiety. Asymptomatic pseudocysts can be managed expectantly, and may resolve spontaneously or persist without complication. Symptomatic or enlarging pseudocysts require treatment, and any presumed pseudocyst without a documented antecedent episode of acute pancreatitis requires investigation to determine the etiology of the lesion. Although pseudocysts comprise roughly two-thirds of all pancreatic cystic lesions, they resemble cystadenomas and cystadenocarcinoma radiographically. An incidentally discovered cystic lesion should be examined by EUS and aspirated to determine whether it is a true neoplasm or a pseudocyst.

The timing and method of treatment requires careful consideration. Pitfalls in the management of pseudocysts result from the incorrect (presumptive) diagnosis of a cystic neoplasm masquerading as a pseudocyst, a failure to appreciate the solid or debris-filled contents of a pseudocyst which appears to be fluid filled on CT scan, and a failure to document true adherence with an adjacent portion of the stomach before attempting transgastric internal drainage. If infection is suspected, the pseudocyst should be aspirated (not drained) by CT- or US-guided fine-needle aspiration, and the contents examined for organisms by Gram stain and culture. If infection is present, and the contents resemble pus, external drainage is employed using either surgical or percutaneous techniques.

If the pseudocyst has failed to resolve with conservative therapy and symptoms persist, internal drainage usually is preferred to external drainage, to avoid the complication of a pancreaticocutaneous fistula. Pseudocysts communicate with the pancreatic ductal system in up to 80 percent of cases, so external drainage creates a pathway for pancreatic duct leakage to and through the catheter exit site. Internal drainage may be performed with either percutaneous catheter-based methods (transgastric puncture and stent placement to create a cystogastrostomy), endoscopic methods (transgastric or transduodenal puncture and multiple stent placements, with or without a nasocystic irrigation catheter), or surgical methods (a true cystoenterostomy, biopsy of cyst wall, and evacuation of all debris and contents). Surgical options include a cystogastrostomy, a Roux-en-Y cystojejunostomy, or a cystoduodenostomy. Cystojejunostomy is the most versatile method, and it can be applied to pseudocysts that penetrate into the transverse mesocolon, the paracolic gutters, or the lesser sac. Cystogastrostomy can be performed endoscopically, laparoscopically, or by a combined laparoscopic-endoscopic method.

Because pseudocysts often communicate with the pancreatic ductal system, two newer approaches to pseudocyst management are based on main duct drainage, rather than pseudocyst drainage per se. Transpapillary stents inserted at the time of ERCP may be directed into a pseudocyst through the ductal communication itself, or can be left across the area of suspected duct leakage to facilitate decompression and cyst drainage, analogous to the use of common bile duct stents in the setting of a cystic duct leak. In a surgical series of patients with chronic pancreatitis, ductal dilatation, and a coexisting pseudocyst, Nealon and Walser showed that duct drainage alone, without a separate cystoenteric anastomosis, was as successful as a combined drainage procedure. Furthermore, the "duct drainage only" group enjoyed a shorter hospital stay and fewer complications than the group who underwent a separate cystoenterostomy. These observations suggest that transductal drainage may be a safe and effective approach to the management of pseudocystic disease. The endoscopic approach seems logical in the treatment of postoperative or posttraumatic pseudocysts when duct disruption is documented, or in those patients with pseudocysts that communicate with the duct. Whether the technique will be as effective for chronic pseudocysts without demonstrable communication with the pancreatic duct remains open to investigation.

The complications of endoscopic or radiologic drainage of pseudocysts often require surgical intervention. Bleeding from the cystoenterostomy, and inoculation of a pseudocyst with failure of resolution and persistence of infection, may require surgical treatment. Bleeding risks may be lessened by the routine use of EUS in the selection of the site for transluminal stent placement. Percutaneous and endoscopic treatment of pseudocysts requires large-bore catheters, multiple stents, and an aggressive approach to management for success to be achieved. Failure of nonsurgical therapy, with subsequent salvage procedures to remove infected debris and establish complete drainage, is associated with increased risks for complications and death. The most experienced therapeutic endoscopists report a complication rate of 17–19 percent for the treatment of sterile pseudocysts, and deaths as a result of endoscopic therapy have occurred. The use of endoscopic methods to treat sterile or infected pancreatic necrosis has a higher complication rate, and is indeed still controversial.

Resection of a pseudocyst is sometimes indicated for cysts located in the pancreatic tail, or when a midpancreatic duct disruption has resulted in a distally located pseudocyst. Distal pancreatectomy for removal of a pseudocyst, with or without splenectomy, can be a challenging procedure in the setting of prior pancreatitis.

Pancreatic ascites and pleural effusion. When a disrupted pancreatic duct leads to pancreatic fluid extravasation that does not become sequestered as a pseudocyst, but drains freely into the peritoneal cavity, pancreatic ascites occurs. Occasionally, the pancreatic fluid tracks superiorly into the thorax, and a pancreatic pleural effusion occurs. Referred to as internal pancreatic fistulae, both complications are seen more often in patients with chronic pancreatitis, rather than after acute pancreatitis. Pancreatic ascites and pleural effusion occur together in 14 percent of patients, and 18 percent have a pancreatic pleural effusion alone. Paracentesis or thoracentesis reveals noninfected fluid with a protein level greater than 25 g/L and a markedly elevated amylase level. Serum amylase may also be elevated, presumably from reabsorption across the parietal membrane. Serum albumin may be low, and patients may have coexisting liver disease. Paracentesis is therefore critical to differentiate pancreatic from hepatic ascites.

ERCP is most helpful to delineate the location of the pancreatic duct leak, and to elucidate the underlying pancreatic ductal anatomy. Pancreatic duct stenting may be considered at the time of ERCP, but if nonsurgical therapy is undertaken and then abandoned, repeat imaging of the pancreatic duct is appropriate to guide surgical treatment.

Antisecretory therapy with the somatostatin analog octreotide acetate, together with bowel rest and parenteral nutrition, is successful in more than half of patients. Reapposition of serosal surfaces to facilitate closure of the leak is considered a part of therapy, and this is accomplished by complete paracentesis. For pleural effusions, a period of chest tube drainage may facilitate closure of the internal fistula. Surgical therapy is reserved for those who fail to respond to medical treatment. If the leak originates from the central region of the pancreas, a Roux-en-Y pancreaticojejunostomy is performed to the site of duct leakage. If the leak is in the tail, a distal pancreatectomy may be considered, or an internal drainage procedure can be performed. The results of surgical treatment are usually favorable if the ductal anatomy has been carefully delineated preoperatively.

Head-of-pancreas mass. In up to 30 percent of patients with advanced chronic pancreatitis, an inflammatory mass develops in the head of the pancreas. The clinical presentation includes severe pain, and frequently includes stenosis of the distal common bile duct, duodenal stenosis, compression of the portal vein, and stenosis of the proximal main pancreatic duct. Treatment in the majority of cases is a duodenum-preserving pancreatic head resection.

Splenic and portal vein thrombosis. Vascular complications of chronic pancreatitis are fortunately infrequent, because they are difficult to treat successfully. Portal vein compression and occlusion can occur as a consequence of an inflammatory mass in the head of the pancreas, and splenic vein thrombosis occurs in association with chronic pancreatitis in 4 to 8 percent of cases. Variceal formation can occur as a consequence of either portal or splenic venous occlusion, and splenic vein thrombosis with gastric variceal formation is referred to as left-sided or sinistral portal hypertension. Although bleeding complications are infrequent, the mortality risk of bleeding exceeds 20 percent. When gastroesophageal varices are caused by splenic vein thrombosis, the addition of splenectomy to prevent variceal hemorrhage is prudent when surgery is otherwise indicated to correct other problems.

Treatment

Medical Therapy

The medical treatment of chronic or recurrent pain in chronic pancreatitis requires the use of analgesics, a cessation of alcohol use, and oral enzyme therapy. Interventional procedures to block visceral afferent nerve conduction or to treat obstructions of the main pancreatic duct are also an adjunct to medical treatment.

Endoscopic Management

Pancreatic duct stenting is used for treatment of proximal pancreatic duct stenosis, decompression of a pancreatic duct leak, and for drainage of pancreatic pseudocysts that can be catheterized through the main pancreatic duct. Pancreatic duct stents can induce an inflammatory response within the duct, so prolonged stenting is usually avoided.

Surgical Therapy

Indications and history. The traditional approach to surgical treatment of chronic pancreatitis and its complications has maintained that surgery should be considered only when the medical therapy of symptoms has failed. The role of surgery in the treatment of chronic pancreatitis, and its timing, is now based on the elucidation of pancreatic ductal disease. Nealon and Thompson published a landmark study in 1993 that showed that the progression of chronic obstructive pancreatitis could be delayed or prevented by pancreatic duct decompression. No other therapy has been shown to prevent the progression of chronic pancreatitis, and this study demonstrated the role of surgery in the early management of the disease. However, small-duct disease or the absence of a clear obstructive component are causes for caution. Major resections have a high complication rate, both early and late, in chronic alcoholic pancreatitis, and lesser procedures often result in symptomatic recurrence. So the choice of operation and the timing of surgery are based on each patient's pancreatic anatomy, the likelihood (or lack thereof) that further medical and endoscopic therapy will halt the symptoms of the disease, and the chance that a good result will be obtained with the lowest risk of morbidity and mortality. Finally, preparation for surgery should include restoration of protein-caloric homeostasis, abstinence from alcohol and tobacco, and a detailed review of the risks and likely outcomes, to establish a bond of trust and commitment between the patient and the surgeon.

ERCP and CT scans are used to differentiate obstructive and sclerotic disease, and this information is used to guide the rational selection of operative procedures. Resection of the pancreatic head (Whipple) is more common in the United States than the Beger procedure. The most common drainage procedure is a longitudinal pancreaticojejunostomy. The Frey procedure combines resection of a portion of the pancreatic head with a longitudinal pancreaticojejunostomy.

Sphincteroplasty. Although endoscopic techniques are now used routinely to perform sphincterotomy of either the common bile duct or pancreatic duct, a true (permanent) sphincteroplasty can only be performed surgically. Transduodenal sphincteroplasty with incision of the septum between the pancreatic duct and common bile duct appears to offer significant relief for patients with obstruction and inflammation isolated to this region.

Drainage procedures. In 1958, Puestow and Gillesby described segmental narrowings and dilatations of the ductal system as a "chain of lakes," and proposed a longitudinal decompression of the body and tail of the pancreas into a Roux limb of jejunum. Four of Puestow and Gillesby's 21 initial cases were side-to-side anastomoses, and 2 years after their report, Partington and Rochelle described a much simpler version of the longitudinal, or side-to-side Roux-en-Y pancreaticojejunostomy that became universally known as the Puestow procedure.

The effectiveness of decompression of the pancreatic duct is dependent on the extent to which ductal hypertension is the etiologic agent for the disease. Thus the diameter of the pancreatic duct is a surrogate for the degree of ductal hypertension, and the Puestow procedure has been shown to be effective for pain relief when the maximum duct diameter exceeds 6 or 7 mm. Results are less impressive in glands with smaller caliber ducts.

Successful pain relief after the Puestow-type decompression procedure has been reported in 75 to 85 percent of patients for the first few years after surgery, but pain recurs in over 20 percent of patients after 5 years, even in patients who are abstinent from alcohol. In 1987, Frey and Smith described the extended lateral pancreaticojejunostomy with excavation of the pancreatic head down to the ductal structures. The Frey procedure provides thorough decompression of the pancreatic head and the body and tail of the gland, and a long-term follow up suggested that improved outcomes are associated with this more extensive decompressive procedure.

The degree and technique of pancreatic head decompression may be critical for good long-term pain relief. The Frey procedure opens the head of the gland down to the proximal ductal system, but was not described as a duct-removing procedure per se. However, an actual excavation of the head of the pancreas, including the ductal system, may provide the best protection against recurrent stenosis.

Resectional Procedure

In 1965, Fry and Child proposed the more radical 95 percent distal pancreatectomy, which was intended for patients with sclerotic (small duct) disease, and which attempted to avoid the morbidity of total pancreatectomy by preserving the rim of pancreas in the pancreaticoduodenal groove, along with its associated blood vessels and distal common bile duct. The operation was found to be associated with pain relief in 60–77 percent of patients long-term, but is accompanied by a high risk of brittle diabetes, hypoglycemic coma, and malnutrition.

Although the operation is seldom used today, there is great interest in combining this procedure with autologous islet transplantation. Avoiding the metabolic consequences of subtotal or total pancreatectomy, although preserving the duodenum and distal bile duct, is an attractive surgical goal for the relief of nonobstructive pancreatic sclerosis.

Pancreaticoduodenectomy, with or without pylorus preservation, has been widely employed for the treatment of chronic pancreatitis. In the three largest modern (circa 2000) series of the treatment of chronic pancreatitis by the Whipple procedure, pain relief 4–6 years after operation was found in 71–89 percent of patients.

Beger and associates described the duodenum-preserving pancreatic head resection (DPPHR) in 1980, and published long-term results with DPPHR for the treatment of chronic pancreatitis in 1985, and more recently in 1999. In 388 patients who were followed for an average of 6 years after DPPHR, pain relief was maintained in 91 percent, mortality was less than 1 percent, and diabetes developed in 21 percent with 11 percent demonstrating a reversal of their preoperative diabetic status. These authors also compared the DPPHR procedure with the pylorus-sparing Whipple procedure in a randomized trial in 40 patients with chronic pancreatitis. The mortality was zero in both groups, and the morbidity was also comparable. Pain relief (over 6 months) was seen in 94 percent of DPPHR patients, but in only 67 percent of Whipple patients. Furthermore, the insulin secretory capacity and glucose tolerance were noted to deteriorate in the Whipple group, but actually improved in the DPPHR patients.

The DPPHR requires the careful dissection of the gastroduodenal artery and the creation of two anastomoses, and carries a similar complication risk as the Whipple procedure because of the risk of pancreatic leakage and intraabdominal fluid collections. Izbicki and associates conducted a randomized trial comparing the Frey procedure with the DPPHR in patients with chronic pancreatitis, and confirmed a reduced morbidity of 9 percent after the Frey procedure, compared to 20 percent after DPPHR. No significant differences were found in postoperative pain relief after the Frey or DPPHR (89 and 95 percent, respectively, over a mean follow up of 1.5 years), nor were there any differences in the ability to return to work, or in endocrine or exocrine function postoperatively.

In a retrospective review of both the DPPHR and Frey procedures performed at Yale, Aspelund and associates found a 25 percent incidence of major complications after the DPPHR, but only a 16 percent incidence after Frey procedures performed for chronic pancreatitis. During the same interval, major complications occurred after 40 percent of Whipple procedures, and new diabetes developed in 25 percent of Whipple patients. New diabetes occurred in only 8 percent of both DPPHR and Frey patients, during a follow-up period of 3 years, and preoperative diabetes improved in an equal number of DPPHR and Frey patients. These results corroborate the findings in the studies from Ulm and Hamburg, and suggest that duodenum-sparing pancreatic head resection, either in the form of the DPPHR (Beger) procedure or the Frey procedure, may provide better outcomes compared to the Whipple procedure for benign disease including chronic pancreatitis.

The decreased incidence of postoperative diabetes after the duodenum-sparing operations may be the result of a preserved β-cell mass in the more conservative resections, and may also be because of the conservation of the pancreatic polypeptide–secreting cells localized to the posterior head and uncinate process. Preservation of near-normal glucose metabolism and the avoidance of pancreatogenic diabetes is a significant benefit of the newer operative procedures.

Autotransplantation of islets. Islet cell transplantation for the treatment of diabetes is an attractive adjunct to pancreatic surgery in the treatment of benign pancreatic disease, but problems because of rejection of allotransplanted islets have plagued this method since its initial clinical application in the early 1970s. However, despite the difficulties in recovering islets from a chronically inflamed gland, Najarian and associates demonstrated the utility of autotransplantation of islets in patients with chronic pancreatitis in 1980. Subsequently, through refinements in the methods of harvesting and gland preservation, and through standardization of the methods by which islets are infused into the portal venous circuit for intrahepatic engraftment, the success of autotransplantation has steadily increased to achieve insulin independence in the majority of patients treated in recent series. Although 2–3 million islets are required for successful engraftment in an allogeneic recipient, the autotransplant recipient usually can achieve long-term, insulin-independent status after engraftment of only 300,000–400,000 islets. However, the ability to recover a sufficient quantity of islets from a sclerotic gland is dependent on the degree of disease present, so the selection of patients as candidates for autologous islet transplantation is important. As success with autotransplantation increases, patients with nonobstructive, sclerotic pancreatitis may be considered for resection and islet autotransplantation earlier in their course, as end-stage fibrosis bodes poorly for transplant success. As the necessary expertise with islet transplantation becomes more widespread, this therapy may become routine in the treatment of chronic pancreatitis.

Denervation procedures. In patients who have persistent and disabling pain, but who are poor candidates for resection or drainage procedures, a denervation procedure may provide symptomatic relief. Neural ablation is a valid treatment strategy to block afferent sympathetic nociceptive pathways. In addition to direct infiltration of the celiac ganglia with long-acting analgesics or neurolytic agents, a variety of true denervation procedures have been described for symptomatic relief in chronic pancreatitis. These include operative celiac ganglionectomy or splanchnicectomy, transhiatal splanchnicectomy, transthoracic splanchnicectomy with or without vagotomy, and videoscopic transthoracic splanchnicectomy. For the patient who is a poor candidate for an abdominal procedure, the transthoracic ablation of the sympathetic chain, either on the left side alone or bilaterally, has been shown to result in pain relief in 60–66 percent of patients. The application of videoscopic techniques to thoracic splanchnicectomy has further reduced the risks and discomfort of these procedures in chronically ill patients, and provides a valuable alternative to a direct attack on the pancreas.

PANCREATIC NEOPLASMS

Neoplasms of the Endocrine Pancreas

Neoplasms of the endocrine pancreas are relatively uncommon, but do occur with enough frequency (five cases per million population) that most surgeons will encounter them in an urban practice. Most pancreatic endocrine neoplasms are functional, secreting peptide products that produce interesting clinical presentations. Special immunohistochemical stains allow pathologists to confirm the peptide products being produced within the cells of a pancreatic endocrine tumor. However, the histologic characteristics of these neoplasms do not predict their clinical behavior, and malignancy is usually determined by the presence of local invasion and lymph node or hepatic metastases. Unfortunately, most pancreatic endocrine tumors are malignant, but the course of the disease is far more favorable than that seen with pancreatic exocrine cancer. The key to diagnosing these rare tumors is recognition of the classic clinical syndrome; confirmation is achieved by measuring serum levels of the elevated hormone. Localization of the tumor can be a challenging step, but once accomplished, the surgery is relatively straightforward. The goals of surgery range from complete resection, often accomplished with insulinomas, to controlling symptoms with debulking procedures, as is the case with most other pancreatic endocrine neoplasms.

As with pancreatic exocrine tumors, the initial diagnostic imaging test of choice for pancreatic endocrine tumors is a dynamic abdominal CT scan with fine cuts through the pancreas. Endoscopic ultrasound also can be valuable in localizing these tumors, which can produce dramatic symptoms despite their small (< 1 cm) size. In contrast to pancreatic exocrine tumors, many of the endocrine tumors have somatostatin receptors that allow them to be detected by a radiolabeled octreotide scan. A radioactive somatostatin analog is injected intravenously, followed by whole-body radionuclide scanning. The success of this modality in localizing tumors and detecting metastases has decreased the use of older techniques such as angiography and selective venous sampling.

Insulinoma

Insulinomas are the most common pancreatic endocrine neoplasms and present with a typical clinical syndrome known as Whipple triad. The triad consists of symptomatic fasting hypoglycemia, a documented serum glucose level less than 50 mg/dL, and relief of symptoms with the administration of glucose. Patients often will present with a profound syncopal episode and will admit to similar less severe episodes in the recent past. They also may admit to palpitations, trembling, diaphoresis, confusion or obtundation, and seizure, and family members may report that the patient has undergone a personality change. Routine laboratory studies will uncover a low blood sugar, the cause of all of these symptoms. The diagnosis is clinched with a monitored fast in which blood is sampled every 4–6 h for glucose and insulin levels until the patient becomes symptomatic. Elevated C-peptide levels rule out the unusual case of surreptitious administration of insulin or oral hypoglycemic agents, because excess endogenous insulin production leads to excess C-peptide. Insulinomas usually are localized with CT scanning and endoscopic ultrasound (EUS). Technical advances in EUS have led to preoperative identification of more than 90 percent of insulinomas. Visceral angiography with venous sampling is rarely required to accurately localize the tumor. Insulinomas are evenly distributed throughout the head, body, and tail of the pancreas. Unlike most endocrine pancreatic tumors, the majority (90 percent) of insulinomas are benign and solitary, with only 10 percent malignant. They are typically cured by simple enucleation. However, tumors located close to the main pancreatic duct and large (> 2 cm) tumors may require a distal pancreatectomy or pancreaticoduodenectomy. Intraoperative ultrasound is useful to determine the tumor's relation to the main pancreatic duct and guide intraoperative decision making. Enucleation of solitary insulinomas and distal pancreatectomy for insulinoma can be performed using a minimally invasive technique.

Ninety percent of insulinomas are sporadic and 10 percent are associated with the MEN-1 syndrome. Insulinomas associated with the MEN-1 syndrome are more likely to be multifocal and have a higher rate of recurrence.

Gastrinoma

Zollinger-Ellison syndrome (ZES) is caused by a gastrinoma, an endocrine tumor that secretes gastrin, leading to acid hypersecretion and peptic ulceration. Many patients with ZES present with abdominal pain, peptic ulcer disease, and severe esophagitis. However, in the era of effective antacid therapy, the presentation can be less dramatic. While most of the ulcers are solitary, multiple ulcers in atypical locations that fail to respond to antacids should raise suspicion for ZES and prompt a work-up. Twenty percent of patients with gastrinoma have diarrhea at the time of diagnosis.

The diagnosis of ZES is made by measuring the serum gastrin level. It is important that patients stop taking proton pump inhibitors for this test. In most patients with gastrinomas, the level is greater than 1000 pg/mL. Gastrin levels can be elevated in conditions other than ZES. Common causes of hypergastrinemia include pernicious anemia, treatment with proton pump inhibitors, renal failure, G-cell hyperplasia, atrophic gastritis, retained or excluded antrum, and gastric outlet obstruction. In equivocal cases, when the gastrin level is not markedly elevated, a secretin stimulation test is helpful.

In 70–90 percent of patients, the primary gastrinoma is found in the Passaro triangle, an area defined by a triangle with points located at the junction of the cystic duct and common bile duct, the second and third portion of the duodenum, and the neck and body of the pancreas. However, because gastrinomas can be found almost anywhere, whole-body imaging is required. The test of choice is somatostatin receptor (octreotide) scintigraphy in combination with CT. The octreotide scan is more sensitive than CT, locating about 85 percent of gastrinomas and detecting tumors smaller than 1 cm. With the octreotide scan, the need for tedious and technically demanding selective angiography and measurement of gastrin gradients has declined. Endoscopic ultrasound is another new modality that assists in the preoperative localization of gastrinomas. It is particularly helpful in localizing tumors in the pancreatic head or duodenal wall, in which gastrinomas are usually less than 1 cm in size. A combination of octreotide scan and EUS detects more than 90 percent of gastrinomas.

Multiple tumors are more common in patients with MEN-1 syndrome. Aggressive surgical treatment is justified in patients with sporadic gastrinomas. If patients have MEN-1 syndrome, the parathyroid hyperplasia is addressed with total parathyroidectomy and implantation of parathyroid tissue in the forearm.

Fifty percent of gastrinomas metastasize to lymph nodes or the liver, and are therefore considered malignant. Patients who meet criteria for operability should undergo exploration for possible removal of the tumor. Although the tumors are submucosal, a full-thickness excision of the duodenal wall is performed if a duodenal gastrinoma is found. All lymph nodes in the Passaro triangle are excised for pathologic analysis. If the gastrinoma is found in the pancreas and does not involve the main pancreatic duct, it is enucleated. Pancreatic resection is justified for solitary gastrinomas with no metastases. A highly selective vagotomy can be performed if unresectable disease is identified or if the gastrinoma cannot be localized. This may reduce the amount of expensive proton pump inhibitors required. In cases in which hepatic metastases are identified, resection is justified if the primary gastrinoma is controlled and the metastases can be safely and completely removed. Debulking or incomplete removal of multiple hepatic metastases is probably not helpful in the setting of MEN-1. Postoperatively, patients are followed with fasting serum gastrin levels, secretin stimulation tests, octreotide scans, and CT scans. Unfortunately, a biochemical cure is achieved in only about one third of the patients operated on for ZES. Despite the lack of success, long-term survival rates are good, even in patients with liver metastases. The 15-year survival rate for patients without liver metastases is about 80 percent, although the 5-year survival rate for patients with liver metastases is 20–50 percent. Pancreatic tumors are usually larger than tumors arising in the duodenum, and more often have lymph node metastases. In gastrinomas, liver metastases decrease survival rates, but lymph node metastases do not. The best results are seen after complete excision of small sporadic tumors originating in the duodenum. Large tumors associated with liver metastases, located outside of Passaro's triangle, have the worst prognosis.

VIPoma

In 1958, Verner and Morrison first described the syndrome associated with a pancreatic neoplasm secreting vasoactive intestinal polypeptide (VIP). The classic clinical syndrome associated with this pancreatic endocrine neoplasm consists of severe intermittent watery diarrhea leading to dehydration, and weakness from fluid and electrolyte losses. Large amounts of potassium are lost in the stool. The VIPoma syndrome also is called the WDHA syndrome because of the presence of watery diarrhea, hypokalemia, and achlorhydria. The massive (5 L/d) and episodic nature of the diarrhea associated with the appropriate electrolyte abnormalities should raise suspicion of the diagnosis. Serum VIP levels must be measured on multiple occasions because the excess secretion of VIP is episodic, and single measurements might be normal and misleading. A CT scan localizes most VIPomas, although as with all islet cell tumors, EUS is the most sensitive imaging method. Electrolyte and fluid balance is sometimes difficult to correct preoperatively and must be pursued aggressively. Somatostatin analogs are helpful in controlling the diarrhea and allowing replacement of fluid and electrolytes. VIPomas are more commonly located in the distal pancreas and most have spread outside the pancreas. Palliative debulking operations can sometimes improve symptoms for a period, along with somatostatin analogs. Hepatic artery embolization also has been reported as a potentially beneficial treatment.

Glucagonoma

Diabetes in association with dermatitis should raise the suspicion of a glucagonoma. The diabetes usually is mild. The classic necrolytic migratory erythema manifests as cyclic migrations of lesions with spreading margins and healing centers typically on the lower abdomen, perineum, perioral area, and feet. The diagnosis is confirmed by measuring serum glucagon levels, which usually are over 500 pg/mL. Glucagon is a catabolic hormone and most patients present with malnutrition. The rash associated with glucagonoma is thought to be caused by low levels of amino acids. Preoperative treatment usually includes control of the diabetes, parenteral nutrition, and octreotide. Like VIPomas, glucagonomas are more often in the body and tail of the pancreas and tend to be large tumors with metastases. Again, debulking operations are recommended in good operative candidates to relieve symptoms.

Somatostatinoma

Because somatostatin inhibits pancreatic and biliary secretions, patients with a somatostatinoma present with gallstones because of bile stasis, diabetes because of inhibition of insulin secretion, and steatorrhea because of inhibition of pancreatic exocrine secretion and bile secretion. Most somatostatinomas originate in the proximal pancreas or the pancreatoduodenal groove, with the ampulla and periampullary area as the most common site (60 percent). The most common presentations are abdominal pain (25 percent), jaundice (25 percent), and cholelithiasis (19 percent). This rare type of pancreatic endocrine tumor is diagnosed by confirming elevated serum somatostatin levels, which are usually above 10 ng/mL. Although most reported cases of somatostatinoma involve metastatic disease, an attempt at complete excision of the tumor and cholecystectomy is warranted in fit patients.

Nonfunctioning Islet-Cell Tumors

Most pancreatic endocrine neoplasms do secrete one or more hormones and are associated with characteristic clinical syndromes. After insulinoma, however, the most common islet-cell tumor is the nonfunctioning islet-cell neoplasm. Because it is clinically silent until its size and location produce symptoms, it is usually malignant when first diagnosed. Some presumably nonfunctional pancreatic endocrine neoplasms stain positive for PP and elevated PP levels are therefore a marker for the lesion. Because clinical manifestations are absent, the tumors are usually large and metastatic at the time of diagnosis, unless they are detected serendipitously on CT scan or sonogram. Nonfunctioning islet-cell tumors also are seen in association with other multiple neoplasia syndromes, such as von Hippel-Lindau syndrome. The tumors grow slowly and 5-year survival is common, as opposed to pancreatic exocrine tumors, for which 5-year survival is extraordinarily rare.

Neoplasms of the Exocrine Pancreas

Epidemiology and Risk Factors

Cancer of the pancreas is the fifth leading cause of cancer death in the United States, with approximately 30,300 new cases and 29,700 deaths reported in 2002. The etiology of pancreatic cancer likely involves a complex interaction of genetic and environmental factors.

A risk factor that is consistently linked to pancreatic cancer is cigarette smoking. Smoking increases the risk of developing pancreatic cancer by at least 2-fold because of the carcinogens in cigarette smoke. Long-standing diabetes may be a risk factor for pancreatic cancer. The new onset of diabetes or a sudden increase in insulin requirement in an older adult patient with preexisting diabetes should provoke concern for the presence of pancreatic cancer. Recent epidemiologic studies have confirmed the fact that patients with chronic pancreatitis have an increased risk of developing pancreatic cancer. Large, retrospective cohort studies of patients with pancreatitis have revealed up to a 20-fold increase in risk for pancreatic cancer. A family history of pancreatic cancer is also a well-recognized risk factor. A family history of pancreatic cancer in a first-degree relative increases the risk of pancreatic cancer by about twofold.

Diagnosis and Staging

Table 32-2 shows the tumor-node-metastasis (TNM) staging of pancreatic cancer. T1 lesions are smaller than 2 cm in diameter and are limited to the pancreas. T2 lesions also are limited to the pancreas, but are larger than 2 cm. T3 lesions extend into the duodenum or extrapancreatic bile duct. T4 lesions extend in to the portal vein, superior mesenteric vein, superior mesenteric artery, stomach, spleen, or colon. T1 and T2 tumors with no lymph node involvement are considered stage I disease, although more extensive invasion, such as that associated with T3 tumors, indicates stage II disease. Any lymph node involvement indicates stage III disease. Stage IV disease is divided into

TABLE 32-2 Staging of Pancreatic Cancer

Primary tumor (T)	
T1	Limited to pancreas, < 2 cm
T2	Limited to pancreas, > 2 cm
T3	Extension into duodenum or bile duct
T4	Extension into portal vein, superior mesenteric vein, superior mesenteric artery, stomach, spleen, colon

Regional lymph nodes (N)	
N0	No nodal metastases
N1	Regional nodal metastases

Distant metastases (M)	
M0	No distant metastases
M1	Distant metastases (liver, lung)

Stage	T	N	M	Description
I	1, 2	0	0	Tumor confined to pancreas
[2pt] II	3	0	0	Tumor invades duodenum and/or bile duct outside pancreas; no lymph node involvement
[2pt] III	1, 2, 3	1	0	Tumor has not spread beyond duodenum or bile duct, but includes regional lymph nodes
[2pt] IVA	4	Any	0	Locally advanced tumor growing into blood vessels, stomach, spleen, and colon, with or without lymph node involvement
[2pt] IVB	Any	Any	1	Distant metastases (liver, lungs) present

patients with locally advanced tumors (T4) without metastatic disease (stage IVA), and patients with metastases to distant sites such as the liver or lungs (stage IVB).

The most critical deficit in the ability to treat pancreatic cancer effectively is the lack of tools for early diagnosis. Ultimately, the majority of patients present with pain and jaundice. On physical exam, weight loss is evident and the skin is icteric; a distended gallbladder is palpable in about one fourth of patients. More fortunate patients have tumors situated such that biliary obstruction and jaundice occurs early and prompts diagnostic tests. Unfortunately, however, the vast majority of patients are not diagnosed until weight loss has occurred—a sign of advanced disease.

Although it often is taught that carcinoma of the pancreas presents with painless jaundice (to help distinguish it from choledocholithiasis), this aphorism is not accurate. Most patients do experience pain as part of the symptom complex of pancreatic cancer, and it is often the first symptom.

Unfortunately, at this time there is no sensitive and specific serum marker to assist in the timely diagnosis of pancreatic cancer. With jaundice, direct hyperbilirubinemia and elevated alkaline phosphatase are expected, but do not serve much of a diagnostic role other than to confirm the obvious. With longstanding biliary obstruction, the prothrombin time will be prolonged because of a depletion of vitamin K, a fat-soluble vitamin dependent on bile flow for absorption.

CA19-9 is a mucin-associated carbohydrate antigen that can be detected in the serum of patients with pancreatic cancer. Serum levels are elevated in about 75 percent of patients with pancreatic cancer; however, CA19-9 also is elevated in about 10 percent of patients with benign diseases of the pancreas, liver, and bile ducts. CA19-9 is thus neither sufficiently sensitive nor specific to allow an earlier diagnosis of pancreatic cancer. Despite the fact that many tumor markers, such as CA19-9, have been studied in an attempt to facilitate early diagnosis, there are still no effective screening tests for pancreatic cancer.

In patients presenting with jaundice, a reasonable first diagnostic imaging study is abdominal ultrasound. If bile duct dilation is not seen, hepatocellular disease is likely. Demonstration of cholelithiasis and bile duct dilation suggests a diagnosis of choledocholithiasis, and the next logical step would be endoscopic retrograde cholangiopancreatography (ERCP) to clear the bile duct. In the absence of gallstones, malignant obstruction of the bile duct is likely and a CT scan rather than ERCP would be the next logical step. For patients suspected of having pancreatic cancer who present without jaundice, ultrasound is not appropriate, and a CT scan should be the first test.

The current diagnostic and staging test of choice for pancreatic cancer is a dynamic contrast-enhanced CT scan, and techniques are constantly improving. The accuracy of CT scanning for predicting unresectable disease is 90–95 percent. CT findings that indicate a tumor is unresectable include invasion of the hepatic or superior mesenteric artery, enlarged lymph nodes outside the boundaries of resection, ascites, distant metastases (e.g., liver), and distant organ invasion (e.g., colon). Invasion of the superior mesenteric vein or portal vein is not in itself a contraindication to resection as long as the veins are patent. In contrast, CT scanning is less accurate in predicting resectable disease. CT scanning will miss small liver metastases and predicting vascular involvement is sometimes difficult.

Currently, CT is probably the single most versatile and cost-effective tool for the diagnosis of pancreatic cancer. Abdominal MRI is rapidly evolving but currently provides essentially the same information as CT scanning. Positron emission tomography (PET) scanning is becoming more widely available and may help distinguish chronic pancreatitis from pancreatic cancer. EUS can be used to detect small pancreatic masses that could be missed by CT scanning, and is commonly used when there is a high suspicion for pancreatic cancer but no mass is identified by the CT scan. EUS is a sensitive test for portal/superior mesenteric vein invasion, although it is somewhat less effective at detecting superior mesenteric artery invasion. When all of the current staging modalities are used, their accuracy in predicting resectability is reported to be about 80 percent, meaning that one in five patients brought to the operating room with the intent of a curative resection will be found at the time of surgery to have unresectable disease.

In an attempt to avoid such futile laparotomies, some surgeons have advocated the use of preliminary laparoscopy for patients with disease felt to be resectable by imaging. Diagnostic laparoscopy with the use of ultrasound is reported to improve the accuracy of predicting resectability to about 98 percent. The technique involves more than simple visualization with the scope, and requires the placement of three ports and manipulation of the tissues. The ultrasound probe is used to examine the liver, porta hepatis, and the portal vein and superior mesenteric artery.

Diagnostic laparoscopy is possibly best applied to patients with pancreatic cancer on a selective basis. Diagnostic laparoscopy will have a higher yield in patients with large tumors (> 2 cm), tumors located in the body or tail, patients with equivocal findings of metastasis or ascites on CT scan, and patients with other indications of advanced disease such as marked weight loss or markedly elevated CA19-9.

Palliative Surgery and Endoscopy

In general, there are three clinical problems in advanced pancreatic cancer that require palliation: pain, jaundice, and duodenal obstruction. The mainstay of pain control is oral narcotics. Sustained-release preparations of morphine sulfate are frequently used. Invasion of retroperitoneal nerve trunks accounts for the severe pain experienced by patients with advanced pancreatic cancer. A celiac plexus nerve block can control pain effectively for a period of months, although the procedure sometimes needs to be repeated. At the time of initial exploration for pancreatic cancer, it is a good practice to think about pain control and consider performing an intraoperative celiac block regardless of whether a resection is performed. The procedure is performed by injecting 50 percent alcohol directly into the tissues along the sides of the aorta just cephalad and posterior to the origin of the celiac trunk. This can be accomplished quite easily with either open surgery or laparoscopic surgery, and does not prolong the operation by more than a few min. If necessary, the procedure can be repeated postoperatively, either percutaneously or with use of endoscopic ultrasound guidance.

Jaundice is present in the majority of patients with pancreatic cancer, and the most troublesome aspect for the patient is the accompanying pruritus. Biliary obstruction may also lead to cholangitis, coagulopathy, digestive symptoms, and hepatocellular failure. In the past, surgeons traditionally performed a biliary bypass when unresectable disease was found at laparotomy. As many patients today already have a bile duct stent in place by the time of operation, it is not clear that operative biliary bypass is required. If an operative bypass is performed, choledochojejunostomy is the preferred approach. Although an easy procedure to perform, choledochoduodenostomy is felt to be unwise because of the proximity of the duodenum to tumor. Some have discouraged the use of the gallbladder for biliary bypass; however, it is suitable as long as the cystic duct clearly enters the common duct well above the tumor.

Duodenal obstruction is usually a late event in pancreatic cancer and occurs in only about 20 percent of patients. Therefore, in the absence of signs or symptoms of obstruction, such as nausea or vomiting, or a tumor that is already encroaching on the duodenum at the time of surgery, the routine use of prophylactic gastrojejunostomy when exploration reveals unresectable tumor is controversial. Although anastomotic leaks are uncommon, gastrojejunostomy is sometimes associated with delayed gastric emptying, the very symptom the procedure is designed to treat.

Whether performing a biliary and enteric bypass or just a biliary bypass, the jejunum is brought anterior to the colon rather than retrocolic, in which the tumor potentially would invade the bowel sooner. Some surgeons use a loop of jejunum with a jejunojejunostomy to divert the enteric stream away from the biliary-enteric anastomosis. Others use a Roux-en-Y limb with the gastrojejunostomy located 50 cm downstream from the hepatico-jejunostomy. Potential advantages of the defunctionalized Roux-en-Y limb include the ease with which it will reach up to the hepatic hilum, probable decreased risk of cholangitis, and easier management of biliary anastomotic leaks. If a gastrojejunostomy is performed, it should be placed dependently and posterior along the greater curvature to improve gastric emptying, and a vagotomy should not be performed. If patients are explored laparoscopically and found to have unresectable disease, palliation of jaundice can be achieved in a minimally invasive fashion with ERCP and placement of a coated, expandable metallic endoscopic biliary stent. Endoscopic stents are definitely not as durable as a surgical bypass. Recurrent obstruction and cholangitis is more common with stents and results in inferior palliation. However, this minimally invasive approach is associated with considerably less initial morbidity and mortality than surgical bypass. Newer, expandable metallic Wallstents demonstrate improved patency and provide better palliation than plastic stents.

If an initial diagnostic laparoscopy reveals a contraindication to the Whipple procedure, such as liver metastases, it is not appropriate to perform a laparotomy simply to create a biliary bypass. In such a patient it is better to place an endoscopic stent. In contrast, if a laparotomy already has been performed as part of the assessment of resectability and the Whipple procedure is not possible, a surgical bypass usually is performed.

Palliative Chemotherapy and Radiation

In patients with unresectable pancreatic cancer, gemcitabine results in symptomatic improvement, improved pain control and performance status, and weight gain. However, survival is improved by only 1–2 months. Although these results may warrant treatment in patients who understand the benefits and risks, the lack of significant survival advantage should encourage physicians to refer motivated patients for experimental protocols because it is only through continued clinical research that more meaningful treatments for pancreatic cancer will be developed.

Surgical Resection: Pancreaticoduodenectomy

In a patient with appropriate clinical and/or imaging indications of pancreatic cancer, a tissue diagnosis prior to performing a pancreaticoduodenectomy is not essential. Although percutaneous CT-guided biopsy is usually safe, complications such as hemorrhage, pancreatitis, fistula, abscess, and even death can occur. Tumor seeding along the subcutaneous tract of the needle is uncommon. Likewise, fine-needle aspiration under endoscopic ultrasound guidance is safe and well tolerated. The problem with preoperative or even intraoperative biopsy is that many pancreatic cancers are not very cellular and contain a significant amount of fibrous tissue, so a biopsy may be misinterpreted as showing chronic pancreatitis if it does not contain malignant glandular cells. In the face of clinical and radiologic preoperative indications of pancreatic cancer, a negative biopsy should not preclude resection. In patients who are not candidates for resection because of metastatic disease, biopsy for a tissue diagnosis becomes important because these patients may be candidates for palliative chemotherapy and radiation therapy trials. It is especially important to make an aggressive attempt at tissue diagnosis prior to surgery in patients whose clinical presentation and imaging studies are more suggestive of alternative diagnoses such as pancreatic lymphoma or pancreatic islet-cell tumors. These patients might avoid surgery altogether in the case of lymphoma, or warrant an aggressive debulking approach in the case of islet-cell carcinoma.

Variations and Controversies in Whipple Procedure

The preservation of the pylorus has several theoretical advantages including prevention of reflux of pancreaticobiliary secretions into the stomach, decreased incidence of marginal ulceration, normal gastric acid secretion and hormone release, and improved gastric function. Patients with pylorus-preserving resections have appeared to regain weight better than historic controls in some studies. Return of gastric emptying in the immediate postoperative period may take longer after the pylorus-preserving operation, and it is controversial whether there is any significant improvement in long-term quality of life with pyloric preservation.

Techniques for the pancreaticojejunostomy include end-to-side or end-to-end and duct-to-mucosa sutures or invagination. Pancreaticogastrostomy also has been investigated. Some surgeons use stents, glue to seal the anastomosis, or octreotide to decrease pancreatic secretions. No matter what combination of these techniques is used, the pancreatic leakage rate is always about 10 percent. Therefore the choice of techniques depends more on the surgeon's personal experience.

Traditionally, most surgeons place drains around the pancreatic and biliary anastomoses because the most dreaded complication of pancreaticoduodenectomy, disruption of the pancreaticojejunostomy, cannot be avoided in 1 out of 10 patients. This complication can lead to the development of an upper abdominal abscess or can present as an external pancreatic fistula. Usually a pure pancreatic leak is controlled by the drains and will eventually seal spontaneously. Combined pancreatic and biliary leaks are cause for concern because bile will activate the pancreatic enzymes. In its most virulent form, disruption leads to necrotizing retroperitoneal infection, which can erode major arteries and veins of the upper abdomen, including the exposed portal vein and its branches or the stump of the gastroduodenal artery. Impending catastrophe often is preceded by a small herald bleed from the drain site. Such an event is an indication to return the patient to the operating room to widely drain the pancreaticojejunostomy and to repair the involved blood vessel. Open packing may be necessary to control diffuse necrosis and infection.

Many patients with pancreatic cancer are malnourished preoperatively and suffer from gastroparesis in the immediate postoperative period. Some surgeons routinely place a feeding jejunostomy tube and gastrostomy tube in all pancreaticoduodenectomies, although others make the decision on a case-by-case basis. Gastrostomy tubes may decrease the length of stay in patients with gastroparesis. Jejunostomy tubes are certainly not benign and can result in leaks and intestinal obstruction. However, parenteral nutrition also is associated with serious complications such as line sepsis, loss of gut mucosal integrity, and hepatic dysfunction.

Because of the high incidence of direct retroperitoneal invasion and regional lymph node metastasis at the time of surgery, it has been argued that the scope of resection for pancreatic cancer should be enlarged to include a radical regional lymphadenectomy and resection of areas of potential retroperitoneal invasion. The "radical pancreaticoduodenectomy" includes extension of the pancreatic resection to the middle body of the pancreas, segmental resection of the portal vein if necessary, resection of retroperitoneal tissue along the right perinephric area, and lymphadenectomy to the region of the celiac plexus. In the hands of experienced surgeons, these techniques are associated with greater blood loss but no increase in mortality; however, improved survival has not been demonstrated. Total pancreatectomy also has been considered in the past. Although pancreatic leaks are eliminated, major morbidity from brittle diabetes and exocrine insufficiency outweigh any theoretical benefit.

Pancreatic cancer usually recurs locally after pancreaticoduodenectomy. Intraoperative radiotherapy (IORT) delivers a full therapeutic dose of radiation to the operative bed at the time of resection. Radiation to surrounding normal areas is minimized, but the radiation is delivered all in one setting, usually about 15 min, rather than in fractionated doses over time. IORT is best performed in a shielded, dedicated, operating room suite rather than by transporting the patient in the middle of an already long and complicated operation. IORT may improve local control and palliate symptoms after pancreaticoduodenectomy. However, IORT has not been shown to be superior to standard external beam radiation therapy, and further randomized trials are needed to determine how this modality should be used.

Complications of Pancreaticoduodenectomy

The operative mortality rate for pancreaticoduodenectomy has decreased to less than 5 percent in "high volume" centers (where more than five cases per year are performed), suggesting that patients in rural areas would benefit from referral to large urban centers. The most common causes of death are sepsis, hemorrhage, and cardiovascular events. Postoperative complications are unfortunately still very common, and include delayed gastric emptying, pancreatic fistula, and hemorrhage. Delayed gastric emptying is common after pancreaticoduodenectomy and is treated conservatively as long as complete gastric outlet obstruction is ruled out by a contrast study. Hemorrhage can occur either intraoperatively or postoperatively. Intraoperative hemorrhage typically occurs during the dissection of the portal vein. A major laceration of the portal vein can occur at a point in the operation at which the portal vein is not yet exposed. Temporary control of hemorrhage is generally possible in this situation by compressing the portal vein and superior mesenteric vein against the tumor with the surgeon's left hand behind the head of the pancreas. An experienced assistant is needed to divide the neck of the pancreas to the left of the portal vein and achieve proximal and distal control. Sometimes the vein can be sutured closed with minimal narrowing. Other times, a patch repair or segmental resection and interposition graft may be needed.

Postoperative hemorrhage can occur from inadequate ligature of any one of numerous blood vessels during the procedure. Hemorrhage also can occur because of digestion of retroperitoneal blood vessels because of a combined biliary-pancreatic leak. Uncommonly, a stress ulcer, or later a marginal ulcer, can result in gastrointestinal hemorrhage. Typically, a vagotomy is not performed when pancreaticoduodenectomy is performed for pancreatic cancer, but patients are placed on proton pump inhibitors.

Outcome and Value of Pancreaticoduodenectomy for Cancer

Survival figures indicate that few, if any, patients are cured indefinitely of pancreatic cancer with pancreaticoduodenectomy. The tumor tends to recur locally with retroperitoneal and regional lymphatic disease. Additionally, most patients also develop hematogenous metastases, usually in the liver. Malignant ascites, peritoneal implants, and malignant pleural effusions are all common. Median survival after pancreaticoduodenectomy is about 12–15 months. Even long-term (5-year) survivors often eventually die because of pancreatic cancer recurrence. Although pancreaticoduodenectomy may be performed with the hope of the rare cure in mind, the operation more importantly provides better palliation than any other treatment, and is the only modality that offers any meaningful improvement in survival. If the procedure is performed without major complications, many months of palliation are usually achieved. It is the surgeon's duty to make sure patients and their families have a realistic understanding of the true goals of pancreaticoduodenectomy.

Adjuvant Chemotherapy and Radiation

Small studies in the 1980s suggested that adjuvant chemotherapy with 5-fluorouracil combined with radiation improves survival by about 9 months after pancreatic resection for pancreatic adenocarcinoma. Subsequent non-controlled studies have reinforced that concept. However, a recent European multicenter trial concluded that there was no value to chemoradiotherapy, although the study suggested the possibility that chemotherapy alone might have survival benefit. Remarkable results in adjuvant therapy have been reported by the Virginia Mason Clinic with combination 5-FU, cisplatinum, interferon-α and external beam radiation. Although the toxicity is high, the promising results have prompted larger confirmatory studies. Nevertheless, pending further study, it is typical in the United States for patients with acceptable functional status to receive adjuvant chemoradiotherapy after surgery.

Neoadjuvant Treatment

There are several potential advantages to the use of chemoradiation prior to an attempt at surgical resection. For example, it avoids the risk that adjuvant treatment is delayed by complications of surgery. Neoadjuvant treatment also may decrease the tumor burden at operation, increasing the rate of resectability and killing some tumor cells before they can be spread intraoperatively. Preoperative chemoradiation has been shown not to increase the perioperative morbidity or mortality of pancreaticoduodenectomy. It may even decrease the incidence of pancreatic fistula. Studies so far indicate that local or regional recurrence is decreased with this technique, but there is no proven survival advantage compared to traditional postoperative therapy.

Management of Periampullary Adenomas

Benign villous adenomas of the ampullary region can be excised locally. This technique is applicable only for small tumors (approximately 2 cm or less) with no evidence of malignancy on biopsy. A longitudinal duodenotomy is made and the tumor is excised with a 2–3-mm margin of normal duodenal mucosa. The edges of the bile duct and pancreatic duct are sewn to the duodenal wall as the excision progresses. A preoperative diagnosis of cancer is a contraindication to transduodenal excision and pancreaticoduodenectomy should be performed. Likewise, if final pathologic examination of a locally excised tumor reveals invasive cancer, the patient should be returned to the operating room for a pancreaticoduodenectomy.

An important subset of patients is one with familial adenomatous polyposis (FAP), who develop periampullary or duodenal adenomas. These lesions have a high incidence of harboring carcinoma, and frequently recur unless the mucosa at risk is resected. A standard (not pylorus-sparing) Whipple is the procedure of choice in FAP patients with periampullary lesions.

Cystic Neoplasms of the Pancreas

Cystic epithelial tumors need to be excluded when patients present with a fluid-containing pancreatic lesion. A variety of cystic neoplasms exist, and include benign serous cystic neoplasms, benign and malignant mucinous cystic neoplasms, and benign and malignant forms of intraductal papillary-mucinous neoplasms (IPMNs). IPMNs can present with a dilated pancreatic duct because of the production of mucin by the lesion. At ERCP or upper endoscopy, mucus may be seen extruding from a gaping ampullary orifice. This confirms the presence of an IPMN, and further investigation is warranted to localize the lesion. It is important to not assume that all fluid-filled pancreatic abnormalities represent pseudocysts, or that a dilated pancreatic duct represents only chronic pancreatitis. The presence of a solid component in a cystic lesion, septations within the cyst, and the absence of a clinical history of pancreatitis are factors that should alert the surgeon to the possible presence of a neoplasm. Even in the absence of these factors, presumed pseudocysts should be biopsied at the time of internal drainage to confirm the absence of malignancy, and dilated pancreatic ducts should be biopsied at the time of a decompression procedure to rule out a ductular neoplasm.

Cystic neoplasms with septations and/or irregular nodularity of the cyst wall are more suspicious for malignancy. In an effort to establish a preoperative diagnosis of malignancy, the cyst fluid can be aspirated using EUS and analyzed. Cysts containing viscous fluid with a low amylase content and an elevated carcinoembryonic antigen level are more likely to be malignant. Cytologic examination of the aspirate also can be performed to aid in the diagnosis.

Cystic pancreatic lesions are usually resected if there is any concern regarding malignant potential. Enucleation of small cystic pancreatic neoplasms that are presumed to be benign may be a valid approach; the use of intraoperative ultrasound in such cases is helpful in avoiding injury to the main pancreatic duct and postoperative fistulas. Laparoscopic distal pancreatectomy with or without splenic preservation may be employed for cystic lesions located in the tail of the pancreas. With limited experience worldwide with laparoscopic pancreatic resection, caution is warranted before application of this technique to potentially malignant lesions.

Small cystic lesions in the head of the pancreas present a difficult challenge. Because of the morbidity and mortality risk of pancreaticoduodenectomy, a more conservative operative approach is attractive in a patient with a premalignant lesion such as a mucinous cystadenoma. The duodenum-preserving pancreatic head resections described earlier may offer a safer option when the lesion does not encroach on the duodenum and appears well delineated.

Pseudopapillary and Papillary-Cystic Neoplasms

An unusual form of exocrine neoplasm occurs predominantly in young women, and is characterized by a large, cystic or partially cystic appearing lesion which contains frond-like papillary elements on histologic examination.

Pseudopapillary and papillary-cystic neoplasms are usually benign, but may assume malignant (metastatic) behavior when they are discovered late in their course. Typically occurring in women from adolescence through the age of menopause, these lesions have been found to express estrogen and progesterone receptors in large numbers. Resection for cure is usually possible despite their typically large size.

Pancreatic Lymphoma

Lymphoma can affect the pancreas. Primary involvement of the pancreas with no disease outside the pancreas also occurs. The clinical presentation often is similar to pancreatic adenocarcinoma, with vague abdominal pain and weight loss. Identification of a large mass often involving the head and body of the pancreas should raise suspicion. Percutaneous or EUS-guided biopsy will confirm the diagnosis in most cases. If the diagnosis cannot be confirmed preoperatively, laparoscopic exploration and biopsy is indicated. There is no role for resection in the management of pancreatic lymphoma. Endoscopic stenting to relieve jaundice followed by chemotherapy is the standard treatment, and long-term remission often is achieved.

Suggested Readings

Steer ML, Saluja AK: Pathogenesis and pathophysiology of acute pancreatitis, in Beger HG, Warshaw AL, Buchler MW, et al (eds): The Pancreas, Vol. 2. London: Blackwell Science Ltd., 1998, p 383.

Whitcomb DC, Gorry MC, Preston RA, et al: Hereditary pancreatitis is caused by a mutation in the cationic trypsinogen gene. Nat Genet 14:141, 1996.

Gross JB: Hereditary pancreatitis, in Go VLW, Gardner JD, Brooks FP et al (eds): The Exocrine Pancreas: Biology, Pathophysiology, and Diseases. New York: Raven Press, 1986, p 829.

Whitcomb DC: Hereditary diseases of the pancreas, in Yamada T, Alpers DH, Laine L, Owyang C, Powell DC (eds): Textbook of Gastroenterology, 4th ed. Philadelphia: Lippincott, Williams & Wilkins, 2002, p 2147.

Nealon WH, Matin S: Analysis of surgical success in preventing recurrent acute exacerbations in chronic pancreatitis. Ann Surg 233:793, 2001.

Bell RH Jr.: Atlas of pancreatic surgery, in Bell RH Jr., Rikkers LF, Mulholland MW (eds): Digestive Tract Surgery. A Text and Atlas. Philadelphia: Lippincott-Raven, 1996, p 963.

Nealon WH, Thompson JC: Progressive loss of pancreatic function in chronic pancreatitis is delayed by main pancreatic duct decompression. A longitudinal prospective analysis of the modified Puestow procedure. Ann Surg 217:458, 1993.

Partington PF, Rochelle REL: Modified Puestow procedure for retrograde drainage of the pancreatic duct. Ann Surg 152:1037, 1960.

Frey CF, Amikura K: Local resection of the head of the pancreas combined with longitudinal pancreaticojejunostomy in the management of patients with chronic pancreatitis. Ann Surg 220:492, 1994.

Jean ME, Lowy AM, Chiao PJ, et al: The molecular biology of pancreatic cancer, in Evans DB, Pisters PWT, Abbruzzese JL (eds): M.D. Anderson Solid Tumor Oncology Series—Pancreatic Cancer. New York: Springer-Verlag, 2002, p 15.

33 | Spleen

Adrian E. Park and Rodrick McKinlay

Until modern times removal of the spleen usually resulted in death of the patient. Pre–nineteenth century splenectomy carried a mortality rate in excess of 90 percent. By 1920 the Mayo Clinic experience with splenectomy reported an 11 percent mortality rate. Currently, the largest series of laparoscopic splenectomies report an overall mortality of 1 percent or less.

EMBRYOLOGY AND ANATOMY

The spleen is the largest reticuloendothelial organ in the body. Arising from the primitive mesoderm as an outgrowth of the left side of the dorsal mesogastrium, by the fifth week of gestation the spleen is evident. The organ continues its differentiation and migration to the left upper quadrant, in which it comes to rest with its smooth, diaphragmatic surface facing posterosuperiorly.

The accessory spleen, the most common anomaly of splenic embryology, is present in up to 20 percent of the population and up to 30 percent of patients with hematologic disease. Over 80 percent of the time, the accessory spleen is found in the splenic hilum and vascular pedicle region.

The abdominal surface of the diaphragm separates the spleen from the lower left lung and pleura and the ninth to eleventh ribs. The spleen's visceral surface faces the abdominal cavity and contains gastric, colic, renal, and pancreatic impressions. A capsule 1–2-mm thick, rich in collagen, and containing elastin fibers contains the spleen. An average adult spleen is 7–11 cm in length and weighs 150 g (range 70–250 g). The term splenomegaly is generally applied to organs weighing 500 mg or more and/or 15 cm or more in length.

Of particular clinical relevance, the spleen is suspended in position by several ligaments and peritoneal folds to the colon (splenocolic ligament); the stomach (gastrosplenic ligament); the diaphragm (phrenosplenic ligament); and the kidney, adrenal gland, and tail of the pancreas (splenorenal ligament). The gastrosplenic ligament contains the short gastric vessels. The remaining ligaments are usually avascular. In cadaveric anatomic series, the tail of the pancreas lies within 1 cm of the splenic hilum 75 percent of the time and actually abuts the spleen in 30 percent of patients.

The spleen derives most of its blood from the splenic artery. Splenic arteries are of two types: the most common (70 percent) distributed type is distinguished by a short trunk with many long branches entering over three fourths of the medial surface of the spleen whereas the less common (30 percent) magistral type has a long main trunk dividing near the hilum into short terminal branches entering over 25–30 percent of the medial surface. The spleen also receives some of its blood supply from the short gastric vessels, which are branches of the left gastroepiploic artery. The splenic vein accommodates the major venous drainage of the spleen.

The splenic parenchyma is composed of two main elements: the red pulp, approximately 75 percent of total splenic volume, and the white pulp. The red pulp is comprised of large numbers of venous sinuses, which ultimately drain into tributaries of the splenic vein and are surrounded and separated by a fibrocellular network, called the reticulum, consisting of collagen fibers and fibroblasts. Within this network or mesh lie splenic macrophages. These

879

intersinusoidal regions appear as splenic cords. The venous sinuses are lined by long, narrow endothelial cells that are variably in close apposition to one another or separated by intercellular gaps in a configuration unique to the spleen. The red pulp serves as a dynamic filtration system, enabling macrophages to remove microorganisms, cellular debris, antigen/antibody complexes, and senescent erythrocytes from circulation.

Around the terminal millimeters of splenic arterioles, a periarticular lymphatic sheath replaces the native adventitia of the vessel. The sheath is comprised of T lymphocytes and intermittent aggregations of B lymphocytes or lymphoid follicles. When antigenically stimulated, the follicles, which are centers of lymphocyte proliferation, develop germinal centers that regress as the stimulus or infection subsides. This white pulp, normally consisting of nodules 1 mm or less in size, can increase to several centimeters in size when nodules coalesce. At the interface between the white and red pulp is the marginal zone, in which lymphocytes are more loosely aggregated. Blood is delivered from this zone to the red pulp, in which lymphocytes and locally produced immunoglobulins ultimately enter the systemic circulation.

PHYSIOLOGY AND PATHOPHYSIOLOGY

Splenic function has historically been summarized as: (1) filtration, (2) host defense, (3) storage, and (4) cytopoiesis. Total splenic inflow of blood is approximately 250–300 mL/min. As blood enters the red pulp, its rate of flow through the spleen can vary greatly. The filtration function of the spleen occurs primarily via the slower circulation. In open circulation, blood percolates through reticular space and splenic cords, gaining access through gaps or slits in the endothelial cell lining to venous sinuses. Blood is thus exposed to extensive contact with splenic macrophages. Plasma is not similarly slowed during its passage through these spaces. Thus, temporary and unique adhesive contact between blood cells and components of the splenic cord may occur. Further evidence of the selective slowing of blood cell flow versus plasma flow is indicated by a concentration of erythrocytes (hematocrit) twice that of the general circulation within the spleen. It is likely during this contact with splenic macrophages that removal of cellular debris and senescent blood cells occurs.

The spleen is the major organ clearing damaged or aged red blood cells and it also plays a role in removing abnormal white blood cells and platelets. During an erythrocyte's 120-day life cycle, a 2-day minimum is spent sequestered in the spleen, in which approximately 20 mL of aged red blood cells are removed daily.

The spleen plays a significant, although not indispensable role in host defense, contributing to both humoral and cell-mediated immunity. Antigens are filtered in the white pulp and presented to immunocompetent centers within the lymphoid follicles, giving rise to the elaboration of immunoglobulins (predominantly IgM). Such an acute IgM response results in the release of opsonic antibodies from the spleen's white pulp. Clearance of the antigen by the splenic and hepatic reticuloendothelial (RE) systems then occurs.

The spleen also produces the opsonins, tuftsin and properdin. Tuftsin, a likely stimulant to general phagocytic function in the host, appears to specifically facilitate clearance of bacteria. Circulating monocytes converted into fixed macrophages with the red pulp account for the spleen's remarkable phagocytic activity.

The spleen also appears to be a major source of properdin, the protein important in the initiation of the alternate pathway of complement activation. The splenic RE system is better able to clear bacteria poorly or inadequately opsonized from the circulation than is the hepatic RE system. There appears to be sufficient physiologic capacity within the complement cascade to withstand the loss of tuftsin and properdin production without increasing patient vulnerability postsplenectomy.

In patients suffering chronic hemolytic disorders, splenic tissue may become permanently hypertrophied. The reticular spaces of the red pulp sometimes become distended with macrophages engorged with the products of erythrocyte breakdown, and as a result the spleen may greatly enlarge (splenomegaly). Splenomegaly alone is an uncommon indication for splenectomy. Hypersplenism or the presence of cytopenia (of one or more blood cell lines) in the context of normally responding bone marrow is one of the most common indications.

Disorders causing hypersplenism in an intrinsically normal spleen can be categorized as either those in which occurs (1) increased destruction of abnormal blood cells or (2) increased sequestration and destruction of normal blood cells.

Hypersplenism may result in neutropenia by sequestration of normal white blood cells or the removal of abnormal ones. Platelets, on the other hand, generally survive in the circulation for 10 days. Under normal circumstances one third of the total platelet pool is sequestered in the spleen. Thrombocytopenia may result from excessive sequestration of platelets and accelerated platelet destruction in the spleen. Splenomegaly may result in sequestration of up to 80 percent of the platelet pool. The spleen may also contribute to the immunologic alteration of platelets, leading to thrombocytopenia in the absence of splenomegaly.

As a site of blood-borne antigen presentation and the initiation of T and B lymphocyte activities involved in humoral and cellular immune responses, the spleen is consistent in immunologic function with other lymphoid organs. Alteration of splenic immune function often gives rise to antibody production, resulting in blood cell destruction.

EVALUATION OF SIZE AND FUNCTION

Before elective splenectomy, imaging of the spleen is frequently indicated to assess size and to determine degree, if any, of splenomegaly.

The sensitivity of ultrasound for detecting textural lesions of the spleen is as high as 98 percent in experienced hands. Computed tomography (CT) scanning affords a high degree of resolution and detail of the spleen and is useful for assessment of splenomegaly, identification of splenic lesions, and guidance for percutaneous procedures. Iodinated contrast material adds diagnostic clarity to CT imaging.

Besides US and CT scan, plain radiography, magnetic resonance imaging (MRI), and radioscintigraphy can be used to image the spleen. Plain radiography, rarely used alone for splenic imaging, can provide an outline of the spleen in the left upper quadrant, suggest splenomegaly, or demonstrate calcifications. MRI offers no advantages in depicting anatomic spleen abnormalities. Radioscintigraphy with 99mTc sulfur colloid demonstrates splenic location and size; there is little benefit to its use as a preoperative scan.

The splenic index (SI) expresses spleen size as a volume in milliliters (mL) and is obtained by multiplying the spleen's length, width, and height as determined by a reliable imaging modality. Normal values for SI range from 120–480 mL. The normal ex vivo weight of the spleen is 150 g.

INDICATIONS FOR SPLENECTOMY

The conditions for which splenectomy is therapeutic include disorders of red blood cells, early cell lines (myeloproliferative disorders), white blood cells, platelets, and miscellaneous disorders and lesions (Table 33-1).

The most common indication for splenectomy is trauma to the spleen, whether iatrogenic or otherwise. Splenectomy for traumatic rupture is addressed in Chapter 6. The most frequent indication for elective splenectomy had been staging for Hodgkin disease, but more recent data suggest it is now idiopathic thrombocytopenic purpura (ITP). In descending order of frequency, other indications include hereditary spherocytosis, autoimmune hemolytic anemia, and thrombotic thrombocytopenic purpura.

TABLE 33-1 Indications for Splenectomy

1. Red cell disorders
    a. Congenital
        i. Hereditary spherocytosis
        ii. Hemoglobinopathies
            1. Sickle cell disease
            2. Thalassemia
            3. Enzyme deficiencies
    b. Acquired
        i. Autoimmune hemolytic anemia
        ii. Parasitic diseases
2. Platelet disorders
    a. Idiopathic thrombocytopenic purpura (ITP)
    b. Thrombotic thrombocytopenic purpura (TTP)
3. White cell disorders
    a. Leukemias
    b. Lymphomas
    c. Hodgkin disease
4. Bone marrow disorders (myeloproliferative disorders)
    a. Myelofibrosis (myeloid metaplasia)
    b. Chronic myeloid leukemia (CML)
    c. Acute myeloid leukemia (AML)
    d. Chronic myelomonocytic leukemia (CMML)
    e. Essential thrombocythemia
    f. Polycythemia vera
5. Miscellaneous disorders and lesions
    a. Infections/abscess
    b. Storage diseases/infiltrative disorders
        i. Gaucher disease
        ii. Niemann-Pick disease
        iii. Amyloidosis
    c. Felty syndrome
    d. Sarcoidosis
    e. Cysts and tumors
    f. Portal hypertension
    g. Splenic artery aneurysm

Red Blood Cell Disorders

Acquired

Autoimmune hemolytic anemia. The autoimmune hemolytic anemias are a set of disorders characterized by autoantibodies against antigens on red blood cells, which decrease the erythrocyte life span. Autoimmune hemolytic anemia (AIHA) is classified into "warm" or "cold" categories, based on the temperature at which the autoantibodies exert their effect. Warm autoantibodies (IgG) bind erythrocytes at 37° C (98.6° F); cold agglutinins (typically IgM) cause erythrocytes to clump at cold temperatures. Warm-antibody is the type of AIHA best treated by splenectomy.

Warm-antibody AIHA. The incidence of warm-antibody AIHA is approximately 1:100,000. More common among women, AIHA occurs at all ages, but is principally seen in mid-life. About one-half of cases are idiopathic. Clinical findings include mild jaundice and symptoms and signs of anemia. Splenomegaly occurs in one third to one half of patients, sometimes enough to result in a palpable spleen on physical examination. Other physical findings may include pallor or slight jaundice. AIHA may develop acutely, with severe symptoms and signs, or gradually, with a relatively asymptomatic presentation. In acute disease, signs of congestive heart failure may be observed.

The diagnosis of AIHA is made by demonstrating hemolysis, followed by performing a direct Coombs test, in which a sample of the patient's blood is mixed with IgG antibody (Coombs reagent). Agglutination represents a positive reaction, indicating the presence of IgG or complement bound to the red blood cell membrane. A positive direct Coombs test confirms the diagnosis of AIHA and distinguishes autoimmune from other forms of hemolytic anemia.

Red blood cells are opsonized by autoantibodies and are destroyed, either directly within the circulation (intravascular hemolysis), or removed from the circulation by tissue macrophages located primarily in the spleen and to a lesser extent in the liver (extravascular hemolysis).

Treatment of AIHA depends on how severe it is and whether it is primary or secondary. Severe anemia (<4 g/dL), causing pulmonary edema, tachycardia, postural hypotension, dyspnea, and angina, demands red blood cell transfusion. Corticosteroids act as the mainstay of treatment for both primary and secondary forms of symptomatic, unstable AIHA. Splenectomy is indicated for failure to respond to steroids, intolerance of steroid side effects, requirement for excessive steroid doses to maintain remission, or inability to receive steroids for other reasons. A favorable response to splenectomy can be expected in up to 80 percent of patients with warm-antibody AIHA.

Congenital

Hereditary spherocytosis. Hereditary spherocytosis (HS) is a disorder of the red blood cell membrane resulting in hemolytic anemia. With an estimated prevalence in Western populations of 1 in 5000, HS is the most common hemolytic anemia for which splenectomy is indicated. The underlying abnormality in HS is an inherited dysfunction or deficiency in one of the erythrocyte membrane proteins (spectrin, ankyrin, band 3 protein, or protein 4.2), resulting in lack of deformability, leading to sequestration and destruction of the spherocytic erythrocytes in the spleen.

Most patients with HS are relatively asymptomatic, although rare fatal crises occur, usually in the setting of infection (e.g., parvovirus). Patients with typical forms of HS may have mild jaundice. Splenomegaly is usually present on physical examination. Spherocytes are readily apparent on peripheral blood film.

Splenectomy is curative for typical forms of HS and serves as the sole mode of therapy. Patients with severe disease usually show a dramatic clinical improvement, even although hemolysis may persist. Because HS may affect children, the timing of splenectomy is important to reduce the very small possibility of overwhelming postsplenectomy sepsis. Most authors recommend delaying the operation until the patient is at least age 4 but before age 7, unless the anemia and hemolysis accelerate. Intractable leg ulcers represent an indication for early splenectomy, because they heal only after removal of the spleen.

Hemoglobinopathies. Sickle cell disease is an inherited chronic hemolytic anemia resulting from the mutant sickle cell hemoglobin (Hb S) within the red blood cell. The prevalence of sickle cell carriers is about 8–10 percent among African Americans in the United States, resulting in 4000–5000 newborns per year at risk for sickle cell disease. In western Africa, by contrast, approximately 120,000 newborns are at risk annually.

The underlying genetic abnormality in sickle cell disease results in the substitution of valine for glutamic acid as the sixth amino acid of the beta-globin chain. Affected B chains lack deformability. This characteristic, in addition to other processes, results in microvascular congestion, which may lead to thrombosis, ischemia, and tissue necrosis. Intermittent painful episodes characterize the disorder.

The most frequent indications for splenectomy among patients with sickle cell disease are hypersplenism and acute sequestration crises, followed by splenic abscess. The occurrence of one major acute sequestration crisis, characterized by rapid painful enlargement of the spleen and circulatory collapse, is generally considered sufficient grounds for splenectomy, as subsequent attacks occur in 40–50 percent of patients, with a mortality rate of 20 percent. The incidence of acute sequestration crises is approximately 5 percent in children with sickle cell disease. Approximately 3 percent of children with sickle cell disease ultimately require splenectomy. Preoperative preparation includes special attention to adequate hydration and avoidance of hypothermia.

Splenectomy does not affect the sickling process, and therapy for sickle cell anemia largely remains palliative. Transfusions are indicated for anemia especially before splenectomy, and for moderately severe episodes of the acute chest syndrome characterized by a new infiltrate on chest radiograph associated with new symptoms, such as fever, cough, sputum production, or hypoxia.

Thalassemia. The thalassemias are a group of inherited disorders of hemoglobin synthesis prevalent among people of Mediterranean extraction, classified according to the hemoglobin chain affected (i.e., α, β, or γ). As a group they are the most common genetic diseases known arising from a single gene defect.

The primary defect in all forms of thalassemia is reduced or absent production of hemoglobin chains. Two significant consequences arise from this abnormality: (1) underproduction of hemoglobin, and (2) excess production of unpaired hemoglobin subunits. Both factors contribute to the morbidity and mortality associated with thalassemia.

The clinical spectrum of the thalassemias is wide. Heterozygous carriers of the disease are usually asymptomatic, but homozygous individuals typically present before 2 years of age with pallor, growth retardation, jaundice, and abdominal swelling because of liver and spleen enlargement. Other characteristics of thalassemia major include intractable leg ulcers, head enlargement, frequent infections, and a requirement for chronic blood transfusions. Untreated individuals usually die in late infancy or early childhood from severe anemia.

Treatment for thalassemia consists of red blood cell transfusions to keep the hemoglobin count greater than 9 mg/dL, along with intensive parenteral chelation therapy with deferoxamine. Splenectomy is indicated for patients with excessive transfusion requirements (> 200 mL/kg per year), discomfort because of splenomegaly, or painful splenic infarction. A careful assessment of the risk-to-benefit ratio for splenectomy is essential, because infectious morbidity following splenectomy in patients with thalassemia is greater than in other patients undergoing splenectomy for hematologic indications.

Bone Marrow Disorders (Myeloproliferative Disorders)

The myeloproliferative disorders are characterized by an abnormal growth of cell lines in the bone marrow. They include chronic myeloid leukemia (CML), acute myeloid leukemia (AML), chronic myelomonocytic leukemia (CMML), essential thrombocythemia (ET), polycythemia vera (PV), and myelofibrosis, also known as agnogenic myeloid metaplasia (see the myelofibrosis section in this chapter). The common underlying problem leading to splenectomy in these disorders is symptomatic splenomegaly. Symptoms because of splenomegaly consist of early satiety, poor gastric emptying, heaviness or pain in the left upper quadrant, and even diarrhea. Hypersplenism, although usually associated with splenomegaly, is a distinct condition. Hypersplenism refers to the presence of one or more peripheral cytopenias in the presence of a normally compensating bone marrow, and can be corrected or improved by splenectomy.

Chronic Myeloid Leukemia

CML is a disorder of the primitive pluripotent stem cell in the bone marrow, resulting in a significant increase in erythroid, megakaryotic, and pluripotent progenitors in the peripheral blood smear. The genetic hallmark is a transposition between the bcr gene on chromosome 9 and the abl gene on chromosome 22. CML is frequently asymptomatic in the chronic phase, but symptomatic patients often present with the gradual onset of fatigue, anorexia, sweating, and left upper quadrant pain and early satiety secondary to splenomegaly. Enlargement of the spleen is found in roughly one half of patients with CML. Splenectomy is indicated to ease pain and early satiety.

Acute Myeloid Leukemia

AML is characterized by a more rapid and dramatic clinical presentation than CML. Death usually results within weeks to months if AML remains untreated. Patients with other myeloproliferative disorders, such as polycythemia vera, primary thrombocytosis, or myeloid metaplasia, are at increased risk for leukemic transformation to AML. Presenting signs and symptoms of AML include a viral-like illness with fever, malaise, and frequently bone pain because of the expansion of the medullary space. Splenomegaly is modest but palpable on physical exam in up to 50 percent of patients. Splenectomy is indicated in AML in the uncommon circumstance that left upper quadrant pain and early satiety become unbearable. Splenectomy in AML adds further risk of infection to patients immunocompromised by neutropenia and chemotherapy.

Chronic Myelomonocytic Leukemia

Chronic myelomonocytic leukemia (CMML) differs from CML in that it is associated with monocytosis in the peripheral smear ($> 1 \times 103/mm^3$) and in the bone marrow. Splenomegaly occurs in one-half of these patients, and splenectomy can result in symptomatic relief.

Essential Thrombocythemia

Essential thrombocythemia (ET) represents abnormal growth of the megakaryocyte cell line, resulting in increased levels of platelets in the bloodstream. Clinical manifestations of ET include vasomotor symptoms, thrombohemorrhagic events, recurrent fetal loss, and the transformation to myelofibrosis with myeloid metaplasia or acute myeloid leukemia. Splenomegaly occurs in one-third to one-half of patients with ET, and its presence may help to distinguish essential from secondary thrombocytosis. Splenectomy is not felt to be helpful in the early stages of ET, and is best reserved for the later stages of disease, in which myeloid metaplasia has developed. Candidates should be chosen selectively, because significant bleeding has been reported to complicate splenectomy.

Polycythemia Vera

Polycythemia vera (PV) is a rare, chronic, progressive myeloproliferative disorder characterized by an increase in red blood cell mass, frequently accompanied by leukocytosis, thrombocytosis, and splenomegaly. Patients affected by PV typically enjoy prolonged survival compared to others affected by hematologic malignancies. Affected patients may present with any number of nonspecific complaints, including headache, dizziness, weakness, pruritus, visual disturbances, excessive sweating, joint symptoms, and weight loss. Physical findings include ruddy cyanosis, conjunctival plethora, hepatomegaly, splenomegaly, and hypertension. Treatment ranges from phlebotomy and aspirin to chemotherapeutic agents. As in ET, splenectomy is not helpful in the early stages of disease and is best reserved for late-stage patients in whom myeloid metaplasia has developed and splenomegaly related symptoms are severe.

Myelofibrosis (Agnogenic Myeloid Metaplasia)

The term myelofibrosis may be used to describe either the generic condition of fibrosis of the bone marrow (which may be associated with a number of benign and malignant disorders) or a specific, chronic, malignant hematologic disease associated with splenomegaly, red blood cell and white blood cell progenitors in the bloodstream, marrow fibrosis, and extramedullary hematopoiesis, otherwise known as agnogenic myeloid metaplasia (AMM). Use of the term myelofibrosis in this chapter will be synonymous with AMM.

In AMM fibrosis of the bone marrow is believed to be a response to a clonal proliferation of hematopoietic stem cells. Marrow failure often ensues, but whether this failure is secondary to the fibrosis itself or to the malignant proliferation of cells is unknown. Clinical manifestations of AMM most frequently relate to anemia, including fatigue, weakness, dyspnea on exertion, and palpitations. About 20 percent of patients, however, are asymptomatic and seek medical attention because of an enlarged spleen on physical exam or an abnormal blood smear. Other clinical manifestations of AMM include bleeding, fever, weight loss, gout/renal stones, night sweats, and symptoms because of an enlarged spleen. Nearly all patients with AMM have splenomegaly, 35 percent of patients have massive splenomegaly, and two thirds have hepatomegaly.

Nucleated red blood cells and immature myeloid elements in the blood are present in 96 percent of cases and strongly suggest the diagnosis. Care must be taken, however, to exclude a history of a primary neoplasm or tuberculosis, because patients with these conditions may develop secondary myelofibrosis.

Asymptomatic patients are closely followed, whereas symptomatic patients undergo therapeutic intervention targeted toward their symptoms. Splenomegaly related symptoms are best treated with splenectomy.

A thorough preoperative workup must precede splenectomy in patients with AMM. The candidate must possess acceptable cardiac, pulmonary, hepatic, and renal reserve for the operation. The coagulation system should be examined, including tests of coagulation factors V and VIII, fibrin split products, platelet count, and bleeding time. Low platelet counts may require adrenal steroids and/or platelet transfusion at the time of surgery. Splenectomy imparts durable, effective palliation for nearly all patients with AMM, although postoperative complications are more common in patients with AMM than in those with other hematologic indications.

White Blood Cell Disorders

Leukemias

Chronic lymphocytic leukemia. Chronic lymphocytic leukemia and hairy cell leukemia (HCL) are the two leukemias most amenable to treatment by splenectomy. Symptoms of CLL are nonspecific and include weakness, fatigue, fever without illness, night sweats, and frequent bacterial and viral infections. Splenomegaly may be massive or barely palpable below the costal margin. Splenectomy is indicated to improve cytopenias. Splenectomy may thus facilitate chemotherapy in patients whose cell counts were prohibitively low prior to spleen removal. Palliative splenectomy also is indicated for symptomatic splenomegaly.

Hairy cell leukemia. Hairy cell leukemia is characterized by splenomegaly, pancytopenia, and large numbers of abnormal lymphocytes in the bone marrow. These lymphocytes contain irregular hair-like cytoplasmic projections identifiable on the peripheral smear. Most patients seek medical attention because of symptoms related to anemia, neutropenia, thrombocytopenia, or splenomegaly.

The most common physical finding is splenomegaly, which occurs in 80 percent of patients with HCL and often is palpable 5 cm below the costal margin. Treatment is indicated for those with moderate to severe symptoms related to cytopenias, such as repeated infections or bleeding episodes, or to splenomegaly. Newer chemotherapeutic agents (the purine analogues 2′ -deoxycoformycin [2′ -DCF] and 2-chlorodeoxyadenosine [2-CdA]) are able to induce durable complete remission in most patients.

Lymphomas

Non–Hodgkin lymphoma. Non–Hodgkin lymphoma (NHL) encompasses all malignancies derived from the lymphoid system except classic Hodgkin disease. Surgical staging is no longer indicated for NHL, as the combination of history and physical examination, chest radiograph and abdominal/pelvic CT scan, biopsy of involved lymph nodes (including laparoscopically directed nodal and liver biopsies), and bone marrow biopsy is sufficient. Splenomegaly exists in various, but not all, forms of NHL, and splenectomy is indicated for symptoms related to an enlarged spleen and to improve cytopenias.

Hodgkin disease. Hodgkin disease (HD) is a disorder of the lymphoid system characterized by the presence of Reed-Sternberg cells, which actually form the minority of the Hodgkin's tumor. The spleen is often an occult site of spread, but massive splenomegaly is not common. Additionally, large spleens do not necessarily signify involvement.

The staging procedure for HD begins with a wedge biopsy of the liver, splenectomy, and the removal of representative nodes in the retroperitoneum, mesentery, and hepatoduodenal ligament. Staging for HD may be performed laparoscopically. A laparoscopic core biopsy of the liver is performed under direct visualization, either using a Tru-cut needle percutaneously or by wedge resection with shears and cautery. Finally, an iliac marrow biopsy is generally included. Refinements of CT scanning and the more liberal use of chemotherapy for patients with HD have significantly reduced the indications for surgical staging of the disease. Current indications for surgical staging include clinical stage I or stage II with nodular sclerosing histology and no symptoms referable to HD. Staging information affects treatment, as early stage patients who have no splenic involvement may be candidates for radiotherapy alone. Those with splenic involvement generally require chemotherapy or multimodality therapy.

Platelet Disorders

Idiopathic Thrombocytopenic Purpura (ITP)

ITP, also called immune thrombocytopenic purpura, is an autoimmune disorder characterized by a low platelet count and mucocutaneous and petechial bleeding. The low platelet count stems from premature removal of platelets opsonized by antiplatelet IgG autoantibodies produced in the spleen. The estimated incidence of ITP is 100 persons per million annually, about one-half of whom are children. Adult-onset and childhood-onset ITP are strikingly different in their clinical course and management.

Patients with ITP typically present with petechiae or ecchymosis, although some will experience major bleeding from the outset. Bleeding may occur from mucosal surfaces in the form of gingival bleeding, epistaxis, menorrhagia, hematuria, or even melena. Patients with platelet counts below 10,000/mm^3 are at risk for internal bleeding. The incidence of major intracranial hemorrhage is about 1 percent, usually occurring early in the disease course. Children often present at a young age (peak age approximately 5 years) with sudden onset of petechiae or purpura several days to weeks after an infectious illness. In contrast, adults experience a more chronic form of disease with an insidious onset. Splenomegaly with ITP is uncommon in both adults and children, and its occurrence should prompt a search for a separate cause of thrombocytopenia.

Diagnosing ITP is based on exclusion of other possibilities (e.g., systemic lupus erythematosus, certain antimicrobials or other drugs) in the presence of a low platelet count and mucocutaneous bleeding. In addition to low platelets, laboratory findings characteristic of ITP consist of large, immature platelets (megathrombocytes) on peripheral blood smear.

Adults generally require treatment at the time of presentation, because up to one half will present with counts below 10,000/mm^3. The usual first line of therapy is oral prednisone at a dose of 1.0–1.5 mg/kg per day. Most responses occur within the first 3 weeks. Response rates range from 50–75 percent, but relapses are common. Intravenous immunoglobulin, given at 1.0 g/kg per day for 2–3 days, is indicated for internal bleeding when counts remain below 5000/mm^3 or when extensive purpura exists. An immediate response is common, but a sustained remission is not. Splenectomy is indicated for failure of medical therapy, for prolonged use of steroids with undesirable effects, or for most cases of first relapse. Splenectomy provides a permanent response without subsequent need for steroids in 75–85 percent of the total number of patients undergoing splenectomy (see the "Splenectomy Outcomes" section of this chapter). Responses usually occur within the first postoperative week. Patients with extremely low platelet counts (< 10,000/mm^3) should have platelets available for surgery, but should not receive them preoperatively. Once the splenic pedicle is ligated, platelets are given to those who continue to bleed.

In children with ITP, the course is self-limited, with durable and complete remission in over 70 percent of patients regardless of therapy. Because of the good prognosis without treatment, children with typical ITP—and certainly those without hemorrhage—are managed principally by observation, with short-term therapy in select cases. Where therapy is indicated, intravenous immune globulin has been shown to shorten the duration of severe thrombocytopenia, and a short course of oral prednisone (4 mg/kg for 4 consecutive days) generally produces excellent results. Splenectomy is reserved for failure of medical therapy in children who have had immune thrombocytopenic purpura for at least 1 year with symptomatic, severe thrombocytopenia. Urgent splenectomy may play a role in the rare circumstance of severe, life-threatening bleeding, in conjunction with aggressive medical therapy, for both children and adults.

Thrombotic Thrombocytopenic Purpura

Thrombotic thrombocytopenic purpura (TTP) is a serious disorder characterized by thrombocytopenia, microangiopathic hemolytic anemia, and neurologic complications. Abnormal platelet clumping occurs in arterioles and capillaries, reducing the lumen of these vessels and predisposing the patient to microvascular thrombotic episodes. TTP is a rare disorder, but its dramatic clinical sequelae and favorable response to early therapy demand an understanding of its clinical presentation to bring about an early diagnosis. Clinical features of the disorder include petechiae, fever, neurologic symptoms, renal failure, and infrequently cardiac symptoms, such as heart failure or arrhythmias. Petechial hemorrhages in the lower extremities are the most common presenting sign. Neurologic changes range from generalized headaches to altered mental status, seizures, and even coma. Generally, however, the mere presence of petechiae and thrombocytopenia are sufficient to lead to the diagnosis of TTP and consideration of treatment.

TTP may be distinguished from autoimmune causes of thrombocytopenia, such as Evans syndrome (ITP and autoimmune hemolytic anemia) or systemic lupus erythematosus, by a negative Coombs test.

The first line of therapy for TTP is plasma exchange. This treatment has dramatically improved survival from less than 10 percent to about 90 percent since its implementation. Splenectomy plays a key role for patients who relapse or require multiple plasma exchanges to control symptoms, and is generally well-tolerated without significant morbidity. Once the spleen is removed, patients typically do not relapse. Platelet transfusions are not recommended in TTP, as severe clinical deterioration has been reported following their administration.

Miscellaneous Disorders and Lesions

Infections and Abscesses

Abscesses of the spleen are uncommon, with an incidence of 0.14–0.7 percent, based on autopsy findings. Five distinct mechanisms of splenic abscess formation have been described: (1) hematogenous infection; (2) contiguous infection; (3) hemoglobinopathy; (4) immunosuppression, including HIV and chemotherapy; and (5) trauma. The most common origins for hematogenous spread are infective endocarditis, typhoid fever, malaria, urinary tract infections, and osteomyelitis. Presentation is frequently delayed. Clinical manifestations include fever, left upper quadrant pain, leukocytosis, and splenomegaly in about one-third of patients. The diagnosis is confirmed by ultrasound or CT scan, which has a 95 percent sensitivity and specificity. On discovery of a splenic abscess, broad-spectrum antibiotics should be started and continued for 14 days. Splenectomy is the operation of choice, but percutaneous or open drainage are options for patients who cannot tolerate splenectomy. Percutaneous drainage is successful for patients with unilocular disease.

Storage Diseases and Infiltrative Disorders

Gaucher's disease. This is an inherited lipid storage disease characterized by the deposition of glucocerebroside in cells of the macrophage-monocyte system. Patients with Gaucher's disease frequently experience symptoms related to splenomegaly—including early satiety and abdominal discomfort—and hypersplenism, including thrombocytopenia, normocytic anemia, and mild leukopenia. Splenectomy alleviates hematologic abnormalities in patients with hypersplenism but does not correct the underlying disease process.

Niemann-Pick disease. This is an inherited disease of abnormal lysosomal storage of sphingomyelin and cholesterol in cells of the macrophage-monocyte system. Types A and B result from a deficiency in lysosomal hydrolase and are the forms most likely to demonstrate splenomegaly with its concomitant symptoms. Splenectomy has been reported to successfully treat symptoms of splenomegaly in these cases.

Amyloidosis. Amyloidosis is a disorder of abnormal extracellular protein deposition. If splenomegaly develops, related symptoms are relieved by splenectomy. Removal of the spleen also has been reported to cure patients of factor X deficiency associated with primary amyloidosis.

Felty Syndrome

The triad of rheumatoid arthritis (RA), splenomegaly, and neutropenia is called Felty syndrome. The spleen in Felty syndrome is four times heavier than normal. Neutropenia causing frequent infections is often the driving force behind the decision for splenectomy. Responses to splenectomy have been excellent, with over 80 percent of patients showing a durable increase in white blood cell count. Besides symptomatic neutropenia, other indications for splenectomy include transfusion-dependent anemia and profound thrombocytopenia. Corticosteroids, hematopoietic growth factors, methotrexate, and splenectomy all have been used to treat the neutropenia of Felty syndrome.

Sarcoidosis

Sarcoidosis is an inflammatory disease of young adults, characterized by noncaseating granulomas in affected tissues. Any organ system may be involved. The most commonly involved organ is the lung, followed by the spleen. Splenomegaly occurs in about 25 percent of patients. Massive splenomegaly (>1 kg) is rare. When splenomegaly occurs and causes symptoms related to size or hypersplenism, splenectomy effectively relieves symptoms and corrects hematologic abnormalities such as anemia and thrombocytopenia.

Cysts and Tumors

Splenic cysts are rare lesions. The most common etiology for splenic cysts worldwide is parasitic infestation, particularly echinococcal. Symptomatic parasitic cysts are best treated with splenectomy, although selected cases may be amenable to percutaneous aspiration, instillation of protoscolicidal agent, and reaspiration. Nonparasitic cysts most commonly result from trauma and are called pseudocysts. The treatment of nonparasitic cysts depends on whether or not they produce symptoms. Asymptomatic nonparasitic cysts may be observed with close ultrasound follow up to exclude significant expansion. Patients should be advised of the risk of cyst rupture with even minor abdominal trauma if they elect nonoperative management for large cysts. Small symptomatic nonparasitic cysts may be excised with splenic preservation, and large symptomatic nonparasitic cysts may be unroofed. Both of these operations may be performed laparoscopically.

The most common primary tumor of the spleen is sarcomatous. Non–Hodgkin lymphoma of the spleen is rare, but splenectomy imparts an excellent prognosis. Lung cancer is the most common tumor to spread to the spleen.

Portal Hypertension

Portal hypertension can result from numerous causes, but usually is because of cirrhosis. Splenomegaly and splenic congestion often accompany portal hypertension. Splenectomy, however, is not indicated for hypersplenism per se in patients with portal hypertension, because no correlation exists between the degree of pancytopenia and long-term survival in these patients.

Portal hypertension secondary to splenic vein thrombosis is potentially curable with splenectomy. Patients with bleeding from isolated gastric varices in the presence of normal liver function tests, especially with a history of pancreatic disease, should be examined for splenic vein thrombosis and treated with splenectomy if positive.

Splenic Artery Aneurysm

Although rare, splenic artery aneurysm (SAA) is the most common visceral artery aneurysm. The aneurysm usually arises in the middle to distal portion of the splenic artery. The risk of rupture is between 3 and 9 percent; however, once rupture occurs, mortality is substantial (35–50 percent). SAA is particularly worrisome when discovered during pregnancy, as rupture imparts a high risk of mortality to both mother (70 percent) and fetus (95 percent). Indications for treatment include presence of symptoms, pregnancy, intention to become pregnant, and pseudoaneurysms associated with inflammatory processes. For asymptomatic patients, size greater than 2 cm constitutes an indication for surgery. Aneurysm resection or ligation alone is acceptable for amenable lesions in the mid-splenic artery, but distal lesions in close proximity to the splenic hilum should be treated with concomitant splenectomy.

PREOPERATIVE CONSIDERATIONS

Splenic Artery Embolization

The use of splenic artery embolization (SAE) as a preoperative technique became available with advances in angiographic technology. Theoretical advantages of SAE include reduced operative blood loss from a devascularized spleen and reduced spleen size for easier dissection and removal. Potential disadvantages of the procedure, however, include acute left-sided pain (although usually of limited duration), pancreatitis, or other embolization-related complications. Not all investigators use or recommend SAE, citing equivalent splenectomy-related blood loss and morbidity. There is currently no consensus on the role of preoperative SAE for elective splenectomy.

Vaccination

Splenectomy imparts a small (<1–5 percent) but definite life-time risk of fulminant, potentially life-threatening infection. Therefore, when elective splenectomy is planned, vaccinations against encapsulated bacteria (e.g., *Streptococcus pneumoniae*, *Haemophilus influenzae* type B, and meningococcus) should be given at least 2 weeks before surgery to protect against such infection. If the spleen is removed emergently (e.g., for trauma), vaccinations should be given as soon as possible following surgery, allowing at least 1–2 days for recovery. Booster injections of pneumococcal vaccine should be considered every 5–6 years regardless of the reason for splenectomy. Additionally, annual influenza immunization is advisable.

Deep Venous Thrombosis Prophylaxis

Deep venous thrombosis (DVT) is not uncommon following splenectomy, especially in cases involving splenomegaly and myeloproliferative disorders (MPD). The risk of portal vein thrombosis (PVT) may be as high as 40 percent for patients with both splenomegaly and MPD. Postsplenectomy PVT typically presents with anorexia, abdominal pain, leukocytosis, and thrombocytosis. A high index of suspicion, early diagnosis with contrast-enhanced CT, and immediate anticoagulation are keys to successful treatment for PVT. Patients undergoing splenectomy should be treated with DVT prophylaxis, including sequential compression devices with subcutaneous heparin (5000 U). Each patient's risk factors for DVT should be evaluated, and where elevated risk exists (obesity, history of prior VTE, known hypercoagulable state, age > 60), a more aggressive antithrombotic regimen, including low-molecular-weight heparin (LMWH), may be pursued.

SPLENECTOMY TECHNIQUES

Patient Preparation

All patients undergoing elective splenectomy should be vaccinated at least 1 week preoperatively with polyvalent pneumococcal, meningococcal, and Haemophilus. Patients' potential need for blood product transfusion must be assessed, and their coagulation status optimized. Anemic patients should be transfused to a hemoglobin of 10 g/dL. For more complex patients, including those with splenomegaly, a type and cross is recommended for at least 2–4 units of blood. Platelet transfusions may transiently correct thrombocytopenia although preferably not preoperatively and ideally not before intraoperative ligation of the splenic artery.

Patients who have been maintained on corticosteroid therapy preoperatively should receive perioperatively parenteral corticosteroid therapy. All splenectomy patients receive deep vein thrombosis (DVT) prophylaxis and intravenous administration of a first-generation cephalosporin. A nasogastric (NG) tube is inserted after endotracheal intubation to decompress the stomach.

Open Splenectomy

Whereas laparoscopic surgery (LS) is increasingly accepted as the standard approach for normosplenic patients, open splenectomy (OS) is still widely practiced. Traumatic rupture of the spleen remains the most common indication for OS, which also may be favored for patients requiring splenectomy who have massive splenomegaly, ascites, portal hypertension, multiple prior operations, extensive splenic radiation, or possible splenic abscess.

Open Splenectomy Technique

In preparation for OS, the patient is placed in the supine position with the surgeon situated on the patient's right. A midline incision is preferable for exposure of a ruptured or massively enlarged spleen or when abdominal access is needed for a staging laparotomy. A left subcostal incision is preferred for most elective splenectomies.

Dividing ligamentous attachments, usually beginning with the splenocolic ligament, mobilizes the spleen. For patients with significant splenomegaly, early ligation of the splenic artery in continuity along the superior border of the pancreas provides for safer manipulation of the spleen and dissection of the splenic hilum, some spleen shrinkage, and an autotransfusion of erythrocytes and platelets. Incising the spleen's lateral peritoneal attachments, most notably the splenophrenic ligament, provides further medial mobilization. The short gastric vessels are then sequentially ligated and divided. Splenic hilar dissection follows with the splenic artery and vein (in that order) dissected and individually ligated prior to division. Care is taken to avoid injuring the tail of the pancreas.

With the spleen excised, the dissection bed is irrigated, suctioned, and inspected meticulously to ensure hemostasis. The splenic bed is not routinely drained. The NG tube is removed at the completion of surgery.

Laparoscopic Splenectomy

LS has supplanted OS as the elective splenectomy approach of choice. Most LS procedures are performed with the patient in the right lateral decubitus position. An angled (30 degrees or 45 degrees) laparoscope (2-mm, 5-mm, or 10-mm) facilitates the lateral approach, in which three or four trocars positioned are routinely used and vital anatomy is exposed in a manner allowing for an intuitive dissection sequence.

The splenocolic ligament and lateral peritoneal attachments are divided, resulting in medial spleen mobilization. The short gastric vessels are divided by individual clip applications, endovascular staples, or hemostatic energy sources. With the lower spleen pole elevated, the splenic hilum is accessible for further clip applications or endovascular stapling. Usually, the splenic artery and vein are separated. With the spleen thus retracted, the surgeon easily visualizes the tail of the pancreas and can avoid its injury.

Once excised, the spleen is placed in a durable nylon sac, then drawn through a 10-mm trocar site. Blunt instruments should be used to morcellate the spleen within the sac for piecemeal extraction.

In patients with splenomegaly, hand-assisted LS can facilitate a safe, expeditious procedure. The surgeon's hand is introduced completely into the peritoneal cavity for palpation of appropriate tissues that allows for identification, retraction, and dissection. Clip, staple, and energy source use achieve hemostasis. The excised specimen is delivered through the hand-access port.

Partial Splenectomy

Certain lipid storage disorders leading to splenomegaly and some forms of traumatic splenic injury are amenable to partial splenectomy. Partial splenectomy is indicated in children to minimize postsplenectomy sepsis risk.

SPLENECTOMY OUTCOMES

Splenectomy results in characteristic changes to blood composition, including the appearance of Howell-Jolly bodies and siderocytes. Leukocytosis and increased platelet counts commonly occur following splenectomy as well.

Complications

Complications of splenectomy may be classified as pulmonary, hemorrhagic, infectious, pancreatic, and thromboembolic. The most common complication is left lower lobe atelectasis, occurring in up to 16 percent of patients following OS. Other pulmonary problems include pleural effusion and pneumonia. Hemorrhage may be intra- or postoperative. Across all elective indications, the need for transfusion arises in 3–5 percent of cases. Infectious complications include subphrenic abscess and wound infection. Pancreatic complications, including pancreatitis, pseudocyst, and pancreatic fistula, may result from intraoperative trauma to the pancreas, especially to the tail, during the dissection of the splenic hilum. Thromboembolic phenomena occur in 5–10 percent of patients undergoing splenectomy.

Hematologic Outcomes

For thrombocytopenia, a long-term response is defined as a platelet count greater than 150,000/mL more than 2 months after surgery without medications. Laparoscopic splenectomy is effective in providing a long-term platelet response in approximately 85 percent of individuals with ITP (Table 33-2). These results are consistent with the success of open splenectomy, which is associated with a long-term success rate of 65–90 percent.

For chronic hemolytic anemias, a rise in hemoglobin levels to above 10 g/dL without the need for transfusion signifies a successful response to splenectomy. By this criterion, splenectomy has been reported to be successful in 60–80 percent of patients with chronic hemolytic anemia. For the subset of patients with spherocytosis, the success rate is usually higher, ranging from 90–100 percent.

TABLE 33-2 Platelet Response Following Laparoscopic Splenectomy for Idiopathic Thrombocytopenic Purpura

Study (lead author)	N	Initial response (%)	Long-term response (%)	Mean follow-up (m)
Szold et al	104	NA	84	36
Katkhouda et al	67	84	78	38
Trias et al	48	NA	88	30
Tanoue et al	35	83	79	36
Friedman et al	31	NA	93	2
Stanton	30	89	89	30
Fass et al	29	90	80	43
Bresler et al	27	93	88	28
Harold et al	27	92	85	20
Lozano-Salazar et al	22	89	88	15
Meyer et al	16	NA	86	14
Watson et al	13	100	83	60
Total/mean	**449**	**90**	**85**	**29**

Surgical and postsurgical outcomes also include the operative time, recovery time, and morbidity and mortality rates of the procedure, which tend to vary according to the hematologic indication.

To date, no prospective, randomized comparisons between laparoscopic and open splenectomy have been published. Numerous retrospective or case-controlled comparisons between LS and OS reveal that the laparoscopic approach typically results in longer operative times, shorter hospital stays, lower morbidity rates, similar blood loss, and similar mortality rates. The laparoscopic approach has emerged as the standard for nontraumatic, elective splenectomy.

Overwhelming Postsplenectomy Infection

Regardless of technique or indication, splenectomy imparts a lifetime risk of severe infection to the patient. The true incidence of postsplenectomy sepsis remains unknown, with estimates varying between less than 1 and 5 percent during a patient's lifetime. Overwhelming postsplenectomy infection (OPSI) is more likely to occur among children compared to adults, and among those with hematologic disorders as compared to splenic trauma.

The loss of the spleen's ability to filter and phagocytose bacteria and parasitized blood cells predisposes the patient to infection by encapsulated bacteria or parasites. Splenectomy also results in the loss of a significant source of antibody production. The most common source of infection reported in the literature is *Streptococcus pneumoniae*, accounting for 50–90 percent of cases. *H. influenzae* type B, meningococcus, and group A streptococci have reportedly accounted for an additional 25 percent of infections.

OPSI is associated with pneumonia or meningitis in roughly one-half of cases, but a substantial number of patients have no clear site of bacterial colonization. OPSI may begin with a relatively mild-appearing prodrome, including fever, malaise, myalgias, headache, vomiting, diarrhea, and abdominal pain. These symptoms may then progress rapidly to fulminant bacteremic septic shock, with accompanying hypotension, anuria, and disseminated intravascular coagulation.

Some risk factors for the development of OPSI have been identified. Patients undergoing splenectomy for hematologic indications carry a higher risk than those who undergo splenectomy for trauma. Individuals with compromised immune systems such as those with Hodgkin disease or those taking chemotherapy or radiation therapy have a higher risk of OPSI than those who do not. OPSI usually develops within the first 2 years after splenectomy, especially in children.

Prudent immunoprophylaxis consists of pneumococcal, meningococcal, and *H. influenzae* type B vaccination at least 7–14 days before splenectomy or as soon as possible after surgery. Pneumococcal vaccine booster injections every 5–6 years should be considered. Annual influenza immunization is advisable. Antibiotic prophylaxis—usually a single daily dose of penicillin or amoxicillin—is recommended for asplenic children for the first 2 years after splenectomy.

Suggested Readings

Katkhouda N, Hurwitz MG, Rivera RT, et al: Laparoscopic splenectomy: Outcome and efficacy in 103 consecutive patients. Ann Surg 228:1, 1998.

Morgenstern L, Skandalakis JE: Anatomy and embryology of the spleen, in Hiatt JR, Phillips EH, Morgenstern L (eds): Surgical Diseases of the Spleen. Berlin-Heidelberg: Springer-Verlag, 1997, p 15.

Schwartz SI: Role of splenectomy in hematologic disorders. World J Surg 20:1156, 1996.

Schwartz RS, Berkman EM, Silberstein LE: Autoimmune hemolytic anemias, in Hoffman R (ed): Hematology: Basic Principles and Practice, 3rd ed. New York: Churchill Livingstone, 2001, p 611.

al-Salem AH, Qaisaruddin S, Nasserallah Z, et al: Splenectomy in patients with sickle-cell disease. Am J Surg 172:254, 1996.

Mesa RA, Elliott MA, Tefferi A: Splenectomy in chronic myeloid leukemia and myelofibrosis with myeloid metaplasia. Blood Rev 14:121, 2000.

Cines DB, Blanchette VS: Immune thrombocytopenic purpura. N Engl J Med 346:995, 2002.

Park AE, Gagner M, Pomp A: The lateral approach to laparoscopic splenectomy. Am J Surg 173:126, 1997.

Park A, Marcaccio M, Sternbach M, et al: Laparoscopic vs open splenectomy. Arch Surg 134:1263, 1999.

Trias M, Targarona EM, Espert JJ, et al: Impact of hematological diagnosis on early and late outcome after laparoscopic splenectomy: An analysis of 111 cases. Surg Endosc 14:556, 2000.

34 | Abdominal Wall, Omentum, Mesentery, and Retroperitoneum

Robert L. Bell, M.D., and Neal E. Seymour, M.D.

ABDOMINAL WALL

Surgical Anatomy

The abdominal wall is an anatomically complex, layered structure with segmentally derived blood supply and innervation. The muscle fibers of the rectus abdominis are encased within an aponeurotic sheath, the anterior and posterior layers of which are fused in the midline at the linea alba. The lateral border of the rectus muscles assumes a convex shape that gives rise to the linea semilunaris.

Lateral to the rectus sheath, there are three muscular layers with oblique fiber orientations relative to one another. The external oblique muscle runs inferiorly and medially, arising from the margins of the lowest eight ribs and costal cartilages and the latissimus dorsi, serratus anterior and the iliac crest. Medially it forms a tendinous aponeurosis, which is contiguous with anterior rectus sheath. The inguinal ligament is the inferior-most edge of the external oblique aponeurosis reflected posteriorly in the area between the anterior superior iliac spine and pubic tubercle. The internal oblique muscle lies immediately deep to the external oblique muscle and arises from the lateral aspect of the inguinal ligament, the iliac crest and the thoracolumbar fascia. Its fibers course superiorly and medially and form a tendinous aponeurosis that contributes to both the anterior and posterior rectus sheath. The lower medial and inferior-most fibers of the internal oblique course may fuse with the lower fibers of the transversus abdominis muscle (the conjoined area). The transversus abdominis muscle is the deepest of the three lateral muscles and, as its name implies, runs transversely.

The complexities of the anterior and posterior aspects of the rectus sheath are best understood in their relationship to the arcuate line (semicircular line of Douglas), which lies roughly at the level of the anterior superior iliac spines. Above the arcuate line, the anterior rectus sheath is formed by the external oblique aponeurosis and the external lamina of the internal oblique aponeurosis whereas the posterior rectus sheath is formed by the internal lamina of the internal oblique aponeurosis, the transversus abdominis aponeurosis, and the transversalis fascia. Below the arcuate line, the anterior rectus sheath is formed by the external oblique aponeurosis, the internal oblique aponeurosis, and the transversus abdominis aponeurosis. There is no aponeurotic posterior covering of this lower portion of the rectus muscles, although the transversalis fascia remains a contiguous structure on the posterior aspect of the anterior abdominal wall.

The majority of the blood supply to the muscles of the anterior abdominal wall is derived from the superior and inferior epigastric arteries. A collateral network of branches of the subcostal and lumbar arteries also contribute the abdominal wall blood supply. Innervation of the rectus muscles, the internal oblique muscles, and the transversus abdominis muscles arises from the anterior rami of spinal nerves at the T6–T12 levels. The overlying skin is innervated by afferent branches of the T4–L1 nerve roots, with the nerve roots of T10 subserving sensation of the skin around the umbilicus.

PHYSIOLOGY

The rectus muscles, the external oblique muscles, and the internal oblique muscles work as a unit to flex the trunk anteriorly or laterally. Rotation of the trunk is achieved by the contraction of the external oblique muscle and the contralateral internal oblique muscle. Additionally, all four muscles (rectus muscles, the external oblique muscles, the internal oblique muscle, and the transversus abdominis muscle) are involved in raising intraabdominal pressure. If the diaphragm is relaxed when the abdominal musculature is contracted, then the pressure exerted by the abdominal muscles results in expiration of air from the lungs. Thus, these abdominal muscles are the primary muscles of expiration. If the diaphragm is contracted when the abdominal musculature is contracted (Valsalva maneuver) the increased abdominal pressure aids in processes such as micturition, defecation, and childbirth.

Congenital Abnormalities

Prominent in the early embryonic abdominal wall is a large central defect through which pass the vitelline (omphalomesenteric) duct connecting the embryonic and fetal midgut to the yolk sac. During the sixth week of development, embryonic midgut herniates into the umbilical cord, and while outside the confines of the developing abdomen, undergoes a 270-degree counterclockwise rotation. At the end of the twelfth week it returns to the abdominal cavity, and attains its final position. Congenital defects in abdominal wall closure may lead to omphalocele or gastroschisis. In omphalocele, viscera protrude through an open umbilical ring and are covered by a sac derived from the amnion. In gastroschisis, the viscera protrude through a defect lateral to the umbilicus and no sac is present.

Persistence of a vitelline duct remnant on the ileal border results in a Meckel diverticulum. Complete failure of the vitelline duct to regress results in a vitelline duct fistula, which is associated with drainage of small intestinal contents from the umbilicus. If both the intestinal and umbilical ends of the vitelline duct regress into fibrous cords, a central vitelline duct (omphalomesenteric) cyst may occur. When diagnosed, vitelline duct fistulas and cysts should be excised along with any accompanying fibrous cord.

Acquired Abnormalities

Rectus Abdominis Diastasis

Rectus abdominis diastasis (or diastasis recti) describes a clinically evident separation of the rectus abdominis muscle pillars, generally as a result of decreased tone of the abdominal musculature. The characteristic bulging of the abdominal wall in the epigastrium is sometimes mistaken for a ventral hernia, despite that fact that the midline aponeurosis is intact and no hernia defect is present. Diastasis is usually easily identified on physical examination. Computed tomography (CT) scanning will differentiate rectus diastasis from a true ventral hernia if clarification is required. Surgical correction of a severe rectus diastasis by plication of the anterior rectus sheath may be undertaken for cosmetic indications, or if it is associated with disability of abdominal wall muscular function.

Rectus Sheath Hematoma

The terminal branches of the superior and inferior epigastric arteries course deep to the posterior aspect of the left and right rectus pillars and penetrate the posterior rectus sheath. An injury to these vessels or any of the collateralizing vessels within the rectus sheath can result in a rectus sheath hematoma. Although there may be a history of significant blunt trauma, less obvious events also have been reported to cause this condition such as sudden contraction of the rectus muscles with coughing, sneezing, or any vigorous physical activity. Spontaneous rectus sheath hematomas have been described in older adults and in those on anticoagulation therapy. Patients frequently describe the sudden onset of unilateral abdominal pain that may be confused with lateralized peritoneal disorders such as appendicitis. Below the arcuate line, a hematoma may cross the midline and cause bilateral lower quadrant pain.

The diagnosis may be suggested by history and physical examination alone. Pain typically increases with contraction of the rectus muscles and a tender mass may be palpated. The ability to appreciate an intraabdominal mass is ordinarily degraded with contraction of the rectus muscles. The Fothergill sign, a palpable abdominal mass that remains unchanged with contraction of the rectus muscles, is classic for rectus hematoma. A hemoglobin/hematocrit level and coagulation studies should be obtained. Abdominal ultrasonography may show a solid or cystic mass within the abdominal wall depending on the chronicity of the bleeding event. Computed tomography is the most definitive study for establishing the correct diagnosis and excluding other intraabdominal disorders.

Specific treatment depends on the severity of the hemorrhage. Small, unilateral, and contained hematomas may be observed without hospitalization. Bilateral or large hematomas will likely require hospitalization and potential resuscitation. The need for red blood cell or coagulation factor transfusion is determined by the clinical circumstances. Reversal of Coumadin anticoagulation may be necessary. Emergent operative intervention or angiographic embolization may be necessary if hematoma enlargement, free bleeding, or clinical deterioration occurs. Surgical therapy consists of evacuation of the hematoma and ligation of any bleeding vessel identified. Mortality in this condition is rare, but has been reported in patients requiring surgical treatment and in the extremely older adult.

Abdominal Wall Hernias

Hernias of the anterior abdominal wall, or ventral hernias represent defects in the abdominal wall fascia and muscle through which intraabdominal or preperitoneal contents can protrude. Ventral hernias may be congenital or acquired. Acquired hernias may develop via slow architectural deterioration of the muscular aponeuroses or they may develop from failed healing of an anterior abdominal wall incision (incisional hernia). The most common finding is a mass or bulge on the anterior abdominal wall, which may increase in size with Valsalva. Ventral hernias may be asymptomatic or cause discomfort, and generally enlarge over time. Physical examination reveals a bulge on the anterior abdomen that may reduce spontaneously, with recumbency, or with manual pressure. A hernia that cannot be reduced is described as incarcerated and may be accompanied by nausea, vomiting, and significant pain. Should the blood supply to the incarcerated bowel be compromised, the hernia is described as strangulated, and the localized ischemia may lead to infarction and perforation.

Primary ventral hernias (nonincisional) also are termed "true" ventral hernias. These are more properly named according to their anatomic location. Epigastric hernias are located in the midline between the xiphoid process and the umbilicus. They are generally small and usually contain omentum or a portion of the falciform ligament.

Umbilical hernias develop at the umbilical ring, and may be present at birth or develop gradually during the life of the individual. Adults with small, asymptomatic umbilical hernias may be followed clinically. Surgical treatment is offered if a hernia is observed to enlarge, is associated with symptoms, or if incarceration occurs.

Spigelian hernias can occur anywhere along the length of the Spigelian line, an aponeurotic band at the lateral border of the rectus abdominus. However, the most frequent location of these rare hernias is at or slightly above the level of the arcuate line. These are not always clinically evident as a bulge, and may come to medical attention because of pain or incarceration.

Incisional hernias result from a healing failure of a prior abdominal wall surgical closure. Although estimates of incidence vary, careful investigation shows that they occur in at least 10–15 percent of all laparotomy incisions. Incisional hernias may be asymptomatic or present with pain, incarceration or strangulation. Risk factors for the development of a ventral incisional hernia include postoperative wound infection, malnutrition, obesity, and immunosuppression.

Several techniques for the repair of ventral hernias have been described, including primary repair, open repair with mesh, and laparoscopic repair with mesh. Primary repair, even for small hernias (abdominal wall defects less than 3 cm) is associated with a high subsequent recurrence rate. Risk factors for recurrence include primary suture repair, postoperative wound infection, prostatism, and surgery for abdominal aortic aneurysm.

Open mesh repair of incisional hernias generally requires overlapping the prosthesis onto the anterior or posterior surfaces of intact abdominal wall fascia for a distance of at least 3–4 cm from defect edge. When properly performed, the peritoneum and hernia sac are dissected away from all fascial defects. A large sheet of polypropylene or polyester (Mersilene) mesh, which is isolated from peritoneal contents, is then secured to the fascia using interrupted nonabsorbable sutures. Polypropylene is an inert substance that induces eventual tissue ingrowth within the interstices of the mesh. This effect is desired in a preperitoneal location, but when exposed to underlying bowel the dense adhesions to mesh can lead to chronic abdominal pain, bowel obstruction, or fistulization. Polytetrafluoroethylene (PTFE) does not become incorporated into surrounding tissues in this way, and does not induce dense adhesions to peritoneal structures such as intestine. It is therefore commonly used in intraperitoneal applications. Other available prosthetic mesh materials include polypropylene/PTFE composites, polyesters with and without adhesion barriers, and most recently engineered tissue replacements from decellularized collagen or cadaveric dermis.

Minimally invasive repair of incisional hernias now are performed at least as often as open repairs. Using this method, the entire undersurface of the abdominal wall can be examined, often revealing multiple defects. In this technique laparoscopic ports are placed laterally for midline defects and contralaterally for lateral defects. Adhesions to the anterior abdominal wall are divided taking great care not to injure the intestines. An appropriate-sized piece of prosthetic mesh (generally PTFE) shaped to allow sufficient overlap (3–4 cm) onto healthy abdominal wall is fixed in place circumferentially with transfascial sutures and spiral tacks according to surgeon preference. With this technique, the 2-year recurrence rate is only 3.4 percent.

Omentum

Anatomy

The greater omentum and lesser omentum are fibrofatty aprons that provide support, coverage and protection of peritoneal contents. In the adult, the greater omentum lies in between the anterior abdominal wall and the hollow viscera and usually extends into the pelvis. The blood supply to the greater omentum is derived from the right and left gastroepiploic arteries.

The lesser omentum also is known as the hepatoduodenal and hepatogastric ligaments. The common bile duct, portal vein, and hepatic artery are located in the inferolateral margin of the lesser omentum, which also forms the anterior margin of the foramen of Winslow.

Physiology

The omentum has been called the "abdominal policeman" because of its tendency to wall off areas of infection and limit the spread of intraperitoneal contamination. Omentum contains a high concentration of tissue factor, which facilitates activation of coagulation at sites of inflammation, ischemia, infection or trauma within the peritoneal cavity. The consequent local production of fibrin contributes to the ability of the omentum to adhere to areas of injury or inflammation.

Omental Infarction

Interruption of the blood supply to the omentum is a rare cause of an acute abdomen that may be secondary to torsion of the omentum, thrombosis or vasculitis of the omental vessels, or omental venous outflow obstruction. Depending on the location of the infarcted omental tissue, this disease process may mimic appendicitis, cholecystitis, diverticulitis, perforated peptic ulcers, or ruptured ovarian cysts. The diagnosis is rarely made before abdominal imaging studies are obtained. Either abdominal CT or ultrasonography will show a localized, inflammatory mass of fat density. Treatment of omental infarction depends on the certainty with which the diagnosis is made. In patients who are not toxic and abdominal imaging is convincing, supportive care is sufficient. However, many cases will be indistinguishable from suppurative appendicitis, cholecystitis or diverticulitis. In these instances, laparoscopy has provided a great advance, providing access to an accurate diagnosis and treatment. Resection of the infarcted tissue results in rapid resolution of symptoms.

Omental Cysts

Cystic lesions of the omentum likely result from lymphatic degeneration. Omental cysts may present as an asymptomatic abdominal mass or may cause abdominal pain or distension. Physical examination reveals a freely mobile intraabdominal mass. Abdominal CT or ultrasonography reveals a well-circumscribed cystic mass lesion arising from the greater omentum. Treatment involves resection of all symptomatic omental cysts.

Malignant Omental Lesions

Primary tumors of the omentum are uncommon. Benign tumors of the omentum include lipomas, myxomas, and desmoid tumors. Primary malignant tumors of the omentum include liposarcomas, leiomyosarcomas, rhabdomyosarcomas, fibrosarcomas, and mesotheliomas. Metastatic tumors involving the omentum are quite common. Metastatic ovarian tumors have a high preponderance of omental involvement. Malignant tumors of the stomach, small intestine, colon, pancreas, biliary tract, uterus, and kidney also may metastasize to the omentum.

Mesentery

The small and large intestinal mesenteries serve as the major pathway for arterial, venous, lymphatic, and neural structures coursing to and from the bowel. Their positions in the abdomen and on the retroperitoneum are determined by the previously described process of intestinal herniation, rotation, and return to the abdominal cavity during fetal development.

Sclerosing Mesenteritis

Sclerosing mesenteritis, also referred to as mesenteric panniculitis or mesenteric lipodystrophy, is a rare chronic inflammatory and fibrotic process that involves a portion of the intestinal mesentery. Sclerosing mesenteritis is most commonly diagnosed in individuals over 50 years of age with no gender or race predominance. The etiology of this process is unknown. Patients typically present with abdominal pain, a nonpainful mass or intestinal obstruction.

Abdominal CT will verify the presence of a mass lesion emanating from the mesentery. CT cannot distinguish sclerosing mesenteritis from a primary or secondary mesenteric tumor. Surgical intervention is usually necessary, if only to establish a diagnosis and rule out malignancy. The extent of the disease process will dictate the aggressiveness of the intervention, which may range from simple biopsy to mesenteric and bowel resection.

Mesenteric Cysts

Cysts of the mesentery are rare, benign lesions that may be asymptomatic or cause symptoms of a mass lesion. When symptomatic, mesenteric cysts usually cause acute or chronic, intermittent abdominal pain. Mesenteric cysts may also be the cause of nonspecific symptoms such as anorexia, nausea, vomiting, fatigue, and weight loss.

Physical examination may reveal a mass lesion which is mobile only to the right and left (Tillaux sign), in contrast to omental cysts which should be freely mobile in all directions. Abdominal CT, ultrasonography, and magnetic resonance imaging all have been used to evaluate patients with mesenteric cysts.

If feasible, simple mesenteric cysts should be surgically excised. Cyst unroofing or marsupialization is not recommended as there is a high propensity to recur after drainage alone. Rarely, adherent mesentery must be sacrificed to achieve complete excision, in which case segmental bowel resection is performed.

Mesenteric Tumors

Primary tumors of the mesentery are rare. Benign tumors of the mesentery include lipoma, cystic lymphangioma, and desmoid tumors. Malignant tumors of the mesentery include liposarcomas, leiomyosarcomas, malignant fibrous histiocytomas, lipoblastomas and lymphangiosarcomas. Treatment of mesenteric malignancies involves wide resection of the mass. Because of the proximity to blood supply to the intestine, such resections may be technically impractical or involve loss of substantial lengths of bowel.

RETROPERITONEUM

Surgical Anatomy

The retroperitoneum is defined as the space between the posterior envelopment of the peritoneum and the posterior body wall. Although technically bounded anteriorly by the posterior reflection of the peritoneum, the anterior border of the retroperitoneum is quite convoluted, extending into the spaces in between the mesenteries of the small and large intestine. Because of the rigidity of the superior, posterior, and inferior boundaries, and the compliance of the anterior margin, retroperitoneal tumors tend to expand anteriorly toward the peritoneal cavity.

Retroperitoneal Infections

The source of retroperitoneal infections is usually an organ contained within or abutting the retroperitoneum. Retrocecal appendicitis, perforated duodenal ulcers, pancreatitis, or diverticulitis may all lead to retroperitoneal infection with or without abscess formation. The substantial space and rather indiscreet boundaries of the retroperitoneum allow some retroperitoneal abscesses to become quite large prior to diagnosis.

Patients with a retroperitoneal abscess usually present with pain, fever, and malaise. The site of the patient's pain may be variable, including the back, pelvis, or thighs. Clinical findings can include tachypnea and tachycardia. A palpable flank or abdominal mass may be present. Laboratory evaluation usually reveals a leukocytosis. The diagnostic imaging modality of choice is abdominal CT, which may demonstrate stranding of the retroperitoneal soft tissues and/or a unilocular or multilocular collection.

Management of retroperitoneal infections includes identification and treatment of underlying conditions, intravenous antibiotics and drainage of all well-defined collections. Whereas unilocular abscesses are usually drained percutaneously under CT guidance, multilocular collections may require operative intervention for adequate drainage. Because of the vastness of the retroperitoneal space, patients with retroperitoneal abscesses do not usually present until the abscess is advanced. Consequently, the mortality rate of retroperitoneal abscess, even when drained, has been reported to be as high as 25 percent.

Retroperitoneal Fibrosis

Retroperitoneal fibrosis is a class of disorders characterized by hyperproliferation of fibrous tissue in the retroperitoneum. Idiopathic retroperitoneal fibrosis (Ormond disease) is a rare disorder primarily affecting individuals in the fourth to sixth decades of life. An allergic or autoimmune mechanism has been postulated for this condition. The fibrotic process begins in the retroperitoneum below the level of the renal arteries and gradually progressed to encase the ureters, inferior vena cava, aorta, mesenteric vessels, and sympathetic nerves. Bilateral involvement is noted in two-thirds of cases.

Retroperitoneal fibrosis may also occur secondary to inflammation or as an allergic reaction to a medication. The associated conditions include abdominal aortic aneurysms, chronic pancreatitis, histoplasmosis, tuberculosis, and actinomycosis. It also has been associated with malignancies (prostate, non–Hodgkin lymphoma, sarcoma, carcinoid tumors, and gastric cancer) and autoimmune disorders (ankylosing spondylitis, systemic lupus erythematosus, Wegener granulomatosis, and polyarteritis nodosa). Although several medications have been linked to retroperitoneal fibrosis (β blockers, hydralazine, α-methyldopa, entacapone), the strongest causal relationship appears to be with Methysergide use. Fibrosis regresses on discontinuation of these medications.

Presenting symptoms depend on the structures affected by the fibrotic process. Initially, patients complain of dull, poorly localized abdominal pain. Sudden or severe abdominal pain may signify acute mesenteric ischemia. Other symptoms and signs may include: unilateral leg swelling, intermittent claudication, oliguria, hematuria, or dysuria.

Findings on physical examination may include hypertension, a palpable abdominal or flank mass, lower extremity edema, and/or diminished lower extremity pulses. Laboratory findings include an elevated erythrocyte sedimentation rate.

Many imaging modalities have been used to aid in the diagnosis of retroperitoneal fibrosis. A lower extremity ultrasound may show deep venous thrombosis, whereas abdominal ultrasonography may identify a mass lesion or hydronephrosis. Intravenous pyelography (IVP) may demonstrate ureteral compression, ureteral deviation toward the midline, and hydronephrosis. The imaging procedure of choice is abdominopelvic CT scan, which demonstrates the size and extent of the fibrotic process. For patients with renal insufficiency, magnetic resonance imaging (MRI) is the procedure of choice.

When a fibrotic mass is identified, biopsy should be performed. Once malignant, drug-induced, and infectious etiologies have been ruled out, treatment of the fibrotic process is instituted. Corticosteroids, with or without surgery, are the mainstay of therapy. Surgical debulking, ureterolysis, or ureteral stenting is required in patients with significant hydronephrosis. Patients with iliocaval thrombosis will require at least 6 months of oral anticoagulation. Cyclosporin, tamoxifen, or azathioprine have been used to treat patients who are recalcitrant to the above regimen. The reported 5-year survival rates in idiopathic retroperitoneal fibrosis are in the range of 90–100 percent.

Suggested Readings

Skandalakis LJ, Colborn GL: Surgical anatomy of the abdominal wall. In: Bendavid R (ed) Prostheses and abdominal wall hernias. Austin, RG Landes Company, 1994.

Zainea GG, Jordan F: Rectus sheath hematomas: their pathogenesis, diagnosis, and management. Am Surg 54:630, 1988.

Bendavid R, Abrahamson J, Arregui ME, Flament JB, Phillips EH (eds): Abdominal Wall Hernias: Principles and Management, 1st ed., New York, Springer-Verlag, 2001.

Anthony T, Bergen PC, et al: Factors affecting recurrence following incisional herniorrhaphy. World J Surg 24:95, 2000.

Luijendijk R, Hop W, et al: A comparison of suture repair with mesh repair for incisional hernia. N Engl J Med 343:392, 2000.

Heniford BT, Park, A, et al: Laparoscopic ventral and incisional hernia repair in 407 patients. J Am Coll Surg 190:645, 2000.

Vanek VW, Phillips AK: Retroperitoneal, mesenteric, and omental cysts. Arch Surg 119:838, 1984.

Pryor JP, Piotrowski E, et al: Early diagnosis of retroperitoneal necrotizing fasciitis. Crit Care Med 29:1071, 2001.

Emory T, Monihan J, et al: Sclerosing mesenteritis, mesenteric panniculitis, and mesenteric lipodystrophy. Am J Surg Path 21:392, 1997.

Kardar AH, Kattan S, et al: Steroid therapy for idiopathic retroperitoneal fibrosis: dose and duration. J Urol 168:550, 2002.

35 | Soft Tissue Sarcomas

Janice N. Cormier and Raphael E. Pollock

INCIDENCE

Sarcomas are a heterogeneous group of tumors that arise predominantly from the embryonic mesoderm. In 2004, approximately 8400 new cases of soft tissue sarcoma were diagnosed in the United States representing less than 1 percent of cancers in adults. Soft tissue sarcomas, the largest of several distinct groups of sarcomas, is the focus of this chapter. Other groups include bone sarcomas (osteosarcomas and chondrosarcomas), Ewing sarcomas, and peripheral primitive neuroectodermal tumors.

Soft tissue sarcomas can occur throughout the body, most commonly in the extremity (59 percent), trunk (19 percent), retroperitoneum (13 percent), and head and neck (9 percent). The most common histologic types of soft tissue sarcoma in adults are malignant fibrous histiocytoma (28 percent), leiomyosarcoma (12 percent), liposarcoma (15 percent), synovial sarcoma (10 percent), and malignant peripheral nerve sheath tumors (6 percent).

EPIDEMIOLOGY

Except for malignant peripheral nerve sheath tumors in patients with neurofibromatosis, sarcomas do not seem to result from the progression or dedifferentiation of benign soft tissue tumors. Despite the variety of histologic subtypes, sarcomas have many common clinical and pathologic features. Overall the clinical behavior of most soft tissue sarcomas is similar and is determined by anatomic location (depth), grade, and size. The dominant pattern of metastasis is hematogenous with metastasis to the lungs. Lymph node metastases are rare.

Radiation Exposure

External radiation therapy is a well-established risk factor for soft tissue sarcoma. An 8-fold to 50-fold increase in the incidence of sarcomas has been reported among patients treated for cancer of the breast, cervix, ovary, testes, and lymphatic system.

Occupational Chemicals

Exposure to some herbicides such as phenoxyacetic acids and wood preservatives containing chlorophenols has been linked to an increased risk of soft tissue sarcoma. Several chemical carcinogens, including thorium oxide (Thorotrast), vinyl chloride, and arsenic, have been associated with hepatic angiosarcomas.

GENETICS

New developments in the field of molecular biology have led to better understanding of the basic cellular processes governed by oncogenes and tumor suppressor genes. Several oncogenes have been identified in association with soft tissue sarcomas, including MDM2, N-myc, c-erbB2, and members of the ras family. Amplification of these genes has been shown to correlate with adverse outcome in several soft tissue sarcomas.

Cytogenetic analysis of soft tissue tumors has identified distinct chromosomal translocations that seem to encode for oncogenes associated with certain histologic subtypes. The best characterized gene rearrangements are found in Ewing sarcoma (EWS—FLI-1 fusion), clear-cell sarcoma (EWS—ATF1 fusion), myxoid liposarcoma (TLS—CHOP fusion), alveolar rhabdomyosarcoma (PAX3—FHKR fusion), desmoplastic small round-cell tumor (EWS—WT1 fusion), and synovial sarcoma (SSX—SYT fusion).

Inactivation of tumor suppressor genes (also known as antioncogenes) can occur through hereditary or sporadic mechanisms. The two genes that are most relevant to soft tissue tumors are the retinoblastoma (Rb) tumor suppressor gene and the p53 tumor suppressor gene. Mutations or deletions in Rb can lead to development of retinoblastoma or sarcomas of soft tissue and bone. Mutations in the p53 tumor suppressor gene are the most common mutations in human solid tumors and have been reported in 30–60 percent of soft tissue sarcomas. Patients with germline mutations in the tumor suppressor gene p53 (the Li-Fraumeni syndrome) have a high incidence of sarcomas.

Neurofibromatosis type 1, also known as von Recklinghausen disease, occurs in approximately one of every 3000 persons, and is because of various mutations in the NF-1 tumor suppressor gene located on chromosome 17. Patients with neurofibromatosis type 1 have an estimated 3–15 percent additional lifetime risk of malignant disease that includes neurofibrosarcoma. Fifty percent of patients with neurofibrosarcomas have a mutation in NF-1.

INITIAL ASSESSMENT

Clinical Presentation

Soft tissue sarcoma most commonly presents as an asymptomatic mass. The size at presentation is usually associated with the location of the tumor. Smaller tumors are generally located in the distal extremities, whereas tumors in the proximal extremities and retroperitoneum can grow quite large before becoming apparent. Often an extremity mass is discovered after a traumatic event that draws attention to a preexisting lesion. Retroperitoneal soft tissue sarcoma almost always presents as a large asymptomatic mass.

The differential diagnosis of a soft tissue mass includes benign lesions including lipomas, lymphangiomas, leiomyomas, and neuromas. In addition to sarcomas, other malignant lesions such as primary or metastatic carcinomas, melanomas, or lymphomas must be considered. Small lesions that have not changed for several years by clinical history may be closely observed. All other tumors should be considered for biopsy to establish a definitive diagnosis.

Diagnostic Imaging

Pretreatment radiologic imaging serves several purposes; it defines the local extent of a tumor, can be used to stage malignant disease, assists in percutaneous biopsy procedures, and aids in the diagnosis of soft tissue tumors (benign versus malignant or low grade versus high grade). Imaging studies also are crucial in monitoring tumor changes after treatment, especially preoperative chemotherapy or radiation therapy, and in detecting recurrences after surgical resection.

Chest radiography should be performed for patients with primary sarcomas to assess for lung metastases. For patients with high-grade lesions or tumors more than 5 cm (T2), computed tomography of the chest should be considered. Both ultrasonography and computed tomography can assist in guiding fine-needle aspiration or core biopsy for initial diagnosis or at recurrence.

Computed tomography (CT) is the preferred technique for evaluating retroperitoneal sarcomas, whereas magnetic resonance imaging (MRI) is often favored for soft tissue sarcomas of the extremities. MRI accurately delineates muscle groups and distinguishes among bone, vascular structures, and tumor. Sagittal and coronal views allow evaluation of anatomic compartments in three dimensions. Soft tissue sarcomas of the extremities usually present on MRI as heterogeneous masses. MRI is also valuable for assessing tumor recurrence after surgery. A baseline image is usually obtained 3 months after surgery.

Biopsy Techniques

Fine-Needle Aspiration

Fine-needle aspiration is an acceptable method of diagnosing most soft tissue sarcomas, particularly when the results correlate closely with clinical and imaging findings. However, fine-needle aspiration biopsy is indicated for primary diagnosis of soft tissue sarcomas only at centers where cytopathologists have experience with these types of tumors. Fine-needle aspiration biopsy is also the procedure of choice to confirm or rule out the presence of a metastatic focus or local recurrence. If tumor grading is essential for treatment planning, fine-needle aspiration biopsy is not the technique of choice.

Superficial lesions are often subjected to fine-needle aspiration biopsies in the clinic setting. Deeper tumors may require an interventional radiologist to perform the technique under sonographic or CT guidance. Diagnostic accuracy rates for fine-needle aspiration biopsy of primary tumors range from 60–96 percent.

Core-Needle Biopsy

Core-needle biopsy is a safe, accurate, and economical diagnostic procedure for diagnosing sarcomas. The tissue sample obtained from a core-needle biopsy is usually sufficient for several diagnostic tests such as electron microscopy, cytogenetic analysis, and flow cytometry. CT guidance can enhance the positive yield rate of a core-needle biopsy by more accurately pinpointing the location of the tumor. Precise localization in the tumor mass is particularly important to avoid sampling nondiagnostic necrotic or cystic areas of the tumor. CT guidance also permits access to tumors in otherwise inaccessible anatomic locations or near vital structures.

Incisional Biopsy

When adequate tissue for diagnosis cannot be obtained by fine-needle aspiration biopsy or core biopsy, an incisional biopsy is indicated for deep tumors or for superficial soft tissue tumors larger than 3 cm. The biopsy incision should be oriented longitudinally along the extremity to allow a subsequent wide local excision that encompasses the biopsy site, scar, and tumor en bloc. Another mandate of surgical technique is that adequate hemostasis must be achieved at the time of biopsy to prevent dissemination of tumor cells into adjacent tissue planes by hematoma.

Pathologic Classification

Some experts have suggested that pathologic classification of soft tissue sarcomas has more prognostic significance than does tumor grade when other pretreatment variables are taken into account. Tumors with limited metastatic potential include desmoids, atypical lipomatous tumors (also called well-differentiated liposarcoma), dermatofibrosarcoma protuberans, and hemangiopericytomas. Tumors with an intermediate risk of metastatic spread usually have a large myxoid component and include myxoid liposarcoma, myxoid malignant fibrous histiocytoma, and extraskeletal chondrosarcoma. Among the highly aggressive tumors that have substantial metastatic potential are angiosarcomas, clear-cell sarcomas, pleomorphic and dedifferentiated liposarcomas, leiomyosarcomas, rhabdomyosarcomas, and synovial sarcomas.

Expert sarcoma pathologists disagree about the specific histologic diagnoses and the criteria for defining tumor grade in 25–40 percent of individual cases. The high rate of discordance emphasizes the need for more objective molecular and biochemical markers to improve conventional histologic assessment.

Staging and Prognostic Factors

The current version of the American Joint Committee on Cancer staging criteria for soft tissue sarcomas relies on histologic grade, tumor size and depth, and the presence of distant or nodal metastases (Table 35-1).

Histologic grade remains the most important prognostic factor for patients with sarcomas. The features that define grade are cellularity, differentiation, pleomorphism, necrosis, and the number of mitoses. In the 2002 American Joint Committee on Cancer staging system, four tumor grades are designated: well differentiated (G1), moderately differentiated (G2), poorly differentiated (G3), and undifferentiated (G4). In this four-tiered system, grades 1 and 2 are considered "low grade" and grades 3 and 4 are considered "high grade."

Tumor size has long been recognized to be an important prognostic variable in soft tissue sarcomas. Sarcomas have classically been stratified into two groups on the basis of size; T1 lesions are 5 cm or smaller and T2 lesions are larger than 5 cm.

The prognostic significance of anatomic tumor location with respect to its association with the investing fascia of the extremity or trunk was incorporated into the American Joint Committee on Cancer staging system in 1998. Soft tissue sarcomas above the superficial investing fascia of the extremity or trunk are designated "a" lesions in the T score, whereas tumors invading or deep to the fascia and all retroperitoneal, mediastinal, and visceral tumors are designated "b" lesions.

Nodal Metastasis

Lymph node metastasis of soft tissue sarcomas is rare; less than 5 percent manifest nodal spread. A few histologic subtypes, including rhabdomyosarcoma, epithelioid sarcoma, and malignant fibrous histiocytoma, have a higher incidence of nodal involvement. Nodal disease is designated as stage IV disease.

Distant Metastasis

Distant metastases occur most often in the lungs. Selected patients with pulmonary metastases may survive for long periods after surgical resection and chemotherapy.

TABLE 35-1 American Joint Committee on Cancer

Primary tumor (T)					

T1	Tumor $\leq$ 5 cm
	   T1a Superficial tumor
	   T1b Deep tumor				

T2	Tumor > 5 cm
	   T2a Superficial tumor
	   T2b Deep tumor				

Regional lymph nodes (N)					
N0	No regional lymph node metastasis				
N1	Regional lymph node metastasis				

Distance metastasis (M)					
M0	No distant metastasis				
M1	Distant metastasis				

Histologic grade (G)					
G1	Well differentiated				
G2	Moderately differentiated				
G3	Poorly differentiated				
G4	Poorly differentiated or undifferentiated				

Stage grouping					
Stage I	T1a, 1b, 2a, 2b	N0	M0	G1–2	G1
Stage II	T1a, 1b, 2a	N0	M0	G3–4	G2–3
Stage III	T2b	N0	M0	G3–4	G2–3
Stage IV	Any T	N1	M0	Any G	Any G
	Any T	N0	M1	Any G	Any G

Source: Reproduced with permission from AJCC.

TREATMENT

For soft tissue sarcomas of the extremities, a multidisciplinary approach to management, including margin-negative resection plus radiotherapy to the tumor bed, has resulted in local control rates up to and exceeding 90 percent. However, patients with abdominal sarcomas continue to have high rates of recurrence and poor overall survival. The overall 5-year survival rate for all stages of soft tissue sarcomas is 50–60 percent. Most patients die of metastatic disease, which becomes evident within 2–3 years of initial diagnosis in 80 percent of cases.

Surgery

Small (< 5 cm) primary tumors with no evidence of distant metastatic disease are managed by local therapy consisting of surgery, alone or in combination with radiation therapy, when wide pathologic margins are limited because of anatomic constraints. The type of surgical resection is determined by several factors, including tumor location, tumor size, depth of invasion, involvement of nearby structures, need for skin grafting or autogenous tissue reconstruction, and the patient's performance status. In 1985, the National Institutes of Health (NIH) developed a consensus statement recommending limb-sparing surgery for most patients with high-grade extremity sarcomas. However, for patients whose tumor cannot be grossly resected with a limb-sparing procedure and preservation of function (<5 percent), amputation remains the treatment of choice.

Wide Local Excision

Wide local excision is the primary treatment strategy for extremity sarcomas. The goal of local therapy for extremity sarcomas is to resect the tumor with a 2-cm margin of surrounding normal soft tissue. In some anatomic areas, negative margins cannot be attained because of the tumor's proximity to vital structures. The biopsy site or tract (if applicable) should also be included en bloc with the resected specimen. With modern surgical and radiotherapy techniques, rates of limb preservation and local control have improved. A currently reported local failure rate of 10 percent after appropriate treatment is typical for soft tissue sarcomas of the extremity.

Amputation is the treatment of choice for patients with the rare 5 percent of tumors that cannot be grossly resected with a limb-sparing procedure and preservation of function.

Isolated Regional Perfusion

Isolated regional perfusion is an investigational approach for treating extremity sarcomas. It has been attempted mainly as a limb-sparing alternative for patients with locally advanced soft tissue sarcomas or as a palliative treatment to achieve local control for patients with distant metastatic disease.

Radiation Therapy

The evidence for adjunctive radiation therapy for patients eligible for conservative surgical resection comes from two randomized trials. In a trial by the National Cancer Institute, 91 patients with high-grade extremity tumors were treated with limb-sparing surgery followed by chemotherapy alone or radiation therapy plus adjuvant chemotherapy. A second group of 50 patients with low-grade tumors were treated with resection alone or resection with radiation therapy. The 10-year rate of local control for all patients receiving radiation therapy was 98 percent, compared with 70 percent for those not receiving radiation therapy. Similarly, in a randomized trial from the Memorial Sloan-Kettering Cancer Center, 164 patients underwent observation or brachytherapy after conservative surgery. The 5-year local control rate for patients with high-grade tumors was 66 percent in the observation group and 89 percent in the brachytherapy group. No significant difference was observed between treatment groups for patients with low-grade tumors.

Until recently, the standard treatment guidelines were to administer radiotherapy as an adjunct to surgery for all patients with intermediate or highly aggressive tumors of any size. However, in general, small tumors (≤5 cm) have not been associated with local recurrence, and radiation therapy may not be necessary.

The optimal mode (external beam or brachytherapy) and timing (preoperative, intraoperative, or postoperative) have yet to be defined. External-beam radiation therapy can be delivered by photons or particle beams (electrons, protons, pions, or neutrons). The optimal margin is not well defined; a radiation margin of 5 to 7 cm is standard, although some centers advocate wider margins for tumors larger than 15 cm. At most institutions the typical preoperative dose is 50 Gy, given in 25 fractions.

Postoperative radiation therapy planning is based on tumor grade, assessment of surgical margins, and institutional preferences. The entire surgical scar and drain sites should be included in the field so that a near-full dose is given to the superficial skin. Metallic clips placed in the tumor bed during surgery can help define the limits of the resection and aid in radiation therapy planning. Doses of 60–70 Gy are usually necessary for postoperative treatment.

No consensus exists on the optimal sequence of radiation therapy and surgery. The available data come largely from single-institution, nonrandomized studies. Proponents of preoperative radiation therapy cite several advantages including multidisciplinary planning with radiation oncologists, medical oncologists, and surgeons is facilitated early in the course of therapy. Additionally, lower doses of preoperative radiation can be delivered to an undisturbed tissue bed that may have improved tissue oxygenation and result in smaller radiation fields with improved functional outcome.

Critics of preoperative radiation therapy cite as deterrents the difficulty of pathologic assessment of margins and the increased rate of wound complications. However, plastic surgery techniques with advanced tissue transfer procedures are being used more often in these high-risk wounds, with better outcomes.

The only randomized comparison of preoperative and postoperative radiation therapy conducted to date was performed by the National Cancer Institute of Canada Clinical Trial Canadian Sarcoma Group. This trial was designed to compare complications and the functional outcome of patients treated with preoperative and postoperative external-beam radiation therapy. At a median follow-up of 3.3 years, wound complications had occurred in 35 percent of patients given preoperative radiotherapy and in 17 percent of patients given postoperative radiation therapy. Both groups had achieved similarly high levels of local control and progression-free survival at 3 years.

Brachytherapy involves the placement of multiple catheters in the tumor resection bed. The primary benefit of brachytherapy is the shorter overall treatment time of 4–6 days, compared with preoperative or postoperative radiation therapy regimens, which generally take 4–6 weeks. Brachytherapy can also be used for recurrent disease previously treated with external-beam radiation. Guidelines established at the Memorial Sloan-Kettering Cancer Center recommend spacing the afterloading catheters in 1-cm increments and leaving a 2-cm margin around the surgical bed. After adequate wound healing is established, usually after the fifth postoperative day, the catheters are loaded with seeds containing iridium-192 that deliver 42–45 Gy of radiation to the tumor bed over 4–6 days. The primary disadvantage of brachytherapy is that it requires an extended inpatient stay and bedrest.

Systemic Therapy

Systemic therapy generally is limited to patients with metastatic disease, those with small-cell sarcomas of any size, or those with large (≥5 cm) high-grade tumors or intermediate-grade tumors larger than 10 cm. Despite improvements in local control rates, metastasis and death remain a significant problem for patients with high-risk soft tissue sarcomas. Patients considered at high risk of death from sarcoma include those presenting with metastatic disease and those presenting with localized sarcomas at nonextremity sites or sarcomas with intermediate- or high-grade histology larger than 5 cm (T2).

Sarcomas encompass a diverse group of cancers that vary greatly in natural history and response to treatment. As a group, sarcomas include histologic subtypes that are very responsive to cytotoxic chemotherapy and subtypes that are universally resistant to current agents. Only three drugs, doxorubicin, dacarbazine, and ifosfamide, have consistently demonstrated response rates of 20 percent or more for advanced soft tissue sarcomas. Doxorubicin and ifosfamide are the two most active agents, with consistently reported response rates of 20 percent or greater.

Integrating Multimodality Therapy

The primary objective of multimodality treatment is cure; when this endpoint is not possible, the goal is palliation of symptoms. Whenever possible, patients with a deep soft tissue mass should be referred, even before a biopsy is performed, to a tertiary treatment center that offers care by a team of specialists. Such multidisciplinary teams typically include oncologists from several disciplines (medicine, pediatrics [if applicable], surgery, and radiation therapy), and a pathologist, radiologist, and ancillary staff.

Adjuvant Chemotherapy

The use of adjuvant chemotherapy for soft tissue sarcomas remains controversial. The average 5-year disease-free survival rate for patients initially presenting with localized disease is only about 50 percent. More than a dozen individual randomized trials of adjuvant chemotherapy have failed to demonstrate improvement in disease-free patients and overall survival in patients with soft tissue sarcomas.

The Sarcoma Meta-Analysis Collaboration analyzed 1568 patients from 14 trials of doxorubicin-based adjuvant chemotherapy to evaluate the effect of adjuvant chemotherapy on localized, resectable soft tissue sarcomas. At a median follow-up of 9.4 years, doxorubicin-based chemotherapy significantly improved the time to local and distant recurrence and recurrence-free survival rates. However, the absolute benefit in overall survival for the sample was only 4 percent, which was not significant.

Subsequent to this meta-analysis, additional randomized controlled trials of more modern (drugs, dose, and schedule) anthracycline/ifosfamide combinations for relatively small numbers of patients have yielded conflicting results. Because the evidence addressing treatment of stage III disease is inconclusive, considerable variation still exists in treatment standards.

Neoadjuvant (Preoperative) Chemotherapy

The rationale for using neoadjuvant and preoperative chemotherapy for soft tissue sarcomas is the belief that only 30–50 percent of patients will respond to standard (postoperative) chemotherapy. Neoadjuvant chemotherapy enables oncologists to identify patients whose disease responds to chemotherapy by assessing that response while the primary tumor is in situ. Patients whose tumors do not respond to short courses of preoperative chemotherapy are thus spared the toxic effects of prolonged postoperative or adjuvant chemotherapy.

Treatment approaches that combine systemic chemotherapy with radiosensitizers and concurrent external-beam radiation may improve disease-free survival by treating microscopic disease and enhancing the treatment of macroscopic disease. Concurrent chemoradiotherapy with doxorubicin-based regimens reportedly produces favorable local control rates for patients with sarcoma. Since those findings were published, several groups have attempted to evaluate the optimal route of administration, alternative chemotherapeutic agents, and the toxicity of combined therapies.

Theoretical advantages of concurrent treatment notwithstanding, use of concurrent local and systemic therapy decreases the total treatment time for patients with high-risk sarcoma. This decrease represents a substantial advantage over current sequential combined-method treatment approaches, for which the total duration of treatment for radiation, chemotherapy, surgery, and rehabilitation frequently exceeds 6–9 months.

SPECIAL SITUATIONS

Retroperitoneal Sarcomas

Fifteen percent of adult soft tissue sarcomas occur in the retroperitoneum. Most retroperitoneal tumors are malignant, and about one third are soft tissue sarcomas. The most common sarcomas occurring in the retroperitoneum are liposarcomas, malignant fibrous histiocytomas, and leiomyosarcomas. Most retroperitoneal sarcomas are liposarcomas or leiomyosarcomas. In contrast to extremity sarcomas, local recurrence and intraabdominal spread are frequent patterns of relapse for retroperitoneal tumors.

Retroperitoneal sarcomas generally present as large masses; nearly 50 percent are larger than 20 cm at the time of diagnosis. They typically do not produce symptoms until they grow large enough to compress or invade contiguous structures.

The overall prognosis for patients with retroperitoneal tumors is worse than that for patients with extremity sarcomas. Tumor stage at presentation, high histologic grade, unresectability, and grossly positive resection margins are strongly associated with increased rates of death from retroperitoneal sarcoma. Survival rates at 5 years are typically reported to be 40–50 percent. The best chance for long-term survival for patients with retroperitoneal sarcoma is achieved with a margin-negative resection.

Radiologic assessment should include CT of the abdomen and pelvis to define the extent of the tumor and its relationship to surrounding structures, particularly vascular structures. Imaging should also encompass the liver for the presence of metastases, the abdomen for discontiguous disease, and the kidneys bilaterally for function. Thoracic CT is indicated to detect lung metastases.

Complete surgical resection is the most effective treatment for primary or recurrent retroperitoneal sarcomas. However, these tumors often involve vital structures, precluding surgical resection. Even if surgical resection can be performed, the margins are often compromised because of anatomic constraints. Chemotherapy has not been shown to be effective against retroperitoneal sarcomas. Protocols are ongoing at several centers to determine whether preoperative chemotherapy and radiation therapy have roles in treating these tumors.

Gastrointestinal Sarcomas

Patients with gastrointestinal sarcomas most often present with nonspecific gastrointestinal symptoms that are determined by the site of the primary tumor. Establishing the diagnosis of a gastrointestinal sarcoma preoperatively is often difficult. Radiologic assessment, including CT of the abdomen or pelvis, is sometimes useful to determine the anatomic location, size, and extent of disease. For tumors involving the stomach, upper endoscopy with endoscopic ultrasonography and biopsy are important diagnostic tests used to distinguish adenocarcinoma from gastrointestinal stromal tumors.

For localized disease, the general recommendation is to perform a margin-negative resection with a 2–4-cm margin of normal tissue. However, some cases may be technically challenging because of the tumor's anatomic location or size. For example, for gastric tumors located near the gastroesophageal junction, achieving adequate surgical margins may not be possible without a total or proximal subtotal gastrectomy. Similarly, large tumors arising from the stomach with invasion of adjacent organs should be resected together with the adjacent involved viscera en bloc.

Segmental bowel resection is the standard treatment for sarcomas of the small or large intestine. For sarcomas originating in the rectum, the technique used for tumor resection is based on the anatomic location and size of the tumor. For small, low rectal lesions, it may be possible to achieve clear margins with a transanal excision. Large or locally invasive lesions may require more extensive operations for complete tumor extirpation.

Gastrointestinal Stromal Tumors

Gastrointestinal stromal tumors (GISTs) constitute the majority of mesenchymal tumors involving the gastrointestinal tract. With an estimated incidence of 2,500–6,000 cases per year in the United States, the clinical presentation of these tumors varies depending on tumor size and anatomic location; however, most tumors are found incidentally at the time of endoscopy or radiologic imaging. GISTs arise most frequently in the stomach (60–70 percent), small intestine (20–25 percent), colon and rectum (5 percent) and esophagus (<5 percent). Most GISTs are sporadic and in 95 percent of cases there is a solitary lesion. Tumor size and mitotic index are the most important prognostic features of these tumors. Surgery remains the primary treatment modality for localized tumors. Until recently, there has been no effective therapy for metastatic or unresectable tumors.

Over the past decade, it has been recognized that GISTs have distinctive immunohistochemical and genetic features. GISTs originate from the intestinal pacemaker cells, the interstitial cells of Cajal (ICC), which are known to express CD117, a transmembrane tyrosine kinase receptor which is the product of the c-KIT proto-oncogene. Expression of CD117 has emerged as an important defining feature in nearly 95 percent of GISTs and the pathogenesis of these tumors is related to c-Kit mutations. Promising preclinical results have provided the driving force for the rapid clinical development of imatinib mesylate (Gleevec [Novartis], formerly known as STI571), a selective tyrosine kinase inhibitor of c-Kit. This novel, molecularly targeted therapy has produced impressive clinical responses in a large percentage of patients with advanced GISTs.

In February 2002, the U.S. Food and Drug Administration (FDA) approved imatinib mesylate for the treatment of GISTs based on promising results seen in patients with metastatic and locally advanced disease. Initial results from clinical trials indicate that about 54 percent of patients with GISTs respond to imatinib therapy and there is no benefit to doses above 400 mg daily. However, little is known about the optimal length of treatment, the duration of benefit, or the long-term toxicity. Given these results in patients with metastatic or locally advanced GISTs, clinical trials are currently underway to study the efficacy of imatinib in the adjuvant and neoadjuvant therapy setting to determine whether it can decrease recurrence rates and prolong disease-specific survival after complete resection.

Pediatric Sarcomas

Soft tissue sarcomas account for 7–8 percent of all pediatric cancers, totaling approximately 600 new cases per year. Associated with skeletal muscle, rhabdomyosarcomas are the most common soft tissue tumors among children younger than 15 years, and they can occur at any site that has striated muscle. These tumors generally present as a painless enlarging mass; about 30 percent arise in the head and neck region, 25 percent in the genitourinary system, and 20 percent in the extremities. About 15–20 percent of cases have metastasis at presentation, most commonly involving the lungs. Several staging systems for rhabdomyosarcoma are available; that of the Intergroup Rhabdomyosarcoma Study Group is based on surgical-pathologic groupings (Table 35-2).

Rhabdomyosarcoma is classified as a small round-cell tumor that demonstrates muscle differentiation on light microscopy and immunohistochemical analysis. Two primary histologic subtypes account for 90 percent of cases, an embryonal subtype (70 percent) and an alveolar subtype (20 percent).

Complete surgical resection is the treatment of choice for rhabdomyosarcoma, when function and cosmesis can be preserved. Patients who are able to undergo a complete tumor resection with negative (group I) or microscopic surgical margins (group II) are able to undergo less intensive systemic therapy with overall survival rates approaching 90 percent. Given the morbidity associated with resections at some anatomic sites surgery is often not undertaken. Recent findings suggest that chemotherapy can adequately control several such tumors without additional local therapy.

Unlike other soft tissue sarcomas, rhabdomyosarcomas have a high propensity for lymph node metastasis, with rates up to 20–30 percent for sites such as the extremities, paratesticular nodes, and prostate. Lymph node sampling and more recently sentinel lymph node mapping have been used to evaluate regional node status in children with rhabdomyosarcoma.

In 1972, the Intergroup Rhabdomyosarcoma Study Committee was established to develop protocols for treating children with rhabdomyosarcomas. The chemotherapy regimens found to be the most active against

TABLE 35-2 Surgical-Pathologic Grouping of Soft Tissue Sarcoma (Intergroup Rhabdomyosarcoma Study Group)

Clinical group	Definition
I	a. Localized, completely resected, confined to site of origin
	b. Localized, completely resected, beyond site of origin
II	a. Localized, grossly resected microscopic residual tumor
	b. Regional disease, involved lymph nodes, completely resected
	c. Regional disease, involved lymph nodes grossly resected with microscopic residual tumor
III	a. Local or regional grossly visible disease after biopsy only
	b. Grossly visible disease after >50% resection of primary tumor
IV	Distant metastases at diagnosis

rhabdomyosarcomas have included vincristine, actinomycin D, and cyclophosphamide. Radiation therapy is given to most patients with microscopic residual disease (group II) after resection.

The prognosis for children with rhabdomyosarcoma is related to tumor site, surgical-pathologic grouping, and tumor histology. The 5-year, disease-free survival rate for all patients has been reported as 65 percent. Disease-free survival by group (see Table 35-2) has been reported as 84 percent, 74 percent, 62 percent, and 23 percent for groups I, II, III, and IV, respectively.

Recurrent Sarcomas

Up to 20 percent of patients with extremity sarcoma develop recurrent disease. The adequacy of surgical resection of sarcomas arising from any anatomic site is clearly related to local recurrence rates. Patients with microscopically positive surgical margins are at increased risk of local recurrence. The effect of local treatment failure on survival and distant disease-free survival is controversial. Many believe that recurrence is a harbinger of distant metastatic disease.

An isolated local recurrence should be treated aggressively with margin-negative resection. For patients with extremity sarcomas, this frequently requires amputation. However, some patients with recurrent extremity sarcoma can undergo function-preserving resection combined with additional radiation therapy, with or without chemotherapy, with acceptable rates of local control.

Retroperitoneal sarcomas recur locally in up to 60 percent of patients. These tumors also can spread diffusely throughout the abdominal cavity and recur as sarcomatosis. The preferred treatment for locally recurrent retroperitoneal tumors is surgical resection, if possible.

Palliative Strategies

Metastases are present at diagnosis in 40–50 percent of patients with intermediate- or high-grade extremity sarcomas, as compared with only 5 percent in patients with low-grade sarcomas. Of those patients who present with high risk localized disease, metastases to distant sites occur within 2–3 years of initial diagnosis. The pattern of recurrence is related to the anatomic site of the primary tumor. Patients with extremity sarcomas generally have recurrence as distant pulmonary metastases, whereas patients with retroperitoneal or intraabdominal sarcomas tend to have local recurrences. Other less common sites of metastasis include bone (7 percent), liver (4 percent), and lymph nodes (<5 percent). Myxoid liposarcoma of the extremity is known to metastasize to the abdomen and pelvis, and requires staging CT of these regions before definitive local therapy.

The primary determinant of survival in patients with soft tissue sarcoma is development of distant metastases. Early recognition and treatment of recurrent, local, or distant disease can prolong survival. A few reports involving small numbers of patients have indicated that salvage after recurrent local disease is possible by performing radical reexcision with or without radiation therapy. Similarly, several groups have reported that survival can be prolonged after resection of pulmonary metastases. These limited data form the basis for the use of aggressive surveillance strategies for all patients with soft tissue sarcoma.

Because most recurrences of soft tissue sarcomas occur in the first 2 years after completion of therapy, it is recommended that patients be evaluated with a complete history and physical examination every 3 months and chest radiography every 6 months during the 2–3-year period. Additionally, most experts recommend that the tumor site be evaluated every 6 months by performing MRI for extremity tumors or CT for intraabdominal or retroperitoneal tumors. In some circumstances, ultrasonography can be used to assess recurrence of tumor in the extremities. Follow-up intervals can be lengthened to every 6 months, with annual imaging, for years 2 through 5. After 5 years, patients should be evaluated and undergo chest radiography annually.

Chemotherapy for Metastatic Sarcoma

The only available treatment for most patients with metastatic disease is chemotherapy. Historically, response rates for patients with stage IV soft tissue sarcoma have been low. Several prognostic factors have been defined for patients undergoing chemotherapy, including performance status, previous response to chemotherapy, younger age, absence of hepatic metastases, low-grade tumors, and long disease-free interval.

CONCLUSION

Soft tissue sarcomas are a family of rare tumors, constituting approximately 1 percent of adult malignancies. The etiology in the vast majority of patients is sporadic. The management of such diverse tumors is complex. Diagnosis by light microscopy is inexact. Molecular diagnosis, although still in its infancy, holds great promise for the future.

Despite these confounding issues, the natural history of soft tissue sarcomas is well established. Approximately two-thirds of cases arise in the extremities, whereas the remaining one-third are distributed between the retroperitoneum, trunk, abdomen, and head and neck. The management algorithm for soft tissue sarcomas is complex and depends on tumor stage, site, and histology. The most common site of metastasis is the lungs, and it generally occurs within 3 years of diagnosis.

The rarity of soft tissue sarcomas creates a challenge for studying the effects of treatment. Collaborative efforts are required to accrue adequate numbers of patients for such studies. Despite these obstacles, progress is being made in understanding these tumors at the molecular level. It can be anticipated that molecular-based therapies will become increasingly incorporated into treatment strategies in the near future.

Suggested Readings

Levine EA: Prognostic factors in soft tissue sarcoma. Semin Surg Oncol 17:23, 1999.

American Joint Committee on Cancer: Cancer Staging Manual. New York: Springer, 2002, p 221.

Yang JC, Chang AE, Baker AR, et al: Randomized prospective study of the benefit of adjuvant radiation therapy in the treatment of soft tissue sarcomas of the extremity. J Clin Oncol 16:197, 1998.

Pisters PW, Harrison LB, Leung DH, et al: Long-term results of a prospective randomized trial of adjuvant brachytherapy in soft tissue sarcoma. J Clin Oncol 14:859, 1996.

O'Sullivan B, Davis AM, Turcotte R, et al: Preoperative versus postoperative radiotherapy in soft-tissue sarcoma of the limbs: A randomised trial. Lancet 359:2235, 2002.

Harrison LB, Franzese F, Gaynor JJ, et al: Long-term results of a prospective randomized trial of adjuvant brachytherapy in the management of completely resected soft tissue sarcomas of the extremity and superficial trunk. Int J Radiat Oncol Biol Phys 27:259, 1993.

Tierney JF: Adjuvant chemotherapy for localised resectable soft-tissue sarcoma of adults: Meta-analysis of individual data. Sarcoma Meta-analysis Collaboration. Lancet 350:1647, 1997.

Catton CN, O'Sullivan B, Kotwall C, et al: Outcome and prognosis in retroperitoneal soft tissue sarcoma. Int J Radiat Oncol Biol Phys 29:1005, 1994.

Demetri GD: Update in the management of gastrointestinal stromal tumor: New guidelines, emerging data. Special Report, 2004, pp 1-8.

Flamant F, Rodary C, Rey A, et al: Treatment of non-metastatic rhabdomyosarcomas in childhood and adolescence. Results of the second study of the International Society of Paediatric Oncology: MMT84. Eur J Cancer 34:1050, 1998.

36 | Inguinal Hernias

Robert J. Fitzgibbons, Jr., and Hardeep S. Ahluwalia

The latter part of the eighteenth century heralded dramatic changes as the anatomy of the groin became better understood. In 1881, a French surgeon, Lucas-Championnière, performed high ligation of an indirect inguinal hernia sac at the internal ring with primary closure of the wound. Edoardo Bassini (1844–1924) is considered the father of modern inguinal hernia surgery. By incorporating the developing disciplines of antisepsis and anesthesia with a new operation that included reconstruction of the inguinal floor along with high ligation of the hernia sac, he was able to substantially reduce morbidity. It is universally agreed that this concept was responsible for the advent of the modern surgical era of inguinal herniorrhaphy and is still valid today. The operation resulted in a recurrence rate one-fifth of that which generally was accepted and was considered the standard criterion for inguinal hernia repair for most of the twentieth century.

Although Bassini's principle of posterior wall reinforcement remains valid in a surgical practice today, his operation has lost its popularity and is used only in selected cases in which prosthetic material is contradicted. This is because of the widespread acceptance of the concept of avoiding tension during herniorrhaphy, championed by Lichtenstein. Lichtenstein theorized that by using a mesh prosthesis to bridge the hernia defect rather than closing it with sutures, as with the Bassini repair and its modifications, tension is avoided ostensibly resulting in a less painful operation. He also felt that the lack of tension reduced the incidence of suture pullout, which would result in a lower recurrence rate. A Lichtenstein type operation has now become the method of choice in the United States.

The preperitoneal space also can be used for repair of an inguinal hernia and has strong proponents because of the mechanical advantage gained from prosthesis placement behind the abdominal wall. Access to the preperitoneal space can be gained through a lower abdominal incision, transabdominally at the time of laparotomy or with the aid of laparoscopic guidance. Irrespective of the mode of entry to the preperitoneal space, a large prosthesis is used that extends far beyond the margins of the myopectineal orifice. This brief overview of the history of inguinal herniorrhaphy provides a background for a comprehensive look at the problem of inguinal herniation.

EPIDEMIOLOGY

Seventy-five percent of all abdominal wall hernias occur in the groin. Indirect hernias outnumber direct hernias by about 2:1, with femoral hernias making up a much smaller proportion. Right-sided groin hernias are more common than those on the left. The male:female ratio for inguinal hernias is 7:1. There are approximately 750,000 inguinal herniorrhaphies performed per year in the United States, compared to 25,000 for femoral hernias, 166,000 for umbilical hernias, 97,000 for incisional hernias, and 76,000 for miscellaneous abdominal wall hernias.

Femoral hernias account for less than 10% of all groin hernias, but 40% of these present as emergencies with incarceration or strangulation. The mortality rate for emergency repair is higher than for elective repair. Femoral hernias are more common in older patients and in men who have previously undergone an inguinal hernia repair. Although the absolute number of femoral hernias in males and females is about the same, the incidence in females is four times that of males because of the lower overall frequency of groin hernia in women.

Estimates of the risk for developing an inguinal hernia vary greatly in the literature, probably because of the lack of a entirely reproducible way to make the diagnose. Self-reporting by patients, audits of routine physical examinations, and insurance company databases are among the diverse sources from which such figures are derived, all of which are known to be notoriously inaccurate. Physician physical examination, even by trained surgeons, also is not dependable because of the difficulty differentiating between lipomas of the cord, a normal expansile bulge and a true groin hernia.

NATURAL HISTORY

Risk factors that are useful in predicting complications in an adult patient with a groin hernia include old age, short duration, femoral hernia and coexisting medical illness. In children, the risk factors are very young age, male sex, short duration and right-sided hernia. A better understanding of the natural history therefore becomes particularly important to identify subgroups that might be at greater risk for a complication.

HERNIA ACCIDENT (INCARCERATION, BOWEL OBSTRUCTION, STRANGULATION)

An incarcerated hernia is by definition an irreducible hernia. However, this should not imply a surgical emergency, as chronic states of incarceration are common because of the size of the neck of the hernia in relationship to its contents or because of adhesions to the hernia sac. The recommended treatment of an incarcerated hernia is surgical repair, but there is no urgency because there is no life threatening complication present.

A patient with an incarcerated inguinal hernia exhibiting signs of a bowel obstruction or one who develops an acute incarceration that remains exquisitely tender represents a completely different clinical scenario. Unlike adhesive small bowel obstructions, partial small bowel obstructions are rare. Therefore, most patients will have had vomiting and absolute constipation (obstipation). In the western world, groin hernia ranks third after adhesive obstruction and cancer as the most common cause of bowel obstruction. In other areas, it remains the most common. It is common for it to be overlooked on clinical examination and therefore must be kept in mind in patients being evaluated for bowel obstruction.

Imaging studies are important in cases in which there is the slightest question about the cause of the patient's obstructive pattern. This is because a distal intestinal obstruction secondary to another cause (e.g., adhesions) may result in distention of a coincidental nonobstructing groin hernia. Should the examiner focus attention exclusively on the hernia, the stage is set for disaster when the hernia is repaired and the real cause of the obstruction is missed. Plain roentgenograms of the abdomen will reveal the usual signs of an intestinal obstruction: dilated loops of bowel with air-fluid levels, absence of bowel gas distal to the obstruction and bowel shadows in the region of the hernia. A lateral view often is useful to demonstrate this more clearly. Computerized tomographic (CT) scans reliably demonstrate the hernia with characteristic features of obstruction and should be considered if the clinical diagnosis is not certain.

The initial treatment, in the absence of signs of strangulation, is taxis. Taxis is performed with the patient sedated and placed in the Trendelenburg position. The hernia sac neck is grasped with one hand with the other applying pressure on the most distal part of the hernia. The goal is to elongate the neck of the hernia so that the contents of the hernia may be guided back into the abdominal cavity with a rocking movement. Taxis should not be performed with excessive pressure. If the hernia is strangulated, gangrenous bowel might be reduced into the abdomen or perforated in the process. One or two gentle attempts should be made at taxis. If this is unsuccessful, the procedure should be abandoned. Rarely, the hernia together with its peritoneal sac and constricting neck may be reduced into the abdomen (reduction en masse). Reduction en masse of a hernia is defined as the displacement of a hernia mass without relief of incarceration or strangulation. This diagnosis has to be considered in all cases of intestinal obstruction after apparent reduction of an incarcerated hernia. Laparoscopy can be both diagnostic and therapeutic and therefore is a particularly good option. Surgeon expertise may make laparotomy a better choice for some.

The most significant complication of either acute incarceration or intestinal obstruction is strangulation. It is a serious, life-threatening condition because the hernia contents have become ischemic and nonviable. The clinical features of a strangulated obstruction are dramatic. In addition to the patient having developed an irreducible hernia and an intestinal obstruction, clinical signs indicate that strangulation has taken place. The hernia is tense, very tender and the overlying skin may be discolored with a reddish or bluish tinge. There are no bowel sounds present within the hernia itself. The patient commonly has a leukocytosis with a left shift, is toxic, dehydrated and febrile. Arterial blood gases may reveal a metabolic acidosis.

Rapid resuscitation with intravenous fluids is essential with electrolyte replacement, antibiotics and nasogastric suction. Urgent surgery is indicated once resuscitation has taken place. The initial surgical approach is to make a conventional inguinal hernia incision. If the bowel is viable, it is reduced into the abdominal cavity prior to repairing the hernia. The neck of the hernia is widened if any difficulty is encountered reducing the hernia. Although rare, the surgeon must be cognizant of the possibility that a nonviable abdominal organ may have been reduced into the abdominal cavity during the course of usual surgical maneuvers before it could be visualized. If such a suspicion is present, the entire GI tract must be evaluated. If the bowel is found to be obviously gangrenous, more bowel must be pulled into the hernia so that viable bowel can be transected and the gangrenous portion removed. In the ideal situation, an end to end anastomosis is performed and the bowel is reduced into the abdominal cavity, followed by hernia repair. The slightest suspicion that the entire process cannot be addressed from the groin mandates exploratory laparoscopy or laparotomy to unequivocally prove that all nonviable tissue has been resected. In the case of a femoral hernia, it is frequently necessary to incise the inguinal ligament anteriorly or the lacunar ligament medially to facilitate reduction.

ETIOLOGY

The cause of an inguinal hernia in a human is far from completely understood but is undoubtedly multifactorial (Table 36-1). Familial predisposition plays a role. However, there is increasing evidence that connective tissue disorders predispose to hernia formation by altering collagen formation. A higher prevalence of inguinal hernias is well known among patients suffering from certain congenital connective tissue disorders. In children with congenital hip dislocation, inguinal hernia occurs five times more often in girls and three times more often in boys compared to children without this disease. The role of physical exertion in the development of inguinal hernia is probably less important than is commonly believed. The cause and effect relationship between a specific lifting episode and the development of an inguinal hernia is present in less than 10 percent except in circumstances in which worker's compensation issues are involved. Additionally, athletes, even weightlifters, do not seem to have an excessive incidence of inguinal hernias. This begs the question whether patients with un-repaired inguinal hernias should be restricted from heavy lifting.

Indirect Inguinal Hernia

The so-called "saccular theory" of indirect inguinal hernia formation proposed by Russell remains popular. Russell's hypothesis that the "presence of a developmental diverticulum associated with a patent processus vaginalis, was essential in every case" is still valid in the minds of many surgeons even today. Russell felt that increased intraabdominal pressure might serve to further stretch and weaken the internal ring allowing additional intraabdominal organs to herniate through the orifice but could not actually cause an indirect inguinal hernia. This does not explain all cases of indirect groin hernias, however. First,

TABLE 36-1 Presumed Causes of Groin Herniation

Coughing
Chronic obstructive pulmonary disease
Obesity
Straining
Constipation
Prostatism
Pregnancy
Birthweight less than 1500 g
Family history of a hernia
Valsalva maneuvers
Ascites
Upright position
Congenital connective tissue disorders
Defective collagen synthesis
Previous right lower quadrant incision
Arterial *aneurysms*
Cigarette *smoking*
Heavy lifting
Physical exertion ?

a patent processus vaginalis can be found at autopsy without clinical evidence of a hernia. Second, there are patients with an obliterated processus vaginalis who have an abdominal wall defect lateral to the epigastric vessels. Third, congenital structural malformations of the transversalis fascia and transversus abdominis aponeurosis can alter the strength and size of the internal inguinal ring. Denervation of the internal oblique muscle by adjacent incisions (e.g., appendectomy) also can be associated with the eventual development of an inguinal hernia.

Excessive fatty tissue involving the cord or round ligament encountered by a surgeon during elective herniorrhaphy traditionally has been referred to as a lipoma of the cord. This term is unfortunate because it implies a neoplastic process but a lipoma of the cord consists of normal fatty tissue. The reason for the term lipoma is that the fatty tissue can easily be separated from the cord structures and reduced into the preperitoneal space "en masse" as if it were a tumor. A lipoma of the cord is important from a clinical standpoint for three reasons: (1) it can cause hernia type symptoms although with less frequency than indirect hernias with a peritoneal sac; (2) it is often difficult to distinguish at physical examination from an indirect hernia with a peritoneal sac; and (3) it can be responsible for an unsatisfactory result because of an unchanged physical examination after elective inguinal herniorrhaphy, especially when a preperitoneal repair is used. For the purposes of the large clinical trials referred to in other parts of this chapter, a lipoma of the cord was classified as an indirect hernia. There is no peritoneal sac by definition because the contents of the indirect hernia (i.e., preperitoneal fat) come from the preperitoneal space rather than the abdominal cavity.

Direct Inguinal Hernias

Two major factors are felt to be important in the development of direct inguinal hernias. The first is increased intraabdominal pressure associated with a variety of conditions listed in Table 36-1. The second factor is relative weakness of the posterior inguinal wall. An abnormally high lying arch of the main body of the transversus abdominis above the superior ramus of the pubis resulting in a large area at risk has been incriminated (see Anatomy). Similarly, a limited insertion of the transversus abdominis muscle onto the pubis, weakness of the iliopubic tract, limited insertion of the iliopubic tract aponeurosis into a Cooper ligament or a combination of these have been reported to contribute.

Femoral Hernias

The size and shape of the femoral ring and increased intraabdominal pressure are factors that contribute to the development of a femoral hernia. The iliopubic tract anteriorly and medially accounts for the variability that allows the development of the hernia. The iliopubic tract normally inserts for a distance of 1–2 cm along the pectinate line between the pubic tubercle and the midportion of the superior pubic ramus. A femoral hernia can result if the insertion is less than 1–2 cm or if it is shifted medially. The net effect of either anatomic subtlety is to widen the femoral ring, predisposing to the hernia. Femoral hernias are particularly dangerous because of the rigid structures that make up the femoral ring. The slightest amount of edema at the ring can produce gangrenous changes of the sac contents continuing distally into the femoral canal and thigh.

Sliding Inguinal Hernia

A sliding inguinal hernia is defined as any hernia in which part of the sac is the wall of a viscus. Approximately 8 percent of all groin hernias present with this finding but the incidence is age related. It rarely is found in patients less than 30 years of age but increases to 20 percent after the age of 70. If the hernia is on the right, the cecum, ascending colon or appendix most commonly are involved; and on the left, the sigmoid colon. The uterus, fallopian tubes, ovaries, ureters and bladder can be involved on either side. The sliding component usually is found on the posterior lateral side of the internal ring. The importance of this condition has lessened considerably in the last several years with the realization that it is not necessary to resect hernia sacs and that simple reduction into the preperitoneal space is sufficient. This eliminates the primary danger associated with sliding hernias, which is injury to the viscus during high ligation and sac excision.

ANATOMY

The anatomy of the groin is best understood when observing from the approach for the herniorrhaphy to be performed. For a conventional operation, this means from the skin to the deeper layers. For the laparoscopic operations or the preperitoneal operations, one should consider the anatomy from the abdominal cavity to the skin. The first layers encountered beneath the skin are the Camper and Scarpa fascia in the subcutaneous tissue. The aponeurosis of the external oblique muscle is the next structure encountered as dissection proceeds through the abdominal wall. The muscle arises from the posterior aspects of the lower eight ribs. The posterior portion of the muscle is orientated vertically and inserts on the crest of the ileum. The anterior portion of the muscle courses inferiorly in an oblique direction toward the midline and pubis. The obliquely oriented anterior-inferior fibers of the aponeurosis of the external oblique muscle fold back on themselves to form the inguinal ligament which attaches laterally to the anterior superior iliac spine. The medial insertion of the inguinal ligament in most individuals is dual. One portion inserts on the pubic tubercle and the pubic bone. The other folds back as the lacunar ligament. It blends laterally with a Cooper (pectineal) ligament. The more medial fibers of the aponeurosis of the external oblique divide into a medial and a lateral crus to form the external or superficial inguinal ring through which the spermatic cord or round ligament and branches of the ilioinguinal and genitofemoral nerves pass.

The internal abdominal oblique muscle fibers fan out following the shape of the iliac crest; the superior fibers course obliquely upward toward the distal ends of the lower three or four ribs whereas the lower fibers orient themselves inferomedially toward the pubis to run parallel to the external oblique aponeurotic fibers. These fibers arch over the round ligament or the spermatic cord forming the superficial part of the internal (deep) inguinal ring.

The first lumbar nerve divides into the ilioinguinal and iliohypogastric nerves. These may divide within the psoas major muscle retroperitoneally or between the internal oblique and transversus abdominis muscles. The ilioinguinal nerve may communicate with the iliohypogastric nerve before innervating the internal oblique. The ilioinguinal nerve then passes through the external inguinal ring to run with the spermatic cord, although the iliohypogastric nerve pierces the external oblique to innervate the skin above the pubis. The cremaster muscle fibers, which are derived from the internal oblique muscle, are innervated by the genitofemoral nerve (L1, L2).

The transversus abdominis muscle arises from the inguinal ligament, the inner side of the iliac crest, the endoabdominal fascia and the lower six costal cartilages and ribs. The medial aponeurotic fibers of the transversus abdominis contribute to the rectus sheath and insert on the pecten pubis and the crest of the pubis forming the falx inguinalis. These fibers are infrequently joined by a portion of the internal oblique aponeurosis; only then is a true conjoined tendon formed.

The myopectineal orifice of Fruchaud refers to an anatomic area in the groin through which all hernias occur. Hesselbach's inguinal triangle is within this orifice and is the site of direct inguinal hernias. When described from the anterior aspect, the inguinal ligament forms the base of the triangle, the edge of the rectus abdominis is the medial border, and the inferior epigastric vessels are the superolateral border. It should be noted, however, that Hesselbach actually described a Cooper ligament as the base.

The transversalis fascia also is important because it forms anatomical landmarks known as analogues or derivatives. The important transversalis fascia analogues for the hernia surgeon are the iliopectineal arch, the iliopubic tract, the crura of the deep inguinal ring and a Cooper (pectineal) ligament. The superior and inferior crura form a transversalis fascia sling, a "monk's hood" shaped structure, around the deep inguinal ring. This sling has functional significance as the crura of the ring are pulled upward and laterally by the contraction of transversus abdominis, resulting in a valvular action that helps to preclude indirect hernia formation. The iliopubic tract is the thickened band of the transversalis fascia that courses parallel to the more superficially located inguinal ligament. It is attached to the iliac crest laterally and inserts on the pubic tubercle medially. The insertion curves inferolaterally for 1–2 cm along the pectinate line to blend with a Cooper (pectineal) ligament, ending at about the midportion of the superior pubic ramus. A Cooper ligament is actually a condensation of periosteum and is not a true analogue of the transversalis fascia.

The femoral ring is bordered by the superior pubic ramus inferiorly and the femoral vein laterally. The iliopubic tract with its curved insertion onto the pubic ramus is the anterior and medial border. The canal normally contains preperitoneal fat, connective tissue and lymph nodes including a Cloquet node at its entrance, the femoral ring.

The Posterior Perspective (Laparoscopic)

An excellent view of the anterior abdominal wall can be obtained from a laparoscopic vantage point. Peritoneal folds are immediately obvious which correspond to important anatomic landmarks in the preperitoneal space. The median umbilical fold extends from the umbilicus to the urinary bladder and covers the urachus, the usually fibrous remnant of the fetal allantois. The lateral umbilical fold covers the inferior epigastric artery as it courses toward the posterior rectus sheath and enters it approximately at the level of the arcuate line.

The fossa formed between the medial and the lateral ligaments is the site of direct inguinal hernias. The lateral fossa is less delineated than the other two. The deep inguinal ring is located in the lateral fossa just lateral to the inferior epigastric vessels.

When the peritoneum is divided and the preperitoneal space entered, the key anatomic elements for a preperitoneal herniorrhaphy can be appreciated.

In the midline behind the pubis, the preperitoneal space is known as the space of Retzius, although laterally it is referred to as the space of Bogros. This space is important because many of the repairs, which are described later, are performed in this area. Perhaps the single most important landmark is the inferior epigastric artery. This branch of the external iliac artery represents the primary blood supply to the deep anterior wall. The veins in this area can be troublesome especially the iliopubic, corona mortis obturator and their tributaries.

Other landmarks that require identification are the internal inguinal ring just lateral to the take off of the inferior epigastric vessels, the internal spermatic artery and vein, and the vas deferens that join to form the spermatic cord just before entering the internal ring. The iliopubic tract, attached to the iliac crest laterally, crosses under the internal ring to make up its inferior border and at the same time contributes to the anterior border of the femoral sheath continuing to its insertion on the pubic tubercle. A Cooper ligament extends from the pubic tubercle inferolateral along the pubic ramus crossing under the femoral vessel. The femoral ring is readily visible from this viewpoint being bordered by the femoral vein laterally, a Cooper ligament inferiorly, and the iliopubic tract superiorly.

The nerves traversing the preperitoneal space are prone to intraoperative injury. They can be damaged when fastening a prosthesis if deep penetration of the fixation device occurs. The genitofemoral nerve may occur as a single trunk lying deep to the peritoneum and fascia on the anterior surface of the psoas muscle or it may divide into its component genital and femoral branches within the muscle. The genital branch travels with the spermatic cord, entering at the deep inguinal ring; it ultimately innervates the cremaster muscle and the lateral scrotum. The femoral branch of the nerve innervates the skin of the proximal mid thigh. The lateral femoral cutaneous nerve crosses the preperitoneal space lateral to the genitofemoral nerve and enters the thigh just beneath the iliopubic tract and the inguinal ligament. This nerve supplies sensory branches for the lateral side of the thigh.

SYMPTOMS

Patients with groin hernias present with a wide range of clinical scenarios ranging from no symptoms at all to the life-threatening condition caused by strangulation of incarcerated hernia contents. Asymptomatic patients may have their hernias diagnosed at the time of a routine physical examination or seek medical attention because of a painless bulge in the groin. Indirect hernias are more likely to produce symptoms than direct hernias. Many describe an annoying heavy feeling or dragging sensation, which tends to be worse as the day wears on. The pain is commonly intermittent and radiation into the testicle is not rare. Others complain of a sharper pain that is either localized or diffuse. Particularly severe patients may need to recline for a short period of time or use other posture altering techniques. Occasionally patients must manually reduce their hernia to obtain relief.

DIAGNOSIS

Physical Examination

Physical examination is the best way to determine the presence or absence of an inguinal hernia. The diagnosis may be obvious by simple inspection

TABLE 36-2 Differential Diagnosis

Malignancy
Lymphoma
Retroperitoneal sarcoma
Metastasis
Testicular tumor
Primary Testicular
Varicocele
Epididymitis
Testicular torsion
Hydrocele
Ectopic testicle
Undescended testicle
Femoral artery aneurysm or pseudoaneurysm
Lymph node
Sebaceous cyst
Hidradenitis
Cyst of the canal of Nuck (Female)
Saphenous varix
Psoas abscess
Hematoma
Ascites

when a visible bulge is present. The differential diagnosis must be considered in questionable cases (Table 36-2). Nonvisible hernias require digital examination of the inguinal canal. Classic teaching is that an indirect hernia will push against the fingertip, whereas a direct hernia will push against the pulp of the finger. Additionally, applying pressure over the mid-inguinal point with the fingertip will control an indirect hernia and prevent it from protruding when the patient strains. A direct hernia will not be effected with this maneuver.

A femoral hernia presents as a swelling below the inguinal ligament and just lateral to the pubic tubercle. Thin patients commonly have prominent bilateral bulges below the inguinal ligament medial to the femoral vessels. They are asymptomatic and disappear spontaneously when the patient assumes a supine position. Operation is not indicated.

Radiological Investigations

Hernias are visualized as abnormal ballooning of the anteroposterior diameter of the inguinal canal and/or simultaneous protrusion of fat or bowel within the inguinal canal. Magnetic resonance imaging (MRI) with the development of the fast imaging scanners that allow dynamic imaging (i.e., performed during straining), shows particular promise for further refinement with the "tweaking" of the best weights for images and the addition of intraperitoneal contrast agents. Both MRI and computerized tomography (CT) may reveal other causes of groin pain because of their ability to visualize related structures in the groin. In a comparative study, the sensitivity and specificity was 74.5 percent and 96.3 percent for physical examination, 92.7 percent and 81.5 percent for ultrasound, and 94.5 percent and 96.3 percent for MRI, respectively.

PREOPERATIVE CARE

Nonoperative Treatment

The term "watchful waiting" is used to describe this treatment recommendation. It is only applicable in asymptomatic or minimally symptomatic hernias. Patients are counseled about the signs and symptoms of complications from their hernia so they might present promptly to their physician in cases in which an adverse event takes place. Definitive data that this recommendation is safe is not available and it is for this reason that standard surgical texts continue to recommend surgical repair of all inguinal hernias at diagnosis. However, a randomized controlled trial is currently underway which should shed some light on this subject in the next few years.

ABDOMINAL WALL SUBSTITUTES

The modern era of herniorrhaphy has seen a progressive decrease in recurrence rate because of improvement in surgical technique and prosthetics. It is apparent that the abdominal wall does not always heal satisfactorily after primary closure and that an irreducible percentage of recurrences is inevitable if one were to insist on pure tissue repairs. The only reasonable solution is the use of a structure that can bridge a defect in certain cases.

Prosthetic Materials

It has now been proven that mesh herniorrhaphy can decrease the recurrence rate by approximately 50 percent when compared to nonmesh repairs. Chronic post herniorrhaphy groin pain occasionally occurs after prosthetic repair and is relieved by prosthesis removal. However, the overall incidence of chronic post herniorrhaphy groin pain is less with a prosthetic repair. The materials that have emerged as suitable for routine use in hernia surgery include polypropylene, either monofilament (Marlex, Prolene) or polyfilament (Surgipro), Dacron (Mersilene) and expanded polytetrafluoroethylene (e-PTFE) (Gore-Tex).

ANESTHESIA FOR GROIN HERNIORRHAPHY

Most inguinal herniorrhaphies can be performed under local or regional anesthesia. Laparoscopic herniorrhaphy is the exception, as general endotracheal anesthesia is primarily mandated by the pneumoperitoneum. This is one of the strongest arguments for conventional herniorrhaphy when compared to laparoscopic herniorrhaphy. Despite this, the best available evidence suggests that the majority of conventional herniorrhaphies are performed under a general anesthetic with local and regional techniques, finding their greatest popularity in specialty clinics. Nevertheless, local anesthesia, when used in adequate doses and far enough in advance of the initial incision, proves very effective when combined with the newer, short-acting amnesic and anxiolytic agents.

One hundred milliliters of 0.5 percent Xylocaine with epinephrine or 0.25 percent bupivacaine with epinephrine or a combination of the two plus or minus sodium bicarbonate is most common. Seventy milliliters of this solution is injected by the surgeon in an adult of normal size prior to prepping and draping the patient. Ten milliliters is placed medial to the anterior superior iliac spine to block the ilioinguinal nerve, and the other 60 mL is used as a field block along the orientation of the eventual incision in the subcutaneous and deeper tissues. Care is taken to inject the areas of the pubic tubercle and a Cooper ligament, both of which can easily be identified by tactile sensation except in the very obese. The remaining 30 mL is reserved for discretionary use during the procedure. With this technique, endotracheal intubation is avoided and the patient can be aroused from sedation at intervals to perform Valsalva maneuvers and test the repair.

INGUINAL HERNIA REPAIRS

Before discussing specific conventional herniorrhaphies, several steps will be described because they are common to all of the conventional operations.

Initial Incision: Classically an oblique skin incision is made between the anterior superior iliac spine and the pubic tubercle. Many surgeons now use a more horizontally placed skin incision in the natural skin lines for cosmetic reasons. Regardless, it is deepened through the Camper and Scarpa fascia and the subcutaneous tissue to expose the external oblique aponeurosis. This structure is incised medially down to and through the external inguinal ring.

Mobilization of the cord structures. The superior flap of the external oblique aponeurosis is bluntly dissected off the internal oblique muscle laterally and superiorly. The iliohypogastric nerve is identified at this time. It can be left in-situ or freed from the surrounding tissue and isolated from the operative field by passing a hemostat under the nerve and grasping the upper flap of the external oblique aponeurosis. Routine division of this nerve along with the ilioinguinal nerve is practiced by some surgeons but not advised by most. The cord structures are then separated from the inferior flap of the external oblique aponeurosis by blunt dissection exposing the shelving edge of the inguinal ligament and the iliopubic tract. The cord structures are lifted en-masse with the fingers of one hand at the pubic tubercle so that the index finger can be passed underneath to meet the index finger of the other hand. Blunt dissection is used to complete mobilization of the cord structures and a Penrose drain is placed around them for retraction during the course of the procedure.

Division of the cremasteric muscle. Complete division of the cremasteric muscle, especially when dealing with an indirect hernia, has been common practice. The purpose is to facilitate sac identification and to lengthen the cord for better visualization of the inguinal floor. However, adequate exposure usually can be obtained by a longitudinal opening of the muscle, which lessens the likelihood of damage to cord structures and avoids the complication of testicular descent. It is probably best not to divide the cremasteric muscle unless the surgeon cannot obtain adequate visualization of the inguinal floor any other way.

High ligation of the sac. The term "high ligation of the sac" will be used frequently as its historical significance has ingrained it in the description of most of the older operations. By convention, high ligation should be considered equivalent to reduction of the sac into the preperitoneal space without excision. Both methods work equally well and are highly effective. Sac inversion, in lieu of excision, does protect intraabdominal viscera in cases of unrecognized incarcerated sac contents or a sliding hernia.

Management of inguinal scrotal hernia sacs. Complete excision of all indirect inguinal hernia sacs is felt to be important by some. The downside to this practice is an excessive rate of ischemic orchitis caused by trauma to the testicular blood supply, especially the delicate venous plexuses. Testicular atrophy is the logical further sequelae although the relationship has not been conclusively proven. A better approach is to divide indirect inguinal hernia sacs in the mid inguinal canal, once confident the hernia is not sliding and there are no abdominal contents. The distal sac is not dissected but the anterior wall is opened as far distally as is convenient. Contrary to popular opinion in the urological literature, this does not result in an excessive rate of postoperative hydrocele formation.

Relaxing incision. A relaxing incision divides the anterior rectus sheath extending from the pubic tubercle superiorly for a variable distance determined by the tension. The relaxing incision works by allowing the various components of the abdominal wall to displace laterally and inferiorly.

Wound closure. The external oblique fascia is closed, serving to reconstruct the superficial (external) ring. The external ring must be loose enough to prevent strangulation of the cord structures yet tight enough to avoid an inexperienced examiner from confusing a dilated ring with a recurrence. The later is sometimes referred to as an "industrial" hernia because historically it has at times been a problem during a preemployment physical. The Scarpa fascia and the skin are closed to complete the operation.

Specific Herniorrhaphies

Bassini

Bassini called his new operation the "radical cure" for an inguinal hernia. The major components of '" this cure" are as follows:

(1) Division of the external oblique aponeurosis over the inguinal canal through the external ring.
(2) Division of the cremaster muscle lengthwise followed by resection so that an indirect hernia is not missed while exposing simultaneously the floor of the inguinal canal to more accurately assess for a direct inguinal hernia.
(3) Division of the floor or posterior wall of the inguinal canal for its full length. This insures adequate examination of the femoral ring from above and exposes the tissue layers that will be used for reconstructing the inguinal floor
(4) High ligation of an indirect sac.
(5) Reconstruction of the posterior wall by suturing the transversalis fascia, the transversus abdominis muscle, the internal oblique muscle (Bassini's famous "triple layer") medially to the inguinal ligament laterally and possibly the iliopubic tract.

Following the initial dissection and reduction or ligation of the sac, attention turns to reconstructing the inguinal floor. Bassini began this part of the operation by opening the transversalis fascia (some prefer to use the term posterior inguinal wall) from the internal inguinal ring to the pubic tubercle, exposing the preperitoneal fat which was bluntly dissected away from the under surface of the superior flap of the transversalis fascia. This allowed him to properly prepare the deepest structure in his famous triple layer (transversalis fascia, transversus abdominis muscle and internal oblique muscle). The first stitch in the repair includes the triple layer superiorly and the periosteum of the medial side of the pubic tubercle along with the rectus sheath. Most surgeons now try to avoid the periosteum of the pubic tubercle to decrease the incidence of osteitis pubis. The repair is continued laterally with nonabsorbable suture securing the triple layer to the reflected inguinal ligament (Poupart ligament). These sutures are continued until the internal ring has been closed on its medial side. A relaxing incision was not part of the original description but is commonly added now.

Shouldice

Local anesthesia with sedation is the rule, and epinephrine is empirically avoided in the event it might contribute to ischemic orchitis. The initial approach is similar to the Bassini repair with particular importance placed on freeing the cord from its surrounding adhesions, resection of the cremaster muscle, high dissection of the hernia sac and division of the transversalis fascia. Continuous nonabsorbable suture is used to repair the floor. Traditionally, this has been monofilament steel wire. The Shouldice surgeons feel a continuous suture distributes tension evenly and prevents defects that could potentially occur between interrupted sutures resulting in a recurrence. The repair is started at the pubic tubercle by approximating the iliopubic tract laterally to the undersurface of the lateral edge of the rectus muscle. The suture is continued laterally, approximating the iliopubic tract to the medial flap that is made up of the transversalis fascia, the internal oblique and transverse abdominis muscles. Eventually four suture lines are developed from the medial flap. The running suture is continued to the internal ring where the lateral stump of the cremaster muscle is picked up, forming a new internal ring. The direction of the suture is reversed back toward the pubic tubercle, approximating the medial edge of the internal oblique and transversus abdominis muscle to Poupart ligament and the wire is tied to itself. Thus, there are two suture lines formed by the first suture. The second wire suture is started near the internal ring and approximates the internal oblique and transversus muscles to a band of external oblique aponeurosis superficial and parallel to the inguinal ligament, in effect creating a second artificial inguinal ligament. This forms the third suture line that ends at the pubic crest. The suture is then reversed and a fourth suture line is constructed in a similar manner, superficial to the third line. At the Shouldice Clinic, the cribriforms fascia always is incised in the thigh, parallel to the inguinal ligament, to make the inner side of the lower flap of the external oblique aponeurosis available for these multiple layers. This step commonly is omitted in general practice.

Conventional Anterior, Prosthetic

Lichtenstein Tension-Free Hernioplasty

At the Lichtenstein Clinic, the procedure is performed under local anesthesia with sedation using 50 mL or less of a 50/50 mixture of 1 percent lidocaine (Xylocaine) and 0.5 percent bupivacaine (Marcaine), with 1/200,000 epinephrine. General or regional anesthesia also can be used. The initial steps are similar to the Bassini repair. After the external oblique aponeurosis has been opened from just lateral to the internal ring through the external ring, the upper leaf is freed from the underlying anterior rectus sheath and internal oblique muscle aponeurosis in an avascular plane from a point at least 2 cm medial to the pubic tubercle to the anterior superior iliac spine laterally. Blunt dissection is continued in this avascular plane from lateral to the internal ring, to the pubic tubercle, along the inguinal ligament and iliopubic tract. Continuing this same motion, the cord with its cremaster covering is swept off the pubic tubercle and separated from the inguinal floor. The ilioinguinal nerve, external spermatic vessels, and the genital branch of the genitofemoral nerve all remain with the cord structures. The effect is to create a large space for the eventual placement of the prosthesis and at the same time providing excellent visualization of the important nerves.

For indirect hernias, the cremasteric muscle is incised longitudinally and the sac dissected free and reduced into the preperitoneal space. A theoretical criticism of this operation is that unless the inguinal floor is opened, an occult femoral hernia may be overlooked. However, an excessive incidence of missed femoral hernias has not been reported. Additionally, it is possible to evaluate the femoral ring by entering the preperitoneal space through a small opening in the canal floor. Direct hernias are separated from the cord and other surrounding structures and reduced back into the preperitoneal space. Dividing the superficial layers of the neck of the sac circumferentially, which in effect opens the inguinal floor, usually facilitates reduction and aids in maintaining it while the prosthesis is placed. This opening in the inguinal floor also can be used to palpate a femoral hernia. Suture can be used to invert the sac but this adds no strength as the purpose is simply to allow the repair to proceed unencumbered by the sac continually protruding into the operative field.

A mesh prosthesis with a minimum size of 15 × 8 cm for an adult is positioned over the inguinal floor. The medial end is rounded to correspond to the patient's anatomy and secured to the anterior rectus sheath a minimum of 2 cm medial to the pubic tubercle. Either nonabsorbable or long acting absorbable suture should be used. The wide overlap of the pubic tubercle is important to avoid the all too common pubic tubercle recurrences seen with other operations. The suture is continued in a running locking fashion laterally, securing the prosthesis to either side of the pubic tubercle (*not into it*) and the shelving edge of the inguinal ligament. The suture is tied at the internal ring.

A slit is made at the lateral end of the mesh creating two tails, a wide one (two thirds) above and a narrower (one-third) below. The tails are positioned around the cord structures and placed beneath the external oblique aponeurosis laterally to about the anterior superior iliac spine with the upper tail being placed on top of the lower. A single interrupted suture is used to secure the lower edge of the superior tail to the lower edge of the inferior tail in effect creating a shutter valve at the internal ring. This step is considered crucial for the prevention of indirect recurrences that are occasionally seen when simple re-approximation of the tails is performed. The surgeons at the Lichtenstein Clinic also include the shelving edge of the inguinal ligament in this shutter valve stitch that serves to buckle the mesh somewhat medially over the direct space, creating a dome like effect to assure there is no tension especially when the patient assumes an upright position. Recently the Lichtenstein group has developed a customized prosthesis with a built in dome-like configuration that they feel makes suturing the approximated tails to the inguinal ligament unnecessary. A few interrupted sutures are used to secure the superior and medial aspects of the prostheses to the underlying internal oblique muscle and rectus fascia. If the iliohypogastric nerve crosses up to the external oblique aponeurosis on the medial side, the prosthesis should be slit to accommodate it. The prosthesis can be trimmed in situ but care should be taken to maintain sufficient laxity to account for a difference between the supine and upright positions and the fact that mesh shrinkage is a reality.

If a femoral hernia is present, the posterior surface of the mesh is sutured to a Cooper ligament after the inferior edge has been attached to the inguinal ligament. This closes the femoral canal and the wound is closed in layers.

Mesh Plug and Patch

The mesh plug technique was developed by Gilbert, and then modified by Rutkow, Robbins, Millikan and others. The groin is entered through a standard anterior approach. The hernia sac is dissected away from surrounding structures and reduced back into the preperitoneal space. A flat sheet of polypropylene mesh is rolled up like a cigarette and held in place with suture. This plug is inserted in the defect and secured to either the internal ring for an indirect hernia or the neck of the defect for a direct hernia using interrupted sutures. The use of a prefabricated, commercially available prosthesis that has the configuration of a flower is recommended by Rutkow and Robbins. The prosthesis is individualized for each patient by removing some of the petals to avoid unnecessary bulk. This step is important, as rarely erosion into a surrounding structure such as the bladder has been reported. Millikan further modified the procedure by recommending that the inside petals be sewn to the ring of the defect. For indirect hernias the inside pedals are sewn to the internal oblique portion of the internal ring which forces the outside of the prosthesis underneath the inner side of the defect making it act like a preperitoneal underlay. For direct hernias, the inside petals are sewn to a Cooper ligament and the shelving edge of the inguinal ligament and the musculoaponeurotic ring of the defect superiorly, again forcing the outside to act as an underlay. The patch portion of the procedure is optional and involves placing a flat piece of polypropylene in the conventional inguinal space widely overlapping the plug in a fashion similar to the Lichtenstein procedure. The difference is that only one or two sutures, or perhaps no sutures are used to secure the flat prosthesis to the underlying inguinal floor. Some surgeons place so many sutures that they have in effect performed a Lichtenstein operation on top of the plug. The euphemism used to describe this is the "plugtenstein." To the credit of its proponents, the plug and patch in all of its varieties has been skillfully presented and has rapidly become a popular repair. Not only is it fast but also easy to teach, making it popular in both private and academic centers.

Conventional Preperitoneal, Prosthetic

The key to the preperitoneal prosthetic repairs is the placement of a large prothesis in the preperitoneal space between the transversalis fascia and the peritoneum. The preperitoneal repair makes use of the abdominal pressure to help fix the prosthetic material against the abdominal wall, adding strength to the repair. The preperitoneal space can be entered from its anterior or posterior aspect. The major difference between the anterior and posterior approaches is that in the latter, the inguinal canal is not entered. Proponents point out that this avoids damage to the cremasteric muscle and lessens the chance of cord injury. If an anterior approach is desirable, a groin incision is used because the space is entered directly through the inguinal floor. Either a lower midline, paramedian, or Pfannenstiel incision without opening the peritoneum can be used for the purposes of entering the preperitoneal space posteriorly as originally popularized by Cheatle, and later by Henry.

The Anterior Approach

Read-Rives. This operation starts like a classical Bassini, including opening the inguinal floor. The inferior epigastric vessels are identified and the preperitoneal space completely dissected. The spermatic cord is "parietalized" by separating the ductus deferens from the spermatic vessels. A 12- × 16-cm piece of mesh is positioned in the preperitoneal space deep to the inferior epigastric vessels and secured with three sutures; one each to the pubic tubercle, a Cooper ligament and the psoas muscle laterally. The transversalis fascia is closed over the prosthesis and the cord structures replaced. The rest of the closure is as described above for the Bassini repair.

The Posterior Approach

Wantz/stoppa/rives (giant prosthetic reinforcement of the visceral sac or GPRVS). These three procedures are grouped together under the heading of GPRVS because there are only minor variations between them. A lower midline, transverse or Pfannenstiel incision can be used according to surgeon preference. If a transverse incision is chosen, it should extend from the midline 8–9 cm in each direction laterally and 2–3 cm below the level of the anterior superior iliac spine but above the internal ring. The anterior rectus sheath and the oblique muscles are incised for the length of the skin incision. The lower flaps of these structures are retracted inferiorly toward the pubis. The transversalis fascia is incised along the lateral edge of the rectus muscle and the preperitoneal space entered. If a lower midline or Pfannenstiel incision is used, the fascia overlying the space of Retzius is opened without violating the peritoneum. A combination of blunt and sharp dissection is continued laterally, posterior to the rectus muscle and the inferior epigastric vessels. The preperitoneal space is completely dissected to a point lateral to the anterior superior iliac spine. The symphysis pubis, a Cooper ligament and the iliopubic tract are identified. Inferiorly the peritoneum is generously dissected away from the vas deferens and the internal spermatic vessels to create a large pocket that will eventually accommodate a prosthesis without the possibility of roll-up. The term "parietalization" of the spermatic cord was popularized by Stoppa and refers to the thorough dissection of the cord to provide enough length to move it laterally.

Direct hernia sacs are reduced during the course of the preperitoneal dissection. When reducing the peritoneum from a direct hernia defect, it is important to stay in the plane between the peritoneum and the transversalis fascia allowing the latter structure to retract back into the hernia defect toward the skin. The transversalis fascia can be thin and if it is inadvertently opened and incorporated with the peritoneal sac during reduction a needless and bloody dissection of the abdominal wall is the result. Indirect sacs are more difficult to deal with than direct as they can be adherent to the cord structures. Care must be taken to minimize trauma to the cord to prevent damage to the vas deferens or the blood supply to the testicle. If it is a small sac it should be mobilized from the cord structures and reduced back into the peritoneal cavity. A larger sac may be difficult to mobilize from the cord without undue trauma if an attempt is made to remove the sac in its entirety. In this situation, the sac should be divided, leaving the distal sac in situ with dissection of the proximal sac away from the cord structures. Division of the sac is easily accomplished by opening the side opposite of the cord structures. A finger can be placed in the sac to facilitate its separation from the cord. Downward traction is placed on the cord structures to reduce excessive amounts of fatty tissue (lipoma of the cord) into the preperitoneal space to preclude the possibility of a "pseudo-recurrence" when the fatty tissue is palpated during physical examination postoperatively.

Management of the abdominal wall defect varies somewhat. Stoppa and Wantz usually leave the defect alone but the transversalis fascia in the defect occasionally is plicated by suturing it to a Cooper ligament to prevent the bulge caused by a seroma in the undisturbed sac.

The next step is the placement of the prosthesis. Dacron mesh is more pliable than polypropylene and is therefore considered particularly suitable for this procedure as it conforms well to the preperitoneal space. For unilateral repairs, the size of the prosthesis is approximately the distance between the umbilicus and the anterior superior iliac spine minus 1 cm for the width, with the height being approximately 14 cm. Wantz recommends cutting the prosthesis excentrically with the lateral side longer than the medial to achieve the best fit in the preperitoneal space. Because of his thorough parietalization of the cord structures, Stoppa indicates that it is not necessary to split the prosthesis laterally to accommodate the cord structures. This avoids the keyhole defect created when the prosthesis is split, which has been incriminated in recurrences. Rignault, on the other hand, prefers a keyhole defect in the mesh to encircle the spermatic cord, feeling that this provides the prosthesis with enough security that fixation sutures or tacks can be avoided. Minimizing fixation in this area is important because of the numerous anatomical elements in the preperitoneal space that may be inadvertently damaged during their placement. For Wantz's technique, three absorbable sutures are used to attach the superior border of the prosthesis to the anterior abdominal wall well above the defect. The three sutures are placed near the linea alba, semilunar line, and the anterior superior iliac spine from medial to lateral. A Reverdin suture needle facilitates this. Three long clamps are placed on each corner and the middle of the inferior border of the prosthesis. The medial clamp is placed in the space of Retzius and held by an assistant. The middle clamp is positioned so that the mesh covers the pubic ramus, obturator fossa and the iliac vessels, and is similarly held by an assistant. The lateral clamp is placed into the iliac fossa to cover the parietalized cord structures and the iliopsoas muscle. Care must be taken to prevent the prosthesis from rolling up as the clamps are removed. Stoppa's technique is most often associated with one large prosthesis for bilateral hernias. The dimensions of this prosthesis are the distance between the two anterior superior iliac spines minus 2 cm for the width and the height is equal to the distance between the umbilicus and the pubis. The prosthesis is cut in a chevron shape and eight clamps are positioned strategically around the prosthesis to facilitate placement into the preperitoneal space. The wound is closed in layers.

Nyhus/Condon (iliopubic tract repair). The names Nyhus and Condon are firmly associated with this preperitoneal repair, especially in North America. The two authorities carried out extensive cadaver dissections and pointed out the importance of the iliopubic tract, which is the reason why their operation is referred to as the Iliopubic Tract Repair. A transverse lower abdominal incision is made two fingerbreadths above the symphysis pubis. The anterior rectus sheath is opened on its lateral side to allow the rectus muscle to be retracted medially and the two oblique and the transversus abdominis muscles are incised exposing the transversalis fascia. A combination of sharp and blunt dissection inferiorly opens the preperitoneal space and exposes the posterior inguinal floor. Direct or indirect defects are similarly repaired after the peritoneal sac has been reduced or divided and closed proximally. The transverse aponeurotic arch is sutured to the iliopubic tract inferiorly, occasionally including a Cooper ligament in the first few medial sutures. If the internal ring is particularly large, a suture is placed lateral to the internal ring. For femoral hernias, the iliopubic tract is sutured to a Cooper ligament to close the canal. Once the defect has been formally repaired, a tailored mesh prosthesis can be sutured to a Cooper ligament and the transversalis fascia for reinforcement. Initially this was only recommended for recurrent hernias but with further patient follow up, it has now become routine for all hernias.

Kugel/Ugahary. These conventional preperitoneal prosthetic repairs were developed to compete with laparoscopy by using a small 2–3-cm skin incision, approximately 2–3 cm above the internal ring. Kugel locates this point by making an oblique incision one third lateral and two thirds medial to a point half way between the anterior superior iliac spine and the pubic tubercle. The incision is carried deep through the external oblique fascia and the internal oblique muscle is bluntly spread. The transversalis fascia is opened vertically approximately 3 cm, but the internal ring is not violated. The preperitoneal space is entered and a blunt dissection performed. The inferior epigastric vessels are identified to assure that the dissection is in the correct plane. These vessels should be left adherent to the overlying transversalis fascia and retracted medially and anteriorly. The iliac vessels, a Cooper ligament, pubic bone, and hernia defect are identified by palpation. Most hernia sacs are simply reduced. The exception is large indirect sacs that often are divided to leave the distal sac in situ with proximal sac closure. The author feels that the cord structures must be thoroughly parietalized to allow adequate posterior dissection if recurrences are to be avoided. The basis of the procedure is a specifically designed 8- × 12-cm prosthesis made of two pieces of polypropylene with a specially extruded single monofilament fiber located near its edge circumferentially. This allows the prosthesis to be formed to fit through the small incision. Once through the incision, it springs open to regain its normal shape to provide a wide overlap of the myopectineal orifice. The prosthesis also has a slit on its anterior surface through which the surgeon places his finger to facilitate postioning.

Ugahary's operation is similar but a special prosthesis is not required. Known as the gridiron technique, the preperitoneal space is prepared through a 3 cm incision in a manner similar to Kugel. The space is held open using a narrow Langenbeck and two ribbon retractors. A 10- × 15-cm piece of polypropylene mesh is rolled onto a long forceps after the edges have been rounded and sutures placed to correspond to various anatomical landmarks. The rolled-up mesh is introduced with forceps into the preperitoneal space and the mesh unrolled using clamps and strategic movements of the ribbon retractors.

Both of these operations have been very successful in some hands and have important proponents, but because they are essentially blind, considerable experience is required to assure that the patch has been placed properly.

Laparoscopic Inguinal Herniorrhaphy

The best indications for a laparoscopic inguinal herniorrhaphy are: (1) a recurrent hernia after a conventional repair because the operation is performed in normal, nonscarred tissue; (2) bilateral hernias, as both sides can easily be repaired using the same small laparoscopic incisions; and (3) the presence of an inguinal hernia in a patient who requires a laparoscopy for another procedure, i.e., a laparoscopic cholecystectomy (assuming the Gram stain of the bile is negative). The more contentious issue is the use of laparoscopy for the uncomplicated unilateral hernia. Meta-analyses have confirmed a significant advantage of the laparoscopic operation over the conventional nonprosthetic repairs in terms of pain, return to activity and recurrence rate. However, there is no difference in recurrence rate when comparing laparoscopy with prosthetic tension free repairs and the laparoscopic operation takes longer. Laparoscopic herniorrhaphy patients return to work quicker and have less persisting pain and numbness. The laparoscopic operation costs more but the difference may be offset by the more rapid recovery. Operative complications are uncommon for both methods but serious complications such as bowel perforation, bowel obstruction, vascular injury or adhesive problems at sites where the peritoneum has been breached or prosthetic material has been placed are seen almost exclusively with laparoscopy.

Absolute contraindications include any sign of intraabdominal infection or coagulopathy. Relative contraindications include intraabdominal adhesions from previous surgery, ascites or previous "Space of Retzius" surgery because of the increased risk of bladder injury. Severe underlying medical illness is also a relative contraindication because of the added risk of general anesthesia. These patients are better suited for a conventional operation under local anesthesia. An incarcerated sliding scrotal hernia is a relative contraindication especially when involving the sigmoid colon because of the risk of perforation because of the traction needed to reduce it.

The two commonly performed laparoscopic herniorrhaphies, the transabdominal preperitoneal (TAPP) and the totally extraperitoneal (TEP) are modeled after the conventional preperitoneal operations described above. The major difference is that the preperitoneal space is entered through three trocar sites rather than a large conventional incision. The ensuing radical dissection of the preperitoneal space with the placement of a large prosthesis is similar to the conventional preperitoneal operation.

Transabdominal Preperitoneal

The operating room setup for the TAPP procedure. The surgeon stands on the opposite side of the table from the hernia. The first assistant stands opposite the surgeon. Three laparoscopic cannulae are placed in a horizontal plane with the umbilicus. After an initial diagnostic laparoscopy, pertinent anatomic landmarks including the median and medial umbilical ligaments, the bladder, the inferior epigastric vessels, the vas deferens, the spermatic vessels, the external iliac vessels and the hernia defect are identified. An incision of the peritoneum is initiated at the medial umbilical ligament at least 2 cm above the hernia defect and extended laterally toward the anterior superior iliac spine. The preperitoneal space is exposed using a combination of blunt and sharp dissection, mobilizing the peritoneal flap inferiorly. The symphysis pubis, a Cooper ligament, the iliopubic tract, and the cord structures are identified. Direct hernia sacs are reduced during this dissection. Indirect sacs are more difficult to deal with as they can be tenaciously adherent to the cord structures. The cord structures must be skeletonized but care must be taken to minimize trauma to prevent damage to the vas deferens or the blood supply to the testicle. The peritoneal flap is dissected inferiorly well proximal to the divergence of the vas deferens and the internal spermatic vessels to assure that the prosthesis will lie flat in the preperitoneal space and will not roll up when the peritoneum is closed.

A large piece of mesh, 15 × 11 cm or greater, is introduced into the abdominal cavity through the umbilical cannula and is positioned over the myopectineal orifice so that it completely covers the direct, indirect and femoral spaces. The landmarks for achieving this goal are the contralateral pubic tubercle and the symphysis pubis for the medial edge, a Cooper ligament or the tissue just above it for the inferior border, and the posterior rectus sheath and transversalis fascia at least 2 cm above the hernia defect superiorly. Some surgeons prefer to slit the mesh to accommodate the cord structures whereas others prefer to simply place the prosthesis over them. Fixation of the mesh is controversial. When closing the peritoneum, it is important to avoid gaps because small bowel has been known to find its way through them resulting in a clinical bowel obstruction.

Totally Extraperitoneal

The preperitoneal space is entered by establishing a plane of dissection outside of the peritoneal cavity between the posterior surface of the rectus muscle and the posterior rectus sheath and peritoneum. An incision is made at the umbilicus as if one were planning to perform open laparoscopy. The rectus sheath is opened on one side and the rectus muscle is retracted laterally. The space is enlarged by blunt or balloon dissection. Once the space is sufficiently enlarged, three additional cannulas are placed in the midline; one at the umbilicus for the optics, another approximately 5 cm above the symphysis pubis and the final cannula midway between the umbilicus and the symphysis pubis. Dissection of the preperitoneal space is now possible under direct vision. The operation then proceeds in an identical fashion to the TAPP procedure described above.

TAPP versus TEP. The Achilles heel of the TAPP procedure is the peritoneal closure. The peritoneum is frequently thin and tears easily once dissected, making it difficult to obtain complete coverage of the prosthesis. This has resulted in major complications. The TEP procedure is more demanding than the TAPP initially because of the limited working space but once mastered completely eliminates the peritoneal closure step, making it faster.

COMPLICATIONS OF GROIN HERNIA REPAIRS (Table 36-3)

Groin Hernias in Females

Groin hernias are much less common in females than males. Less than 10 percent of all elective inguinal hernia repairs are performed in women. Nevertheless, given the overall frequency of the condition, the absolute number is still significant. Femoral hernias are ten times more common in women than men (10 percent in females vs. 1 percent in males), giving rise to the false notion that it is the most common groin hernia. In fact, indirect hernias are much more common. Direct hernias are rare almost to the point of being reportable. Occult inguinal hernias are a significant problem in women because the skin of the labium majus does not allow easy examination of the inguinal canal. There is insufficient skin redundancy to invert and allow the examining finger to coapt directly to the inguinal floor. The extensive differential diagnosis of groin pain makes the definitive diagnosis of an occult hernia difficult.

TABLE 36-3 Complications

Recurrence	C) Infection
Chronic Groin Pain	D) Rejection
Nociceptive	E) Fracture
A) Somatic	Laparoscopic
B) Visceral	Vascular injury
	A) Intra-abdominal
Neuropathic	B) Retroperitoneal
A) Iliohypogastric	C) Abdominal wall
B) Ilioinguinal	D) Gas embolism
C) Genitofemoral	Visceral injury
D) Lateral Cutaneous	A) Bowel perforation
E) Femoral	B) Bladder perforation
Cord and testicular	Trocar Site Complications
A) Hematoma	A) Hematoma
B) Ischemic orchitis	B) Hernia
C) Testicular atrophy	C) Wound infection
D) Dysejaculation	D) Keloid
E) Division of vas deferens	Bowel Obstruction
F) Hydrocele	A) Trocar or peritoneal closure site hernia
G) Testicular descent	B) Adhesions
Bladder Injury	Miscellaneous
Wound Infection	A) Diaphragmatic dysfunction
Seroma	B) Hypercapnia
Hematoma	General
A) Wound	Urinary
B) Scrotal	Paralytic ileus
C) Retroperitoneal	Nausea and vomiting
Osteitis pubis	Aspiration pneumonia
Prosthetic Complications	Cardiovascular
A) Contraction	Respiratory insufficiency
B) Erosion	

The indications for surgery are similar in males and females. There is no place for a strategy of watchful waiting for femoral hernias as the incidence of incarceration and/or strangulation is far too high to justify such a recommendation. The choice of procedure is not unique to females and is largely left to the surgeon based on experience and training. Resection of the round ligament simplifies many of the repairs because complete closure of the internal ring is then possible. Groin hernias become evident during pregnancy (1:1000–3000 pregnancies). They are best managed expectantly and repaired after gestation is complete.

PEDIATRIC HERNIAS

Most inguinal hernias in children are indirect, related to a persistent patent processes vaginalis. Approximately 1–5 percent of children are born with or develop an inguinal hernia. However, the incidence rises in preterm infants and those with low birth weights (13 percent of patients born before 32 weeks and 30 percent of patients with a birth weight less than 1,000 g). Overall, right-sided hernias are twice as common as left, and about 10 percent of hernias diagnosed at birth are bilateral. However, this varies greatly on the basis of numerous risk factors, the most important of which is age. The right-sided

TABLE 36-4 Conditions Associated with an Increased Incidence
of Pediatric Hernia

Family history
Undescended testis
Hypospadias/epispadias
Ventriculoperitoneal shunt
Peritoneal dialysis
Cryptorchism
Prematurity
Other abdominal wall defect
Cystic fibrosis
Ascites
Intersex conditions
Connective tissue disorders
Hunter-Hurler syndrome
Ehlers-Danlos syndrome

predominance is felt by most authorities to be related to the later descent of the right testicle during gestation. There are several conditions which predispose a child to develop an inguinal hernia in Table 36-4.

Infants or children may present with a mass in the groin or scrotum. The diagnosis may be obvious but one must be careful to differentiate the mass from other cord and testicular abnormalities such as a hydrocele, undescended testicle, varicocele or even a testicular tumor. Commonly no hernia is able to be demonstrated when the patient presents to the surgeon. Some surgeons rely on the so called "silk glove sign" which reflects the way the hernia sac feels as it is palpated over the cord structures. The finding is controversial and there is some evidence that what is actually being felt is hypertrophied cremasteric muscle. In the end, the diagnosis commonly hinges on the observation of the referring physician or a parent. Most surgeons feel the risk/benefit ratio favors this as an acceptable indication for operation when the source seems reliable rather than taking the chance of strangulation.

Incarceration is a more serious problem in the pediatric patient than in the adult, with large series reporting rates up to 20 percent. The patient presents with a hard, tender groin mass. In 75–80 percent of these, they can be successfully reduced initially using sedation, Trendelenburg position, ice packs and gentle taxis. A reasonable attempt at conservative management of an incarcerated pediatric hernia before proceeding to emergency surgery is in the patient's best interest because the complication rate compared to elective herniorrhaphy is twenty fold, including irreversible abnormalities such as testicular infarction or atrophy. If no progress in reduction is made within 6 h, or if the patient exhibits signs of peritonitis or systemic toxicity, immediate operation is appropriate.

Most pediatric inguinal hernias are repaired using the principle of high ligation of the sac. The external oblique aponeurosis is opened for a short distance beginning at the external ring and proceeding laterally. The sac is then gently dissected away from the cord structures proximally until the internal ring is reached, twisted, suture ligated and amputated. If the sac extends into the scrotum, it can be divided leaving the distal sac in situ. Care must be taken to exclude abdominal contents such as the tube and ovary before suture ligation. Occasionally, a Marcy repair of the internal ring is added if the structure is unusually large.

Exploration of the opposite groin remains controversial. As an alternative, ultrasound examination has become popular at some centers, however, it is largely dependent on the expertise and/or interest of the ultrasonographer. The size of the internal ring and the presence of bowel or fluid in the spermatic cord are diagnostic criteria indicative of a positive exam. Another alternative is laparoscopy using either a rigid or a flexible endoscope placed through the hernia sac to inspect the opposite side. The accuracy is high for properly trained laparoscopists, such that it is considered the gold standard in studies using both ultrasonography and laparoscopy. The disadvantage of laparoscopy is cost and potential intraabdominal complications.

Suggested Readings

Rutkow IM: Epidemiologic, economic, and sociologic aspects of hernia surgery in the United States in the 1990s. Surg Clin North Am 78:941, 1998.

van den Berg JC, de Valois JC, Go PM, Rosenbusch G: Detection of groin hernia with physical examination, ultrasound, and MRI compared with laparoscopic findings. Invest Radiol 34:739, 1999.

Read RC: Prosthesis in abdominal wall hernia surgery in prosthesis and abdominal wall hernias, in Bendavid R (ed): Title?. Austin, TX: RG Landes Co, 1994, p 2.

EU Hernia Trialists Collaboration: Repair of groin hernia with synthetic mesh: meta-analysis of randomized controlled trials. Ann Surg 235:322, 2002.

Castrini G, Pappalardo G, Trentino P, et al: The original Bassini technique in the surgical treatment of inguinal hernia. Int Surgery 71:141, 1986.

Millikan KW, Cummings B, Doolas A: A prospective study of mesh plug hernioplasty. Am Surg 67:285, 2001.

Stoppa RE: The midline preperitoneal approach and prosthetic repair of groin hernias, in Fitzgibbons Jr. RJ, Greenburg AG (eds): Nyhus and Condon's Hernia, 5th ed. Philadelphia: Lippincott Williams & Wilkins, 2002, p 199.

The EU Hernia Trialists Collaboration: Laparoscopic compared with open methods of groin hernia repair: systematic review of randomized controlled trials. Br J Surg 87:860, 2000.

Bringman S, Ramel S, Heikkinen TJ, et al: Tension-free inguinal hernia repair: TEP versus mesh-plug versus Lichtenstein: a prospective randomized controlled trial. Ann Surg 237:142, 2003.

Bendavid R: Compications of groin hernia surgery. Surg Clin North Am 78:1089, 1998.

Bendavid R: Femoral hernias in females: Facts, figures, and fallacies, in Bendavid R (ed): Prostheses and Abdominal Wall Hernias. Austin, TX: Landes Publishing, 1994, p 82.

Kurkchubasche AG, Tracy TF: Unique features of groin hernia repair in infants and children, in Fitzgibbons RJ Jr., Greenburg AG (eds): Nyhus and Condon's Hernia, 5th ed. Philadelphia: Lippincott Williams & Wilkins, 2002, p 435.

Chen KC, Chu CC, Chou TY, et al: Ultrasonography for inguinal hernias in boys. J Pediatr Surg 34:1890, 1999.

37 | Thyroid, Parathyroid, and Adrenal

Geeta Lal and Orlo H. Clark

THYROID

Embryology

The thyroid gland arises as an outpouching of the primitive foregut around the third week of gestation, originating at the base of the tongue in the vicinity of the foramen cecum. Endoderm cells in the floor of the pharyngeal anlage thicken to form the medial thyroid anlage that descends in the neck anterior to structures that form the hyoid bone and larynx and gives rise to the thyroid follicular cells. Paired lateral anlages (of neuroectodermal origin) originate from the fourth branchial pouch, fuse with the median anlage at approximately the fifth week of gestation and provide the calcitonin producing parafollicular or C cells.

Developmental Abnormalities

Thyroglossal Duct Cyst and Sinus

During the fifth week of gestation, the thyroglossal duct, which connects the thyroid with the foramen cecum, starts to obliterate. Thyroglossal duct cysts may occur anywhere along the migratory path of the thyroid, although 80 percent are found in juxtaposition to the hyoid bone. They are usually asymptomatic, but occasionally become infected by oral bacteria. Sinuses result from infection of the cyst secondary to spontaneous or surgical drainage and are accompanied by minor inflammation of the surrounding skin. The diagnosis is usually established by observing smooth, well-defined midline neck mass that moves upward with tongue protrusion. Routine thyroid imaging is not necessary. Treatment involves the "Sistrunk operation," which consists of en bloc cystectomy and excision of the central hyoid bone to minimize recurrence.

Lingual Thyroid

This represents failure of the median thyroid anlage to descend normally and may be the only thyroid tissue present. Some patients are hypothyroid and intervention becomes necessary for obstructive symptoms such as choking, dysphagia, airway obstruction, and hemorrhage. Treatment options include administration of exogenous thyroid hormone to treat hypothyroidism or to suppress thyroid-stimulating hormone (TSH), radioactive iodine, or surgical excision.

Ectopic thyroid. Normal thyroid tissue may be found anywhere in the central neck compartment and also has been observed adjacent to the aortic arch, in the aortopulmonary window, within the upper pericardium, and in the interventricular septum. Thyroid tissue situated lateral to the carotid sheath and jugular vein, previously termed "lateral aberrant thyroid," almost always represents metastatic thyroid cancer in lymph nodes.

943

Pyramidal lobe. In approximately 50 percent of individuals, the distal end of the thyroglossal duct that connects to the thyroid persists as a pyramidal lobe projecting up from the isthmus, lying just to the left or right of the midline.

Thyroid Anatomy

The adult thyroid gland is brown in color, weighs about 20 g, and is located posterior to the strap muscles. The thyroid lobes are located adjacent to the thyroid cartilage and are connected in the midline by an isthmus. The thyroid is enveloped by loosely connecting fascia that is formed from the partitioning of the deep cervical fascia into anterior and posterior divisions. The thyroid capsule is condensed into the posterior suspensory or Berry ligament near the cricoid cartilage and upper tracheal rings. The gland is well vascularized by two major sets of arteries. The superior thyroid arteries arise from the ipsilateral external carotid arteries. The inferior thyroid arteries are derived from the thyrocervical trunk shortly after their origin from the subclavian arteries. The inferior thyroid arteries travel upward in the neck posterior to the carotid sheath to enter the thyroid lobes at their midpoint. A thyroidea ima artery arises directly from the aorta or innominate in 1–4 percent of individuals, to enter the isthmus or replace a missing inferior thyroid artery. Venous drainage of the thyroid gland occurs via multiple small surface veins, which coalesce to form three sets of veins—the superior, middle, and inferior thyroid veins.

The left recurrent laryngeal nerve (RLN) arises from the vagus nerve where it crosses the aortic arch, loops around the ligamentum arteriosum and ascends medially in the neck within the tracheoesophageal groove. The right RLN arises from the vagus at its crossing with the right subclavian artery, and passes posterior to the artery before ascending in the neck. The RLNs may branch, and pass anterior, posterior or interdigitate with branches of the inferior thyroid artery and terminate by entering the larynx posterior to the cricothyroid muscle. The RLNs innervate all the intrinsic muscles of the larynx, except the cricothyroid muscles.

The superior laryngeal nerves also arise from the vagus nerves and travel along the internal carotid artery. The internal branch is sensory to the supraglottic larynx, whereas the external branch of the superior laryngeal nerve lies on the inferior pharyngeal constrictor muscle and descends alongside the superior thyroid vessels before innervating the cricothyroid muscle.

The thyroid gland is endowed with an extensive network of lymphatics. Regional lymph nodes include pretracheal, paratracheal, perithyroidal, recurrent laryngeal nerve, superior mediastinal, retropharyngeal, esophageal, and upper, middle, and lower jugular chain nodes.

Thyroid Histology

Microscopically, the thyroid is divided into lobules that contain 20–40 follicles averaging 30 μm in diameter. Each follicle is lined by cuboidal epithelial cells and contains a central store of colloid secreted from the epithelial cells under the influence of the pituitary hormone, TSH. C cells or parafollicular cells, which secrete calcitonin, are found as individual cells or clumped in the interfollicular stroma.

THYROID PHYSIOLOGY

Thyroid Hormone Synthesis, Secretion, and Transport

The average daily iodine requirement is 0.1 mg. Dietary iodine is rapidly converted to iodide and absorbed into the bloodstream. Iodide is actively transported into the thyroid follicular cells by an ATP-dependent process. The synthesis of thyroid hormone consists of several steps: (1) iodide trapping which involves ATP-dependent transport of iodide across the basement membrane of the thyrocyte via the Na+/I- symporter (NIS); (2) oxidation of iodide to iodine and iodination of tyrosine residues on Thyroglobulin (Tg), a 660-kDa glycoprotein, which is present in thyroid follicles, to form monoiodotyrosines (MITs) and diiodotyrosines (DITs)—both processes are catalyzed by thyroid peroxidase; (3) coupling of two DIT molecules to form tetraiodothyronine or thyroxine (T4), and one DIT molecule with one MIT molecule to form 3,5,3′-triiodothyronine (T3) or reverse 3,3′,5′-triiodothyronine (rT3); (4) hydrolysis of Tg to release free iodothyronines (T3 and T4) and mono- and diiodotyrosines; and (5) deiodination of mono and diiodotyrosines to yield iodide, which is reused in the thyrocyte.

In the euthyroid state, T4 is the predominant hormone produced by the thyroid. Most T3 (80 percent) is produced by extrathyroidal, peripheral deiodination (removal of 5′-iodine from the outer ring) of T4 in the liver, muscles, kidney, and anterior pituitary, a reaction that is catalyzed by 5′-monodeiodinase. Some T4 is converted to rT3, the metabolically inactive compound, by deiodination of the inner ring of T4. Thyroid hormones are transported in serum bound to carrier proteins such as thyroxine-binding globulin (TBG), thyroxine-binding prealbumin (TBPA), and albumin. Only a small fraction (0.02 percent) of thyroid hormone (T3 and T4) is free (unbound) and is the physiologically active component. The secretion of thyroid hormone is controlled by the hypothalamic–pituitary–thyroid axis.

EVALUATION OF PATIENTS WITH THYROID DISEASE

Tests of Thyroid Function

No single test is sufficient to assess thyroid function in all situations and the results must be interpreted in the context of the patient's clinical condition.

Serum TSH – (normal 0.5 to 5 μU/mL) Serum TSH levels reflect the ability of the anterior pituitary to detect free T4 levels. There is an inverse relationship between the free T4 level and the logarithm of the TSH concentration—small changes in free T4 lead to a large shift in TSH levels. Thus, the ultrasensitive TSH assay has become the most sensitive and specific test for the diagnosis of hyper- and hypothyroidism and for optimizing T4 replacement and suppressive therapy.

Total T4 and Total T3 – Total T4 (reference range: 55–150 nmol/L) and T3 (reference range: 1.5–3.5 nmol/L) levels are measured by radioimmunoassay and measure both the free and bound components of the hormones. Total T4 levels reflect the output from the thyroid gland, whereas T3 levels in the nonstimulated thyroid gland are more indicative of peripheral thyroid hormone metabolism.

Free T4 and Free T3 – These radioimmunoassay-based tests are a sensitive and accurate measurement of biologically active thyroid hormone. Free T4 (reference range: 12 to 28 pmol/L) measurement is confined to cases of early hyperthyroidism in which total T4 levels may be normal but free T4 levels are raised. In patients with end-organ resistance to T4 (Refetoff syndrome), T4 levels are increased, but TSH levels usually are normal. Free T3 (reference range: 3 to 9 pmol/L) is most useful in confirming the diagnosis of early hyperthyroidism, in which levels of free T4 and free T3 rise before total T4 and T3.

Thyroid Antibodies – Thyroid antibodies include antithyroglobulin (anti-Tg), antimicrosomal or antithyroid peroxidase (anti-TPO) and thyroid-stimulating immunoglobulin (TSI). Anti-Tg and anti-TPO antibody levels do not determine thyroid function; instead, they indicate the underlying disorder, usually an autoimmune thyroiditis.

Serum Thyroglobulin – Thyroglobulin is not normally released into the circulation in large amounts, but increases dramatically in thyroiditis or Graves disease and toxic multinodular goiter. The most important use for serum thyroglobulin levels is in monitoring patients with differentiated thyroid cancer for recurrence. Because only thyroid tissues produce thyroglobulin, the levels of this protein should be low after total thyroidectomy.

Thyroid Imaging

Radionuclide imaging. Both iodine-123 (123I) and iodine-131 (131I) are used to image the thyroid gland. The former emits low-dose radiation, has a half-life of 12–14 h, and is used to image lingual thyroids or goiters. In contrast, 131I use leads to higher-dose radiation exposure and has a half-life of 8–10 days. Therefore, this isotope is used to screen and treat patients with differentiated thyroid cancers for metastatic disease. Areas that trap less radioactivity than the surrounding gland are termed "cold" whereas areas that demonstrate increased activity are termed "hot". The risk of malignancy is higher in "cold" lesions (15–20 percent) than in "hot" or "warm" lesions (< 5 percent). Technetium-99m (99mTc) pertechnetate is taken up by the thyroid gland, but is not organified. It also has the advantage of having a shorter half-life and minimizes radiation exposure. It is particularly sensitive for nodal metastases. More recently, 18F-fluorodeoxyglucose positron emission tomography (FDG PET) has been used to screen for metastases in thyroglobulin-positive patients with thyroid cancer, in whom other imaging studies are negative.

Ultrasound. Ultrasound is helpful in the evaluation of thyroid nodules, distinguishing solid from cystic ones, and providing information about size and multicentricity. Ultrasound also can be used to assess for cervical lymphadenopathy and to guide fine-needle aspiration (FNA) biopsy.

CT/MRI scan. These studies are primarily used in evaluating the extent of large, fixed, or substernal goiters and their relationship to the airway and vascular structures.

BENIGN THYROID DISORDERS

Hyperthyroidism

Graves Disease

Graves disease is, by far, the most common cause of hyperthyroidism in North America, accounting for 60–80 percent of cases. It is an autoimmune disorder of unknown cause with a strong familial predisposition, female preponderance

(5:1), and peak incidence between the ages of 40 and 60 years. It is characterized by thyrotoxicosis, diffuse goiter, and extrathyroidal manifestations, including ophthalmopathy, dermopathy (pretibial myxedema), thyroid acropachy, gynecomastia, and others.

Etiology, pathogenesis, and pathology. The exact etiology of the initiation of the autoimmune process in Graves disease is unknown. However, conditions such as the postpartum state, iodine excess, lithium therapy, and bacterial and viral infections have been suggested as possible triggers. Graves disease also is associated with certain human leukocyte antigen (HLA) haplotypes and polymorphisms of the cytotoxic T-lymphocyte antigen 4 (CTLA-4) gene. Once initiated, the process causes sensitized T-helper lymphocytes to stimulate B lymphocytes, which produce antibodies directed against the thyroid hormone receptor (TRAbs). Thyroid stimulating immunoglobulins (TSI), and TSH-binding inhibiting immunoglobulins (TSIIs) have been described. These antibodies stimulate the thyrocytes to grow and synthesize excess thyroid hormone, which is a hallmark of Graves disease.

Clinical features. Symptoms of hyperthyroidism include heat intolerance, increased sweating and thirst, and weight loss despite adequate caloric intake. Symptoms of increased adrenergic stimulation include palpitations, nervousness, fatigue, emotional lability, hyperkinesis, and tremors. Female patients often develop amenorrhea, decreased fertility, and an increased incidence of miscarriages. Children experience rapid growth with early bone maturation, whereas older patients present with cardiovascular complications. On physical examination, weight loss and facial flushing may be evident. The skin may be warm and moist. Tachycardia or atrial fibrillation, a fine tremor, muscle wasting, and proximal muscle group weakness with hyperactive tendon reflexes often are present.

Approximately 50 percent of patients with Graves disease also develop clinically evident ophthalmopathy. Eye symptoms include lid lag (von Graefe sign), spasm of the upper eyelid revealing the sclera above the corneoscleral limbus (Dalrymple sign), and a prominent stare as a consequence of catecholamine excess. True infiltrative eye disease results in periorbital edema, conjunctival swelling and congestion (chemosis), proptosis, limitation of upward and lateral gaze, keratitis, and even blindness. The etiology of Graves ophthalmopathy is not completely known. Dermopathy occurs in 1–2 percent of patients and is characterized by deposition of glycosaminoglycans leading to thickened skin in the pretibial region. The thyroid is usually diffusely and symmetrically enlarged. There may be an overlying bruit or thrill and loud venous hum in the supraclavicular space.

Diagnostic tests. The diagnosis of hyperthyroidism is made by a suppressed TSH with or without an elevated free T4 or T3 level. In the absence of eye findings, an 123I uptake and scan should be performed. An elevated uptake, with a diffusely enlarged gland confirms the diagnosis of Graves disease and helps to differentiate it from other causes of hyperthyroidism. Anti-Tg and anti-TPO antibodies are elevated in up to 75 percent of patients, but are not specific. Elevated thyroid-stimulating hormone receptor (TSH-R) or TSAb are diagnostic of Graves disease and are increased in approximately 90 percent of patients. MRI scans of the orbits are useful in evaluating ophthalmopathy.

Treatment

Antithyroid drugs. These are generally administered in preparation for radioactive iodine ablation or surgery. The medications commonly used are propylthiouracil (PTU, 100–300 mg three times daily) and methimazole (10–30 mg three times daily). Methimazole has a longer half-life and can be dosed once daily. Both drugs reduce thyroid hormone production by inhibiting the organic binding of iodine and the coupling of iodotyrosines. Additionally, PTU also inhibits the peripheral conversion of T4 to T3. Both drugs can cross the placenta, inhibiting fetal thyroid function, and are excreted in breast milk, although PTU has a lower risk of transplacental transfer. Side effects of treatment include reversible granulocytopenia, skin rashes, fever, peripheral neuritis, polyarteritis, vasculitis, and, rarely, liver failure, agranulocytosis, and aplastic anemia.

Most patients have improved symptoms in 2 weeks and become euthyroid in about 6 weeks. Treatment with antithyroid medications is associated with a high relapse rate when these drugs are discontinued. Therefore, treatment for curative intent is reserved for patients with small, nontoxic goiters (< 40 g) and mildly elevated thyroid hormone levels. The catecholamine hyperthyroidism response can be alleviated by administering β-blocking agents. These drugs have the added effect of decreasing the peripheral conversion of T4 to T3. Propranolol is the most commonly prescribed medication in doses of about 20–40 mg four times daily.

Radioactive iodine therapy. Radioactive iodine (RAI; 131I) forms the mainstay of Graves disease treatment in North America. Antithyroid drugs are discontinued to maximize drug uptake. The 131I dose is calculated after a preliminary uptake and scan, and usually consists of 8–12 mCi administered orally. However, RAI is associated with the progressive development of hypothyroidism (over 70 percent at 11 years), requiring lifelong thyroxine replacement therapy and also has been shown to lead to progression of ophthalmopathy. Consequently, RAI therapy most often is used in older patients with small or moderate-size goiters, in patients who have relapsed after medical or surgical therapy, and in patients in whom antithyroid drugs or surgery are contraindicated.

Surgical treatment. In North America, surgery is recommended in patients who (1) have coexistent, confirmed cancer or suspicious thyroid nodules, (2) are young, (3) are pregnant or desire to conceive soon after treatment, (4) have allergies to antithyroid medications, (5) have large goiters causing compressive symptoms, and (6) are reluctant to undergo RAI therapy. Relative indications for thyroidectomy include patients, particularly smokers, with moderate to severe Graves ophthalmopathy, patients who desire rapid control of hyperthyroidism with a chance of being euthyroid, and patients who demonstrate poor compliance with antithyroid medications. The goal of thyroidectomy for Graves disease should be the complete and permanent control of the disease with minimal morbidity related to RLN injury or hypoparathyroidism.

Patients are rendered euthyroid before operation with antithyroid drugs that should be continued up to the day of surgery. Lugol iodide solution or supersaturated potassium iodide (SSKI) is administered preoperatively—3 drops twice daily beginning 10 days preoperatively—to reduce vascularity of the gland and decrease the risk of precipitating thyroid storm. The extent of thyroidectomy to be performed is controversial and is determined by the desired outcome (risk of recurrence versus euthyroidism) and surgeon experience. Patients with coexistent thyroid cancer, and those patients who refuse RAI therapy, who have severe ophthalmopathy, or who have life-threatening reactions to antithyroid medications should undergo total or near-total thyroidectomy, which can be performed with minimal morbidity by an experienced thyroid surgeon. A subtotal thyroidectomy, leaving a 4–7-g remnant, is recommended for all remaining patients.

Toxic Multinodular Goiter

Toxic multinodular goiters usually occur in individuals older than 50 years of age who often have a prior history of a nontoxic multinodular goiter. Over several years, enough thyroid nodules become autonomous to cause hyperthyroidism. Symptoms and signs of hyperthyroidism are similar to Graves disease, but are less severe and extrathyroidal manifestations are absent.

Diagnostic studies and treatment. TSH is suppressed with elevated free T4 or T3 levels. RAI uptake also is increased, showing multiple nodules with increased uptake and suppression of the remaining gland. Surgical resection is the preferred treatment method, with subtotal thyroidectomy being the standard procedure. RAI therapy is reserved for older adult patients who represent very poor operative risks, provided there is no airway compression from the goiter and thyroid cancer is not a concern.

Plummer Disease (Toxic Adenoma)

Hyperthyroidism from a single hyperfunctioning nodule typically occurs in younger patients who note recent growth of a long-standing nodule along with the symptoms of hyperthyroidism. Most hyperfunctioning nodules have attained a size of at least 3 cm before hyperthyroidism occurs. RAI scanning shows a "hot" nodule with suppression of the rest of the thyroid gland. These nodules are rarely malignant. Smaller nodules may be managed with antithyroid medications and RAI, surgery (lobectomy and isthmusectomy) is recommended to treat young patients and those with larger nodules.

Thyroiditis

Thyroiditis is defined as an inflammatory disorder of the thyroid gland and usually is classified into acute, subacute, and chronic forms, each associated with a distinct clinical presentation and histology. Chronic and subacute thyroiditis are usually managed medically, but surgical treatment is occasionally needed for these conditions, and for acute suppurative thyroiditis.

Goiter

Most nontoxic goiters result from iodine deficiency and/or TSH stimulation secondary to inadequate thyroid hormone synthesis and other paracrine growth factors. Goiters may be diffuse, uninodular, or multinodular. Familial goiters result from inherited deficiencies in enzymes necessary for thyroid hormone synthesis. The term endemic goiter refers to the occurrence of a goiter in a significant proportion of individuals in a particular geographic region. In the past, dietary iodine deficiency was the most common cause of endemic goiter. This condition has largely disappeared in North America as a consequence of routine use of iodized salt and iodination of fertilizers, animal feeds, and preservatives. However, in areas of iodine deficiency, such as Central Asia,

South America, and Indonesia, up to 90 percent of the population have goiters. Other dietary goitrogens include cassava and cabbage. In many sporadic goiters, no obvious cause can be identified, but in some patients, it is familial.

Clinical Features

Most patients with nontoxic goiters are asymptomatic. As the goiters become very large compressive symptoms, such as dyspnea and dysphagia, ensue. Dysphonia from recurrent laryngeal nerve injury is rare, except when malignancy is present. Obstruction of venous return at the thoracic inlet from a substernal goiter results in a positive Pemberton sign—facial flushing and dilatation of cervical veins on raising the arms above the head. Sudden enlargement of nodules because of hemorrhage or cysts may cause acute pain. Physical examination may reveal a soft, diffusely enlarged gland (simple goiter) or nodules of various size and consistency in case of a multinodular goiter. Tracheal deviation with or without compression is common.

Diagnostic Tests and Treatment

Patients are usually euthyroid with normal TSH and low-normal or normal free T4 levels. If some nodules develop autonomy, patients have suppressed TSH levels or become hyperthyroid. FNA biopsy is recommended in euthyroid patients who have a dominant nodule or one that is painful or enlarging.

Most euthyroid patients with small, diffuse goiters do not require treatment. Some physicians give patients with large goiters exogenous thyroid hormone to reduce the TSH stimulation of gland growth; this treatment may result in a decrease and/or stabilization of goiter size. Endemic goiters are treated by iodine administration, but its use is controversial. Surgical resection is reserved for goiters that (1) continue to increase despite T4 suppression, (2) cause obstructive symptoms, (3) have substernal extension, (4) are suspected to be malignant or are proven malignant by FNA biopsy, and (5) are cosmetically unacceptable. Total lobectomy on the side of the dominant nodule and subtotal resection of the contralateral side is the treatment of choice and patients require lifelong T4 therapy to prevent recurrence.

SOLITARY THYROID NODULE

Solitary thyroid nodules are present in approximately 4 percent of the population, whereas thyroid cancer has a much lower incidence of 40 new cases per 1 million. Therefore, it is of utmost importance to determine which patients with solitary thyroid nodule would benefit from surgery.

History

Details regarding the nodule, such as time of onset, change in size, and associated symptoms, such as pain, dysphagia, dyspnea, or choking, should be elicited. Pain is an unusual symptom and when present, should raise suspicion for intrathyroidal hemorrhage in a benign nodule, thyroiditis, or malignancy. A history of hoarseness is worrisome because it may be secondary to malignant involvement of the recurrent laryngeal nerves. Most importantly, patients should be questioned regarding risk factors for malignancy, such as exposure to ionizing radiation and family history of thyroid and other malignancies associated with thyroid cancer.

Physical Examination

Thyroid masses move with swallowing, and failure to observe the patient swallowing may lead one to miss a large substernal goiter. Nodules that are hard, gritty, or fixed to surrounding structures, such as to the trachea or strap muscles, are more likely to be malignant. The ipsilateral and contralateral jugular and posterior triangle lymph nodes should be assessed.

Diagnostic Tests

A fine-needle aspiration biopsy is the most important diagnostic test. After FNA biopsy, the majority of nodules can be categorized into: benign (65 percent), suspicious (20 percent), malignant (5 percent), and nondiagnostic (10 percent). The incidence of false-positive results is approximately 1 percent and false-negative results occur in approximately 3 percent of patients. Benign lesions include cysts and colloid nodules. The risk of malignancy in this setting is less than 3 percent. The risk of malignancy in the setting of a suspicious cytology is anywhere from 10–20 percent. Most of these lesions are follicular or Hürthle cell neoplasms. In this situation, diagnosis of malignancy relies on demonstrating capsular or vascular invasion, features that cannot be determined via FNA biopsy. FNA biopsy also is less reliable in patients who have a history of head and neck irradiation or a family history of thyroid cancer, because of a higher likelihood of cancer and coexistent benign and malignant lesions. Most patients with thyroid nodules are euthyroid. Determining the blood TSH level is helpful although most patients are euthyroid. If a patient with a nodule is found to be hyperthyroid, the risk of malignancy is approximately 1 percent.

Ultrasound is helpful for detecting nonpalpable thyroid nodules, for differentiating solid from cystic nodules, for diagnosing suspicious nodules with microcalcifications and for identifying adjacent lymphadenopathy. Computed tomography (CT) and magnetic resonance imaging (MRI) are unnecessary in the routine evaluation of thyroid tumors, except for large, fixed, or substernal lesions. 123I or 99mTc is rarely necessary, unless evaluating patients for "hot" or autonomous thyroid nodules.

Management

Malignant tumors are generally treated by total or near-total thyroidectomy. Simple thyroid cysts resolve with aspiration in approximately 75 percent of cases. If the cyst persists after three attempts at aspiration, unilateral thyroid lobectomy is recommended. Lobectomy also is recommended for cysts greater than 4 cm in diameter and for complex cysts with solid and cystic components, because the latter have a higher incidence of malignancy (15 percent). When FNA biopsy is used in complex nodules, the solid portion should be sampled. If a colloid nodule is diagnosed by FNA biopsy, patients should still be observed with serial ultrasound and Tg measurements. If the nodule enlarges, repeat FNA biopsy often is indicated. Although controversial, L-thyroxine in doses sufficient to maintain a serum TSH level between 0.1 and 1.0 μU/mL also may be administered. Approximately 50 percent of these nodules decrease in size in response to the TSH suppression of this regimen, and others may not continue to grow, but it is most effective for nodules smaller than 3 cm. Thyroidectomy should be performed if a nodule enlarges on TSH suppression, causes compressive symptoms, or for cosmetic reasons. An exception to this general rule is the patient who has had previous irradiation of the thyroid gland or who has a family history of thyroid cancer. In these patients total or near-total thyroidectomy is recommended because of the high incidence of thyroid cancer ($\geq$ 40 percent) and decreased reliability of FNA biopsy in this setting.

MALIGNANT THYROID DISEASE

In the United States, thyroid cancer accounts for less than 1 percent of all malignancies (3 percent of women and 0.5 percent of men). Thyroid cancer is responsible for six deaths per 1 million persons annually. However, it is the most rapidly increasing cancer in women.

Molecular Genetics of Thyroid Tumorigenesis

Several oncogenes and tumor-suppressor genes are involved in thyroid tumorigenesis. The RET proto-oncogene, located on chromosome 10, plays a significant role. It encodes a receptor tyrosine kinase, which binds several growth factors. Germline mutations in the RET proto-oncogene are known to predispose to multiple endocrine neoplasia type 2A (MEN 2A), MEN 2B, and familial medullary thyroid cancers; and somatic mutations have been demonstrated in tumors derived from the neural crest, such as MTCs (30 percent) and pheochromocytomas. The tyrosine kinase domain of RET can fuse with other genes by rearrangement. These fusion products also function as oncogenes and have been implicated in the pathogenesis of papillary thyroid cancers. At least 15 RET/PTC rearrangements have been described and appear to be early events in tumorigenesis. Up to 70 percent of papillary cancers in children exposed to the radiation fallout from the 1986 Chernobyl disaster carry RET/PTC rearrangements. BRAF (B-type Raf kinase) mutations have recently been identified in about 40 percent of papillary thyroid cancers. Mutated ras oncogenes have been identified in up to 40 percent of thyroid follicular adenomas and carcinomas, multinodular goiters, and papillary and anaplastic carcinomas. Mutations in the TSH-R and gsp oncogenes have been noted in toxic adenomas. Mutations of p53 tumor suppressor are rare in PTCs, but are common in undifferentiated thyroid cancers and thyroid cancer cell lines. An oncogene resulting from the fusion of the DNA binding domain of the thyroid transcription factor PAX8 gene to the peroxisome proliferator-activated receptor gamma 1 (PPARγ1) has been noted to play an important role in the development of follicular neoplasms, including follicular cancers.

Specific Tumor Types

Papillary Carcinoma

Papillary carcinoma accounts for 80 percent of all thyroid malignancies in iodine-sufficient areas and is the predominant thyroid cancer in children and individuals exposed to external radiation. Papillary carcinoma occurs more often in women, with a 2:1 female-to-male ratio; the mean age at presentation is 30–40 years. Most patients are euthyroid and present with a slow-growing painless mass in the neck. Dysphagia, dyspnea, and dysphonia are usually associated with locally advanced invasive disease. Lymph node metastases are common, especially in children and young adults, and may be the presenting complaint. The so-called "lateral aberrant thyroid" almost always denotes a cervical lymph node metastases. Suspicion of thyroid cancer often originates through physical examination of the patient and a review of the patient's history. Diagnosis is established by FNA biopsy of the thyroid mass or lymph node.

Distant metastases are uncommon at initial presentation, but may ultimately develop in up to 20 percent of patients. The most common sites are the lungs, followed by bone, liver, and brain.

Pathology. Calcification, necrosis, or cystic change may be apparent grossly. Histologically, papillary carcinomas may exhibit papillary projections, a mixed pattern of papillary and follicular structures, or a pure follicular pattern (follicular variant). The diagnosis is established by characteristic cellular features. Cells are cuboidal with pale, abundant cytoplasm, "grooving," crowded nuclei, and intranuclear cytoplasmic inclusions, leading to the designation of Orphan Annie nuclei, which allows diagnosis by FNA biopsy. Psammoma bodies, which are microscopic, calcified deposits representing clumps of sloughed cells, may be present. Mixed papillary–follicular tumors and follicular variant of papillary carcinoma are classified as papillary carcinomas because they act biologically as papillary carcinomas. Multifocality is common in papillary carcinoma and may be present in up to 85 percent of cases on microscopic examination. Multifocality is associated with an increased risk of cervical nodal metastases and these tumors may rarely invade adjacent structures such as the trachea, esophagus, and recurrent laryngeal nerves. Other variants of papillary carcinoma including tall cell, columnar, diffuse sclerosing, clear cell, trabecular, Hurthle cell variant and poorly differentiated types. These variants account for approximately 1 percent of all papillary carcinomas and are generally associated with a worse prognosis.

Macroscopically, there are three recognized forms of papillary carcinoma, each based on the size and extent of the primary disease. Minimal or occult/microcarcinoma tumors are defined as tumors of 1 cm or less in size with no evidence of local invasiveness or lymph node metastases. They are nonpalpable and usually are incidental findings at operative, histologic, or autopsy examination. Occult papillary thyroid cancer is present in 2–36 percent of thyroid glands removed at autopsy. Intrathyroidal tumors are confined to the thyroid gland, with no evidence of extrathyroid invasion. Extrathyroidal tumors invade through the thyroid capsule and/or into adjacent structures. All types of primary thyroid cancers can be associated with lymph node metastases and invasion into intrathyroidal blood vessels or occasionally distant metastases. Long-term prognosis is better for patients with small, intrathyroidal lesions.

Prognostic indicators. In general, patients with papillary carcinoma have an excellent prognosis with a greater than 95 percent 10-year survival rate. Several prognostic indicators have been incorporated into various staging systems, which enable patients to be stratified into low-risk and high-risk groups.

The AGES scoring system incorporates age, histologic grade, extrathyroidal invasion and metastases, and tumor size to predict the risk of dying from papillary cancer. The MACIS scale is similar but incorporates completeness of original surgical resection with size of original lesion, invasion and metastases. The AMES system is a simpler classificstion that divides differentiated thyroid tumors into low- and high-risk groups using age (men < 40 years, women < 50 years), metastases, extrathyroidal spread, and size of tumors (< or > 5 cm). Another classification system is the TNM system, (tumor, nodal status, metastases; Table 37-1), used by most medical centers in North America. Unfortunately, all of these classification systems rely on data that is not available preoperatively.

TABLE 37-1 TNM Classification of Thyroid Tumors

Papillary or follicular tumors	
Stage	TNM
Younger than age 45 years	
I	Any T, Any N, M0
II	Any T, Any N, M1
Age 45 years and older	
I	T1, N0, M0
II	T2, N0, M0
III	T3, N0, M0; T1-3, N1a, M0
IVA	T4a, N0-1a, M0; T1-4a, N1b, M0
IVB	T4b, Any N, M0
IVC	Any T, Any N, M1

Medullary thyroid cancer	
Stage	TNM
I	T1, N0, M0
II	T2-3, N0, M0
III	T1-3, N1a, M0
IVA	T4a, N0-1a, M0; T1-4a, N1b, M0
IVB	T4b, any N, M0
IVC	Any T, Any N, M1

Anaplastic cancer	
Stage	TNM
IVA	T4a, Any N, M0
IVB	T4b, Any N, M0
IVC	Any T, Any M, M1

Definitions:
Primary tumor (T)

TX	Primary tumor cannot be assessed
T0	No evidence of primary tumor
T1	Tumor ≤ 2 cm in diameter, limited to thyroid
T2	Tumor > 2 cm but < 4 cm in diameter, limited to thyroid
T3	Tumor > 4 cm in diameter, limited to thyroid, or any tumor with minimal extrathyroidal invasion
T4a	Any size tumor extending beyond capsule to invade subcutaneous soft tissue, larynx, trachea, esophagus, or recurrent laryngeal nerve, or intrathyroidal anaplastic cancer
T4b	Tumor invading prevertebral fascia, or encasing carotid artery or mediastinal vessels, or extrathyroidal anaplastic cancer

Regional lymph nodes (N) include central, lateral, cervical, and upper mediastinal nodes

Nx	Regional lymph nodes cannot be assessed
N0	No regional lymph node metastasis
N1	Regional lymph node metastasis
N1a	Metastases to level VI (pretracheal, paratracheal, and prelaryngeal/Delphian lymph nodes)
N1b	Metastases to unilateral, bilateral, or contralateral cervical or superior mediastinal lymph nodes

Distant metastasis (M)

MX	Distant metastases cannot be assessed
M1	No distant metastasis

Source: Reproduced with permission from *AJCC Cancer Staging Manual*, 6th ed. New York: Springer-Verlag, 2002.

Surgical treatment. Most authors agree that patients with high-risk tumors (judged by any of the classification systems discussed above) or bilateral tumors should undergo total or near-total thyroidectomy. When patients are found to have a minimal papillary thyroid carcinoma in a thyroid specimen removed for other reasons, unilateral thyroid lobectomy and isthmusectomy is usually considered to be adequate treatment, unless the tumor has evidence of angioinvasion, multifocality, or positive margins. The optimal surgical strategy in the majority of patients with low-risk (small, unilateral) cancers remains controversial. The focus of the debate centers around outcome data and risks associated with either lobectomy or total thyroidectomy in this group of patients.

Proponents of total thyroidectomy argue that the procedure (1) enables one to use RAI to effectively detect and treat residual thyroid tissue or metastatic disease; (2) makes the serum Tg level a more sensitive marker of recurrent or persistent disease; (3) eliminates the contralateral occult cancers as sites of recurrence (because up to 85 percent of tumors are multifocal); (4) reduces the risk of recurrence and improves survival; (5) decreases the 1 percent risk of progression to undifferentiated or anaplastic thyroid cancer; and (6) reduces the need for reoperative surgery with its attendant risk of increased complication rates.

Investigators that favor lobectomy argue that (1) total thyroidectomy is associated with a higher complication rate than lobectomy; (2) recurrence in the remaining thyroid tissue is unusual (5 percent) and most are curable by surgery; (3) tumor multicentricity seems to have little prognostic significance; and (4) patients who have undergone lesser procedures, such as lobectomy, still have an excellent prognosis. However, it is known that a significant proportion (33–50 percent) of patients who develop a recurrence die from their disease, and even though the data are retrospective, long-term, follow-up studies suggest that recurrence rates are lowered, and that survival is improved in patients undergoing near-total or total thyroidectomy. Additionally, diminished survival is noted in patients with so-called low-risk disease (mortality rates of 5 percent at 10–20 years) and it is not possible to accurately risk stratify patients preoperatively. Given the above, it is recommended that even patients with low-risk tumors undergo total or near-total thyroidectomy, provided complication rates are low (< 2 percent).

Consequently, most patients with thyroid nodules should have FNA biopsy performed. When PTC is diagnosed, the definitive operation can be done without confirming the diagnosis by frozen section during the operation. Patients with a nodule that may be papillary cancer should be treated by thyroid lobectomy, isthmusectomy, and removal of any pyramidal lobe or adjacent lymph nodes. If intraoperative frozen-section examination of a lymph node or of the primary tumor confirms carcinoma, completion of total or near-total thyroidectomy should be performed. If a definitive diagnosis cannot be made, or if the surgeon is concerned about the viability of the parathyroid glands or the status of the RLN, the operation should be terminated. For patients who have minimal papillary thyroid cancer confined to the thyroid gland without angioinvasion, no further operative treatment is recommended.

During thyroidectomy, enlarged ipsilateral central neck nodes should be removed. Lymph node metastases in the lateral neck in patients with papillary carcinoma are usually managed with modified radical or functional neck dissection. Dissection of the posterior triangle and suprahyoid dissection are usually not necessary unless there is extensive metastatic disease in levels 2,

3, and 4, but should be performed when appropriate. Prophylactic neck node dissection is not necessary in patients with papillary thyroid cancer, because these cancers do not appear to metastasize systemically from lymph nodes and micrometastases appear to be ablated with RAI therapy.

Follicular Carcinoma

Follicular carcinomas account for 10 percent of thyroid cancers and occur more commonly in iodine-deficient areas. The overall incidence of this tumor is declining in the United States, probably as a result of iodine supplementation and improved histologic classification. Women have a higher incidence of follicular cancer, with a female:male ratio of 3:1, and a mean age at presentation of 50 years. Follicular cancers usually present as solitary thyroid nodules. Unlike papillary cancers, cervical lymphadenopathy is uncommon at initial presentation (approximately 5 percent), although distant metastases may be present. In less than 1 percent of cases, follicular cancers may be hyperfunctioning. FNA biopsy is unable to distinguish benign follicular lesions from follicular carcinomas. Therefore, preoperative diagnosis of cancer is difficult unless distant metastases are present. Large follicular tumors (> 4 cm) in older men are more likely to be malignant.

Pathology. Follicular carcinomas are usually solitary lesions, the majority of which are surrounded by a capsule. Histologically, follicles are present, but the lumen may be devoid of colloid. Malignancy is defined by the presence of capsular and vascular invasion. Minimally invasive tumors appear grossly encapsulated but have evidence of microscopic invasion through the tumor capsule and/or invasion into small- to medium-size vessels (venous caliber) in or immediately outside the capsule, but not within the tumor. On the other hand, widely invasive tumors demonstrate evidence of large-vessel invasion and/or broad areas of tumor invasion through the capsule. They may, in fact, be unencapsulated. However, there is a wide variation of opinion among clinicians and pathologists with respect to the above definitions.

Surgical treatment and prognosis. Patients diagnosed by FNA biopsy as having a follicular lesion should undergo thyroid lobectomy because at least 80 percent of these patients will have benign adenomas. Some surgeons recommend total thyroidectomy in older patients with follicular lesions larger than 4 cm as there is a higher risk of cancer in this setting (50 percent). Total thyroidectomy should be performed when thyroid cancer is diagnosed. There is debate among experts about whether patients with minimally invasive follicular cancers should undergo completion thyroidectomy because the prognosis is so good in these patients. A diagnosis of frankly invasive carcinoma necessitates completion of total thyroidectomy. Total thyroidectomy in patients with angioinvasion is also recommended. Prophylactic nodal dissection is not needed but in the unusual patient with nodal metastases, therapeutic neck dissection is recommended. The cumulative mortality rate from follicular thyroid cancer is approximately 15 percent at 10 years and 30 percent at 20 years.

Hürthle Cell Carcinoma

Hürthle cell carcinomas account for approximately 3 percent of all thyroid malignancies. Under the World Health Organization classification, Hürthle cell carcinomas are considered to be a subtype of follicular thyroid cancer. Like follicular cancers, Hürthle cell cancers are characterized by vascular or capsular invasion, and therefore cannot be diagnosed by FNA biopsy. Tumors contain sheets of eosinophilic cells packed with mitochondria, which are derived from the oxyphilic cells of the thyroid gland. Hürthle cell tumors also differ from follicular carcinomas in that they are more often multifocal and bilateral (approximately 30 percent), usually do not take up RAI (approximately 5 percent), are more likely to metastasize to local nodes (25 percent) and distant sites, and are associated with a higher mortality rate (approximately 20 percent at 10 years). Hence, they are considered to be a separate class of tumors by some surgeons.

Management is similar to that of follicular neoplasms, with lobectomy and isthmusectomy being sufficient surgical treatment for unilateral Hürthle cell adenomas. When Hürthle cell neoplasms are found to be invasive on intraoperative, frozen-section, or definitive paraffin-section histology, then total thyroidectomy should be performed. These patients should also undergo routine central neck node removal, similar to patients with MTC, and modified radical neck dissection when lateral neck nodes are palpable. Although RAI scanning and ablation usually are ineffective, they probably should be considered for ablation of any residual normal thyroid tissue and, occasionally, for ablation of tumors, because there is no other good therapy.

Postoperative Management of Differentiated Thyroid Cancer

Thyroid hormone.   TSH suppression reduces tumor recurrence rates, particularly in young patients with papillary and follicular thyroid cancer. Thyroxine should be administered to ensure that the patient remains euthyroid, with circulating TSH levels at about 0.1 μU/L in low-risk patients, or less than 0.1 μU/mL in high-risk patients. The risk of tumor recurrence must be balanced with the side effects associated with prolonged TSH suppression, including osteopenia and cardiac problems, particularly in older patients.

Thyroglobulin measurement.   Thyroglobulin levels in patients who have undergone total thyroidectomy should be below 2 ng/mL when the patient is taking T4, and below 5 ng/mL when the patient is hypothyroid. A Tg level above 2 ng/mL after total thryoidectomy is highly suggestive of metastatic disease or persistent normal thyroid tissue.

Thyroglobulin and anti-Tg antibody levels should be measured initially at 6-month intervals and then annually if the patient is clinically disease free. High-risk patients should also have an ultrasound of the neck and CT or MRI scan of the neck and mediastinum for early detection of any persistent or recurrent disease.

Radioiodine therapy.   Long-term cohort studies suggest that postoperative RAI therapy reduces recurrence and provides a small improvement in survival, even in low-risk patients. Screening and treatment are facilitated by the removal of all normal thyroid tissue, which effectively competes for iodine uptake. Metastatic differentiated thyroid carcinoma can be detected and treated by 131I in approximately 75 percent of patients. Generally, T4 therapy is discontinued for approximately 6 weeks prior to scanning with 131I. Patients should receive T3 during this time period to decrease the period of hypothyroidism. A low-iodine diet is also recommended during the 2-week period when all thyroid hormone has been discontinued. After a total thyroidectomy, radioactive uptake should be less than 1 percent. If there is significant uptake, then a therapeutic dose of 131I should be administered to patients (low-risk patients: 30–100 mCi; high-risk patients: 100–200 mCi). The maximum dose of radioiodine that can be administered at one time without performing dosimetry is approximately 200 mCi with a cumulative dose of 1000–1500 mCi. Up to 500 mCi can be given with proper pretreatment dosimetry. If follow-up RAI scans are negative, but Tg levels remain elevated, other imaging studies such as neck ultrasound, MRI scan, and FDG-PET scans should be considered.

External beam radiotherapy and chemotherapy. External beam radiotherapy is occasionally required to control unresectable, locally invasive or recurrent disease and to treat metastases in support bones to decrease the risk of fractures. Single and multidrug chemotherapy has been used with little success in disseminated thyroid cancer. Adriamycin and Taxol are the most frequently used agents.

Medullary Carcinoma

These tumors account for about 5 percent of thyroid malignancies and arise from the parafollicular or C cells of the thyroid, which are concentrated superolaterally in the thyroid lobes. C cells secrete calcitonin, a 32-amino-acid polypeptide. In some animals, especially those that lay eggs with shells, calcitonin is a significant regulator of calcium metabolism, but in humans, it has only minimal physiologic effects. Most medullary carcinomas occur sporadically. However, approximately 25 percent occur within the spectrum of several inherited syndromes such as familial medullary thyroid cancer, MEN2A, and MEN2B—all of which result secondary to germline mutations in the RET proto-oncogene.

Patients with medullary carcinoma often present with a neck mass that may be associated with palpable cervical lymphadenopathy (15–20 percent). Local invasion produces symptoms of dysphagia, dyspnea, or dysphonia. Distant blood-borne metastases to the liver, bone (frequently osteoblastic), and lung occur later in the disease. The female:male ratio is 1.5:1. Most patients present between 50 and 60 years of age, although patients with familial disease present at a younger age. Medullary thyroid tumors secrete not only calcitonin and carcinoembryonic antigen (CEA), but also calcitonin gene-related peptide (CGRP), histaminadases, prostaglandins E_2 and $F_2\alpha$, serotonin and ACTH.

Pathology. The tumors are typically unilateral, but are multicentric in familial cases. Familial cases also are associated with C-cell hyperplasia, which is considered a premalignant lesion. Microscopically, tumors are composed of sheets of infiltrating neoplastic cells separated by collagen and amyloid. The presence of amyloid is a diagnostic finding, but immunohistochemistry for calcitonin is more commonly used as a diagnostic marker.

Diagnosis. The diagnosis of medullary carcinoma is established by history, physical examination, raised serum calcitonin or CEA levels, and FNA cytology of the thyroid mass. Attention to family history is important because approximately 25 percent of patients with MTC have familial disease. All new patients with MTC should be screened for RET point mutations, pheochromocytoma, and hyperparathyroidism. It is important to rule out a coexisting pheochromocytoma to avoid precipitating a hypertensive crisis and death.

Treatment. If patients are found to have a pheochromocytoma, this must be operated on first. Total thyroidectomy is the treatment of choice for these patients because of the high incidence of multicentricity, the more aggressive course, and 131I therapy is not usually effective. The central compartment nodes are frequently involved early in the disease process, so that a bilateral central neck node dissection should be routinely performed. In patients with palpable cervical nodes or involved central neck nodes, ipsilateral or bilateral, modified radical neck dissection is recommended. Similarly, patients with tumors larger than 1.5 cm should undergo ipsilateral prophylactic modified radical neck dissection, because greater than 60 percent of these patients have nodal metastases. Approximately 30 percent of these patients will also have contralateral nodal metastases. In the case of locally recurrent or metastatic disease, tumor debulking is advised.

In patients who have hypercalcemia at the time of thyroidectomy, only obviously enlarged parathyroid glands should be removed. The other parathyroid glands should be preserved and marked in patients with normocalcemia as only approximately 20 percent of patients with MEN 2A develop hyperparathyroidism. Total thyroidectomy is indicated in RET mutation carriers and should be performed before age 6 years in MEN 2A patients and prior to age 1 year in MEN 2B patients.

Prognosis. Prognosis is related to disease stage and type. It is best in patients with non-MEN familial medullary cancer, followed by patients with MEN 2A, and then by patients with sporadic disease. Patients with MEN 2B have the worst prognosis.

Anaplastic Carcinoma

Anaplastic carcinoma accounts for approximately 1 percent of all thyroid malignancies in the United States and is the most aggressive of thyroid tumors. The majority of tumors present in the seventh and eighth decades of life. The typical patient has a long-standing neck mass, which rapidly enlarges and may be painful. Associated symptoms, such as dysphonia, dysphagia, and dyspnea are common. Lymph nodes usually are palpable at presentation. Evidence of metastatic spread also may be present. Diagnosis is confirmed by FNA biopsy revealing characteristic giant and multinucleated cells. Foci of more differentiated thyroid tumors may be seen, suggesting that anaplastic tumors arise from more well-differentiated tumors. Incisional biopsy is occasionally needed to confirm the diagnosis and isthmusectomy is performed to alleviate tracheal compression.

Treatment and prognosis. This tumor is one of the most aggressive thyroid malignancies. If anaplastic carcinoma presents as a resectable mass, thyroidectomy may lead to a small improvement in survival. Combined radiation and chemotherapy in an adjuvant setting in patients with resectable disease has been associated with prolonged survival. Tracheostomy may be needed to alleviate airway obstruction.

Lymphoma

Lymphomas account for less than 1 percent of thyroid malignancies, are mostly of the non–Hodgkin B-cell type and tend to develop in patients with chronic lymphocytic thyroiditis. Patients usually present with symptoms similar to anaplastic carcinoma, although the rapidly enlarging neck mass often is painless. Patients may present with acute respiratory distress. The diagnosis usually is suggested by FNA biopsy, although needle-core or open biopsy may be necessary for definitive diagnosis. Staging studies should be obtained to assess the extent of extrathyroidal spread.

Treatment and prognosis. Patients respond rapidly to chemotherapy (CHOP—cyclophosphamide, doxorubicin, vincristine, and prednisone), which also is associated with improved survival. Thyroidectomy and nodal resection are reserved for patients who do not respond quickly to the above regimens, or in patients who have completed the regimen prior to diagnosis.

Metastatic Carcinoma

The thyroid gland is a rare site of metastases from other cancers, including kidney, breast, lung, and melanoma. Resection of the thyroid, usually lobectomy, may be helpful in many patients, depending on the status of their primary tumor.

THYROID SURGERY

Preoperative Preparation

Patients with any recent or remote history of altered phonation or prior neck surgery should undergo vocal cord assessment by direct or indirect laryngoscopy prior to thyroidectomy. The patient is positioned supine, with a sandbag between the scapulae. The head is placed on a donut cushion and the neck is extended and supported to provide maximal exposure without hyperextension. A Kocher transverse collar incision, typically 4–5 cm in length, is placed in or parallel to a natural skin crease 1 cm below the cricoid cartilage. Subplatysmal flaps are raised superiorly to the level of the thyroid cartilage and inferiorly to the suprasternal notch. The strap muscles are divided in the midline and the thyroid gland is exposed. The straps are then dissected off the underlying thyroid by a combination of sharp and blunt dissection, thus exposing the middle thyroid veins. The thyroid lobe is retracted medially and anteriorly and the lateral tissues are swept posterolaterally using a peanut sponge. The middle thyroid veins are ligated and divided. Attention is then turned to the midline where Delphian nodes and the pyramidal lobe are identified. Some surgeons divide the isthmus early for patients with benign or indeterminate disease. The superior thyroid pole is identified by retracting the thyroid first inferiorly and medially, and then the upper pole of the thyroid is mobilized caudally and laterally. The dissection plane is kept as close to the thyroid as possible and the superior pole vessels are individually identified, skeletonized, ligated, and divided low on the thyroid gland, to avoid injury to the external branch of the superior laryngeal nerve.

The recurrent laryngeal nerve can then be identified, most consistently at the level of the cricoid cartilage. The parathyroids can usually be identified within 1 cm of the crossing of the inferior thyroid artery and the RLN. If not present in this location, the lower glands may be found in the thyrothymic ligament or the upper thymus. The lower pole of the thyroid gland should be mobilized by gently sweeping all tissues dorsally. The inferior thyroid vessels are dissected, skeletonized, ligated, and divided as close to the surface of the thyroid gland as possible. The RLN is most vulnerable to injury in the vicinity of the ligament of Berry. Any bleeding in this area should be controlled with gentle pressure before carefully identifying the vessel and ligating it. Use of the electrocautery should be avoided in proximity to the RLN. Once the ligament is divided, the thyroid can be separated from the underlying trachea by sharp dissection. The pyramidal lobe, if present, must be dissected in a cephalad direction to above the level of the notch in the thyroid cartilage or higher in continuity with the thyroid gland. If a lobectomy is to be performed, the isthmus is divided flush with the trachea on the contralateral side and suture ligated. The procedure is repeated on the opposite side for a total thyroidectomy.

Parathyroid glands that cannot be dissected from the thyroid with a good blood supply, or have been inadvertently removed during the thyroidectomy, should be resected, confirmed as parathyroid tissue by frozen section, divided into 1-mm fragments, and reimplanted into individual pockets in the sternocleidomastoid muscle. The sites should be marked with silk sutures and a clip. If a subtotal thyroidectomy is to be performed, once the superior pole vessels are divided and the thyroid lobe mobilized anteriorly, the thyroid lobe is cross-clamped with a Mayo clamp, leaving approximately 4 g of the posterior portion of the thyroid. The thyroid remnant is suture ligated, taking care to avoid injury to the recurrent laryngeal nerve. Routine drain placement is rarely necessary. After adequate hemostasis is obtained, the strap muscles are reapproximated in the midline using absorbable sutures. The platysma is approximated in a similar fashion. The skin can be closed with subcuticular sutures or clips.

Several approaches to minimally invasive thyroidectomy, such as video-assisted thyroidectomy and endoscopic thyroidectomy via axillary incisions, have been proposed. These methods are feasible, but clear benefits over the "traditional" open approach have not been established.

Surgical Removal of Intrathoracic Goiter

A goiter is considered mediastinal if at least 50 percent of the thyroid tissue is located intrathoracically. Mediastinal goiters can be primary or secondary. Primary mediastinal goiters (1 percent) arise from accessory (ectopic) thyroid tissue located in the chest. These goiters are supplied by intrathoracic blood vessels and do not have any connection to thyroid tissue in the neck. Secondary goiters arise from downward extension of cervical thyroid tissue along the fascial planes of the neck and derive their blood supply from thyroid arteries. Virtually all intrathoracic goiters can be removed via a cervical incision. Patients who have invasive thyroid cancers, have had previous thyroid operations (may have developed parasitic mediastinal vessels), or have primary mediastinal goiters with no thyroid tissue in the neck, may require a median sternotomy for removal.

Neck Dissection for Nodal Metastases

A modified radical (functional) neck dissection can be performed via the cervical incision used for thyroidectomy, which can be extended laterally (MacFee extension). The procedure involves removal of all fibrofatty tissue along the internal jugular vein (levels II, III, and IV) and the posterior triangle (level V). In contrast to a radical neck dissection, the internal jugular vein, the spinal accessory nerve, the cervical sensory nerves, and the sternocleidomastoid muscle are preserved unless they are adherent to or invaded by tumor. The procedure begins by opening the plane between the strap muscles medially and the sternocleidomastoid muscle laterally. The anterior belly of the omohyoid muscle is retracted laterally and the dissection is carried posteriorly until the carotid sheath is reached. The internal jugular vein is retracted medially with a vein retractor and the fibrofatty tissue and lymph nodes are dissected away from it by a combination of sharp and blunt dissection. The lateral dissection is carried along the posterior border of the sternocleidomastoid muscle, removing the tissue from the posterior triangle. The deep dissection plane is the anterior scalenus muscle, the phrenic nerve, the brachial plexus, and the medial scalenus muscle.

Complications of Thyroid Surgery

Injury to the RLN may occur by severance, ligation, or undue traction, but should occur in less than 1 percent of patients undergoing thyroidectomy by experienced surgeons. The RLN is most vulnerable to injury during the last 2–3 cm of its course. If the injury is recognized intraoperatively, most surgeons advocate primary reapproximation of the perineurium using nonabsorbable sutures. Approximately 15 percent of patients are at risk of injury to the external branches of the superior laryngeal nerve, especially if superior pole vessels are ligated en masse. The cervical sympathetic trunk is at risk of injury in the rare scenario of retroesophageal goiter extension and might result in Horner syndrome. Transient hypocalcemia (from surgical injury or inadvertent removal of parathyroid tissue) has been reported in up to 50 percent of cases, but permanent hypoparathyroidism occurs less than 2 percent of the time. Postoperative hematomas or bleeding may also complicate thyroidectomies, and rarely necessitate emergency reoperation to evacuate the hematoma. Bilateral vocal cord dysfunction with respiratory difficulty can require immediate reintubation or tracheostomy. Seromas may need aspiration to relieve patient discomfort. Wound cellulitis and infection, and injury to surrounding structures, such as the carotid artery, jugular vein, thoracic duct and esophagus are infrequent.

PARATHYROID

Embryology

In humans, the superior parathyroid glands are derived from the fourth branchial pouch, which also gives rise to the thyroid gland. The third branchial pouches give rise to the inferior parathyroid glands and the thymus. The parathyroids remain closely associated with their respective branchial pouch derivatives. The position of normal superior parathyroid glands is more consistent, with 80 percent of these glands being found near the posterior aspect of the upper and middle thyroid lobes, at the level of the cricoid cartilage. Approximately 1 percent of normal upper glands may be found in the paraesophageal or retroesophageal space. Truly ectopic superior parathyroid glands are rare, but may be found in the middle or posterior mediastinum, commonly in the aortopulmonary window. As the embryo matures, the thymus and inferior parathyroids migrate together caudally in the neck. The most common location for inferior glands is within a distance of 1 cm from a point centered where the inferior thyroid artery and recurrent laryngeal nerve cross. Approximately 15 percent of inferior glands are found in the thymus. The position of the inferior glands, however, tends to be more variable as a consequence of their longer migratory path. Undescended inferior glands may be found near the skull base, angle of the mandible, or superior to the superior parathyroid glands, along with an undescended thymus. The frequency of intrathyroidal glands varies in the literature from 0.5–3 percent. Although some authors consider upper parathyroid glands more likely to be intrathyroidal, because of the close embryologic association of the upper glands and the lateral thyroid anlage, they may also be lower glands.

ANATOMY AND HISTOLOGY

Most patients have four parathyroid glands. Normal parathyroid glands are gray and semitransparent in newborns, but appear golden-yellow to light-brown in adults. They are located in loose tissue or fat and are ovoid and measure 5–7 mm in size (weight 40–50 mg each). The parathyroid glands derive most of their blood supply from branches of the inferior thyroid artery, although branches from the superior thyroid artery supply at least 20 percent of upper glands; venous drainage is via the ipsilateral superior, middle, and inferior thyroid veins. Akerstrom and associates, in an autopsy series of 503 cadavers, found four parathyroid glands in 84 percent of cases. Supernumerary glands were present in 13 percent of patients, most commonly in the thymus. Only 3 percent of patients had less than four glands.

Histologically, parathyroid glands are composed of chief cells (which produce PTH) and oxyphil cells arranged in trabeculae, within a stroma composed primarily of adipose cells. A third group of cells, known as water-clear cells (rich in glycogen), also are derived from chief cells. Although most, but not all, oxyphil and water-clear cells retain the ability to secrete PTH, their functional significance is unknown.

PARATHYROID PHYSIOLOGY AND CALCIUM HOMEOSTASIS

Calcium is the most abundant cation in human beings, and has several crucial functions. Calcium is absorbed from the small intestine in its inorganic form. Extracellular calcium (900 mg) accounts for only 1 percent of the body's calcium stores, the majority of which is sequestered in the skeletal system. Approximately 50 percent of the serum calcium is in the ionized form, which is the active component. The remainder is bound to albumin (40 percent) and organic anions such as phosphate and citrate (10 percent). The total serum calcium levels range from 8.5–10.5 mg/dL (2.1–2.6 mmol/L) and ionized calcium levels range from 4.4–5.2 mg/dL (1.1–1.3 mmol/L). Total serum calcium levels must always be considered in the context of serum albumin levels.

Parathyroid Hormone

Parathyroid cells rely on a G-protein-coupled membrane receptor, the calcium-sensing receptor (CASR), to regulate PTH secretion. PTH secretion is also stimulated by low levels of 1,25-dihydroxy vitamin D, catecholamines, and hypomagnesemia. The PTH gene is located on chromosome 11. PTH is synthesized as a precursor hormone, preproparathyroid hormone, which is cleaved first to proparathyroid hormone and then to the final 84-amino-acid PTH. Secreted PTH has a half-life of 2–4 min.

PTH increases the resorption of bone by stimulating osteoclasts and promotes the release of calcium and phosphate into the circulation. At the kidney, PTH acts to limit calcium excretion at the distal convoluted tubule via an active transport mechanism. PTH also inhibits phosphate and bicarbonate reabsorption and enhances 1-hydroxylation of 25-hydroxyvitamin D, which is responsible for its indirect effect of increasing intestinal calcium absorption.

Calcitonin

Calcitonin inhibits osteoclast-mediated bone resorption. Its production is stimulated by calcium and pentagastrin, and also by catecholamines, cholecystokinin, and glucagon. It produces hypocalcemia, when administered intravenously to experimental animals but plays a minimal, if any, role in the regulation of calcium levels in humans.

Vitamin D

Vitamin D2 and vitamin D3 are produced by photolysis of naturally occurring sterol precursors. Vitamin D is metabolized in the liver to its primary circulating form, 25-hydroxy vitamin D. Further hydroxylation in the kidney results in 1,25-dihydroxy vitamin D, which is the most metabolically active form of vitamin D. Vitamin D stimulates the absorption of calcium and phosphate from the gut.

HYPERPARATHYROIDISM

Hyperfunction of the parathyroid glands may be classified as primary, secondary, or tertiary. Primary hyperparathyroidism (PHPT) arises from increased PTH production from abnormal parathyroid glands and results from a disturbance of normal feedback control exerted by serum calcium. Elevated PTH levels may also occur as a compensatory response to hypocalcemic states resulting from chronic renal failure or gastrointestinal malabsorption of calcium. This state is referred to as secondary hyperparathyroidism (HPT) and can be reversed by correction of the underlying problem, (e.g., kidney transplantation for chronic renal failure). However, chronically stimulated glands may occasionally become autonomous, resulting in persistence or recurrence of hypercalcemia after successful renal transplantation, resulting in tertiary HPT.

Primary Hyperparathyroidism

PHPT is a common disorder, affecting 0.1–0.3 percent of the general population and is more common in women (1:500) than in men (1:2000). Increased PTH production leads to hypercalcemia via increased gastrointestinal absorption of calcium, increased production of vitamin D3 and reduced renal calcium clearance. PHPT is characterized by increased parathyroid cell proliferation and PTH secretion which is independent of calcium levels.

Etiology

The exact cause of PHPT is unknown, although exposure to low-dose therapeutic ionizing radiation and familial predisposition account for some cases. Various diets and intermittent exposure to sunshine may also be related. Other causes include renal leak of calcium and declining renal function with age, and alteration in the sensitivity of parathyroid glands to suppression by calcium. PHPT results from the enlargement of a single gland or parathyroid adenoma in approximately 80 percent of cases, multiple adenomas or hyperplasia in 15–20 percent of patients and parathyroid carcinoma in 1 percent of patients.

Genetics

Although most cases of PHPT are sporadic, PHPT also occurs within the spectrum of a number of inherited disorders such as MEN1, MEN 2A, isolated familial HPT, and familial HPT with jaw-tumor syndrome. All of these syndromes are inherited in an autosomal dominant fashion. Primary HPT is the earliest and most common manifestation of MEN1 and develops in 80–100 percent of patients by age 40 years. These patients also are prone to pancreatic neuroendocrine tumors, pituitary adenomas, and less commonly to adrenocortical tumors, lipomas, skin angiomas, and carcinoid tumors of the bronchus, thymus, or stomach. MEN1 has been shown to result from germline mutations in the MEN1 gene, a tumor-suppressor gene located on chromosome 11q12-13. Hyperparathyroidism develops in approximately 20 percent of patients with MEN 2A and is generally less severe. Patients with the familial HPT with jaw-tumor syndrome have an increased predisposition to parathyroid carcinoma. This syndrome maps to a tumor-suppressor locus HRPT2, on chromosome 1.

Approximately 25–40 percent of sporadic parathyroid adenomas and some hyperplastic parathyroid glands have loss of heterozygosity at 11q13, the site of the MEN1 gene. The parathyroid adenoma 1 oncogene (PRAD1), which encodes cyclin D1, a cell-cycle control protein, is overexpressed in approximately 18 percent of parathyroid adenomas. Sporadic parathyroid cancers are characterized by uniform loss of the tumor-suppressor gene RB, and mutations of HRPT2 and p53.

Clinical Manifestations

Patients with PHPT formerly presented with the "classic" pentad of symptoms (i.e., kidney stones, painful bones, abdominal groans, psychic moans, and fatigue overtones). With the advent and widespread use of automated blood analyzers in the early 1970s, there has been an alteration in the "typical" patient with PHPT, who is more likely to be minimally symptomatic or asymptomatic. Currently, most patients present with weakness, fatigue, polydipsia, polyuria, nocturia, bone and joint pain, constipation, decreased appetite, nausea, heartburn, pruritus, depression, and memory loss. Truly "asymptomatic" PHPT appears to be rare. Complications of HPT are described below.

Renal disease. Approximately 80 percent of patients with PHPT have some degree of renal dysfunction or symptoms. Kidney stones or nephrocalcinosis were previously found in up to 80 percent of patients, but now occur in approximately 20–25 percent. The calculi are typically composed of calcium phosphate or oxalate. In contrast, primary HPT is found to be the underlying disorder in only 3 percent of patients presenting with nephrolithiasis. The incidence of hypertension is variable.

Bone disease. Bone disease, including osteopenia, osteoporosis, and osteitis fibrosa cystica, is found in approximately 15 percent of patients with PHPT. Advanced PHPT and/or vitamin D deficiency leads to osteitis fibrosa cystica, a condition which now occurs in less than 5 percent of patients. It is characterized by pathognomonic radiologic findings, which are best seen on radiographs of the hands that demonstrate subperiosteal resorption (most apparent on the radial aspect of the middle phalanx of the second and third fingers), bone cysts, and tufting of the distal phalanges. The skull may also be affected and appears mottled (salt and pepper) with a loss of definition of the inner and outer cortices. Brown or osteoclastic tumors and bone cysts may also be present. Hyperparathyroidism typically results in a loss of bone mass at sites of cortical bone, such as the radius and relative preservation of cancellous bone such as that located at the vertebral bodies.

Gastrointestinal complications. PHPT has been associated with peptic ulcer disease, pancreatitis and cholelithiasis.

Neuropsychiatric manifestations. Severe hypercalcemia may lead to various neuropsychiatric manifestations such as florid psychosis, obtundation, or coma. Other findings, such as depression, anxiety, and fatigue, are more commonly observed in patients with only mild hypercalcemia.

Other features. Primary HPT also can lead to fatigue and muscle weakness, which is prominent in the proximal muscle groups. Patients also have an increased incidence of chondrocalcinosis and pseudogout. Calcification at ectopic sites such as blood vessels, cardiac valves and skin, also has been reported, as has hypertrophy of the left ventricle independent of the presence of hypertension. Several large studies from Europe also suggest that PHPT is associated with increased death rates from cardiovascular disease and cancer, even in patients with mild HPT, although this finding was not substantiated in other studies.

Physical Findings

Parathyroid tumors are seldom palpable, except in patients with profound hypercalcemia. A palpable neck mass in a patient with PHPT is more likely to be thyroid in origin or a parathyroid cancer. Patients may also demonstrate evidence of band keratopathy, a deposition of calcium in Bowman membrane just inside the iris of the eye.

Differential Diagnosis

Hypercalcemia may be caused by a multitude of conditions (Table 37-2). PHPT and malignancy account for more than 90 percent of all cases of hypercalcemia. PHPT is more common in the outpatient setting, whereas malignancy is the leading cause of hypercalcemia in hospitalized patients. PHPT can virtually always be distinguished from other diseases causing hypercalcemia by a combination of history, physical examination, and appropriate laboratory investigations. Hypercalcemia of malignancy is known to be mediated primarily by parathyroid hormone-related peptide (PTHrP). Benign familial hypocalciuric hypercalcemia (BFHH) is a rare autosomal dominant condition with nearly 100 percent penetrance and results from inherited heterozygous mutations in the CASR gene located on chromosome 3. Patients with BFHH have lifelong hypercalcemia, which is not corrected by parathyroidectomy.

Diagnostic Investigations

Biochemical studies. The presence of an elevated serum calcium and intact PTH (iPTH) or two-site PTH levels establishes the diagnosis of PHPT with

TABLE 37-2 Differential Diagnosis of Hypercalcemia

Hyperparathyroidism
Malignancy—hematologic (multiple myeloma), solid tumors (caused by PTHrP)
Endocrine diseases—hyperthyroidism, addisonian crisis, VIPoma
Granulomatous diseases—sarcoidosis, tuberculosis, berylliosis, histoplasmosis
Milk–alkali syndrome
Drugs—thiazide diuretics, lithium, vitamin A or D intoxication
Benign familial hypocalciuric hypercalcemia
Paget disease
Immobilization

PTHrP = parathyroid hormone-related protein; VIPoma = vasoactive intestinal peptide-secreting tumor.

virtual certainty. These sensitive PTH assays employ immunoradiometric or immunochemiluminescent techniques, and can reliably distinguish primary HPT from other causes of hypercalcemia. Furthermore, they do not cross-react with PTHrP. In patients with metastatic cancer and hypercalcemia, iPTH levels help to determine whether the patient also has concurrent PHPT. Patients with PHPT also typically have decreased serum phosphate (approximately 50 percent) and elevated 24-hour urinary calcium concentrations (approximately 60 percent). A mild hyperchloremic metabolic acidosis also is present (80 percent), thereby leading to an elevated chloride:phosphate ratio (> 33). Urinary calcium levels need not be measured routinely, except in patients who have not had previously documented normocalcemia, or who have a family history of hypercalcemia, to rule out BFHH (24-h urinary calcium excretion < 100 mg/day). Furthermore, in these patients, the serum calcium to creatinine clearance ratio is usually less than 0.01, whereas it is typically greater than 0.02 in patients with primary hyperparathyroidism. Elevated levels of alkaline phosphatase may be found in approximately 10 percent of patients with PHPT. Occasionally, patients present with normocalcemic PHPT caused by vitamin D deficiency, a low serum albumin, excessive hydration, a high phosphate diet, or a low normal blood calcium set-point.

Radiologic tests. Routine hand radiographs are only recommended for patients with an elevated alkaline phosphatase level. Bone mineral density studies using dual-energy absorptiometry are, however, being increasingly used to assess the effects of PHPT on bone. Abdominal ultrasound examination is used selectively to document renal stones.

Treatment

Rationale for parathyroidectomy and guidelines for operative treatment. Most authorities agree that patients who have developed complications such as kidney stones, osteoporosis, or renal dysfunction, have the "classic" symptoms of PHPT, or who are younger than age 50 years, should undergo parathyroidectomy. However, the treatment of patients with asymptomatic PHPT has been the subject of controversy, partly because there is little agreement on what constitutes an "asymptomatic" patient. At the National Institutes of Health (NIH) consensus conference in 1990, "asymptomatic" PHPT was defined as "the absence of common symptoms and signs of PHPT, including no bone, renal, gastrointestinal, or neuromuscular disorders." The panel advocated nonoperative management of these patients with mild PHPT based on observational studies, which suggested relative stability of biochemical parameters over time. However, the consensus panel considered certain asymtomatic patients to be candidates for surgery. These guidelines were reassessed at a second NIH workshop in 2002. Parathyroidectomy is now recommended for patients with (1) smaller elevations in serum calcium levels (< 1 mg/dL above the upper limit of normal), (2) a greater than 30 percent decline in creatinine clearance, (3) urinary calcium greater than 400g/day, (4) bone mineral density measured at any of three sites (radius, spine, or hip) is greater than 2.5 SD below those of gender- and race-matched, but not age-matched, controls (i.e., peak bone density or T-score [rather than Z-score] < 2.5) and (5) age less than 50 years. The panel still recommends exercising caution in using neuropsychologic abnormalities, cardiovascular disease, gastrointestinal symptoms, menopause, and elevated serum or urine indices of increased bone turnover as sole indications for parathyroidectomy.

Although bisphosphonates and calcimimetics show promise in the treatment of patients with PHPT, these therapies are experimental, long-term outcome data is lacking, and their routine use is not advocated. Parathyroidectomy also is more cost-effective than medical follow up within 5 years of initial treatment. Therefore, it is recommended that parathyroidectomy should be offered to virtually all patients, except those in whom the operative risks are prohibitive. Patients who do not undergo surgery should undergo routine follow-up consisting of biannual calcium measurements and annual measurements of bone mineral density and serum creatinine.

Preoperative localization tests. The diagnosis of PHPT is a metabolic one and localization studies should not be used to make or confirm it. Most endocrine surgeons agree that localization studies are mandatory and invaluable prior to any redo-parathyroid surgery, but their utility prior to initial neck exploration continues to be controversial. There also is little consensus on which localization studies should be used. 99m Technetium-labeled sestamibi is the most widely used and accurate modality, with a sensitivity greater than 80 percent for detection of parathyroid adenomas. Sestamibi scans are generally complemented by neck ultrasound, which can identify adenomas with greater than 75 percent sensitivity in experienced centers, and is most useful in identifying intrathyroidal parathyroids. Single-photon emission computed tomography (SPECT), when used with planar sestamibi, has particular utility in the evaluation of ectopic parathyroid adenomas, such as those located deep in the neck or in the mediastinum. Specifically, SPECT can indicate whether an adenoma is located in the anterior or posterior mediastinum (aortopulmonary window), thus enabling the surgeon to modify the operative approach accordingly. CT and MRI scans are less sensitive than sestamibi scans, but are helpful in localizing mediastinal glands. Intraoperative parathyroid hormone was initially introduced in 1993, and is used to determine the adequacy of parathyroid resection. According to one commonly used criterion, when the PTH falls by 50 percent or more in 10 min after removal of a parathyroid tumor, as compared to the highest preremoval value, the test is considered positive and the operation is terminated. Although preoperative localization studies and intraoperative PTH have become widely used since their inception, long-term outcome data and cost-effectiveness studies are needed before their routine use can be recommended.

Operative Approaches

When unilateral parathyroid exploration was first carried out, the choice of side to be explored was random, but the introduction of preoperative localization studies has enabled a more directed approach. The focused approach identifies only the enlarged parathyroid gland and no attempts are made to locate other normal parathyroid glands. Unilateral neck explorations have several advantages over bilateral neck exploration, including reduced operative times and complications, such as injury to the recurrent laryngeal nerve and hypoparathyroidism. However, most existing studies comparing the two approaches are retrospective and do not analyze the results on an intention-to-treat basis. The issues relating to optimal approach will only be resolved by a large, prospective, multicenter study or by improved molecular analytic techniques. Similarly, although various videoscopic and video-assisted techniques of parathyroidectomy currently are in use, they also are associated with increased operating times, often require more personnel, are expensive, and have, in general, not been useful for patients with multiglandular disease.

The practice of these authors involves obtaining both a sestamibi scan and neck ultrasound in patients with PHPT. Studies show that if both studies independently identify the same enlarged parathyroid gland, and no other gland, it is indeed the abnormal gland in approximately 95 percent of cases. These patients with sporadic PHPT are candidates for a focused neck exploration. A standard bilateral neck exploration is planned if parathyroid localization studies or intraoperative parathyroid hormone are not available; if the localizing studies fail to identify any abnormal parathyroid gland, or identify multiple abnormal glands, in patients with a family history of PHPT, MEN1, or MEN 2A; or if there is a concomitant thyroid disorder that requires bilateral exploration.

Conduct of Parathyroidectomy (Standard Bilateral Exploration)

The procedure is usually performed under general anesthesia. For a bilateral exploration, the neck is explored via a 3–4-cm incision just caudal to the cricoid cartilage. The initial dissection and exposure is similar to that used for thyroidectomy. After the strap muscles are separated in the midline, one side of the neck is chosen for exploration. During parathyroidectomy, the dissection is maintained lateral to the thyroid, making it easier to identify the parathyroid glands and not disturb their blood supply.

Identification of the parathyroid glands. A bloodless field is important to enable identification of parathyroid glands. The middle thyroid veins are ligated and divided, thus enabling medial and anterior retraction of the thyroid lobe. This may be facilitated by a peanut sponge or placement of 2-0 silk sutures into the thyroid substance. The space between the carotid sheath and thyroid is then opened by gentle sharp and blunt dissection, from the cricoid cartilage superiorly to the thymus inferiorly and the RLN is identified. Approximately 85 percent of the parathyroid glands are found within 1 cm of the junction of the inferior thyroid artery and recurrent laryngeal nerves. Parathyroid glands are partly surrounded by fat, therefore, any fat lobule at typical parathyroid locations should be explored, because the normal or abnormal parathyroid gland may be concealed in the fatty tissue. The thin fascia overlying a "suspicious" fat lobule should be incised using a sharp, curved hemostat and scalpel. This maneuver often causes the parathyroid gland to "pop" out. Alternatively, gentle, blunt peanut sponge dissection between the carotid sheath and the thyroid gland often reveals a "float" sign, suggesting the site of the abnormal parathyroid gland.

Several characteristics, such as size (> 7 mm), weight, and color, are used to distinguish normal from hypercellular parathyroid glands. Hypercellular glands are generally darker, more firm, and more vascular than normocellular glands. Because no single method is 100 percent reliable, the parathyroid surgeon must rely on experience, and sometimes a good pathologist, to help distinguish normal from hypercellular glands. Although several molecular studies have shown utility in distinguishing parathyroid adenomas from hyperplasia, this determination must also be made by the surgeon intraoperatively by documenting the presence of a normal parathyroid gland.

Location of parathyroid glands. The majority of lower parathyroid glands are found in proximity to the lower thyroid pole. If not found at this location, the thyrothymic ligament and thymus should be mobilized and explored. The carotid sheath should also be opened from the bifurcation to the base of the neck if the parathyroid tumor cannot be found. If these maneuvers are unsuccessful, an intrathyroidal gland should be sought by using intraoperative ultrasound, incising the thyroid capsule on its posterolateral surface, or by performing an ipsilateral thyroid lobectomy and "bread-loafing" the thyroid lobe. Preoperative or intraoperative ultrasonography can be useful for identifying intrathyroidal parathyroid glands. Rarely, the third branchial pouch may maldescend and be found high in the neck (undescended parathymus), anterior to the carotid bulb, along with the missing parathyroid gland. Upper parathyroid glands are more consistent in position and are usually found near the junction of the upper and middle thirds of the gland, at the level of the cricoid cartilage. Ectopic upper glands may be found in the carotid sheath, tracheoesophageal groove, in the retroesophageal, or in the posterior mediastinum. Treatment depends on the number of abnormal glands.

A single adenoma is presumed to be the cause of a patient's primary HPT if only one parathyroid tumor is identified and the other parathyroid glands are normal, a situation present in approximately 80 percent of patients with PHPT. Adenomas typically have an atrophic rim of normal parathyroid tissue, but this characteristic may be absent. If two abnormal and two normal glands are identified, the patient has double adenomas. Triple adenomas are present if three glands are abnormal and one is normal. Multiple adenomas are more common in older patients with an incidence of up to 10 percent in patients more than 60 years old. The abnormal glands should be excised, provided the remaining glands are confirmed as such, thus excluding asymmetric hyperplasia, after biopsy and frozen section.

If all parathyroid glands are enlarged or hypercellular, patients have parathyroid hyperplasia, which has been shown to occur in approximately 15 percent of patients in various series. These glands are often lobulated, usually lack the rim of normal parathyroid gland seen in adenomas, and may be variable in size. It is often difficult to distinguish multiple adenomas from hyperplasia with variable gland size. Hyperplasia may be of the chief cell (more common), mixed, or clear-cell type. Patients with hyperplasia may be treated by subtotal parathyroidectomy or by total parathyroidectomy and autotransplantation. Initial studies demonstrated equivalent cure rates and postoperative hypocalcemia for the two techniques, with the latter having the added advantage of avoiding recurrence in the neck. However, subtotal parathyroidectomy is preferred because autotransplanted tissue may fail to function in approximately 5 percent of cases.

For patients with hyperplasia, a titanium clip is placed across the most normal gland, leaving a 50-mg remnant and taking care to avoid disturbing the vascular pedicle. If the remnant appears to be viable, the remaining glands are resected. If there is any question regarding the viability of the initially subtotally resected gland, another gland is chosen for subtotal resection and the initial remnant is removed. Bilateral upper cervical thymectomy also is routinely performed because supernumerary glands occur in up to 20 percent of patients. Whenever multiple parathyroids are resected, it is preferable to cryopreserve tissue. Parathyroid tissue usually is transplanted into brachioradialis muscle of the nondominant forearm. Pockets are made in the belly of the muscle and one to two pieces of parathyroid tissue, measuring 1 mm each, are placed into each pocket. Twelve to 14 pieces are transplanted.

Indications for Sternotomy

A median sternotomy may be necessary to locate a missing gland only after a complete search has been conducted in the neck. A sternotomy is not usually recommended at the initial operation, unless the calcium level is greater than 13 mg/dL. Rather, it is preferred to biopsy the normal glands and subsequently close the patient's neck and obtain localizing studies, if they were not obtained previously.

Special Situations

Parathyroid carcinoma. Parathyroid cancer accounts for approximately 1 percent of the cases of PHPT. It may be suspected preoperatively by the presence of severe symptoms, serum calcium levels greater than 14 mg/dL, significantly elevated PTH levels, and a palpable parathyroid gland. Local invasion is common, as are lymph node and distant metastases. Intraoperatively, parathyroid cancer is suggested by the presence of a large, gray-white to gray-brown parathyroid tumor that is adherent to or invasive into surrounding tissues such as muscle, thyroid, recurrent laryngeal nerve, trachea, or esophagus. Enlarged lymph nodes also may be present. Accurate diagnosis necessitates histologic examination, which reveals local tissue invasion, vascular or capsular invasion, trabecular or fibrous stroma, and frequent mitoses.

Treatment of parathyroid cancer consists of bilateral neck exploration, with en bloc excision of the tumor and the ipsilateral thyroid lobe. Modified radical neck dissection is recommended in the presence of lymph node metastases. Radiation and chemotherapy can be considered in patients with unresectable disease. Bisphosphonates and calcimimetic drugs may also be effective in long-term palliation.

Familial HPT. These patients generally have a higher incidence of multiglandular disease, supernumerary glands, and recurrent or persistent disease. Therefore, they warrant a more aggressive approach and are not candidates for various focused surgical approaches. Localization studies can be obtained to identify potential ectopic glands. A standard bilateral neck exploration is performed, along with a bilateral cervical thymectomy, regardless of the results of localization studies. Both subtotal parathyroidectomy and total parathyroidectomy with autotransplantation are appropriate, and parathyroid tissue should also be cryopreserved. If an adenoma is found in patients with familial HPT, the adenoma and the ipsilateral normal parathyroid glands are resected. The normal-appearing glands on the contralateral side are biopsied and marked, so that only one side of the neck will need to be explored in the event of recurrence. In patients with MEN 2A, HPT is less aggressive. Hence, only abnormal parathyroid glands need to be resected at neck exploration.

Parathyromatosis. Parathyromatosis is a rare condition characterized by the finding of multiple nodules of hyperfunctioning parathyroid tissue throughout the neck and mediastinum, usually following a previous parathyroidectomy. The true etiology of parathyromatosis is not known. Parathyromatosis represents a rare cause of persistent or recurrent HPT and can be identified intraoperatively. Aggressive local resection of these deposits can result in normocalcemia, but is rarely curative. Some studies suggest that these patients have low-grade carcinoma because of invasion into muscle and other structures distant from the resected parathyroid tumor.

Persistent and Recurrent Hyperparathyroidism

Persistence is defined as hypercalcemia that fails to resolve after parathyroidectomy and is more common than recurrence, which refers to HPT occurring after an intervening period of at least 6 months of biochemically documented normocalcemia. The most common causes for both these states include ectopic parathyroids, unrecognized hyperplasia, supernumerary glands, subtotal resection of a parathyroid tumor, parathyroid cancer, and parathyromatosis. More rare causes include parathyroid carcinoma, missed adenoma in a normal position, incomplete resection of an abnormal gland, and an inexperienced surgeon. The most common sites of ectopic parathyroid glands in patients with persistent or recurrent HPT are paraesophageal (28 percent), mediastinal (26 percent), intrathymic (24 percent), intrathyroidal (11 percent), carotid sheath (9 percent), and high cervical or undescended (2 percent).

Once the diagnosis of persistent or recurrent HPT is suspected, it should be confirmed by the necessary biochemical tests. In particular, a 24-hour urine collection should be performed to rule out benign familial hypocalciuric hypercalcemia (BFHH). In redo parathyroid surgery, the glands are more likely to be in ectopic locations and postoperative scarring tends to make the procedure more technically demanding. Cure rates are generally lower (80–90 percent as compared with 95–99 percent for initial operation) and risk of injury to RLNs and permanent hypocalcemia are higher. Therefore, an evaluation of severity of HPT and the patient's anesthetic risk is important. High-risk patients whose tumors cannot be identified by localization studies may benefit from nonoperative management such as calcimimetic drugs or angiographic embolization.

Preoperative localization studies are routinely performed. Noninvasive studies, such as a sestamibi scan, ultrasound, and MRI, are recommended and reportedly have a combined accuracy of approximately 85 percent for these studies in cases of persistent or recurrent HPT. If these studies are negative or equivocal, highly selective venous catheterization for PTH levels is performed. Previous operative notes and pathology reports should be carefully reviewed and reconciled with the information obtained from localization studies. Generally, these patients are approached with a focused exploration with intraoperative PTH measurement to reduce the risk of complications.

Hypercalcemic Crisis

Patients with primary HPT may occasionally present acutely with nausea, vomiting, fatigue, muscle weakness, confusion and a decreased level of consciousness; a complex referred to as hypercalcemic crisis. This condition results from severe hypercalcemia from uncontrolled PTH secretion, worsened by polyuria, dehydration, and reduced kidney function, and may occur with other conditions causing hypercalcemia. Calcium levels are markedly elevated and may be as high as 16–20 mg/dL. Parathyroid glands are always large or multiple, and the tumor may be palpable. Patients with parathyroid cancer or familial HPT are more likely to present with hyperparathyroid crisis. Treatment consists of therapies to lower serum calcium levels followed by surgery to correct hyperparathyroidism.

Secondary Hyperparathyroidism

Secondary HPT commonly occurs in patients with chronic renal failure but may also occur in those with hypocalcemia secondary to inadequate calcium or vitamin D intake, or malabsorption. The pathophysiology of HPT in chronic renal failure is complex and is thought to be related to hyperphosphatemia (and resultant hypocalcemia), deficiency of 1,25-dihydroxy vitamin D as a result of loss of renal tissue, low calcium intake, decreased calcium absorption, and abnormal parathyroid cell response to extracellular calcium or vitamin D in vitro and in vivo. Patients are generally hypocalcemic or normocalcemic. These patients are generally treated medically with a low-phosphate diet; phosphate binders; adequate intake of calcium and 1,25-dihydroxyvitamin D; and a high-calcium, low-aluminum dialysis bath. Calcimimetics control parathyroid hyperplasia and osteitis fibrosa cystica associated with secondary HPT in animal studies, and decrease plasma PTH and total and ionized calcium levels in humans.

Surgical treatment is indicated and recommended for patients with bone pain, pruritus, and (1) a calcium-phosphate product greater than or equal to 70, (2) Ca greater than 11 mg/dL with markedly elevated PTH, (3) calciphylaxis, (4) progressive renal osteodystrophy, and (5) soft-tissue calcification and tumoral calcinosis. Calciphylaxis is a rare, limb- and life-threatening complication of secondary HPT characterized by painful (sometimes throbbing), violaceous and mottled lesions, usually on the extremities, which often become necrotic and progress to nonhealing ulcers, gangrene, sepsis, and death.

Patients should undergo routine dialysis to correct electrolyte abnormalities, especially in serum potassium levels. Localizations studies are unnecessary but can identify ectopic parathyroid glands. A bilateral neck exploration is indicated. The parathyroid glands in secondary HPT are characterized by asymmetric enlargement and nodular hyperplasia. These patients may be treated by subtotal resection, leaving about 50 mg of the most normal parathyroid gland or total parathyroidectomy and autotransplantation of parathyroid tissue into the brachioradialis muscle of the nondominant forearm. Upper thymectomy usually is performed because 15–20 percent of patients have one or more parathyroid glands situated in the thymus or perithymic fat.

Tertiary Hyperparathyroidism

Tertiary hyperparathyroidism is seen most commonly in patients with long-standing renal dysfunction who undergo successful renal transplantation. Generally, renal transplantation is an excellent method of treating secondary HPT, but some patients develop autonomous parathyroid gland function and tertiary HPT. Tertiary HPT can cause problems similar to PHPT, such as pathologic fractures, bone pain, renal stones, peptic ulcer disease, pancreatitis, and mental status changes. The transplanted kidney is also at risk.

Operative intervention is indicated for symptomatic disease or if autonomous PTH secretion persists for more than 1 year after a successful transplant. All parathyroid glands should be identified. The traditional surgical management of these patients consisted of subtotal or total parathyroidectomy with autotransplantation. However, more recent studies suggest that these patients derive similar benefit from excision of only obviously enlarged glands, although avoiding the higher risks of hypocalcemia associated with the former approach. It is recommended that all parathyroid glands be identified. If one gland is distinctly abnormal and others minimally abnormal, the abnormal gland and the more-normal gland on the same side should be resected with the remaining parathyroids marked. If all the glands are abnormal, a subtotal parathyroidectomy should be performed with upper thymectomy.

COMPLICATIONS OF PARATHYROID SURGERY

Parathyroidectomy can be accomplished successfully in greater than 95 percent of patients with minimal mortality and morbidity, provided the procedure is performed by a surgeon experienced in parathyroid surgery. General complications are similar to those for thyroidectomy. Specific complications include transient and permanent vocal cord palsy and hypoparathyroidism. The latter is more likely to occur in patients who undergo four-gland exploration with biopsies, subtotal resection with an inadequate remnant, or total parathyroidectomy with a failure of autotransplanted tissue. Furthermore, hypocalcemia is more likely to occur in patients with high turnover bone disease as evidenced by elevated preoperative alkaline phosphatase levels. Vocal cord paralysis and hypoparathyroidism are considered permanent if they persist for more than 6 months. Fortunately, these complications are rare, occurring in approximately 1 percent of patients undergoing surgery by experienced parathyroid surgeons.

Patients with symptomatic hypocalcemia or those with calcium levels less than 8 mg/dL are treated with oral calcium supplementation (up to 1–2 g every 4 h). 1,25-Dihydroxy vitamin D (Rocaltrol 0.25–0.5 μg bid) may also be required, particularly in patients with severe hypercalcemia and elevated serum alkaline phosphatase levels preoperatively and with osteitis fibrosa cystica. Intravenous calcium supplementation is rarely needed, except in cases of severe, symptomatic hypocalcemia. Caution should be exercised in its administration because extravasation from the vein can cause extensive tissue necrosis.

HYPOPARATHYROIDISM

The parathyroid glands may be congenitally absent in the DiGeorge syndrome, which also is characterized by lack of thymic development, and, therefore, a thymus-dependent lymphoid system. Hyperparathyroidism in pregnant women can lead to hypoparathyroidism in neonates from suppression of fetal parathyroid tissue. By far, the most common cause of hypoparathyroidism is thyroid surgery, particularly total thyroidectomy with a concomitant central neck dissection. Patients often develop transient hypocalcemia as a result of bruising or damage to the vascular supply of the glands; permanent hypoparathyroidism is uncommon. Hypoparathyroidism may also occur after parathyroid surgery, which is more likely if patients have parathyroid hyperplasia and undergo a subtotal resection or total parathyroidectomy with parathyroid autotransplantation. Parathyroid tissue should be cryopreserved in any patient who could develop hypoparathyroidism, but is only needed in approximately 2 percent of patients.

Acute hypocalcemia results in decreased ionized calcium and increased neuromuscular excitability. Patients initially develop circumoral and fingertip numbness and tingling. Mental symptoms include anxiety, confusion, and depression. Physical examination reveals positive Chvostek sign (contraction of facial muscles elicited by tapping on the facial nerve anterior to the ear) and Trousseau sign (carpopedal spasm, which is elicited by occluding blood flow to the forearm with a blood pressure cuff for 2–3 min). Tetany, which is characterized by tonic–clonic seizures, carpopedal spasm, and laryngeal stridor, may prove fatal. Most patients with postoperative hypocalcemia can be treated with oral calcium and vitamin D supplements. Intravenous calcium infusion rarely is required.

ADRENAL/EMBRYOLOGY

The adrenal glands consist of an outer cortex and an inner medulla. The cortex originates around the fifth week of gestation from mesodermal tissue near the gonads on the adrenogenital ridge. Therefore, ectopic adrenocortical tissue may be found in the ovaries, spermatic cord, and testes. In contrast, the adrenal medulla is ectodermal in origin and arises from the neural crest. At around the same time as cortical development, neural crest cells migrate to the para-aortic and paravertebral areas and toward the medial aspect of the developing cortex to form the medulla. Adrenal medullary tissue may also be found in neck, urinary bladder, and para-aortic regions.

ANATOMY

The adrenal glands are paired, retroperitoneal organs located superior and medial to the kidneys at the level of the eleventh ribs. The normal adrenal gland measures $5 \times 3 \times 1$ cm and weighs 4–5 g. Each gland is supplied by three groups of vessels: the superior adrenal arteries derived from the inferior phrenic artery, the middle adrenal arteries derived from the aorta, and the inferior adrenal arteries derived from the renal artery. Other vessels originating from the intercostal and gonadal vessels may also supply the adrenals. These arteries branch into about 50 arterioles to form a rich plexus beneath the glandular capsule. In contrast to the arterial supply, each adrenal usually is drained by a single, major adrenal vein. The right adrenal vein usually is short and drains into the inferior vena cava, whereas the left adrenal vein is longer and empties into the left renal vein after joining the inferior phrenic vein. Accessory veins occur in 5–10 percent of patients.

The adrenal cortex accounts for approximately 80–90 percent of the gland's volume and is divided into three zones: zona glomerulosa (site of aldosterone production), zona fasciculata, and zona reticularis. The latter zones are the site of production of glucocorticoids and adrenal androgens. The adrenal medulla constitutes up to 10–20 percent of the gland's volume and produces the catecholamine hormones epinephrine and norepinephrine. The cells of the adrenal medulla often are referred to as chromaffin cells because they stain specifically with chromium salts.

PHYSIOLOGY

Cholesterol, derived from the plasma or synthesized in the adrenal, is the common precursor of all steroid hormones derived from the adrenal cortex. Cholesterol is initially cleaved within mitochondria to 5-δ-pregnenolone, which, in turn, is transported to the smooth endoplasmic reticulum where it forms the substrate for various biosynthetic pathways leading to steroidogenesis.

The major adrenal mineralocorticoid hormones are aldosterone, 11-deoxycorticosterone (DOC), and cortisol. Cortisol has minimal effects on the kidney because of hormone degradation. Aldosterone secretion is regulated primarily by the renin–angiotensin system. Decreased renal blood flow, decreased plasma sodium and increased sympathetic tone, all stimulate the release of renin from juxtaglomerular cells. Renin, in turn, leads to the production of angiotensin I from its precursor angiotensinogen. Angiotensin I is cleaved by pulmonary angiotensin-converting enzyme (ACE) to angiotensin II, which is not only a potent vasoconstrictor, but also leads to increased aldosterone synthesis and release. Hyperkalemia is another potent stimulator of aldosterone synthesis, whereas ACTH, pituitary pro-opiomelanocortin (POMC), and antidiuretic hormone (ADH) are weak stimulators. Aldosterone functions mainly to increase sodium reabsorption and potassium and hydrogen ion excretion at the level of the renal distal convoluted tubule.

The secretion of cortisol, the major adrenal glucocorticoid, is regulated by ACTH secreted by the anterior pituitary, which in turn, is under the control of corticotrophin-releasing hormone (CRH) secreted by the hypothalamus. ACTH secretion may be stimulated by pain, stress, hypoxia, hypothermia, trauma, and hypoglycemia. ACTH secretion fluctuates, thus, there is a diurnal variation in the secretion of cortisol with peak cortisol excretion also occurring in the early morning and declining during the day to its lowest levels in the evening. Cortisol controls the secretion of both CRH and ACTH via a negative-feedback loop. Cortisol is transported in plasma bound primarily to cortisol-binding globulin (75 percent) and albumin (15 percent). Most of the cortisol metabolites are conjugated with glucuronic acid in the liver, thus facilitating their renal excretion. A small amount of unmetabolized cortisol is excreted unchanged in the urine. Cortisol also binds the mineralocorticoid receptor with an affinity similar to aldosterone. However, the specificity of mineralocorticoid action is maintained by the production of 11β-hydroxysteroid dehydrogenase, an enzyme that inactivates cortisol to cortisone in the kidney. Glucocorticoids have important functions in intermediary metabolism, but also affect growth and development and the connective tissue, immune, cardiovascular, renal, and central nervous systems.

Adrenal androgens are produced from 17-hydroxypregnenolone in response to ACTH stimulation. The adrenal androgens include dehydroepiandrosterone (DHEA) and its sulfated counterpart (DHEAS), androstenedione, and small amounts of testosterone and estrogen. Adrenal androgens exert their major effects by peripheral conversion to the more potent testosterone and dihy-drotestosterone, but also have weak intrinsic androgen activity. During fetal development, adrenal androgens promote the formation of male genitalia, and are responsible for the development of secondary sexual characteristics at puberty.

Catecholamine hormones (epinephrine, norepinephrine, and dopamine) are produced both in the central and sympathetic nervous system and in the adrenal medulla from the substrate tyrosine. Phenylethanolamine-N-methyltransferase, which converts norepinephrine to epinephrine, is only present in the adrenal medulla and the organ of Zuckerkandl. Therefore, the primary catecholamine produced can be used to distinguish adrenal medullary tumors from those situated at extra-adrenal sites. Catecholamines are cleared by several mechanisms including reuptake by sympathetic nerve endings, periph-eral inactivation by catechol-O-methyltransferase (COMT) and monoamine oxidase (MAO), and direct excretion by the kidneys. Metabolism of cat-echolamines leads to the formation of metabolites such as metanephrines, normetanephrines, and vanillylmandelic acid.

DISORDERS OF THE ADRENAL CORTEX

Hyperaldosteronism (Conn Syndrome)

Primary hyperaldosteronism results from autonomous aldosterone secretion, which, in turn, leads to suppression of renin secretion. Primary aldosteronism usually occurs in individuals between the ages of 30 and 50 years and ac-counts for 1 percent of cases of hypertension. It is usually associated with hypokalemia; however, more patients with Conn syndrome are being diag-nosed with normal potassium levels. Most cases result from a solitary func-tioning adrenal adenoma (approximately 70 percent) and idiopathic bilateral hyperplasia (30 percent). Adrenocortical carcinoma and glucocorticoid suppressible hyperaldosteronism are rare, each accounting for less than 1 percent of cases.

Symptoms and Signs

Patients typically present with hypertension, which is long-standing, moderate to severe, and may be difficult to control despite multiple-drug therapy. Other symptoms include muscle weakness, polydipsia, polyuria, nocturia, headaches, and fatigue.

Diagnostic Studies

Laboratory studies. Hyperaldosteronism must be suspected in any hypertensive patient who presents with coexisting spontaneous hypokalemia (K < 3.2 mmol/L), or hypokalemia (< 3 mmol/L) while on diuretic therapy, despite potassium replacements. However, up to 40 percent of patients may be normokalemic. Patients have an elevated plasma aldosterone concentration (PAC) level with a suppressed plasma renin activity (PRA); a PAC:PRA ratio of 25–30:1 is strongly suggestive of the diagnosis. Patients with primary hyperaldosteronism also fail to suppress aldosterone levels with sodium loading. This test can be performed by performing a 24-h urine collection for cortisol, sodium, and aldosterone after 5 days of a high-sodium diet, or, alternatively, by giving the patient a load of 2 L of saline while in the supine position, 2–3 days after being on a low-sodium diet. Plasma aldosterone levels less than 8.5 ng/mL or a 24-h urine aldosterone less than 14 μg after saline loading essentially rules out primary hyperaldosteronism. Further evaluation should be directed at determining which patients have a unilateral aldosteronoma and will thus benefit from surgery.

Radiologic studies. CT scans with 0.5-cm cuts in the adrenal area can localize aldosteronomas with a sensitivity of 90 percent. A unilateral 0.5–2-cm adrenal tumor with a normal-appearing contralateral gland confirms an aldosteronoma in the presence of appropriate biochemical parameters. MRI scans are less sensitive, but more specific, particularly if opposed-phase chemical-shift images are obtained. Selective venous catheterization with adrenal vein sampling for aldosterone is 95 percent sensitive and 90 percent specific in localizing the aldosteronoma. A greater than 4-fold difference in the aldosterone:cortisol ratios between the adrenal veins indicates the presence of a unilateral tumor. Most groups advocate use of this modality selectively in ambiguous cases, when the tumor cannot be localized, and in patients with bilateral adrenal enlargement. Scintigraphy with 131I-6β-iodomethyl noriodocholesterol (NP-59) may also be used for the same purpose.

Treatment

Preoperatively, control of hypertension and adequate potassium supplementation (to keep K > 3.5 mmol/L) are important. Patients are generally treated with spironolactone (an aldosterone antagonist), amiloride (a potassium-sparing diuretic that blocks sodium channels in the distal nephron), nifedipine (a calcium channel blocker), or captopril (an ACE inhibitor). Unilateral tumors producing aldosterone are best managed by adrenalectomy, either by a laparoscopic approach (preferred) or via a posterior open approach, unless a carcinoma is suspected. For patients with bilateral hyperplasia, medical therapy with spironolactone, amiloride, or triamterene is the mainstay of management, with adrenalectomy reserved for patients with the most refractory cases. Patients who respond to spironolactone therapy, and those with a shorter duration of hypertension with minimal end-organ (renal) damage, are more likely to achieve improvement in hypertension, whereas male patients, those older than age 50 years, and those with multiple adrenal nodules are least likely to benefit from adrenalectomy.

Cushing Syndrome

The term Cushing syndrome refers to a complex of symptoms and signs resulting from hypersecretion of cortisol. In contrast, Cushing disease refers to a pituitary tumor, usually an adenoma, which leads to bilateral adrenal hyperplasia and hypercortisolism. Cushing syndrome (endogenous) is a rare disease, affecting 10 in 1 million individuals. It is more common in adults, but may occur in children. Women are more commonly affected than men (male-to-female ratio 1:8).

Cushing syndrome may be classified as ACTH-dependent or ACTH-independent (Table 37-3). Patients with major depression, alcoholism, pregnancy, chronic renal failure, or stress may also have elevated cortisol levels and symptoms of hypercortisolism. However, these manifestations resolve with treatment of the underlying disorder (pseudo-Cushing syndrome).

Primary adrenal hyperplasia may be micronodular, macronodular, or massively macronodular. Adrenal hyperplasia resulting from ACTH stimulation is usually macronodular (3-cm nodules). Primary pigmented nodular adrenocortical disease is a rare cause of ACTH-independent Cushing's syndrome, which is characterized by the presence of small (< 5 mm), black adrenal micronodules. Primary pigmented nodular adrenocortical disease may be associated with Carney complex (atrial myxomas, schwannomas, and pigmented nevi) and is thought to be immune related.

Symptoms and Signs

Progressive truncal obesity is the most common symptom, occurring in up to 95 percent of patients. Fat deposition also occurs in unusual sites, such as the supraclavicular space and posterior neck region, leading to the so-called buffalo hump. Purple striae often are visible on the protuberant abdomen. Rounding of the face secondary to thickening of the facial fat leads to moon facies, and thinning of subcutaneous tissue leads to plethora. There is an increase in fine

TABLE 37-3 Etiology of Cushing Syndrome

ACTH-dependent (70%)
Pituitary adenoma or Cushing disease ($\sim$ 70%)
Ectopic ACTH production[a] ($\sim$ 10%)
Ectopic CRH production (< 1%)
ACTH-independent (20–30%)
Adrenal adenoma (10–15%)
Adrenal carcinoma (5–10%)
Adrenal hyperplasia—pigmented micronodular cortical hyperplasia or gastric inhibitory peptide-sensitive macronodular hyperplasia (5%)
Other
Pseudo-Cushing syndrome
Iatrogenic—exogenous administration of steroids

[a]From small-cell lung tumors, pancreatic islet cell tumors, medullary thyroid cancers, pheochromocytomas, and carcinoid tumors of the lung, thymus, gut, pancreas, and ovary.

hair growth on the face, upper back, and arms, although true virilization is more commonly seen with adrenocortical cancers. Endocrine abnormalities include glucose intolerance, amenorrhea, and decreased libido or impotence. Large, purple striae on the abdomen or proximal extremities are most reliable for making the diagnosis. In children, Cushing syndrome is characterized by obesity and stunted growth. Patients with Cushing disease may also present with headaches, visual field defects, and panhypopituitarism. Hyperpigmentation of the skin, if present, suggests an ectopic ACTH-producing tumor with high levels of circulating ACTH.

Diagnostic Tests

The aims of these studies are 2-fold: to confirm the presence of Cushing syndrome and to determine its etiology.

Laboratory studies. The secretion of cortisol is episodic and has a diurnal variation, therefore a single measurement of the plasma cortisol level is unreliable in diagnosing Cushing syndrome. The overnight low-dose dexamethasone suppression test is used to screen patients—1 mg of a synthetic glucocorticoid (dexamethasone) is given at 11 PM and plasma cortisol levels are measured at 8 AM the following morning. Normal adults suppress cortisol levels less than 3 μg/dL, whereas most patients with Cushing syndrome do not. False-negative results may be obtained in patients with mild disease, therefore some authors consider the test positive only if cortisol levels are suppressed to less than 1.8 μg/dL. In patients with a negative test, but a high clinical suspicion, the classic low-dose dexamethasone (0.5 mg every 6 h for 8 doses, or 2 mg over 48 h) suppression test or urinary cortisol measurement should be performed. A urinary free cortisol excretion of less than 100 μg/dL (in most laboratories) rules out hypercortisolism. Salivary cortisol measurements using commercially available kits are being increasingly used.

Once a diagnosis is established, further testing is aimed at determining the cause by measurement of plasma ACTH levels using immunoradiometric assay (normal 10–100 pg/mL). Elevated ACTH levels indicate adrenal hyperplasia as a result of Cushing disease (15–500 pg/mL) or CRH-secreting tumors, but the highest levels are found in patients with ectopic sources of ACTH (> 1000 pg/mL). In contrast, ACTH levels are characteristically suppressed (< 5 pg/mL) in patients with primary cortisol-secreting adrenal tumors. The high-dose dexamethasone suppression test is used to distinguish between the causes of ACTH-dependent Cushing syndrome (pituitary vs. ectopic). Bilateral petrosal vein sampling also is helpful for determining whether the patient has Cushing disease or ectopic Cushing syndrome. The CRH test also is helpful in determining the etiology of Cushing syndrome. Patients with a primary adrenal cause of hypercortisolism exhibit a blunted response (ACTH peak < 10 pg/mL), whereas those with ACTH-dependent Cushing syndrome demonstrate a higher elevation of ACTH (> 30 pg/mL).

Radiologic studies. CT and MRI scans of the abdomen can identify adrenal tumors with 95 percent sensitivity. They also are helpful in distinguishing adrenal adenomas from carcinomas. Adrenal adenomas appear darker than the liver on T2-weighted imaging. Radioscintigraphic imaging of the adrenals using NP-59 also can be used to distinguish adenoma from hyperplasia. Adrenal adenomas show increased uptake of NP-59 with suppression of uptake in the contralateral gland, whereas hyperplastic glands demonstrate bilateral uptake.

NP-59 scanning is most useful in identifying patients with adrenal source of hypercortisolism and primary pigmented micronodular hyperplasia.

Contrast-enhanced MRI scans of the brain are better than CT scans for identifying pituitary tumors (sensitivity 33–67 percent), although small microadenomas may still escape detection. Inferior petrosal sinus sampling for ACTH before and after injection of CRH has been helpful in this regard, and has a sensitivity approaching 100 percent. In patients suspected of having an ectopic tumor–producing ACTH, CT or MRI scans of the chest and anterior mediastinum should be performed first, followed by imaging of the neck, abdomen, and pelvis if the initial studies are negative.

Treatment

Unilateral laparoscopic adrenalectomy is the treatment of choice for patients with adrenal adenomas. Open adrenalectomy is reserved for large tumors ($\geq$ 6 cm) or those suspected to be adrenocortical cancers. Bilateral adrenalectomy is curative for primary adrenal hyperplasia. The treatment of choice in patients with Cushing disease is transsphenoidal excision of the pituitary adenoma, although pituitary irradiation has been used for patients with persistent or recurrent disease after surgery. Stereotactic radiosurgery, which uses CT guidance to deliver high doses of radiotherapy to the tumor (photon or gamma knife) is being increasingly used. Patients who fail to respond to either treatment are candidates for pharmacologic therapy with adrenal inhibitors such as ketoconazole, metyrapone, or aminoglutethimide, or bilateral adrenalectomy. Patients with ectopic ACTH production are best managed by treating the primary tumor, including recurrences, if possible. Medical or surgical adrenalectomy also has been shown to be safe and effective in the management of patients with Cushing disease whose ectopic ACTH-secreting tumor cannot be localized.

Adrenocortical Cancer

Adrenal carcinomas are rare neoplasms with a worldwide incidence of 2 per 1 million. These tumors have a bimodal age distribution, with an increased incidence in children and in adults in the fourth and fifth decades of life. Functioning tumors are more common in women, whereas men are more likely to develop nonfunctioning carcinomas. The majority are sporadic, but adrenocortical carcinomas also occur in association with germline mutations of p53 (Li-Fraumeni syndrome) and MENIN (multiple endocrine neoplasia 1) genes. Loci on 11p (Beckwith-Wiedemann syndrome), 2p (Carney complex), and 9q also have been implicated.

Symptoms and Signs

Approximately 50 percent of adrenocortical cancers are nonfunctioning. The remaining secrete cortisol (30 percent), androgens (20 percent), estrogens (10 percent), aldosterone (2 percent), or multiple hormones (35 percent). Patients with functioning tumors often present with the rapid onset of Cushing syndrome accompanied by virilizing features. Nonfunctioning tumors more commonly present with an enlarging abdominal mass and abdominal pain. Rarely, weight loss, anorexia, and nausea may be present.

Diagnostic Tests

Diagnostic evaluation of these patients begins with measurement of serum electrolyte levels to rule out hypokalemia, an overnight 1-mg dexamethasone suppression test and a 24-hour urine collection for cortisol, 17-ketosteroids, and catecholamines (to rule out pheochromocytomas). CT and MRI scans are used to image these tumors. The size of the adrenal mass on imaging studies is the single most important criterion to help diagnose malignancy. In the series reported by Copeland and associates, 92 percent of adrenal cancers were greater than 6 cm in diameter. CT imaging characteristics suggesting malignancy include tumor heterogeneity, irregular margins and the presence of hemorrhage and adjacent lymphadenopathy or liver metastases. Moderately bright signal intensity on T2-weighted images (adrenal mass-to-liver ratio 1.2:2.8), significant lesion enhancement, and slow washout after injection of gadolinium contrast also indicate malignancy, as does evidence of local invasion into surrounding structures such as the liver, blood vessels (inferior vena cava), and distant metastases.

Pathology

On gross examination, areas of hemorrhage and necrosis are often evident. Microscopically, cells are hyperchromatic and typically have large nuclei and prominent nucleoli. It is very difficult to distinguish benign adrenal adenomas from carcinomas by histologic examination alone. Other criteria supporting malignancy include invasion, distant metastases, the presence of aneuploidy, increased mitotic figures and production of androgens and 11-deoxysteroids.

Treatment

The most important predictor of survival in patients with adrenal cancer is the adequacy of resection. Therefore, adrenocortical carcinomas are treated by excision of the tumor en bloc, with any contiguously involved lymph nodes or organs, such as the diaphragm, kidney, pancreas, liver, or inferior vena cava. This is best accomplished by open adrenalectomy via a generous incision. Mitotane or o, p-DDD or 1,1-dichloro-2-(o-chlorophenyl)-2-(p-chlorophenyl) ethane, which is a derivative of the insecticide DDT, has adrenolytic activity and has been used in the adjuvant setting and for the treatment of unresectable or metastatic disease. Treatment with replacement doses of steroids is essential in patients receiving mitotane. The therapeutic effectiveness of these agents is conflicting and consistent improvement in survival rates are lacking.

Adrenocortical tumors commonly metastasize to the liver, lung, and bone. Surgical debulking is recommended for isolated, recurrent disease and has been demonstrated to prolong survival. Systemic chemotherapeutic agents used in this tumor include etoposide, cisplatin, doxorubicin, and, more recently, paclitaxel, but consistent responses are rare. Adrenocortical cancers also are relatively insensitive to conventional external beam radiation therapy. Ketoconazole, metyrapone, or aminoglutethimide may also be useful in controlling steroid hypersecretion.

Sex Steroid Excess

Adrenal adenomas or carcinomas that secrete adrenal androgens lead to virilizing syndromes. Although women with virilizing tumors develop hirsutism, amenorrhea, infertility, and other signs of masculinization, men with these tumors are more difficult to diagnose and hence usually present with disease in advanced stages. Children with virilizing tumors have accelerated growth, premature development of facial and pubic hair, acne, genital enlargement, and deepening of their voice. Feminizing adrenal tumors are less common and occur in men in the third to fifth decades of life.

Virilizing tumors produce excessive amounts of the androgen precursor, DHEA, which can be measured in plasma or urine as 17-ketosteroids. Patients with feminizing tumors also have elevated urinary 17-ketosteroids, in addition to increased estrogen levels. These tumors are treated by adrenalectomy. Malignancy is difficult to diagnose histologically, but is suggested by the presence of local invasion, recurrence, or distal metastases. Adrenolytic drugs, such as mitotane, aminoglutethimide, and ketoconazole, may be useful in controlling symptoms in patients with metastatic disease.

Congenital Adrenal Hyperplasia

This refers to a group of disorders that result from deficiencies, or complete absence, of enzymes involved in adrenal steroidogenesis. 21-Hydroxylase (CYP21A2) deficiency is the most common enzymatic defect, accounting for more than 90 percent of cases of CAH. This deficiency prevents the production of 11-deoxyxortisol and 11-deoxycorticosterone from progesterone precursors. Deficiency of glucocorticoids and aldosterone leads to elevated ACTH levels and overproduction of adrenal androgens and corticosteroid precursors such as 17-hydroxyprogesterone and δ4-androstenedione. These compounds are converted to testosterone in the peripheral tissues, thereby leading to virilization. Complete deficiency of 21-hydroxylase presents at birth with virilization, diarrhea, hypovolemia, hyponatremia, hyperkalemia, and hyperpigmentation. Partial enzyme deficiency may present at birth or later with virilizing features. These patients are less prone to the salt-wasting that characterizes complete enzyme deficiency.

The particular enzyme deficiency can be diagnosed by karyotype analysis and measurement of plasma and urinary steroids. Absence of 21-hydroxylase leads to increased plama 17-hydroxyprogesterone and progesterone levels, because these compounds cannot be converted to 11-deoxycortisol and 11-deoxycorticosterone, respectively. CT, MRI, and iodocholesterol scans are generally used to localize the tumors.

These patients have traditionally been managed medically, with cortisol and mineralocorticoid replacement to suppress the hypothalamic–pituitary–adrenal axis. However, this often leads to iatrogenic hypercortisolism. More recently, bilateral laparoscopic adrenalectomy has been proposed as an alternative treatment for this disease and has been successfully performed in a limited number of patients.

DISORDERS OF THE ADRENAL MEDULLA

Pheochromocytomas

Pheochromocytomas are rare tumors with prevalence rates ranging from 0.3–0.95 percent in autopsy series, and approximately 1.9 percent in series using biochemical screening. They can occur at any age and have no gender predilection. Extra-adrenal tumors may be found at sites of sympathetic ganglia in the organ of Zuckerkandl, neck, mediastinum, abdomen, and pelvis. Pheochromocytomas often are called the "10 percent tumor," because 10 percent are bilateral, 10 percent are malignant, 10 percent occur in pediatric patients, 10 percent are extra-adrenal, and 10 percent are familial.

Pheochromocytomas occur in families with MEN 2A and MEN 2B, in approximately 50 percent of patients. Both syndromes are inherited in an autosomal dominant fashion and are caused by germline mutations in the RET proto-oncogene. Another familial cancer syndrome with an increased risk of pheochromocytomas includes von Hippel-Lindau disease, which also is inherited in an autosomal dominant manner. The incidence of pheochromocytomas in the syndrome is approximately 14 percent, but varies depending on the series. The gene causing von Hippel-Lindau disease has been mapped to chromosome 3p and is a tumor-suppressor gene. Pheochromocytomas also are included within the tumor spectrum of neurofibromatosis type 1 and other neuroectodermal disorders (Sturge-Weber syndrome and tuberous sclerosis), Carney syndrome and, rarely, in the MEN1 syndrome.

Symptoms and Signs

Headache, palpitations, and diaphoresis constitute the "classic triad" of pheochromocytomas. Symptoms such as anxiety, tremulousness, paresthesias, flushing, chest pain, shortness of breath, abdominal pain, nausea, vomiting, and others are nonspecific and may be episodic in nature. Cardiovascular complications may ensue. These symptoms can be incited by a range of stimuli including exercise, micturition, and defecation. The most common clinical sign is hypertension, which may be paroxysmal with intervening normotension, sustained with paroxysms, or sustained hypertension alone.

Diagnostic Tests

Pheochromocytomas are diagnosed by testing 24-h urine samples for catecholamines and their metabolites, and by determining plasma metanephrine levels. Urinary metanephrines are 98 percent sensitive and are also highly specific for pheochromocytomas, whereas vanillylmandelic acid (VMA) measurements are slightly less sensitive and specific. Because extra-adrenal sites lack phenylethanolamine-N-methyltransferase, these tumors secrete norepinephrine, whereas epinephrine is the main hormone secreted from adrenal pheochromocytomas. Recent studies have shown that plasma metanephrines are the most reliable tests to identify pheochromocytomas.

CT scans are 85–95 percent sensitive and 70–100 percent specific for pheochromocytomas and should image the region from the diaphragm to the aortic bifurcation so as to image the organ of Zuckerkandl. MRI scans are 95 percent sensitive and almost 100 percent specific for pheochromocytomas because these tumors have a characteristic appearance on T2-weighted images or after gadolinium. 131I radiolabeled MIBG is useful for localizing pheochromocytomas, especially those in ectopic positions.

Treatment

Alpha blockers such as phenoxybenzamine are started 1–3 weeks before surgery at doses of 10 mg twice daily, which may be increased to 300–400 mg/day. Beta blockers, such as propranolol at doses of 10–40 mg every 6–8 h, often need to be added preoperatively in patients who have persistent tachycardia and arrhythmias, but only after adequate α blockade and hydration to avoid the effects of unopposed alpha stimulation, i.e., hypertensive crisis and congestive heart failure. Patients should also be volume repleted preoperatively.

Adrenalectomy is the treatment of choice. The chief goal of surgery is to resect the tumor completely with minimal tumor manipulation or rupture of the tumor capsule. Surgery should be performed with both noninvasive and invasive monitors, including an arterial line and central venous lines. The common medications used for intraoperative blood pressure control include nitroprusside, nitroglycerin, and phentolamine. Intraoperative arrhythmias are best managed by short-acting beta blockers such as esmolol. Pheochromocytomas less than 5 cm in diameter are currently safely resected laparoscopically, others require open adrenalectomy. In case of hereditary pheochromocytomas, unilateral adrenalectomy is recommended in the absence of obvious lesions in the contralateral adrenal gland, because the high incidence of an addisonian crisis in patients undergoing bilateral adrenalectomy. For patients with tumors in both adrenal glands, cortical-sparing subtotal adrenalectomy may be offered to preserve adrenocortical function and avoid the morbidity of bilateral total adrenalectomy.

THE ADRENAL INCIDENTALOMA

Adrenal lesions discovered during imaging performed for unrelated reasons are referred to as incidentalomas. The incidence of these lesions identified by CT scans ranges from 0.4–4.4 percent. Table 37-4 lists a multitude of lesions that are included in the differential diagnosis. Nonfunctional cortical adenomas account for the majority (36–94 percent) of adrenal incidentalomas in patients without a history of cancer. By definition, patients with incidentalomas do not have clinically overt Cushing syndrome, but subclinical Cushing syndrome is estimated to occur in approximately 8 percent of patients. Examination of the natural history of subclinical Cushing syndrome indicates that although most patients of this disorder remain asymptomatic, some do progress to clinically evident Cushing syndrome. The adrenal is a common site of metastases of lung and breast tumors, melanoma, renal cell cancer, and lymphoma.

Diagnostic Investigations

The diagnostic work-up of an adrenal incidentaloma is aimed at identifying functioning tumors and those at increased risk of being malignant. It is not necessary for asymptomatic patients whose imaging studies are consistent with obvious cysts, hemorrhage, myelolipomas, or diffuse metastatic disease to undergo additional investigations. All other patients should be tested for underlying hormonally active tumors by (1) low-dose (1 mg) overnight dexamethasone suppression test or 24-h urine cortisol to rule out subclinical Cushing syndrome; (2) a 24-h urine collection for catecholamines, metanephrines, vanillylmandelic acid, or plasma metanephrine to rule out pheochromocytoma; and (3) in hypertensive patients, serum electrolytes, plasma aldosterone, and plasma renin to rule out an aldosteronoma. Confirmatory tests can be performed based on the results of the initial screening studies.

TABLE 37-4 Differential Diagnosis of Adrenal Incidentaloma

Functioning lesions	Nonfunctioning lesions
Benign	*Benign*
Aldosteronoma	Cortical adenoma
Cortisol-producing adenoma	Myelolipoma
Sex-steroid-producing adenoma	Cyst
Pheochromocytoma	Ganglioneuroma
	Hemorrhage
Malignant	*Malignant*
Adrenocortical cancer	Metastasis
Malignant pheochromocytoma	

Determination of the malignant potential of an incidentaloma is more complicated. The risk of malignancy in an adrenal lesion is related to its size. Lesions greater than 6 cm in diameter have a risk of malignancy of approximately 35 percent. However, this size cutoff is not absolute because adrenal carcinomas also have been reported in lesions smaller than 6 cm. This has led to increased use of the imaging characteristics of incidentalomas on CT scan and MRI to predict malignancy. Unfortunately, these are not 100 percent reliable either. FNA biopsy has gained widespread use for the diagnosis of many endocrine lesions, but cannot be used to distinguish adrenal adenomas from carcinomas. This being said, FNA biopsy is useful in the setting of a patient with a history of cancer and a solitary adrenal mass. The positive predictive value of FNA biopsy in this situation has been shown to be almost 100 percent, although false-negative rates of up to 33 percent have been reported. Pheochromocytomas should be excluded prior to the procedure.

Management

Patients with functional tumors, as determined by biochemical testing, or with obviously malignant lesions, should undergo adrenalectomy. Operative intervention also is advised in patients with subclinical Cushing syndrome with suppressed plasma ACTH levels and elevated urinary cortisol levels because these patients are at high risk for progression to overt Cushing syndrome. Adrenalectomy also should be considered in patients with normal ACTH and urinary free cortisol if they are younger than 50 years old or have recent weight gain, hypertension, diabetes, or osteopenia.

For nonfunctional lesions that do not meet any of the above criteria, the risk of malignancy or malignant potential needs to be balanced with operative morbidity and mortality. Lesions larger than 6 cm, or those with suspicious features on imaging studies such as heterogeneity, irregular capsule, or adjacent nodes, should be treated by adrenalectomy because of the increased prevalence of malignancy in this group. Nonoperative therapy, with close periodic follow up is advised for lesions less than 4 cm in diameter with benign imaging characteristics. However, the management of lesions 4–6 cm in size with benign imaging features remains controversial; i.e., this group of patients can be treated with observation or surgery. Recommendations from various groups of endocrine surgeons regarding this "intermediate" group of patients are variable, with some advising adrenalectomy for tumors at cutoff sizes of 3, 4, or 5 cm.

However, several important points must be considered in the management of these patients. First, size criteria for malignancy are not definitive and are derived from a selected series of patients. Second, the actual size of adrenal tumors can be underestimated by at least 1 cm by modalities such as CT scans, because tumors are larger in a cephalocaudal axis. Third, the natural history of incidentalomas is variable and depends on the underlying diagnosis, age of the study population, and the size of the mass. The current recommendation of these authors concerning size threshold for adrenalectomy is 3–4 cm in young patients with no comorbidity, and 5 cm in older patients with significant comorbidity. Lesions that grow during follow up also are treated by adrenalectomy. Resection of solitary adrenal metastases in patients with a history of nonadrenal cancer, especially non–small cell lung and renal cancers, has been demonstrated to lead to prolonged patient survival. Suspected adrenal metastases also may be resected for diagnosis or for palliation, if large and symptomatic in good-risk patients.

ADRENAL INSUFFICIENCY

Adrenal insufficiency may be primary, resulting from adrenal disease, or secondary, as a result of a deficiency of ACTH. The most commonly encountered causes of primary adrenal insufficiency are autoimmune disease, infections, and metastatic deposits. Spontaneous adrenal hemorrhage can occur in patients with fulminant meningococcal septicemia, and in this context is referred to as the Waterhouse-Friderichsen syndrome. It also can occur secondary to trauma, severe stress, infection, and coagulopathies. Exogenous glucocorticoid therapy with suppression of the adrenal glands is the most common cause of secondary adrenal insufficiency.

Symptoms and Signs

Acute adrenal insufficiency should be suspected in stressed patients with any of the relevant risk factors. It may mimic sepsis and presents with fever, nausea, vomiting, lethargy, mild abdominal pain, or severe hypotension. Chronic adrenal insufficiency may be more subtle, with symptoms such as fatigue, salt-craving, weight loss, nausea, vomiting, abdominal pain, and diarrhea. These patients may also appear hyperpigmented.

Diagnostic Studies and Treatment

Characteristic laboratory findings include hyponatremia, hyperkalemia, eosinophilia, mild azotemia, and fasting or reactive hypoglycemia. The peripheral blood smear may demonstrate eosinophilia in approximately 20 percent of patients. Adrenal insufficiency is diagnosed by the ACTH stimulation test. ACTH (250 μg) is infused intravenously, and cortisol levels are measured at 0, 30, and 60 min. Peak cortisol levels less than 20 μg/dL suggest adrenal insufficiency. ACTH levels also enable one to distinguish primary from secondary causes. Treatment measures should begin based on clinical suspicion alone, and initiated even before test results are obtained or the patient is unlikely to survive. Management includes volume resuscitation with at least 2–3 L of a 0.9 percent saline solution or 5 percent dextrose in saline solution. Dexamethasone (4 mg) should be administered intravenously. Hydrocortisone (100 mg IV every 6 h) may also be used, but it interferes with testing of cortisol levels. Once the patient has been stabilized, underlying conditions, such as infection, should be sought, identified, and treated. The ACTH stimulation test should be performed to confirm the diagnosis. Glucocorticoids can then be tapered to maintenance doses. Mineralocorticoids (fludrocortisone 0.05–0.1 mg daily) may be required once the saline infusions are discontinued.

ADRENAL SURGERY

Choice of Procedure

Adrenalectomy may be performed via an open or laparoscopic technique. In either approach, the gland may be approached anteriorly, laterally, or posteriorly via the retroperitoneum. Laparoscopic adrenalectomy has rapidly become the standard procedure of choice for the excision of most benign-appearing adrenal lesions less than 6 cm in diameter. The role of laparoscopic adrenalectomy in the management of adrenocortical cancers is controversial. Although laparoscopic adrenalectomy appears to be feasible and safe for solitary adrenal metastasis (provided there is no local invasion and the tumor can be resected intact), open adrenalectomy is the safest option for suspected or known adrenocortical cancers and malignant pheochromocytomas.

Laparoscopic Adrenalectomy

Lateral Transabdominal Approach

The patient is placed in the lateral decubitus position and the operating table is flexed at the waist to open the space between the lower rib cage and the iliac crest. The surgeon and assistant both stand on the same side, facing the front of the patient. After pneumoperitoneum is created, four 10-mm trocars are placed between the mid-clavicular line medially and the anterior axillary line laterally, 1–2 fingerbreadths below the costal margin. A 30-degree laparoscope is inserted through the second port.

For a right adrenalectomy, a fan retractor is inserted through the most medial port to retract the liver. An atraumatic grasper and an L-hook cautery are inserted via the two lateral ports for the dissection. The right triangular ligament is divided and the liver is rotated medially. Rarely, the hepatic flexure of the colon may need mobilization during a right adrenalectomy. The right kidney is identified visually and by palpation with an atraumatic grasper. The adrenal gland is identified on the superomedial aspect of the kidney. Gerota fascia is incised with the hook cautery. Dissection of the adrenal is started superomedially and then proceeds inferiorly, dissecting around the adrenal in a clockwise manner. The peri-adrenal tissues are grasped or moved with a blunt grasper to facilitate circumferential dissection. Although early identification of the adrenal vein is helpful to facilitate mobilization and prevent injury, it can be dissected whenever it is safe to do so. The right adrenal vein is identified at its junction with the inferior vena cava, ligated with clips and divided using endoscopic scissors. There may be a second adrenal vein on the right. Generally, two clips are left on the vena cava side. Early ligation of the adrenal vein makes it easier to mobilize the gland, but may make subsequent dissection more difficult because of venous congestion. The arterial branches to the adrenal gland can be electrocoagulated, if small, or clipped and divided.

For a left adrenalectomy, the fan retractor is used to retract the spleen. The splenic flexure is mobilized early and the lateral attachments to the spleen and the tail of the pancreas are divided using the electrocautery. Gravity allows the spleen and the pancreatic tail to fall medially. The remainder of the dissection proceeds similar to that described for the right adrenal. In addition to the adrenal vein, the inferior phrenic vein, which joins the left adrenal vein medially, also needs to be dissected, doubly clipped, and divided. Once the dissection is complete, the area of the adrenal bed can be irrigated and suctioned. A drain is rarely necessary. The gland is placed in a nylon specimen bag, which is brought out via one of the ports after morcellation, if necessary.

Complications of Adrenal Surgery

General complications associated with laparoscopic adrenalectomy include wound and infection, urinary tract infections, and deep vein thrombosis. Patients with Cushing syndrome are more prone to infectious (incisional and intraabdominal abscess) and thrombotic complications. Specific complications arising from the creation of pneumoperitoneum include injury to various organs from Veress needle and trocar insertion, subcutaneous emphysema, pneumothorax, and hemodynamic compromise. Excessive retraction and dissection may lead to bleeding from injury to the inferior vena cava and renal vessels, or from injury to surrounding organs, such as the liver, pancreas, spleen, and stomach. Postoperative hemodynamic instability may be evident in patients with pheochromocytomas and patients are at risk of adrenal insufficiency after bilateral adrenalectomy and sometimes after unilateral adrenalectomy (unrecognized Cushing syndrome or, very rarely, Conn syndrome). Long-term morbidity results mainly from injury to nerve roots during trocar insertion, which can lead to chronic pain syndromes or muscle weakness, although this is more of an issue in case of open procedures.

Approximately 30 percent of patients who undergo bilateral adrenalectomy for Cushing disease are at risk of developing Nelson syndrome from progressive growth of the preexisting pituitary tumor. This leads to increased ACTH levels, hyperpigmentation, visual field defects, headaches, and extraocular muscle palsies. Transsphenoidal pituitary resection is the initial mode of therapy, and external beam radiotherapy is used in patients with residual tumor or extrasellar invasion.

Suggested Readings

Bouknight AL: Thyroid physiology and thyroid function testing. Otolaryngol Clin North Am 36:9, 2003.

Streetman DD, Khanderia U: Diagnosis and treatment of Graves' disease. Ann Pharmacother 37:1100, 2003.

Muller PE, Bein B, Robens E, et al: Thyroid surgery according to Enderlen-Hotz or Dunhill: A comparison of two surgical methods for the treatment of Graves' disease. Int Surg 86:112, 2001.

Pasieka JL: Hashimoto's disease and thyroid lymphoma: Role of the surgeon. World J Surg 24:966, 2000.

Mazzaferri EL, Massoll N: Management of papillary and follicular (differentiated) thyroid cancer: New paradigms using recombinant human thyrotropin. Endocr Relat Cancer 9:227, 2002.

Mazzaferri EL, Robbins RJ, Spencer CA, et al: A consensus report of the role of serum thyroglobulin as a monitoring method for low-risk patients with papillary thyroid carcinoma. J Clin Endocrinol Metab 88:1433, 2003.

Bilezikian JP, Potts JT Jr., El-Hajj Fuleihan G, et al: Summary statement from a workshop on asymptomatic primary hyperparathyroidism: A perspective for the 21st century. J Clin Endocrinol Metab 87:5353, 2002.

Wells SA Jr., Debenedetti MK, Doherty GM: Recurrent or persistent hyperparathyroidism. J Bone Miner Res 17:N158, 2002.

Ng L, Libertino JM: Adrenocortical carcinoma: Diagnosis, evaluation and treatment. J Urol 169:5, 2003.

Brunt LM, Moley JF: Adrenal incidentaloma. World J Surg 25:905, 2001.

38 | Pediatric Surgery

David J. Hackam, Kurt Newman, and Henri R. Ford

In his 1953 classic textbook entitled "The Surgery of Infancy and Childhood," Dr. Robert E. Gross summarized the essential challenge of pediatric surgery: "Those who daily operate on adults, even with the greatest of skill, are sometimes appalled—or certainly are not at their best—when called on to operate on and care for a tiny patient. Something more than diminutive instruments or scaled-down operative manipulations are necessary to do the job in a suitable manner." To this day, surgical residents often approach the pediatric surgical patient with a mix of fear and anxiety. Nonetheless, they generally complete their pediatric surgical experience with a clear sense of the enormous ability of children to tolerate large operations, and with a true appreciation for the precision required in their care both in the operating room and during the peri-operative period. The specialty has evolved considerably in its ability to care for the smallest of patients with surgical disorders, so that in-utero surgery is now an option in certain circumstances. Similarly, our understanding of the pathophysiology of the diseases that pediatric surgeons face has increased greatly to the point in which our focus has shifted from the developmental process defining the molecular or cellular signaling pathways that regulate tissue growth and differentiation. There are few specialties in all of medicine that provide the opportunity to intervene in such a positive manner in such a wide array of diseases, and to receive the most heartfelt appreciation possible from another human being—that of a parent whose child's life has forever been improved.

GENERAL CONSIDERATIONS

Fluid and Electrolyte Balance

In managing the pediatric surgical patient, an understanding of fluid and electrolyte balance is critical, as the margin between dehydration and fluid overload is small. Several surgical diagnoses such as gastroschisis or short-gut syndrome, for instance, are characterized by a predisposition to fluid loss. Others require judicious restoration of intravascular volume to prevent cardiac failure; as in patients with congenital diaphragmatic hernia and associated pulmonary hypertension. It is important to realize that the infant's physiologic day is approximately eight h in duration. A careful assessment of the individual patient's fluid balance tally—showing fluid intake and output fluid out for the previous eight h—will prevent dehydration or fluid overload. Clinical signs of dehydration include tachycardia, reduced urine output, and a depressed fontanelle, lethargy, and poor feeding. Fluid overload is often manifested by the onset of new oxygen requirement, respiratory distress, tachypnea and tachycardia.

The infant is born with a surplus of body water, which is normally excreted by the end of the first week of life. At birth, fluid requirements are 65 mL/kg (750 to mL/m^2) and increase to 100 mL/kg (1000 mL/m^2) by the end of the first week. Daily maintenance fluids for most children can be estimated using the formula: 100 mL/kg for the first 10 kg plus 50 mL/kg for 11 to 20 kg plus 25 mL/kg for each additional kilogram of body weight thereafter. Because intravenous (I.V.) fluid orders are written as mL per h, this can be conveniently converted to

4 mL/kg/h up to 10 kg, add 2 mL/kg/h for 11 to 20 kg, and add 1 mL/kg/h for each additional kilogram body weight thereafter. For example, a 26-kg child has an estimated maintenance fluid requirement of $(10 \times 4) + (10 \times 2) + (6 \times 1) = 66$ mL/h in the absence of massive fluid losses or shock. Fluid for maintenance is generally provided as 5 percent dextrose in one-fourth normal saline. For short-term intravenous therapy, sodium 5 mEq/kg/day and potassium 2 mEq/kg/day will satisfy the daily need. Fluid and electrolyte losses secondary to protracted vomiting or diarrhea are corrected by modifying this formula according to the measured losses. In the infant the normal serum osmolarity is between 280 and 290 mO/L. Newborns have the ability to concentrate their urine well by the fifth day of life; thus urine concentration and output must be considered when ordering intravenous (IV) fluids postoperatively. If the child has a significant ongoing fluid loss (e.g., from a nasogastric tube), it is best to properly replace that loss with IV fluids at least every 4h. A typical replacement formula is D5 one-half normal saline + 20 mEq KCl/Liter. Whatever the formula used to calculate fluid replacement for the infant or small child, the optimal strategy is to analyze serum electrolytes and fluid losses, and to replace the appropriate constituents precisely.

Blood Volume and Blood Replacement

A useful guideline for estimation of blood volume for the newborn infant is 85 mL/kg of body weight. When packed red blood cells (PRBC) are used, the transfusion requirement is calculated as 10 mL/kg, which roughly is equivalent to a 500-mL transfusion for a 70-kg adult. At our institution, the following formula is used to estimate the volume of blood to be replaced in ml:

$$(\text{Target Hematocrit} - \text{Current Hematocrit}) \times \text{weight (kg)} \times 80/65$$

In the child, coagulation deficiencies may assume clinical significance rapidly after extensive blood transfusion. It is advisable to have fresh frozen plasma and platelets available if more than 30 mL/kg have been transfused. Plasma is given in a dose of 10–20 mL/kg and platelets are given in a dose of 1 unit/5 kg. Each unit of platelets consists of 40–60 mL of fluid and the platelets can be spun down to a platelet "button" for infants who require restricted fluid administration. Following transfusion of PRBC to neonates with tenuous fluid balance, a single dose of a diuretic (such as furosemide 1mg/kg) may help to facilitate excretion of the extra fluid load.

Venous Access

Obtaining reliable vascular access in an infant or child is a major responsibility of the pediatric surgeon. The goal should always be to place the catheter in the least invasive, least risky, and least painful manner, and in a location that is most accessible and facilitates use of the catheter without complications for as long as needed. In infants, our general approach is to place a central venous catheter using a cutdown approach, either in the antecubital fossa, external jugular vein, facial vein, or proximal saphenous vein. If the internal jugular vein is used, we recommend placing a purse-string suture at the venotomy site if possible, to prevent venous occlusion. In infants over 2 kg and in older children, percutaneous access of the subclavian, internal jugular or femoral veins is possible in most cases, and central access is achieved using the Seldinger technique. The catheters are tunneled to an exit site separate from the venotomy site. Regardless of whether the catheter is placed by a cutdown or percutaneous approach, a chest radiograph to confirm central location of the catheter tip and to exclude the presence of a pneumothorax or hemothorax is mandatory. When discussing the placement of central venous catheters with parents, it is important to note that the complication rate for central venous lines in children is high. The incidence of catheter-related sepsis or infection approaches 10 percent in many series. Superior or inferior vena caval occlusion is a significant risk, particularly in the smallest premature patients.

NECK MASSES

The management of neck masses in children is determined by their location and the length of time that they have been present. Neck lesions are found either in the midline or lateral compartments. Midline masses include thyroglossal duct remnants, thyroid masses, thymic cysts, or dermoid cysts. Lateral lesions include branchial cleft remnants, cystic hygromas, vascular malformations, salivary gland tumors, torticollis and lipoblastoma (a rare benign mesenchymal tumor of embryonal fat occurring in infants and young children). Enlarged lymph nodes and rare malignancies such as rhabdomyosarcoma can occur either in the midline or laterally.

RESPIRATORY SYSTEM

Congenital Diaphragmatic Hernia (Bochdalek)

Pathology

During formation of the diaphragm, the pleural and coelomic cavities remain in continuity by means of the pleuroperitoneal canal. The posterolateral communication is the last to be closed by the developing diaphragm. Failure of diaphragmatic development leaves a posterolateral defect known as a Bochdalek hernia. This anomaly is encountered more commonly on the left (80–90 percent). Incomplete development of the posterior diaphragm allows the abdominal viscera to fill the chest cavity. The abdominal cavity is small and underdeveloped and remains scaphoid after birth. Both lungs are hypoplastic, with decreased bronchial and pulmonary artery branching. Lung weight, lung volume, and deoxyribonucleic acid (DNA) content are also decreased, but these findings are more striking on the ipsilateral side. In many instances, evidence suggests that a paucity of surfactant is present, which compounds the degree of respiratory insufficiency. Amniocentesis with karyotypes may show chromosomal defects, especially trisomy 18 and 21. Associated anomalies, once thought to be uncommon, are identified in 40 percent of these infants, and most commonly involve the heart, brain, genitourinary system, craniofacial structures, or limbs.

Prenatal ultrasonography is successful in making the diagnosis of congenital diaphragmatic hernia (CDH) as early as 15 weeks gestation. Ultrasound findings include herniated abdominal viscera, abnormal anatomy of the upper abdomen, and mediastinal shift away from the herniated viscera. Accurate prenatal prediction of outcome for fetuses with CDH is very difficult. A useful index of severity for patients with left CDH is the lung-to-head ratio (LHR), which is the product of the length and the width of the right lung at the level of the cardiac atria divided by the head circumference (all measurements in millimeters). An LHR value of less than 1.0 is associated with a very poor prognosis, whereas an LHR greater than 1.4 predicts a more favorable outcome.

Following delivery, the diagnosis of CDH is made by chest radiograph. The differential diagnosis includes congenital cystic adenomatoid malformation, in which the intrathoracic loops of bowel may be confused with multiple lung cysts. The vast majority of infants with CDH develop immediate respiratory distress, which is because of the combined effects of three factors. First, the air-filled bowel in the chest compresses the mobile mediastinum which shifts to the opposite side of the chest, compromising air exchange in the contralateral lung. Second, pulmonary hypertension develops. This phenomenon results in persistent fetal circulation, with resultant decreased pulmonary perfusion, and impaired gas exchange. Finally, the lung on the affected side is often markedly hypoplastic, such that it is essentially nonfunctional. Varying degrees of pulmonary hypoplasia on the opposite side may compound these effects. As a result, neonates with CDH are extremely sick, and the overall mortality in most series is approximately 50 percent.

Treatment

Many infants are symptomatic at birth because of hypoxia, hypercarbia, and metabolic acidosis. Prompt cardiorespiratory stabilization is mandatory. It is interesting that the first 24–48 h after birth are often characterized by a period of relative stability with high levels of PaO_2 and relatively good perfusion. This has been termed the "honeymoon period," and is often followed by progressive cardiorespiratory deterioration in the majority of patients. In the past, correction of the hernia was felt to be a surgical emergency; therefore, these patients underwent surgery shortly after birth. It is now accepted that the presence of persistent pulmonary hypertension that results in right-to-left shunting across the open foramen ovale or the ductus arteriosus, and the degree of pulmonary hypoplasia, are the leading causes of cardiorespiratory insufficiency. Current management therefore is directed toward preventing or reversing the pulmonary hypertension, and minimizing barotrauma while optimizing oxygen delivery. To achieve this goal, infants are placed on mechanical ventilation using relatively low or "gentle" settings that prevent overinflation of the noninvolved lung. Levels of $PacO_2$ in the range of 50–60 mmHg or higher are accepted as long as the pH remains greater than or equal to 7.25. If these objectives cannot be achieved using conventional ventilation, high frequency oscillatory ventilation (HFOV) may be employed to avoid the injurious effects of conventional tidal volume ventilation. Echocardiography is used to assess the degree of pulmonary hypertension, and to identify the presence of a coexisting cardiac anomaly. To minimize the degree of pulmonary hypertension, inhaled nitric oxide may be used. In certain patients, this agent significantly improves pulmonary perfusion, as manifested by improved oxygenation. Nitric oxide is administered into the ventilation circuit, and is used in concentrations up to 40 parts per million. Correction of acidosis using bicarbonate solution may minimize the degree of pulmonary hypertension. As the degree of pulmonary hypertension becomes hemodynamically significant, right sided heart failure develops and systemic perfusion is impaired. Administration of excess intravenous fluid will compound the degree of cardiac failure, and lead to marked peripheral edema. Inotropic support using epinephrine is therefore useful in optimizing cardiac contractility and maintaining mean arterial pressure.

Infants with CDH who remain severely hypoxic despite maximal ventilatory support may be candidates for treatment of their respiratory failure by extracorporeal membrane oxygenation (ECMO). Venovenous or venoarterial bypass is used. Venovenous bypass is established with a single cannula through the internal jugular vein, with blood removed from, and infused into, the right atrium via separate ports. Venoarterial bypass is used preferentially by some centers because it provides the cardiac support that is often needed. The right atrium is cannulated by means of the internal jugular vein and the aortic arch through the right common carotid artery. As much of the cardiac output is shunted through the membrane oxygenator as needed to provide oxygenated blood to the infant and remove carbon dioxide. The infant is maintained on bypass until the pulmonary hypertension is reversed and lung function, as measured by compliance, is improved. This is usually seen within 7–10 days, but in some infants it may take up to 3 weeks to occur. The use of ECMO is associated with significant risk. Because patients require systemic anticoagulation, bleeding complications are the most significant. Bleeding may occur intracranially or at the site of cannula insertion, and may be life threatening. Systemic sepsis is a significant problem that may force early decannulation. Criteria for placing infants on ECMO include the presence of normal cardiac anatomy by echocardiography, the absence of fatal chromosome anomalies, and the expectation that the infant would die without ECMO. Traditionally, a threshold weight greater than 2.5 kg and gestational age older than 34 weeks have been used to select patients for ECMO, although success has been achieved at weights as low as 1.8 kg. It is important to emphasize that although ECMO may salvage a population of neonates with refractory pulmonary hypertension, the use of this technique remains controversial. A strategy that does not involve the use of ECMO but instead emphasizes the use of permissive hypercapnia and the avoidance of barotrauma may provide similar overall outcome in patients with CDH. This observation likely reflects the fact that mortality in infants with CDH is related to the degree of pulmonary hypoplasia and the presence of congenital anomalies, neither of which can be corrected by ECMO.

The timing of CDH repair is controversial. In patients that are not placed on ECMO, most surgeons perform repair the defect once the hemodynamic status has been optimized. In neonates that are on bypass, some surgeons perform early repair on bypass; others wait until the infant's lungs are fully recovered, repair the diaphragm and discontinue bypass within h of surgery. Still others repair the diaphragm only after the infant is off bypass. Operative repair of the diaphragmatic hernia is best accomplished by an abdominal approach. Through a subcostal incision, the abdominal viscera are withdrawn from the chest, exposing the defect in the diaphragm. Care must be taken when reducing the spleen and liver, as bleeding from these structures can be fatal. The anterior margin is often apparent, although the posterior muscular rim is attenuated. If the infant is heparinized on bypass, minimal dissection of the muscular margins is performed. Electrocautery is used liberally to minimize postoperative bleeding. Most infants who require ECMO support prior to hernia repair have large defects, often lacking the medial and posterior margins. Prior to the availability of ECMO therapy, most of these infants died. About three fourths of infants repaired on bypass require prosthetic material to patch the defect, suturing it to the diaphragmatic remnant or around ribs or costal cartilages for the large defects. If there is adequate muscle for closure, a single layer of nonabsorbable suture is used to close the defect. Just before the repair is complete, a chest tube may be positioned in the thoracic cavity. We tend to reserve the use of chest tubes for patients who are repaired on ECMO, as these patients are at risk for developing a hemothorax which can significantly impair ventilation. Anatomic closure of the abdominal wall may be impossible after reduction of the viscera. Occasionally a prosthetic patch of Gore-Tex or Surgisis may be sutured to the fascia to facilitate closure. The prosthetic patch can be removed at a later time and the ventral hernia closed at that time.

If the diaphragm has been repaired on ECMO, weaning and decannulation are accomplished as soon as possible. All infants are ventilated postoperatively to maintain preductal arterial oxygenation of 80–100 torr. Very slow weaning from the ventilator may be necessary to avoid recurrent pulmonary hypertension. Oscillatory ventilation may be switched to conventional ventilation as part of the process of weaning.

Congenital Lobar Emphysema

Congenital lobar emphysema (CLE) is characterized by progressive hyperexpansion of one or more lobes of the lung. It is diagnosed during the first few months of life and can be life-threatening in the newborn period; but in the older infant, it causes less respiratory distress. Air entering during inspiration is trapped in the lobe. On expiration, the lobe cannot deflate and progressively overexpands, causing atelectasis of the adjacent lobe or lobes. This hyperexpansion eventually shifts the mediastinum to the opposite side and compromises the other lung. CLE usually occurs in the upper lobes of the lung (left greater than right), followed next in frequency by the right middle lobe, but it also can occur in the lower lobes. It is caused by intrinsic bronchial obstruction from poor bronchial cartilage development or extrinsic compression. Approximately 14 percent of children with this condition have cardiac defects, with an enlarged left atrium or a major vessel compressing the ipsilateral bronchus. Symptoms range from mild respiratory distress to full-fledged respiratory failure with tachypnea, dyspnea, cough, and late cyanosis. These symptoms may be stationary or they may progress rapidly and result in recurrent pneumonia. Occasionally, infants with CLE present with failure to thrive, which likely reflects the increased work associated with the overexpanded lung. Diagnosis is made by chest radiograph, which shows a hyperlucent affected lobe with adjacent lobar compression and atelectasis with varying degrees of shift of the mediastinum to the opposite side and compression of the contralateral lung. If definitive diagnosis is unclear by chest radiograph, CT scan may be helpful. Unless foreign body or mucous plugging is suspected as a cause of hyperinflation, bronchoscopy is not advisable because it can produce more air trapping and cause life-threatening respiratory distress in a stable infant. Treatment consists of resection of the affected lobe. Unless symptoms necessitate urgent surgery, resection can usually be performed after the infant is several months of age. The prognosis is excellent.

Congenital Cystic Adenomatoid Malformation

This malformation consists of cystic proliferation of the terminal airway, producing cysts lined by mucus-producing respiratory epithelium, and elastic tissue in the cyst walls without cartilage formation. There may be a single cyst with a wall of connective tissue containing smooth muscle. Cysts may be large and multiple (type I), smaller and more numerous (type II), or they may resemble fetal lung without macroscopic cysts (type III). Most congenital cystic adenomatoid malformation (CCAM) frequently occur in the left lower lobe. However, this lesion can occur in any lobe and may occur in both lungs simultaneously. In the left lower lobe, type I may be confused at birth with a congenital diaphragmatic hernia. Clinical symptoms may range from none at all to severe respiratory failure at birth. The cyst(s), whether single or multiple, can produce air trapping and may be confused with congenital lobar emphysema, pneumatoceles or even pulmonary sequestrations. They can also be involved with repeated infections and produce fever and cough in older infants and children. Prenatal ultrasound may suggest the diagnosis. At birth, the diagnosis often can be confirmed by chest radiograph; in certain cases, ultrasound or CT scan may be definitive. In the newborn period, ultrasound may also be useful, especially to distinguish between CCAM and congenital diaphragmatic hernia. Resection is curative and may need to be performed urgently in the infant with severe respiratory distress. Lobectomy is usually required. Prognosis is excellent.

Pulmonary Sequestration

Pulmonary sequestration is uncommon and consists of a mass of lung tissue, usually in the left lower chest, occurring without the usual connections to the pulmonary artery or tracheobronchial tree, yet with a systemic blood supply from the aorta. There are two kinds of sequestration. Extralobar sequestration consists of a small area of nonaerated lung separated from the main lung mass, with a systemic blood supply located immediately above the left diaphragm. It is commonly found in cases of CDH. Intralobar sequestration more commonly occurs within the parenchyma of the left lower lobe but can occur on the right. There is no major connection to the tracheobronchial tree, but a secondary connection may be established, perhaps through infection or via adjacent intrapulmonary shunts. The blood supply originates from the aorta, frequently below the diaphragm. Venous drainage of both types can be systemic or pulmonary. The cause of sequestration is unknown but most probably involves an abnormal budding of the developing lung that picks up a systemic blood supply and never becomes connected with the bronchus or pulmonary vessels. Extralobar sequestration is asymptomatic and is usually discovered incidentally on chest radiograph. Diagnosis of intralobar sequestration, on the other hand, is usually made after repeated infections manifested by cough, fever, and consolidation in the posterior basal segment of the left lower lobe. Increasingly the diagnosis is being made in the early months of life by ultrasound, and color Doppler often can be helpful in delineating the systemic arterial supply. Removal of the entire left lower lobe is usually necessary because the diagnosis often is made late after multiple infections. Occasionally the sequestered part of the lung can be removed segmentally. Prognosis is excellent.

Bronchogenic Cyst

Bronchogenic cysts can occur anywhere along the respiratory tract from the neck to the lung parenchyma. They can present at any age. Histologically, they are hamartomatous and usually consist of a single cyst lined with respiratory epithelium, containing cartilage and smooth muscle. They are probably embryonic rests of foregut origin that have been pinched off from the main portion of the developing tracheobronchial tree and are closely associated in causation with other foregut duplication cysts arising from the esophagus. Bronchogenic cysts may be seen on prenatal ultrasound but are discovered most often incidentally on postnatal chest radiograph. Although they may be completely asymptomatic, bronchogenic cysts may, however, produce symptoms, depending on their anatomic location. In the paratracheal region of the neck they can produce airway compression and respiratory distress. In the lung parenchyma, they may become infected and present with fever and cough. In addition they may cause obstruction of the bronchial lumen with distal atelectasis and infection. They may also cause mediastinal compression. Rarely, rupture of the cyst can occur. Chest radiograph usually shows a dense mass, and computed tomography (CT) scan or magnetic resonance imaging (MRI) delineates the precise anatomic location of the lesion. Treatment consists of resection of the cyst, which may need to be undertaken in emergency circumstances for airway or cardiac compression. Resection can be performed either as an open procedure, or using a thoracoscopic approach.

ESOPHAGUS

Esophageal Atresia and Tracheoesophageal Fistula

Esophageal atresia (EA) with tracheoesophageal fistula (TEF) is one of the most gratifying pediatric surgical conditions to treat. In the distant past, nearly all infants born with EA and TEF died. In 1939, Ladd and Leven performed the first successful repair by ligating the fistula, placing a gastrostomy and reconstructing the esophagus at a later time. Subsequently, Dr. Cameron Haight in Ann Arbor, Michigan, performed the first successful primary anastomosis for esophageal atresia, which remains the current approach for treatment of this condition. Despite the fact that there are several common varieties of this anomaly and the underlying cause remains obscure, a careful approach consisting of meticulous perioperative care and attention to the technical detail of the operation can result in an excellent prognosis in most cases.

Anatomic Varieties

There are five major varieties of EA and TEF. The most commonly seen variety is esophageal atresia with distal tracheoesophageal fistula (Type C), which occurs in approximately 85 percent of the cases in most series. The next most frequent is pure esophageal atresia (Type A), occurring in 8–10 percent of patients, followed by tracheoesophageal fistula without esophageal atresia (Type E). This type occurs in 8 percent of cases, and is also referred to as an H-type fistula, based on the anatomic similarity to that letter. Esophageal atresia with fistula between both proximal and distal ends of the esophagus and trachea (Type D) is seen in approximately 2 percent of cases, and type B, esophageal atresia with tracheoesophageal fistula between distal esophagus and trachea, is seen in approximately 1 percent of all cases.

Etiology and Pathologic Presentation

The esophagus and trachea share a common embryologic origin. They typically divide into separate tubes by approximately 36 days gestation. Failure to separate can result in a spectrum of anomalies. Recent studies have shed light on some of the molecular mechanisms underlying this condition. Mice deficient in the Sonic-hedgehog signaling pathway develop a phenotype which includes EA-TEF, suggesting a role for this molecule in the pathogenesis of the anomaly in humans. In support of this theory, Sonic-hedgehog transcripts were absent in human esophageal samples obtained from infants with TEF. Similarly, tissue obtained from the fistula tract were found to express Thyroid transcription factor one (TTF-1) and fibroblast growth factor FGF-10), suggesting that the fistula is of respiratory origin. Although a genetic basis for EA-TEF has not been definitively established, reports indicate that this anomaly may occur in several generations of the same family. Twin studies also demonstrate the presence of esophageal atresia in sets of dizygotic twins.

Other congenital anomalies frequently occur in association with EA-TEF. These defects are known by the acronym VATER or VACTERRL syndrome, which refers to vertebral (missing vertebra) and anorectal (imperforate anus) anomalies, cardiac defects (severe congenital cardiac disease), tracheoesophageal fistula, renal anomalies (renal agenesis, renal anomalies), and radial limb hyperplasia. In nearly 20 percent of the infants born with esophageal atresia, some variant of congenital heart disease occurs.

Clinical presentation of infants with esophageal atresia and tracheoesophageal fistula. The anatomic variant of infants with EA-TEF predicts the clinical presentation. When the esophagus ends either as a blind pouch or as a fistula into the trachea (as in Types A, B, C, or D), infants present with excessive drooling, followed by chocking or coughing immediately after feeding is initiated as a result of aspiration through the fistula tract. As the neonate coughs and cries, air is transmitted through the fistula into the stomach, resulting in abdominal distention. As the abdomen distends, it becomes increasingly more difficult for the infant to breathe. This leads to further atelectasis, which compounds the pulmonary dysfunction. In patients with type C and D varieties, the regurgitated gastric juice passes through the fistula, where it collects in the trachea and lungs and leads to a chemical pneumonitis, which further exacerbates the pulmonary status. In many instances, the diagnosis is actually made by the nursing staff who attempt to feed the baby and notice the accumulation of oral secretions.

The diagnosis of esophageal atresia is confirmed by the inability to pass an orogastric tube into the stomach. The dilated upper pouch may be occasionally seen on a plain chest radiograph. If a soft feeding tube is used, the tube will coil in the upper pouch, which provides further diagnostic certainty. An important alternative diagnosis that must be considered when an orogastric tube does not enter the stomach is that of an esophageal perforation. This problem can occur in infants after traumatic insertion of a nasogastric or orogastric tube. In this instance, the perforation classically occurs at the level of the piriform sinus, and a false passage is created which prevents the tube from entering the stomach. Whenever there is any diagnostic uncertainty, a contrast study will confirm the diagnosis of EA and occasionally document the TEF. The presence of a tracheoesophageal fistula can be demonstrated clinically by finding air in the gastrointestinal tract. This can be proven at the bedside by percussion of the abdomen, and confirmed by obtaining a plain abdominal radiograph. Occasionally, a diagnosis of EA-TEF can be suspected prenatally on ultrasound evaluation. Typical features include failure to visualize the stomach and the presence of polyhydramnios. These findings reflect the absence of efficient swallowing by the fetus.

In a child with esophageal atresia, it is important to identify whether co-existing anomalies are present. These include cardiac defects in 38 percent, skeletal defects in 19 percent, neurological defects in 15 percent, renal defects in 15 percent, anorectal defects in 8 percent, and other abnormalities in 13 percent. Examination of the heart and great vessels with echocardiography is important to exclude cardiac defects, as these are often the most important predictors of survival in these infants. The echocardiogram also demonstrates whether the aortic arch is left sided or right sided, which may influence the approach to surgical repair. Vertebral anomalies are assessed by plain radiography, and a spinal ultrasound is obtained if any are detected. A patent anus should be confirmed clinically. The kidneys in a newborn may be assessed clinically by palpation. An ultrasound of the abdomen will demonstrate the presence of renal anomalies, which should be suspected in the child who fails to make urine. The presence of extremity anomalies is suspected when there are missing digits, and confirmed by plain radiographs of the hands, feet, forearms and legs. Rib anomalies may also be present. These may include the presence of a thirteenth rib.

Initial management. The initial treatment of infants with EA-TEF includes attention to the respiratory status, decompression of the upper pouch, and appropriate timing of surgery. Because the major determinant of poor survival is the presence of other severe anomalies, a search for other defects including congenital cardiac disease is undertaken in a timely fashion. The initial strategy after the diagnosis is confirmed is to place the neonate in an infant warmer with the head elevated at least 30 degrees. A sump catheter is placed in the upper pouch on continuous suction. Both of these strategies are designed to minimize the degree of aspiration from the esophageal pouch. When saliva accumulates in the upper pouch and is aspirated into the lungs, coughing, bronchospasm and desaturation episodes can occur, which may be minimized by ensuring the patency of the sump catheter. Intravenous antibiotic therapy is initiated, and warmed electrolyte solution is administered. Where possible, the right upper extremity is avoided as a site to start an intravenous line, as this location may interfere with positioning of the patient during the surgical repair.

The timing of repair is influenced by the stability of the patient. Definitive repair of the EA-TEF is rarely a surgical emergency. If the child is hemodynamically stable and is oxygenating well, definitive repair may be performed within 1–2 days after birth. This allows for a careful determination of the presence of coexisting anomalies, and for selection of an experienced anesthetic team.

Management of esophageal atresia and tracheoesophageal fistula in the preterm infant. The ventilated, premature neonate with EA-TEF and associated hyaline membrane disease represents a patient who may develop severe pulmonary disease. The tracheoesophageal fistula can worsen the fragile pulmonary status as a result of recurrent aspiration through the fistula, and of increased abdominal distention which impairs lung expansion. Moreover, the elevated airway pressure that is required to ventilate these patients can worsen the clinical course by forcing air through the fistula into the stomach, thereby exacerbating the degree of abdominal distention and compromising lung expansion. In this situation, the first priority is to minimize the degree of positive pressure needed to adequately ventilate the child. This can be accomplished using high frequency oscillatory ventilation (HFOV). If the gastric distention becomes severe, a gastrostomy tube should be placed. This procedure can be performed at the bedside under local anesthesia, if necessary. The dilated, air filled stomach can easily be accessed through an incision in the left-upper quadrant of the abdomen. Once the gastrostomy tube is placed, and the abdominal pressure is relieved, the pulmonary status can paradoxically worsen. This is because the ventilated gas may pass preferentially through the fistula, which is the path of least resistance, and bypass the lungs thereby worsening the hypoxemia. To correct this problem, the gastrostomy tube may be placed under water seal, elevated or intermittently clamped. If these maneuvers are to no avail, ligation of the fistula may be required. This procedure can be performed in the neonatal intensive care unit if the infant is too unstable to be transported to the operating room. These interventions allow for the infant's underlying hyaline membrane disease to improve, for the pulmonary secretions to clear, and for the infant to reach a period of stability so that definitive repair can be performed.

Primary Surgical Correction

In a stable infant, definitive repair is achieved through performance of a primary esophago-esophagostomy. The infant is brought to the operating room, intubated, and placed in the lateral decubitus position with the right side up in preparation for a right posterolateral thoracotomy. If a right-sided arch was determined previously by echocardiography, consideration is given to performing the repair through the left chest, although most surgeons believe that the repair can be performed safely from the right side as well. Bronchoscopy may be performed to exclude the presence of additional, upper pouch fistulae in cases of esophageal atresia. This permits differentiation of types B, C and D variants, and identification of a laryngotracheoesophageal cleft.

The operative technique for primary repair is as follows: A retropleural approach is generally used, as this technique prevents widespread contamination of the thorax if a postoperative anastomotic leak occurs. The sequence of steps includes:

1. Mobilization of the pleura to expose the structures in the posterior mediastinum.
2. Division of the fistula and closure of the tracheal opening.
3. Mobilization of the upper esophagus sufficiently to permit an anastomosis without tension, and to determine whether a fistula is present between the upper esophagus and the trachea. Forward pressure by the anesthesia staff on the sump drain in the pouch can greatly facilitate dissection at this stage of the operation. Care must be taken when dissecting posteriorly to avoid violation of the lumen of either the trachea or esophagus.
4. Mobilization of the distal esophagus. This needs to be performed judiciously to avoid devascularization, because the blood supply to the distal esophagus is segmental from the aorta. Most of the esophageal length is obtained from mobilizing the upper pouch, because the blood supply travels via the submucosa from above.
5. Performing a primary esophago-esophageal anastomosis. Most surgeons perform this procedure in a single layer using 5-0 sutures. If there is excess tension, the muscle of the upper pouch can be circumferentially incised without compromising blood supply to increase its length. Many surgeons place a transanastomotic feeding tube to institute feeds in the early postoperative period.
6. A retropleural drain is placed, and the incision is closed in layers.

Postoperative Course

The postoperative management strategy of patients with EA-TEF is influenced to a great degree by the preference of the individual surgeon and the institutional culture. Many surgeons prefer not to leave the infants intubated postoperatively, to avoid the effects of positive pressure on the site of tracheal closure. However, extubation may not be possible in babies with underlying lung disease either from prematurity or pneumonia, or when there is vocal cord edema. When a transanastomotic tube is placed, feeds are begun slowly in the postoperative period. Some surgeons institute parenteral nutrition for several days, using a central line. The retropleural drain is assessed daily for the presence of saliva, indicating an anastomotic leak. Many surgeons obtain a contrast swallow 1 week after repair to assess the caliber of the anastomosis and to determine whether a leak is present. If there is no leak, feedings are started.

Complications of surgery. Anastomotic leak occurs in 10–15 percent of patients and may be seen either in the immediate postoperative period, or after several days. Early leakage is manifested by a new pleural effusion, pneumothorax and sepsis, and requires immediate exploration. In these circumstances, the anastomosis may be completely disrupted, possibly because of excessive tension. Revision of the anastomosis may be possible. If not, cervical esophagostomy and gastrostomy placement is required, with a staged procedure to re-establish esophageal continuity. Anastomotic leakage that is detected after several days usually heals without intervention, particularly if a retropleural approach is used. Under these circumstances, broad spectrum antibiotics, pulmonary toilet and optimization of nutrition are important. After approximately a week, a repeat contrast swallow should be performed to determine if the leakage has resolved.

Strictures are not infrequent (10–20 percent), particularly if a leak has occurred. A stricture may become apparent at any time, from the early postoperative period to months or years later. It may present as choking, gagging, or failure to thrive, but often becomes clinically apparent with transition to eating solid food. A contrast swallow or esophagoscopy is confirmatory, and simple dilatation is usually corrective. Occasionally, repeated dilatations are required. These may be performed pneumatically or in a retrograde fashion, during which a silk suture is placed into the oropharynx and delivered from the esophagus through a gastrostomy tube. Tucker dilators are then tied to the suture and passed in a retrograde fashion from the gastrostomy tube and delivered out of the oropharynx. Increasing sizes are used, and the silk is replaced at the end of the procedure in which it is taped to the side of the face at one end, and to the gastrostomy tube at the other.

"Recurrent" tracheoesophageal fistula may represent a missed upper pouch fistula or a true recurrence. This may occur after an anastomotic disruption, during which the recurrent fistula may heal spontaneously. Otherwise, re-operation may be required. Recently, the use of fibrin glue has been successful in treating recurrent fistulas, although long-term follow up is lacking. Gastroesophageal reflux commonly occurs after repair of EA-TEF, potentially because of alterations in esophageal motility and the anatomy of the gastroesophageal junction. The clinical manifestations of such reflux are similar to those seen in other infants with primary gastroesophageal reflux disease (GERD). A loose antireflux procedure, such as a Nissen fundoplication, is used to prevent further reflux, but the child may have feeding problems after antireflux surgery as a result of the innate dysmotility of the distal esophagus. The fundoplication may be safely performed laparoscopically in experienced hands, although care should be taken to ensure that the wrap is not excessively tight.

Special Circumstances

Patients with type E tracheoesophageal fistulas (also called H-type) most commonly present beyond the newborn period. Presenting symptoms include recurrent chest infections, bronchospasm and failure to thrive. The diagnosis is suspected using barium esophagography, and confirmed by endoscopic visualization of the fistula. Surgical correction is generally possible through a cervical approach, and requires mobilization and division of the fistula. Outcome is usually excellent.

Patients with duodenal atresia and EA-TEF may require urgent treatment because of the presence of a closed obstruction of the stomach and proximal duodenum. In stable patients, treatment consists of repair of the esophageal anomaly and correction of the duodenal atresia if the infant is stable during surgery. If not, a staged approach should be used consisting of ligation of the fistula and placement of a gastrostomy tube. Definitive repair can then be performed at a later point in time.

Primary esophageal atresia (type A) represents a challenging problem, particularly if the upper and lower ends are too far apart for an anastomosis to be created. Under these circumstances, treatment strategies include placement of a gastrostomy tube and performing serial bougienage to increase the length of the upper pouch. Occasionally, when the two ends cannot be brought safely together, esophageal replacement is required using either a gastric pull-up or colon interposition (see below).

Outcome

Various classification systems have been used to predict survival in patients with EA-TEF and to stratify treatment. A system devised by Waterston in 1962 was used to stratify neonates based on birth weight, the presence of pneumonia, and the identification of other congenital anomalies. In response to advances in neonatal care, the surgeons from the Montreal Children's Hospital proposed a new classification system in 1993. In the Montreal experience only two characteristics independently affected survival: preoperative ventilator dependence and associated major anomalies. Pulmonary disease as defined by ventilator dependence appeared to be more accurate than pneumonia. When the two systems were recently compared, the Montreal system more accurately identified children at highest risk. Spitz and colleagues recently analyzed risk factors in infants who died with EA-TEF. Two criteria were found to be important predictors of outcome: birth weight less than 1,500 g and the presence of major congenital cardiac disease. A new classification for predicting outcome in esophageal atresia was therefore proposed: group I: birth weight $\geq$ 1,500 g, without major cardiac disease, survival 97 percent (283 of 293); group II: birth weight < 1,500 g, or major cardiac disease, survival 59 percent (41 of 70); and group III: birth weight < 1,500 g, and major cardiac disease, survival 22 percent (2 of 9).

In general, surgical correction of EA-TEF leads to a satisfactory outcome with nearly normal esophageal function in most patients. Overall survival rates of greater than 90 percent have been achieved in patients classified as stable, in all the various staging systems. Unstable infants have an increased mortality (40–60 percent survival) because of potentially fatal associated cardiac and chromosomal anomalies or prematurity. However, the use of a staged procedure also has increased survival in even these high-risk infants.

GASTROINTESTINAL TRACT

Hypertrophic Pyloric Stenosis

Clinical Manifestations

Timely diagnosis and treatment of infants with hypertrophic pyloric stenosis (HPS) is extremely gratifying; it is one of the few instances in surgery where a relatively simple operation can have such a dramatic long-term effect. HPS occurs in approximately 1 in 300 live births and classically presents in a first-born male between 3 and 6 weeks of age. However, children outside of this age range are commonly seen, and the disease is by no means restricted to either males or first born children. The cause of HPS has not been determined. Studies have shown that HPS is found in several generations of the same family, suggesting a familial link. Administration of erythromycin in early infancy has been linked to the subsequent development of HPS, although the cause is unclear.

Infants with HPS present with nonbilious vomiting that becomes increasingly projectile over the course of several days to weeks. Eventually, the infant develops almost complete gastric outlet obstruction, and is no longer able to tolerate even clear liquids. Despite the recurrent emesis, the child normally has a voracious appetite, leading to a cycle of feeding and vomiting that invariably results in severe dehydration, if untreated. Jaundice may occur in association with HPS, although the reason for this finding is unclear. Particularly perceptible caregivers will mention that their infant is passing less flatus, which provides a further clue that gastric outlet obstruction is complete.

Infants with HPS develop a hypochloremic, hypokalemic metabolic alkalosis. The urine pH level is high initially, but eventually drops because hydrogen ions are preferentially exchanged for sodium ions in the distal tubule of the kidney as the hypochloremia becomes severe. The diagnosis of pyloric stenosis usually can be made on physical examination by palpation of the typical "olive" in the right upper quadrant and the presence of visible gastric waves on the abdomen. When the olive cannot be palpated, ultrasound can diagnose the condition accurately in 95 percent of patients. Criteria for ultrasound diagnosis include a channel length of over 16 mm and pyloric thickness over 4 mm.

Treatment

Pyloric stenosis is never a surgical emergency, although the dehydration and electrolyte abnormalities may present a medical emergency. Fluid resuscitation with correction of electrolyte abnormalities and metabolic alkalosis is essential before induction of general anesthesia for operation. For most infants, fluid containing 5 percent dextrose and 0.45 percent saline with added potassium of 2–4 mEq/kg over 24 h at a rate of approximately 150–175 mL/kg for 24 h will correct the underlying deficit. It is important to ensure that the child has an adequate urine output (>1 mL/kg/h) as further evidence that rehydration has occurred. After resuscitation, a Fredet-Ramstedt pyloromyotomy is performed. It may be performed using an open or laparoscopic approach. The open pyloromyotomy is performed through either an umbilical or a right upper quadrant transverse abdominal incision. The former route is cosmetically more appealing, although the transverse incision provides easier access to the antrum and pylorus. In recent years, the laparoscopic approach has gained great popularity. Whether done through an open or laparoscopic approach, the operation involves splitting the pyloric muscle until the submucosa is seen bulging upwards. The incision begins at the pyloric vein of Mayo and extends onto the gastric antrum; it typically measures between 1 and 2 cm in length. Postoperatively, intravenous fluids are continued for several h after which Pedialyte followed by formula or breast milk are offered and are gradually increased to 60 mL every 3 h. Most infants can be discharged home within 24–48 h following surgery. Recently, several authors have shown that ad lib feeds are safely tolerated by the neonate and result in a shorter hospital stay.

The complications of pyloromyotomy include perforation of the mucosa (1–3 percent), bleeding, wound infection, and recurrent symptoms because of inadequate myotomy. When perforation occurs, the mucosa is repaired with a stitch that is placed to tack the mucosa down and re-approximate the serosa in the region of the tear. A nasogastric tube is left in place for 24 h. The outcome is generally very good.

Intestinal Obstruction in the Newborn

The cardinal symptom of intestinal obstruction in the newborn is bilious emesis. Prompt recognition and treatment of neonatal intestinal obstruction can truly be life saving.

Intestinal obstruction can be thought of as either proximal or distal to the ligament of Treitz. Proximal obstruction presents as bilious vomiting, with minimal abdominal distention. In cases of complete obstruction, either there may be a paucity of gas, or no distal air may be seen on the supine and upright films of the abdomen. In this case, the diagnosis of malrotation and midgut volvulus must be excluded. Distal obstruction presents with abdominal distention and bilious emesis. The physical examination will determine whether the anus is patent. Calcifications on the abdominal plain film may indicate meconium peritonitis; pneumatosis and/or free abdominal air indicates necrotizing enterocolitis (NEC) with or without intestinal perforation. A contrast enema will show whether there is a microcolon indicative of jejuno-ileal atresia or meconium ileus. If a microcolon is not present, then the diagnoses of Hirschsprung disease, small left colon syndrome, or meconium plug syndrome should be considered. In all cases of intestinal obstruction, it is vital to obtain abdominal films in the supine and upright (lateral decubitus) views. This is the only way to assess the presence of air-fluid levels or free air, and to characterize the obstruction as proximal or distal. Moreover, it is important to realize that in the absence of contrast, it is difficult to determine whether a loop of dilated bowel is either part of the small or large intestine, as the neonatal bowel lacks typical features, such haustra or plicae circulares, that characterize these loops in older children or adults. For this reason, care must be taken to take a complete prenatal history, to perform a thorough physical examination, and to judiciously determine the need for further contrast studies versus immediate abdominal exploration.

Duodenal Obstruction

Whenever the diagnosis of duodenal obstruction is entertained, malrotation and midgut volvulus must be excluded. This topic is covered in further detail below. Other causes of duodenal obstruction include duodenal atresia, duodenal web, stenosis, annular pancreas or duodenal duplication cyst. Duodenal obstruction is easily diagnosed on prenatal ultrasound, which demonstrates the fluid-filled stomach and proximal duodenum as two discrete cystic structures in the upper abdomen. Associated polyhydramnios is common and presents in the third trimester. In 85 percent of infants with duodenal obstruction, the entry of the bile duct is proximal to the level of obstruction, such that vomiting is bilious. Abdominal distention is typically not present because of the proximal level of obstruction. In those infants with obstruction proximal to the bile duct entry, the vomiting is nonbilious. The classic finding on abdominal radiography is the "double bubble" sign, which represents the dilated stomach and duodenum. In association with the appropriate clinical picture, this finding is sufficient to confirm the diagnosis of duodenal obstruction. However, if there is any uncertainty, particularly when a partial obstruction is suspected, a contrast upper gastrointestinal series is diagnostic.

Treatment

An orogastric tube is inserted to decompress the stomach and duodenum and the infant is given intravenous fluids to maintain adequate urine output. If the infant appears ill, or if abdominal tenderness is present, a diagnosis of malrotation and midgut volvulus should be considered, and surgery should not be delayed. Typically, the abdomen is soft and the infant is very stable. Under these circumstances, the infant should be evaluated thoroughly for other associated anomalies. Approximately one-third of newborns with duodenal atresia have associated Down syndrome (trisomy 21). These patients should also be evaluated for associated cardiac anomalies. Once the work-up is complete and the infant is stable, he or she is taken to the operating room and the abdomen is entered through a transverse right upper quadrant supraumbilical incision under general endotracheal anesthesia. Associated anomalies should be searched for at the time of the operation. These include malrotation, anterior portal vein, a second distal web, and biliary atresia. The surgical treatment of choice for duodenal obstruction because of duodenal stenosis or atresia or annular pancreas is a duodeno-duodenostomy. This procedure can be most easily performed using a proximal transverse-to-distal longitudinal (diamond shaped) anastomosis. In cases in which the duodenum is extremely dilated, the lumen may be tapered using a linear stapler with a large Foley catheter (24-F or greater) in the duodenal lumen. It is important to emphasize that an annular pancreas is never divided. Treatment of duodenal web includes vertical duodenotomy, excision of the web, oversewing of the mucosa and horizontal closure of the duodenotomy. Gastrostomy tubes are not placed routinely. Recently reported survival rates exceed 90 percent. Late complications from repair of duodenal atresia occur in approximately 12–15 percent of patients and include megaduodenum, intestinal motility disorders and gastroesophageal reflux.

Intestinal Atresia

Obstruction because of intestinal atresia can occur at any point along the intestinal tract. Most cases are believed to be caused by in utero mesenteric vascular accidents leading to segmental loss of the intestinal lumen. The incidence of intestinal atresia has been estimated to be between 1 in 2000 to 1 in 5000 live births, with equal representation of the sexes. Infants with jejunal or ileal atresia present with bilious vomiting and progressive abdominal distention. The more distal the obstruction, the more distended the abdomen becomes, and the greater the number of obstructed loops on upright abdominal films.

In cases in which the diagnosis of complete intestinal obstruction is ascertained by the clinical picture and the presence of staggered air-fluid levels on plain abdominal films, the child can be brought to the operating room after appropriate resuscitation. In these circumstances, there is little extra information to be gained by performing a barium enema. By contrast, when there is diagnostic uncertainty, or when distal intestinal obstruction is apparent, a barium enema is useful to establish whether a microcolon is present, and to diagnose the presence of meconium plugs, small left colon syndrome, Hirschsprung disease or meconium ileus. Judicious use of barium enema is therefore required to safely manage neonatal intestinal obstruction, based on an understanding of the expected level of obstruction.

Surgical correction of the small intestinal atresia should be performed urgently. At laparotomy, one of several types of atresia will be encountered. In type I there is a mucosal atresia with intact muscularis. In type 2 the atretic ends are connected by a fibrous band. In type 3A the two ends of the atresia are separated by a V-shaped defect in the mesentery. Type 3B is an "apple-peel" or "Christmas tree" deformity in which the bowel distal to the atresia receives its blood supply in a retrograde fashion from the ileocolic or right colic artery. In type 4 atresia, there are multiple atresias with a "string of sausage" or "string of beads" appearance. Disparity in lumen size between the proximal distended bowel and the small diameter of collapsed bowel distal to the atresia has led to a number of innovative techniques for anastomosis. However, under most circumstances, an anastomosis can be performed using the end-to-back technique in which the distal, compressed loop is "fish-mouthed" along its antimesenteric border. The proximal distended loop can be tapered as described above. Because the distended proximal bowel rarely has normal motility, the extremely dilated portion should be resected prior to performing the anastomosis.

Occasionally the infant with intestinal atresia will develop ischemia or necrosis of the proximal segment secondary to volvulus of the dilated, bulbous, blind-ending proximal bowel. Under these conditions, an end ileostomy and mucus fistula should be created, and the anastomosis should be deferred to another time after the infant stabilizes.

Malrotation and Midgut Volvulus

Embryology

During the sixth week of fetal development, the midgut grows too rapidly to be accommodated in the abdominal cavity and therefore prolapses into the umbilical cord. Between the tenth and twelfth week, the midgut returns to the abdominal cavity, undergoing a 270-degree counterclockwise rotation around the superior mesenteric artery. Because the duodenum also rotates caudal to the artery, it acquires a C-loop, which traces this path. The cecum rotates cephalad to the artery, which determines the location of the transverse and ascending colon. Subsequently, the duodenum becomes fixed retroperitoneally in its third portion and at the ligament of Treitz, although the cecum becomes fixed to the lateral abdominal wall by peritoneal bands. The takeoff of the branches of the superior mesenteric artery elongates and becomes fixed along a line extending from its emergence from the aorta to the cecum in the right lower quadrant.

If rotation is incomplete, the cecum remains in the epigastrium, but the bands fixing the duodenum to the retroperitoneum and cecum continue to form. This results in (Ladd) bands extending from the cecum to the lateral abdominal wall and crossing the duodenum, which creates the potential for obstruction. The mesenteric takeoff remains confined to the epigastrium, resulting in a narrow pedicle suspending all the branches of the superior mesenteric artery and the entire midgut. A volvulus may therefore occur around the mesentery. This twist not only obstructs the proximal jejunum but also cuts off the blood supply to the midgut. Intestinal obstruction and complete infarction of the midgut occur unless the problem is promptly corrected surgically.

Presentation and Management

Midgut volvulus can occur at any age, although it is seen most often in the first few weeks of life. Bilious vomiting is usually the first sign of volvulus and all infants with bilious vomiting must be evaluated rapidly to insure that they do not have intestinal malrotation with volvulus. The child with irritability and bilious emesis should raise particular suspicion for this diagnosis. If left untreated, vascular compromise of the midgut initially causes bloody stools, but eventually results in circulatory collapse. Additional clues to the presence of advanced ischemia of the intestine include erythema and edema of the abdominal wall, which progresses to shock and death. It must be reemphasized that the index of suspicion for this condition must be high, because abdominal signs are minimal in the early stages. Abdominal films show a paucity of gas throughout the intestine with a few scattered air-fluid levels. When these findings are present, the patient should undergo immediate fluid resuscitation to ensure adequate perfusion and urine output followed by prompt exploratory laparotomy.

Often the patient will not appear ill, and the plain films may suggest partial duodenal obstruction. Under these conditions, the patient may have malrotation without volvulus. This is best diagnosed by an upper gastrointestinal series that shows incomplete rotation with the duodenojejunal junction displaced to the right. The duodenum may show a corkscrew effect diagnosing volvulus, or complete duodenal obstruction, with the small bowel loops entirely in the right side of the abdomen. Barium enema may show a displaced cecum, but this sign is unreliable; especially in the small infant in whom the cecum is normally in a somewhat higher position than in the older child. When volvulus is suspected, early surgical intervention is mandatory if the ischemic process is to be avoided or reversed. Volvulus occurs clockwise and it is therefore untwisted counterclockwise. This can be remembered using the memory aid "turn back the hands of time." Subsequently, a Ladd procedure is performed. This operation does not correct the malrotation, but does broaden the narrow mesenteric pedicle to prevent volvulus from recurring. This procedure is performed as follows: The bands between the cecum and the abdominal wall and between the duodenum and terminal ileum are divided sharply to splay out the superior mesenteric artery and its branches. This maneuver brings the straightened duodenum into the right lower quadrant and the cecum into the left lower quadrant. The appendix is removed to avoid diagnostic errors in later life. No attempt is made to suture the cecum or duodenum in place. With advanced ischemia, reduction of the volvulus without the Ladd procedure is accomplished, and a "second look" 24–36 h later often will show some vascular recovery. A plastic transparent silo may be placed to facilitate constant evaluation of the intestine, and to plan for the timing of re-exploration. Frankly necrotic bowel can then be resected conservatively. With early diagnosis and correction the prognosis is excellent. However, diagnostic delay can lead to mortality, or to short-gut syndrome requiring intestinal transplantation.

A subset of patients with malrotation will demonstrate chronic obstructive symptoms. These symptoms may result from the Ladd bands across the duodenum, or occasionally, from intermittent volvulus. Symptoms include intermittent abdominal pain, and intermittent vomiting which may occasionally be bilious. Infants with malrotation may demonstrate failure to thrive, and they may be diagnosed initially as having gastroesophageal reflux disease. Surgical correction using the Ladd procedure as described above can prevent volvulus from occurring and improve symptoms in many instances.

Meconium Ileus

Pathogenesis and Clinical Presentation

Infants with cystic fibrosis have characteristic pancreatic enzyme deficiencies and abnormal chloride secretion in the intestine that result in the production of viscous, water-poor meconium. Meconium ileus occurs when this thick, highly viscous meconium becomes impacted in the ileum and leads to high grade intestinal obstruction. Meconium ileus can be either uncomplicated, in which there is no intestinal perforation, or complicated, in which prenatal perforation of the intestine has occurred or vascular compromise of the distended ileum develops. Antenatal ultrasound may reveal the presence of intraabdominal or scrotal calcifications, or distended bowel loops. These infants present shortly after birth with progressive abdominal distention and failure to pass meconium with intermittent bilious emesis. Abdominal radiographs show dilated loops of intestine. Because the enteric contents are so viscous, air-fluid levels do not form, even when obstruction is complete. Small bubbles of gas become entrapped in the inspissated meconium in the distal ileum, where they produce a characteristic "ground glass" appearance.

The diagnosis of meconium ileus is confirmed by a contrast enema which typically demonstrates a microcolon. In patients with uncomplicated meconium ileus, the terminal ileum is filled with pellets of meconium. In patients with complicated meconium ileus, intraperitoneal calcifications form, producing an eggshell pattern on plain abdominal radiograph.

Management

The treatment strategy depends on whether the patient has complicated or uncomplicated meconium ileus. Patients with uncomplicated meconium ileus can be treated nonoperatively. Dilute water soluble contrast is advanced through the colon under fluoroscopic control into the dilated portion of the ileum. Because these contrast agents act partially by absorbing fluid from the bowel wall into the intestinal lumen, maintaining adequate hydration of the infant during this maneuver is extremely important. The enema may be repeated at 12-h intervals over several days until all the meconium is evacuated. Failure to reflux the contrast into the dilated portion of the ileum signifies the presence of an associated atresia or complicated meconium ileus, and thus warrants exploratory laparotomy. If surgical intervention is required because of failure of contrast enemas to relieve obstruction, operative irrigation with dilute contrast agent, N-acetyl cysteine (Mucomyst) or saline through a purse-string suture may be successful. Alternatively, resection of the distended terminal ileum is performed and the meconium pellets are flushed from the distal small bowel.

At this point, ileostomy and mucous fistula may be created from the proximal and distal ends respectively.

Necrotizing Enterocolitis

Clinical Features

Necrotizing enterocolitis (NEC) is the most frequent and lethal gastrointestinal disorder affecting the intestine of the stressed, preterm neonate. Over 25,000 cases of NEC are reported annually. The overall mortality ranges between 10 percent and 50 percent. Advances in neonatal care such as surfactant therapy and improved methods of mechanical ventilation have resulted in increasing numbers of low birth weight infants surviving neonatal hyaline membrane disease. An increasing proportion of survivors of neonatal respiratory distress syndrome will therefore be at risk for developing NEC. Consequently, it is estimated that NEC soon will surpass respiratory distress syndrome as the principal cause of death in the preterm infant.

Multiple risk factors have been associated with the development of NEC. These include prematurity, initiation of enteral feeding, bacterial infection, intestinal ischemia resulting from birth asphyxia, umbilical artery cannulation, persistence of a patent ductus arteriosus, cyanotic heart disease and maternal cocaine abuse. Nonetheless, the mechanisms by which these complex interacting etiologies lead to the development of the disease remain undefined. The only consistent epidemiologic precursors for NEC are prematurity and enteral alimentation, representing the commonly encountered clinical situation of a stressed infant who is fed enterally. Of note, there is some debate regarding the importance of enteral alimentation in the pathogenesis of NEC. A prospective randomized study showed no increase in the incidence of NEC despite an aggressive feeding strategy, and up to 10 percent of infants with NEC have never received any form of enteral nutrition.

The indigenous intestinal microbial flora has been postulated to play a central role in the pathogenesis of NEC. Bacterial colonization may be a prerequisite for the development of this disease, as oral prophylaxis with vancomycin or gentamicin reduced the incidence of NEC. The importance of bacteria in the pathogenesis of NEC is further supported by the finding that NEC occurs in episodic waves that can be abrogated by infection control measures, and the fact that NEC usually develops at least 10 days postnatally, when the GI tract is colonized by coliforms. Common bacterial isolates from the blood, peritoneal fluid and stool of infants with advanced NEC include *Escherichia coli*, Enterobacter, Klebsiella, and occasionally, coagulase-negative Staphylococcus species.

NEC may involve single or multiple segments of the intestine, most commonly the terminal ileum, followed by the colon. The gross findings in NEC include bowel distention with patchy areas of thinning, pneumatosis, gangrene or frank perforation. The microscopic features include the appearance of a "bland infarct" characterized by full thickness necrosis.

Pathogenesis of NEC

The exact mechanisms that lead to the development of NEC remain incompletely understood. However, current thinking suggests that in the setting of an episode of perinatal stress, such as respiratory distress syndrome, the premature infant suffers a period of intestinal hypoperfusion. This is followed by a period of reperfusion, and the combination of ischemia and reperfusion lead to mucosal injury. The damaged intestinal mucosa can then be readily breached by indigenous microorganisms that translocate across it. The translocated bacteria then initiate an inflammatory cascade that involves the release of various proinflammatory mediators which in turn may be responsible for further epithelial injury and the systemic manifestations of NEC. It is postulated that maintenance of the gut barrier is essential for the protection of the host against NEC, and that impairment of the mechanisms that normally repair the damaged mucosal barrier may facilitate propagation of the mucosal injury and thus, NEC.

Clinical Manifestations

Infants with NEC present with a spectrum of disease. In general, the infants are premature and may have sustained one or more episodes of stress, such as birth asphyxia, or they may have congenital cardiac disease. The clinical picture of NEC has been characterized as progressing from a period of mild illness to that of severe, life threatening sepsis by Bell and colleagues. Although not all infants progress through the various "Bell stages," this classification scheme provides a useful format to describe the clinical picture associated with the development of NEC. In the earliest stage (Bell Stage I), infants present with formula intolerance. This is manifested by vomiting or by finding a large residual volume from a previous feeding in the stomach at the time of the next feeding. Following appropriate treatment, which consists of bowel rest and intravenous antibiotics, many of these infants will not progress to more advanced stages of NEC. These infants are colloquially described as suffering from a "NEC scare," and represent a population of neonates that are at risk of developing more severe NEC if a more prolonged period of stress supervenes.

Infants with Bell Stage II have established NEC that is not immediately life threatening. Clinical findings include abdominal distention and tenderness, bilious nasogastric aspirate, and bloody stools. These findings indicate the development of intestinal ileus and mucosal ischemia respectively. Abdominal examination may reveal a palpable mass indicating the presence of an inflamed loop of bowel, diffuse abdominal tenderness, cellulitis and edema of the anterior abdominal wall. The infant may appear systemically ill, with decreased urine output, hypotension, tachycardia and noncardiac pulmonary edema. Hematologic evaluation reveals either leukocytosis or leukopenia, an increase in the number of bands, and thrombocytopenia. An increase in the blood urea nitrogen and plasma creatinine level may be found, which signify the development of renal dysfunction. The diagnosis of NEC may be confirmed by abdominal radiography. The pathognomonic radiographic finding in NEC is pneumatosis intestinalis, which represents invasion of the ischemic mucosa by gas producing microbes. Other findings include the presence of ileus or portal venous gas. The latter is a transient finding that indicates the presence of severe NEC with intestinal necrosis. A fixed loop of bowel may be seen on serial abdominal radiographs, which suggests the possibility that a diseased loop of bowel, potentially with a localized perforation, is present. Although these infants are at risk of progressing to more severe disease, with timely and appropriate treatment, they often recover.

Infants with Bell Stage III have the most advanced form of NEC. Abdominal radiographs often demonstrate the presence of pneumoperitoneum, indicating that intestinal perforation has occurred. These patients may develop a fulminant course with progressive peritonitis, acidosis, sepsis, disseminated intravascular coagulopathy, and death.

Treatment

In all infants suspected of having NEC, feedings are discontinued, a nasogastric tube is placed, and broad spectrum parenteral antibiotics are given. The infant is resuscitated, and inotropes are administered to maintain perfusion as needed. Intubation and mechanical ventilation may be required to maintain oxygenation. Total parenteral nutrition is started. Subsequent treatment may be influenced by the particular stage of NEC that is present. Patients with Bell I are closely monitored, and generally remain "nothing by mouth" (NPO) and on intravenous antibiotics for 7–10 days, prior to re-initiating enteral nutrition. After this time, provided that the infant fully recovers, feedings may be re-initiated.

Patients with Bell II disease merit close observation. Serial physical examinations are performed looking for the development of diffuse peritonitis, a fixed mass, progressive abdominal wall cellulitis or systemic sepsis. If infants fail to improve after several days of treatment, consideration should be given to exploratory laparotomy. Paracentesis may be performed, and if the gram stain demonstrates multiple organisms and leukocytes, perforation of the bowel should be suspected, and patients should be treated as Bell III patients.

In the most severe form of NEC (Bell III), patients have definite intestinal perforation, or have not responded to nonoperative therapy. Two schools of thought direct further management. One group favors exploratory laparotomy. At laparotomy, frankly gangrenous or perforated bowel is resected, and the intestinal ends are brought out as stomas. When there is massive intestinal involvement, marginally viable bowel is retained and a "second-look" procedure is carried out after the infant stabilizes (24–48 h). Patients with extensive necrosis at the second look may be managed by placing a proximal diverting stoma, resecting bowel that is definitely not viable, and leaving questionably viable bowel behind distal to the diverted segment. When the intestine is viable except for a localized perforation without diffuse peritonitis and if the infant's clinical condition permits, intestinal anastomosis may be performed either proximal or distal to the divided segment. In cases in which the diseased, perforated segment can not be safely resected, drainage catheters may be left in the region of the diseased bowel, and the infant is allowed to stabilize.

An alternative approach to the management of infants with perforated NEC involves drainage of the peritoneal cavity. This may be performed under local anesthesia at the bedside, and can be an effective means of stabilizing the desperately ill infant by relieving increased intraabdominal pressure and allowing ventilation. When successful, this method also allows for drainage of perforated bowel by establishing a controlled fistula. Approximately one-third of infants treated with drainage alone survive without requiring additional operations. Infants that do not respond to peritoneal drainage alone after 48–72 h should undergo laparotomy. This procedure allows for the resection of frankly necrotic bowel diversion of the fecal stream and facilitates more effective drainage.

Outcome

Survival in patients with NEC is dependent on the stage of disease, the extent of prematurity, and the presence of associated comorbidities. Survival by stage has recently been shown to be approximately 85 percent, 65 percent and

35 percent for stages I, II and III respectively. Strictures develop in 20 percent of medically or surgically treated patients, and a contrast enema is mandatory before re-establishing intestinal continuity. If all other factors are favorable, the ileostomy is closed when the child is between 2 and 2.5 kg. At the time of stoma closure, the entire intestine should be examined to search for areas of NEC. Patients that developed massive intestinal necrosis are at risk of developing short-gut syndrome, particularly when the total length of the viable intestinal segment is below 40 cm. These patients require TPN to provide adequate calories for growth and development, and may develop TPN-related cholestasis and hepatic fibrosis. In a significant number of these patients, transplantation of the liver and small bowel may be required.

Intussusception

Intussusception is the leading cause of intestinal obstruction in the young child. It refers to the condition whereby a segment of intestine becomes drawn into the lumen of the more proximal bowel. The process usually begins in the region of the terminal ileum, and extends distally into the ascending, transverse or descending colon. Rarely, an intussusception may prolapse through the rectum.

The cause of intussusception is not clear, although current thinking suggests that hypertrophy of the Peyer patches in the terminal ileum from an antecedent viral infection acts as a lead point. Peristaltic action of the intestine then causes the bowel distal to the lead point to invaginate into itself. Idiopathic intussusception occurs in children between the ages of approximately 6 and 24 months of age. Beyond this age group, one should consider the possibility that a pathologic lead point maybe present. These include polyps, malignant tumors such as lymphoma, enteric duplication cysts or Meckel diverticulum. Such intussusceptions are rarely reduced by air or contrast enema, and thus the lead point is identified when operative reduction of the intussusception is performed.

Clinical Manifestations

Because intussusception is frequently preceded by a gastrointestinal viral illness, the onset may not be easily determined. Typically, the infant develops paroxysms of crampy abdominal pain and intermittent vomiting. Between attacks, the infant may act normally, but as symptoms progress, increasing lethargy develops. Bloody mucus ("currant-jelly" stool) may be passed per rectum. Ultimately, if reduction is not accomplished, gangrene of the intussusceptum occurs, and perforation may ensue. On physical examination, an elongated mass is detected in the right upper quadrant or epigastrium with an absence of bowel in the right lower quadrant (Dance sign). The mass may be seen on plain abdominal radiograph but is more easily demonstrated on air or contrast enema.

Treatment

Patients with intussusception should be assessed for the presence of peritonitis and for the severity of systemic illness. Following resuscitation and administration of intravenous antibiotics, the child is assessed for suitability to proceed with radiographic versus surgical reduction. In the absence of peritonitis, the child should undergo radiographic reduction. If peritonitis is present, or if the child appears systemically ill, urgent laparotomy is indicated.

In the stable patient, the air enema is both diagnostic and often curative. It constitutes the preferred method of diagnosis and nonoperative treatment of intussusception. Air is introduced with a manometer and the pressure that is administered is carefully monitored. Under most instances, this should not exceed 120 mmHg. Successful reduction is marked by free reflux of air into multiple loops of small bowel and symptomatic improvement as the infant suddenly becomes pain free. Unless both of these signs are observed, it cannot be assumed that the intussusception is reduced. If reduction is unsuccessful, and the infant remains stable, the infant should be brought back to the radiology suite for a repeat attempt at reduction after a few h. This strategy has improved the success rate of nonoperative reduction in many centers. Additionally, hydrostatic reduction with barium may be useful if pneumatic reduction is unsuccessful. The overall success rate of radiographic reduction varies based on the experience of the center, and is typically between 60 and 90 percent.

If nonoperative reduction is successful, the infant may be given oral fluids after a period of observation. Failure to reduce the intussusception mandates surgery. Two approaches are used. In an open procedure, exploration is carried out through a right lower quadrant incision, delivering the intussuscepted mass into the wound. Reduction usually can be accomplished by gentle distal pressure, where the intussusceptum is gently milked out of the intussuscipiens. Care should be taken not to pull the bowel out, as this can cause damage to the bowel wall. The blood supply to the appendix is often compromised, and appendectomy is performed. If the bowel is frankly gangrenous, resection and primary anastomosis is performed. In experienced hands, laparoscopic reduction may be performed, even in very young infants. Intravenous fluids are continued until the postoperative ileus subsides. Patients are started on clear liquids, and their diet is advanced as tolerated. Of note, recurrent intussusception occurs in 5–10 percent of patients, independent of whether the bowel is reduced radiographically or surgically. Patients present with recurrent symptoms in the immediate postoperative period. Treatment involves repeat air enema, which is successful in most cases. In patients who experience three or more episodes of intussusception, the presence of a pathologic lead point should be suspected and carefully evaluated using contrast studies. After the third episode of intussusception, many pediatric surgeons will perform an exploratory laparotomy to reduce the bowel and to resect a pathologic lead point if identified.

Appendicitis

Presentation

Correct diagnosis of appendicitis in children can be one of the most humbling and challenging tasks faced by the pediatric surgeon. The classical presentation is known to all students and practitioners of surgery: generalized abdominal pain that localizes to the right lower quadrant followed by nausea, vomiting, fever, and localized peritoneal irritation in the region of McBurney's point. When children present in this manner, there should be little diagnostic delay. The child should be made NPO, administered intravenous fluids and broad spectrum antibiotics, and brought to the operating room for an appendectomy. However, children often do not present in this manner. The co-existence of viral syndromes, and the inability of young children to describe the location and quality of their pain, often result in diagnostic delay. As a result, children with appendicitis often present with perforation, particularly those who are younger than 5 years of age. Perforation increases the length of hospital stay, and makes the overall course of the illness significantly more complex.

Diagnosis of Appendicitis in Children

Controversy exists regarding the role of radiographic studies in the diagnosis of acute appendicitis. Because children have less peri-appendiceal fat than adults, computerized tomography is less reliable in making the diagnosis. Additionally, radiation exposure resulting from the CT scan may have potentially long-term adverse effects. Likewise, ultrasonography is neither sufficiently sensitive nor specific to accurately make the diagnosis of appendicitis, although it is very useful for excluding ovarian causes of abdominal pain. Therefore, the diagnosis of appendicitis remains largely clinical, and each clinician should develop his or her own threshold to operate or to observe the patient. A reasonable practice guideline is as follows: when the diagnosis is clinically apparent, appendectomy should obviously be performed with minimal delay. Localized right lower quadrant tenderness associated with low grade fever and leukocytosis in boys should prompt surgical exploration. In girls, ovarian or uterine pathology must also be considered. When there is diagnostic uncertainty, the child may be observed, rehydrated and reassessed. In girls of menstruating age, an ultrasound may be obtained to exclude ovarian pathology (cysts, torsion or tumor). If all studies are negative, yet the pain persists and the abdominal findings remain equivocal, diagnostic laparoscopy may be employed to determine the etiology of the abdominal pain. The appendix should be removed even if it appears to be normal, unless another pathologic cause of the abdominal pain is definitively identified and the appendectomy would substantially increase morbidity.

Management of the child with perforated appendicitis. The signs and symptoms of perforated appendicitis can closely mimic those of gastroenteritis and include abdominal pain, vomiting and diarrhea. Alternatively, the child may present with symptoms of intestinal obstruction. An abdominal mass may be present in the lower abdomen. When the symptoms have been present for more than 4 or 5 days, and an abscess is suspected, it is reasonable to obtain a computerized tomogram of the abdomen and pelvis with intravenous, oral and rectal contrast to visualize the appendix and the presence of an associated abscess, phlegmon or fecalith.

An individualized approach is necessary for the child who presents with perforated appendicitis. When there is evidence of generalized peritonitis, intestinal obstruction or systemic toxicity, the child should undergo appendectomy. This should be delayed only for as long as is required to ensure adequate fluid resuscitation and administration of broad spectrum antibiotics. The operation can be performed through an open procedure through a laparoscopic approach. One distinct advantage of the laparoscopic approach is that it provides excellent visualization of the pelvis and all four quadrants of the abdomen. At the time of surgery, adhesions are gently lysed, abscess cavities are drained and the appendix is removed. Drains are seldom used, and the skin incisions can be closed primarily. If a fecalith is identified outside the appendix on computerized tomography, every effort should be made to retrieve it and to remove it along with the appendix, if at all possible. Often, the child in whom symptoms have been present for more than 4 or 5 days will present with an abscess cavity without evidence of generalized peritonitis. Under these circumstances, it is appropriate to perform image-guided percutaneous drainage of the abscess followed by broad spectrum antibiotic therapy. The inflammation will generally subside within several days, and the appendix can be safely removed as an outpatient 6–8 weeks later. If the child's symptoms do not improve, or if the abscess is not amenable to percutaneous drainage, then laparoscopic or open appendectomy and abscess drainage is required. Patients who present with a phlegmon in the region of a perforated appendix may be managed in a similar manner. In general, children who are younger than 4 or 5 years of age do not respond as well to initial nonoperative approach, because their bodies do not localize or isolate the inflammatory process. Thus, these patients are more likely to require early surgical intervention. Patients who have had symptoms of appendicitis for no more than four days should probably undergo "early" appendectomy, because the inflammatory response is not as excessive during that initial period and the procedure can be performed safely.

Intestinal Duplications

Duplications represent mucosa-lined structures that are in continuity with the gastrointestinal tract. Although they can occur at any level in the gastrointestinal tract, these anomalies are found most commonly in the ileum within the leaves of the mesentery. Duplications may be long and tubular, but usually are cystic masses. In all cases, they share a common wall with the intestine. Symptoms associated with enteric duplication cysts include recurrent abdominal pain, emesis from intestinal obstruction, or hematochezia. Such bleeding typically results from ulceration in the duplication or in the adjacent intestine if the duplication contains ectopic gastric mucosa. On examination, a palpable mass is often identified. Children may also develop intestinal obstruction. Torsion may produce gangrene and perforation. Computerized tomography, ultrasonography and technetium pertechnetate scanning can be very helpful in diagnosis. Occasionally, a duplication is seen on small bowel follow through or barium enema. In the case of short duplications, resection of the cyst and adjacent intestine with end-to-end anastomosis can be performed in a straightforward fashion. If resection of long duplications would compromise intestinal length, multiple enterotomies and mucosal stripping in the duplicated segment will allow the walls to collapse and become adherent. An alternative method is to divide the common wall using the GIA stapler, forming a common lumen. Patients with duplications who undergo complete excision without compromise of the length of remaining intestine have an excellent prognosis.

Meckel Diverticulum

A Meckel diverticulum is a remnant of a portion of the embryonic omphalomesenteric (vitelline) duct. It is located on the antimesenteric border of the ileum, usually within 2 ft of the ileocecal valve. It may be found incidentally at surgery or may present with inflammation masquerading as appendicitis. Perforation of a Meckel diverticulum may occur if the outpouching becomes impacted with food, leading to distention and necrosis. Occasionally, a band of scar tissue (omphalomesenteric band) may extend from the Meckel diverticulum to the anterior abdominal wall and result in an internal hernia. This is an important cause of intestinal obstruction in the older child who has a scarless abdomen. Similar to duplications, ectopic gastric mucosa may produce ileal ulcerations that bleed and lead to the passage of maroon-colored stools. Pancreatic mucosa may also be present. Diagnosis may be made by technetium pertechnetate scans when the patient presents with bleeding. Treatment is surgical. If the base is narrow and there is no mass present in the lumen of the diverticulum, a wedge resection of the diverticulum with transverse closure of the ileum can be performed. A linear stapler is especially useful in this circumstance. When a mass of ectopic tissue is palpable, if the base is wide, or when there is inflammation, it is preferable to perform a resection of the involved bowel and end-to-end ileo-ileostomy.

Hirschsprung Disease

Pathogenesis

In his classic textbook titled "Pediatric Surgery" Dr. Orvar Swenson—who is eponymously associated with one of the classic surgical treatments for Hirschsprung disease—described this condition as follows: "congenital megacolon is caused by a malformation in the pelvic parasympathetic system which results in the absence of ganglion cells in Auerbach's plexus of a segment of distal colon. Not only is there an absence of ganglion cells, but the nerve fibers are large and excessive in number, indicating that the anomaly may be more extensive than the absence of ganglion cells." This narrative of Hirschsprung disease is as accurate today as it was nearly 50 years ago, and summarizes the essential pathologic features of this disease: absence of ganglion cells in Auerbach plexus and hypertrophy of associated nerve trunks. The cause of Hirschsprung disease remains incompletely understood, although current thinking suggests that the disease results from a defect in the migration of neural crest cells, which are the embryonic precursors of the intestinal ganglion cell. Under normal conditions, the neural crest cells migrate into the intestine from cephalad to caudad. The process is completed by the twelfth week of gestation, but the migration from midtransverse colon to anus takes 4 weeks. During this latter period, the fetus is most vulnerable to defects in migration of neural crest cells. This may explain why most cases of aganglionosis involve the rectum and rectosigmoid. The length of the aganglionic segment of bowel is therefore determined by the most distal region that the migrating neural crest cells reach. In rare instances, total colonic aganglionosis may occur.

Clinical presentation. The incidence of sporadic Hirschsprung disease is 1 in 5000 live births. There are reports of increased frequency of Hirschsprung disease in multiple generations of the same family. Occasionally such families have mutations in the genes described above, including the Ret gene. Because the aganglionic colon does not permit normal peristalsis to occur, the presentation of children with Hirschsprung disease is characterized by a functional distal intestinal obstruction. In the newborn period, the most common symptoms are abdominal distention, failure to pass meconium, and bilious emesis. Any infant who does not pass meconium beyond 48 h of life must be investigated for the presence of Hirschsprung disease. Occasionally, infants present with a dramatic complication of Hirschsprung disease called enterocolitis. This pattern of presentation is characterized by abdominal distention and tenderness, and is associated with manifestations of systemic toxicity that include fever, failure to thrive and lethargy. Infants are often dehydrated, and demonstrate a leukocytosis or increase in circulating band forms on hematologic evaluation. On rectal examination, forceful propulsion of foul smelling liquid feces is typically observed, and represents the accumulation of stool under pressure in an obstructed distal colon. Treatment includes rehydration, systemic antibiotics, nasogastric decompression and rectal irrigations while the diagnosis of Hirschsprung disease is being confirmed. In children that do not respond to nonoperative management, a decompressive stoma is required. It is important to ensure that this stoma is placed in ganglion-containing bowel, which must be confirmed by frozen section at the time of stoma creation.

In approximately 20 percent of cases, the diagnosis of Hirschsprung disease is made beyond the newborn period. These children have severe constipation, which has usually been treated with laxatives and enemas. Abdominal distention and failure to thrive may also be present at diagnosis.

Diagnosis

The definitive diagnosis of Hirschsprung disease is made by rectal biopsy. Samples of mucosa and submucosa are obtained at 1 cm, 2 cm, and 3 cm from the dentate line. This can be performed at the bedside in the neonatal period without anesthesia, as samples are taken in bowel that does not have somatic innervation and is thus not painful to the child. In older children, the procedure should be performed using intravenous sedation. The histopathology of Hirschsprung disease is the absence of ganglion cells in the myenteric plexuses, increased staining of a acetyl cholinesterase staining and the presence of hypertrophied nerve bundles.

It is important to obtain a barium enema in children in whom the diagnosis of Hirschsprung disease is suspected. This test may demonstrate the location of the transition zone between the dilated ganglionic colon and the distal constricted aganglionic rectal segment. Our practice is to obtain this test before instituting rectal irrigations, so that the difference in size between the proximal and distal bowel is preserved. Although the barium enema can only suggest, but not reliably establish, the diagnosis of Hirschsprung disease, it is very useful in excluding other causes of distal intestinal obstruction. These include small left colon syndrome (as occurs in infants of diabetic mothers), colonic atresia, meconium plug syndrome or the unused colon observed in infants after the administration of magnesium or tocolytic agents. The barium enema in total colonic aganglionosis may show a markedly shortened colon. Some surgeons have found the use of rectal manometry helpful, particularly in older children, although it is relatively inaccurate.

Treatment

The diagnosis of Hirschsprung disease requires surgery in all cases. The classic surgical approach consisted of a multiple stage procedure. This included a colostomy in the newborn period, followed by a definitive pull-through operation after the child was over 10 kg. There are three viable options for the definitive pull through procedure that are currently used. Although individual surgeons may advocate one procedure over another, studies have demonstrated that the outcome after each type of operation is similar. For each of the operations that is performed, the principles of treatment include confirming the location in the bowel where the transition zone between ganglionic and aganglionic bowel exists, resecting the aganglionic segment of bowel and performing an anastomosis of ganglionated bowel to either the anus or a cuff of rectal mucosa.

Recently, it has been shown that a primary pull-through procedure can be performed safely—even in the newborn period. This approach follows the same treatment principles as a staged procedure, and saves the patient from an additional surgical procedure. Many surgeons perform the intraabdominal dissection using the laparoscope. This approach is especially useful in the newborn period, as this provides excellent visualization of the pelvis. In children with significant colonic distention, it is important to allow for a period of decompression using a rectal tube if a single staged pull through is to be performed. In older children with very distended, hypertrophied colon, it may be prudent to perform a colostomy to allow the bowel to decompress, prior to performing a pull through procedure. However, it should be emphasized that there is no upper age limit for performing a primary pull through.

Of the three pull-through procedures performed for Hirschsprung disease, the first is the original Swenson procedure. In this operation, the aganglionic rectum is dissected in the pelvis and removed down to the anus. The ganglionic colon is then anastomosed to the anus via a perineal approach. In the Duhamel procedure, dissection outside the rectum is confined to the retrorectal space, and the ganglionic colon is anastomosed posteriorly just above the anus. The anterior wall of the ganglionic colon and the posterior wall of the aganglionic rectum are anastomosed, using a stapler. Although both of these procedures are extremely effective, they are limited by the possibility of damage to the parasympathetic nerves that are adjacent to the rectum. To circumvent this potential problem, the Soave procedure involves dissection entirely within the rectum. The rectal mucosa is stripped from the muscular sleeve, and the ganglionic colon is brought through this sleeve and anastomosed to the anus. This operation may be performed completely from below. In all cases, it is critical that the level at which ganglionated bowel exists be determined. Most surgeons believe that the anastomosis should be performed at least 5 cm from the point at which ganglion cells are determined. This avoids performing a pull-through in the transition zone, which is associated with a high incidence of complications because of inadequate emptying of the pull-through segment. Up to one-third of patients who undergo a transition zone pull through will require a re-operation.

The main complications of all procedures include postoperative enterocolitis, constipation and anastomotic stricture. As mentioned, long-term results with the three procedures are comparable and generally excellent in experienced hands. These three procedures also can be adapted for total colonic aganglionosis in which the ileum is used for the pull-through segment.

JAUNDICE

The Approach to the Jaundiced Infant

Jaundice is present during the first week of life in 60 percent of term infants and 80 percent of preterm infants. There is usually accumulation of unconjugated bilirubin, but there may also be deposition of direct bilirubin. During fetal life, the placenta is the principal route of elimination of unconjugated bilirubin. In the newborn infant, bilirubin is conjugated through the activity of glucuronyl transferase. In the conjugated form, bilirubin is water soluble, which results in its excretion into the biliary system, then into the gastrointestinal tract. Newborns have a relatively high level of circulating hemoglobin, and relative immaturity of the conjugating machinery. This results in a transient accumulation of bilirubin in the tissues, which is manifested as jaundice. Physiologic jaundice is evident by the second or third day of life, and usually resolves within approximately 5–7 days. By definition, jaundice that persists beyond 2 weeks is considered pathologic.

Pathologic jaundice may be because of biliary obstruction, increased hemoglobin load or to liver dysfunction. The work-up of the jaundiced infant therefore should include a search for the following possibilities: (1) obstructive disorders, including biliary atresia, choledochal cyst and inspissated bile syndrome; (2) hematologic disorders, including ABO incompatibility, Rh incompatibility, spherocytosis; (3) metabolic disorders, including alpha$_1$ antitrypsin deficiency, galactosemia; pyruvate kinase deficiency; and (4) congenital infection, including syphilis and rubella.

Biliary Atresia

Pathogenesis

The most important surgical cause of jaundice in the newborn period is biliary atresia. The incidence of this disease is approximately 1 in 20,000. This disease is characterized by an obliterative process of the extrahepatic bile ducts, and is associated with hepatic fibrosis. The etiology is unknown. In the classic textbook, "Abdominal Surgery of Infancy And Childhood," Ladd and Gross described the cause of biliary atresia as an "arrest of development during the solid stage of bile duct formation." More recent evidence suggests an acquired basis for this disease, and studies in both animals and humans have implicated a role for the immune system and systemic viral infections in its pathogenesis.

Clinical Presentation

Jaundice, a constant finding, is usually present at birth or shortly thereafter but may go undetected or may be regarded as "physiologic" until the child is 2 or 3 weeks old. The infant demonstrates acholic, grey appearing stools, secondary to obstructed bile flow. Infants with biliary atresia also manifest progressive failure to thrive, and if untreated, progress to develop stigmata of liver failure and portal hypertension; particularly splenomegaly and esophageal varices.

The obliterative process involves the common duct, cystic duct, one or both hepatic ducts, and the gallbladder, in a variety of combinations. Approximately 25 percent of the patients have coincidental malformations, often associated with polysplenia and may include intestinal malrotation, preduodenal portal vein, and intrahepatic vena cava.

Diagnosis

Generally, a combination of investigations is required to ascertain the diagnosis of biliary atresia, as no single test is sufficiently sensitive or specific. In many centers the nuclear medicine scan using technetium–99m IDA (DISIDA), performed after pretreatment of the patient with phenobarbital, has proven to be an accurate and reliable study. If radionuclide appears in the intestine, extrahepatic bile duct patency is ensured and the diagnosis of biliary atresia is excluded. If radiopharmaceutical is normally concentrated by the liver but not excreted despite treatment with phenobarbital, and the metabolic screen, particularly alpha$_1$-antitrypsin determination, is normal, the presumptive diagnosis is biliary atresia. An ultrasound may be performed to assess for the presence of other causes of biliary tract obstruction including choledochal cyst. The presence of a gallbladder is also evaluated, although it is important to emphasize that the presence of a gallbladder does not exclude the diagnosis of biliary atresia. In approximately 10 percent of patients, the distal biliary tract is patent and a gall bladder may be visualized, even though the proximal ducts are atretic. It is worth noting that the intrahepatic bile ducts are never dilated in the patient with biliary atresia. A percutaneous liver biopsy may, at times, differentiate biliary atresia from neonatal hepatitis. When these tests point to a diagnosis of biliary atresia, surgical exploration is warranted. At surgery, a cholangiogram is performed, using the gallbladder as a conduit. This demonstrates the anatomy of the biliary tree, determines whether extrahepatic bile duct atresia is present and evaluates whether there is distal bile flow into the duodenum. The cholangiogram may demonstrate hypoplasia of the extrahepatic biliary system. This condition is associated with hepatic parenchymal disorders that cause severe intrahepatic cholestasis, including alpha1-antitrypsin deficiency and arteriohepatic dysplasia (Alagille syndrome).

The presentation of biliary atresia closely mimics that of inspissated bile syndrome. This term is applied to patients with normal biliary tracts who have persistent obstructive jaundice. Increased viscosity of bile and obstruction of the canaliculi are implicated as causes. The condition has been seen in infants receiving parenteral nutrition, but it is also encountered in conditions associated with hemolysis, or in cystic fibrosis. In some instances, no etiologic factors can be defined. Neonatal hepatitis may present in a similar fashion to biliary atresia. This disease is characterized by persistent jaundice because of acquired biliary inflammation without obliteration of the bile ducts. There may be a viral etiology, and the disease is usually self limited.

Treatment

If the intraoperative cholangiogram confirms the presence of biliary atresia, then surgical correction should be immediately undertaken. The most effective surgical treatment for biliary atresia is the hepatoportoenterostomy, as described by Kasai. The purpose of this procedure is to promote bile flow into the intestine. The procedure is based on Kasai's observation that the fibrous tissue at the porta hepatis invests microscopically patent biliary ductules that, in turn, communicate with the intrahepatic ductal system. Transecting this fibrous tissue, invariably encountered cephalad to the bifurcating portal vein, opens these channels and establishes bile flow into a surgically constructed intestinal conduit, usually a Roux-en-Y limb of jejunum. Some authors believe that an intussuscepted antireflux valve is useful in preventing retrograde bile reflux, although the data suggest that it does not impact outcome. A liver biopsy is performed at the time of surgery to determine the degree of hepatic fibrosis that is present. The likelihood of surgical success is increased if the procedure is accomplished before the infant attains the age of 8 weeks. Although the outlook is less favorable for patients after the twelfth week, it is reasonable to proceed with surgery even beyond this time point, as the alternative is certain liver failure. It is noteworthy that a significant number of patients do have favorable outcomes when operated on at this time point.

Bile drainage is anticipated when the operation is carried out early; however, bile flow does not necessarily imply cure. Approximately a third of patients remain symptom-free after portoenterostomy, the remainder require liver transplantation because of progressive liver failure. Independent risk factors that predict failure of the procedure include bridging liver fibrosis at the time of surgery and postoperative cholangitic episodes. A recent review of the data of the Japanese Biliary Atresia Registry (JBAR), which includes the results of

1,381 patients, showed that the 10-year survival rate was 53 percent without transplantation, and with transplantation was 66.7 percent. A common postoperative common is cholangitis. There is no effective strategy to completely eliminate this complication, and the effectiveness of long-term prophylactic antibiotics has not been fully resolved.

DEFORMITIES OF THE ABDOMINAL WALL

Embryology of the Abdominal Wall

The abdominal wall is formed by four separate embryologic folds—cephalic, caudal, and right and left lateral folds—each of which is composed of somatic and splanchnic layers. Each of the folds develops toward the anterior center portion of the coelomic cavity, joining to form a large umbilical ring that surrounds the two umbilical arteries, the vein, and the yolk sac or omphalomesenteric duct. These structures are covered by an outer layer of amnion, and the entire unit composes the umbilical cord. Between the fifth and tenth weeks of fetal development the intestinal tract undergoes a rapid growth outside the abdominal cavity within the proximal portion of the umbilical cord. As development is completed, the intestine gradually returns to the abdominal cavity. Contraction of the umbilical ring completes the process of abdominal wall formation.

Failure of the cephalic fold to close results in sternal defects such as congenital absence of the sternum. Failure of the caudal fold to close results in exstrophy of the bladder and, in more extreme cases, exstrophy of the cloaca. Interruption of central migration of the lateral folds results in omphalocele. Gastroschisis, originally thought to be a variant of omphalocele, probably results from a fetal accident in the form of intrauterine rupture of a hernia of the umbilical cord.

Umbilical Hernia

Failure of the umbilical ring to close results in a central defect in the linea alba. The resulting umbilical hernia is covered by normal umbilical skin and subcutaneous tissue, but the fascial defect allows protrusion of abdominal contents. Hernias less than a cm in size at the time of birth usually will close spontaneously by four years of life. Sometimes the hernia is large enough that the protrusion is disfiguring and disturbing to both the child and the family. In such circumstances early repair may be advisable.

Repair of uncomplicated umbilical hernia is performed under general anesthesia as an outpatient procedure. A small curving incision that fits into the skin crease of the umbilicus is made, and the sac is dissected free from the overlying skin. The fascial defect is repaired with permanent or long-lasting absorbable, interrupted sutures that are placed in a transverse plane. The skin is closed using subcuticular sutures.

Omphalocele

Presentation

Omphalocele refers to a congenital defect of the abdominal wall in which the bowel and solid viscera are covered by peritoneum and amniotic membrane. The umbilical cord inserts into the sac. The abdominal wall defect measures 4 cm or more in diameter. The incidence is approximately 1 in 5000 live births, and occurs in association with special syndromes such as exstrophy of the cloaca (vesicointestinal fissure), the Beckwith-Wiedemann constellation of anomalies (macroglossia, macrosomia, hypoglycemia, and visceromegaly and omphalocele) and the Cantrell Pentology (lower thoracic wall malformations [cleft sternum], ectopia cordis, epigastric omphalocele, anterior midline diaphragmatic hernia and cardiac anomalies). The size of the defect may be very small or large enough that it contains most of the abdominal viscera. There is a 60–70 percent incidence of associated anomalies, especially cardiac (20–40 percent of cases) and chromosomal abnormalities. Chromosomal anomalies are more common in children with smaller defects. Omphalocele is associated with prematurity (10–50 percent of cases) and intrauterine growth restriction (20 percent of cases).

Treatment

Immediate treatment of an infant with omphalocele consists of attending to the vital signs and maintaining the body temperature. The omphalocele should be covered with saline-soaked gauze and the trunk should be wrapped circumferentially. No pressure should be placed on the omphalocele sac in an effort to reduce its contents, as this maneuver may increase the risk of rupture of the sac, or may interfere with abdominal venous return. Prophylactic antibiotics should be administered in case of rupture. Whenever possible, a primary repair of the omphalocele should be undertaken. This involves resection of the omphalocele membrane and closure of the fascia. A layer of prosthetic material may be required to achieve closure.

Occasionally, an infant will have a giant omphalocele (defect greater than 7 cm in diameter) that cannot be closed primarily because there is simply no room to reduce the viscera into the abdominal cavity. Other, infants may have associated congenital anomalies that complicate surgical repair. Under these circumstances, a nonoperative approach can be used. The omphalocele sac can be treated with desiccating substances such as Silvadene. It typically takes two to three months before re-epithelialization occurs. In the past, mercury compounds were used, but they have been discontinued because of associated systemic toxicity.

Gastroschisis

Presentation

Gastroschisis represents a congenital defect characterized by a defect in the anterior abdominal wall through which the intestinal contents freely protrude. Unlike the omphalocele, there is no overlying sac and the size of the defect is much smaller (< 4 cm). The abdominal wall defect is located at the junction of the umbilicus and normal skin, and is almost always to the right of the umbilicus. The umbilicus becomes partly detached, allowing free communication with the abdominal cavity. The appearance of the bowel provides some information with respect to the in utero timing of the defect. The intestine may be normal in appearance, suggesting that the rupture occurred relatively late during the pregnancy. More commonly however, the intestine is thick, edematous, discolored, and covered with exudate, implying a more longstanding process.

Unlike infants born with omphalocele, associated anomalies seen with gastroschisis consist mostly of intestinal atresia. This defect can readily be diagnosed on prenatal ultrasound. There is no advantage in performing a cesarian section over a vaginal delivery. Even though the thickness of the peel on the surface of the bowel indicates that a shorter gestational time would be less injurious, there is no benefit to early versus late delivery.

Treatment

All infants born with gastroschisis require urgent surgical treatment. In many instances, the intestine can be returned to the abdominal cavity, and a primary surgical closure of the abdominal wall is performed. Techniques that facilitate primary closure include mechanical stretching of the abdominal wall, thorough orogastric suctioning with foregut decompression, rectal irrigation and evacuation of all the meconium. Care must be taken to prevent increased abdominal pressure during the reduction, which would lead to compression of the inferior vena cava, respiratory embarrassment and result in abdominal compartment syndrome. To avoid this complication, it is helpful to monitor the bladder or airway pressure during reduction. In infants whose intestine has become thickened and edematous, it may be impossible to reduce the bowel into the peritoneal cavity in the immediate post natal period. Under such circumstances, a plastic spring-loaded silo can be placed onto the bowel and secured beneath the fascia. The silo covers the bowel and allows for graduated reduction on a daily basis as the edema in the bowel wall decreases. Surgical closure can usually be accomplished within approximately one week. A prosthetic piece of material (Gore-Tex, Surgisis) may be required to bring the edges of the fascia together. If an atresia is noted at the time of closure, it is prudent to reduce the bowel at the first operation, then to return after several weeks once the edema has resolved, to correct the atresia. Intestinal function does not typically return for several weeks in patients with gastroschisis. This is especially true if the bowel is thickened and edematous. As a result, these patients will require central line placement and institution of total parenteral nutrition to grow.

Inguinal Hernia

An understanding of the management of pediatric inguinal hernias is a central component of modern pediatric surgical practice. Inguinal hernia repair represents one of the most common operations performed in children. The presence of an inguinal hernia in a child is an indication for surgical repair. The operation to perform an inguinal hernia is termed a herniorrhaphy because it involves closing the patent processus vaginalis. This is to be contrasted with the hernioplasty that is performed in adults, which requires a reconstruction of the inguinal floor.

Embryology

To understand how to diagnose and treat inguinal hernias in children, it is critical to understand the embryologic origin. It is very useful to describe these events to the parents, who often are under the misconception that the hernia was somehow caused by their inability to console their crying child, or the child's high activity level. Inguinal hernia results from a failure of closure of the processus vaginalis; a finger-like projection of the peritoneum that accompanies the testicle as it descends into the scrotum. Closure of the processus vaginalis normally occurs a few months prior to birth. This explains the high incidence of inguinal hernias in premature infants. When the processus vaginalis remains completely patent, a communication persists between the peritoneal cavity and the groin, resulting in a hernia. Partial closure can result in entrapped fluid, which results in the presence of a hydrocele. A communicating hydrocele refers to a hydrocele that is in communication with the peritoneal cavity, and can therefore be thought of as a hernia. Using the classification system that is typically applied to adult hernias, all congenital hernias in children are by definition indirect inguinal hernias. Children also present with direct inguinal and femoral hernias, although these are much less common.

Clinical Manifestation

Inguinal hernias occur more commonly in males than females (10:1), and are more common on the right side than the left. Infants are at high risk for incarceration of an inguinal hernia because of the narrow inguinal ring. Patients most commonly present with a groin bulge that is noticed by the parents as they change the diaper. Older children may notice the bulge themselves. On examination, the cord on the affected side will be thicker, and pressure on the lower abdomen usually will display the hernia on the affected side. The presence of an incarcerated hernia is manifested by a firm bulge that does not spontaneously resolve, and may be associated with fussiness and irritability in the child. The infant that has a strangulated inguinal hernia will manifest an edematous, tender bulge in the groin, occasionally with overlying skin changes. The child will eventually develop intestinal obstruction, peritonitis and systemic toxicity.

Usually an incarcerated hernia can be reduced. Occasionally this may require light sedation. Gentle pressure is applied on the sac from below in the direction of the internal inguinal ring. Following reduction of the incarcerated hernia, the child may be admitted for observation, and herniorrhaphy is performed within the next 24 h to prevent recurrent incarceration. Alternatively, the child may be scheduled for surgery at the next available time slot. If the hernia cannot be reduced, or if evidence of strangulation is present, emergency operation is necessary. This may require a laparotomy and bowel resection.

When the diagnosis of inguinal hernia is made in an otherwise normal child, operative repair should be planned. Spontaneous resolution does not occur and therefore a nonoperative approach can not be ever justified. An inguinal hernia in a female frequently contains an ovary rather than intestine. Although the gonad usually can be reduced into the abdomen by gentle pressure, it often prolapses in and out until surgical repair is carried out. In some patients, the ovary and fallopian tube constitute one wall of the hernia sac (sliding hernia), and in these patients the ovary can be reduced effectively only at the time of operation. If the ovary is irreducible, prompt hernia repair is indicated to prevent ovarian torsion or strangulation.

When a hydrocele is diagnosed in infancy and there is no evidence of a hernia, observation is proper therapy until the child is older than 12 months. If the hydrocele has not disappeared by 12 months, invariably there is a patent processus vaginalis, and hydrocelectomy with excision of the processus vaginalis is indicated. When the first signs of a hydrocele are seen after 12 months of age, the patient should undergo elective hydrocelectomy, which in a child is always performed through a groin incision. Aspiration of hydroceles is discouraged, because almost all without a patent processus vaginalis will resorb spontaneously, and those with a communication to the peritoneum will recur and require operative repair eventually.

Surgical Repair

The repair of a pediatric inguinal hernia can be extremely challenging, particularly in the premature child with incarceration. A small incision is made in a skin crease in the groin directly over the internal inguinal ring. The Scarpa fascia is seen and divided. The external oblique muscle is dissected free from overlying tissue, and the location of the external ring is confirmed. The external oblique aponeurosis is then opened along the direction of the external ring. The undersurface of the external oblique is then cleared from surrounding tissue. The cremasteric fibers are separated from the cord structures and hernia sac, and these are then elevated into the wound. Care is taken not to grasp the vas deferens. The hernia sac is then dissected up to the internal ring and doubly suture ligated. The distal part of the hernia sac is opened widely to drain any hydrocele fluid. When the hernia is very large and the patient very small, tightening of the internal inguinal ring or even formal repair of the inguinal floor may be necessary, although the vast majority of children do not require any treatment beyond high ligation of the hernia sac.

Controversy exists regarding the role for exploration of an asymptomatic opposite side in a child with an inguinal hernia. Several reports indicate that frequency of a patent processus vaginalis on the side opposite the obvious hernia is approximately 30 percent, although this figure decreases with increasing age of the child. Management options include never exploring the opposite side, to exploring only under certain conditions such as in premature infants or in patients in whom incarceration is present. The opposite side may be explored laparoscopically. To do so, a blunt 4-mm trocar is placed into the hernia sac of the affected side. The abdominal cavity is insufflated, and the 4-mm, 70-degree camera is placed through the trocar such that the opposite side is visualized. The status of the processus vaginalis on the opposite side can be visualized. However, the presence of a patent processus vaginalis by laparoscopy does not always imply the presence of a hernia.

Several authors have now reported a completely laparoscopic approach in the management of inguinal hernias in children. This technique requires insufflation through the umbilicus, and the placement of an extraperitoneal suture to ligate the hernia sac. Proponents of this procedure emphasize the fact that no groin incision is used and there is a decreased chance of injuring cord structures. The long term results of this technique remain to be established.

Inguinal hernias in children recur in less than 1 percent of patients, and recurrences usually result from missed hernia sacs at the first procedure, a direct hernia, or a missed femoral hernia. All children should have local anesthetic administered either by caudal injection or by direct injection into the wound. Spinal anesthesia in preterm infants decreases the risk of postoperative apnea when compared with general anesthesia.

GENITALIA

Undescended Testis

Embryology

The term undescended testicle (cryptorchidism) refers to the interruption of the normal descent of the testis into the scrotum. The testicle may reside in the retroperineum, in the internal inguinal ring, in the inguinal canal, or even at the external ring. The testicle begins as a thickening on the urogenital ridge in the fifth to sixth week of embryologic life. In the seventh and eighth months the testicle descends along the inguinal canal into the upper scrotum, and with its progress the processus vaginalis is formed and pulled along with the migrating testicle. At birth, approximately 95 percent of infants have the testicle normally positioned in the scrotum.

A distinction should be made between the undescended testicle and the ectopic testicle. An ectopic testis, by definition, is one that has passed through the external ring in the normal pathway and then has come to rest in an abnormal location overlying either the rectus abdominis or external oblique muscle, or the soft tissue of the medial thigh, or behind the scrotum in the perineum. A congenitally absent testicle results from failure of normal development or an intrauterine accident leading to loss of blood supply to the developing testicle.

Clinical Presentation

The incidence of undescended testes is approximately 30 percent in preterm infants and 1–3 percent at term. For diagnosis, the child should be examined in the supine position, where visual inspection may reveal a hypoplastic or poorly rugated scrotum. Usually a unilateral undescended testicle can be palpated in the inguinal canal or in the upper scrotum. Occasionally, the testicle will be difficult or impossible to palpate, indicating either an abdominal testicle or congenital absence of the gonad. If the testicle is not palpable in the supine position, the child should be examined with his legs crossed while seated. This maneuver diminishes the cremasteric reflex and facilitates identification of the location of the testicle.

It is now established that cryptorchid testes demonstrate an increased predisposition to malignant degeneration. Additionally, fertility is decreased when the testicle is not in the scrotum. For these reasons, surgical placement of the testicle in the scrotum (orchidopexy) is indicated. It should be emphasized that this procedure does improve the fertility potential, although it is never normal. Similarly, the testicle is still at risk of malignant change, although its location in the scrotum facilitates potentially earlier detection of a testicular malignancy. Other reasons to consider orchidopexy include the risk of trauma to the testicle located at the pubic tubercle, and increased incidence of torsion, and the psychological impact of an empty scrotum in a developing male. The reason for malignant degeneration is not established, but the evidence points to an inherent abnormality of the testicle that predisposes it to incomplete descent and malignancy rather than malignancy as a result of an abnormal environment.

Treatment

Males with bilateral undescended testicles are often infertile. When the testicle is not within the scrotum, it is subjected to a higher temperature, resulting in decreased spermatogenesis. Mengel and coworkers studied 515 undescended testicles by histology and demonstrated a decreasing presence of spermatogonia after 2 years of age. Consequently it is now recommended that the undescended testicle be surgically repositioned by 2 years of age at the latest. Despite orchidopexy, the incidence of infertility is approximately two times higher in men with unilateral orchidopexy compared to men with normal testicular descent.

The use of chorionic gonadotropin occasionally may be effective in patients with bilateral undescended testes, suggesting that these patients are more apt to have a hormone insufficiency than children with unilateral undescended testicle. If there is no testicular descent after a month of endocrine therapy, operative correction should be undertaken. A child with unilateral cryptorchidism should have surgical correction of the problem. The operation is typically performed through a combined groin and scrotal incision. The cord vessels are fully mobilized, and the testicle is placed in a dartos pouch within the scrotum. An inguinal hernia often accompanies a cryptorchid testis. This should be repaired at the time of orchidopexy.

Patients with a nonpalpable testicle present a challenge in management. The current approach involves laparoscopy to identify the location of the testicle. If the spermatic cord is found to traverse the internal ring or the testis is found at the ring and can be delivered into the scrotum, a groin incision is made and an orchidopexy is performed. If an abdominal testis is identified which is too far to reach the scrotum, a two staged Fowler-Stephens approach is used. In the first stage, the testicular vessels are clipped laparoscopically. The orchidopexy is then performed through the groin approximately 6 months later, after which time collateral flow supplies the testicle. It is preferable to preserve the testicular vessels whenever possible. When the testicle is within one or two centimeters from the ring, its blood supply may be preserved by mobilizing the testicular vessels up to the renal hilum, then releasing the peritoneal attachments. This often provides sufficient length to allow an orchidopexy to be performed through the groin.

Some patients who have an absent testis are greatly bothered by this anatomic deficiency. Prostheses of all sizes are now available and can be simply inserted into the scrotum, achieving normal appearance and a normal structure for palpation. Any patient who has an undescended testicle corrected surgically should be examined yearly by the surgeon until his mid-teen years. At that time, the individual should undergo thorough explanation about the possibility of malignant degeneration and be instructed in self-examination, which should be carried out at least twice a year for life.

Ovarian Cysts and Tumors

Pathologic Classification

Ovarian cysts and tumors may be classified as nonneoplastic or neoplastic. Nonneoplastic lesions include cysts (simple, follicular, inclusion, paraovarian, or corpus luteum), endometriosis, and inflammatory lesions. Neoplastic lesions are classified based on the three primordia that contribute to the ovary: mesenchymal components of the urogenital ridge; germinal epithelium overlying the urogenital ridge; and germ cells migrating from the yolk sac. The most common variety is germ cell tumors. Germ cell tumors are classified based on the degree of differentiation and the cellular components involved. The least differentiated tumors are the dysgerminomas, which share features similar to the seminoma in males. Although these are malignant tumors, they are extremely sensitive to radiation and chemotherapy. The most common lesions are the teratomas, which may be mature, immature, or malignant. The degree of differentiation of the neural elements of the tumor determines the degree of immaturity. The sex cord stromal tumors arise from the mesenchymal components of the urogenital ridge. These include the granulose-theca cell tumors and the Sertoli-Leydig cell tumors. These tumors often produce hormones that result in precocious puberty or hirsutism respectively. Although rare, epithelial tumors do occur in children. These include serous and mucinous cystadenomas.

Clinical Presentation

Children with ovarian lesions usually present with abdominal pain. Other signs and symptoms include a palpable abdominal mass, evidence of urinary obstruction, symptoms of bowel obstruction, and endocrine imbalance. The surgical approach depends on the appearance of the mass at operation, i.e., whether it is benign-appearing or is suspicious for malignancy. In the case of a simple ovarian cyst, surgery depends on the size of the cyst and the degree of symptoms it causes. In general, large cysts (over 4–5 cm) in size should be resected, as they are unlikely to resolve, may be at risk of torsion, and may mask an underlying malignancy. Resection may be performed laparoscopically, and ovarian tissue should be spared in all cases.

Surgical Management

For ovarian lesions that appear malignant, it is important to obtain tumor markers including alpha fetoprotein (teratomas), LDH (dysgerminoma), beta human chorionic gonadotropin (choriocarcinoma) and CA-125 (epithelial tumors). Although the diagnostic sensitivity of these markers is not always reliable, they provide material for postoperative follow up and indicate the response to therapy. When a malignancy is suspected, the patient should undergo a formal cancer operation. This procedure is performed through either a midline incision or a Pfannenstiel approach. Ascites and peritoneal washings should be collected for cytologic study. The liver and diaphragm are inspected carefully for metastatic disease. An omentectomy is performed if there is any evidence of tumor present. Pelvic and paraaortic lymph nodes are biopsied and the primary tumor is resected completely. Finally, the contralateral ovary is carefully inspected and if a lesion is seen it should be biopsied. Dysgerminomas and epithelial tumors may be bilateral in up to 15 percent of cases. It is occasionally possible to preserve the ipsilateral fallopian tube. More radical procedures are not indicated.

Ovarian Cysts in the Newborn

An increasing number of ovarian cysts are being detected by prenatal ultrasound. In the past, surgical excision was recommended for all cysts greater than 5 cm in diameter because of the perceived risk of ovarian torsion. More recently, it has become apparent from serial ultrasound examinations that many of these lesions will resolve spontaneously. Therefore, asymptomatic, simple cysts may be observed, and surgery can be performed only when they fail to decrease in size or become symptomatic. Typically, resolution occurs by approximately 6 months of age. A laparoscopic approach may be used. By contrast, complex cysts of any size require surgical intervention at presentation.

PEDIATRIC MALIGNANCY

Cancer is the second leading cause of death in children after trauma, and accounts for approximately 11 percent of all pediatric deaths in the United States. Several features distinguish pediatric from adult cancers, including the presence of tumors that are predominantly seen in children, such as neuroblastoma and germ cell tumors, and the favorable response to chemotherapy observed for many pediatric solid malignancies, even in the presence of metastases.

Wilms Tumor

Clinical Presentation

Wilms tumor is the most common primary malignant tumor of the kidney in children. There are approximately 500 new cases annually in the United States, and most are diagnosed between 1 and 5 years of age, with the peak incidence at age 3 years. Advances in the care of patients with Wilms tumor have resulted in an overall cure rate of roughly 90 percent, even in the presence of metastatic spread. The tumor usually develops in otherwise healthy children as an asymptomatic mass in the flank or upper abdomen. Frequently, the mass is discovered by a parent while bathing or dressing the child. Other symptoms include hypertension, hematuria, obstipation or weight loss. Occasionally the mass is discovered following blunt abdominal trauma.

Genetics of Wilms tumor. Wilms tumor can arise from both germline and somatic mutations, and can occur in the presence or absence of a family history. Nearly 97 percent of Wilms tumors are sporadic in that they occur in the absence of a heritable or congenital cause or risk factor. When a heritable risk factor is identified, the affected children often present at an earlier age, and are frequently bilateral. Most of these tumors are associated with germline mutations. It is well established that there is a genetic predisposition to Wilms tumor in the WAGR syndrome, which consists of Wilms tumor, aniridia, genitourinary abnormalities, and mental retardation. Additionally, there is an increased incidence of Wilms tumor in certain overgrowth conditions, particularly Beckwith–Wiedemann syndrome and hemi-hypertrophy. The WAGR syndrome has been shown to result from the deletion of one copy each of the Wilms tumor gene, WT1 and the adjacent aniridia gene, PAX6 on chromosome 11p13. Beckwith–Wiedemann syndrome is an overgrowth syndrome that is characterized by visceromegaly, macroglossia and hyperinsulinemic hypoglycemia. It arises from mutations at the 11p15.5 locus. There is evidence to suggest that analysis of the methylation status of several genes in the 11p15 locus could predict the individual risk to the development of Wilms tumor. Importantly, most patients with Wilms tumor do not have mutations at these genetic loci.

Surgical treatment. Before operation, all patients suspected of Wilms tumor should undergo abdominal and chest CT. These studies characterize the mass, identify the presence of metastases, and provide information on the opposite kidney. CT scanning also indicates the presence of nephrogenic rests, which are precursor lesions to Wilms tumor. An abdominal ultrasound should be performed to demonstrate the presence of renal vein or vena caval extension.

The management of patients with Wilms tumor has been carefully evaluated within the context of large studies involving thousands of patients. These studies have been coordinated by the National Wilms' Tumor Study Group (NWTSG) in North America and the International Society of Pediatric Oncology (SIOP), mainly involving European countries. Significant differences in the approach to patients that present with Wilms tumor have been highlighted by these studies. NWTSG supports a strategy of surgery followed by chemotherapy in most instances, whereas the SIOP approach is to shrink the tumor using preoperative chemotherapy. There are instances where preoperative chemotherapy is supported by both groups, including the presence of bilateral involvement or inferior vena cava involvement that extends above the hepatic veins and involvement of a solitary kidney by Wilms tumor. The NWTSG proponents argue that preoperative therapy in other instances results in a loss of important staging information, and therefore places patients at higher risk for recurrence, alternatively it may lead to overly aggressive treatment in some cases. However, the overall survival rates are not different between the NWTSG and SIOP approaches.

The goals of surgery include complete removal of the tumor. It is crucial to avoid tumor rupture or injury to contiguous organs. A sampling of regional lymph nodes should be included and all suspicious nodes should be sampled. Typically a transverse abdominal incision is made, and a transperitoneal approach is used. The opposite side is carefully inspected to ensure that there is no disease present. A radical nephroureterectomy is then performed with control of the renal pedicle as an initial step. If there is spread above the hepatic veins, an intrathoracic approach may be required. If bilateral disease is encountered, both lesions are biopsied, and chemotherapy is administered followed by a nephron-sparing procedure.

Neuroblastoma

Clinical presentation. Neuroblastoma is the third most common pediatric malignancy, and accounts for approximately 10 percent of all childhood cancers. The vast majority of patients have advanced disease at the time of presentation, and unlike Wilms tumor, the overall survival is less than 30 percent. Over 80 percent of cases present before the age of 4 years, and the peak incidence is 2 years of age. Neuroblastomas arise from the neural crest cells and show different levels of differentiation. The tumor originates most frequently in the adrenal glands, posterior mediastinum, neck, or pelvis but can arise in any sympathetic ganglion. The clinical presentation depends on the site of the primary and the presence of metastasis.

Two-thirds of these tumors are first noted as an asymptomatic abdominal mass. The tumor may cross the midline, and a majority of patients will already show signs of metastatic disease. Occasionally, children may present with pain from the tumor mass or to bone pain from metastases. Proptosis and periorbital ecchymosis may occur because of the presence of retrobulbar metastasis. Because they originate in paraspinal ganglia, neuroblastomas may invade through neural foramina and compress the spinal cord, causing muscle weakness or sensory changes. Rarely, children may have severe watery diarrhea because of the secretion of vasoactive intestinal peptide by the tumor, or with paraneoplastic neurologic findings including cerebellar ataxia or opsoclonus/myoclonus.

Diagnostic Evaluation

Because these tumors derive from the sympathetic nervous system, catecholamines and their metabolites will be produced at increased levels. These include elevated levels of serum catecholamines (dopamine, norepinephrine) or urine catecholamine metabolites: vanillylmandelic acid (VMA) or homovanillic acid (HVA). Measurement of VMA and HVMA in serum and urine aids in the diagnosis and in monitoring adequacy of future treatment and recurrence. The minimum criterion for a diagnosis of neuroblastoma is based on 1 of the following: (1) An unequivocal pathologic diagnosis made from tumor tissue by light microscopy (with or without immunohistology, electron microscopy, or increased levels of serum catecholamines or urinary catecholamine metabolites); (2) The combination of bone marrow aspirate or biopsy containing unequivocal tumor cells and increased levels of serum catecholamines or urinary catecholamine metabolites as described above.

The patient should be evaluated by abdominal computerized tomography, which usually shows displacement and occasionally obstruction of the ureter of an intact kidney. Prior to the institution of therapy, a complete staging work-up should be performed. This includes radiograph of the chest, bone marrow biopsy, and radionuclide scans to search for metastases. Any abnormalities on chest radiograph should be followed up with computerized tomography of the chest.

Prognostic Indicators

A number of biologic variables have been studied in children with neuroblastoma. An open biopsy is required to obtain sufficient tissue for this analysis. Hyperdiploid tumor DNA is associated with a favorable prognosis, and N-myc amplification is associated with a poor prognosis regardless of patient age. The Shimada classification describes tumors as either favorable or unfavorable histology based on the degree of differentiation, the mitosis-karyorrhexis index, and the presence or absence of schwannian stroma. In general, children of any age with localized neuroblastoma and infants younger than 1 year of age with advanced disease and favorable disease characteristics have a high likelihood of disease free survival. By contrast, older children with advanced-stage disease, have a significantly decreased chance for cure despite intensive therapy. For example, aggressive multiagent chemotherapy has resulted in a 2-year survival rate of approximately 20 percent in older children with stage IV disease. Neuroblastoma in the adolescent has a worse long-term prognosis regardless of stage or site and, in many cases, a more prolonged course.

Surgery

The goal of surgery is complete resection. However, this is often not possible because of the extensive locoregional spread of the tumor at the time of presentation. Under these circumstances, a biopsy is performed and preoperative chemotherapy is provided based on the stage of the tumor. After neoadjuvant treatment has been administered, surgical resection is performed. The principal goal of surgery is to obtain at least a 95 percent resection, without compromising major structures. Abdominal tumors are approached through a transverse incision. Thoracic tumors may be approached through a posterolateral thoracotomy or through a thoracoscopic approach. These may have an intraspinal component.

Neuroblastoma in Infants

Spontaneous regression of neuroblastoma has been well described in infants, especially in those with Stage 4S disease. Regression generally occurs only in tumors with a near triploid number of chromosomes that also lack N-myc amplification and loss of chromosome 1p. Recent studies indicate that infants with asymptomatic, small, low-stage neuroblastoma detected by screening, may have tumors that spontaneously regress. These patients may be observed safely without surgical intervention or tissue diagnosis.

TRAUMA IN CHILDREN

Injury is the leading cause of death among children older than 1 year. In fact, trauma accounts for almost half of all pediatric deaths; more than cancer, congenital anomalies, pneumonia, heart disease, homicide, and meningitis combined. Death from unintentional injury accounts for 65 percent of all injury deaths in children younger than 19 years. From 1972–1992, motor vehicle collisions were the leading cause of death in people aged 1–19 years, followed by homicide or suicide (predominantly with firearms) and drowning. Each year, approximately 20,000 children and teenagers die as a result of injury in the United States. For every child who dies from an injury, it is calculated that 40 others are hospitalized and 1120 are treated in emergency departments. An estimated 50,000 children acquire permanent disabilities each year, most of whom are the result of head injuries. Thus, pediatric trauma continues to be one of the major threats to the health and well-being of children.

Specific considerations apply to trauma in children that influence management and outcome. These relate to the mechanisms of injury, the anatomic variations in children compared to adults and the physiologic responses.

Mechanisms of Injury

Most pediatric trauma is blunt. Penetrating injuries are seen in the setting of gun violence, falls onto sharp objects, or penetration by glass after falling through windows. Age and gender significantly influence the patterns of injury. Male children younger than 18 years are exposed to contact sports and drive motor vehicles. As a result, they have a different pattern of injury than younger children, characterized by higher injury severity scores. In the infant and toddler age group, falls are a common cause of severe injury. Injuries in the home are extremely common. These include falls, near-drownings, caustic ingestion and nonaccidental injuries.

Initial Management

The goals of managing the pediatric trauma patient are similar to that of adults, and follow Advanced Trauma Life Support guidelines as established by the American College of Surgeons. Airway control is the first priority. In a child, respiratory arrest can proceed quickly to a cardiac arrest. It is important to be aware of the anatomic differences between the airway of the child and the adult. The child has a shorter neck, smaller and anterior larynx, floppy epiglottis, short trachea, and large tongue. The child's fifth digit can provide an estimate of the size of the endotracheal tube. Alternatively, the formula (age + 16)/4 may be used. It is preferable to use uncuffed endotracheal tubes in children younger than 8 years to minimize tracheal trauma. After evaluation of the airway, breathing is assessed. It is important to consider that gastric distention from aerophagia can severely compromise respirations. A nasogastric tube should therefore be placed early in the resuscitation. Pneumothorax or hemothorax should be treated promptly. When evaluating the circulation, it is important to recognize that tachycardia is usually the earliest measurable response to hypovolemia. Other signs of impending hypovolemic shock in children include changes in mentation, delayed capillary refill, skin pallor, and hypothermia. Intravenous access should be rapidly obtained once the patient arrives in the trauma bay. The first approach should be to use the antecubital fossae. If this is not possible, a cut-down onto the saphenous at the groin can be performed quickly and safely. Intraosseous cannulation can provide temporary access in infants until intravenous access is established. Percutaneous neck lines should be generally avoided. Blood is drawn for cross-match and evaluation of liver enzymes, lipase, amylase and hematologic profile after the intravenous lines are placed.

In patients who show signs of volume depletion, a 20 mL/kg bolus of saline or lactated Ringer should be promptly given. If the patient does not respond to three boluses, blood should be transfused (10 mL/kg). The source of bleeding should be established. Common sites include the chest, abdomen, pelvis, extremity fractures or large scalp wounds. These should be carefully sought. Care is taken to avoid hypothermia, by infusing warmed fluids and by using external warming devices.

Evaluation of Injury

All patients should receive a radiograph of the c-spine, chest, and abdomen with pelvis. All extremities that are suspicious for fracture should also be evaluated by radiograph. Screening blood work that includes AST, ALT, and amylase/lipase is useful for the evaluation of liver and pancreatic injures. Significant elevation in these tests require further evaluation by CT scanning. The child with significant abdominal tenderness and a mechanism of injury that could cause intraabdominal injury should undergo abdominal CT scanning using intravenous and oral contrast in all cases. There is a limited role for diagnostic peritoneal lavage (DPL) in children as a screening test. However, this can be very useful in the child that is brought emergently to the operating room for management of significant intracranial hemorrhage. At the time of craniotomy, a DPL can be performed concurrently, to identify abdominal bleeding. Although abdominal ultrasound is extremely useful in the evaluation of adult abdominal trauma, it has not been widely accepted in the management of pediatric injury. In part this relates to the widespread use of nonoperative treatment for most solid-organ injuries, which would result in a positive abdominal ultrasound scan.

Thoracic Injuries

The pediatric thorax is pliable because of incomplete calcification of the ribs and cartilages. As a result, blunt chest injury commonly results in pulmonary contusion, although rib fractures are infrequent. Diagnosis is made by chest radiograph and may be associated with severe hypoxia requiring mechanical ventilation. Pulmonary contusion usually resolves with careful ventilator management and judicious volume resuscitation. Children who have sustained massive blunt thoracic injury may develop traumatic asphyxia. This is characterized by cervical and facial petechial hemorrhages or cyanosis associated with vascular engorgement and subconjunctival hemorrhage. Management includes ventilation and treatment of coexisting central nervous system (CNS) or abdominal injuries. Penetrating thoracic injuries may result in damage to the lung, or to major disruption of the bronchi or great vessels.

Abdominal Injuries

In children, the small rib cage and minimal muscular coverage of the abdomen can result in significant injury after seemingly minor trauma. The liver and spleen in particular are relatively unprotected, and are often injured after direct abdominal trauma. Duodenal injuries are usually the result of blunt trauma, which may arise from child abuse or injury from a bicycle handlebar. Duodenal hematomas usually resolve without surgery. Small intestinal injury usually occurs in the jejunum in the area of fixation by the ligament of Treitz. These injuries are usually caused by rapid deceleration in the setting of a lap belt. There may be a hematoma on the anterior abdominal wall caused by a lap belt, the so-called "seat belt sign." This finding should alert the caregiver to the possibility of an underlying small bowel injury, and a lumbar spine fracture (Chance fracture).

The spleen is injured relatively commonly after blunt abdominal trauma in children. The extent of injury to the spleen is graded, and the management is governed by the injury grade. Current treatment involves a nonoperative approach in most cases, even for grade 4 injuries, provided that the patient is hemodynamically stable. This approach avoids surgery in most cases. All patients should be placed in a monitored unit, and type specific blood should be available for transfusion. When nonoperative management is successful, as it is in most cases, an extended period of bed rest is prescribed. This optimizes the chance for healing, and minimizes the likelihood of re-injury. A typical guideline is to keep the children on restricted activity for two weeks longer than the grade of spleen injury (i.e., a child with a grade 4 spleen injury receives 6 weeks of restricted activity). In children that have an ongoing fluid requirement, or when a blood transfusion is required, exploration should not be delayed. At surgery, the spleen can often be salvaged. If a splenectomy is performed, prophylactic antibiotics and immunizations should be administered to protect against overwhelming postsplenectomy sepsis. The liver is also commonly injured after blunt abdominal trauma. A grading system is used to characterize hepatic injuries, and nonoperative management is usually successful. Recent data have shown that associated injuries are more significant predictors of outcome in children with liver injuries rather than the actual injury grade. Criteria for surgery are similar to those for splenic injury, and primarily involve hemodynamic instability. The intraoperative considerations in the management of massive hepatic injury are similar in children and adults. Renal contusions may occur after significant blunt abdominal trauma. Nonoperative management is usually successful, unless patients are unstable because of active renal bleeding. It is important to confirm the presence of a normal contralateral kidney at the time of surgery.

Suggested Readings

Ahuja AT, King AD, et al: Thyroglossal duct cysts: sonographic appearances in adults. AJNR Am J Neuroradiol 20:579, 1999.

Andersen B, Kallehave F, et al: Antibiotics versus placebo for prevention of postoperative infection after appendicectomy. Cochrane Database Syst Rev 2:CD001439.

Azarow K, Messineo A, et al: Congenital diaphragmatic hernia—a tale of two cities: The Toronto experience. J Pediatr Surg 32:395, 1997.

Bohn D: Congenital diaphragmatic hernia. Am J Respir Crit Care Med 166:911, 2002.

Boloker J, Bateman DA, et al: Congenital diaphragmatic hernia in 120 infants treated consecutively with permissive hypercapnea/spontaneous respiration/elective repair. J Pediatr Surg 37:357, 2002.

Bratton S, Annich G: Packed red blood cell transfusions for critically ill pediatric patients: When and for what conditions? J Pediatr 142:95, 2003.

Cotterill SJ, Pearson ADJ, et al: Clinical prognostic factors in 1277 patients with neuroblastoma: Results of The European Neuroblastoma Study Group 'Survey' 1982-1992. Eur J Cancer 36:901, 2000.

Geisler DP, Jegathesan S, et al: Laparoscopic exploration for the clinically undetected hernia in infancy and childhood. Am J Surg 182:693, 2001.

Georgeson K: Laparoscopic-assisted pull-through for Hirschsprung's disease. Semin Pediatr Surg 11:205, 2002.

Gollin Ga, Abarbanell Aa, et al: Peritoneal drainage as definitive management of intestinal perforation in extremely low-birth-weight infants. J Pediatr Surg 38:1814, 2003.

Guthrie S, Gordon P, et al: Necrotizing enterocolitis among neonates in the United States. J Perinatol 23:278, 2003.

Hackam DJ, Superina R, et al: Single-stage repair of Hirschsprung's disease: A comparison of 109 patients over 5 years. J Pediatr Surg 32:1028, 1997.

Hackam DJ, Filler R, et al: Enterocolitis after the surgical treatment of Hirschsprung's disease: Risk factors and financial impact. J Pediatr Surg 33:830, 1998.

Hackam DJ, Reblock K, et al: The influence of Down's syndrome on the management and outcome of children with Hirschsprung's disease. J Pediatr Surg 38:946, 2003.

Hackam DJ, Potoka D, et al: Utility of radiographic hepatic injury grade in predicting outcome for children after blunt abdominal trauma. J Pediatr Surg 37:386, 2002.

Hirschl RB, Philip WF, et al: A prospective, randomized pilot trial of perfluorocarbon-induced lung growth in newborns with congenital diaphragmatic hernia. J Pediatr Surg 38:283, 2003.

Kalapurakal J, Li S, et al: Influence of radiation therapy delay on abdominal tumor recurrence in patients with favorable histology Wilms' tumor treated on NWTS-3 and NWTS-4: A report from the National Wilms' Tumor Study Group. Int J Radiat Oncol Biol Phys 57:495, 2003.

Kim HB, Lee PW, et al: Serial transverse enteroplasty for short bowel syndrome: A case report. J Pediatr Surg 38:881, 2003.

Konkin D, O'hali W, et al: Outcomes in esophageal atresia and tracheoesophageal fistula. J Pediatr Surg 38:1726, 2003.

Langer J, Durrant A, et al: One-stage transanal Soave pullthrough for Hirschsprung disease: A multicenter experience with 141 children. Ann Surg 238:569, 2003.

Levitt MA, Ferraraccio D, et al: Variability of inguinal hernia surgical technique: A survey of North American pediatric surgeons. J Pediatr Surg 37:745, 2002.

Lintula H, Kokki H, et al: Single-blind randomized clinical trial of laparoscopic versus open appendicectomy in children. Br J Surg 88:510, 2001.

Lipshutz G, Albanese C, et al: Prospective analysis of lung-to-head ratio predicts survival for patients with prenatally diagnosed congenital diaphragmatic hernia. J Pediatr Surg 32:1634, 1997.

Little D, Rescorla F, et al: Long-term analysis of children with esophageal atresia and tracheoesophageal fistula. 38:852, 2003.

Molik KA, West KW, et al: Portal venous air: The poor prognosis persists. J Pediatr Surg 36:1143, 2001.

Nadler E, Stanford A, et al: Intestinal cytokine gene expression in infants with acute necrotizing enterocolitis: Interleukin-11 mRNA expression inversely correlates with extent of disease. J Pediatr Surg 36:1122, 2001.

Pedersen A, Petersen O, et al: Randomized clinical trial of laparoscopic versus open appendicectomy. Br J Surg:200, 2001.

Potoka D, Schall L, et al: Improved functional outcome for severely injured children treated at pediatric trauma centers. J Trauma 51:824, 2001.

Potoka DA, Schall LC, et al: Risk factors for splenectomy in children with blunt splenic trauma. J Pediatr Surg 37:294, 2002.

Puapong D, Kahng D, et al: Ad libitum feeding: Safely improving the cost-effectiveness of pyloromyotomy. J Pediatr Surg 37:1667, 2002.

Rozmiarek AJ, Qureshi FG, Cassidy L, Ford HR, et al: How low can you go? Effectiveness and safety of extracorporeal membrane oxygenation in low-birth-weight neonates. J Pediatr Surg 39:845, 2004.

Rozmiarek AJ, Qureshi FG, Cassidy L, Ford HR, et al: Factors influencing survival in newborns with congenital diaphragmatic hernia: The relative role of timing of surgery. J Pediatr Surg 39:821, 2004.

Sandler A, Ein S, et al: Unsuccessful air-enema reduction of intussusception: is a second attempt worthwhile? Pediatr Surg Int 15:214, 1999.

Schier F, Montupet P, et al: Laparoscopic inguinal herniorrhaphy in children: A three-center experience with 933 repairs. J Pediatr Surg 37:395, 2002.

Shamberger R, Guthrie K, et al: Surgery-related factors and local recurrence of Wilms tumor in National Wilms Tumor Study 4. Ann Surg 229:292, 1999.

Shimada H, Ambros I, et al: The International Neuroblastoma Pathology Classification (the Shimada system). Cancer 86:364, 1999.

Teitelbaum D, Coran A: Reoperative surgery for Hirschsprung's disease. Semin Pediatr Surg 12:124, 2003.

Tolia V, Wureth A, et al: Gastroesophageal Reflux Disease: Review of Presenting Symptoms, Evaluation, Management, and Outcome in Infants. Digestive Diseases & Sciences 48:1723, 2003.

Wildhaber B, Coran A, et al: The Kasai portoenterostomy for biliary atresia: A review of a 27-year experience with 81 patients. J Pediatr Surg 38:1480, 2003.

Wilson J, Lund D, et al: Congenital diaphragmatic hernia—a tale of two cities: the Boston experience. J Pediatr Surg 32:401, 1997.

39 | Urology

Hyung L. Kim and Arie Belldegrun

ANATOMY

The Kidney and Ureter

The organs of the urinary system, which include the kidney, ureter, and bladder, are located in the retroperitoneum. The kidneys are paired organs surrounded by perirenal fat and the Gerota fascia. The superior aspect of the kidney is contained within the lower thoracic cavity at the level of the tenth rib.

The blood supply to the kidney comes from the renal artery. The right and left renal arteries come off the aorta just inferior to the takeoff of the superior mesenteric artery. The renal veins are anterior to the renal arteries and drain into the inferior vena cava. In the kidney, the arteries are end-arteries, although the veins anastomose freely. The left adrenal vein and left gonadal vein drain into the left renal vein, although on the right, these same vessels drain directly into the vena cava.

Adrenal Gland

The adrenal glands are endocrine organs that lie superomedial to the kidneys. They are surrounded by the perirenal fat and contained within the Gerota fascia. The right adrenal gland is positioned posterolateral to the inferior vena cava and tends to be more superior in relation to the left adrenal gland. The arterial blood supply to the adrenal glands is provided primarily by the inferior phrenic artery. On the right, the primary venous drainage is directly to the inferior vena cava. On the left, the primary venous drainage is to the left renal vein.

Bladder and Urethra

The bladder is a hollow, muscular organ adapted for storing and expelling urine. When it is empty, it lies posterior to the pubic symphysis in the pelvis and is extraperitoneal. The dome of the bladder is covered with peritoneum, and when the bladder is full, it can rise into the abdomen and is palpable on physical examination. The normal bladder can store approximately 350–450 mL. The arterial blood supply to the bladder comes from the superior, middle, and inferior vesical arteries, which are all branches of the internal iliac artery. The venous return from the bladder drains into the internal iliac vein.

Prostate and Seminal Vesicle

The prostate gland and the seminal vesicles are part of the male reproductive system. Secretions from these two organs make up part of the male semen. The prostate surrounds the proximal urethra. The gland can be divided into several zones. Most prostate cancers form in the peripheral zone. The central zone surrounds the ejaculatory ducts as they empty into the urethra at the verumontanum. Benign prostatic hyperplasia (BPH) is caused by enlargement of the transition zone surrounding the urethra. BPH, which is common in the older adult population, can lead to increased urinary resistance and voiding symptoms.

Testis

The volume of an average testis is approximately 20 mL. The testicles have two important functions: androgen and sperm production. The Leydig cells in the testis produce testosterone. The Sertoli cells support the maturation of spermatogenic cells into sperm. The Sertoli cells also are responsible for establishing a blood–testis barrier.

The testicles are surrounded by several fascial layers that are embryologically derived from the same layers comprising the anterior abdominal wall. The external spermatic fascia is analogous to the external oblique. The cremasteric muscle envelops the spermatic cord and is analogous to the internal oblique and transversus abdominis. The internal spermatic fascia is analogous to the transversalis fascia. The visceral and parietal layers of the tunica vaginalis testis represent peritoneum that surrounded the testicle during its descent into the scrotum.

The blood supply to the testicles is provided by three arteries: gonadal, cremasteric, and vasal. The gonadal artery branches directly from the aorta. The cremasteric artery branches from the inferior epigastric artery, and the vasal artery branches from the superior vesical artery. The venous drainage from the testicles forms the pampiniform plexus at the level of the spermatic cord. At the internal inguinal ring, the pampiniform plexus coalesces to form the gonadal vein, which drains into the inferior vena cava on the right and into the renal vein on the left.

Penis

The penis is formed by three corpora bodies: two corpora cavernosa and a corpus spongiosum. The corpus spongiosum surrounds the male urethra. The three corpora bodies are covered by the tunica albuginea. The common penile artery is the terminal branch of the internal pudendal artery. It divides into three branches that supply blood to the penis. Venous drainage from the penis is provided by the dorsal and cavernous veins, which join to form the internal pudendal vein. Sensory innervation is carried by the dorsal nerves that run with the dorsal vessels. Autonomic innervation is provided by the cavernous nerves that pierce the tunica albuginea to innervate the smooth muscles found in the corpora cavernosa.

SIGNS AND SYMPTOMS

Symptoms Related to Voiding

Symptoms related to voiding can be broadly categorized as irritative or obstructive. Specific irritative symptoms include dysuria, frequency, and urgency. These symptoms generally imply inflammation of the urethra, prostate, or bladder. Although irritative voiding symptoms are commonly caused by infection, they also can be caused by malignancy, and in patients with symptoms that persist after treatment with appropriate antibiotics, malignant processes such as transitional cell carcinoma must be ruled out.

Specific obstructive voiding symptoms include a weak urinary stream, urgency, frequency, hesitancy, intermittency, nocturia, and sense of incomplete emptying. The most common cause of obstructive voiding in men is benign prostatic hyperplasia. Urethral strictures may also obstruct the bladder outlet and often are secondary to trauma, urethritis, or previous instrumentation of the bladder.

Urinary Incontinence

Urinary incontinence can be categorized as stress, urge, total, and overflow. Stress incontinence refers to incontinence associated with an increase in intraabdominal pressure. Patients often report leakage of urine when coughing, laughing, or during physical exertion. Urge incontinence is secondary to an involuntary contraction of the bladder and is accompanied by a sudden sense of needing to void. Urge incontinence may be secondary to inflammation and irritation of the bladder, or it may result from neurologic disorders such as a stroke or spinal cord injury.

Total incontinence refers to a continuous leakage of urine and implies a fistula between the skin or vagina and the urinary tract, proximal to the sphincter mechanism. Overflow incontinence is secondary to an obstruction of the lower urinary tract. As urine builds up in the bladder, the intravesical pressure increases and overcomes the resistance provided by the urinary sphincter. All patients at risk for urinary tract obstruction who develop new-onset incontinence should be checked for urinary retention by postvoid bladder ultrasound or catheterization of the bladder.

Hematuria

Patients with gross or microscopic hematuria, in the absence of obvious evidence of a urinary tract infection, need to be evaluated with upper and lower tract studies. On microscopic examination of the urine, more than five red blood cells per high power field in spun urine or more than two red blood cells per high power field in unspun urine is considered significant microscopic hematuria. Because hematuria can be intermittent, even a single documented episode of significant microscopic hematuria warrants a complete evaluation. The upper tract, which includes the kidney and ureter, should be evaluated with an intravenous pyelogram, computed tomography (CT) scan, or retrograde pyelogram. The CT scan should be performed with intravenous contrast and delayed images should be obtained once the excreted contrast has filled the upper tract collecting system. The lower tract, which includes the bladder and urethra, should be evaluated by cystoscopy.

The differential diagnosis for hematuria includes malignancies, infections, kidney stones, and trauma. Malignancies of the kidney and bladder classically present with painless hematuria. Patients with gross painless hematuria should be considered to have a urinary tract malignancy until proven otherwise. Infections involving the bladder or urethra generally are associated with symptoms of irritative voiding. Pyelonephritis is a clinical diagnosis based on findings of irritative voiding symptoms, fever, and flank pain. Kidney stones are associated with a colicky pain. The localization of the pain depends on the level of obstruction by the stone. An obstruction at the ureteropelvic junction will cause flank pain while obstruction of the lower ureter can produce colicky pain referred to the lower abdomen or groin.

LABORATORY EXAMINATION

Examination of the Urine

The complete urinalysis includes testing with a dipstick impregnated with an array of chemical reagents and a microscopic examination of urinary sediments obtained by centrifugation. Most standard dipsticks will test for urinary pH, specific gravity, protein, glucose, ketones, bilirubin, urobilinogen, hemoglobin, leukocytes, and nitrites. Usually the urine pH will reflect the pH of the serum. Exceptions to this rule occur in patients with renal tubular acidosis or a urinary tract infection involving a urea-splitting organism.

The specific gravity of the urine reflects the hydration status of the patient and the concentrating ability of the kidney. Proteinuria detected on dipstick may indicate intrinsic renal pathology or the presence of excess protein in the serum. Persistent proteinuria determined using a dipstick should be confirmed by a 24-h urine collection for protein. Testing for urinary glucose and ketones is useful in screening for diabetes. Urinary glucose usually will be detected when serum glucose levels are greater than 180 mg/dL. A small amount of urobilinogen can normally be detected in the urine. However, a positive test for bilirubin and high levels of urobilinogen may indicate liver disease or hemolysis. Presence of hemoglobin, myoglobin, and red blood cells in the urine can produce a positive result on dipstick tests for blood. Therefore, a positive dipstick test should be confirmed by microscopy.

A positive urinalysis for leukocytes and nitrites suggests inflammation, which most commonly is caused by a bacterial infection. The dipstick tests for leukocyte esterase, which is an enzyme found in neutrophils. The urine may be positive for leukocytes in the presence of both hematuria and pyuria. Therefore, suspected pyuria should be confirmed by microscopic examination of the urine. Normal urine does not contain nitrites. However, in the presence of urea-splitting organisms, urinary nitrates are converted to nitrites, which can be detected by the dipstick test. Urea-splitting bacteria include the Proteus, Klebsiella, Pseudomonas, Enterococcus, and Morganella species. It should be noted that this list does not include Escherichia, which is the most common cause of urinary infections.

Urine Culture

It is important to keep in mind that the urinalysis results may be normal in patients with a urinary tract infection. A urine culture is the most definitive test for symptomatic patients. Greater than 105 organisms/mL of urine is consistent with a urinary tract infection. However, in patients who have irritative voiding symptoms, such as frequency and dysuria, 100 organisms/mL of a known urinary pathogen is sufficient evidence of a bacterial infection.

Tests of Kidney Function

Several simple tests can be used to estimate kidney function. Urine-specific gravity can be measured in the office by using a dipstick. As renal function decreases, the ability of the kidney to concentrate urine decreases. This is reflected by a proportional change in specific gravity. Serum creatinine level is a better approximation of kidney function. Creatinine is an end-product of muscle creatine metabolism and is excreted by the kidney. Serum creatinine levels are less affected by hydration status. However, creatinine does not reflect early loss of renal function, as serum creatinine levels remain in the normal range until approximately 50 percent of the kidney function is lost.

The best measure of kidney function that does not involve infusion of exogenous substances is the endogenous creatinine clearance rate. Creatinine clearance is defined as the volume of plasma from which creatinine is completely removed per unit of time and is a clinical approximation of the glomerular filtration rate (GFR) and renal function. Creatinine clearance is calculated from a 24-h urine collection according to the following formula:

$$\text{Clearance} = UV/P$$

In this formula, U and P represent the urine and plasma concentrations of creatinine, respectively, and V represents the urine flow rate. Normal creatinine clearance is 90–110 mL/min.

The gold standard for measuring GFR involves infusing and measuring the clearance of inulin. Inulin is an ideal substance for measuring GFR because it is completely filtered by the kidney without being secreted or reabsorbed by the tubules. In contrast, creatinine is secreted in small amounts by the proximal tubule. Therefore, creatinine clearance will slightly overestimate GFR at all levels of kidney function.

RADIOLOGIC STUDIES OF THE URINARY SYSTEM

Imaging of Kidney and Ureter

With recent improvements in CT technology, CT scans have become the study of choice for general imaging of the kidney and ureter. On a CT scan, kidney stones that are radiolucent on plain radiograph are readily visible. Uptake of contrast by the renal parenchyma during the nephrogram phase of the CT scan provides a rough estimate of the kidney function. After the contrast is excreted by the kidney into the collecting system, the collecting system can be evaluated for subtle filling defects and hydronephrosis.

CT scans are useful when renal or ureteral malignancy is suspected. When a CT scan is performed for evaluation of hematuria, the study should be performed with and without intravenous (IV) contrast, and delayed images should be obtained after the contrast has been excreted into the renal pelvis and ureter. Renal cell carcinomas classically appear as solid, enhancing masses. The degree of enhancement can be determined by comparing the images with and without contrast. Transitional cell tumors of the renal pelvis and ureter often present as filling defects on delayed images.

Although CT scan is the study of choice in most settings, an intravenous pyelogram (IVP) is a better test when the primary goal is to evaluate the collecting system. To obtain an IVP, radiologic contrast is infused and a series of plain radiographs are taken of the abdomen and pelvis. When an IVP is not diagnostic, or if the patient is allergic to IV contrast, a retrograde pyelogram can be performed. A magnetic resonance image (MRI) obtained with contrast medium such as gadolinium generally can be used in place of a CT scan when renal insufficiency or contrast allergy prohibits the use of CT contrast.

The least-invasive imaging modality for the kidney is a renal ultrasound. Many common renal pathologies have a characteristic appearance on ultrasound. Kidney stones are identified as a hyperechoic lesion associated with hypoechoic "shadowing" behind the stone. On ultrasound, fluid is hypoechoic, therefore renal cysts and hydronephrosis are readily identified. Renal masses appear as hyperechoic lesions and generally warrant further evaluation with a CT scan. In the pediatric population, a renal ultrasound is the first screening test obtained when a congenital abnormality of the urinary system is suspected.

Imaging of the Bladder and Urethra

A urethrogram should be performed when a urethral stricture or a traumatic urethral disruption is suspected. A Foley catheter is inserted just beyond the tip of the meatus and the catheter balloon is inflated with approximately 0.5 mL of fluid. Radiologic contrast is injected in a retrograde fashion and a plain radiograph is taken. Alternatively, the urethra is visualized during the injection using fluoroscopy.

An antegrade urethrogram also can be performed during a voiding cystourethrogram (VCUG). For a VCUG, a small-diameter catheter is inserted into the bladder and a cystogram is obtained. The patient is then asked to void the contrast and a urethrogram is taken. In the pediatric population, a VCUG is most commonly performed to rule out ureteral reflux or a posterior urethral valve.

Testicular Ultrasound

A testicular ultrasound most commonly is performed to evaluate testicular pain or a palpable lesion noted on physical examination. On Doppler ultrasound, the absence of blood flow is consistent with a testicular torsion, although increased blood flow suggests epididymal orchitis. Solid masses in the testicle or in the epididymis should be considered a malignancy until proven otherwise and an orchiectomy should be performed to make a definitive diagnosis.

Renal Scan

A renal scan is a nuclear medicine study used to determine renal function and evaluate drainage of the renal pelvis and ureter. An agent such as technetium-99m mercaptoacetyltriglycine (MAG-3) is administered intravenously, and is both filtered by the glomeruli and secreted by the tubules. Therefore, it is well suited for imaging the renal cortex, estimating differential renal function, and evaluating drainage of the renal pelvis.

BENIGN PROSTATIC HYPERPLASIA

Etiology

Benign prostatic hyperplasia (BPH) refers to the stromal and epithelial proliferation in the prostate gland that may eventually result in voiding symptoms. BPH occurs primarily in the transition zone of the prostate gland.

Natural History

Patients with BPH can present with both obstructive and irritative voiding symptoms, which often are referred to collectively as lower urinary tract symptoms (LUTS). Patients may complain of a decreased urinary stream, frequency, nocturia, urgency, hesitancy, intermittency, and a sense of incomplete emptying.

Medical Therapy

BPH is not always progressive. Patients with mild symptoms can be managed by watchful waiting. Patients with more severe symptoms should be treated based on the degree of bother. Absolute indications for treatment include urinary retention, bladder stones, upper tract dilation, and renal failure. Relative indications for treatment include large postvoid residuals, hematuria, and recurrent urinary tract infections.

The smooth muscles at the bladder outlet are under α_1-adrenergic innervation. The first line therapy for BPH is an α blocker. Tamsulosin is an example of a selective alpha blocker that targets the α_1a-adrenoceptor subtype, which is predominately found in the prostate. Patients in urinary retention require emergent catheterization and the catheter should be left in place for at least 24 h to allow the acutely distended bladder to remain decompressed.

Surgical Management

Surgery should be recommended for patients who continue to be bothered by their symptoms or who experience urinary retention despite medical therapy. Surgery also should be recommended for patients with upper tract dilation, renal insufficiency secondary to BPH, or bladder stones. Surgery for BPH most commonly is performed endoscopically; however, if the prostate gland is greater than 80–100 g, an open prostatectomy should be performed.

The standard endoscopic procedure for BPH is a transurethral resection (TUR) of the prostate. TUR is performed with a nonhemolytic fluid such as 1.5 percent glycine. Saline cannot be used because electrolytes in the irrigation fluid will dissipate the electric current used to resect the prostate. During the resection some of the irrigation fluid is absorbed through venous channels in the prostate. If enough fluid is absorbed, TUR syndrome may develop from the resulting hypervolemia and dilutional hyponatremia. Patients with TUR syndrome may experience hypertension, bradycardia, nausea, vomiting, visual disturbance, mental status changes, and even seizures. Patients with evidence of TUR syndrome should be treated with diuretics, and electrolyte imbalances should be corrected.

UROLOGIC ONCOLOGY

Renal Cell Carcinoma

Epidemiology

Each year more than 30,000 new cases of renal cell carcinoma are diagnosed in the United States, resulting in approximately 12,000 deaths. With the increased use of ultrasonography and CT scanning, incidental detection of early renal cell carcinoma has accounted, at least in part, for a 3 percent increase in incidence each year since the 1970s. However, the mortality rate for renal cell carcinoma also has been increasing, suggesting that other factors are involved. Currently, renal cell carcinoma represents approximately 3 percent of all malignancies. The male-to-female ratio is approximately 3:2. At the time of diagnosis, approximately one third of patients have metastatic disease.

Presentation and Prognosis

Before the widespread use of radiologic studies, patients often presented with advanced disease with findings of a palpable mass, flank pain, and hematuria. Today, most renal tumors are incidentally discovered on ultrasounds and CT scans performed for unrelated disorders. Patients with renal cell carcinoma also can present with paraneoplastic manifestations such as anemia, hepatic dysfunction (Stauffer syndrome), cachexia, polycythemia, and hypercalcemia. Paraneoplastic findings result from soluble substances released by the tumor or by immune cells in response to the tumor. Paraneoplastic findings resulting from localized disease resolve following a nephrectomy.

Work-Up

All patients with a history of gross or microscopic hematuria should undergo a cystoscopy and an upper tract imaging study such as a CT scan, MRI, or renal ultrasound. A solid, enhancing mass in the kidney has a 90 percent chance of being a renal cell carcinoma. Except in select cases, a renal biopsy is unnecessary. A renal biopsy is associated with a high false-negative rate because of potential sampling error and difficulty interpreting the pathology from a biopsy sample. Therefore, a negative or nondiagnostic biopsy does not obviate the need for surgical removal of the mass. A biopsy may be helpful in patients with a history of another primary malignancy or in patients with metastatic disease in whom the primary site is unknown. In these patients, a biopsy is performed to determine whether the renal mass is a primary tumor or a metastatic deposit.

A simple cyst in the kidney is a common, benign finding. However, a complex cyst may harbor a malignant tumor. Several features of a renal cyst are suggestive of a malignant component. These features include multiple septations, irregular cyst wall, calcifications, and wall or septations that enhance with IV contrast on CT or MRI.

The most common benign tumors in the kidney are oncocytomas and angiomyolipomas. Oncocytomas do not have a characteristic radiologic appearance and the diagnosis is made histologically following a nephrectomy. Angiomyolipomas are benign lesions common in patients with tuberous sclerosis. They have a characteristic appearance on CT scan, and nephrectomy is generally not necessary to confirm the diagnosis. Large angiomyolipomas, however, have a high risk of bleeding and embolization should be considered for lesions larger than 4 cm.

Several histologic subtypes of renal cell carcinoma have been defined. Approximately 80 percent of renal cell carcinomas are clear cell tumors and approximately 75 percent of sporadic clear cell tumors have a mutation of the von Hippel-Lindau (VHL) gene found on chromosome 3. The papillary subtype represents 10–15 percent of renal cell carcinomas and is associated with activation of the MET proto-oncogene or cytogenetic abnormalities involving chromosomes 7 and 17.

All patients with a renal mass should undergo a metastatic work-up that includes a check of serum electrolyte levels, liver function tests, chest radiograph, and imaging of the abdomen and pelvis with a CT scan or MRI. The CT scan or MRI should be performed with and without IV contrast. If there is any suspicion of renal vein or inferior vena cava involvement by a tumor thrombus, a vena cavagram or MR angiogram with coronal sections should be performed to evaluate the extent of caval involvement. Patients with metastatic lesions on imaging of the chest, abdomen, and pelvis should undergo a bone scan and a head CT as well.

Treatment

The standard treatment for localized renal cell carcinoma remains a radical nephrectomy. The classic radical nephrectomy involves removal of the kidney, the ipsilateral adrenal gland, and all the fat contained within the Gerota fascia. However, it has been shown that if there is no evidence of adrenal involvement by the tumor on the CT scan, the adrenal gland can be spared. A radical nephrectomy can be performed using either an open or a laparoscopic approach. The laparoscopic approach is associated with less postoperative pain and a more rapid return to normal activities.

Metastatic renal cell carcinoma is resistant to radiation and standard chemotherapies. There are several important principles to guide the treatment of metastatic disease. Any metastatic lesion to the central nervous system can become rapidly symptomatic and should be addressed by the radiation oncologist and neurosurgeon prior to initiating any further treatment. Patients with a relatively good prognosis, as determined by a good performance status and a limited number of metastatic sites, are candidates for a cytoreductive nephrectomy and interleukin-2 or interferon-based immunotherapy. The combination of neoadjuvant nephrectomy and immunotherapy represents the current standard of care for patients with metastatic renal cell carcinoma.

Bladder Cancer

Epidemiology

In the United States, approximately 56,000 new cases of bladder cancer are diagnosed each year, resulting in approximately 13,000 deaths. Bladder cancer represents 7 percent of all newly diagnosed cancers in men and 2 percent of all newly diagnosed cancers in women. The majority of patients with bladder cancer have superficial disease, which is associated with long-term survival. Therefore, there is a cohort of 300,000–400,000 patients with bladder cancer in the United States at all times.

In Western countries, more than 90 percent of bladder cancers are transitional cell carcinomas (TCCa), approximately 5 percent are squamous cell carcinomas, and less than 2 percent are adenocarcinomas. In the developing countries, 75 percent of bladder cancers are squamous cell carcinomas and most of these are secondary to Schistosoma haematobium infection. TCCa is strongly linked to environmental exposures. Smoking accounts for more than 50 percent of bladder cancers, and 2-naphthylamine and 4-aminobiphenyl are likely the most significant carcinogens found in cigarette smoke that lead to TCCa. The development of bladder cancer also has been associated with industrial exposure to aromatic amines in dyes, paints, solvents, leather dust, inks, combustion products, rubber, and textile. Prior radiation treatments to the pelvis and acrolein, a urinary metabolite of cyclophosphamide, increase the risk of bladder cancer.

Presentation

The classic presentation of bladder cancer is painless hematuria. Eighty-five percent of patients with bladder cancer present with hematuria. Hematuria, whether gross or microscopic, requires a urologic evaluation. Microscopic hematuria as a result of bladder cancer may be intermittent, therefore, bladder cancer cannot be ruled out with a repeat negative urinalysis. Persistent, irritative voiding symptoms may be a result of carcinoma in situ (CIS) or muscle-invasive bladder cancer. Therefore, irritative voiding symptoms that do not resolve with treatment for a urinary tract infection require further evaluation. A urologic work-up for hematuria includes cystoscopy and radiographic imaging of the upper urinary tract as previously discussed.

Work-Up

At the time of clinic cystoscopy, a bladder wash for cytology can be sent. Bladder cytology is 95 percent accurate for diagnosing high-grade tumors and CIS, however, its accuracy for diagnosing low-grade carcinoma is only 10–50 percent. Newer assays for the detection and surveillance of TCCa in voided urine include the BTA-Stat, NMP-22, and FDP tests. However, because of high false-positive rates and high false-negative rates, it is unlikely that these tests will obviate the need for cystoscopy. Patients with an abnormal cystoscopic exam or suspicious bladder wash cytology should be further evaluated with an operating room cystoscopy. In the operating room, all suspicious lesions should be endoscopically biopsied. Blood effluxing from either ureteral orifice should be further investigated with a retrograde pyelogram and possibly ureteroscopy.

Both tumor grade and stage correlate independently with prognosis. Transitional cell cancer most commonly is graded on a scale between 1 and 3, representing well, moderate, and poorly differentiated tumors. The TNM system, developed by the International Union Against Cancer and the American Joint Committee on Cancer Staging, is used to stage bladder cancer. Tumors that involve the bladder mucosa (Ta and CIS) or lamina propria (T1) are considered superficial cancers. CIS is a unique designation that signifies a flat, high-grade tumor confined to the mucosa, and CIS generally implies a higher risk of recurrence following treatment. Tumors that invade the muscular layer of the bladder wall (T2) or beyond (T3 and T4) are considered muscle invasive.

Approximately 25 percent of patients with bladder cancer have muscle-invasive disease at the time of diagnosis. Patients with muscle-invasive bladder cancer should undergo a metastatic work-up, which includes a CT scan of the abdomen and pelvis, chest radiograph, serum chemistries, and liver function tests. If the patients are asymptomatic with normal calcium and alkaline phosphatase, bone scans are unnecessary. Approximately 15 percent of all patients have metastatic disease at the time of initial presentation. The life expectancy for most patients with overt metastatic disease is less than 2 years; however, approximately 25 percent of patients with only limited regional lymph node metastases discovered during cystectomy and pelvic lymph node dissection may survive beyond 5 years.

Treatment of Superficial Bladder Cancer (Ta, T1, CIS)

Most superficial bladder cancers are adequately treated by endoscopic resection and fulguration of the bladder tumor. No further metastatic work-up is indicated if the pathology confirms a low-grade, superficial TCCa. However, bladder cancer is considered a polyclonal, field-change defect and continued surveillance is mandatory. In other words, the underlying genetic changes that resulted in the bladder cancer have occurred in the entire urothelium, making the entire urothelium susceptible to future tumor formation. The risk of recurrence following the treatment of superficial bladder cancer is approximately 70 percent within 5 years.

The risk of disease progression, defined as a subsequent increase in tumor grade or stage, depends on the initial tumor grade. The risk of progression for TCCa grades I, II, and III is 10–20 percent, 19–37 percent, and 33–67 percent, respectively. Carcinoma in situ alone or in association with Ta or T1 papillary tumor carries a poorer prognosis, with a recurrence rate of 63–92 percent. Patients with a history of superficial TCCa should undergo surveillance with cystoscopy and bladder wash cytology every 3 months for 2 years. If they are disease free during this period, the follow-up intervals can be gradually increased.

Intravesical therapy is effective for patients with high-risk, superficial TCCa in reducing the risk of recurrence. The most effective intravesical therapy is bacille Calmette-Guérin (BCG), which is a live, attenuated strain of *Mycobacterium bovis*. BCG is recommended for carcinoma in situ, T1 tumors, and high-risk Ta tumors (large, high-grade, recurrent, or multifocal tumors). The beneficial effects of intravesical BCG is thought to be mediated by a nonspecific immune cytokine response. Because BCG is a live, attenuated organism, it can cause tuberculosis-like symptoms if it is absorbed into the blood stream. Contraindications for BCG treatment include active hematuria, immunodeficiency, and active urinary tract infection. BCG therapy reduces recurrence and some studies suggest it may reduce the risk of progression as well.

Treatment of Muscle-Invasive Bladder Cancer (T2, T3, T4)

The gold standard for organ-confined, muscle-invasive bladder cancer (T2 and T3) is radical cystoprostatectomy in men and anterior pelvic exenteration in women. In men, radical cystectomy involves the removal of the bladder, prostate, and pelvic lymph nodes. A total urethrectomy also is performed if the urethral margin is positive. In women, a classic anterior pelvic exenteration includes the removal of the bladder, urethra, uterus, ovaries, and anterior vaginal wall. However, in a female patient, if the bladder neck margin is negative, the urethra and anterior vaginal wall may be spared. With treatment, the 5-year survival rates for pathologic T2, T3, T4a, and N + tumors are 63–80 percent, 19–57 percent, 0–36 percent, and 15–44 percent, respectively.

After cystectomy, the urine is diverted using segments of bowel. The various types of urinary diversions can be separated into continent and incontinent diversions. The most commonly performed incontinent diversion is the ileal conduit. A small segment of ileum is taken out of continuity with the GI tract while maintaining its mesenteric blood supply. The ureters are anastomosed to one end of the conduit and the other end is brought out to the abdominal wall as a stoma. The urine continuously collects in an external collection device worn over the stoma.

There are two commonly performed continent urinary diversions. An Indiana pouch is a urinary reservoir created from detubularized right colon and an adjacent limb of terminal ileum. The terminal ileum is plicated and brought to the abdominal wall, creating a catheterizable stoma. The native ileocecal valve provides the continence mechanism. The Indiana pouch is emptied by clean intermittent catheterization of the stoma 4–6 times per day. An orthotopic neobladder is a similar reservoir that is connected to the urethra. Various segments of intestine, including small and large bowel, may be used in constructing the orthotopic neobladder. The orthotopic neobladder most closely restores the natural storage and voiding function of the native bladder. Patients have volitional control of urination and void by Valsalva maneuver.

Prostate Cancer

Epidemiology

Prostate cancer is the most common cancer in men and the second most common cause of cancer-related death in the United States. Each year, approximately 189,000 cancers are diagnosed, representing approximately 30 percent of all cancers diagnosed in men, and approximately 30,000 deaths results from prostate cancer. It is estimated that in the United States, one in six men will be diagnosed with prostate cancer during their lifetime. Because the widespread use of screening prostate-specific antigen (PSA) in the late 1980s, the incidence of prostate cancer has dramatically increased; however, after about 1990, the death rate from prostate cancer has been declining. It often is suggested that this decline in prostate cancer mortality has resulted from increased screening and early detection of prostate cancer.

Family history, race, and environmental factors determine the risk of prostate cancer. The risk of prostate cancer is directly related to the number of affected family members and if three first-degree relatives are affected, the relative risk may be as high as 11. In the United States, the risk of prostate cancer also is related to race. African Americans have a higher incidence of prostate cancer than do whites, although Hispanics and Asians have a lower incidence than whites. Environmental factors also affect the risk of prostate cancer. There is scientific evidence suggesting that the risk of prostate cancer can be lowered by a low-fat diet, and by various nutritional supplements including lycopene, vitamin E, and selenium.

Prostate Cancer Screening

Until prostate cancer metastasizes or becomes locally advanced, it does not generally cause symptoms. Most prostate cancers are diagnosed based on an elevated PSA or an abnormal digital rectal examination (DRE) of the prostate. PSA is a serine protease that is synthesized by the prostate epithelium and is elevated in prostate cancer. A PSA greater than 4 ng/mL is considered abnormal. Approximately 25 percent of patients with a PSA greater than 4 ng/mL will have a positive prostate biopsy, which establishes the diagnosis of prostate cancer. Approximately 50 percent of patients with both an elevated PSA and an abnormal DRE will have a biopsy positive for prostate cancer.

The American Cancer Society recommends offering annual prostate cancer screening to men starting at 50 years of age who have at least a 10-year life expectancy. Additionally, the society recommends offering PSA screening at 45 years of age in African American men and in men with a family history of prostate cancer. However, the value of screening is debated within the medical community, and this debate is reflected by the conflicting guidelines published by various medical and health care organizations.

Work-Up

Despite the controversy surrounding prostate cancer screening, it is important to point out that most cancers detected as a result of an elevated PSA or abnormal DRE are clinically significant cancers that should be treated in men with at least a 10-year life expectancy. The diagnosis of prostate cancer is made by biopsy. Using transrectal ultrasound guidance, the biopsy needles are directed at the peripheral zones in which prostate cancer tends to develop. Prostate cancer is graded by the pathologist using the Gleason system. The two most predominant histologic patterns of the prostate cancer are assigned a Gleason grade, on a scale from 1–5. The two Gleason grades are added to give a Gleason score, on a scale from 2–10.

Tumors with Gleason scores of 8–10 are considered high-grade tumors, and tumors with Gleason scores of 5–7 are considered intermediate-grade tumors. High-grade prostatic intraepithelial neoplasia (PIN) is considered a premalignant lesion that may indicate the presence of adjacent cancer. Given the possibility for sampling error, the presence of PIN in a biopsy that is negative for prostate cancer is an indication for repeating the biopsy; a repeat biopsy will be positive for prostate cancer in approximately 40 percent of cases.

Prostate cancer is most commonly staged using the TNM system. The most common sites of metastasis for prostate cancer are the axial bones and pelvic lymph nodes. For the majority of patients diagnosed with prostate cancers, no formal metastatic work-up is necessary. However, a PSA greater than 20 ng/mL or a PSA greater than 10 ng/mL in a patient with a Gleason score 8–10 tumor is associated with an increased risk of metastatic disease, and a bone scan and pelvic CT scan should be performed. Additionally, any patient complaining of bone pain should undergo a bone scan.

Treatment

Localized prostate cancer. Prostate cancer tends to progress slowly and have a long, natural history. Therefore, treatment for localized prostate cancer generally is offered to patients with at least a 10-year life expectancy. Patients with high-grade tumors (Gleason score of 8–10) may represent an exception to this rule; without treatment, they are at a significantly higher risk of developing symptomatic disease and dying from their disease. Therefore, in these patients, curative therapy should be considered regardless of life expectancy. The treatment options for localized prostate cancer can be broadly categorized as involving surgery or radiation therapy.

The most commonly performed surgical procedure is a radical retropubic prostatectomy (RRP). A pelvic lymph node dissection is generally performed for staging purposes at the time of surgery. The most significant complications associated with surgery are urinary incontinence and erectile dysfunction, which occur in approximately 5–10 percent and 14–30 percent of cases, respectively. During RRP, care should be taken to avoid injuring the urinary sphincter located just distal to the apex of the prostate. The neurovascular bundles that run along the posterolateral border of the prostate contain the cavernous nerves, which are responsible for erectile function. Care should be taken to separate the neurovascular bundle from the prostate and preserve it during surgery.

Options for radiation therapy include external radiation therapy (XRT) and brachytherapy. With most XRT protocols, 60–80 Gy is delivered by conformal radiotherapy. The primary genitourinary side effects following XRT include frequency, dysuria, hematuria, and decreased bladder capacity. The primary gastrointestinal side effects include diarrhea, rectal pain, and rectal bleeding. The sexual dysfunction following XRT develops gradually and 40–50 percent of previously potent men are impotent 5 years following treatment. Brachytherapy involves the percutaneous placement of radioactive seeds into the prostate. Although the side effects associated with brachytherapy are generally less severe than those associated with XRT, brachytherapy is less effective than XRT for treatment of high-risk prostate cancer.

Metastatic prostate cancer. The first-line therapy for metastatic prostate cancer is androgen-ablative hormone therapy. Since Charles Huggins won the Nobel Prize in 1966 for discovering the therapeutic effects of androgen ablation on metastatic prostate cancer, the fundamental principles for treating metastatic prostate cancer have not changed. Androgen-ablation is accomplished by performing bilateral orchiectomies or by administering gonadotropin-releasing hormone (GnRH) agonist. Testosterone synthesis by the Leydig cell in the testicles is stimulated by luteinizing hormone (LH) from the pituitary. The release of LH requires a pulsatile discharge of GnRH. Therefore, a constant GnRH stimulation paradoxically results in inhibition of LH and testosterone. Nonsteroidal antiandrogens such as flutamide and bicalutamide often are added to block the low levels of androgens produced by the adrenal medulla.

Testis Cancer

Testicular cancer is the most common cancer in men between the ages of 20 and 35 years. There are approximately 7000 new cases and 400 deaths related to testis cancer per year. For more than 90 percent of patients, testicular cancer is curable. Any patient with a solid testicular mass, which has been confirmed on ultrasound, is considered to have testicular cancer until proven otherwise, and should undergo a radical orchiectomy to make a definitive diagnosis. Prior to surgery, serum markers for testicular cancer should be obtained. The two markers used in routine clinical practice are human chorionic gonadotropin (hCG) and follicle-stimulating hormone (FSH).

When performing a radical orchiectomy, the surgery should be performed by an inguinal approach rather than a scrotal approach. The metastatic spread of testicular cancer is ordered and predictable. The primary metastatic landing sites for left and right testicular cancers are the para-aortic and the interaortocaval nodes in the retroperitoneum, respectively. The lymphatic drainage of the scrotum, on the other hand, is to the inguinal nodes. If the scrotum is surgically violated by performing a scrotal orchiectomy, metastatic spread to both the retroperitoneal and the inguinal nodes becomes possible.

Penile Cancer

Penile cancer is rare in the United States, representing less than 1 percent of all tumors in men. However, in certain regions of Africa and South America, penile cancer represents 10–20 percent of all malignancies. The majority of penile malignancies are squamous cell carcinomas. The diagnosis is made on biopsy. The primary lesion should be completely resected, whenever possible, to prevent the morbidities associated with local invasion.

UROLOGIC INFECTIONS

Cystitis

Cystitis is inflammation of the bladder mucosa and usually is caused by bacterial organisms. *Escherichia coli* is the most common cause of urinary tract infection (UTI), including cystitis. Other common causative organisms include Proteus, Klebsiella, Enterococcus, and *Staphylococcus saprophyticus*. Women are at a higher risk for UTI than men because their urethra is shorter. Fecal flora contaminating the vaginal mucosa can ascend through the female urethra. Certain bacterial factors, such as type 1 pili found on some strains of *E. coli*, mediate adhesion and are more likely to cause UTI. Additionally, certain host factors such as vaginal pH, can promote vaginal colonization and UTI.

Symptoms of cystitis include urinary frequency, urgency, and dysuria. Uncomplicated cystitis generally does not cause fevers or leukocytosis. Patients with voiding symptoms can be worked up with a urinalysis. However, a urine culture provides a more definitive diagnosis of a UTI than a urinalysis. Important considerations when obtaining a urine culture have been previously discussed in this chapter. Bacterial UTI in women should be treated with 3 days of antibiotics. In men, bacterial UTI should be treated with 7 days of antibiotics and younger men should be evaluated for correctable structural anomalies with an IVP or CT scan with IV contrast, and a cystoscopy.

Asymptomatic bacteriuria occurs in approximately 30 percent of older adult nursing home residents and in 5 percent of sexually active women. Asymptomatic bacteriuria is the rule in patients with chronic indwelling Foley catheters. Most asymptomatic bacteriuria does not need to be treated. However, asymptomatic patients with urea-splitting organisms should be treated with antibiotics. Pregnant women with bacteriuria should also be treated as they are at an increased risk for developing pyelonephritis.

Pyelonephritis

Pyelonephritis refers to inflammation of the renal parenchyma and collecting system. It is a clinical diagnosis that is made based on the presence of fever, flank pain, and infected urine. Older patients and young children may present with less-specific symptoms such as mental status changes, abdominal discomfort, and low-grade fevers. The most common causative agents are gram-negative bacteria such as *E. coli*, Proteus, Pseudomonas, and Klebsiella. Most bacterial agents gain access to the urinary system through the urethra and ascend to the kidney. Therefore, women generally are more susceptible to UTI and pyelonephritis because of the shorter urethra in females compared to males.

Patients presenting with signs and symptoms of pyelonephritis should have a urine culture and serial blood cultures. The results of the urine culture may not be available for 48 h; therefore, a urinalysis can be used to support a presumptive diagnosis of pyelonephritis. Healthy adults with no significant comorbidities can be treated as an outpatient; however, most patients diagnosed with pyelonephritis are admitted to the hospital. Broad-spectrum IV antibiotics, such as ampicillin and gentamicin, should be started until the results of the urine culture are available and a more selective antibiotic can be identified. When patients are afebrile, they can be discharged on oral antibiotics. Uncomplicated pyelonephritis should be treated for a total of 14 days while pyelonephritis associated with structural or functional abnormalities should be treated for 21 days.

In select patients with pyelonephritis, the upper tracts should be imaged at the time of presentation. In selecting patients for early radiologic study, the most important principle to keep in mind is that an obstructed and infected urinary system is a surgical emergency that requires prompt intervention to establish drainage. Therefore, the upper tracts should be studied in any patient with a history of kidney stones, anatomic abnormalities such as a ureteropelvic junction obstruction, or malignancies that may cause extrinsic compression of the urinary system. Options for emergently draining an obstructed kidney include percutaneous nephrostomy tube placement and cystoscopic placement of a ureteral stent. Bladder outlet obstruction causing bilateral hydronephrosis can be relieved by the placement of a Foley catheter.

Other findings on CT scan and MRI may require surgical intervention. Small renal and perirenal abscesses can be conservatively managed with antibiotics in clinically stable patients. However, if there is inadequate clinical improvement or if the abscess is large, the infectious collection should be immediately drained. Drainage is preferably accomplished percutaneously.

Emphysematous pyelonephritis often is seen in older diabetic patients and represents a medical emergency. Air bubbles produced by gas-forming organisms can be seen in the renal parenchyma on radiograph or CT scan. Emphysematous pyelonephritis should be promptly treated with percutaneous drainage; if there is no evidence of clinical improvement, an urgent nephrectomy should be performed.

In adult patients, there is no permanent sequela following successful treatment of pyelonephritis. However, pyelonephritis in an infant kidney that is still developing can be devastating. Pyelonephritis can lead to permanent parenchymal scarring and loss of renal function. The most common abnormality resulting in pyelonephritis in infants and children is ureteral reflux. Ureteral reflux can carry an infectious organism from the bladder to the kidney, and severe reflux can cause hydronephrosis and urinary stasis. Therefore, pediatric patients with cystitis or pyelonephritis should be worked up with a renal ultrasound and a voiding cystourethrogram. Any pediatric patient at risk for pyelonephritis should be treated with long-term antibiotic prophylaxis.

TRAUMA

Kidney and Ureter

Approximately 10 percent of traumas involve the urologic system, most commonly the kidneys. The best study for evaluating the kidneys is a helical abdominal CT scan with IV contrast. A CT scan should be performed for all penetrating traumas. For adult patients with blunt trauma, a CT scan should be obtained in patients with gross hematuria, or with microscopic hematuria and systolic blood pressure less than 90 mmHg at any point during the transport and resuscitation. Approximately one third of renovascular injuries present with complete absence of hematuria, and, therefore, mechanism of injury and associated clinical findings, such as flank contusions and lower rib fractures, should also prompt a CT scan. Pediatric patients are able to maintain blood pressure despite an almost 50 percent loss of circulating volume. Therefore, hypotension is a poor indicator for radiologic work-up. All pediatric patients with gross hematuria should have a CT scan, and all pediatric patients with microscopic hematuria and potential renal trauma based on the mechanism of injury should have a CT scan.

The most commonly applied staging system for renal injury was developed by the American Association for the Surgery of Trauma (Table 39-1). Approximately 95 percent of renal traumas are grade 1. Approximately 98 percent of renal injuries can be managed nonoperatively. The only absolute indications for surgical management of a renal injury are persistent bleeding resulting in hemodynamic instability or an expanding perirenal hematoma. Relative indications for surgical management include major urinary extravasation, vascular injury, and devitalized parenchymal tissue. Studies show that even large urinary extravasations will resolve with conservative management. Smaller vascular injuries resulting in devitalized tissue also can be managed without surgery; however, if the amount of devitalized tissue exceeds 20 percent of the renal tissue, surgical management leads to quicker resolution of the injury and to fewer subsequent complications.

Patients managed nonoperatively should be placed on bedrest until resolution of gross hematuria. After resuming ambulation, the patient should be carefully monitored for recurrence of gross hematuria, which requires reinstitution of bedrest. Surgical exploration should be performed following CT

TABLE 39-1 Staging System for Renal Injury Developed by the American Association for the Surgery of Trauma

Grade	Description of Injury
1	Contusion or nonexpanding subcapsular hematoma No laceration
2	Nonexpanding perirenal hematoma Cortical laceration <1 cm deep without extravasation
3	Cortical laceration >1 cm without urinary extravasation
4	Laceration: through corticomedullary junction into collecting system *or* Vascular: segmental renal artery or vein injury with contained hematoma
5	Laceration: shattered kidney *or* Vascular: renal pedicle injury or avulsion

Source: From Moore EE, Shackford SR, Pachter HL, et al: Organ & injury scaling: Spleen, liver, and kidney. *J Trauma* 29:1664, 1989.

staging when possible. If the patient requires immediate exploration for hemodynamic instability and a CT scan cannot be performed, a one-shot intravenous pyelogram (1 mL/kg of body weight of 30 percent contrast administered 10 min before radiograph) should be performed intraoperatively to evaluate the kidneys and confirm the presence of a functioning contralateral kidney. If surgical exploration of a kidney is required, the presence of a contralateral kidney should be confirmed. Surgical exploration should be performed through a midline approach. The renal vessels should be identified and controlled prior to opening the Gerota fascia, to allow the vessels to be rapidly occluded if massive bleeding is encountered. Injuries to the collecting system should be repaired by a watertight closure. Devitalized tissue should be excised and meticulous hemostasis should be obtained by ligating open segmental vessels. If bleeding cannot be controlled or only minimal vitalized tissue remains, a nephrectomy should be performed.

Ureteral injuries are rare, with the majority of injuries resulting from penetrating trauma. The diagnosis of ureteral injuries can be challenging as they often present without hematuria. Ureteral injuries often are discovered during radiographic work-up or abdominal exploration for related injuries. If a ureteral injury is suspected, an intravenous pyelogram, a retrograde pyelogram, or a contrast CT scan should be obtained. When performing a CT scan, delayed images should be obtained after the contrast has entered the collecting system. Surgical repair depends on the level of injury and the length of the injured segment. Important principles for surgical repair include a tension-free, water-tight closure after widely débriding the injured segment. For coverage of large ureteral defects, interposition of intestinal segments or bladder flaps may be required to achieve a tension-free repair. The adventitia surrounding the ureter should be carefully preserved to maintain the tenuous, ureteral blood supply.

Bladder

Hematuria, gross or microscopic, is the hallmark of bladder injury. The vast majority of bladder injuries are found in patients with pelvic fractures. More than 90 percent of patients diagnosed with bladder injury have a pelvic fracture and approximately 10 percent of pelvic fractures are associated with bladder ruptures. Therefore, radiographic imaging should be obtained in all patients with hematuria and pelvic fractures, or in patients with penetrating trauma to the pelvis and lower abdomen. Rarely, bladder injury can occur in the absence of a pelvic fracture. Therefore, radiographic imaging also should be considered if pelvic contusions or urethral injuries are present.

A retrograde cystogram is the most accurate test for ruling out a bladder rupture. When performing a retrograde cystogram, it is critical to adequately distend the bladder (400 mL or 40 cm H_2O) and obtain a postdrainage film to look for extravasation of contrast. An alternative study is a CT cystogram, which can be obtained at the same time the abdomen and pelvis are imaged for related injuries. The management of bladder injury depends on the site of rupture. Extraperitoneal ruptures usually can be managed conservatively with prolonged catheter drainage; however, intraperitoneal ruptures should be explored and surgically repaired.

Urethra

Patients with urethral injury resulting from trauma classically present with blood at the meatus and inability to void. Other potential findings include a perineal hematoma and a "high-riding" prostate on digital rectal exam. If any of these findings are present, a retrograde urethrogram should be performed before attempting to catheterize the bladder. To perform a retrograde urethrogram, a small Foley catheter is placed just inside the meatus and the Foley balloon is inflated with 1–2 mL of water. Lateral decubitus films are taken while 30–50 mL of radiographic contrast is gently injected through the catheter. When feasible, performing the study under fluoroscopy is preferred. Urethral injuries are categorized as posterior or anterior injuries.

Posterior Urethra

Trauma to the posterior urethral, which includes the prostatic and membranous urethra, occurs in the context of pelvic fractures. The statistics are similar to that of bladder trauma. More than 90 percent of posterior urethral injuries occur in patients with a pelvic fracture and approximately 10 percent of pelvic fractures are associated with urethral injuries. Although a suprapubic tube provides effective urinary drainage without risking further disruption of the urethra, a urethral Foley catheter should be placed across the injury when possible.

The anterior urethra includes the bulbous and penile urethral. Anterior urethral traumas usually are isolated injuries that most commonly result from a straddle injury. Anterior urethral injury also can occur as a result of direct trauma to the penis. Pelvic fractures are rare in patients with anterior urethral injuries. More distal injuries are contained by the Buck fascia and resulting hematomas dissect along the penile shaft. More proximal injuries to the anterior urethra may be contained by the Colles fascia and produce a perineal hematoma.

The treatment of choice for most blunt and penetrating injuries is immediate exploration, débridement, and direct repair. An exception is an anterior urethral injury resulting from a high-velocity gunshot, which should be managed with a suprapubic cystostomy and delayed repair after clear demarcation of injured tissues. Proximal injuries to the anterior urethra can be approached through a perineal incision, and more distal injuries can be approached by making a circumferential, subcoronal incision and degloving the penis.

Penis

Penetrating injuries to the penis are rare. Injuries to the penile corporal should be repaired by closing ruptures of the tunica albuginea. Blunt or penetrating penile injuries resulting from an accident should be evaluated with a urethrogram. Urethral injuries should be managed as described in the section on urethral trauma.

Testis

The most common causes of testicular injury are assaults and sports injuries. Blunt trauma to the scrotum can disrupt the vessels surrounding the testicles and result in a hematocele. Small traumatic hematoceles do not require surgical intervention. An ultrasound should be performed to confirm that the testicles are intact. Rupture of the testicle itself is rare and requires immediate exploration and surgical repair. The testicles should be immediately explored with no need for an ultrasound if physical findings such as a large hematocele, large hematoma, or gross disruption of the testicular wall are found, suggesting testicular rupture. At the time of surgery, the hematoma should be evacuated and the tunica albuginea should be closed. Penetrating scrotal injuries should be explored, and amputated testicles often can be successfully reimplanted when warm ischemia time is less than 6 h.

STONE DISEASE

Etiology

Stone disease is one of the most common urologic diseases, affecting one in eight white men by age 70 years. Stone disease is most common in 20–40-year-olds and is three times more common in men than in women. The prevalence of urinary tract stone disease has been estimated at 2–3 percent. For patients developing a stone, the risk of recurrent stone formation within 5 years may be as high as 50 percent. Therefore, successful treatment of stone disease not only involves management of the acute stone, but also long-term medical management to prevent future stone formation.

Acute Kidney Stone

Presentation

An acute stone is defined as a urinary stone obstructing the kidney or ureter, and causing symptoms. The classic symptoms of an obstructing kidney stone include colicky flank pain and hematuria, often accompanied by nausea and vomiting. If the stone moves down the ureter, the pain may localize to the ipsilateral lower abdomen. A stone impacted in the distal, intramural ureter may produce pain referred to the inguinal and perineal areas. On physical exam, costovertebral angle tenderness usually can be appreciated. The hematuria accompanying stone disease may be microscopic or gross. However, approximately 15 percent of acute renal stones present without hematuria. Patients with a superimposed urinary tract infection may present with fever and irritative voiding symptoms. Patients with an infected urinary system and a completely impacted stone may even present with signs and symptoms of sepsis.

Radiologic Work-Up

The diagnosis of a urinary stone can be confirmed radiologically. A plain radiograph of the abdomen and pelvis is the simplest test to obtain; however, radiolucent stones, such as uric acid stones and cystine stones, may not be visualized, and stool in the colon may make it difficult to identify smaller stones in the ureter. The test of choice at most centers for diagnosing an acute stone is a noncontrast, helical CT scan. All stones, regardless of composition, are visualized on CT scan with the exception of a small percentage of indinavir stones. Indinavir stones form in human immunodeficiency virus (HIV)-positive patients treated with the protease inhibitor indinavir sulfate.

Management

The majority of renal stones will pass spontaneously. Only 10 percent of patients presenting with an acute renal stone require hospital admission. Patients with any of the following presentations should be managed as an inpatient: intractable pain, severe nausea with inability to tolerate oral intake, urinary infection, or renal insufficiency. All other patients can be managed on an outpatient basis.

Patients with obstructing stones and no evidence of urinary infection can safely be given up to 4 weeks to spontaneously pass their stone. No detectable renal damage occurs within 4 weeks of even complete ureteral obstruction. However, in the presence of a urinary infection, emergent intervention is indicated. A percutaneous nephrostomy tube or a ureteral stent should be placed to establish drainage of the obstructed urinary system. Following treatment of the urinary infection, the stone can be treated electively. Stones 4–5 mm in diameter have at least a 40–50 percent chance of passing spontaneously; however, stones greater than 6 mm in diameter have less than 5 percent chance of passing. Therefore, patients with larger stones should be considered for early intervention.

Surgical management. The least-invasive treatment option for renal stones is extracorporeal shock wave lithotripsy (ESWL). Shock waves are generated outside the body and focused on the stone. The shock waves harmlessly propagate through intervening tissue and attain sufficient intensity to fragment the stone only when it reaches the calculus. The stone is placed in the focal point of the shock waves by using ultrasound or fluoroscopy.

Endoscopic options for the surgical treatment of upper tract stone disease include retrograde ureteroscopy and percutaneous nephroscopy. Selection of the specific approach depends on the size and location of the stone. For example, a large stone filling multiple renal calyces is best treated using a percutaneous approach to directly access the kidney through the flank.

Once the stone is endoscopically visualized through a nephroscope or a ureteroscope, small stones can be snared and removed with a number of specialized instruments, such as a stone basket or a three-prong grasper. Larger stones can be fragmented intracorporeally by using a variety of energies, including laser, ultrasound, or mechanical force. Energy is applied to the stone through the working port of the scope and the stone is fragmented under direct vision.

SEXUAL DYSFUNCTION

Priapism

Priapism refers to an erection that is unrelated to sexual activity or persists beyond sexual activity. Priapism can be classified as low-flow (ischemic) or high-flow (nonischemic). The two forms of priapism can be distinguished by assessing the blood gas drawn from the penile corpora. The blood gas from a normal penis that is erect or a penis affected by high-flow priapism is similar to an arterial blood gas. However, in low-flow priapism, the blood gas will be similar to that of venous blood. Low-flow priapism results from venous occlusion. It is associated with severe pain. It is essentially a compartment syndrome of the penis and should be treated as a medical emergency. Most priapisms are idiopathic; however, specific causes of low-flow priapism include sickle cell disease, pelvic tumors, leukemia, spinal cord injury, penile injections for erectile dysfunction, antidepressants, and antipsychotics, especially chlorpromazine.

The management of low-flow priapism should be dictated by the duration of the priapism. Within 36 h of onset of low-flow priapism, intracorporal irrigation with an alpha-adrenergic agonist may be effective. A variety of protocols exist. One example of a protocol for intracorporal irrigation involves diluting 5 mg of phenylephrine in 500 mL of normal saline and repeatedly aspirating 20 mL of blood and injecting 20–30 mL of the phenylephrine solution through a 21-gauge butterfly needle.

If this is ineffective, or if the priapism has been present for more than 36 h, a distal shunt should be performed under anesthesia. A commonly performed distal shunt is the Winter shunt, in which a biopsy needle is inserted through the penile glans into the corpora cavernosa to create a shunt. If this procedure is unsuccessful, a more proximal shunting procedure, between the corpora cavernosum and the corpora spongiosum, should be performed. The rationale for these shunting procedures is that the glans of the penis and the corporal spongiosum are flaccid during priapism and unaffected by the veno-occlusive process. Therefore, a shunt will allow the occluded blood in the corpora cavernosa to drain.

Priapism resulting from sickle cell disease or leukemia should initially be managed medically. Patients with sickle cell disease tend to have recurrence of priapism, and, therefore, a trial of conservative therapy directed at preventing additional sickling is warranted. Medical therapy should include hydration, oxygenation, and alkalinization. Transfusions or exchange transfusions should be considered. Patients with leukemia should be promptly treated with chemotherapy rather than surgery.

High-flow priapism generally is painless, and because tissue ischemia is not a feature, treatment is less urgent. Nonischemic priapism results from an arterial-venous fistula that is most commonly secondary to trauma. The diagnosis of high-flow priapism can be confirmed by color Doppler ultrasound. The arterial-venous fistula can be identified by angiography and selectively embolized. If this fails, the fistula can be surgically ligated.

PEDIATRIC UROLOGY

Hydronephrosis

Hydronephrosis, or dilation of the upper urinary tract, may signify a congenital anomaly with the potential for adversely impacting renal function. Fetal hydronephrosis is diagnosed in 1 of 500 routine prenatal ultrasounds. The majority of fetal hydronephrosis resolves by birth or within the first year of life. Fetal intervention rarely is necessary, and should only be considered in cases of bilateral hydronephrosis and severe oligohydramnios. Following birth, severe hydronephrosis may be appreciated as a palpable abdominal mass.

In cases of bilateral hydronephrosis, a renal ultrasound and a VCUG should be obtained shortly after birth. For unilateral hydronephrosis, both studies can be obtained electively at approximately 1 month of life. Because neonates with hydronephrosis are at a higher risk for pyelonephritis, all neonates diagnosed with unilateral or bilateral hydronephrosis should be started on antibiotic prophylaxis (i.e., amoxicillin, 10 mg/kg per 24 h). Pyelonephritis during the first year of life, when the kidney is still immature, leads to permanent deterioration in renal function.

Ureteropelvic Junction Obstruction

Ureteropelvic junction (UPJ) obstruction is the most common cause of hydronephrosis in neonates. The precise etiology is poorly defined. UPJ obstructions may result from abnormal development of the smooth muscle at the UPJ. In some cases, an aberrant lower pole vessel crosses the UPJ, possibly resulting in extrinsic compression. Most neonates are asymptomatic, whereas older children often present with symptoms, such as flank or abdominal pain.

Initial evaluation should include a renal ultrasound and a VCUG to rule out coexisting reflux. If a UPJ obstruction is suspected, a nuclear renal scan should be performed to assess differential function in the right and left kidneys, and to assess renal pelvic drainage by timing the washout of nuclear isotope following Lasix administration. Mild to moderate hydronephrosis resulting from a UPJ obstruction can be safely observed and usually will resolve by 2 years of age. Antibiotic prophylaxis should be continued until the UPJ obstruction resolves completely.

Surgical repair should be performed for a UPJ obstruction associated with severe hydronephrosis, diminished renal function, high-grade obstruction or breakthrough infections while on antibiotic prophylaxis. The most commonly performed surgical repair is a dismembered pyeloplasty. The dyskinetic segment of the collecting system at the UPJ is resected, and the ureter and renal pelvis are brought over any crossing vessels that may be present and then anastomosed. The ureter in older patients may readily accommodate endoscopic instruments and a UPJ obstruction may be incised using either a percutaneous or a ureteroscopic approach. Kidneys with minimal function may best be treated with a simple nephrectomy.

Vesicoureteral Reflux

Vesicoureteral reflux is the second most common cause of hydronephrosis and may be found in as many as 70 percent of infants presenting with a urinary tract infection. For vesicoureteral reflux detected after birth, there is a female preponderance, with 85 percent of cases diagnosed in females. Vesicoureteral reflux is often an inherited anomaly. It is ten times more common in whites than in blacks and up to 45 percent of siblings of children with reflux also have reflux. Primary reflux is a congenital anomaly caused by a deficiency of the longitudinal bladder muscle surrounding the intramural portion of the ureter. Secondary reflux results from bladder outlet obstruction and an increase in intravesical pressure. Secondary reflux is corrected by addressing the underlying bladder outlet obstruction.

Vesicoureteral reflux is diagnosed by demonstrating ureteral reflux on VCUG. The degree of reflux can be graded according to the International Classification System devised in 1981 by the International Reflux Study Committee. As the infant bladder grows and the bladder wall thickens, most low-grade refluxes resolve. Approximately 85 percent of all grades I and II reflux will spontaneously resolve, although 30–40 percent of grades III and IV reflux and 9 percent of grade V reflux will resolve. Given that some high-grade reflux will eventually resolve, it is reasonable to conservatively follow children with reflux, regardless of the grade. However, it is critical that patients managed conservatively are maintained on antibiotic prophylaxis.

Surgical repair should be performed in all patients with a breakthrough infection while on antibiotic prophylaxis. Although there is some controversy surrounding this issue, most practitioners recommend surgical correction before the onset of puberty for girls with persistent reflux. The rationale for this recommendation is based on the observation that after the cessation of longitudinal growth, the likelihood of spontaneous resolution of reflux is small, and during pregnancy, reflux places women at a higher risk of pyelonephritis and miscarriage. Boys are at a lower risk of infection secondary to reflux. Therefore, most practitioners recommend stopping antibiotic prophylaxis after early childhood and continuing to observe persistent reflux.

Ureterocele

A ureterocele is a cystic dilation of the distal ureter associated with a stenotic ureteral opening. Ureteroceles occur four times more frequently in girls than in boys and occur almost exclusively in whites. Approximately 80 percent are associated with the upper-pole moiety of a duplicated ureter.

Posterior Urethral Valve

Posterior urethral valves are obstructive urethra lesions usually diagnosed in male newborns and infants. The valves are thin, membranous folds located in the prostatic urethra. Posterior urethra valves are the most common cause of bilateral hydronephrosis detected on prenatal ultrasound.

The Penis

Hypospadias

Hypospadias results from incomplete fusion of the urethral plate during development of the male penis. Hypospadias occurs in 1 in 300 males. The risk for hypospadias is increased by history of maternal estrogen or progestin use during pregnancy. Hypospadias are classified by the location of the urethral opening. Approximately 70 percent of hypospadias occur on the corona or distal shaft of the penis. Neonates with a hypospadias are not at increased risk for having other congenital abnormalities of the urinary tract.

For psychologic reasons, the hypospadias should be repaired before 2 years of age. Newborns diagnosed with a hypospadias should not be circumcised. The foreskin may be needed for future corrective surgery. The goals of surgical treatment include correction of any penile curvature, moving the urethral opening to the tip of the glans, and producing a cosmetically satisfactory result.

Phimosis

Phimosis is the inability to retract the foreskin past the glans of the penis. In most neonates, a physiologic phimosis exists. By 3 years of age, 90 percent of males are able to retract their foreskin.

Paraphimosis

Paraphimosis occurs when the foreskin that has been retracted past the glans of the penis cannot be reduced to its normal position. Constriction of the distal penis by the foreskin leads to venous congestion and swelling, making reduction of the foreskin even more difficult. As swelling and edema worsen, arterial supply to the glans may be compromised, resulting in ischemia, and even necrosis of the glans. Paraphimosis should be reduced emergently.

The Testicle

Testicular Torsion

Testicular torsion occurs when the testicle rotates and strangulates its blood supply at the level of the spermatic cord. Testicular torsion is a medical emergency that requires prompt surgical attention. Torsion occurring in the neonatal and prenatal period is extravaginal—the testicle and both layers of the tunica vaginalis rotate. Testicular torsion in neonates may not produce symptoms and is usually only noted after the testicle has atrophied. Torsion in children and young adults is intravaginal—the testicle and the inner layer of the tunica vaginalis rotate.

Intravaginal torsion is most common in 12–18-year-olds, with peak incidence at age 13 years. Adolescents presenting with testicular torsion complain of severe pain. The differential diagnosis includes epididymo-orchitis and torsion of the appendix testis. Epididymo-orchitis is rare in adolescents and is accompanied by pyuria. When evaluating a patient with torsion, manual detorsion can be attempted. If this fails, the patient should be immediately taken to the operating room.

Surgery performed within 4–6 h of onset of pain has better than a 90 percent testicular salvage rate. Therefore, unless the evidence for a competing diagnosis is overwhelming, surgery should not be delayed by diagnostic studies. At the time of surgery, an orchiopexy should be performed by fixing the testicle to the scrotal wall at three different points. The anatomic predisposition to torsion affects both testicles; therefore, the contralateral testicle should be similarly repaired. In select cases in which the diagnosis is uncertain and testicular torsion is unlikely, Doppler ultrasound or nuclear scintigraphy can be performed to more definitively rule out testicular torsion.

Hydrocele

In infants, hydroceles are fluid collections within the tunica vaginalis or processus vaginalis. During development, the testicles are enveloped by a double layer of peritoneum, which becomes the tunica vaginalis. With normal development, the processus vaginalis, which connects the tunica vaginalis with the peritoneum, becomes obliterated. If the process vaginalis persists, peritoneal fluid can track into the space surrounding the testicles, creating a communicating hydrocele. If bowel tracks down the same space, an indirect inguinal hernia is the result. If the processus vaginalis obliterates and traps fluid in the tunica vaginalis, a noncommunicating hydrocele is the result.

Suggested Readings

Walsh PC, Retik AB, Vaughan ED, et al (eds): Campbell's Urology, 8th ed. Philadelphia: W.B. Saunders, 2002.

Tanagho EA, McAninch JW (eds): Smith's General Urology, 16th ed. New York: McGraw-Hill, 2003.

Marshall FF (eds): Textbook of Operative Urology. Philadelphia: W.B. Saunders, 1996.

McConnell JD, Barry MJ, Bruskewitz RC, et al: Benign Prostatic Hyperplasia: Diagnosis and Treatment. Clinical Practice Guideline, No. 8. Rockville, MD: Agency for Health Care Policy and Research, Public Health Service, US Department of Health and Human Services, 1994.

Flanigan RC, Salmon SE, Blumenstein BA, et al: Nephrectomy followed by interferon alfa-2b compared with interferon alfa-2b alone for metastatic renal-cell cancer. N Engl J Med 345:1655, 2001.

Carroll P (ed): Urothelial Carcinoma Cancers of the Bladder Ureter and Renal Pelvis, 14th ed. Norwalk, CT: Appleton and Lange, 1995.

Dupont MC, Albo ME, Raz S: Diagnosis of stress urinary incontinence. An overview. Urol Clin North Am 23:407, 1996.

Santucci RA, McAninch JW: Diagnosis and management of renal trauma: Past, present, and future. J Am Coll Surg 191:443, 2000.

Coe FL, Parks JH, Asplin JR: The pathogenesis and treatment of kidney stones. N Engl J Med 327:1141, 1992.

Medical versus surgical treatment of primary vesicoureteral reflux: Report of the International Reflux Study Committee. Pediatrics 67:392, 1981.

40 | Gynecology

Gregory P. Sutton, Robert E. Rogers, William W. Hurd, and Martina F. Mutone

DIAGNOSIS

Diagnostic Procedures

Cervical Cytology

An annual cervical cytology (Papanicolaou [Pap] smear) and pelvic examination should be scheduled for all women who are or who have been sexually active or who have reached 18 years of age. After a woman has had three or more consecutive, satisfactory, annual cytologic examinations with normal findings, the Pap test may be performed less frequently on a low-risk woman at the discretion of her physician (ACOG Committee Opinion Number 186, September 1997).

After removal of the uterus and cervix for benign disease, the Pap test is not required more often than every three years as a part of the periodic examination. The practitioner should expect a report from the laboratory in the format of the Bethesda classification (Table 40-1) for cervical cytologic reporting. The Bethesda system for reporting cervical cytologic diagnoses was developed in 1988 and improved in 1991; it replaced the original Papanicolaou reporting system and provides a uniform format for cytopathology reports.

Vaginal Discharge

The patient's complaint of abnormal vaginal discharge should be investigated. Vaginal fluid is prepared by placing a small amount of the saline suspension on a microscopic slide with a cover slip and examining it under magnification. The examiner may note motile trichomonads, indicative of *Trichomonas vaginalis*; characteristic "clue cells," indicative of bacterial vaginosis; or pus cells, which may be indicative of gonorrhea, chlamydial, or other bacterial infections.

Potassium hydroxide enables the practitioner to appreciate the presence of mycelia characteristic of *Candida vaginitis*.

Cultures

Vaginal and cervical cultures are most useful for the detection of sexually transmitted disease. Although the diagnosis of gonorrhea might be suspected when Gram-negative intracellular diplococci are found on a vaginal smear stained by Gram stain, culture should be obtained to prove the infection. Gonorrhea is cultured on a chocolate agar plate and incubated in a reduced oxygen atmosphere. Cultures are most conveniently collected on a Thayer-Martin medium in a bottle containing a carbon dioxide atmosphere.

Chlamydial infection is suggested by the finding of a characteristic thick, yellow mucus (mucopus) in the cervical canal. Mucopus should be collected with a calcium alginate–tipped swab and sent to the laboratory in transport media specifically designated for Chlamydia. Some laboratories are now offering urine tests for gonorrhea and Chlamydia using the ligase chain reaction (LCR).

TABLE 40-1 The Bethesda Classification for the Classification of Pap Smear Abnormalities

Adequacy of the specimen	*Epithelial cell abnormalities*
Satisfactory for evaluation	Squamous cell
Satisfactory for evaluation but limited by ... (specify)	Atypical squamous cells of undetermined significance
Unsatisfactory ... (specify)	Low-grade squamous intraepithelial lesion encompassing human papillomavirus
General categorization	High-grade squamous intraepithelial lesion encompassing moderate dysplasia, severe dysplasia, carcinoma in situ
Within normal limits	
Benign cellular changes: see descriptive diagnosis	
Epithelial cell abnormality: see descriptive diagnosis	Squamous cell carcinoma
	Glandular cell
Descriptive diagnosis	Endometrial cells, cytologically benign in postmenopause
Benign cellular changes	
Trichomonas vaginalis	Atypical glandular cells of undetermined significance
Fungus organisms	
Predominence of coccobacilli	Endocervical adenocarcinoma
Consistent with *Actinomyces* sp.	Endometrial adenocarcinoma
Consistent with herpes simplex virus	Extrauterine adenocarcinoma
Reactive changes	*Adenocarcinoma, NOS*
Changes associated with inflammation	*Other malignant neoplasms (specify)*
Atrophy with inflammation	*Hormonal evaluation (applies to vaginal smears only)*
Radiation	Hormonal pattern compatible with age and history
Intrauterine contraceptive device	Hormonal pattern incompatible with age and history
	Hormonal evaluation not possible due to ... (specify)

Source: From the International Federation of Gynecology and Obstetrics.

Pregnancy Tests

These tests measure increased amounts of the beta subunit of human chorionic gonadotropin (hCG) in urine. These urine tests are very sensitive and specific, measuring hCG as low as 20 mIU/mL. Serum tests are more accurate and sensitive, and have an advantage in that they can be quantitated to give an hCG level. Serial hCG levels are helpful in circumstances in which it is important to determine that hCG levels are increasing or decreasing, such as in the management of threatened abortion, ectopic pregnancy, or trophoblastic disease.

Abnormal Bleeding

After the first menstrual period (menarche), cyclic bleeding is considered the norm but is subject to great variation. Menstrual interval varies from 21–45 days (time from the beginning of one menstrual period until the beginning of another). Menstrual duration varies from 1–7 days. The menstrual flow is a subjective assessment and varies from light to heavy. Some women experience bleeding at midcycle at the time of ovulation. Abnormal genital bleeding falls into six categories.

Bleeding Associated with Pregnancy

The availability of extremely sensitive pregnancy tests has made it possible to confirm pregnancy in the early days of gestation. Although bleeding can occur in up to 25 percent of all normally pregnant women, this symptom must be considered a threatened abortion until the bleeding is otherwise clarified. In the presence of threatened abortion, the pregnancy test is positive, the cervix is closed, and the uterus generally is consistent with the history of gestation. An abortion is considered inevitable when the cervix accommodates ring forceps and fetal tissue appears at the cervical os. Abortion is incomplete after a portion of the products of conception has been expelled; it is considered complete after all the products of conception have been expelled. Inevitable and incomplete abortion generally is treated by dilatation and curettage.

Ectopic pregnancy must be considered in any patient with a positive pregnancy test, pelvic pain, and abnormal uterine bleeding. Approximately 20 percent of patients with ectopic pregnancy have no bleeding, but others might complain of vaginal spotting or, occasionally, of hemorrhage.

Gestational trophoblastic disease also causes abnormal bleeding associated with a positive pregnancy test. Most gestational trophoblastic disease is represented by hydatidiform mole (see below).

Dysfunctional Uterine Bleeding

This type of bleeding abnormality is characterized by irregular menses with occasional extended intervals of amenorrhea. When bleeding does occur after one of these periods of amenorrhea, it tends to be extremely heavy. The combination of a period of amenorrhea and extremely heavy bleeding occasionally suggests spontaneous abortion. In the majority of instances, the problem is secondary to failure to ovulate. Evaluation of these patients should include a pregnancy test, which should be negative. Endometrial sampling usually reveals a nonsecretory or proliferative endometrium. In the presence of extremely heavy bleeding, dilatation and curettage is occasionally required, but in most instances, the condition can be managed with cyclic estrogen/progesterone treatment.

Trauma

The bleeding associated with genital trauma may be diagnosed secondary to a history of rape or genital injury. In the presence of genital bleeding secondary to trauma, the lesion must be evaluated carefully and repaired in the operating room under anesthesia if necessary.

In infants and premenarchal patients, the vaginal canal should be examined carefully for foreign bodies.

Bleeding Secondary to Neoplasm

Tumors, both benign and malignant, involving the genital tract from the vulva to the ovary, can produce abnormal bleeding.

The most common cause of abnormal bleeding in reproductive-age women is the presence of leiomyomas (fibroids). Leiomyomas are a common cause of heavy noncyclic bleeding (menometrorrhagia). Pelvic ultrasound is helpful in the diagnosis of uterine fundal tumors.

Pain

Pain associated with menses is the most common office complaint. Cyclic pain limited to that period just before or with the onset of menses is referred to as dysmenorrhea. Pain occurring without a demonstrable pathologic lesion is referred to as primary dysmenorrhea and is a common feature of ovulatory menstrual cycles. This condition is usually treated satisfactorily with nonsteroidal antiinflammatory analgesics. In some cases producing periodic disability, the use of ovarian suppression with oral contraceptives may be considered. Secondary dysmenorrhea commonly is associated with endometriosis, cervical stenosis, and pelvic inflammation. Acute pelvic pain may have its origin in abnormal pregnancy, benign or malignant neoplasia, or a variety of nongynecologic diseases. Pregnancy disorders include threatened abortion, inevitable abortion, incomplete abortion, and ectopic pregnancy.

Neoplasms cause acute pain through degeneration of a myoma or torsion of a myoma or ovarian neoplasm. The spontaneous rupture of an ovarian cyst can produce severe pelvic pain. Common causes of acute pain are salpingitis and endometriosis. Pain secondary to inflammatory conditions is associated with fever and other evidence of infection in most cases. Pelvic infection secondary to *C. trachomatis* is the exception to this rule. The possibility of a nongynecologic condition as the cause of pain must always be considered.

Pelvic Mass

The clinician must be aware that several physiologic conditions cause enlargement of pelvic organs. Pregnancy should be considered in all cases of uterine enlargement in reproductive-age women. Ovarian enlargement, as a result of ovulation and corpus luteum hematomas, produces masses that are easily palpable and that may persist for several weeks. In addition to a carefully performed pelvic examination, vaginal ultrasonography is a useful tool. Simple cysts associated with a normal CA125 are virtually never malignant.

Pelvic ultrasonography, computed tomography (CT), magnetic resonance (MR) and PET scanning all provide clues to the origin of pelvic tumors. Uterine enlargement may suggest pregnancy, uterine myomata, adenomyosis, or malignancy, such as endometrial cancer or sarcoma. Tubal tumors may represent a tubal pregnancy, inflammatory conditions of the tube and hydrosalpinx formation, or a primary fallopian tumor. Ovarian enlargement may suggest endometriosis, ectopic pregnancy, tuboovarian abscess, or benign or malignant tumor of the ovary. The decision to operate is predicated on the patient's age, clinical presentation, and character and clinical course of the mass. If the differential diagnosis points to a strong possibility of ovarian malignancy, the patient should be explored under conditions that will allow for the treatment of a pelvic cancer.

INFECTIONS

Vulvar and Vaginal Infections

Mycotic Infection

The most common cause of vulvar pruritus is candidal vulvovaginitis. The infection is most common in patients who are diabetic, pregnant, or on antibiotics. The majority of cases are caused by *C. albicans*, although other species may be incriminated. Diagnosis is confirmed by examination of the vaginal secretions and recognition of the characteristic pseudomycelia. Systemic treatment is possible through the oral use of fluconazole 150-mg tablet in a single dose.

Parasitic Infections

Pin worms (*Enterobius vermicularis*), which are common in young girls, cause vulvitis. Diagnosis is made by finding the adult worms or recognizing the ova on microscopic examination of perianal material collected on adhesive tape. A number of antihelmintic agents are available; mebendazole therapy is commonly used.

Trichomonas vaginalis causes primarily a vaginal infection, but the copious vaginal discharge causes secondary vulvitis. Diagnosis is made by recognizing the motile flagellates on microscopic examination. Treatment consists of metronidazole 250 mg given three times daily for 7 days.

The vulvar skin is a frequent site for infestation by *Phthirus pubis* (crab lice) and *Sarcoptes scabiei* (scabies, itch mites). The primary symptom of both these infestations is severe pruritus. The adult and immature forms are recognized on close inspection of the skin. Treatment consists of Kwell. The use of this agent is contraindicated in pregnancy.

Bacterial Infections

Bacterial vaginosis is the most common bacterial pathogen. The vaginal discharge found with this condition is not unlike that found with trichomonal vaginitis. The discharge is thin and gray-green in color. Diagnosis is made by microscopic study of the vaginal secretions to identify characteristic "clue cells." The condition is treated with metronidazole orally or with metronidazole or clindamycin topical creams.

Viral Infections

A number of viral infections affect the vulva and vagina, the most common of these being condyloma acuminatum. The causative organism is the human papillomavirus. The lesions are characteristic wart-like growths that begin as single lesions but can grow to huge confluent lesions that distort the normal structures. The lesions enlarge rapidly in pregnancy. Diagnosis is suspected on the basis of appearance and may be confirmed by biopsy. Treatment depends on the destruction of the lesions with caustic agents, imiquimod, cryocautery, laser ablation, or electrocautery.

Herpes simplex infection causes painful vesicles followed by ulceration of the vulva, vagina, or cervix. Initial infection usually is widespread, but recurrent infection usually involves a single lesion. Cytologic evaluation of lesions in the vagina is helpful; culture is confirmatory for herpes infection. Once a patient is infected, there is a tendency for the lesions to recur at various intervals for the life of the patient. The attacks may be aborted and the interval between attacks lengthened through the use of acyclovir (400 mg orally three times daily for 7–10 days). Active infection in pregnancy carries the risk of newborn infection if the patient delivers vaginally. Cesarean section is recommended in patients in labor with vulvar or vaginal ulceration as a result of herpes simplex infection.

Molluscum contagiosum causes groups of small pruritic nodules with an umbilicated center. The lesions are treated by ablation by cautery, curettage, or corrosive medication.

Pelvic Inflammatory Disease

It is estimated that there are approximately 1.5 million cases of pelvic inflammatory disease in the United States each year. The condition might produce infertility in 10 percent of the cases that occur; 3 percent or more of patients will have ectopic pregnancy, and chronic pain is a problem in many others.

Several factors have been recognized as placing the patient at risk: age younger than 20 years, multiple sexual partners, nulliparity, and previous pelvic inflammatory disease.

Pelvic inflammatory disease is classified as acute or chronic. The most common organisms that produce the condition are *N. gonorrhoeae* and Chlamydia, but numerous other organisms have been incriminated. The classic signs include fever, lower abdominal pain with pelvic tenderness, and purulent vaginal discharge. Some patients, however, will have minimal or absent symptomatology, particularly in the presence of a chlamydial infection. In patients requiring further study, pelvic ultrasonography may be helpful in confirming a diagnosis. When pelvic inflammatory disease is present, laparoscopy will confirm it by finding tubal edema, erythema, and exudate. The presence of a tuboovarian abscess can be confirmed in this manner.

Treatment

Women with pelvic inflammatory disease with evidence of peritonitis, high fever, or suspected tuboovarian abscess should be admitted to the hospital for observation and intravenous antibiotics.

The Centers for Disease Control and Prevention (CDC) recommends one of the following oral regimens: ofloxacin 400 mg orally twice a day for 14 days or levofloxacin 500 mg orally once daily for 14 days with or without metronidazole 500 mg orally twice daily for 14 days.

Recommendations from the CDC for parenteral treatment include cefotetan 2.0 g intravenously (IV) every 12 h or cefoxitin 2 g IV every 6 h plus doxycycline 100 mg orally or IV every 12 h. This regimen is continued for at least 24 h after the patient shows clinical improvement. Doxycycline 100 mg orally twice daily is given to complete a total of 14 days of therapy. The use of broad-spectrum antibiotics, which must include an antibiotic with anaerobic activity, will result in cures of some pelvic abscesses.

Surgical Therapy

Surgery becomes necessary under the following conditions: (1) the intraperitoneal rupture of a tuboovarian abscess; (2) the persistence of a pelvic abscess despite antibiotic therapy; and (3) chronic pelvic pain.

In young women whose reproductive goals have not been achieved, especially in the presence of unilateral disease, a unilateral salpingo-oophorectomy may be more appropriate than total hysterectomy with removal of both ovaries and fallopian tubes.

The rupture of a tuboovarian abscess is a true surgical emergency. Rupture most frequently is associated with a sudden severe increase in abdominal pain. A shock-like state commonly accompanies rupture. Leukocyte counts are not necessarily increased, and some patients are afebrile. With prompt surgical intervention and intensive medical management, the mortality rate today is less than 5 percent.

The patient with a ruptured abscess must be explored promptly through an adequate incision. Hysterectomy and oophorectomy are commonly indicated.

Operation may be technically difficult because of the distortion and edema secondary to the inflammatory process. Before the extirpation of any pelvic organ, adhesions must be lysed and normal structures, such as ureters and the large and small bowel, identified. At the conclusion of the procedure, the abdomen should be liberally irrigated. If the uterus is removed, the vaginal cuff should be left open for drainage.

ENDOMETRIOSIS

It has been estimated that endometriosis will be demonstrated in approximately 20 percent of all women in the reproductive age group. Although the condition occurs in teenage women, it is found most often in the third and fourth decades of life.

The most common theory for endometriosis is that it is initiated by retrograde menstruation. The most common lesions of endometriosis can be recognized as bluish or black lesions, sometimes raised, sometimes puckered, giving them a "gunpowder burn" appearance. Although many patients are asymptomatic even with widespread endometriosis, others have severe pain, particularly dysmenorrhea, and dyspareunia. Other signs and symptoms depend on the location and depth of endometriotic implants. Infertility and abnormal bleeding are common problems.

Pain is associated most often with the menstrual period; deep pelvic dyspareunia is commonly associated with this disease, particularly in those individuals with implants involving the uterosacral ligaments or the rectovaginal septum.

The finding of a pelvic mass and tender nodularity of the uterosacral ligament strongly suggests endometriosis. The mass usually represents an ovarian endometrioma, often referred to as a "chocolate cyst" because of its dark-brown fluid contents.

Treatment

Patients with minimal endometriosis who are asymptomatic can be cared for through simple observation and management with cyclic oral contraceptives and simple analgesia.

Pseudomenopause is currently the most common medical treatment for endometriosis. The most common medications used today for this purpose are the gonadotropin-releasing hormone agonists (GnRHa).

Conservative surgical therapy for endometriosis has become much more common with the advancement of laparoscopic surgery. Until menopause, extirpative surgery is the only permanent cure for endometriosis.

ECTOPIC PREGNANCY

The most common complaint of patients with ectopic pregnancy is pain, frequently associated with irregular vaginal bleeding. Approximately 80 percent of affected women will recall a missed menstrual period. An adnexal mass may be palpated in approximately 50 percent of patients. As a result of the intraperitoneal bleeding, some patients present in shock.

Laboratory examination of β-hCG enables the surgeon to confirm the pregnant state in patients at risk for ectopic pregnancy. Once the physician is assured that the patient is pregnant, it must be determined that the pregnancy is in the uterus. Vaginal ultrasonography important in differentiating uterine gestations from ectopic gestations.

In those patients who do not desire to continue the pregnancy, curettage of the uterus with examination of the tissue can be diagnostic. In the event that fetal tissue is not found, a diagnostic laparoscopy usually is required in the symptomatic patient for definitive diagnosis.

Treatment

Laparoscopic Procedures

Linear salpingostomy is the treatment of choice for ectopic pregnancies less than 4 cm in diameter that occur in the distal third (ampullary) segment of the tube. To aid in hemostasis, the mesentery below the involved tubal segment is infiltrated with a dilute vasopressin solution. The tube may then be opened in its long axis along the antimesenteric side with laser or a cutting cautery. The conceptus is then aspirated, and any bleeding is electrocoagulated. Partial or total salpingectomy is indicated when the pregnancy is located in the isthmic portion of the tube.

Medical Therapy

Conservative criteria for treatment of ectopic pregnancy with methotrexate include serum β-hCG levels less than 3500 IU/L and vaginal ultrasound that reveals the tubal pregnancy to be less than 3.5 cm in diameter with no visible fetal cardiac motion and no sign of hemoperitoneum. In this situation intramuscular methotrexate will result in complete resolution of the ectopic pregnancy in 96 percent of the cases. Subsequent tubal patency on the affected side can be documented in approximately 85 percent of the patients so treated. The risk of rupture and intraperitoneal hemorrhage must be made clear to the patient.

PELVIC FLOOR DYSFUNCTION

Pelvic Organ Prolapse

Female pelvic floor dysfunction is common. It includes many clinical conditions, the most prevalent of which are pelvic organ prolapse and urinary incontinence. Race, collagen metabolism, vaginal delivery, chronic constipation, chronic lung disease, and smoking are among the factors thought to be associated with the development of pelvic floor dysfunction (Bump).

Pelvic organ prolapse is the descent of the pelvic organs into or through the vagina because of deficient support of the vaginal walls. The standardization report of the International Continence Society in 1996 names "anterior vagina," "posterior vagina," and "vaginal apex" as reference points in the description of pelvic organ prolapse. This terminology, known as the Pelvic Organ Prolapse Quantification (POP-Q) system, quantifies prolapse according to the positions of those reference points relative to the hymen. The POP-Q has replaced the arbitrary grading systems that have been used in the past, improving the quality of description of the examination findings and facilitating communication among practitioners.

Patients with symptomatic pelvic organ prolapse report pelvic pressure and heaviness or a bulge protruding through the vagina. Patients may report difficulty with bowel or bladder emptying which requires them to push the prolapsed tissue back in manually. Obstructed voiding may occur, predisposing to urinary tract infection, urinary frequency and urgency, or, in rare cases, hydroureter and hydronephrosis. Because of shared risk factors, many patients with prolapse also have urinary incontinence. However, the relationship between urinary incontinence and prolapse is complex. Advanced prolapse may be associated with paradoxical continence, in which kinking of the urethra by the prolapse masks symptoms of stress incontinence that would otherwise occur because of a defective urethral closure mechanism.

Reconstructive surgery is indicated for symptomatic pelvic organ prolapse. Symptoms requiring surgery may include discomfort, irritation, or disturbance of bowel and bladder function. It is important to carefully define which of the patient's symptoms can be reasonably expected to improve with an operation. A pessary trial may be recommended for patients who are not surgical candidates. The reconstructive pelvic surgeon must recognize pelvic organ prolapse as a quality-of-life issue. This means that surgical goals and outcomes are measured not only by restoration of anatomy, but by relief of the specific symptoms with which the patient presents.

Urinary Incontinence

Urinary incontinence is defined as involuntary leakage of urine. Stress urinary incontinence is leakage of urine on exertion or effort, or with sneezing or coughing, which can be objectively demonstrated. It results from a dynamic urethral closure mechanism which is insufficient to overcome increases in abdominal pressure. Urge incontinence is characterized by urine leakage which is accompanied or immediately preceded by urgency. Urge incontinence is thought to result from inappropriate activation of the micturition reflex ("overactive bladder"). Stress incontinence, but not urge incontinence, is amenable to surgical therapy.

A baseline physical examination for a patient complaining of urinary incontinence includes a standing stress (cough) test, pelvic examination—including prolapse staging and evaluation for pelvic mass—urinalysis, and post void residual determination. Urethral mobility may be evaluated using the cotton swab ("Q-tip") test. Urethral hypermobility often serves as a focus for repair in continence operations. It is important to note, however, that urethral hypermobility is not specific for, nor causative of, urinary incontinence.

A patient presenting with uncomplicated stress urinary incontinence may be a candidate for surgical therapy. Potential complicating factors include: history of previous incontinence or prolapse surgery; prolapse greater than Stage II; elevated postvoid residual or abnormal voiding function; urinary urgency, frequency, or symptoms of urge incontinence; hematuria; neurologic disease; and previous pelvic radiation or radical pelvic surgery. Such patients should undergo complex urodynamic studies and evaluation by a pelvic floor specialist prior to consideration of an incontinence operation.

Stress urinary incontinence may be treated conservatively or surgically. Commonly used conservative treatments include pelvic muscle rehabilitation and vaginal obstructive devices. Estrogen supplementation and $\alpha 1$-adrenergic medications have been advocated for the treatment of stress incontinence, but their efficacy remains unproven.

Continence is a dynamic, complex function which surgery attempts to restore by unnatural means. The goal of a continence operation is to improve the ability of the urethra to close with increases in abdominal pressure, yet avoid interfering with voiding function. Surgical treatments for urinary incontinence have been performed since the beginning of the 20th century, pioneered by Howard Kelly and other gynecologic surgeons. Hundreds of different of operations have been developed, a fact which testifies to the difficulty of consistently achieving satisfactory and long-lasting outcomes.

SURGERY FOR PELVIC ORGAN PROLAPSE

Many factors are important in determining which reconstructive operation is optimal for a given patient. Variations of operative techniques have been described. Surgical decisions often are based on case series and expert opinions which may not have universal applicability. The few controlled studies that have been published suggest that, in general, failure rates for vaginal procedures are higher than those for abdominal procedures. This difference may relate to the use of graft materials, a concept that has been well established in the general surgery literature regarding abdominal wall hernia repair.

Vaginal Procedures

Colporrhaphy

The oldest type of vaginal reconstructive operation is colporrhaphy. This type of procedure involves the destruction or excision of vaginal epithelium. Anterior colporrhaphy begins with incision of the anterior vaginal epithelium in a midline sagittal direction. The epithelium is sharply dissected away from the underlying vaginal muscularis. The vaginal muscularis is plicated with interrupted delayed absorbable stitches, following which the epithelium is trimmed and reapproximated. Posterior colporrhaphy is performed in a similar manner, often including the distal pubococcygeus muscles in the plication.

Sacrospinous fixation. The sacrospinous ligament may be used for suspension of the prolapsed vaginal vault. The procedure begins with entry into the rectovaginal space. The rectal pillar is penetrated to gain access to the pararectal space. Two nonabsorbable monofilament sutures are placed in the sacrospinous ligament, at least two fingerbreadths medial to the ischial spine. Structures at risk of injury in this area include the inferior gluteal neurovascular bundle, lumbosacral plexus, and sciatic nerve. The stitches are anchored to the vaginal apex and tied without suture bridging. The remainder of the epithelial incision is closed.

Uterosacral ligament suspension. This approach is based on the original description of posterior culdoplasty by McCall in 1957. The uterosacral ligaments are exposed with an intraperitoneal approach. Multiple delayed absorbable or permanent sutures are used to attach the lateral-most portion of the vaginal cuff to the distal-most portion of the ligament and the medial cuff to the proximal ligament. Intraoperative evaluation of the lower urinary tract is important to confirm the absence of ureteral compromise.

Colpocleisis. Colpocleisis is the term applied to a class of vaginal prolapse operations that involves removal of part or all of the vaginal epithelium. The main benefits of colpocleisis operations are their simplicity, speed, and—in the case of total colpocleisis—high efficacy.

The LeFort colpocleisis for complete uterovaginal prolapse requires preoperative screening of the cervix and endometrium for malignancy. The procedure involves denudation of a rectangular portion of vaginal epithelium on both the anterior and posterior vaginal walls, followed by suture reapproximation of the exposed submucosal surfaces. The uterus is left in situ. Lateral drainage canals remain for drainage of uterine secretions. Total colpocleisis involves excision of the entire vaginal epithelium, followed by pursestring closure and inversion of the vaginal muscularis with complete obliteration of the vaginal vault.

Abdominal Procedures

Sacral Colpopexy

Pelvic reconstructive surgery by the abdominal approach allows for the use of graft material to support the vaginal apex. Suspension of the vaginal vault to the anterior surface of the sacrum using graft material was first reported in 1962. The procedure may be modified to include the anterior and posterior vaginal walls, and the perineal body, in the suspension.

Abdominal sacral colpoperineopexy begins with the attachment of graft material to the perineal body. The rectovaginal space is opened, and an allograft or xenograft is anchored to the levator ani muscles bilaterally and the perineal body distally using delayed absorbable or permanent monofilament suture in interrupted fashion. Laparotomy is then performed and the graft is retrieved. A strip of synthetic mesh is fixed to the remainder of the posterior vaginal wall directly and another to the anterior wall. The peritoneum overlying the presacral area is opened, and the anterior surface of the sacrum is skeletonized. Two to four permanent sutures are placed through the anterior longitudinal ligament. The sutures are passed through both leaves of the graft at the appropriate location which supports the vaginal vault under no tension. The peritoneum is then closed. The most dangerous potential complication of sacral colpopexy is life-threatening sacral hemorrhage.

SURGERY FOR STRESS URINARY INCONTINENCE

The choice of an incontinence operation for a given patient depends on many factors. Incontinence operations fall into three categories: needle suspension, retropubic urethropexy, and suburethral sling. Anterior vaginal wall plication, or anterior colporrhaphy, is no longer advocated for the surgical treatment of stress incontinence.

In cases of uncomplicated stress incontinence accompanied by urethral hypermobility, retropubic urethropexy most commonly is used. In the presence of intrinsic sphincter deficiency, success rates with colposuspension may be less than 50 percent. Therefore, intrinsic sphincter deficiency (ISD) with urethral hypermobility is best treated with suburethral sling procedures. ISD without urethral hypermobility is treated with suburethral slings, periurethral bulk injections, or rarely artificial sphincters.

Needle Suspension

Variations of this technique include the Pereyra, Stamey, Gittes, and Raz procedures. After an anterior colpotomy is made, the space of Retzius is entered bilaterally. Through a small transverse suprapubic incision, a long angled needle is passed through the space of Retzius to bring up the ends of a suture that has been secured to the periurethral vaginal muscularis. Variations exist regarding the way in which suture is attached to the periurethral tissue and the method of abdominal wall fixation. The utility of these procedures is limited by high long-term failure rates.

Retropubic Colposuspension

The first retropubic colposuspension was described in 1949 and modified in 1961.

Marshall-Marchetti-Krantz (MMK) procedure. Permanent suture is placed lateral to the urethra bilaterally and tied to the periosteum of the pubic ramus or perichondrium of the symphysis pubis. The surgical objective is to appose the urethra to the posterior surface of the symphysis pubis.

Burch procedure, Tanagho modification. Two pairs of large caliber delayed absorbable suture are placed through the periurethral vaginal wall, one pair at the midurethra and one at the urethrovesical junction. Each stitch is then anchored to the ipsilateral Cooper (iliopectineal) ligament. The sutures are tied to give preferential support to the urethrovesical junction relative to the anterior vaginal wall. Long-term outcome studies up to 10 years have shown cure rates of 80–85 percent for the Burch procedure.

Suburethral Sling

Suburethral sling procedures for stress incontinence have been in use since the beginning of the 20th century. Currently, the most commonly used sling materials include autografts (rectus fascia) and processed cadaveric allografts (fascia lata). The procedure is performed by a combined abdominovaginal approach, using a small transverse suprapubic skin incision. The anterior vaginal epithelium is incised and dissected from the underlying muscularis. The space of Retzius is entered. A Bozeman clamp or long angled ligature carrier is used to perforate the rectus fascia, passing it through the space of Retzius to retrieve the arms of the sling. The sling arms are fixed in place with suture. The base of the sling is positioned at the urethrovesical junction. Cure rates for the many different types of sling procedures described in the literature range from 75–95 percent.

Tensionless Sling

The tension free vaginal tape procedure was introduced in 1996. It is a modified sling using a strip of polypropylene mesh. Unlike traditional sling procedures, the mesh is positioned at the midurethra, not the urethrovesical junction, and is not sutured or otherwise fixed into place. Advantages of tension-free vaginal tape (TVT) include the ability to perform the procedure under local anesthesia and on an outpatient basis. Through an anterior vaginal wall incision, small subepithelial tunnels are made bilaterally to the descending pubic rami using sharp dissection. A specialized conical metal needle coupled to a handle is used to drive each end of the sling through the perineal membrane, space of Retzius, and suprapubic skin. The mesh is positioned at the midurethra without tension. The 7-year cure rate of TVT for stress incontinence is 82–85 percent.

Bulking Agent Injection

Glutaraldehyde cross-linked (GAX) bovine dermal collagen is currently the most widely used injectable. A transurethral or periurethral technique may be used, using a 30-degree operating female cystourethroscope to directly visualize the injection. The material is injected underneath the urethral mucosa at the bladder neck and proximal urethra, usually at the 4 and 8 o'clock positions, until mucosal apposition is seen. The long-term cure rate is 20–30 percent, with an additional 50–60 percent of patients demonstrating improvement. Repeat injections are frequently necessary because of migration and dissolution of the collagen material.

Surgical Complications

The most common complication of incontinence surgery is voiding dysfunction. Complete urinary retention may be transient or permanent, depending on the procedure and the way it is performed. There is also a spectrum of voiding difficulties related to partial urethral obstruction. Because of the 1–3 percent risk of injury to bladder or ureters, intraoperative evaluation of the urinary tract is recommended whenever incontinence surgery is performed. Other potential complications include urinary tract infection, retropubic hemorrhage or abscess, intestinal tract injury, ilioinguinal or other nerve injury, enterocele formation, foreign body complications because of graft materials, and inflammatory or infectious processes involving the pubic bones.

BENIGN TUMORS

Ovarian Tumors

Nonneoplastic Cysts

By definition, a cystic enlargement of the ovary should be at least 2.5 cm in diameter to be termed a cyst.

Wolffian duct remnants. These are small unilocular cysts. They may enlarge or twist and infarct.

Müllerian duct remnants. These can appear as paraovarian cysts or as small cystic swellings at the fimbriated end of the fallopian tube (hydatids of Morgagni).

Nonfunctioning Tumors

Cystadenomas. Many fluid-containing cystic tumors of the ovary are also accompanied by papillary projections and are known as papillary serous cystadenomas or mucinous cystadenomas. Approximately 20 percent of the serous tumors and 5 percent of the mucinous tumors are bilateral.

Mature teratoma. The tumors often contain calcified masses, and, occasionally, either teeth or pieces of bone can be seen on abdominal radiographs. Mature teratomas occur at any age but are more frequent in patients between 20 and 40 years old. If a teratoma (dermoid) is encountered in a young woman, it is preferable to shell it out from the ovarian stroma, preserving functioning tissue in the affected ovary. The opposite ovary should be inspected, but no further operative procedure is performed if the opposite ovary appears normal. In approximately 12 percent of patients, these tumors are bilateral.

Meigs syndrome. This pertains to ascites with hydrothorax, seen in association with benign ovarian tumors with fibrous elements, usually fibromas. Meigs syndrome can be cured by excising the fibroma.

Functioning Tumors

Granulosa-theca cell tumor. Pure theca cell tumors (thecomas) are benign, but those with granulosa cell elements are low-grade malignancies. Usually, granulosa cell tumors elaborate estrogen, but some of these tumors have no hormone production. In young girls, they are characteristically manifested by isosexual precocity, and in older adult women, they are sometimes associated with postmenopausal bleeding or endometrial carcinoma. The tumor can occur at all ages from childhood to the postmenopausal period, but it is most common in later life, with maximal occurrence between the ages of 40 and 60 years. If the tumor is discovered in the reproductive years and confined to one ovary without signs of surface spread or dissemination, a simple oophorectomy may be sufficient therapy. If it is discovered in later life, removal of both ovaries with the uterus is indicated. These tumors produce $\bar{\beta}$inhibin, which may be measured in the peripheral circulation.

Struma ovarii. This term refers to the presence of grossly detectable thyroid tissue in the ovary, usually as the predominant element in dermoid cysts. This tissue occasionally may produce the clinical picture of hyperthyroidism and is rarely malignant.

Uterine Tumors

Leiomyomas

Uterine leiomyomas are the most common benign tumor in the female pelvis. It is estimated that up to 50 percent of all women at some time in their life have one or more of these tumors.

Treatment. Most symptomatic leiomyomata can be managed expectantly. When symptoms indicate surgical treatment, consideration must be given to the age of the patient, the number of children she desires, and her reaction to possible loss of reproductive and menstrual function. Surgery should be fitted to the needs and desires of the patient. Therapeutic options may include myomectomy, embolization, and hysterectomy.

Vulvar Lesions

In many instances, chronically irritated areas of the vulva will show sclerosing atrophy of the skin (lichen sclerosus). Lichen sclerosus is a pruritic lesion that does not appear to be premalignant. Hyperplastic lesions termed hypertrophic dystrophies are found that may be benign (epithelial hyperplasia) or that may show atypia, in which case dysplastic changes can be observed. The pruritic symptoms can be helped by topical application of testosterone, clobetasol or tacrolimus ointments.

MALIGNANT TUMORS

Ovarian Tumors

Ovarian Carcinoma

Ovarian carcinomas are divided histologically into epithelial, germ cell, and stromal malignancies. The majority of the 27,000 or more cases of ovarian cancer diagnosed annually in the United States are of the epithelial type. The median age at diagnosis for epithelial ovarian cancer is 61 years, and the overall 5-year survival rate for epithelial cancers is 37 percent. Approximately 15,000 women die of this disease in the United States annually.

Although the etiology of ovarian cancer is uncertain, approximately 10 percent of patients with epithelial tumors come from families in which one or more first-degree relatives also have this disease or breast cancer. In such families, prophylactic oophorectomy may be considered at the completion of childbearing, especially if specific BRCA1 or BRCA2 mutations are identified. Testing for these mutations is now readily available in the United States. Primary peritoneal carcinomatosis has been reported in women who have undergone prophylactic surgery, however. Life-long screening with CA 125 levels, pelvic examination, and vaginal ultrasonography of women from affected families is important.

Table 40-2 outlines the International Federation of Gynecology and Obstetrics (FIGO) staging system for ovarian cancer. Early lesions are largely asymptomatic, and advanced tumors may produce only nonspecific symptoms such as early satiety, abdominal distention, and vague gastrointestinal symptoms. Although an annual pelvic examination is valuable in detecting early

TABLE 40-2 FIGO (1988) Staging System for Ovarian Cancer

Stage	Characteristic
I	Growth limited to the ovaries
IA	Growth limited to one ovary; no ascites; no tumor on the external surfaces, capsule intact
IB	Growth limited to both ovaries; no ascites; no tumor on the external surfaces, capsule intact
IC	Tumor either stage IA or stage IB but with tumor on the surface of one or both ovaries, or with capsule ruptured, or with ascites containing malignant cells or with positive peritoneal washings
II	Growth involving one or both ovaries on pelvic extension
IIA	Extension or metastases to the uterus or tubes
IIB	Extension to other pelvic tissues
IIC	Tumor either stage IIA or IIB with tumor on the surface of one or both ovaries, or with capsule(s) ruptured, or with ascites containing malignant cells or with positive peritoneal washings
III	Tumor involving one or both ovaries with peritoneal implants outside the pelvis or positive retroperitoneal or inguinal nodes; superficial liver metastases equals stage III; tumor is limited to the true pelvis but with histologically verified malignant extension to small bowel or omentum
IIIA	Tumor grossly limited to the true pelvis with negative nodes but with histologically confirmed microscopic seeding of abdominal peritoneal surfaces
IIIB	Tumor of one or both ovaries; histologically confirmed implants of abdominal peritoneal surfaces, none exceeding 2 cm in diameter; nodes negative
IIIC	Abdominal implants greater than 2 cm in diameter or positive retroperitoneal or inguinal nodes
IV	Growth involving one or both ovaries with distant metastases; if pleural effusion is present, there must be positive cytologic test results to allot a case to stage IV; parenchymal liver metastases equals stage IV

Source: From the International Federation of Gynecology and Obstetrics.

ovarian cancer, efforts to establish other cost-effective screening programs using serum markers such as CA 125 and vaginal ultrasound examination are being developed. Vaginal ultrasound is a promising technology that is not presently cost-effective in mass screening programs, because the yield is no more than 1 ovarian cancer per 1000 asymptomatic postmenopausal women screened. Currently, more than 70 percent of women with epithelial cancer have stage III tumors at the time of diagnosis. Widespread peritoneal dissemination, omental involvement, and ascites are the rule, rather than the exception, in these women.

Treatment.   In general, therapy for epithelial ovarian cancer consists of surgical resection and appropriate staging followed by adjuvant chemotherapy. Women with low-grade early stage (IA or IB) cancers who have undergone appropriate surgical staging may be treated with surgery without adjuvant therapy. If the lesion is bilateral (stage IB), abdominal hysterectomy and bilateral salpingo-oophorectomy are sufficient. It is in the limited group of patients with unilateral histologic grade 1 or 2 lesions that fertility can be preserved by performing adnexectomy and staging biopsies without removing the uterus or contralateral ovary and fallopian tube. In all other patients (stage IA, grade 3, and stage IC and above), appropriate initial surgery includes bilateral salpingo-oophorectomy, abdominal hysterectomy if the uterus has not been removed on a prior occasion, appropriate staging, and tumor resection.

Staging.   Thorough staging is imperative in determining appropriate treatment for patients with ovarian cancer. Among patients whose cancer is confined to one or both ovaries at the time of gross inspection, occult metastases can be identified by careful surgical staging in one third. If staging is improperly performed and adjuvant therapy omitted in patients whose tumors are apparently confined to the ovary, 35 percent will suffer preventable relapse.

Epithelial ovarian cancers disseminate along peritoneal surfaces and by lymphatic channels. The first site of spread is the pelvic peritoneum. Later the abdominal peritoneal surfaces and diaphragms are involved. The omentum is a common site for metastases, as are both the para-aortic and pelvic lymph nodes. It is paramount that surgery for ovarian malignancies be performed through a full-length midline abdominal incision. After the peritoneal cavity is entered, the visceral and parietal surfaces are inspected for metastatic disease, and any suspicious areas are biopsied. If ascites is present, it should be aspirated and cytologic evaluation performed. If no ascites is found, peritoneal washings with balanced salt solution or lactated Ringer solution are obtained from the abdominal cavity and submitted for cytologic evaluation after centrifugation and fixation.

Appropriately staged patients with histologic grade 1 or grade 2 tumors confined to one or both ovaries (stage IA or IB) require no postoperative therapy. Five-year survival in this group of patients exceeds 90 percent.

Those patients who have stage I, grade 3 lesions, stage IC tumors (malignant peritoneal washings, rupture of tumor, surface excrescences, or ascites), or stage II cancers that are completely resected may be treated equally well with systemic chemotherapy, radiotherapy of the whole abdomen, or a single instillation of intraperitoneal radioactive chromic phosphate. Five-year survival approaches 75 percent in this group of patients.

Women with stages III and IV disease require systemic chemotherapy with cisplatin or carboplatin, generally in combination with a taxane such as paclitaxel. Survival at 5 years in such patients may exceed 20 percent, although this rate drops as low as 10 percent at 10 years.

It is widely accepted that patients in whom little or no residual disease remains after initial operation, on average, live longer than those in whom a great deal of tumor remains unresected. Because of the survival advantage, every effort should be made to resect as much disease at the time of laparotomy as is possible. Because many patients with advanced ovarian cancer are older adults and nutritionally depleted, surgical enthusiasm must be tempered by proper preoperative evaluation and support with appropriate central monitoring and hyperalimentation when indicated. Occasionally, it is more prudent to obtain confirmation of the diagnosis, treat with neoadjuvant chemotherapy, and then perform definitive surgery when the tumor has diminished in size and the patient has been nutritionally resuscitated.

Resection of nodules involving the small or large bowel is warranted if it results in complete removal of all observed disease. Such procedures are probably not indicated if tumor remains at other sites. After surgical extirpation of the tumor, patients with ovarian cancers must be treated with chemotherapy. Approximately 80 percent of these tumors will respond to platinum-based combination therapy; 40 percent of all patients will experience a complete clinical response, or complete resolution of tumor identified on physical examination or radiographic or serologic study.

Disease on the right diaphragm may be resected by transecting the falciform ligament and retracting the liver inferiorly. If it serves to remove all remaining tumor, splenectomy may be performed. Resection of small and large bowel may be performed if the operation removes all residual disease. Use of the ultrasound aspirator and argon beam coagulator have resulted in an increased ability to completely remove tumors, including those that are implanted on the serosal surfaces and mesentery of the bowel. With diligence it often is possible to remove all appreciable disease with these instruments.

Palliative surgery. In most cases of advanced ovarian cancer, death is associated with bowel dysfunction or frank obstruction. Although invasion of the small bowel and colon is unusual, growth of the tumor adjacent to the bowel leads to mesenteric compromise and dysfunction usually heralded by distention, nausea, and vomiting. When bowel obstruction occurs early in the clinical course of ovarian cancer, particularly if it occurs before the administration of chemotherapy, surgical intervention is warranted and should be aggressive. Resection or bypass of the involved bowel is indicated; colonic resection also may be indicated. It is important to perform adequate radiographic studies preoperatively so that obstructed small bowel is not decompressed into a compromised colon.

When bowel obstruction occurs after chemotherapy, the prognosis is unfavorable. Women who develop such difficulties have a limited survival following surgical correction. Surgery is often difficult to perform because of extensive tumor. Laparotomy may be complicated by intestinal injury or fistula. Often the best approach in these patients is the use of a percutaneous or endoscopically positioned gastrostomy tube and intravenous fluids or conservative nutritional support. Such a procedure may limit the length of hospitalization and allow the patient to remain in a supportive home environment for a greater period of time.

Laparoscopy in ovarian cancer. At present, our ability to resect large ovarian cancers successfully using laparoscopic equipment is limited. Several investigators have developed successful methods of performing both pelvic and para-aortic lymphadenectomies using endoscopic equipment. Additionally, ultrasonographic and serologic criteria are evolving that will allow the surgeon to more successfully distinguish between benign and malignant neoplasms of the ovary. Caution must be exercised when dealing with potentially malignant unresected ovarian tumors using the laparoscope.

Tumors of Low Malignant Potential

These are epithelial tumors of malignant potential intermediate between benign lesions and frank malignancies. Histologically, most are of the serous type. Although these tumors may be associated with epithelial budding, atypia, mitoses, and stratification, they are distinguished from invasive cancers microscopically by lack of stromal invasion. The median age of diagnosis is approximately 10 years younger than that of patients with epithelial cancers. The vast majority occur in stage I and have a favorable prognosis. Surgery should include abdominal hysterectomy and bilateral salpingo-oophorectomy unless fertility is to be preserved in patients with unilateral lesions. These patients may undergo unilateral salpingo-oophorectomy. Ovarian cystectomy or nonextirpative resections commonly result in recurrences.

Patients with stages III and IV lesions have 5-year survival rates that approach 85 percent after complete surgical resection. There is little evidence that either chemotherapy or radiotherapy administered after surgery improves survival; on the other hand, deaths from chemotherapy-induced leukemia are not uncommon.

Germ Cell Tumors

These tumors occur in women in the first three decades of life and typically grow rapidly, producing symptoms of distention and abdominal fullness. Torsion may occur, producing an acute abdomen. Most are unilateral, and all have a tendency to spread to the para-aortic lymph nodes, and throughout the peritoneal cavity. Although they are similar in many ways to testicular cancer in the male, there are some differences.

Dysgerminoma, the female equivalent of testicular seminoma, is composed of pure, undifferentiated germ cells. It is bilateral in 10–15 percent of patients and occasionally is associated with elevated levels of hCG or lactate dehydrogenase (LDH). It is the most common ovarian malignancy diagnosed during pregnancy. Patients bearing dysgerminomas should undergo appropriate staging at the time of the primary resection but need not undergo hysterectomy (if fertility is to be preserved) or removal of the opposite ovary if it is normal in appearance. Secondary operations solely for staging purposes are unwarranted. Adjuvant therapy is unnecessary unless there is evidence of extraovarian spread. Either radiotherapy encompassing the whole abdomen or systemic chemotherapy can be given to patients with metastases. This tumor is exquisitely sensitive to either type of treatment, and the cure rate exceeds 90 percent even in patients with metastases. Chemotherapy has the advantage of preserving ovarian function, whereas radiotherapy results in ovarian failure.

The other germ cell tumors, in order of frequency, are immature teratoma; endodermal sinus, or "yolk sac," tumor; mixed tumors; embryonal carcinomas; and choriocarcinomas. The first may be associated with elevated levels of alpha-fetoprotein (AFP). Elevated AFP levels are found in all patients with endodermal sinus tumors and mixed tumors that contain this component.

Embryonal carcinomas are associated with abnormal levels of both AFP and hCG, and choriocarcinomas secrete hCG.

These tumors are invariably unilateral but may spread by peritoneal, hematogenous, or lymphatic routes. Surgical therapy involves unilateral oophorectomy and appropriate staging. Except for those with completely resected stage I, grade 1 immature teratomas and those with stage I dysgerminoma, all patients with germ cell tumors require systemic chemotherapy. Three courses of a platinum and etoposide-containing combination suffice in those patients whose tumors are completely resected. Cure rates in these patients approach 90 percent. In women with incompletely resected nondysgerminomatous germ cell tumors, cure may still be expected in more than 50 percent, but prolonged chemotherapy may be necessary. These tumors are not sensitive to radiotherapy.

Carcinoma of the Cervix

Carcinoma of the cervix accounts for about 16,000 cases and 5000 deaths annually in the United States. Risk factors include multiple sexual partners, early age at first intercourse, and early first pregnancy. Deoxyribonucleic acid (DNA) related to that found in the human papillomavirus has been identified in cervical dysplasia and carcinoma in situ, both precursor lesions, and in invasive cancers and lymph node metastases. Cigarette smoking is highly associated with an increased risk of cervical cancer and may impair the activity of T lymphocytes.

In no other cancer has widespread screening had as profound an impact on mortality as it has in carcinoma of the cervix. Georges Papanicolaou developed the cytologic smear that bears his name in 1943. Since then, screening programs have dramatically reduced the rate of invasive cervical cancer in countries in which this test is widely available. Use of the Pap smear has shifted the frequency of cervical abnormalities toward the premalignant intraepithelial diseases, dysplasia, and carcinoma in situ. Although there are histologic grades of dysplasia leading to carcinoma in situ, all intraepithelial lesions are noninvasive and can be treated successfully using conservative methods.

Eighty percent of all cervical cancers are squamous cell in type and arise from the squamocolumnar junction of the cervix. This epithelial transition zone is found on the face of the cervix or ectocervix in adolescence, and, through a process of squamous metaplasia, gradually moves into the endocervical canal as menopause is passed. Dysplasia represents a disordered metaplasia and gives rise to epithelial cells that contain increased mitotic rates and nuclear atypia and that lack appropriate maturation within the epithelium. Identification and eradication of intraepithelial lesions before invasion can occur are the goals of cervical cancer screening.

The remainder of cervical malignancies arise in the endocervical canal and are either adenocarcinomas or adenosquamous carcinomas. Although adenocarcinomas are very similar in their clinical behavior to squamous cancers, there is some evidence that adenosquamous cancers are more aggressive. Other rare histologic varieties associated with poor prognosis are neuroendocrine small cell carcinomas and clear cell cancers. The latter are frequently associated with maternal exposure to diethylstilbestrol.

Staging

Cervical cancers spread predominantly by lymphatic channels. The first lymph nodes involved are those in the tissues immediately lateral to the cervix. This region is referred to as the paracervical or parametrial area. The next lymph nodes to be involved, in order, are those in the obturator fossa, the internal and external iliac chain, the common iliac chain, and the para-aortic lymph nodes. Direct vaginal extension may occur. The lymph nodes in the presacral area may be involved in early stage lesions, and the supraclavicular lymph nodes are the most common site of distant nodal metastases.

FIGO staging for cervical cancer is based on clinical examination, intravenous pyelography, and chest radiography. CT or MRI findings do not affect the clinical stage. Table 40-3 illustrates the FIGO staging system. Note that the presence of hydronephrosis connotes stage IIIB even if there is no clinical evidence of extracervical spread. Except for selected patients with stage IVA lesions and those with distant metastases, all patients with stage IIB cancer and above are treated primarily with radiotherapy in the United States.

TABLE 40-3 FIGO Staging System for Cervical Cancer

Stage	Characteristic
0	Carcinoma in situ
I	The carcinoma is strictly confined to the cervix (extension to the corpus should be disregarded)
IA	Preclinical carcinomas of the cervix; that is, those diagnosed only by microscopy
IA_1	Minimal microscopically evident stromal invasion
IA_2	Lesions detected microscopically that can be measured. The upper limit of the measurement should not show a depth of invasion of more than 5 mm taken from the base of the epithelium, either surface or glandular, from which it originates, and a second dimension, the horizontal spread, must not exceed 7 mm. Larger lesions should be staged as IB
IB	Lesions of greater dimensions than Stage IA_2 whether seen clinically or not. Preformed space involvement should not alter the staging but should be specifically recorded so as to determine whether it should affect treatment decisions in the future
IB_1	Tumor size no greater than 4 cm
IB_2	Tumor size greater than 4 cm
II	Involvement of the vagina but not the lower third, or infiltration of the parametria but not out to the sidewall
IIA	Involvement of the vagina but no evidence of parametrial involvement
IIB	Infiltration of the parametria but not out to the sidewall
III	Involvement of the lower third of the vagina or extension to the pelvic sidewall
IIIA	Involvement of the lower third of the vagina but not out to the pelvic sidewall if the parametria are involved
IIIB	Involvement of one or both parametria out to the sidewall
III (urinary)	Obstruction of one or both ureters on intravenous pyelogram (IVP) without the other criteria for stage III disease
IV	Extension outside the reproductive tract
IVA	Involvement of the mucosa of the bladder or rectum
IVB	Distant metastasis or disease outside the true pelvis

Source: From the International Federation of Gynecology and Obstetrics.

Treatment

Intraepithelial or preinvasive disease. Abnormal Pap smears must be evaluated by colposcopy and biopsy. Colposcopy is the examination of the cervix with a low-power ($10–50\times$) microscope after application of dilute acetic acid to the cervix. The acid solution is mucolytic and serves to desiccate the epithelium, a process that brings out subtle epithelial patterns referred to as white epithelium, punctation, mosaicism, and abnormal vasculature. Abnormal areas must undergo mechanical biopsy or wide excision with a wire loop electrode and are examined histologically. If loop excision is not performed, the endocervical canal should be curetted to exclude epithelial abnormalities in this area, which is difficult to visualize colposcopically.

Once the diagnosis of an intraepithelial process is made and stromal invasion excluded, local therapy can be performed. If there are abnormal cells on the endocervical curettage specimen, a diagnostic cone biopsy or loop electrosurgical excision procedure (LEEP) is indicated to exclude the possibility of an invasive or microinvasive lesion in the endocervical canal.

Cervical intraepithelial neoplasia is treated in a number of ways. In general, the larger the lesion and the higher the grade of dysplasia, the greater the failure rate. Similarly, more aggressive therapy yields lower failure rates at increased risk of complications. The most definitive treatment for cervical intraepithelial neoplasia is vaginal or abdominal hysterectomy. This operation is associated with a rate of subsequent dysplasia at the vaginal apex of 1–2 percent. This major operation is usually reserved, however, for patients with extensive or high-grade lesions, those with recurrent disease after conservative treatment, those in whom adequate follow up is unlikely, and those with other indications for hysterectomy, such as prolapse, abnormal uterine bleeding, pain, or a pelvic mass. Cervical cone biopsy is curative in most cases of cervical intraepithelial neoplasia. In patients in whom the surgical margins of the cone specimen are uninvolved, the risk of recurrence is less than 5 percent. If the surgical margins are involved, half of such patients will develop recurrent disease. This is an outpatient procedure and is associated with few serious risks. It may, however, require general anesthesia.

More conservative methods of treating cervical intraepithelial neoplasia include wire loop excision, laser vaporization, and cryosurgery. Loop excision can be done under local anesthesia (paracervical block) in the outpatient setting. The advantage of loop excision is that it removes the diseased area and provides a diagnostic biopsy specimen. The main disadvantage is the relatively large amount of cervical stroma that is taken with the involved epithelium. In cases of cervical intraepithelial neoplasia confined to the ectocervix, such deep excision is probably unnecessary.

Laser vaporization usually is performed with a carbon dioxide laser, but other laser instruments may be used. The ectocervical transformation zone is ablated to a depth of about 7 mm to ensure the removal of endocervical glandular epithelium. This is a convenient outpatient procedure that results in a clearly visible squamocolumnar junction at the site of treatment. Risks of bleeding and infection are small. Cryotherapy is an inexpensive outpatient procedure that produces a frostbite injury to the ectocervical epithelium. When the cervix reepithelializes, the dysplasia generally does not recur. This is a simple technique that should not be applied to patients with endocervical lesions. The main disadvantage of cryotherapy is obliteration of the squamocolumnar junction, making subsequent colposcopic examination somewhat difficult.

In patients with very localized mild dysplasias or low-grade cervical intraep-ithelial neoplasia, local excision or electrocautery may be sufficient to eradicate the disease.

Microinvasive cervical cancer. FIGO (see Table 40-3) subdivides microinva-sive cancers into those with "early" invasion (stage IA1) and those in which the tumor measurements are less than 5 mm in thickness and 7 mm in lateral extent (stage IA2). This aspect of the FIGO staging system for cervical cancer fails to distinguish adequately between stages IA2 and IB, however, because both may have occult lymph node metastases requiring regional therapy.

Many prefer the original system of the Society of Gynecologic Oncologists, in which stage IA (microinvasive) tumors may invade to no more than 3 mm and must lack capability of lymphatic space invasion. Stage IB includes all other cancers clinically confined to the cervix, even if they cannot be visualized on examination. The advantage of this system is that it clearly divides stage I cancer into two treatment groups. Few patients with stage IA cervical cancer have metastases to the lymph nodes. Simple, or extrafascial, hysterectomy without lymphadenectomy is therefore adequate therapy. Five-year survival rates approach 100 percent in these patients. In exceptional patients, cervical cone biopsy or electrosurgical excision may be sufficient treatment, provided close surveillance is possible.

Early invasive cervical cancer (stages IB and IIA). Stages IB and IIA tumors are associated with a risk of pelvic lymph node metastases of 10–15 percent and a risk of spread to the para-aortic nodes of about 5 percent. Treatment must include the regional lymph nodes in these patients. Radical hysterectomy with pelvic lymphadenectomy or definitive radiotherapy is effective treatment in this stage cancer. Prognosis with either modality depends on the size of the primary lesion, the presence or absence of lymph–vascular space involvement, spread to the regional lymph nodes, and status of the surgical margins.

Women with stage IB2 cervical cancers (exceeding 4 cm in diameter), espe-cially those endocervical primaries that distend the cervix circumferentially, may require a combination of radiotherapy and surgery. These large endocer-vical tumors are referred to as "barrel" lesions and are refractory to surgery or radiotherapy alone. Isodose curves from cesium sources may not encompass the entire tumor. Cure rates with either treatment may be as low as 50 percent.

One current approach to these tumors is the administration of pelvic radio-therapy followed by a cesium implant and subsequent simple hysterectomy. This technique may reduce the number of patients who have persistent invasive cancer in the cervix after radiotherapy and consequently improve survival.

Stage IB1 lesions and early stage IIA cancers may be treated successfully with radical hysterectomy and pelvic lymphadenectomy. This operation was pioneered in the U.S. by John Clark in 1895. Radical surgery was transiently eclipsed by the first use of radium in the treatment of cervical cancer by Sjögren and Stenbeck in 1899, and subsequent establishment of the first radium hospital in Stockholm, Sweden, in 1910.

Radical surgery reemerged in the treatment of early carcinoma of the cervix with the advent of the Pap smear and increased diagnosis of early stage tumors in young women. Because early cervical cancer so rarely spreads to the ovaries, radical hysterectomy need not include oophorectomy. Ovarian preservation is one of the strongest arguments for the use of surgery over radiotherapy, because the latter inevitably results in the premature loss of ovarian function. Sexual function also is preserved.

Locally advanced carcinoma of the cervix (stages IIB–IVA). These cancers are treated primarily with radiotherapy, with cisplatin as a radiosensitizer. Treatment consists of a combination of external therapy to the pelvis (teletherapy) from a high-energy source such as a linear accelerator and a local dose delivered to the cervix and parametrial tissue (brachytherapy) using a cesium applicator such as a Fletcher-Suite tandem and ovoids. Combination therapy is essential because doses adequate to control cervical tumors exceeding about 1 cm in diameter cannot be given using teletherapy alone. Bladder and rectal tolerances are approximately 6000 rads; higher doses can only be attained by combination therapy. The addition of cisplatin as a weekly radiosensitizer has resulted in improved survival with no apparent increase in toxicity when compared with radiation alone.

Cure rates for stage IIB cervical cancers approach 70 percent, and those for stage IIIB approach 40 percent. Because the risk of pelvic sidewall lymph node involvement increases with advancing stage, the dose of radiotherapy to this area is advanced with increasing stage. When para-aortic metastases are present in either stage, survival is significantly impaired. Survival for patients with stage IIB carcinoma of the cervix and para-aortic metastases is poorer than that for those with stage IIIB disease and negative para-aortic lymph nodes. Gross para-aortic lymph node metastases may be detected by CT, MRI, lymphangiography, or PET scanning.

Microscopic nodal metastases are best detected by retroperitoneal common iliac and para-aortic lymphadenectomy, a relatively simple procedure performed through a "hockey stick" or paramedian incision. The fascial layers are divided, sparing the peritoneum, which is reflected medially to expose the lymph node–bearing areas overlying the major blood vessels. Laparoscopic staging and pelvic and para-aortic lymph node dissection may be used by appropriately trained surgeons.

The finding of metastases in the common iliac or para-aortic chain indicates the need for extended-field radiotherapy encompassing these areas in addition to the pelvis. Even with such therapy, 5-year survival rates are low, seldom exceeding 20 percent. Many consider the presence of para-aortic lymph node metastases to be an indicator of systemic disease, although supraclavicular metastases are present in fewer than 25 percent of such patients.

Recurrent cervical cancer. As a rule, patients who develop local recurrences after primary surgical therapy are treated most effectively with external and internal beam radiotherapy. Although those with lymph node failures may not be curable in this setting, those with vaginal recurrences often can be saved with such an approach. Patients who suffer recurrences at sites distant from the pelvis may be treated with palliative local radiotherapy or chemotherapy with limited success.

Women who develop recurrent cancer following primary radiotherapy are generally not candidates for curative therapy. If, however, recurrence is small, the interval to failure is a year or more, and the lesion is unaccompanied by symptoms such as back or leg pain or edema, surgical resection may be possible. Because radiotherapy results in fibrosis of the connective tissues surrounding the cervix, radical hysterectomy is impractical. The risk of vesicovaginal or rectovaginal fistulas approaches 50 percent. Additionally, surgical margins may be compromised by limited resection in such a situation.

Most gynecologic oncologists prefer to perform pelvic exenteration in such circumstances. Often, an anterior exenteration with en bloc removal of the bladder, cervix, uterus, and upper vagina is feasible. These operations require urinary diversion. Because of radiation exposure, however, an ileal conduit may be associated with urinary leakage from ureteroileal anastomoses. The preferred method of diversion in these patients is the creation of a sigmoid urostomy or transverse colon conduit. Other surgical options include a Koch pouch or the Indiana reservoir, both of which provide a means of urinary continence without an external appliance.

In the case of extensive local recurrences, sigmoid resection may be required in addition to removal of the bladder. A total pelvic exenteration is performed. The sigmoid colon may be brought to the skin as a colostomy or reanastomosed to the rectal stump. Pelvic exenterations may be subclassified as supralevator or infralevator depending on whether this muscular diaphragm is broached. Supralevator exenterations generally are associated with less operative morbidity. An infralevator exenteration is required if the tumor involves the middle or lower third of the vagina or the vulva. Vaginal reconstruction in these extensive procedures with gracilis or rectus abdominis myocutaneous flaps is highly satisfactory.

In general, about half the patients thought to be candidates for pelvic exenteration are found to have intraperitoneal spread or nodal metastases at the time of exploratory laparotomy, and, in most centers, do not undergo resection. Laparoscopy may be a useful way of excluding such patients from laparotomy. Of the remaining patients in whom surgery is possible, 30–50 percent will develop a second, nearly always fatal, recurrence after surgery. This complex operation should thus be undertaken only in carefully selected patients.

Endometrial Cancer

Endometrial cancer is the most common female genital malignancy, accounting for 34,000 cases annually in the United States. It is a highly treatable cancer, with approximately only 6000 deaths reported each year.

Risk factors for endometrial cancer include obesity, diabetes mellitus, hypertension, low parity, early menarche, and late menopause. Prolonged or unopposed exposure to estrogens is implicated in the genesis of endometrial cancer and its precursor, endometrial hyperplasia. Women who take estrogens in the menopausal years are known to have a 6-fold increase in the risk of endometrial cancer if progestational agents are not taken as well. There is also an increase in the incidence of endometrial lesions in women with a history of chronic anovulation (Stein-Leventhal syndrome) and in those with estrogen-producing ovarian stromal neoplasms, such as granulosa cell tumors, and in those who take tamoxifen.

Endometrial hyperplasia may be divided into classifications of simple and complex, depending on the microscopic architecture, and into those with or without atypia. These hyperplasias are thought to be estrogen-dependent. Atypical complex hyperplasias are most likely to give rise to frank adenocarcinomas. They occur in women at an average age that is 5–10 years younger than those with frank carcinomas. Simple hysterectomy is the preferred method of treatment for the hyperplasias. In women with underlying health problems that preclude surgical therapy, therapy with progestational agents such as megestrol or medroxyprogesterone acetate may be used with success. Careful monitoring with endometrial biopsy or curettage or vaginal ultrasound is required in these patients, however.

Treatment

Endometrial cancer is staged according to the FIGO criteria detailed in Table 40-4. Many patients have stage I disease and can be managed successfully with abdominal hysterectomy and bilateral salpingo-oophorectomy. Adjuvant radiotherapy may be required, primarily to reduce the risk of vaginal recurrence. This can be given preoperatively with external therapy or a Fletcher-Suite implant or intrauterine packing (Heyman or Simon capsules).

TABLE 40-4 FIGO (1988) Staging System for Endometrial Cancer

Stages	Characteristics
IA G123	Tumor limited to endometrium
IB G123	Invasion to < 1/2 myometrium
IC G123	Invasion to > 1/2 myometrium
IIA G123	Endocervical glandular involvement only
IIB G123	Cervical stromal invasion
IIIA G123	Tumor invades serosa or adnexae or positive peritoneal cytology
IIIB G123	Vaginal metastases
IIIC G123	Metastases to pelvic or para-aortic lymph nodes
IVA G123	Tumor invasion bladder and/or bowel mucosa
IVB	Distant metastases including intra-abdominal and/or inguinal lymph node

Histopathology—Degree of Differentiation
Cases should be grouped by the degree of differentiation
of the adenocarcinoma:

G1	5% or less of a nonsquamous or nonmorular solid growth pattern
G2	6%–50% of a nonsquamous or nonmorular solid growth pattern
G3	More than 50% of a nonsquamous or nonmorular solid growth pattern

Notes on Pathologic Grading
Notable nuclear atypia, inappropriate for the architectural grade, raises the grade of a grade I or grade II tumor by I.

In serous adenocarcinomas, clear cell adenocarcinomas, and squamous cell carcinomas, nuclear grading takes precedence.

Adenocarcinomas with squamous differentiation are graded according to the nuclear grade of the glandular component.

Rules Related to Staging
Because corpus cancer is now surgically staged, procedures previously used for determination of stages are no longer applicable, such as the finding of fractional D&C to differentiate between stage I and II. It is appreciated that there may be a small number of patients with corpus cancer who will be treated primarily with radiation therapy. If that is the case, the clinical staging adopted by FIGO in 1971 would still apply but designation of that staging system would be noted.

Ideally, width of the myometrium should be measured along with the width of tumor invasion.

Some clinicians prefer to deliver radiotherapy postoperatively after the uterus has been evaluated thoroughly. Either external beam therapy or vaginal cesium may be used.

Pelvic lymph node metastases occur in about 12 percent of patients with endometrial cancer apparently confined to the uterus. Lymph node metastases have a significant negative impact on survival. Risk factors associated with lymph node spread include high histologic grade (grade 2 or 3), low levels of progesterone receptor, deep myometrial or lymphatic channel invasion, spread to the adnexa, endocervical extension, and unusual histologic variants, such as papillary serous or clear cell carcinomas. Patients should have pelvic and para-aortic lymph nodes sampled at the time of hysterectomy. Therapeutic lymphadenectomy is advocated. Those with a high likelihood of spread to pelvic lymph nodes (grade 3, the outer one-third myometrial or uterine serosal involvement, and those with high-risk histologic subtypes) should undergo sampling of the common iliac and para-aortic lymph nodes, because these areas lie outside the usual fields of pelvic radiotherapy. Patients with papillary serous tumors may present with metastases in the abdominal cavity or omentum much as those with ovarian epithelial tumors; omentectomy, diaphragmatic, and peritoneal biopsies should be obtained.

Another important element of staging endometrial cancer is the evaluation of peritoneal lavage fluid for the presence of malignant cells. Approximately 12 percent of patients are found to have malignant peritoneal cytology; one half have other evidence of extrauterine spread of the disease, but the remainder have no other associated risk factors.

Vaginal hysterectomy occasionally is useful in patients with early endometrial cancer when lymph node metastases are thought to be unlikely. This operation is particularly well suited for massively obese parous patients in whom an abdominal incision would be prohibitive.

In patients with large stage IIB and III lesions, consideration generally is given to preoperative pelvic radiotherapy, because surgery may be otherwise difficult or impossible. These tumors should receive appropriate surgical staging or thorough radiographic evaluation if primary radiotherapy is used.

Radiotherapy alone may be the treatment of choice in patients at excessive risk for operative intervention. Radiotherapy alone produces results inferior to those of surgery or surgery and adjuvant radiotherapy; therefore patients treated without hysterectomy should be selected carefully. Advanced or recurrent endometrial cancer is responsive to progestin or tamoxifen therapy in 30 percent of unselected patients. Lesions that are well differentiated contain higher levels of progesterone receptor and respond more frequently. Only 10 percent of poorly differentiated cancers respond to hormonal treatment. Local radiotherapy or chemotherapy with paclitaxel, doxorubicin, topotecan, platinum compounds, or combinations may be of benefit in some cases as well.

Vulvar Cancer

Vulvar cancer accounts for approximately 5 percent of all gynecologic cancers. Although uncommon histologic types such as malignant melanoma and adenocarcinoma of the Bartholin's gland occur, more than 90 percent of vulvar malignancies are squamous carcinomas.

Although the etiology of this cancer is not well understood, it is likely that the human papillomavirus plays an important role, especially in younger women.

Spread of squamous carcinoma of the vulva is primarily via the lymphatics of the vulva. Lesions arising in the anterior aspect of the vulva drain preferentially to the inguinal lymph nodes, and posterior lesions may drain directly to the lymph nodes of the pelvis.

The 1988 FIGO staging system for vulvar cancer (Table 40-5) is currently accepted. This system requires surgical evaluation of the inguinal lymph nodes and provides a schema in which prognosis and therapy are closely linked with stage.

Treatment

Pelvic lymphadenectomy is probably not indicated in vulvar cancer except in those patients found to have grossly enlarged pelvic lymph nodes on preoperative CT or MRI. Patients with inguinal node metastases are best treated with inguinal and pelvic radiotherapy following resection of the inguinal lymph nodes. In the case of large vulvar primaries or suspicious inguinal lymph nodes, this approach yields better survival rates than those obtained when pelvic lymphadenectomy alone is performed.

Because extended radical vulvectomy is associated with long hospital stays and significant morbidity from wound breakdown and infectious complications, there has been a long-standing interest in more conservative surgery

TABLE 40-5 FIGO Staging of Vulvar Cancer

Stage 0	
Tis	Carcinoma in situ, intraepithelial carcinoma.
Stage I	
T1 N0 M0	Tumor confined to the vulva and/or perineum—2 cm or less in greatest dimension. No nodal metastasis.
Stage IA	$\leq$ 1 mm invasion + other criteria
Stage IB	> 1 mm invasion + other criteria
Stage II	
T2 N0 M0	Tumor confined to the vulva and/or perineum—more than 2 cm in greatest dimension. No nodal metastasis.
Stage III	
T3 N0 M0	Tumor of any size with
T3 N1 M0	1) adjacent spread to the lower urethra and/or the vagina, or the anus, and/or
T1 N1 M0	2) unilateral regional lymph node metastasis.
T2 N1 M0	
Stage IV A	
T1 N2 M0	Tumor invades any of the following:
T2 N2 M0	Upper urethra, bladder mucosa, rectal mucosa, pelvic bone, and/or bilateral regional node metastasis.
T3 N2 M0	
T4 Any N M0	
Stage IV B	
Any T, Any N, M1	Any distant metastasis, including pelvic lymph nodes.

for early vulvar cancer. The first efforts to this end were made in the 1960s. Several investigators introduced the concept of radical vulvectomy and inguinal lymphadenectomy through separate incisions. This approach not only reduces hospital time but also results in fewer major wound complications. This approach, has been widely embraced by gynecologic oncologists. Because inguinal node metastases are the result of an embolic process rather than infiltration or direct extension, the approach is rational. Early concerns regarding recurrence in the skin bridge between the vulvar and groin incisions have been largely allayed by experience with this approach. Recurrence in the skin bridge usually is associated with preexisting large inguinal metastases.

Another area of progress in the surgical management of vulvar carcinoma has been the use of conservative surgery for early lesions of the vulva. Although specific criteria vary, most investigators recognize that squamous cancers of the vulva less than 2 cm in diameter and no more than 1 mm thick, and that are of histologic grade 1 or 2, are associated with a very small risk of inguinal metastases. Such lesions are adequately treated with deep, wide excision, provided skin margins of 8 mm are obtained and the dissection is carried to the level of the superficial transverse perineal muscles. Inguinal lymphadenectomy can be omitted in such patients.

In patients with intermediate lesions located on the labium minus or majus that do not cross the midline or involve midline structures such as the clitoris, perineal body, or perianal area, modified hemivulvectomy and ipsilateral inguinofemoral lymphadenectomy have been used successfully. This approach should be considered if the primary lesion is less than 2 cm in diameter and 5 mm or less in thickness. Lymph node metastases are uncommon in this group of patients and the groin nodes may be evaluated by frozen section at the time of surgery. Sentinal lymph node biopsy is being evaluated in vulvar cancer. Although it was once believed that superficial inguinal lymph nodes were "sentinel," it has been demonstrated that vulvar cancer often involves the deep femoral lymph nodes primarily as well. A conservative groin incision can also be used to sample these lymph nodes. If "sentinel" lymph nodes are free of tumor, the risk of involvement of other groin or pelvic lymph nodes is probably small. This excision site may be closed primarily with good results.

Another controversial area in the management of squamous carcinomas of the vulva is that of the patient with locally advanced disease. When extensive vulvar cancer involves more than the distal urethra, the vagina or rectovaginal septum, or the anal musculature, ultraradical surgery may be required. Anterior, posterior, or total pelvic exenteration may be necessary to resect such lesions successfully. The presence of fixed, matted, or ulcerating inguinal lymph nodes presents another problem that may require extensive surgical excision. Following such extirpative procedures, reconstruction of the vulva and groins is accomplished using myocutaneous flaps based on the gracilis, sartorius, or tensor fasciae latae muscles. Approximately 50 percent of patients are cured by such surgical procedures.

In recent years, such locally advanced lesions of the vulva also have been treated successfully with external beam radiotherapy combined with radiosensitizing drugs such as cisplatin. At the completion of combination therapy, the areas of involvement are excised widely or biopsied. This approach is associated with results as good as or better than those achieved with ultraradical surgery and generally results in less morbidity. The need for urinary and fecal diversion also is obviated.

Uncommon Vulvar Tumors

Melanoma. Traditional surgical therapy for malignant melanoma of the vulva has included en bloc radical vulvectomy and inguinofemoral lymphadenectomy. It is now known that lesions less than 1 mm thick or Clark level II lesions may be treated conservatively with wide local excision. The value of inguinofemoral lymphadenectomy is controversial in lesions of greater depth, although primary surgical cure occasionally is achieved in patients with microscopic nodal metastases. Melanomas of the urethra or vagina usually are diagnosed in advanced stages and may require pelvic exenteration for successful management.

Intraepithelial disease. Intraepithelial disease (Bowen disease, bowenoid papulosis, vulvar intraepithelial neoplasia, carcinoma in situ) may be treated successfully by removing the involved epithelium. Characteristically, this is a raised, velvety lesion with sharply demarcated borders that may contain gray, brown, or red pigmentation. Removal is accomplished by simple vulvectomy, where the plane of dissection is limited to the epithelium, or by wide excision. In the case of diffuse intraepithelial disease, a so-called skinning vulvectomy and split-thickness skin graft may be required. This approach is associated with prolonged hospital stays, however, and should be reserved for exceptional cases. Also effective in the treatment of intraepithelial disease are the carbon dioxide laser and the electrosurgical loop.

Paget disease is an unusual epithelial or invasive process characterized by the presence of distinct "Paget cells" in the involved epithelium. Grossly, the lesion is confluent, raised, red, and waxy in appearance. This lesion also can be excised widely, although the microscopic extent of the disease may exceed the visible margins. Intravenous fluorescein dye and ultraviolet light highlight areas that cannot be detected by the naked eye, and this assists in excision. Frozen-section examination of the surgical margins also is helpful but time-consuming. Paget disease occasionally is associated with an underlying invasive adenocarcinoma; careful pelvic examination and proctoscopy are indicated in patients with this process.

GYNECOLOGIC OPERATIONS

Dilatation and Curettage

The patient is placed on the operating table in a lithotomy position, and the vagina and cervix are prepared as for any vaginal operation. The cervix is grasped on the anterior lip with a tenaculum. The cervix is gently pulled toward the outlet of the vagina. Some traction on the cervix is necessary to reduce the angulation between the cervical canal and the uterine cavity. A sound is inserted into the uterine cavity, and the depth of the uterus is noted. The cervical canal is then systematically dilated beginning with a small cervical dilator. Most operations can be performed after the cervix is dilated to accommodate a number 8 or 9 Hegar dilator or its equivalent. Dilatation is accomplished by firm, constant pressure with a dilator directed in the axis of the uterus.

After the cervix is dilated to admit the curette, the endocervical canal should be curetted and the sample submitted separate from the endometrial curettings. The endometrial cavity is then systemically scraped with a uterine curette.

In recent years, suction curettage for incomplete abortion, hydatid mole, and therapeutic abortion has become popular. Suction machines fitted with cannulas that vary from 4–12 mm in diameter evacuate the uterus in less time and with less blood loss.

Endoscopic Surgery

Endoscopic surgery, including both laparoscopy and hysteroscopy, has assumed a major role in gynecology. Although the limits of what is possible continue to be defined, the relative safety of some of these techniques in general use remains uncertain.

Laparoscopy

Tubal Sterilization Procedures

As in diagnostic laparoscopy, a one- or two-port technique can be used. Tubes are occluded in the mid-isthmic section (approximately 3 cm from the cornua) using clips, elastic bands, or bipolar electrosurgery. With electrosurgery, approximately 2 cm of tube should be desiccated. Pregnancy rates after any of these techniques have been reported in the range of 3 per 1000 women.

Fulguration of endometriosis. Conservative laparoscopic treatment of endometriosis increases fertility and often helps with pelvic pain. This condition and the various approaches to treatment were considered earlier in this chapter (see "Endometriosis").

Treatment of ectopic pregnancy. Laparoscopy has established itself as the primary treatment approach for ectopic pregnancies, a condition considered earlier in this chapter (see "Ectopic Pregnancy, Treatment").

Ovarian cystectomy. The laparoscopic removal of ovarian cysts less than 6 cm in diameter in premenopausal women has become common. Using a multiple-port technique, the peritoneal cavity is inspected for signs of malignancy, including ascites, peritoneal or diaphragmatic implants, and liver involvement. In the absence of signs of malignancy, pelvic washings are obtained, and the ovarian capsule is excised with scissors or a power instrument. The cyst is shelled out carefully and placed in a bag, intact if possible. The bag opening is brought through the lower port incision along with the 10-mm port. The cyst is then drained and the cyst wall removed. Hemostasis of the ovary is achieved with bipolar electrosurgery, but the ovary usually is not closed, because this may increase postoperative adhesion formation. Except in the obvious cases of simple cysts, endometriomas, or dermoid cysts, the cyst wall should be sent for frozen section to verify the absence of the malignancy. If malignancy is detected, immediate definitive surgery, usually by laparotomy, is recommended. All cyst walls are sent for permanent section and pathologic diagnosis.

In many cases the cyst will rupture prior to removal. This is always the case with an endometrioma that contains "chocolate" fluid. On rupture, the cyst contents are thoroughly aspirated, and the cyst wall is removed and sent for pathologic evaluation. The peritoneal cavity is copiously rinsed with Ringer lactate solution. This is especially important when a dermoid cyst is ruptured, because the sebaceous material can cause a chemical peritonitis unless all the visible oily substance is carefully removed.

Ovarian cysts larger than 6 cm and those discovered in postmenopausal women also can be removed laparoscopically. Because of the increased risk of malignancy associated with these situations, laparotomy is more commonly used. Laparoscopy may be a reasonable alternative in select patients if standard methods for staging are used in conjunction with appropriate frozen-section evaluation and expedient definitive therapy when indicated.

Removal of adnexa. Occasionally, all or part of an adnexa must be removed. This may be the case with a large tubal pregnancy, a large hydrosalpinx, or when a small but growing cyst is found in a postmenopausal woman. Using a multiple-port technique, the vascular supply to the tissue is first desiccated with bipolar cautery and then divided with scissors. Alternatively, the ovarian vessels in the infundibulopelvic ligament can first be occluded with one of the techniques described earlier. Special care should be taken to identify and avoid the ureter, which lies retroperitoneally as it crosses the ovarian vessels and courses along the ovarian fossa.

Once the adnexa has been excised and hemostasis is achieved, attention is turned to removing the tissue from the peritoneal cavity. Small specimens can be removed using a retrieval bag via a 12-mm port. The port is removed with the sack, and the fascial incision is enlarged, if required.

For larger specimens, the opening of the sack is exposed outside the abdomen whereas the specimen remains in the abdomen. A cyst can be aspirated, and the remaining specimen can be removed piecemeal, taking care not to allow intraperitoneal spillage.

In difficult cases, the specimen can be removed via a colpotomy incision. For this procedure, a 12-mm port is placed through the posterior cul-de-sac under direct visualization. A retrieval sack is placed through the port, and the port and specimen in the sack are removed together. The distensible peritoneum and vaginal wall will allow the removal of a large specimen through a relatively small defect, which can then be closed with a running suture vaginally. Prophylactic antibiotics may decrease the risk of infection.

Myomectomy. Uterine leiomyomas often are approachable via the laparoscope. Hemostasis is assisted by intrauterine injection of dilute vasopressin (10 U in 50 mL) at the site of incision. Pedunculated leiomyomas can be excised at the base using scissors or a power instrument. Intramural leiomyomas require deep dissection into the uterine tissue, which must be closed subsequently with laparoscopic suturing techniques. Because myomectomies are associated with considerable postoperative adhesion formation, barrier techniques are used to decrease adhesion formation.

Removing the specimen can be difficult. In general, morcellation is required, and power morcellators have been developed that significantly expedite this technique.

Hysterectomy. Laparoscopy was first used to restore normal anatomy prior to vaginal hysterectomy. More recently, laparoscopy has been used to perform some or all of the actual hysterectomy to avoid laparotomy in patients with known pelvic adhesions, endometriosis, or in whom the uterus is enlarged by leiomyoma. Although multiple variations in technique exist, there are three basic laparoscopic approaches for hysterectomy: laparoscopic-assisted vaginal hysterectomy (LAVH), laparoscopic hysterectomy (LH), and laparoscopic supracervical hysterectomy (LSH). Although basic techniques for each of these methods have become somewhat standardized, the indications and relative risk for each remain controversial.

The most technically simple, and probably the most widely applied, is the LAVH. The round ligaments are occluded and divided, and the uterovesical peritoneum is incised. Next, the proximal uterine blood supply is occluded and divided. When the ovaries are removed, the infundibulopelvic ligaments are divided. If the ovaries are conserved, the utero-ovarian ligament and blood vessels are divided and occluded. In some cases, the posterior cul-de-sac also is incised laparoscopically. The remainder of the case is performed vaginally, including dissection of the bladder from the anterior uterus, ligation of the uterine vessels, removal of the specimen, and closure of the vaginal cuff.

A LH differs from an LAVH in that almost the entire hysterectomy is performed laparoscopically. This procedure is used for the indications listed above and also when lack of uterine descent makes the vaginal approach impossible.

LH is begun in a manner identical to LAVH. But after the proximal uterine blood supply is divided, the bladder is dissected from the anterior uterus. This is followed by a retroperitoneal dissection in which the ureter is identified along its entire pelvic course and the uterine vessels are selectively occluded and divided. The uretero sacral ligaments are likewise divided and the posterior cul-de-sac incised. The specimen is removed vaginally, and the vaginal cuff is closed. The drawback to this approach is the reported increased risk of bladder and ureter injuries as compared to both abdominal and vaginal approach for hysterectomy.

The third common laparoscopic approach is the LSH. This procedure has been advocated for all benign indications for hysterectomy. Technically, it is begun in a manner identical to the first two approaches. However, after the proximal vessels are divided and the bladder is dissected from the anterior uterus, the ascending branches of the uterine arteries are occluded and the entire uterine fundus is removed from the cervix. The endocervix is either cauterized or cored out with a special instrument. The fundus is then morcellated and removed through a 12-mm abdominal port or through a special transcervical morcellator. The end result is an intact cervix and cuff, with no surgical dissection performed near the uterine artery and adjacent ureter. This approach avoids both a large abdominal incision and a vaginal incision. According to its advocates, this approach minimizes operating time, recovery time, and risk of both infection and ureteral injury. LSH has yet to be widely applied, in part out of concern for the subsequent risk of developing cancer in the residual cervical stump.

A guiding principle is that the same care must be rendered laparoscopically that would be performed by laparotomy with the same or less risk of complications. Until the relative risk of complications and effect on prognoses have been established for these approaches compared with laparotomy, application of the laparoscopic approach in gynecologic oncology will remain highly controversial.

Hysteroscopy

Hysteroscopy, like laparoscopy, has gained widespread support as a very useful technique for both diagnosis and treatment of intrauterine pathology and for ablation of the endometrium as an alternative to hysterectomy for the treatment of abnormal uterine bleeding.

General Hysteroscopic Techniques

Type of instruments.   Hysteroscopes can be divided into the categories of diagnostic, operative, and hysteroresectoscope. The lens for all three is identical. This is usually a fiberoptic lens and light source with an outside diameter of

3 mm and an objective lens that is offset up to 30 degrees from the long axis of the instrument. In contrast, the sleeves for the three types of hysteroscopes vary considerably. The diagnostic sleeve usually has an external diameter of 5 mm and a single-direction flow. Because outflow is limited, bleeding may impede a clear intrauterine view.

The operative sleeve, with an external diameter usually less than 10 mm, has a flow-through design with separate channels for input and outflow of distention media. A separate channel is available for placement of fine operating instruments.

The final type of sleeve is the hysteroresectoscope. This is also of a flow-through design and has an integral unipolar resecting loop identical to a urologic resectoscope. The loop can be replaced with a roller bar for endometrial ablation.

Distention media and pumps. Several distention media have found widespread use for hysteroscopy. For diagnostic hysteroscopy, CO_2 gives excellent clarity. Although it is extremely safe in general use, fatal gas embolisms have been reported when CO_2 was used after cervical dilatation or intrauterine surgery. To minimize this risk, CO_2 should be used for diagnostic hysteroscopy only with specifically designed pumps that are relatively high pressure (80–90 mmHg) and low flow. More importantly, the use of CO_2 should be avoided after cervical dilatation or any uterine instrumentation.

For operative hysteroscopy, one of the first fluid media used was 32 percent dextran and 70 percent dextrose. This syrup-like substance is usually introduced by hand with a large syringe. The advantage is simplicity and low cost. The view is excellent in the absence of bleeding. The disadvantage is the difficulty in completely removing the substance from the instruments. If this solution is allowed to dry in critical movable points, the instrument may "freeze up," and it is very difficult to remove. Additionally, intravascular intravasation can result in pulmonary edema.

More recently, aqueous solutions with pressure-controlled pumps have been used. For operative hysteroscopy, where electrosurgery is not being used, it is safest to use a balanced salt solution, such as Ringer lactate solution. Moderate fluid intravasation will be of no consequence in a healthy individual. However, intravasation of larger volumes can result in fluid overload, especially in a patient with any cardiac compromise. To minimize this risk, the use of a fluid-medium pump is recommended rather than gravity or a pressure cuff. This allows the maximal pressure to be limited to approximately 80 mmHg to prevent excess intravasation of distention media.

When electrosurgery is used for hysteroresectoscope excision of leiomyomas or roller-blade endometrial ablation, a nonconducting solution such as glycine must be used. Significant vascular intravasation can cause hyponatremia, potentially resulting in cerebral edema, coma, or even death. For this reason, protocols must be followed rigorously to detect and treat significant intravasation whenever these solutions are used. Intraoperatively, differences in distention medium input and output should be calculated every 15 min. If the difference is greater than 500 mL, a diuretic should be given. If the difference is greater than 1000 mL, the procedure also should be terminated. Whenever significant intravasation is suspected, serum sodium level should be checked immediately postoperatively and a few h later because later hyponatremia, presumably because of transperitoneal absorption, has been reported.

Hysteroscopic Procedures

Diagnostic hysteroscopy. This common procedure often is performed prior to uterine curettage to identify any focal abnormalities such as an endometrial polyp or a malignancy. This procedure usually is performed in the operating room with either general or regional anesthesia, although it has been performed by some as an office procedure with minimal analgesia.

After determining the position of the uterus, the anterior cervix is grasped with a tenaculum and traction placed to straighten the cervical canal. The lens and diagnostic sleeve are placed into the cervix, and distention medium is introduced with a pressure of 80–90 mmHg. The hysteroscope is advanced slowly and carefully toward the fundus, using tactile and visual cues to avoid perforation. The entire uterine cavity is inspected, and any abnormal anatomy is documented. As the hysteroscope is withdrawn, the uterocervical junction and the endocervix are examined.

Directed endometrial biopsy. If a focal abnormality of the endometrium is observed, directed biopsy may be more accurate than a simple uterine curettage. The cervix is dilated to allow passage of an 8–10-mm flow-through operating hysteroscope, and a balanced salt solution is used for distention. Once the hysteroscope is positioned in the uterine cavity, the area of interest is biopsied under direct visualization.

Polypectomy. If an intrauterine polyp is discovered, the base of the polyp is incised with hysteroscopic scissors, and the polyp is grasped with grasping forceps. The hysteroscope, sleeve, and polyp are removed simultaneously, because most polyps will not fit through the operating channel. Extremely large polyps may have to be removed piecemeal. Any residual base of the polyp may be removed with biopsy forceps.

Uterine septum resection. A septum may be resected with scissors, electro-surgery, or laser. Scissors are used most commonly in light of the minimal vascularity of septa and the decreased potential for bowel injury should inad-vertent uterine perforation occur. An operating hysteroscope is placed into the uterine cavity, which will appear to be two tubular structures rather than the broad uterine fundus usually encountered. The septum is then evenly divided across the fundus. If scissors are used, rather than a power cutting instrument, the presence of bleeding indicates that the level of resection is shifting from the avascular septum to the vascular myometrium. After surgery, no special device is placed in the uterus because intrauterine synechiae formation is uncommon.

Removal of intrauterine synechiae. Intrauterine synechiae almost always are associated with previous uterine curettage, especially when performed in the immediate postpartum period. These synechiae may result in amenorrhea or infertility.

The removal of synechiae is performed in a manner similar to that described above for a uterine septum, with some differences. The first is that the anatomy, and thus the visual cues for location of normal uterine wall, are completely unpredictable from patient to patient. Preoperative hysterosalpingography usu-ally is very helpful. Findings can vary from a few small synechiae to complete obliteration of the cavity.

In difficult cases, simultaneous transabdominal ultrasound is extremely helpful in guiding the direction and limits of hysteroscopic resection. Standby laparoscopy should be available in the event of perforation, which is a significant risk in these patients. However, once pneumoperitoneum is achieved, abdominal ultrasound is no longer possible.

Following surgery, some type of intrauterine splint, such as an intrauterine device or a balloon catheter, often is placed to avoid synechia re-formation. Patients usually are placed on estrogen supplementation for a month and prophylactic antibiotics until the intrauterine splint is removed 1–2 weeks later.

Intrauterine myomectomy. Pedunculated or submucosal leiomyoma can be removed safely hysteroscopically with subsequent improvement in both abnormal uterine bleeding and infertility. Because myoma tissue is relatively dense, a power cutting instrument is required. The choices are either laser or, more commonly, electrosurgery. For argon or Nd-to-YAG laser, a fiber is placed through the operating channel of the operating hysteroscope, and a balanced salt solution is used for distention. When electrosurgery is used via a hysteroresectoscope, an electrolyte-free solution, such as glycine or sorbitol, must be used because a balanced salt solution will dissipate the current and prevent cutting. Use of an electrolyte-free solution requires a thorough understanding of the potential risk and prevention of hyponatremia, because fatal complications have been reported with its use (see "Fluid Overload and Hyponatremia" below).

Both pedunculated and submucosal fibroids are shaved into small pieces with either the laser fiber or the hysteroresectoscope. In the case of a pedunculated fibroid, the urge to simply transect the stalk as a first step should be resisted unless the fibroid is 10 mm or less in size. Fibroids that are larger than this are difficult to remove in one piece without excessive cervical dilatation. Morcellation is much easier when the stalk is still attached for stability.

When the field of view is obscured by multiple pieces of tissue, the hysteroresectoscope is removed and the tissue collected in the urologic pouch. The hysteroscope is replaced in the uterus, and the procedure is repeated until the pedunculated fibroid and its stalk are completely removed, or the submucosal fibroid is shaved flush to the adjacent wall of the uterine cavity. After surgery, some gynecologists will treat the patient with estrogen or place an intrauterine splint as described above (see "Removal of Intrauterine Synechiae" above).

Risks of Hysteroscopy

Gas embolism. Gas embolism has been reported when using CO_2 for distention after intrauterine surgery. It is recommended that CO_2 not be used for any operative procedure or after significant dilation of the cervix. If symptoms of massive gas embolism occur during diagnostic hysteroscopy, the procedure should be stopped and the patient treated as described elsewhere.

Fluid overload and hyponatremia. During operative hysteroscopy, significant intravasation of distention medium can occur through venous channels opened during surgery or transperitoneally as a result of any fluid forced through the tubes. Symptomatic fluid overload has been reported with all fluid distention media, including 32 percent dextran 70 in dextrose. The volume of distention medium introduced through the operating hysteroscope or hysteroresectoscope should always be compared with the volume retrieved using a urologic collection drape. When using a balanced salt solution (e.g., Ringer lactate solution), symptomatic fluid overload is treated effectively with diuretics.

When electrolyte-free solutions are used for electrosurgery, the potential exists for serious and even fatal hyponatremia, even without significant fluid overload. Electrolyte-free solutions should not be used for hysteroscopy when electrosurgery is not required. When these solutions are used, careful monitoring of fluid balance should be performed every 15 min to detect intravasation.

Uterine perforation and bowel injury. Uterine perforation is a common risk of uterine dilation prior to hysteroscopy. If it is not possible to distend the uterine cavity when the hysteroscope is placed in the uterus, perforation should be suspected. If no sharp instrument or power source has been placed through the defect, expectant outpatient management is appropriate. Occasionally, perforation will occur during resection of a septum or leiomyoma or other operative procedures. If any chance of bowel injury exists, laparoscopy to evaluate contiguous bowel for injury is a reasonable precaution.

Intrauterine synechia. The formation of adhesions between the anterior and posterior uterine walls, referred to as synechiae, is an uncommon complication after intrauterine surgery. Although intrauterine devices, intrauterine catheters, and high-dose estrogen therapy have been advocated to decrease the risk of this complication, the efficacy of these treatments remains uncertain.

Abdominal Procedures

Incisions

There are several incisions used in pelvic surgery. The midline incision is the most useful. It is simple and tends to bleed less than incisions made off the midline. The midline incision provides excellent exposure of the pelvis, and, when necessary, the entire abdomen is accessible for operation. This incision is more susceptible to hernia formation and is somewhat more uncomfortable than the transverse incision. The resulting scar occasionally is thicker than incisions made along the Langer lines, resulting in a less-desirable cosmetic result.

Transverse incisions are used more often by a pelvic surgeon because the entire incision is centered over the area of operative interest. The incisions are more comfortable postoperatively and heal with a lower incidence of dehiscence or hernia formation. The most common transverse incision is the Pfannenstiel incision. The skin is incised transversely approximately 2 cm above the symphysis pubis, and the incision is taken down to the rectus fascia, which is entered transversely. The rectus fascia is dissected bluntly away from the underlying rectus muscles in both a superior and inferior direction. The rectus muscles are separated in the midline, and the peritoneum is opened in the vertical midline.

The Maylard incision carries with it the advantages of a transverse incision but affords more exposure of the pelvis than that provided by the Pfannenstiel. The skin is incised transversely approximately 4–6 cm above the symphysis pubis, and the rectus fascia is opened transversely but not separated from the underlying rectus muscles. The rectus muscles are cut directly under the fascial incision, and several small bleeders in the body of the rectus muscles are clamped and coagulated. The epigastric artery and vein located just below the lateral edge of the rectus muscles are ligated and cut; the peritoneum is then opened transversely to afford good visualization and access to the entire pelvis.

The Cherney incision provides the advantages of a transverse incision and all the visibility provided by the Maylard incision. The incision is made in the transverse direction in the lower abdomen approximately 2 cm above the symphysis, the rectus fascia is opened transversely, the lower portion of the rectus sheath is dissected free of the rectus muscle, and the insertion of the rectus muscles on the symphysis pubis is visualized. The tendon of the rectus muscle is then cut free of the symphysis pubis, and the muscle is allowed to retract upward. The peritoneum is opened transversely. This incision is repaired by simply sewing the rectus tendon to the lower aspect of the rectus sheath just above the symphysis before closing the rectus sheath at the completion of the operation.

Hysterectomy for Benign Disease

The abdomen is entered through an appropriate incision. The upper abdomen is examined for evidence of extrapelvic disease, and a suitable retractor is placed in the abdominal wound. The bowel is packed out of the pelvis and held in place with a retractor. The uterus is grasped at either cornu and elevated. The round ligament is identified and suture ligated and cut or electrocautorized. If the ovaries are to be removed, the peritoneal incision is extended from the round ligament lateral to the infundibulopelvic ligament for approximately 2.5 cm. The retroperitoneal space is bluntly opened. The ureter is identified on the medial leaf of the broad ligament. The infundibulopelvic ligament is isolated, clamped, and cut, and ligated. A similar procedure is carried out on the opposite side.

In the event that the ovaries are not to be removed, after ligating the round ligament, an avascular area in the broad ligament is chosen and the broad ligament bluntly fractured with a finger, producing an opening below the ovarian ligament and fallopian tube. The fallopian tube and ovarian ligament are clamped, cut, and ligated.

Upward traction is placed on the uterus. The peritoneum in the anterior cul-de-sac is opened between the ligated round ligaments. The bladder is mobilized by sharply dissecting it free of the anterior surface of the uterus and cervix. The uterine vessels are skeletonized by transilluminating the fold of the broad ligament and dissecting the avascular tissue off the uterine vessels. The peritoneum on the posterior surface of the uterus is dissected free of the uterus and then cut. Clamps are placed on the uterine vessels at the cervicouterine junction. The vessels are cut and the clamps replaced with suture ligatures. The bladder is again examined to ensure that it has been mobilized sufficiently from the vagina near the cervix. The cardinal ligaments are clamped, cut, and ligated. Following division of the cardinal ligaments, the uterus is elevated and the vagina entered with scissors or a knife. The uterus and cervix are cut free of the vagina. Sutures are placed at each lateral angle of the vagina, and the cardinal ligament is sutured to either lateral vaginal angle. The central portion of the vagina is left open after repairing it with a running absorbable suture. Pelvic reperitonealization is not necessary. The rectosigmoid colon is allowed to return to the pelvis. The pelvic packs are removed and the small bowel is allowed to return to the pelvis. The omentum is placed over the bowel and under the abdominal wound. The abdominal wound is closed in an appropriate manner. In some circumstances, uterine myomata interfere with the operative procedure and myomectomy or supracervical hysterectomy might be accomplished before removing the cervix. Control of vascular pedicles may also be accomplished using linear stapling devices or bipolar cautery.

Myomectomy

Myomectomy should be performed through an incision that will allow good visibility of the pelvis. Hemostasis for the procedure is aided by the placement of a Penrose drain around the base of the uterus and pulled through small perforations in the broad ligament lateral to the uterine blood supply on either side. This "uterine tourniquet" is held in place with a clamp.

Further hemostasis may be obtained by placing bulldog or rubber-shod clamps on the infundibulopelvic ligament to control the utero-ovarian blood supply. When possible, the uterine incision should be made in the anterior surface of the uterus to reduce the incidence of postoperative adhesions. An incision is made through the uterine musculature into the myoma. The pseudo-capsule surrounding the tumor is identified and the tumor is bluntly dissected out with scissors, a knife handle, or a finger. After the tumor is freed of its lateral attachments, it can be twisted to expose a pedicle that frequently contains its major blood supply. On occasion, several myomas may be removed through a single incision. The uterine wounds are closed with absorbable sutures to obliterate the dead space and provide hemostasis. The uterine serosa is closed with a 000 absorbable suture placed subserosally if possible. Adhesion barriers may be used.

Radical Hysterectomy (Modified from Okabayashi)

The patient is placed in a modified lithotomy position with legs in obstetric stirrups, hips abducted 45 degrees and flexed 15 degrees. The peritoneal cavity is entered through a Maylard incision after ligating and dividing the inferior epigastric vessels. The Maylard incision permits unequaled exposure of structures on the lateral pelvic sidewall. Access to the retroperitoneum is obtained by dividing the round ligaments. A U-shaped incision is carried from one lateral abdominal gutter to the other, including the peritoneum of the bladder reflection. The pararectal and paravesical spaces are opened using blunt digital or instrument dissection, and narrow rigid retractors are placed to maintain exposure. Pelvic lymphadenectomy is performed by removing lymph nodes from the external, internal, and common iliac vessels, and the obturator fossa. If there are no pelvic lymph node metastases, para-aortic lymph node sampling is unnecessary. Isolation of the superior vesicle artery by lateral retraction of the obliterated umbilical artery brings the uterine artery into view; this vessel is skeletonized and clipped at its origin from the anterior division of the internal iliac artery. Next, the structures inferior to the uterine artery in the cardinal ligament are clamped and divided; freeing the cervix and upper vagina from the lateral pelvic sidewall. A linear stapling device may expedite this portion of the procedure.

At this point, the proper ovarian ligaments and the proximal fallopian tubes may be transected between clamps. After the ovarian vessels are mobilized, the ovaries may be marked with vascular clips and suspended in the lateral abdominal gutters above the pelvic brim. This measure protects the ovaries if postoperative pelvic radiotherapy is to be given. The ureters are carefully detached from the posterior leaves of the broad ligament for a short distance and retracted laterally before the posterior cul-de-sac is entered and the rectovaginal space developed bluntly; the uterosacral ligaments are divided. Upward traction on the uterus facilitates dissection of the bladder inferiorly away from the underlying cervix and upper vagina. The ureters are freed from their investment in the paracervical tissue, allowing the bladder and ureters to be displaced inferolaterally, exposing the upper vagina and paravaginal tissues. The tissues are clamped and cut, taking care to remove a 3–4-cm margin of vagina with the cervix. The vagina is closed, a suprapubic catheter is inserted, and the abdominal incision is repaired.

Radical hysterectomy is associated with 85–90 percent cure rates in patients without lymph node, parametrial, or marginal involvement, and with 65–70 percent cure rates in those with spread to the regional nodes. The primary morbidity is bladder denervation, which occurs to some extent in almost all women undergoing this procedure. Generally, loss of bladder sensation is the only deficit, although inability to void is not uncommon in the immediate postoperative period. Rectal dysfunction may result in difficult defecation. Ureterovaginal fistulas occur in approximately 1 percent of all patients in recent studies.

Postoperative external beam radiotherapy may be elected if nodal metastases, positive surgical margins, or parametrial tissue involvement is found. Because bladder and ureteral complications are more common in women undergoing postoperative radiotherapy, surgical candidates must be chosen with care.

Resection of Ovarian Cancer

Radical or modified radical hysterectomy is indicated in the treatment of epithelial ovarian cancer only if peritoneal tumor nodules obliterate the posterior cul-de-sac or extend to the retroperitoneal spaces. Generally, extrafascial (simple or conservative) hysterectomy suffices in the resection of these tumors.

When hysterectomy and salpingo-oophorectomy are completed, the omentum should be removed by reflecting the fatty organ superiorly, isolating and dividing the right and left gastroepiploic vessels, and dissecting through the avascular posterior leaf before isolating and dividing the vessels in the anterior leaf of the omentum. If the omentum contains a large amount of disease, the gastrocolic omentum should be removed by isolating and dividing the short gastric vessels along the greater curvature of the stomach. In cases of extensive omental involvement, care must be taken not to injure the spleen, stomach, or transverse colon. Generous peritoneal biopsies should be obtained from the right hemidiaphragm, both lateral abdominal gutters, and the anterior and posterior peritoneum of the pelvis.

If gross intraperitoneal tumor is completely resected, the lymph nodes should be evaluated. The left para-aortic lymph nodes may be exposed by reflecting the sigmoid colon medially. These lymph nodes should be liberally sampled, keeping in mind that the primary venous drainage of the left ovary is the left renal vein and that of the right ovary is the inferior vena cava at the level of the renal vein. Metastases are more common above than below the inferior mesenteric artery. The right para-aortic lymph nodes may be sampled transperitoneally or by mobilizing the ileocecal area and reflecting it superiorly.

Pelvic lymph node sampling is also an important aspect of surgical staging in ovarian cancer and is completed by removing lymph nodes from the distribution of the external and internal iliac vessels and obturator space above the level of the obturator nerve. This part of the staging procedure is facilitated by first opening the paravesical and pararectal spaces as described for radical hysterectomy above. Lymph node sampling is primarily a diagnostic procedure in the management of early ovarian cancers. Complete lymphadenectomy may extend disease-free interval, but does not affect survival in patients with advanced disease.

Vaginal Procedures

Hysterectomy

The removal of the uterus through the vagina is preferred in many cases of myoma, uterine prolapse, intraepithelial neoplasia, and uterine bleeding disorders. Patients are more comfortable and operative time, hospital stay, and recovery time are shorter than in cases of abdominal operation. Vaginal hysterectomy is an acceptable approach in those patients in whom the uterus descends, the bony pelvis allows vaginal operation, the uterine tumors are small enough to permit vaginal removal, and the patient is amenable to vaginal operation. The patient is placed in a high lithotomy position, and the pelvis is examined under anesthesia. This examination should confirm previous findings and provide assurance that the operation is possible through the vaginal route. The bladder is not catheterized before operation unless it is greatly distended. A weighted vaginal speculum is placed in the posterior vagina, and the cervix is grasped with a tenaculum and pulled in the axis of the vagina. The posterior cul-de-sac is identified and entered with scissors. Mayo scissors are used to circumcise the cervix, and the mucosa is cut down to the pubocervical-vesical fascia. The vaginal mucosa and the bladder are sharply and bluntly dissected free of the cervix and the lower portion of the uterus. When the peritoneum of the anterior cul-de-sac is identified, it is entered with the scissors, and a retractor is placed in the defect. The uterosacral ligaments are identified, doubly clamped, cut, and ligated. Serial clamps are placed on the parametrial structures above the uterosacral ligament; these pedicles are cut, and the clamps are replaced with ties. At the cornu of the uterus, the tube, round ligament, and suspensory ligament of the ovary are doubly clamped and cut. The procedure is carried out on the opposite side, and the uterus is removed. The first clamp is replaced with a free tie; the second clamp is replaced with a suture ligature that is transfixed. The second suture ligature is held long. The pelvis is inspected for hemostasis; all bleeding must be meticulously controlled at this point.

The pelvic peritoneum is closed with a running purse-string suture incorporating those pedicles which were held. This exteriorizes those areas which might tend to bleed. The sutures attached to the ovarian pedicles are cut. The vagina may be closed with interrupted mattress stitches, incorporating the uterosacral ligaments into the corner of the vagina with each lateral stitch. The vaginal cuff is inspected again for hemostasis. In most cases, no vaginal packing is required. A catheter is left in the bladder until the patient has fully awakened and is ambulatory.

On occasion, the uterus, which is initially too large to remove vaginally, may be reduced in size by morcellation. After the uterine vessels have been clamped and ligated, serial wedges are taken from the central portion of the uterus to reduce the uterine mass. This procedure will allow the vaginal delivery of even very large uterine leiomyomas.

Suggested Readings

Baggish MS, Sze EH: Endometrial ablation: A series of 568 patients treated over an 11-year period. Am J Obstet Gynecol 174:908, 1966. Copeland LJ: Textbook for Gynecology. St. Louis: CV Mosby, 1993.

Herbst AL, Michell D, et al: Comprehensive Gynecology, 2d ed. St. Louis: CV Mosby, 1992.

Hoskins WJ, Perez. CA, Young RC (eds): Gynecologic Oncology. 3rd ed. Philadelphia: JB Lippincott, 2004.

Hurd WW, Bude RO, et al: The location of abdominal wall blood vessels in relationship to abdominal landmarks apparent at laparoscopy. Am J Obstet Gynecol 171:642, 1994.

Kurman RJ: Blaustein's Pathology of the Female Genital Tract, 4th ed. New York: Springer-Verlag, 1994.

Lee RH: Atlas of Gynecologic Surgery. Philadelphia: WB Saunders, 1992.

Nichols DH: Gynecologic and Obstetric Surgery. St Louis: CV Mosby, 1993.

Rubin SC, Sutton GP (eds): Ovarian Cancer, 2nd ed. New York: McGraw-Hill, 2002.

Saidi MH, Sadler RK, et al: Diagnosis and management of serious urinary complications after major operative laparoscopy. Obstet Gynecol 87:272, 1996.

Shingleton HM, Fowler WC, et al (eds): Gynecologic Oncology. Philadelphia: WB Saunders, 1996.

Singer A, Monaghan JM: Lower Genital Tract Precancer. Boston: Blackwell Scientific, 1994.

Speroff L, Glass RH, Kase NG: Clinical Gynecologic Endocrinology and Infertility, 5th ed. Baltimore: Williams and Wilkins, 1994.

Steege JF: Laparoscopic approach to the adnexal mass. Clin Obstet Gynecol 37:392, 1994.

Thompson JD, Rock JA (eds): TeLinde's Operative Gynecology, 7th ed. Philadelphia: JB Lippincott, 1992.

Bump RC, Norton PA. Epidemiology and natural history of pelvic floor dysfunction. Obstet Gynecol Clin N Am 1998;25(4):723–747.

Urinary Incontinence Guideline Panel. Urinary incontinence in adults: clinical practice guidelines. Rockville, MD: US Department of Health and Human Services. AHCPR Publication no. 92-0038, March 1992.

Abrams P, Cardozo L, Fall M et al. The standardisation of terminology of lower urinary tract function: report from the Standardisation Sub-committee of the International Continence Society. Neurourol Urodyn 2002;21:167–178.

41 | Neurosurgery

Michael L. Smith and M. Sean Grady

Neurologic surgery is a discipline of medicine and the specialty of surgery that provides the operative and nonoperative management including prevention, diagnosis, evaluation, treatment, critical care, and rehabilitation of disorders of the central, peripheral, and autonomic nervous systems, including their supporting structures and vascular supply; the evaluation and treatment of pathologic processes that modify the function or activity of the nervous system, including the hypophysis; and the operative and nonoperative management of pain. As such, neurologic surgery encompasses the treatment of adult and pediatric patients with disorders of the nervous system. These disorders include those of the brain, meninges, skull and skull base, and their blood supply, including surgical and endovascular treatment of disorders of the intracranial and extracranial vasculature supplying the brain and spinal cord; disorders of the pituitary gland; disorders of the spinal cord, meninges, and vertebral column, including those that may require treatment by fusion, instrumentation, or endovascular techniques; and disorders of the cranial and spinal nerves throughout their distribution (courtesy of the American Board of Neurological Surgeons).

An accurate history is the first step toward neurologic diagnosis. A history of trauma or of neurologic symptoms is of obvious interest, but general constitutional symptoms also are important. Neurologic disease may have systemic effects, although diseases of other symptoms may affect neurologic function. The patient's general medical ability to withstand the physiologic stress of anesthesia and surgery should be understood. A detailed history from the patient and/or family, along with a reliable physical examination will clarify these issues.

NEUROANATOMY

The cerebral hemispheres consist of the cerebral cortex, underlying white matter, the basal ganglia, hippocampus, and amygdala. The cerebral cortex is the most recently evolved part of the nervous system. The frontal areas are involved in executive function, decision making, and restraint of emotions. The motor strip, or precentral gyrus, is the most posterior component of the frontal lobes, and is arranged along a homunculus with the head inferior and lateral to the lower extremities superiorly and medially. The motor speech area (Broca area) lies in the left posterior inferior frontal lobe in almost all right-handed people and in up to 90 percent of left-handed people. The parietal lobe lies between the central sulcus anteriorly and the occipital lobe posteriorly. The postcentral gyrus is the sensory strip, also arranged along a homunculus. The visual cortex is arrayed along the medial surfaces of the occipital lobes. The temporal lobes lie below the sylvian fissures. The hippocampus, amygdala, and lower optic radiations (Meyer loops) are important components of the temporal lobe.

Lying deep to the cerebral hemispheres the thalamus and hypothalamus. The thalamus is a key processor and relay circuit for most motor and sensory information going to or coming from the cortex. The hypothalamus, at the base of the brain, is a key regulator of homeostasis, via the autonomic and neuroendocrine systems.

The brain stem consists of the midbrain, pons, and medulla. Longitudinal fibers run through the brain stem, carrying motor and sensory information between the cerebral hemispheres and the spinal cord. The nuclei of cranial nerves III through XII are also located within the brain stem. The cerebellum arises from the dorsal aspect of the brain stem.

The ventricular system is a cerebrospinal fluid (CSF)-containing contiguous space inside the brain, continuous with the subarachnoid space outside the brain. There are two lateral ventricles, and the third and fourth ventricle. Choroid plexus creates the CSF, mostly in the lateral ventricles. The average adult has an approximate CSF volume of 150 mL and creates approximately 500 mL per day.

The spinal cord starts at the bottom of the medulla and extends through the spinal canal down to approximately the first lumbar vertebra. It transmits motor (efferent) and sensory (afferent) information between the brain and the body. Paired nerves exit the spinal cord at each level. There are 31 pairs: 8 cervical, 12 thoracic, 5 lumbar, 5 sacral, and 1 coccygeal. The C5–T1 spinal nerves intersect in the brachial plexus and divide to form the main nerve branches to the arm, including the median, ulnar, and radial nerves. The L2–S4 spinal nerves intersect in the lumbosacral plexus and divide to form the main nerve branches to the leg, including the common peroneal, tibial, and femoral nerves.

The autonomic nervous system (ANS) carries messages for homeostasis and visceral regulation from the central nervous system (CNS) to target structures such as arteries, veins, the heart, sweat glands, and the digestive tract. The ANS is divided into the sympathetic, parasympathetic, and enteric systems. The sympathetic system drives the "fight or flight" response, and uses epinephrine to increase heart rate, blood pressure, blood glucose, and temperature, and to dilate the pupils. The parasympathetic system promotes the "rest and digest" state, and uses acetylcholine to maintain basal metabolic function under nonstressful circumstances. The enteric nervous system controls the synchronization of the digestive tract. It can run autonomously, but is under the regulation of the sympathetic and parasympathetic systems.

NEUROLOGIC EXAMINATION

Mental status is assessed first. A patient may be awake, lethargic, stuporous, or comatose. Cranial nerves may be thoroughly tested in the awake patient, but pupil reactivity, eye movement, facial symmetry, and gag are the most relevant when mental status is impaired. Motor testing is based on maximal effort of major muscle groups in those able to follow commands, although reaction to pain may be all that is possible for stuporous patients. Characteristic motor reactions to pain in patients with depressed mental status include withdrawal from stimulus, localization to stimulus, flexor (decorticate) posturing, extensor (decerebrate) posturing, or no reaction (in order of worsening pathology). Light touch, proprioception, temperature, and pain testing may be useful in awake patients. It is critical to document sensory patterns in spinal cord injury patients. Muscle stretch reflexes should be checked for symmetry and amplitude. Check for ankle-jerk clonus or up-going toes (the Babinski test). Presence of either is pathologic and signifies upper motor neuron disease.

Diagnostic Studies

Plain Films

Plain radiographs of the skull may demonstrate fractures, osteolytic or osteoblastic lesions, or pneumocephaly (air in the head). Plain spine films are used to assess for fracture, soft-tissue swelling, spinal deformities, osteolytic, or osteoblastic processes.

Computed Tomography (CT)

The noncontrast head CT scan of the head is useful in the setting of new focal neurologic deficit, decreased mental status, or trauma. It is very sensitive for hemorrhage. A contrast-enhanced CT scan will help show neoplastic or infectious processes. Spine CT scans are helpful for defining bony anatomy and pathology, and is usually done after an abnormality is seen on plain films. New high-speed scanners allow CT-angiography (CT-A). CT-A does not reliably detect lesions such as cerebral aneurysms less than 3 mm across, but can provide detailed morphologic data of larger lesions.

Magnetic Resonance Imaging (MR)

MRI provides better soft tissue imaging than does CT. Several MRI sequences are available. T1 with and without gadolinium are useful for detecting neoplastic and infectious processes. T2 sequences facilitate assessment of neural compression in the spine by the presence or absence of bright T2 CSF signals around the cord or nerve roots. Diffusion-weighted images (DWI) can detect ischemic stroke earlier than CT. Time-of-flight (TOF) images can be reformatted to build MR-angiograms (MR-A) and MRI-venograms (MR-V).

Angiography

Transarterial catheter-based angiography remains the standard criterion for evaluation of vascular pathology of the brain and spine because of its ability to detect smaller lesions and give dynamic flow information.

Electromyography and Nerve Conduction Studies (EMG/NCS)

These studies evaluate the function of peripheral nerves. EMG records muscle activity in response to stimulation of a motor nerve. NCS records the velocity and amplitude of the nerve action potential. EMG/NCS is typically performed 3–4 weeks after an acute injury.

Invasive Monitoring

Intracranial monitors are used in patients with intracranial pathology without a reliable neurologic exam.

External ventricular drain (EVD, ventriculosomy). A catheter is inserted into the frontal horn of the lateral ventricle. ICP can be transduced, and CSF drained to reduce ICP or for laboratory studies.

Intraparenchymal fiberoptic pressure transducer ("bolt"). It allows ICP monitoring, and is smaller and less invasive than a ventriculostomy.

Brain tissue oxygen sensors. Patients with brain trauma or aneurysmal hemorrhage may have insufficient brain oxygen tension with relatively normal ICPs. Oxygen sensors can provide additional management information.

NEUROLOGIC AND NEUROSURGICAL EMERGENCIES

Raised Intracranial Pressure

ICP normally varies between 4 and 14 mmHg. Sustained ICP levels above 20 mmHg can injure the brain. The Monro-Kellie doctrine states that the cranial vault is a rigid structure, and therefore the total volume of the contents determines ICP. The three normal contents of the cranial vault are brain, blood, and CSF. The brain can swell because of traumatic brain injury (TBI), stroke, or reactive edema. Intravascular (vasodilation) or extravascular (hematoma) blood volume can increase. CSF volume increases in the setting of hydrocephalus. Addition of a fourth element, such as a tumor or abscess, will also increase ICP.

Increased ICP often presents with headache, nausea, vomiting, and mental status decline. Cushing triad is the classic presentation of ICH: hypertension, bradycardia, and irregular respirations. This triad is usually a late manifestation. Patients with these symptoms should have an urgent head CT.

Brain Stem Compression

Mass effect in the posterior can rapidly kill by occluding the fourth ventricle causing acute obstructive hydrocephalus, or directly crushing the brain stem. Both cause rapid mental status decline and death but are treatable if caught immediately.

Stroke

Patients who present with acute focal neurologic deficits for whom the time of onset of symptoms can be clearly defined must be evaluated rapidly. A patient with a clinical diagnosis of acute stroke younger than 3 h old, without hemorrhage on CT, may be a candidate for thrombolytic therapy with tissue plasminogen activator (t-PA).

Seizure

Seizures may be because of a tumor, hematoma, or intrinsic brain disorder. A seizing patient is at risk for neurologic damage if the seizure is not stopped, and airway and ventilation problems. Any patient with new-onset seizure should have imaging of the brain, such as a head CT scan, after the seizure is controlled and the patient resuscitated.

TRAUMA

Trauma is a leading cause of death and disability in children and young adults. The three main areas of neurosurgic interest in trauma are traumatic brain injury (TBI), spine and spinal cord injury (SCI), and peripheral nerve injury.

Head Trauma

Glasgow Coma Scale (GCS) Score

Neurosurgical evaluation begins as part of "D" after "ABC" in the primary evaluation with assessment of the Glasgow Coma Scale. Table 41-1 describes how the GCS is determined.

TABLE 41-1 The Glasgow Coma Scale (GCS) Score[a]

Motor response (M)		Verbal response (V)		Eye-opening response (E)	
Obeys commands	6	Oriented	5	Opens spontaneously	4
Localizes to pain	5	Confused	4	Opens to speech	3
Withdraws from pain	4	Inappropriate words	3	Opens to pain	2
Flexor posturing	3	Unintelligible sounds	2	No eye opening	1
Extensor posturing	2	No sounds	1		
No movement	1	Intubated	T		

[a]Add the three scores to obtain the Glasgow Coma Scale score, which can range from 3 to 15. Add "T" after the GCS if intubated and no verbal score is possible. For these patients, the GCS can range from 2T to 10T.

Scalp Injury

The scalp is densely vascularized and can contribute to significant blood loss. Lacerations should be irrigated and sutured closed, either in one layer if simple or two layers (galea and skin) if long and complex.

Skull Fractures

A closed fracture is covered by intact skin. A compound fracture is associated with open skin. The fracture lines may be single (linear), multiple and radiating from a point (stellate), multiple, creating fragments of bone (comminuted), or pushed into the brain (depressed). Closed skull fractures do not normally require specific treatment. Open fractures require repair of the scalp. Depressed fractures may require craniotomy to elevate the bone, evacuate associated blood clots, and stop bleeding.

Skull base fractures are common in TBI patients. They indicate significant impacts and are generally apparent on CT. If asymptomatic, they require no treatment. Symptoms from skull base fractures include cranial nerve deficits (anosmia, facial palsy) and CSF leaks (rhinorrhea, otorrhea). Many CSF leaks will heal with elevation of the head of the bed for several days although some require a lumbar drain or direct surgical repair. There is no proven efficacy of antibiotic coverage for preventing meningitis in patients with CSF leaks. Traumatic cranial neuropathies are generally followed conservatively. Steroids may help facial nerve palsies.

Closed Head Injury

Closed head injury (CHI) is the most common type of TBI. There are two components of CHI and TBI in general. The initial impact causes the primary injury, defined as the immediate injury to neurons from transmission of the force of impact. Prevention strategies, such as wearing helmets, remain the best means to decrease disability from primary injury. Subsequent neuronal damage because of hypotension, hypoxia, hematomas, or increased ICP is referred to as secondary injury.

Initial assessment. Hypoxia and hypotension worsen outcome in TBI (secondary injury), so cardiopulmonary stabilization is critical. Patients who cannot follow commands require intubation for airway protection and ventilatory control. Spontaneous movements and responsiveness to voice commands or pain gives an initial indication of severity of injury.

Medical management. Phenytoin prophylaxis may decrease the incidence of early post-TBI seizures. Blood glucose and body temperature should be kept normal. Peptic ulcers occurring in patients with head injury or high ICP are referred to as Cushing ulcers, and may be reduced with H_2-blockers. Compression stockings should be used when the patient cannot be mobilized rapidly.

Classification. TBI can be classified as mild (GCS 14–15), moderate (GCS 9–13), or severe (GCS 3–8).

TBI patients who are asymptomatic; have only headache, dizziness, or scalp lacerations or abrasions; or did not lose consciousness have a low risk for intracranial injury and may be discharged home without a head CT. Patients with a history of altered or lost consciousness, amnesia, progressive headache, skull or facial fracture, vomiting, or seizure have a moderate risk for intracranial injury and should undergo prompt head CT. If the CT is normal, and the neurologic exam has returned to baseline (excluding amnesia of the event), then the patient can be discharged to the care of a responsible adult.

Patients with depressed consciousness, focal neurologic deficits, penetrating injury, depressed skull fracture, or changing neurologic exam have a high risk for intracranial injury. These patients should undergo immediate head CT and admission for observation or intervention as needed.

Concussion. Temporary neuronal dysfunction after TBI. The CT is normal and deficits resolve over min to h. Amnesia is very common. The brain remains in a hypermetabolic state for up to a week after injury and is more susceptible to injury from even minor head trauma in the first 1–2 weeks after concussion (second-impact syndrome). Patients should be informed that even after mild head injury they may experience memory difficulties or persistent headaches.

Contusion. A contusion is a bruise of the brain, and occurs when the force from trauma is sufficient to cause breakdown of small vessels and extravasation of blood into the brain. The contused areas appear bright on CT scan. They may be under the area of impact (coup injury) or opposite the area of impact (contrecoup injury). They frequently do not require direct treatment unless they enlarge or hemorrhage and cause mass effect.

Diffuse axonal injury. Diffuse axonal injury is caused by damage to axons throughout the brain, because of rotational acceleration and then deceleration. Axons may be completely disrupted and then retract, forming axon balls. Small hemorrhages can be seen in more severe cases, especially on MRI. Hemorrhage is classically seen in the corpus callosum and the dorsolateral midbrain (Duret hemorrhage).

Penetrating injury. The two main subtypes are missile injury (e.g., bullets) and nonmissile injury (e.g., knives). Skull radiographs and CT scans are useful in assessing the nature of the injury. Cerebral angiography must be considered if the object passes near a major artery or dural venous sinus. Operative exploration is necessary to remove any object extending out of the cranium, and for débridement, irrigation, hemostasis, and definitive closure. Small objects contained within brain parenchyma often are left in place to avoid iatrogenic secondary brain injury.

Traumatic Intracranial Hematomas

The various traumatic intracranial hematomas contribute to death and disability secondary to head injury. Hematomas can expand rapidly and cause brain shifting and subsequent herniation.

Epidural hematoma (EDH). Tearing of the middle meningeal artery results in accumulation of blood between the skull and the dura. CT reveals a bright biconvex (lentiform) clot. EDH has a classic three-stage clinical presentation with immediate loss of consciousness (concussion), a lucid interval, and then lethargy and herniation as the hematoma expands. This is probably seen in only 20 percent of cases. Treatment of symptomatic EDH is craniotomy.

Acute subdural hematoma (SDH). Tearing of a bridging vein from the cerebral cortex to the dural sinuses leads to subdural blood accumulation. CT reveals a bright crescent-shaped (lunate) clot. Craniotomy is indicated for any acute SDH more than 1 cm in thickness, or smaller hematomas that are symptomatic. Symptoms may be as subtle as a contralateral pronator drift, or as dramatic as coma. Smaller hematomas may stabilize and eventually reabsorb, or become chronic SDHs. The prognosis for functional recovery is significantly worse for acute SDH than EDH because it is associated with greater primary injury to brain parenchyma from high-energy impacts.

Chronic subdural hematoma. Small acute SDHs may not resorb and may evolve from blood clots to a dark motor-oil-like fluid that may expand and cause delayed symptoms. A chronic SDH thicker than 1 cm, or any symptomatic SDH should be surgically drained via a burr hole.

Intraparenchymal hemorrhage. Isolated hematomas within the brain parenchyma may be due TBI but hypertensive hemorrhage, arteriovenous malformations, or underlying tumors are more likely.

Vascular Injury

Trauma to the head or neck may cause dissection of the carotid or vertebrobasilar arteries. The newly created space within the vessel wall is referred to as the false lumen. Dissection can cause ischemia or thromboembolism in supplied tissues. Diagnosis is by four-vessel angiography, which may reveal stenosis of the true lumen, visible intimal flaps, or the appearance of contrast in the false lumen. Neurology may assist with antiplatelet or anticoagulation therapies. Endovascular options include vessel occlusion or stenting.

Carotid dissection. Carotid dissection may result from neck extension combined with lateral bending to the opposite side, or trauma from an incorrectly placed shoulder belt tightening across the neck in a motor vehicle accident. Symptoms of cervical carotid dissection include contralateral neurologic deficit from brain ischemia, headache, and ipsilateral Horner syndrome from disruption of the sympathetic tracts ascending from the stellate ganglion into the head on the surface of the carotid artery. Traumatic vessel wall injury to the portion of the carotid artery running through the cavernous sinus may result in a carotid-cavernous fistula (CCF). These present with pulsatile proptosis (the globe pulses outward with arterial pulsation), retro-orbital pain, and decreased visual acuity or loss of normal eye movement (because of damage to cranial nerves III, IV, and VI in the cavernous sinus). Symptomatic CCFs should be treated by balloon occlusion to preserve eye function.

Vertebrobasilar dissection. Vertebrobasilar dissection may result from sudden rotation or flexion/extension of the neck, chiropractic manipulation, or a direct blow to the neck. Common symptoms are neck pain, headache, brain stem stroke, or subarachnoid hemorrhage.

Brain Death

Brain death occurs when there is an absence of signs of brain stem function or motor response to deep central pain in the absence of pharmacologic or systemic medical conditions that could impair brain function.

Clinical examination. Two exams consistent with brain death 12 h apart, or one exam consistent with brain death followed by a consistent confirmatory study is generally sufficient to declare brain death. The patient must be normotensive, euthermic, oxygenating well, and not be under the effects of sedating or paralytic drugs.

Documentation of no brain stem function includes the following: nonreactive pupils; lack of corneal blink, oculocephalic (doll's eyes), or oculovestibular (cold calorics) reflexes; and loss of drive to breathe (apnea test). The apnea test demonstrates failure of spontaneous breathing when $Paco_2$ is allowed to rise above 60 mmHg.

Deep central painful stimulus is provided by forceful twisting pinch of the sensitive skin above the clavicle. Pathologic responses such as flexor or extensor posturing are not compatible with brain death. Spinal reflexes to peripheral pain, such as triple flexion of the lower extremities, are compatible with brain death.

Confirmatory studies. Lack of cerebral blood flow consistent with brain death may be documented by cerebral angiography, technetium radionuclide study, and transcranial Doppler ultrasonography. An electroencephalogram (EEG) documenting electrical silence is not favored because there is often artifact or noise on the recording.

Spine Trauma

Damage to the bone or soft tissues of the spine can reduce its stability and its ability to protect the spinal cord and nerve roots. Spine trauma may occur with or without neurologic injury. Neurologic injury may be incomplete, if there is some residual motor or sensory neurologic function below the level of the lesion, or complete, if there is no residual neurologic function below the level of the lesion. A patient with 24 h of complete neurologic dysfunction has a low probability of return of function in the involved area.

The Mechanics of Spine Trauma

Flexion/extension. Bending the head and body forward into a fetal position flexes the spine. Arching the neck and back extends the spine. Extension loads the spine posteriorly and distracts the spine anteriorly.

Compression/distraction. Force applied along the spinal axis (axial loading) compresses the spine. A pulling force in line with the spinal axis distracts the spine.

Rotation. Force applied tangential to the spinal axis rotates the spine.

Patterns of Injury

Remember that a patient with a spine injury at one level is at significant risk for additional injuries at other levels.

Cervical. The cervical spine is more mobile than the thoracolumbar spine. Stability comes primarily from the multiple ligamentous connections of adjacent vertebral levels. Disruption of the cervical ligaments can lead to instability in the absence of fracture.

Jefferson fracture. Bursting fracture of the ring of C1 (the atlas) because of compression forces. There are usually two or more fractures through the ring of C1. The open-mouth odontoid view may show lateral dislocation of the lateral masses of C1. The rule of Spence states that 7 mm or greater combined dislocation indicates disruption of the transverse ligament and the potential need for surgical stabilization.

Odontoid fractures. The odontoid process, or dens, is the large ellipse of bone arising anteriorly from C2 (the axis) and projecting up through the ring of C1 (the atlas). Odontoid fractures usually result from flexion forces. Odontoid fractures are classified as type I, II, or III. A type I fracture involves the tip only. A type II fracture passes through the base of the odontoid process. A type III fracture passes through the body. Type II fractures are most likely to need surgery.

Hangman's fracture. Either hyperextension/distraction or hyperextension/compression. The part of C2 bridging C1–C3 is broken. Most hangman's fractures heal well with external immobilization.

Jumped facets. The facet joints of the cervical spine slope forward, and the facet from the level above can slide up and forward over the facet from the level below if the joint capsule is torn. Patients with a unilateral injury are usually neurologically intact, although those with bilateral injury usually have spinal cord compression.

Thoracolumbar. The thoracic spine is significantly stabilized by the rib cage. The lumbar spine has comparatively very large vertebrae. Thus the thoracolumbar spine has a higher threshold for injury than the cervical spine. The three-column model is useful for categorizing thoracolumbar injuries. The anterior longitudinal ligament and the anterior half of the vertebral body constitute the anterior column. The posterior half of the vertebral body and the posterior longitudinal ligament constitute the middle column. The pedicles, facet joints, laminae, spinous processes, and interspinous ligaments constitute the posterior column.

Compression fracture. Compression/flexion injury causing failure of the anterior column only. It is stable and not associated with neurologic deficit, although the patient may have significant pain.

Burst fracture. Axial compression injury causing failure of the anterior and middle columns. It is unstable, and perhaps patients may have neurologic deficit because of retropulsion of bone fragments.

Chance fracture. Flexion-distraction injury causing failure of the middle and posterior columns. It is unstable and is often associated with neurologic deficit.

Fracture-dislocation. Flexion/distraction, shear, or compression injuries causing failure of the anterior, middle, and posterior columns. They are unstable and often associated with neurologic deficit.

Initial Assessment and Management

The possibility of a spine injury must be considered in all trauma patients. A patient with no symptoms referable to neurologic injury, a normal neurologic exam, no neck or back pain, and a known mechanism of injury unlikely to cause spine injury is at minimal risk for significant injury to the spine. Victims of moderate or severe trauma, especially those with injuries to other organ systems, usually fail to meet these criteria or cannot be assessed adequately. The latter is often because of impaired sensorium or significant pain. Because of the potentially catastrophic consequences of failure to diagnose spine instability in a neurologically intact patient, spine precautions should be maintained until fully evaluated.

Studies

Plain radiographs provide initial assessment of spinal alignment but are often inadequate for full evaluation. CT and MR scans are useful adjuncts.

Definitive Management

Spinal-dose steroids. The National Acute Spinal Cord Injury Study (NASCIS) I and II papers provide controversial evidence of improved outcome in spinal cord injury patients if they are given high-dose methylprednisolone acutely.

Orthotic devices. External stabilization by decreasing range of motion and minimizing stress transmitted through the spine. Philadelphia and Miami-J hard collars stabilize the neck. Cervical collars are poor for C1, C2, or cervicothoracic instability. Halo-vest assemblies provide the most external cervical stabilization. Four pins driven into the skull lock the halo ring in position. Four posts arising from a tight-fitting rigid plastic vest immobilize the halo ring. Lumbar stabilization may be provided by thoracolumbosacral orthoses (TLSOs).

Surgery. Neurosurgical intervention has two goals. First is the decompression of the spinal cord or nerve roots in patients with incomplete neurologic deficits. These patients should be decompressed expeditiously if there is evidence of neurologic deterioration over time. Second is the stabilization of injuries judged too unstable to heal with external orthotics only. Surgical stabilization can allow early mobilization, aggressive nursing care, and physical therapy and may decrease the need for burdensome orthotics.

Continued Care

Regional spinal cord injury centers with nurses, respiratory therapists, pulmonologists, physical therapists, physiatrists, and neurosurgeons specifically trained in caring for these patients may improve outcomes. Acute issues include hypotension and aspiration pneumonia. Chronic issues include deep venous thrombosis, autonomic hyperreflexia, and decubitus ulcer formation. Patients should be transferred to spinal cord injury rehabilitation centers after stabilization of medical and surgical issues.

Peripheral Nerve Trauma

The peripheral nervous system extends throughout the body and is subject to injury from a wide variety of traumas. Peripheral nerves transmit motor and sensory information between the CNS and the body.

The four major mechanisms of injury to peripheral nerves are laceration (knives, bullets), stretch (hematomas, fracture), compression (casts, external blow), and contusion (shock wave from bullet).

The following four characteristics make a nerve segment more vulnerable to injury: proximity to a joint, superficial course, passage through a confined space, and fixed position.

The Seddon Classification

Neurapraxia. (Least severe) Temporary failure of nerve function without physical axonal disruption. Axon degeneration does not occur. Return of normal axonal function occurs over h to months, often in the 2–4-week range.

Axonotmesis. Disruption of axons and myelin. The surrounding connective tissues, including endoneurium, are intact. The axons degenerate proximally and distally (Wallerian degeneration) from the area of injury. Axon regeneration within the connective tissue pathways can occur at a rate of 1 mm per day. Recovery may occur for up to 18 months. Scarring at the site of injury from connective tissue reaction can form a neuroma and interfere with regeneration.

Neurotmesis. (Most severe) Disruption of axons and endoneurial tubes. Peripheral collagenous components, such as the epineurium, may or may not be intact. Proximal and distal axonal degeneration occurs.

Management of Peripheral Nerve Injury

The sensory and motor deficits should be documented. Deficits are usually immediate. Clean and sharp or progressing injuries may benefit from early exploration and repair. Most other peripheral nerve injuries should be observed and be tested by EMG/NCS after 3–4 weeks if deficits persist. If there is no improvement over 3 months the injury should be explored. Surgical techniques include nerve grafting and neuroma excision. The tissue structure of the graft provides a pathway for axon regrowth.

Patterns of Injury

Brachial plexus. Susceptible to injury during parturition, falls, and motorcycle accidents by stetching or shoulder dislocation. A lung apex tumor, known as a Pancoast tumor, can cause compression injury to the plexus. Two well-known patterns of plexus injury are Erb palsy and Klumpke palsy. Injury high in the plexus to the C5 and C6 roots resulting from glenohumeral dislocation causes Erb palsy with the characteristic "bellhop's tip" position. The arm hangs at the side, internally rotated. Hand movements are not affected. Injury low in the plexus, to the C8 and T1 roots, resulting from stretch or compression injury, causes Klumpke palsy with the characteristic "claw hand" deformity. There is weakness of the intrinsic hand muscles, similar to that seen with ulnar nerve injury.

Radial nerve. Susceptible to injury from improper crutch use, humerus fractures, or improper sleeping position (Saturday night palsy). The key finding is wrist drop (weakness of hand and finger extensors). Axillary (proximal) injury causes tricep weakness in addition to wrist drop.

Common peroneal nerve. Susceptible to injury from car bumpers in the lateral knee where it wraps superficially around the fibular neck. The key finding is foot drop (weakness of the tibialis anterior) and numbness over the anterolateral surface of the lower leg and dorsum of the foot.

CEREBROVASCULAR DISEASE

This is the most frequent cause of nontraumatic acute neurologic deficit. Common medical problems including diabetes, high cholesterol, hypertension, and smoking contribute to vascular disease by such mechanisms as atheroma deposition causing luminal stenosis, endothelial damage promoting thrombogenesis, and weakening of the vessel wall resulting in aneurysm formation or dissection. The most common cerebrovascular diseases are carotid stenosis, ischemic and hemorrhagic stroke, and aneurysm formation.

Ischemic Diseases

Ischemic stroke accounts for approximately 85 percent of acute cerebrovascular events. Arterial occlusion leads to ischemia in the neural tissues supplied by that vessel. This leads to immediate dysfunction and eventual tissue death. Symptoms depend on which area of the brain is ischemic. Collateral blood supply minimizes ischemia in some situations.

A transient ischemic attack (TIA) resolves within 24 h. A reversible ischemic neurologic deficit (RIND) resolves within one week. A stroke, i.e., a cerebrovascular accident, or CVA, indicates permanent neurologic deficit.

Thromboembolic Disease

Thombi that form in the heart, aorta, or carotid arteries can break off and embolize to the brain, causing vessel blockage and tissue ischemia. Thrombosis also can completely occlude the carotid artery and cause ischemia without embolus.

Management

Thrombus formation can be treated medically with anticoagulation and antiplatelet agents. Chronic atrial fibrillation is an indication for coumadin therapy. Patients with symptomatic carotid stenosis with 70–99 percent occlusion should undergo carotid endarterectomy. Certain asymptomatic carotid lesions also should be considered for surgery.

Patients with suspected stroke should have an immediate head CT to evaluate for hemorrhage. Management of ischemic stroke includes maintaining good cerebral perfusion pressure, aspirin, hydration, and careful neurologic monitoring on the neurology service.

Common Types of Strokes

Anterior cerebral artery stroke. The ACA supplies the medial frontal and parietal lobes, including the motor strip, as it courses into the interhemispheric fissure. ACA stroke results in contralateral leg weakness.

Middle cerebral artery stroke. The MCA supplies the lateral frontal and parietal lobes and the temporal lobe. MCA stroke results in contralateral face and arm weakness. Dominant-hemisphere MCA stroke causes language deficits. Proximal MCA occlusion causing ischemia and swelling in the entire MCA territory can lead to significant intracranial mass effect and midline shift and may benefit from decompressive hemicraniectomy (removing half of the skull).

Posterior cerebral artery stroke. The PCA supplies the occipital lobe. PCA stroke results in a contralateral homonymous hemianopsia.

Posterior inferior cerebellar artery stroke. The PICA supplies the lateral medulla and the inferior half of the cerebellar hemispheres. PICA stroke results in nausea, vomiting, nystagmus, dysphagia, ipsilateral Horner syndrome, and ipsilateral limb ataxia. The constellation of symptoms resulting from PICA occlusion is referred to as lateral medullary syndrome or Wallenberg's syndrome.

Hemorrhagic Diseases

Intracranial hemorrhage (ICH) from abnormal or diseased vascular structures accounts for approximately 15 percent of acute cerebrovascular events. Hypertension and amyloid angiopathy account for most intraparenchymal hemorrhages. Aneurysms and ateriovenous malformations (AVMs) are the most common causes of nontraumatic subarachnoid hemorrhage (SAH). Tumors and venous sinus thrombosis also can cause ICH.

Hypertension

Hypertension increases the relative risk of ICH by approximately 4-fold, likely because of chronic degenerative vasculopathy. Hypertensive hemorrhages often present in the basal ganglia, thalamus, or pons, and result from breakage of small perforating arteries that branch off of much larger parent vessels. Surgery often causes more injury than benefit.

Amyloid Angiopathy

Amyloid deposition in the media of small cortical vessels compromises vessel integrity and predisposes to more superficial (lobar) hemorrhages. Patients may have multiple hemorrhages over time. These occasionally benefit from surgery because they are more superficial than hypertensive hemorrhages.

Cerebral Aneurysm

Aneurysms are focal dilatation of the vessel wall that usually occur at branch points of major vessels. They may be saccular (balloon-like) or fusiform (elongated). They have thin, weakened walls and are prone to rupture, causing subarachnoid hemorrhage (SAH). Symptoms range from sudden "thunderclap" headache to coma or death. The Hunt-Hess grading system categorizes patients clinically (Table 41-2). Patients with suspected SAH should have a head CT immediately. If the CT is negative but clinical suspicion is high, a lumbar puncture should be performed to look for xanthochromia. If either is positive the patient should have a four-vessel cerebral angiography within 24 h to assess for aneurysms or other vascular malformations.

SAH patients should be resuscitated as needed and admitted to the neurologic ICU. Ruptured aneurysms require occlusion by surgical clipping or endovascular coiling according to the neurosurgeon's judgment. Certain aneurysms are more appropriate for one approach or the other. The International Subarachnoid Aneurysm Trial (ISAT) researchers suggested that endovascular occlusion resulted in better outcomes for certain types of cerebral aneurysms, however, this trial was marred by poor selection and randomization

TABLE 41-2 The Hunt-Hess Clinical Grading System for Subarachnoid Hemorrhage

Hunt-Hess grade	Clinical presentation
0	Unruptured aneurysm
1	Awake; asymptomatic or mild headache; mild nuchal rigidity
2	Awake; moderate to severe headache, cranial nerve palsy (e.g., CN III or IV), nuchal rigidity
3	Lethargic; mild focal neurologic deficit (e.g., pronator drift)
4	Stuporous; significant neurologic deficit (e.g., hemiplegia)
5	Comatose; posturing

techniques and the validity of its conclusions have been questioned. Debate also continues regarding optimal care for unruptured intracranial aneurysms.

SAH patients often require 1–3 weeks of ICU care after aneurysm occlusion for medical complications that accompany neurologic injury. In addition to routine ICU concerns, SAH patients also are at risk for cerebral vasospasm, which is pathologic vessel constriction 4–21 days after SAH, potentially causing ischemia and stroke.

Arteriovenous Malformations

AVMs are abnormal, dilated arteries and veins without an intervening capillary bed. They may bleed or cause seizures. AVMs hemorrhage at an average rate of 2–4 percent a year.

Three therapeutic modalities for AVMs are currently in common use: microsurgical excision, endovascular glue embolization, and stereotactic radiosurgery. Each has limitations so they are often used in combination.

TUMORS OF THE CENTRAL NERVOUS SYSTEM

A wide variety of tumors affect the brain and spine. Primary benign and malignant tumors arise from the various elements of the CNS, including neurons, glia, and meninges. Tumors metastasize to the CNS from many primary sources. Presentation and prognosis vary widely depending on location and histology.

Brain Tumors

Brain tumors may be clinically silent and found incidentally or cause symptoms from mass effect or seizures. Supratentorial tumors commonly present with focal neurologic deficit, such as contralateral limb weakness or visual field deficit, or headache or seizure. Infratentorial tumors often cause increased ICP because of hydrocephalus because of compression of the fourth ventricle, leading to headache, nausea, vomiting, or diplopia. Cerebellar hemisphere or brain stem dysfunction can lead to ataxia, nystagmus, or cranial nerve palsies. Infratentorial tumors rarely cause seizures. Patients with such symptoms should undergo head CT or brain MRI with contrast.

Metastatic Tumors

The sources of most cerebral metastases are (in decreasing frequency) the lung, breast, kidney, gastrointestinal (GI) tract, and melanoma. Lung and breast cancers account for more than half of cerebral metastases. Metastases often are very well circumscribed, round, and multiple.

Craniotomy for resection of 1–3 metastases followed by whole brain radiation can improve survival. Stereotactic radiosurgery also is an option.

Glial Tumors

Glial cells provide the anatomic and physiologic support for neurons and their processes in the brain. The several types of glial cells (astrocytes, oligo-dendrocytes, ependymal and choroid cells) give rise to distinct primary CNS neoplasms.

Astrocytomas

Astrocytomas are the most common primary CNS neoplasm. They are graded from I–IV. Grades I and II are referred to as low-grade astrocytoma (LGA), grade III as anaplastic astrocytoma (AA), and grade IV as glioblastoma multiforme (GBM). Hypercellularity, nuclear atypia, neovascularity, and necrosis characterize higher grades. Median survival for LGA is 8 years, AA is 2–3 years, and GBM is 1 year. GBMs account for almost two-thirds of all astrocytomas, AAs account for two-thirds of the rest, and LGAs the remainder.

The treatment for GBMs and AAs is surgical resection followed by brain radiation. Management of LGAs is less clear and may involve stereotactic biopsy, resection, radiation, or observation. Adjuvant chemotherapy remains disappointing but clinical trials are ongoing. Brachytherapy with carmustine wafers provides a small increase in length of survival for GBMs.

Oligodendroglioma

These account for approximately 10 percent of gliomas. They often present with seizures and demonstrate calcifications and hemorrhage on CT. Oligo-dendrogliomas also are graded from I–IV; grade portends prognosis. Prognosis is slightly better overall than for astrocytomas. Median survival ranges from 2–7 years for highest and lowest grade tumors, respectively. Aggressive resection improves survival. Chemotherapy, and occasionally radiation, are adjuvants.

Ependymoma

The lining of the ventricular system consists of cuboidal/columnar ependymal cells from which ependymomas may arise. They arise from the lateral, third, and fourth ventricles and often cause symptomatic hydrocephalus. They may metastasize within the CNS. Two main histologic subtypes are papillary ependymomas and anaplastic ependymomas, with the latter characterized by increased mitotic activity and areas of necrosis. Gross total resection can result in cure. Radiation is usually administered postoperatively.

Choroid Plexus Papilloma and Carcinoma

The choroid plexus is composed of many small vascular tufts covered with cuboidal epithelium. Choroid plexus papillomas and carcinomas arise from these cells. They are uncommon. Papillomas are well circumscribed and vividly enhance because of extensive vasculature. They often present with hydrocephalus. Treatment is surgical excision; total surgical excision is curative.

Neural Tumors and Mixed Tumors

Neural and mixed tumors are a diverse group that includes tumors variously containing normal or abnormal neurons and/or normal or abnormal glial cells. Primitive neuroectodermal tumors (PNETs) arise from bipotential cells, capable of differentiating into neurons or glial cells.

Medulloblastoma

Medulloblastoma is the most common malignant pediatric brain tumor. They are usually midline in the posterior fossa and present with hydrocephalus. Histologic characteristics include densely packed small round cells with large nuclei and scant cytoplasm. They are generally not encapsulated, frequently disseminate within the CNS, and should undergo surgical resection followed by radiation therapy and chemotherapy.

Ganglioglioma

Ganglioglioma is a mixed tumor in which both neurons and glial cells are neoplastic. They present in the first three decades of life with seizures. They are usually circumscribed masses in the medial temporal lobe, often with cysts or calcium. Patients have a good prognosis after complete surgical resection.

Neural Crest Tumors

Multipotent neural crest cells develop into a variety of disparate cell types, including smooth muscle cells, sympathetic and parasympathetic neurons, melanocytes, Schwann cells, and arachnoid cap cells. They migrate in early development from the primitive neural tube throughout the body.

Miscellaneous Tumors

Meningioma

Meningiomas are derived from arachnoid cap cells of the arachnoid mater. They appear to arise from the dura mater grossly and on MRI, and so are commonly referred to as dural-based tumors. The most common intracranial locations are along the falx, the convexities (over the cerebral hemispheres), and the sphenoid wing. Less common locations include the foramen magnum, olfactory groove, and inside the lateral ventricle. Most are slow growing, encapsulated, benign tumors. Aggressive atypical or malignant meningiomas may invade adjacent bone or into the cortex. Previous cranial irradiation increases the incidence of meningiomas. Approximately 10 percent of patients with a meningioma have multiple meningiomas. Total resection is curative, although involvement with small perforating arteries or cranial nerves may make total resection of skull base tumors impossible without significant neurologic deficit. Small, asymptomatic meningiomas can be followed until symptoms present or growth is documented. Atypical and malignant meningiomas may require postoperative radiation. Patients may develop recurrences from the surgical bed or distant de novo tumors.

Vestibular Schwannoma (VS or Acoustic Neuroma)

VSs arise from the superior half of the vestibular portion of the vestibulocochlear nerve (cranial nerve VIII). They present with progressive hearing loss, tinnitus, or balance difficulty. Large tumors may cause brain stem compression and obstructive hydrocephalus. Bilateral VSs are pathognomonic for neurofibromatosis type 2, a syndrome resulting from chromosome 22 mutation associated with an increased incidence of meningiomas and gliomas.

Vestibular schwannomas may be treated with microsurgical resection or with stereotactic radiosurgery. The main complication of either treatment is damage to the facial nerve (cranial nerve VII), which runs through the internal auditory canal with the vestibulocochlear nerve. Risk of facial nerve dysfunction increases with increasing tumor diameter.

Pituitary Adenoma

Pituitary adenomas arise from the anterior pituitary gland. They are microadenomas if less than 1 cm in diameter, macroadenomas if larger, functional if they secrete endocrinologically active compounds, or nonfunctional (silent) if they do not. Functional tumors are often diagnosed when quite small because of endocrine symptoms. The most common endocrine syndromes are Cushing disease because of adrenocorticotropic hormone (ACTH) secretion, Forbes-Albright syndrome because of prolactin secretion, and acromegaly because of growth hormone secretion. Nonfunctional tumors commonly present when larger because of mass effect (visual field deficits because of compression of the optic chiasm, panhypopituitarism because of compression of the gland). Pituitary apoplexy is hemorrhage into an adenoma causing abrupt headache, visual disturbance, decreased mental status, and endocrine dysfunction. It may require urgent decompressive surgery. Surgical resection is indicated to eliminate symptomatic mass effect or to attempt endocrine cure in medically refractory cases. Prolactinomas usually shrink with dopaminergic therapy. Most pituitary tumors are approached through the nose by the transsphenoidal approach. Endoscopic sinus surgery techniques may be helpful and are increasingly being used.

Hemangioblastoma

Hemangioblastomas occur almost exclusively in the posterior fossa. Twenty percent occur in patients with von Hippel-Lindau (vHL) disease, a multisystem neoplastic disorder associated with renal cell carcinoma, pheochromocytoma, and retinal angiomas. Many appear as cystic tumors with an enhancing mural (wall) nodule. Surgical resection of the nodule is curative for sporadic (non-vHL) tumors.

Lymphoma

CNS lymphoma may arise primarily in the CNS or secondary to systemic disease. Increasing incidence may be because of increasing numbers of immunocompromised people in the transplant and acquired immune deficiency syndrome (AIDS) populations. Presenting symptoms include mental status changes, headache because of increased ICP, and cranial nerve palsy because of lymphomatous meningitis (analogous to carcinomatous meningitis). Surgical excision has little role. Diagnosis often is made by stereotactic needle biopsy. Subsequent treatment includes steroids, whole brain radiation, and chemotherapy. Intrathecal methotrexate chemotherapy is an option.

Embryologic Tumors

Embryologic tumors result from embryonal remnants that fail to involute completely or differentiate properly during development.

Craniopharyngioma

Craniopharyngiomas are cystic, usually calcified lesions with bimodal incidence peaks in childhood and the fifth decade of life. Symptoms include visual field defects, endocrine dysfunction, or hydrocephalus from mass effect on the optic chiasm, pituitary, or third ventricle. Treatment is primarily surgical. These are histologically benign but clinically more malignant because of difficult resection frequently causing neurologic injury (visual loss, panhypopituitarism, diabetes insipidus, and cognitive impairment from basal frontal injury).

Epidermoid

These are cystic lesions with stratified squamous epithelial walls from trapped ectodermal cell rests that grow slowly and linearly by desquamation into the cyst cavity. The cysts contain keratin, cholesterol, and cellular debris. They occur most frequently in the cerebellopontine angle and may cause symptoms because of brain stem compression. Recurrent bouts of aseptic meningitis may occur because of release of irritating cyst contents into the subarachnoid space (Mollaret meningitis). Treatment is surgical drainage and removal of cyst wall. Intraoperative spillage of cyst contents leads to severe chemical meningitis and must be avoided by containment and aspiration.

Dermoid

Dermoids are less common than epidermoids. They contain hair follicles and sebaceous glands in addition to a squamous epithelium. Dermoids are more commonly midline structures and are associated with other anomalies than are epidermoids. They may be traumatic, as from a lumbar puncture that drags skin structures into the CNS. Bacterial meningitis may occur when associated with a dermal sinus tract to the skin. Treatment of symptomatic lesions is surgical resection, again with care to control cyst contents.

Teratoma

Teratomas are germ cell tumors that arise in the midline, often in the pineal region. They contain elements from all three embryonal layers: ectoderm, mesoderm, and endoderm. Teratomas may contain skin, cartilage, GI glands, and teeth. Teratomas with more primitive features are more malignant, although those with more differentiated tissues are more benign. Surgical excision may be attempted. Prognosis for malignant teratoma is very poor.

Spinal Tumors

A wide variety of tumors affect the spine. Approximately 20 percent of CNS tumors occur in the spine. The majority of spinal tumors are histologically benign. Understanding the concepts of spinal stability and neural compression facilitates understanding of the effects of spinal tumors. Destruction of bones or ligaments can cause spinal instability and lead to deformities such as kyphosis or subluxation and possible subsequent neural compression. Tumor growth in the spinal canal or neural foramina can cause direct compression of the spinal cord or nerve roots resulting in neurologic deficit.

Extradural Tumors

Extradural tumors comprise 55 percent of spinal tumors. This category includes tumors arising within the bony structures of the vertebrae and in the epidural space. Destruction of the bone can lead to instability and fractures, leading to pain and/or deformity. Epidural expansion can lead to spinal cord or nerve root compression with myelopathy or radiculopathy, respectively.

Metastatic tumors. Metastatic tumors are the most common extradural tumors. Spinal metastases most commonly occur in the thoracic and lumbar vertebral bodies because the greatest volume of red bone marrow is found therein. The most common primary tumors are lymphoma, lung, breast, and prostate. Other sources include renal, colon, thyroid, sarcoma, and melanoma. Most spinal metastases create osteolytic lesions. Osteoblastic, sclerotic lesions suggest prostate cancer in men and breast cancer in women. Patients with progressing neurologic dysfunction or debilitating pain should undergo urgent surgery or radiation therapy. Preoperative neurologic function correlates with postoperative function. Patients may lose function over h. These patients should be given high-dose intravenous dexamethasone, taken immediately to MRI, and then to the operating room or radiation therapy suite, as appropriate.

Primary tumors. Hemangiomas are benign tumors found in 10 percent of people at autopsy. They occur in the vertebral bodies of the thoracolumbar spine and are frequently asymptomatic. They are often vascular and may hemorrhage, causing pain or neurologic deficit. Large hemangiomas can destabilize the body and predispose to fracture. Osteoblastic lesions include osteoid osteoma and osteoblastoma. The latter tends to be larger and more destructive. Aneurysmal bone cysts are nonneoplastic, expansile, lytic lesions containing thin-walled blood cavities that usually occur in the lamina or spinous processes of the cervicothoracic spine. They may cause pain or sufficiently weaken the bone to lead to fracture. Cancers arising primarily in the bony spine include Ewing sarcoma, osteosarcoma, chondrosarcoma, and plasmacytoma.

Intradural Extramedullary Tumors

Intradural extramedullary tumors comprise 40 percent of spinal tumors and arise from the meninges or nerve root elements. They may compress the spinal cord, causing myelopathy, or the nerve roots, causing radiculopathy. Most are benign, slow growing, and well circumscribed. Rare epidural masses include arachnoid cysts, dermoids, epidermoids, metastases, and gliomas.

Meningioma. Meningiomas arise from the arachnoid mater. They enhance on MRI, appear to have a "dural tail," and are most frequent in the thoracic spine. Treatment is surgery.

Schwannoma. Schwannomas are derived from peripheral nerve sheath Schwann cells. They are benign, encapsulated, and tend to grow out of the parent nerve. Two-thirds are entirely intradural, one sixth are entirely extradural, and one sixth are intra- and extra-dural ("dumb-bell" shaped). Treatment is surgery to alleviate symptoms and rule-out malignant disease. Patients with multiple schwannomas likely have neurofibromatosis type 2 (NF-2).

Neurofibroma. Neurofibromas tend to be more fusiform and grow within the parent nerve, rather than forming an encapsulated mass off the nerve, as with schwannomas. They are benign but not encapsulated. Treatment is by surgery, but salvage of the parent nerve is more challenging than with schwannomas. Thoracic and high cervical nerve roots may be sacrificed, with no or minimal deficit, to improve likelihood of total resection. Patients with multiple neurofibromas likely have von Recklinghausen neurofibromatosis (NF-1).

Intramedullary Tumors

Intramedullary tumors comprise 5 percent of spinal tumors. They arise within the parenchyma of the spinal cord. Common presenting symptoms are local or radicular pain, sensory loss, weakness, or sphincter dysfunction. Patients with such symptoms should undergo MRI.

Ependymoma. Ependymomas are the most common intramedullary tumors in adults. There are several histologic variants. The myxopapillary type occurs in the conus medullaris and has a better prognosis. The cellular type occurs more frequently in the cervical cord. Many have cystic areas and may contain hemorrhage. They are more likely than astrocytomes to have a clean surgical margin. Treatment is surgery and adjuvant radiation.

Astrocytoma. Astrocytomas are the most common intramedullary tumors in children. They may be associated with a dilated central canal, referred to as syringomyelia (syrinx). They are most commonly in the cervical cord and are usually low grade. Treatment is surgery and radiation but complete excision is rarely possible because of the nonencapsulated, infiltrative nature of the tumor. As such, patients with astrocytomas fare worse overall than patients with ependymomas.

Other tumors. Other types of rare tumors include high-grade astrocytomas, dermoids, epidermoids, teratomas, hemangiomas, hemangioblastomas, and metastases. Patients usually present with pain. Prognosis depends generally on preoperative function and the histologic characteristics of the lesion.

SPINE

The spine is a complex structure subject to a wide variety of pathologic processes, including degeneration, inflammation, infection, neoplasia, and trauma. Please refer to the sections on trauma, tumor, and infection for discussions of how these processes impact the spine.

The spine consists of a series of stacked vertebrae, intervening discs, and longitudinal ligaments. The vertebrae consist of the vertebral body anteriorly and the pedicles, articular facets, laminae, and spinous processes posteriorly. The intervertebral discs are composed of the tough, fibrous outer ring (annulus fibrosus) and the spongy central material (nucleus pulposus). They cushion adjacent vertebral bodies, absorb forces transmitted to the spine, and allow some movement. The ligaments stabilize the spine by limiting the motion of adjacent vertebrae.

Two concepts critical to understanding the mechanics and pathologic processes affecting the spine are stability and neural compression.

Stability

The spinal column is the principal structural component of the axial spine. It bears significant load. The vertebrae increase in size from the top to the bottom of the spine, correlating with the increased loads the lower spine must bear. The cervical spine is the most mobile. Cervical stability depends greatly on the integrity of the ligaments that run from level to level. The thoracic spine is the least mobile, because of the rib cage. The lumbar spine has large vertebrae, supports heavy loads, and has intermediate mobility. The sacral spine (sacrum) is fused together and has no intrinsic mobility. The load borne by the lumbar spine is transmitted to the pelvis via the sacrum. The coccyx is the inferiormost segment of the spine and does not contribute to load bearing or mobility.

A stable spine is one that can bear normal physiologic forces resulting from body mass, movement, and muscle contraction, although protecting the spinal cord and nerve roots by maintaining normal structure and alignment.

Radiographs and CT scans are good for detecting bony defects such as fractures or subluxation; MRI is better for detecting disruption of the ligaments and discs.

Neural Compression

Besides providing a stable central element of the body's support structure, the spine must also protect the spinal cord in the central canal and the nerve roots in the neural foramena. The spinal cord and nerve roots are normally suspended in CSF, free of mechanical compression. Degenerative disease, mass lesions, or traumatic movement can impinge on the CSF spaces and cause myelopathy (cord dysfunction,) or radiculopathy (nerve root dysfunction).

Myelopathy

Cord compression can lead to crush injury or ischemia because of reduced perfusion. Histopathologic changes can include edema, demyelination, gliosis (scarring), and necrosis, leading to impairments in motor, sensory, and/or autonomic function below the level of injury. Myelopathy leads to upper-motor neuron symptoms below the injury, including hyperreflexia and spasticity.

Radiculopathy

Nerve root compression causing radiculopathy can cause lower motor neuron signs (hyporeflexia, atrophy, and weakness) and sensory disturbances such as numbness, tingling sensations (paresthesias), burning sensations (dysesthesias), and shooting pain. Myelopathy and radiculopathy often present together in diseases that involve the central canal and the neural foramina. This can lead to lower motor neuron dysfunction at the level of disease, and upper motor neuron dysfunction below that level.

Patterns of Disease

Cervical Radiculopathy

The cervical nerve roots exit the central canal above the pedicle of the same-numbered vertebra and at the level of the higher adjacent intervertebral disc. Therefore a C5–C6 disc herniation will cause C6 radiculopathy. Most patients with acute disc herniations will improve without surgery. Progressive numbness, weakness, and/or refractory pain are indications for surgery. Nerves can be decompressed anteriorly by discectomy and fusion or posteriorly by hemilaminotomy.

Cervical Spondylotic Myelopathy

The term spondylosis refers to diffuse degenerative and hypertrophic changes of the discs, intervertebral joints, and ligaments. Spondylosis can cause myelopathy from cord compression, a syndrome called cervical spondylotic myelopathy (CSM). CSM presents with spasticity and hyperreflexia because of corticospinal tract dysfunction, upper extremity weakness and atrophy from degeneration of the motor neurons in the anterior horns of the spinal gray matter, and loss of lower extremity proprioception because of dorsal column injury. Patients complain of difficulty ambulating and using buttons and utensils. Treatment is operative decompression by cervical laminectomy or anterior decompression and fusion. Patients may have significant recovery or only prevention of further worsening.

Care must be taken to avoid misdiagnosing amyotrophic lateral sclerosis (ALS, Lou Gehrig disease) as CSM because both have similar upper and lower motor neuron findings. Two findings help differentiate CSM from ALS: cranial nerve dysfunction such as dysphagia (not caused by cervical spine disease) and sensory disturbance (not found in ALS).

Thoracic Disc Herniation

Thoracic disc herniation accounts for less than 1 percent of herniated discs. They may present with radicular pain leg spasticity because of thoracic myelopathy. Discectomy often requires an anterior approach via thoracotomy.

Lumbar Radiculopathy

The anatomy of the lumbar spine is such that a disc herniation compresses the passing nerve root that exits at the next lower level. Therefore, an L4–L5 disc herniation compresses the exiting L5 nerve root. Herniated lumbar discs normally cause pain lancing down the leg (sciatica). Most improve without surgery. Lumbar discectomy is indicated for symptoms persisting more than 6–8 weeks, progressive motor deficit (e.g., foot drop), or for patients with incapacitating pain not manageable with analgesics. After lumbar discectomy, approximately two thirds of patients will have complete relief of pain, and up to 85 percent will have significant improvement.

Neurogenic Claudication

Neurogenic claudication is low back and leg pain that occurs while walking and is relieved by stopping, leaning forward, or sitting. It is caused by lumbar spinal stenosis. It must be distinguished from vascular claudication, which tends to resolve quickly with cessation of walking without need to change position, be in a stocking distribution rather than a dermatomal distribution, and be associated with cold, pale feet. Lumbar laminectomy is offered when the pain causes unacceptable functional impairment.

Cauda Equina Syndrome

Lumbar disc herniation, epidural hematoma, epidural abscess, tumor, or traumatic subluxation from trauma can cause compression of the cauda equina (the lumbar and sacral nerve roots in the thecal sac below the end of the spinal cord at L1–L2). Symptoms are urinary retention, saddle anesthesia (numbness in the perineum, genitals, inner thighs), or progressing leg weakness. The patient should have an urgent MRI and surgical decompression.

Spine Fusion Surgery

Patients who have unstable spines (because of disease or surgery) often need restabilization by fusion. Fusion occurs when a solid mass of bone grows from one vertebral body to the next. This is called arthrodesis and is the same process of bone growth and remodeling that occurs to heal a fractured bone. Movement across a spine fusion site hinders solid fusion. External orthotics (hard collars, braces) and internal fixation with wires, screws, rods, and hooks minimize movement for the 2-4 months required for solid fusion. The arthodesis is the permanent cure; braces and fixation devices will all eventually fail if fusion does not occur.

PERIPHERAL NERVE

Common pathologic processes that compromise function of the peripheral nervous system include mechanical compression, ischemia, inflammation, and neoplasia.

Peripheral Nerve Tumors

Most peripheral nerve tumors are benign. Pain suggests malignancy. Treatment for peripheral nerve tumors is surgical resection to establish diagnosis and evaluate for signs of malignancy.

Schwannoma

Schwannomas are the most common peripheral nerve tumors. They arise from Schwann cells, which form myelin in peripheral nerves. They tend to grow slowly and eccentrically on the parent nerve and can usually be dissected free of the parent nerve for complete resection.

Neurofibroma

Neurofibromas arise within the nerve and tend to be fusiform masses. Neurofibromas are often difficult to resect completely without sacrifice of the parent nerve. Neurofibromas have a higher incidence of malignant transformation, so patients with known residual tumors require close observation.

Malignant Nerve Sheath Tumors

Patients with malignant peripheral nerve tumors typically complain of constant pain, rather than pain only on palpation, and are more likely to have motor and sensory deficits in the distribution of the parent nerve. Treatment for these tumors is radical excision, often requiring sacrifice of the parent nerve.

Entrapment Neuropathies

Neurologic dysfunction in nerves passing through a pathologically narrowed space. Typical symptoms are pain, numbness, and muscle atrophy.

Ulnar Neuropathy

The ulnar nerve is susceptible to injury in its passage posterior to the medial epicondyle in the elbow. Disease causes numbness/pain in the medial digits and intrinsic hand muscle weakness. If splinting and behavior modification fail the nerve should be surgically decompressed at the elbow.

Carpal Tunnel Syndrome

The median nerve is susceptible to injury in its passage through the carpal tunnel at the base of the palm. Disease causes numbness/pain in the lateral digits and thenar wasting. As with ulnar neuropathy, the patient should have surgical division of the flexor retinaculum if conservative measures fail.

INFECTION

Cranial

Osteomyelitis

The skull is highly vascular and resistant to infections. Paranasal sinus disease, craniotomy, or traumatic contamination can lead to osteomyelitis of the skull. Staphylococcus aureus and epidermidis are the most frequent organisms. Treatment is surgical débridement of involved bone followed by 2–4 months of antibiotics.

Subdural Empyema

Subdural empyema is a rapidly progressive pyogenic infection with fever and meningeal signs followed quickly by coma and death. Streptococci and staphylococci are the most frequently found organisms. Neurologic deficit results from inflammation of cortical blood vessels, leading to thrombosis and stroke. The treatment is urgent surgery, for lavage and microbiologic diagnosis, followed by culture-directed antiobiotic therapy. Rapid intervention may minimize the chance of permanent neurologic deficit or death.

Brain Abscess

Bacteria may invade the brain by hematogenous (endocarditis) or local (sinus) routes. Cerebritis (infected brain tissue) evolves into a walled-off abscess. Typical therapy is open or needle aspiration followed by antibiotics.

Spine

Pyogenic Vertebral Osteomyelitis

Destructive bacterial infection of the vertebrae that can result from hematogenous spread or local extension. *Staphylococcus aureus* and Enterobacter spp. are the most frequent etiologic organisms. Patients usually present with fever and back pain. There is increased incidence in diabetics, intravenous (IV) drug abusers, and dialysis patients. Most cases can be treated successfully with antibiotics alone, although surgery may be indicated for diagnosis, medical failure, or spinal stabilization.

Tuberculous Vertebral Osteomyelitis (Pott disease)

Tuberculous vertebral osteomyelitis is a more indolent infection. It rarely involves the intervertebral disc space. Treatment is with long-term antibiotics. Again, surgery may be indicated for diagnosis or spinal stabilization.

Discitis

Discitis is most commonly a postoperative infection. Spontaneous discitis occurs more commonly in children. *S. epidermidis* and *S. aureus* account for most cases. Patients may have back pain and fevers. Persistent cases require antibiotics. Surgery is generally unnecessary.

Epidural Abscess

Epidural abscesses present with back pain, fever, and neurologic deficit. S. aureus and Streptococcus spp. are the most common organisms. The source may be hematogenous spread, local extension, or operative contamination.

Surgery is indicated for diagnosis and neural decompression. Antibiotics are then administered.

FUNCTIONAL NEUROSURGERY

Epilepsy Surgery

Patients with recurrent seizures (epilepsy) refractory to medical managements may be candidates for epilepsy surgery. Surgery can cure seizures or allow better seizure control with less and fewer medication. Epilepsy surgery may be underused, given the relatively low risk of the procedures and the crippling effects of poorly controlled epilepsy.

Anterior Temporal Lobectomy

This is preformed for complex partial seizures (CPS) originating in the medial temporal lobe. Many patients with CPS have poor seizure control on medications and can improve significantly after surgery. Risks include visual field deficit, language or memory problems, and depression, but many patients will recover.

Corpus Callosotomy

This procedure "splits" the brain and can prevent seizure activity in one hemisphere from spreading to the other. Loss of consciousness requires bilateral seizure activity. A common indication is atonic seizures with drop attacks. The posterior one-third of the callosum is spared to minimize disconnection syndrome, which is the inability to match objects in the opposite visual hemifields, to identify objects held in one hand with the other hemifield, to write with the left hand, or to name objects held in the left hand (in left hemisphere–dominant patients).

Hemispherectomy

Children with intractable epilepsy, structural anomalies in one hemisphere, and contralateral hemiplegia, may have improved seizure control after resection of the hemisphere (anatomic hemispherectomy) or disruption of all connections to the hemisphere (functional hemispherectomy).

Deep Brain Stimulators (DBS)

Fine electrical leads placed in deep brain structures can modify pathologic signals that contribute to abnormal motor activity. The stimulators are placed by MRI-guided stereotaxic systems involving fixing a rigid cage around the head with skull pins.

Essential Tremor

Essential tremors are action tremors of 4–8 Hz rhythmic oscillation that often affect one arm or the head, start in the third or fourth decade, and may respond to beta blockers. Placement of a DBS in the contralateral ventrointermediate nucleus (VIN) of the thalamus can dramatically help refractory cases.

Parkinson Disease (Paralysis Agitans)

Parkinson's disease is a progressive disorder characterized by rigidity, bradykinesia, and resting tremor because of loss of dopamine-secreting neurons in the substantia nigra and locus ceruleus. Dopaminergic and anticholinergic agents minimize symptoms. Refractory cases can benefit from DBSs in the subthalamic nuclei (STN) or globus pallidus pars interna (GPi) with durable symptom control and decreased medication use.

Trigeminal Neuralgia (Tic Douloureux)

This is a syndrome of repetitive, unilateral, sharp and lancinating pains in the distribution of one of the three branches of the trigeminal nerve (cranial nerve V). This seems to result from pulsatile irritation of the root entry zone by a loop of the superior cerebellar artery. The pain is excruciating and can be debilitating. Medical therapy, including carbamazepine and amitriptyline, may reduce the frequency of events. Options for medically refractory cases include percutaneous injection of glycerol into the path of the nerve, peripheral transection of the nerve branches, stereotactic radiosurgery, and microvascular decompression (MVD). MVD involves a craniotomy to move the artery away from the root entry zone of the nerve to relieve compression. It remains the first definitive management option because stereotactic radiosurgery is associated with a high incidence of facial numbness.

STEREOTACTIC RADIOSURGERY (SRS)

SRS refers to techniques that allow delivery of high-dose radiation that conforms to the shape of the target and has rapid isodose fall-off, minimizing damage to adjacent neural structures. The two most common devices for this are the LINAC (linear accelerator) and the gamma knife.

Arteriovenous Malformations

SRS is an effective therapy for AVMs up to 3 cm in diameter. SRS is best for lesions that are difficult to access surgically. SRS is not effective for lesions larger than 3 cm and is associated with a 2–4 percent hemorrhage risk per year in the 2 years it takes for AVM obliteration. There are reports of late AVM recanalization and hemorrhage. SRS may be used as an adjuvant in lesions that cannot be completely resected surgically.

Vestibular Schwannomas

SRS is an alternative to microsurgical resection for vestibular schwannomas up to 2.5 cm in maximum diameter. It seems to be associated with lower incidence of early postoperative facial nerve palsy but an increased incidence of delayed palsies. Long-term follow up is now becoming available on this modality to compare it with microsurgery.

Intracranial Metastases

Patients with solitary or multiple intracranial metastases may be treated primarily with SRS. SRS plus whole-brain radiation therapy (WBRT) seems to be similar to craniotomy plus WBRT. SRS is being explored as a treatment for multiple metastases (up to seven) because surgery is usually inappropriate for these patients. Patients with multiple intracranial metastases have almost zero long-term survival, and most will die of their intracranial disease. These patients live 3–6 months on average with medical care and WBRT. This can be extended to 9–16 months with SRS or surgery, depending on tumor type, age, and patient condition.

CONGENITAL AND DEVELOPMENTAL ANOMALIES

Dysraphism

Dysraphisms are defects of fusion of the neural tube in the spine or cranium involving the neural tube or overlying bone or skin. Neural tube defects are among the most common congenital abnormalities but can be reduced with prenatal vitamins.

Spina Bifida Occulta

Spina bifida occulta is the congenital absence of posterior vertebral elements, including the spinous processes and the laminae. Patients are neurologically normal. It is common (25 percent incidence), but asymptomatic.

Spina Bifida with Myelomeningocele

Spina bifida with myelomeningocele (MM) describes congenital absence of posterior vertebral elements with protrusion of the meninges through the defect, and underlying neural structural abnormalities. Common findings are weakness and atrophy of the lower extremities, gait disturbance, urinary incontinence, and deformities of the foot. MMs arising from the high lumbar cord usually cause total paralysis and incontinence, although those arising from the sacral cord may have only clawing of the foot and partial urinary function. MM patients always have Chiari II malformations (abnormal downward herniation of the cerebellum and brain stem through the foramen magnum) and frequently have hydrocephalus. Treatment is closure of dura, fascia and skin over the defect.

Encephalocele

Herniation of brain encased in meninges through the skull that forms an extracranial mass is referred to as encephalocele. Most occur over the convexity of the skull. Treatment is excision of the herniated tissue and closure of the defect. Most patients with encephaloceles and meningoceles have impaired cognitive development. Patients with greater amounts of herniated neural tissue tend to have more severe cognitive deficits.

Craniosynostosis

Craniosynostosis is the abnormal early fusion of a cranial suture line with resultant restriction of skull growth in the affected area and compensatory bulging at the other sutures. Skull growth occurs at the cranial sutures for the first 2 years of life, at the end of which the skull has achieved over 90 percent of its eventual adult size. Fusion may involve any of the various sutures individually or in combination and results in characteristic patterns of abnormal head shapes. Treatment involves resection of the fused sutures and cranial remodeling as needed.

Hydrocephalus

Excess CSF in the brain that results in enlarged ventricles is known as hydrocephalus (HCP). The adult forms approximately 500 mL of CSF per day. CSF flows from the lateral to third to fourth ventricles and then to the subarachnoid space, where it is absorbed into the venous blood through the arachnoid granulations. Treatment for symptomatic HCP is shunting the CSF to the peritoneum, pleura, or right atrium.

Communicating Hydrocephalus

Obstruction at the level of the arachnoid granulations causes communicating HCP. This usually causes dilation of the lateral, third, and fourth ventricles equally. The most common causes in adults are meningitis and subarachnoid hemorrhage.

Obstructive Hydrocephalus

Obstruction of CSF pathways is known as obstructive HCP. Ventricles proximal to the obstruction dilate, although those distal to the obstruction remain normal in size. It is frequently caused by periventricular tumors or cerebellar hemorrhage. Obstructive hydrocephalus may present precipitously and require urgent ventriculostomy to prevent herniation.

Chiari I Malformation

Chiari I malformation is the caudal displacement of the cerebellar tonsils below the foramen magnum. It is often asymptomatic and found incidentally. Symptomatic patients usually present with headache, neck pain, or symptoms of myelopathy, including numbness or weakness in the extremities. The brain stem and lower cranial nerves are usually normal in Chiari I malformations. Symptomatic patients may be treated with suboccipital craniectomy to remove the posterior arch of the foramen magnum and the posterior ring of C1. Removal of these bony structures relieves the compression of the cerebellar tonsils and cervicomedullary junction, and may allow reestablishment of normal CSF flow patterns.

Suggested Readings

Ingebrigtsen R, Romner B: Routine early CT scan is cost-saving after minor head injury. Acta Neurol Scand 93:207, 1996.

Howard MA, Gross AS, Dacey RG, et al: Acute subdural hematomas: An age-dependent clinical entity. J Neurosurg 71:856, 1989.

Bracken MB, Shepard MJ, Collins WF, et al: Methylprednisolone or naloxone treatment after acute spinal cord injury: 1-Year follow up data. J Neurosurg 76:23, 1992.

North American Symptomatic Carotid Endarterectomy Trial Collaborators: Beneficial effects of carotid endarterectomy in symptomatic patients with high-grade carotid stenosis. N Engl J Med 325:445, 1991.

Monylneux A, Kerr R, Stratton I, et al: International Subarachnoid Aneurysm Trial (ISAT) of neurosurgical clipping versus endovascular coiling in 2143 patients with ruptured intracranial aneurysms: A randomised trial. Lancet 360:1267, 2002.

Benbadis S, Heriaud L, Tatum WO, et al: Epilepsy surgery, delays and referral patterns—are all your epilepsy patients controlled? Seizure 12:167, 2003.

Rausch R, et al: Early and late cognitive changes following temporal lobe surgery for epilepsy. Neurology 60:9551, 2003.

Rehncrona S, et al: Long-term efficacy of thalamic deep brain stimulation for tremor: Double-blind assessments. Move Disord 18:163, 2003.

Pan D, Guo WY, Chung WY, et al: Gamma knife radiosurgery as a single treatment modality for large cerebral AVMs. J Neurosurg 93:113, 2000.

Gerosa M, Nicolato A, Foroni R, et al: Gamma knife radiosurgery for brain metastases: A primary therapeutic option. J Neurosurg 97:515, 2002.

42 | Orthopaedics

Dempsey Springfield

SKELETAL GROWTH AND PHYSIOLOGY

The skeletal system is initially formed as cartilage with the exception of the craniofacial bones and clavicle. These bones do not have a cartilaginous analogue and are formed directly from membranous tissue. The process of bone formation without an intermediate cartilage form is called intramembranous bone formation. The majority of an adult's bone is formed by intramembranous bone formation because diaphyseal bone grows circumferentially by the apposition of bone by the surrounding periosteum without cartilage being produced. Enchondral ossifications is the formation of bone through the initial formation of a cartilage model that then becomes bone. The skeletal system is formed in utero as cartilage; however, prior to birth, some of these prebone structures are well on their way to bone formation. This happens first in the middle of the diaphysis, known as the primary center of ossification. Later, at the secondary ossification center, bone will begin to form at the ends of the prebone structures. The secondary center of ossification has articular cartilage surrounding it on the side facing the joint and epiphyseal cartilage on the side facing the primary ossification center. The bone grows in length through the epiphyseal growth plate, which produces cartilage that undergoes enchondral ossification.

The epiphyseal growth plate is made up of proliferating cartilage cells that eventually die. After the cartilage cells die, osteoblasts line the calcified cartilage matrix previously produced by the chondrocytes, thus forming bone. The epiphyseal growth plate is divided into zones. The number of zones often varies in the literature dependent on the author; however, a general consensus specifies five zones. The first zone is the resting or reserve zone, followed by the proliferative zone, the maturation zone, the degeneration zone, and the zone of calcification. The zones of maturation, degeneration, and calcification often are referred to as the hypertrophic zone. The initial bone formed consists of spicules of bone with a calcified cartilaginous core and is call the primary spongiosa. The calcified cartilage will be removed entirely as the bone continues to remodel. The area of the bone with the primary spongiosa is called the metaphysis. This bone remodels to become the narrower diaphysis. The initial bone formed during this process is referred to as woven bone. This bone is unorganized both grossly and microscopically. As it remodels and matures, it becomes lamellar bone. It can be either cortical bone with a blood supply and a Haversian system, or trabecular bone, which does not have a Haversian system.

Osteoporosis is defined as a loss of bone per unit of volume. A more strict definition is bone with a bone mineral density (BMD) as measured by a dual-energy x-ray absorptiometry (DEXA) scan of more than 2.5 below the norm. The norm is based on a series of bone mineral density analyses done on healthy women who were at the peak bone mass. Osteomalacia (disorder in adults) and rickets (disorder in children) are the inadequate mineralization of bone. Osteopenia is the term used to describe the radiographic appearance of a bone with less density than expected. Osteoporosis should be prevented by having young persons, especially women, take adequate amounts of calcium and vitamin D, and exercise to build their skeletal to its maximum. Osteomalacia is treated by restoring a normal calcium metabolism. Abnormal calcium metabolism may be caused by a congenital disorder, dietary abnormalities, gastrointestinal disorders, by-pass surgery, parathyroid dysfunction, or renal disease.

JOINT ANATOMY AND PHYSIOLOGY

A diarthrodial joint is one in which a complete separation between the connecting parts is present. The diarthrodial joint contains synovial fluid, which lubricates the two articular cartilage-covered surfaces that rub against one another. The amount of articular cartilage achieved on completing growth (mid-teenage years) is the total amount a person will possess for the remainder of life. Once damaged, it cannot be replaced. Repair cartilage (fibrocartilage) can look similar and even have similar (not identical) properties, but does not have the mechanical properties to withstand the high demands placed on a joint surface. Articular cartilage is composed of hyaline cartilage, which is between 60 and 80 percent water. The remaining composition consists of macromolecules—collagen, proteoglycans, and noncollagenous proteins—which are all composed of amino acids and sugars. Type II collagen accounts for approximately 95 percent of the collagen in articular cartilage. Articular cartilage is organized into four zones or layers; superficial or gliding, middle or transitional, deep or radial, and calcified. Each has its own organization, collagen and proteoglycan contents, and function. Disruption of any layer causes the articular cartilage to malfunction. There are many other minor proteins in articular cartilage that are critical to the normal function of the cartilage.

Degenerative arthritis or osteoarthritis is the wearing away of articular cartilage. It can occur secondary to an injury, from malalignment leading to abnormal forces, from numerous conditions that interfere with the synovial lining from doing its job, or for no apparent reason. Idiopathic or osteoarthritis of old age is the most common form. The hallmark of degenerative arthritis is a loss of articular cartilage.

The synovium is critical to the normal function of the joint as it provides synovial fluid that surrounds the joint that is necessary to maintain the extremely low coefficient of friction between the articular surfaces. The synovial fluid also contains the nutrients needed for chondrocytes in the articular cartilage to survive. Normal synovial fluid is viscous, slightly yellow, and has no white blood cells, erythrocytes, or clotting factors. However, a traumatic or nonspecific reactive synovitis produces synovial fluid with decreased viscosity that can contain as many as 10,000 white blood cells. A synovitis associated with an inflammatory, noninfectious condition can have a white blood cell count of up to 50,000. Synovial fluid associated with an infectious process usually will have a white blood cell count of over 50,000 (Table 42-1).

Joints are stabilized by a combination of ligaments and muscles that cross the joint. These ligaments are subject to injury when stretched, resulting in a sprain. The degree of the injury is usually reflected in the severity of the local swelling and pain. Ligaments heal as does other collagenous tissue. Often the ligaments need surgical repair to assure that they are properly tensioned.

TUMORS OF THE MUSCULOSKELETAL SYSTEM

General Considerations

Primary tumors of the musculoskeletal system are rare. Most histogenetic tumor types have variable levels of aggressiveness and occur in benign and

TABLE 42-1 Synovial Fluid Analysis

Clinical example	Normal	Noninflammatory (osteoarthrosis)	Inflammatory (rheumatoid)	Septic (bacterial)
Color	Clear	Clear yellow	Opalescent yellow	Turbid yellow to green
Viscosity	High	High	Low	Low
WBC/mm^3	200	200–2000	200–100,000	> 100,000
% PMM leukocytes	< 25%	< 25%	> 50%	> 75%
Culture	Negative	Negative	Negative	Positive
Mucin clot	Firm	Firm	Friable	Friable
Glucose (% of serum glucose)	100%	100%	50–75%	< 50%
Total protein	Normal	Normal	Elevated	Elevated

malignant forms. Table 42-2 illustrates the range of incidence and histogenesis of musculoskeletal neoplasms. The biologic behavior of tumors can vary, as reflected by the pathologic grade of the tumor. Although various grading systems exist for different tumors, in general the simplified system adopted by the Musculoskeletal Tumor Society reflects overall gross behavior differences, with benign, low-grade malignant, and high-grade malignant forms.

Characteristics. Musculoskeletal neoplasms are characterized by initial centrifugal growth from a single focus, pseudoencapsulation (formation of a zone of reactive tissue around the expanding lesion, which in malignant lesions can be focally invaded by the tumor), and a tendency to respect anatomic boundaries early in the evolution of the lesion. These tumors thus tend to spread along fascial planes and tend to remain contained in anatomic compartments, a crucial characteristic in strategies for staging and surgical treatment of these lesions.

Metastasis. Metastasis of malignant musculoskeletal neoplasms is associated with a poor prognosis. Metastases are most often pulmonary, although some tumors tend also to involve regional lymph nodes, and bony metastases also occur. Brain and visceral metastases are unusual, generally occurring only in terminal end-stage disseminated disease.

Staging. Table 42-3 shows the most widely used staging system for musculoskeletal neoplasms.

Clinical manifestations. Patients typically present with a history of pain that is often worse at night and usually is not activity related. A mass or swelling may be present, but constitutional symptoms (weight loss, fevers, night sweats, malaise) usually are absent, except in cases with disseminated disease. Lesions adjacent to joints can cause effusion, contractures, and pain with motion. Soft-tissue tumors often are painless unless there is involvement of neurovascular structures. Patients may also present with a pathologic fracture as a manifestation of benign or malignant intraosseous lesions, with bone destruction and subsequent mechanical failure.

Radiographic findings. The plain radiograph is the single most useful study in differential diagnosis of bone lesions. Considerations include the following:

TABLE 42-2 Incidence of Bone Tumors (After Dahlin)

Histology	Benign	% Cases	Malignant	% Cases
Hemopoietic (28%)			Myeloma	24.7
			Lymphoma	3.1
Chondrogenic (27%)	Osteochondroma	12.0	Primary chondrosarcoma	8.7
	Enchondroma	4.3		
	Chondroblastoma	0.7	Secondary chondrosarcoma	0.8
	Chondromyxoid fibroma	0.6		
Osteogenic (25%)	Osteoid osteoma	2.5	Osteosarcoma	9.9
	Osteoblastoma	0.7	Chondroblastic osteosarcoma	6.0
			Fibroblastic osteosarcoma	4.6
			Parosteal osteosarcoma	0.9
Unknown origin (12%)	Giant cell tumor	4.8	Ewing's sarcoma	6.2
			Giant cell tumor	0.5
			Adamantinoma	0.2
Fibrogenic (4%)	Fibroma	1.5	Fibrosarcoma	2.5
Notochordal (3.5%)			Chordoma	3.5
Vascular (0.8%)	Hemangioma	0.6	Hemangioen-dothelioma	0.1
	Hemangio-pericytoma	0.1		
Lipogenic (0.1%)	Lipoma	0.1		
Neurogenic (<1%)	Neurilemmoma	< 0.1		

1. Evidence of matrix production (bone formation, calcification)
2. Pattern of growth (permeative, geographic, moth-eaten, loculated, expansile, exophytic)
3. Presence of bony reaction to the lesion (periosteal reaction, sclerotic margination)
4. Zone of transition between the host bone and lesion (narrow or well marginated versus wide or poorly defined)
5. Age of the patient
6. Bone involved (flat bone, long bone, skull, vertebrae, acral bone)
7. Location within the bone (epiphyseal, metaphyseal, diaphyseal)
8. Associated soft-tissue mass, clinical symptoms
9. Presence of solitary versus multiple lesions

Using these criteria, an accurate differential diagnosis can be formulated in most cases. Infection (osteomyelitis) must always be considered given its highly variable radiographic appearance. Metabolic, inflammatory, dysplastic, traumatic, congenital, and degenerative conditions also always are considered.

TABLE 42-3 Surgical Staging System for Musculoskeletal Tumors (After Enneking)

Stage	Characteristics	Metastases
Benign		
1	Latent	No
2	Active	No
3	Aggressive	No
Malignant		
IA	Low grade; intracompartmental	No
IB	Low grade; extracompartmental	No
IIA	High grade; intracompartmental	No
IIB	High grade; extracompartmental	No
III	Low or high grade; intra or extracompartmental	Yes

Source: Enneking WF: *Musculoskeletal tumor surgery,* London: Churchill–Livingston, 1983.

Soft-tissue lesions are better evaluated by magnetic resonance imaging (MRI) than any other type of radiographic study.

Diagnostic evaluation. Routine laboratory studies include complete blood count and differential; erythrocyte sedimentation rate; serum alkaline phosphatase, calcium, and phosphate levels, renal and liver function studies, and urinalysis. If multiple myeloma is within the differential diagnostic possibilities, determination of serum protein level or immunoelectrophoresis should also be performed.

Biopsy. For lesions with a radiographically benign appearance, imaging studies of the lesion usually are unnecessary, and the appropriate next step is tissue diagnosis by biopsy. For any potentially malignant lesion, three-dimensional imaging studies (computed tomography [CT] or, preferably, MRI) before biopsy are recommended to fully assess the extent of the lesion and to plan the biopsy procedure, minimizing potential contamination of compartments, which could compromise subsequent definitive surgery. Depending on the experience of the surgeon and pathologist, needle or trocar biopsy is appropriate for the majority of soft-tissue and bone tumors. General principles of the biopsy procedure include the following:

1. Biopsy incisions should always be longitudinal on extremities.
2. Needle biopsy tracts and incisional biopsy should be placed so that they can be excised en bloc at the time of resection.
3. Radiographic localization should be done to ensure accuracy.
4. Frozen-section examination should be done to be sure that adequate tissue has been obtained.
5. Cultures and appropriate microbiologic studies should be performed.
6. The bone biopsy cortical window should be as small as possible and oval in shape to minimize the risk of pathologic fracture.
7. Central or necrotic areas should be avoided; biopsy at the periphery of the lesion is most helpful.
8. Exposure of any major neurovascular structures should be avoided.
9. Hemostasis must be obtained to prevent hematoma, which could seed other compartments; for bone lesions suspected of malignancy, the biopsy site should be plugged with methacrylate cement to prevent hematoma.
10. Tourniquet use is helpful for intraoperative accuracy of dissection.

11. Use of a drain with its tract in line with the biopsy incision and near it will facilitate later en bloc resection.
12. Contamination of any uninvolved compartment must be avoided.
13. In general, the surgeon providing definitive treatment should also perform the biopsy whenever possible; this would usually involve a tertiary care referral center.

Treatment. In the treatment of benign and nonmetastatic malignant musculoskeletal tumors the primary goal is eradication of the disease; preservation of limb function is an important but secondary consideration. Long-term results have improved dramatically in the past two decades, and the treatment approach for malignant lesions has changed, with a shift away from amputations and toward limb salvage procedures. The specific treatment varies with the lesion but usually includes a combination of several modalities: surgery, chemotherapy, and radiotherapy.

Specific Musculoskeletal Tumors

Osteoid osteoma. This benign bone-forming lesion primarily affects patients under 30 years of age and has a male preponderance. Patients present with local pain, which can be quite severe and often is relieved by aspirin. Radiographically, a small (less than 1 cm) lucent lesion (nidus) is seen, typically surrounded by marked reactive sclerosis. Sometimes areas of radiodensity are seen within the lucent lesion, corresponding histologically to disorganized woven bone formation. The lesion gradually regresses over a period of 5–10 years, but most patients are unable to tolerate the symptoms and opt for surgical resection of the lesion, which usually is curative if the entire nidus is removed.

Osteosarcoma. Osteosarcoma is the most common primary bone malignancy apart from multiple myeloma, although it is nonetheless a rare disease (incidence 2.8/1,000,000). Patients 10–25 years of age most often are affected, and the most common sites are areas of maximal bone growth (distal femur—52 percent; proximal tibia—20 percent; proximal humerus—9 percent). Usually the lesions are metaphyseal. Although any bone can be involved, the disease seldom occurs in the small bones of the distal extremities and in the spine. This disease has a number of variants:, (1) "classic" central or medullary high-grade osteosarcoma; (2) periosteal osteosarcoma; (3) parosteal osteosarcoma; (4) osteosarcoma secondary to malignant degeneration of Paget disease, fibrous dysplasia, or radiation; and (5) telangiectatic osteosarcoma.

Osteosarcoma exhibits a blastic radiographic appearance in most cases because of the neoplastic woven bone formation. The periosteum may be raised off the bone by the tumor mass, causing a fusiform swelling with reactive periosteal bone at the periosteal margins (Codman triangle). The malignant bone formation may have a sunburst appearance, with invasion into adjacent compartments. Pathologic fractures can occur but are unusual.

Histologically, the tumor consists of small pleomorphic spindle cells, with osteoid and woven bone formation, and there is often cartilage formation as well. Cartilage formation is a prominent feature of periosteal and parosteal variants of osteosarcoma. Telangiectatic variants are lytic and expansible, resembling an aneurysmal bone cyst, and have prominent vascular spaces and relatively sparse bone formation.

Patients present with pain that often is nocturnal and a mass or swelling. Metastatic spread usually is pulmonary, and evaluation of the chest by CT is necessary. Serum alkaline phosphatase levels may be markedly elevated, but laboratory studies are otherwise usually negative. Evaluation also should include bone scan to rule out bone metastases, and CT or, preferably, MRI of the region for surgical planning. Most osteosarcomas present as stage IIB lesions.

Osteosarcoma is not particularly sensitive to radiation, but it does typically respond well to combination chemotherapy. Depending on the extent and location of the lesion, treatment typically involves wide surgical resection or amputation, usually after preoperative (neoadjuvant) chemotherapy. Bone resected in limb salvage operations can be reconstructed by custom prosthetic replacement, arthrodesis, or allografting. Results of combination chemotherapy with resection are better than even radical surgical amputation without adjuvant therapy, with 50–70 percent 5-year survival rates and usually better than 90 percent local control (compared with a 20 percent 5-year survival rate with radical surgery alone). Pathologic fracture, with contamination of all compartments, can preclude limb salvage surgery. Chemotherapy is continued after surgery for 1 year. Prosthetic designs that can be periodically lengthened by a minor surgical procedure allow limb salvage even in relatively young children with osteosarcoma, in whom progressive limb length discrepancy might otherwise be a severe problem. Preoperative intraarterial chemotherapy and radiotherapy have been used instead of neoadjuvant systemic chemotherapy, and results appear to be comparable.

Osteochondroma (exostosis). This lesion is a common exophytic benign lesion that occurs during childhood, usually in the metaphyses of the long bones. It is thought to result from an aberrant fragment of the growth plate that is left behind and undergoes spontaneous growth. The lesions have a bony base with a cartilaginous cap, from which the growth occurs as it does in normal growth plates during childhood. A multiple hereditary form occurs and was discussed earlier. There is a familial condition called multiple hereditary exostosis in which patients have many osteochondroma. It has a variable penetrance. The lesions may cause pain from impingement on tendons, nerves, or muscle and frequently require surgical excision. Growth of the lesion, although not of concern in children, may indicate malignant transformation in adults. A cartilaginous cap thickness of more than 1 cm (assessed by CT or MRI) should arouse suspicion of malignancy. In solitary lesions the risk of malignant degeneration is less than 1 percent, although in multiple lesions it may be as high as 15 percent. Marginal to wide excision of benign or malignant lesions usually is curative if all the cartilage is removed.

Enchondroma. Enchondromas are intramedullary cartilage lesions, often exhibiting calcification and expansion of the bone. The small bones of the hands and feet are commonly involved, but long bone involvement also occurs. The disease occurs in solitary and multiple forms. Patients may present with pain or pathologic fracture. The usual treatment is intralesional resection (curettage) and bone grafting. The most serious concern is the possibility of malignant degeneration, and careful sampling at the time of biopsy is necessary to exclude the possibility of chondrosarcoma.

Chondroblastoma. This is one of the few epiphyseal tumors and occurs most often in the first and second decades of life, when the growth plate is still open. Patients present with pain, joint effusions, or contractures, and radiographs show a lytic lesion with calcifications in the epiphysis. The lesion is composed of chondroblasts, cartilage, giant cells, and vascular stroma. Treatment is by curettage and bone grafting and often is challenging because of the intraarticular location of the lesions. A rare malignant epiphyseal cartilage tumor in older adults, clear cell chondrosarcoma, probably represents the malignant degenerative counterpart of chondroblastoma.

Chondrosarcoma. Chondrosarcoma can be primary or secondary (as discussed above) and affects a broad age range (age 20–60 years). The pelvis, femur, tibia, and other long bones can be involved, and lesions closer to the axial skeleton are more likely to be malignant. Intramedullary calcifications are usually evident. Differential diagnosis includes bone infarction and enchondroma. Features of cortical destruction and pain are important indicators of possible malignancy. The tumors are graded as low, intermediate, or high grade of malignancy on the basis of cytologic features and presence of matrix production. Lower-grade lesions can be treated by wide resection, but with high-grade lesions metastatic disease is frequent and the prognosis is poor. Limb salvage surgery often is feasible, but adjuvant treatments are not particularly helpful because these lesions tend to be resistant to chemotherapy and radiotherapy.

Unicameral (solitary) bone cyst. This lesion occurs in children in the metaphysis of the long bones adjacent to the growth plate, most often the humerus or femur, although the radius, calcaneus, and tibia also can be affected. Usually the lesions are painless and may present with a pathologic fracture as the initial manifestation of the disease. The lesions are lytic, expansile, and well marginated, and may be found in the diaphysis in older children as a result of continued growth of the growth plate away from the lesion. In young children fractures heal, but the lesions usually recur, causing recurrent fractures during childhood. The cyst fluid contains high levels of bone resorptive cytokines, presumably produced by the living tissue and accounting for the aggressive bone resorption in these lesions. At skeletal maturity the cysts tend gradually to disappear. In older children and young adults, the lesions become latent (stage I) and do not progress. Recurrence rates in active (stage II) lesions in younger children after surgical treatment (curettage and bone grafting) average 50 percent. Partial or complete healing of the majority of these lesions has been obtained after intraosseous injection of methylprednisolone, currently the preferred treatment (70–90 percent effective with up to three sequential injections). In older children or adults with latent cysts, curettage and bone grafting is effective, and steroid injections appear to have little effect.

Aneurysmal bone cyst. This tumor, found most often in children or young adults, consists of a cystic lesion with large vascular spaces, characterized by aggressive, expansile lysis of bone. The tumor is composed of fibrous tissue, vascular spaces with a lining resembling endothelium, giant cells, and reactive bone formation at the periphery. Aneurysmal cysts can arise as a secondary degenerative vascular lesion within another primary benign or malignant bone tumor, such as giant cell tumor or chondroblastoma; however, about half are thought to represent primary lesions. Because recurrence is relatively frequent with simple curettage, local resection with bone grafting is preferable. Embolization has been used successfully in unresectable spinal or pelvic lesions, as has intermediate-dose radiation treatment. Preoperative embolization of large lesions is helpful in decreasing the risk of hemorrhage.

Round Cell Tumors

Ewing sarcoma. Ewing sarcoma is a highly malignant primary bone tumor of children (age range 5–15 years) that tends to arise in the diaphyses of long bones. The spine and pelvis also may be primary sites. The radiographic appearance usually is that of an aggressive lesion, with a permeative pattern of bone lysis and periosteal reaction. Often there is an associated large soft-tissue mass, and patients have systemic symptoms (fever, weight loss) in addition to local pain, which tends to be worse at night. A soft-tissue variant of Ewing sarcoma, primitive neuroectodermal tumor (PNET), occurs as well, usually exhibiting evidence of neural differentiation immunohistochemically. Differential diagnosis includes osteomyelitis, lymphoma, and eosinophilic granuloma. Diagnostic evaluation includes chest and abdominal CT scans and bone scan to rule out metastases. Treatment consists of a combination of local radiation therapy and systemic chemotherapy. Five-year survival rates with this approach are around 50 percent. A multimodality treatment that uses adjuvant surgery (wide or marginal resection) has resulted in 5-year survival rates of 75 percent. In young children amputation may be necessary because of the severe compromise of bone growth that can result from the effect of the required levels of radiation on the growth plates.

Giant cell tumor of bone. These tumors arise in the epiphyses of young adults, most commonly in the proximal tibia, distal femur, proximal femur, and distal radius. Characteristically the lesion is radiographically purely lytic, well circumscribed, and occasionally expansile with cortical destruction. The lesion often extends to the subchondral surface and can even invade the joint. Although usually benign, a malignant variant occurs in a small proportion of cases, and even the benign lesions are stage III tumors, with local aggressive behavior and a high tendency to recur after surgical treatment. Patients usually present with pain, and pathologic fracture may occur. The tumor consists of monocytic stromal cells, vascular tissue, and sheets of large, multi-nucleated osteoclast-like cells. The key feature in differentiating these tumors from other tumors that can contain large numbers of giant cells (eosinophilic granuloma, brown tumor of hyperparathyroidism, aneurysmal bone cyst, chondroblastoma, osteoblastoma, nonossifying fibroma) is that the oval nuclei of the monocytic stroma resemble those of the giant cells, suggesting a common origin. The most common cause of malignant giant cell tumors is prior radiation therapy for a benign giant cell tumor, which was a former mode of treatment and can be associated with malignant recurrence in up to 10 percent of cases. Because of this radiation is no longer used in the treatment of giant cell tumors except in dire circumstances (such as unresectable lesions in the spine with threat of neurologic deficit).

The most common treatment of a giant cell tumor, curettage of the lesion, is associated with recurrences in 25–50 percent of cases. Alternative treatments therefore have included wide resection (usually reserved for recurrent cases) and adjuvant local treatments such as cryotherapy with liquid nitrogen or phenol and, most recently, filling the defect with methyl methacrylate. The lowest recurrence rates have been with cryotherapy and methyl methacrylate cementation. Cementation causes a thermal kill of tissue within several millimeters of the margin in bone as a result of the exothermic reaction that occurs during polymerization of the cement. If local recurrence occurs after cementation, it is readily detectable radiographically as a lucency next to the cement. With bone grafting, remodeling changes in the graft can obscure signs of recurrence.

Because these are epiphyseal lesions, the presence of cement next to the articular cartilage may predispose to cartilage degeneration, and in young patients, some advise removal of the cement and bone grafting after 2 years if the patient remains free of recurrence. Given an incidence of joint degeneration of only 15–20 percent in long-term follow-up studies, the indications for cement removal are controversial. Control of the lesion with this treatment approach has been successful in 90 percent of cases.

Vascular Tumors

Metastatic Bone Tumors

Carcinomas often metastasize to the skeleton, and metastatic lesions are much more common than primary bone lesions in general orthopaedic practice. The five primary cancers with a strong propensity to metastasize to bone are those originating in the breast, prostate, lung, kidney, and thyroid. Multiple myeloma, although technically a primary bone tumor, also must be considered in this group because of its similar age distribution (patients over age 50 years), radiographic presentation, and orthopaedic problems and treatment (pathologic fractures). Over 90 percent of patients with metastatic breast or prostate carcinoma have at least microscopic bone involvement.

The axial skeleton, including the skull, thoracic spine, ribs, lumbar spine, and pelvis, is most commonly involved. The proximal long bones, particularly the humerus and femur, also are affected frequently. Acral (distal) metastases are uncommon and are almost always secondary to lung carcinoma when they do occur. The predilection of particular tumors for bone, and for particular regions of specific bones, is thought to be caused by cytokines, local growth factors, or matrix components that attract and support growth of these lesions in specific areas. Lesions can be blastic (breast, prostate), lytic (breast, lung, myeloma, kidney, thyroid), or mixed (breast, lung) in radiographic appearance. Blastic or sclerotic lesions are less prone to pathologic fractures.

EVALUATION OF THE MUSCULOSKELETAL SYSTEM

History and Physical Examination

Collecting a thorough history and performing a physical examination is the foremost priority when examining a patient who has a musculoskeletal condition. The physical examination is concentrated on the musculoskeletal system, including its neurologic aspects, but a complete general examination is also important. The patient's chief complaint should direct the nature of history taking. Because the most common complaint is pain, it is important to note its location, duration, its intensity, how long it lasts, what makes it worse, what makes it better, and what they do to relieve it. It is also important to know what past treatments have been employed and their results. In conjunction with a past medical and familial history, a social history is often important for conditions of the musculoskeletal system because many problematic musculoskeletal system conditions are a result of the patient's occupation or hobby. Additionally, decisions about treatment should take the patient's expectations and physical requirements into consideration.

The initial aspect of the physical examination is to observe the patient's general condition. The patient should be wearing a minimal amount of clothing. Observe how the patient moves about, examining their gait pattern. An antalgic gait indicates pain. Its feature is marked by a shortened period of time with the extremity bearing weight. A Trendelenburg gait or gluteus medius limp is caused by malfunction of the hip abductor mechanism. A positive indicator for Trendelenburg sign is if the patient leans toward the affected side when the opposite extremity is raised off the floor. The following questions may help to elucidate additional musculoskeletal dysfunctions: Is the alignment of the lower extremities symmetric? Do the upper extremities move symmetrically? Does the patient stand straight? Additionally, the patient's range-of-motion (ROM) of all joints should be measured and areas of interest palpated. Joints should be inspected for effusion. A check of the vascular supply and a neurologic examination should also be performed.

Virtually all patients with musculoskeletal complaints should have plain radiographs. The minimum is two views taken perpendicular to one another. Once these have been examined, a differential diagnosis can be made which usually includes only a few conditions. Additional diagnostic tests may be needed before a treatment plan can be finalized.

The evaluation of a patient who has sustained acute trauma requires a slightly different approach, which involves collecting a detailed summary of the events of the injury. The following questions may be helpful in this effort: What was the patient doing when the patient was injured? Was the twist internal rotation or external rotation? Can the patient estimate the height from which the patient fell? Was the patient a pedestrian, cyclist, or passenger in or driver of an automobile? Was the patient wearing a seatbelt? Did the patient lose consciousness? Was the patient ejected from the vehicle? Answers to questions such as these can provide clues to the degree of injury and indicate possible associated injuries that should be looked for.

The measurement of joint motion is important and can be ascertained with the help of a goniometer. Comparing the affected side to the unaffected side is useful. In general, 0 degrees is the neutral anatomic position. Movements into the plane anterior to the body are flexion and movements into the plane posterior to the body are extension. Rotation (internal and external), abduction, and adduction are also important indicators to the measurement of motion. In general, flexion and extension are maintained longer than rotation, abduction, and adduction. Loss of motion can be from pathology intrinsic or extrinsic to the joint. For example, a patient with loss of flexion, rotation, and abduction in the hip might have degenerative disease of the hip joint or the patient might have muscular contractures. A careful analysis of the patient should distinguish between intrinsic and extrinsic causes.

Joint stability is important and ligaments are examined by stressing the joint in various directions. The knee, shoulder, elbow, and ankle are all joints commonly associated with injuries that lead to ligamentous disruption. The specifics for each of these joints are described in their respective sections.

The vascular supply to the extremity should be determined. If the patient has good pulses of the dorsalis pedis, posterior tibial, radial, and ulnar arteries, significant vascular injury or arterial disease is unlikely. Those patients without peripheral pulses should be examined more thoroughly to determine the status of the vascular supply. Edema should be noted if present.

After physical examination, plain radiographs are the single-most important diagnostic tool for evaluating a patient with a complaint related to the musculoskeletal system. Before obtaining a computerized tomography (CT scan) or an MRI, a plain radiograph should always be taken. A minimum of two views at right angles to one another should be obtained. Obliques are often useful to visualize certain aspects of the skeletal anatomy. The quality of the radiograph is important; the bone should be clearly seen and the soft tissues, although visible, should not interfere with visualization of the bone.

Nuclear studies often are used to evaluate the skeletal system. Technetium-99 (99Tc) bone scans are the most commonly used study. The 99Tc is tagged to phosphorus, which attaches itself to the bone. The amount of 99Tc attached to the bone is directly related to bone formation. Therefore, any reactivity of the bone is seen as a "hot" spot. The patient is injected with the 99Tc and approximately 2 h later images are taken. The scan is sensitive but not specific. Indium (In) scans are used primarily to determine if there is an infection. White blood cells from the patient are tagged with Indium and injected into the patient. Because the tagged white blood cells concentrate at the site of an infection, the scan has a "hot" spot. Thallium scans also are occasionally used to identify soft-tissue inflammatory lesions.

Computed axial tomography (CAT) is the best method to use for visualizing the details of bone and calcifications. It is often used to evaluate fractures, especially comminuted ones and those involving an articular surface. Three-dimensional reconstructions can be done to better evaluate the injury. Computed tomography is useful in the evaluation of patients with suspected herniated nucleus pulposus, although MRI is probably better.

MRI is most valuable for the examination of soft tissues. It is particularly valuable in examining the soft tissue around joints. Torn ligaments and meniscus can usually be seen on an MRI. It is also an excellent means of examining the soft tissues of the extremities and the spine. The spinal canal is visible and damage to the spinal cord can be seen easily.

DISORDERS OF THE MUSCULOSKELETAL SYSTEM

Osteomyelitis

Osteomyelitis is an infection of the bone that most commonly occurs secondary to an open wound with an associated or compound fracture. However, osteomyelitis also can occur spontaneously, presumably as a consequence of circulating bacteria in the bloodstream, and is known as hematogenous osteomyelitis. Hematogenous osteomyelitis is an infection that predominantly occurs in children. The most common causative organism is Staphylococcus, but any bacteria can produce osteomyelitis. Less-common infectious agents include viruses, fungi, and mycobacteria. Osteomyelitis is divided into "acute" and "chronic" categories. Although the time limits delineating one category from the other are somewhat arbitrary, as a rule, infections up to 3 months' duration are termed acute, although those enduring longer than 3 months are termed chronic. In general, acute osteomyelitis is associated with systemic findings of an infection with fever, malaise, elevated white blood cell count, erythrocyte sedimentation rate (ESR), and C-reactive protein (CRP). The site of the infection is tender and the patient often does not want to move the extremity involved. Patients with chronic osteomyelitis usually are not systemically sick. They are more likely to have a draining sinus, necrotic bone (a sequestrum) surrounded by reactive bone (an involucrum).

Hematogenous osteomyelitis often is associated with an infection within a joint, or pyarthrosis. Joint infections also can occur without bone involvement and should be recognized and treated as soon as possible to reduce damage to the articular cartilage.

Arthritis

There are a variety of pathways by which a joint is transformed from an efficient, mobile, low-friction, shock-absorbing, and energy-conserving structure to one that is painful and stiff. One common pathway involves greater or lesser degrees of destruction of articular cartilage.

Osteoarthritis

Osteoarthritis (OA) is the most common form of arthritis, with up to 40 million people in the United States having been diagnosed with it. Also known as degenerative joint disease, OA generally has been considered to be noninflammatory. Some prefer to refer to this disease as osteoarthrosis, changing the suffix -itis to -osis to emphasize the noninflammatory degenerative nature of this aliment. In fact, the same cytokines and interleukins seen in inflammatory arthritis also are seen in osteoarthritis, although in lesser quantity.

Typical findings on a radiographic examination reveal loss of articular cartilage, osteophytes, and subchondral cysts.

Physical examination reveals pain on walking (an antalgic gait pattern) or motion of the involved joint. Patients have some degree of limitation of motion, pain and/or crepitus with that motion. There usually is an effusion in the joint.

The initial treatment includes activity modification, weight reduction if indicated, the use of a cane for lower-extremity problems, and nonsteroidal anti-inflammatory and nonnarcotic analgesics medications if required. Patients should be encouraged to maintain their joint motion and muscular strength. If they cannot do this on their own, they should be referred to a physical therapist. Joint replacement is recommended to relieve pain and restore function to the arthritic joint for the patient whose symptoms persist despite nonoperative management.

Rheumatoid Arthritis

Rheumatoid arthritis is the most common form of inflammatory arthritis. It is an apparent autoimmune response that involves synovium, articular cartilage, and soft tissue. The joints of the hand are most commonly involved, but wrists, feet, knees, and hips are frequently affected. This disease is often symmetric, (i.e., both knees and both hands). Patients frequently suffer from morning stiffness. Subcutaneous nodules may be palpated, especially at the proximal ulna. The rheumatoid arthritis (RA) factor is positive in approximately 80 percent of patients.

Typical radiographs show loss of articular cartilage, osteopenia, and periarticular erosions. A typical hip deformity of the femoral protruding medially into the pelvis (protrusio acetabulum) is not uncommon. These patients can have vasculitis, pericarditis, and pulmonary involvement.

Lyme disease is a tick-borne (deer tick, *Ixodes dammini*) illness caused by the spirochete *Borrelia burgdorferi*. Affected patients may have intermittent attacks of swelling in one or more large joints, accompanied by a characteristic skin rash (*erythema chronicum migrans*) that often precedes the arthritis. The knee is the most effected joint. A serum Lyme titer is diagnostic. Treatment includes tetracycline, penicillin, or erythromycin.

Gout results from abnormalities in the metabolism of urate that causes deposition of urate crystals in joints, kidneys, and musculoskeletal soft tissues.

When deposited in the synovium, the urate crystals may cause an acute inflammatory reaction. The patient often presents with acute onset of pain, swelling, and erythema of a single joint. The most commonly effected joint is the first metatarsophalangeal (MP) joint of the foot. The patient has elevated serum uric acid levels and urate crystals are seen on an analysis of the joint fluid. The crystals are long and thin. Colchicine has been used since the days of Hippocrates. A 0.65-mg dose is given orally every 1–2 h until the pain subsides or diarrhea begins. For less-painful episodes, nonsteroidal antiinflammatory medication can be used. Patients with gout should be treated to lower their serum urate levels.

Calcium pyrophosphate deposition disease (CPPD or pseudogout) is also an inflammatory synovial disorder caused by crystals. The crystals of CPPD are calcium pyrophosphate. The presentation is similar to gout but usually not as painful. Calcifications are often seen in the cartilage or meniscus. The crystals can be seen on analysis of the joint fluid. They are short and rectangular. Nonsteroidal antiinflammatory medication usually is sufficient treatment.

Infectious Arthritis

Infectious arthritis, also known as septic arthritis or pyarthrosis, is relatively uncommon. It most often is seen in patients younger than age 5 years or older than age 80 years. However, both morbidity and mortality rates can be relatively high. The knee and hip are the joints most typically infected. *Staphylococcus aureus*, streptococci, and gonococci are the organisms most typically involved. Viruses, mycobacteria, fungal agents, and Lyme disease are other causes. Early diagnosis and treatment limits joint destruction and preserves function. Early joint drainage and lavage are the mainstays of treatment, followed by intravenous antibiotics. Hematogenous seeding during a transient or persistent bacteremia is believed to be the most common mechanism in septic arthritis. The American College of Rheumatology defines septic arthritis as a synovial fluid aspirate that demonstrates a minimum of 50,000 white blood cells (WBC) per high-powered field and at least 80 percent neutrophils on differential count. In patients with previous total joint replacements, much lower counts can be diagnostic (see Table 42-1).

TRAUMA

Initial Assessment

The initial evaluation of the injured patient should be geared toward identifying life-threatening injuries. Injuries to the chest, head, abdomen, and major vessels may require emergent treatment and take precedence over most musculoskeletal injuries. Patients in shock must be treated aggressively with volume replacement. Unstable pelvic fractures often require some type of stabilization to control hemorrhage. Occult arterial bleeding requires emergency arteriography and embolization.

The trauma surgeon, in conjunction with the orthopaedic surgeon, should make the assessment of skeletal injuries. Evaluation of all open injuries, long-bone fractures, and spinal injuries is imperative. The patient should not be mobilized until appropriate radiographs of the spine have been taken and evaluated. Anterior and posterior radiographs of the cervical spine are the minimal requirement. The extremities need to be evaluated for neurovascular compromise, soft-tissue and bony injuries, and ligamentous injuries. Sensory and motor examinations, including peripheral pulses and capillary refill, should be evaluated and carefully documented.

Injured extremities need to be splinted for soft-tissue management and mobilization of the patient. Skeletal traction should be considered for long-bone fractures when the patients are not going directly to the operating room, but femur fractures in multiply injured patients require stabilization as soon as possible.

An open fracture is defined as any fracture that is exposed to the outside environment. This can result from a penetrating injury that has caused a fracture or from a displaced fragment of bone that has violated the skin. Open fractures often are caused by high-energy injuries and associated injuries should be sought.

The early goals of treatment should include immediate irrigation and débridement combined with skeletal stabilization to prevent infection and to facilitate soft-tissue healing. Vascular injuries, larger wounds, greater comminution, and soft-tissue loss all are associated with increased risk of osteomyelitis. Once osteomyelitis has been established, it may be extremely difficult to eradicate. Therefore, early treatment should include aggressive and immediate débridement of the wound and fracture site in an operative environment and intravenous antibiotic therapy. Repeat intraoperative débridement is recommended when significant soft-tissue damage or contamination is present. Primary closure of wounds is controversial. Open wounds with fractures are classified to indicate the degree of damage and allow easy communication of injury level (Table 42-4). Low-grade, open wounds often are closed and sometimes not emergently débrided. This remains controversial and should not be the standard for surgeons inexperienced in dealing with open fractures. Higher-grade, open wounds will need surgical evaluation by a plastic surgeon as soon as possible. The orthopaedic surgeon and the plastic surgeon must work together to achieve soft-tissue closure, to prevent infection, and to achieve bony union. Ultimately, a prolonged course of rehabilitation will be necessary to ensure the best possible function for these patients.

The first principle of treatment involves reduction of the fracture. If a fracture is truly nondisplaced, then no reduction is necessary. For displaced fractures and dislocations, a reduction maneuver usually is performed. For extra-articular fractures, this often is unnecessary. Guidelines for determining what an adequate reduction is exist as a range of parameters; however, these parameters may differ among surgeons. In general, lower extremities require more precise reduction. Intraarticular fractures require an almost anatomic reduction. The second principle of treatment is to maintain the reduction. There is an arsenal of treatment methods available to the orthopaedic surgeon, including internal fixation and external fixation. External fixation includes casts or skeletal external fixation with percutaneous pins and external fixators. Internal fixation includes screw fixation, plate fixation, intramedullary fixation, and other types of metals or absorbable materials for fixation. In some cases,

TABLE 42-4 Grading of Open Wounds

Type I	Low energy, <1 cm
Type II	Modest energy, >1 cm
Type III	High energy, usually >10 cm
A	No vascular involvement
B	Vascular injury

a suture fixation is all that is necessary. Surgeons with different training can successfully treat the same fracture by totally different, but equally acceptable, methods. It is important to remember that the goal of treatment is function and how the reduction is maintained is simply a means to the end.

Terminology

It is useful for surgeons of all disciplines to understand some basic orthopaedic terminology. Orthopaedic surgeons use different terms to facilitate communication. Understanding these concepts and terms will help the physician communicate with the orthopaedist. A fracture is determined to be open when the fracture communicates with the outside environment. Fortunately, most fractures are closed and the soft-tissue envelope is intact. However, the internal soft-tissue injury can be quite variable and attempts have been made to classify the soft-tissue injury with closed fractures. The orthopaedic surgeon is aware that there are low-energy closed fractures and high-energy closed fractures. High-energy closed fractures generally are more difficult to treat because they tend to be more "displaced." Displacement is defined as fracture ends that are no longer contiguous. The authors describe displacement based on the distal segment. The distal segment can be medial or lateral on an anteroposterior radiograph. The distal segment can be anterior or posterior on a lateral radiograph.

Fractures are often "angulated." Angulation is described by the vertex of the angulation. The authors measure angulation by the deviation from normal alignment. If the vertex points anterior, then "anterior angulation" is present. Anterior and posterior angulation can be seen on lateral radiographs. Anterior/posterior radiographs can show "varus" or "valgus" angulation. If the fracture has a vertex that points medially, the fracture is in "valgus." If the vertex points laterally, the fracture is in "varus."

Rotational malalignment is sometimes difficult to determine on plain radiographs. Often this is quite evident by the clinical appearance of the extremity. If the distal portion of the extremity is rotated externally, then "external rotation" is present. Conversely, if the distal portion of the extremity is rotated internally, the fracture is described as being "internally rotated." Radiographically, a joint should be viewed from above and below to see the rotational alignment. This visualization of the joints, above and below the fracture, also is necessary to determine if there has been a joint injury associated with the fracture.

If a long bone is displaced 100 percent, it is said that "shortening" of the fracture has occurred. Shortening can be seen on either anteroposterior (AP) or lateral radiographs. The amount of shortening will not change from AP to lateral radiographs. However, two radiographs in planes 90 degrees to each other are necessary to visualize translation and angulation.

Pelvic Fractures

Injuries to the pelvic ring should be differentiated between the low-energy, stable fractures and the high-energy, life-threatening injuries. The former are commonly seen in older adult osteoporotic patients who may have sustained isolated fractures of the pubic rami or nondisplaced fractures of the acetabuli or sacrum from a fall. These fractures usually do not have disruption of the pelvic ring or weight-bearing segments and are considered stable.

High-energy injuries are the result of automobile collisions, pedestrians and cyclists being struck by motor vehicles, or falls from significant heights.

These injuries are caused by direct crush, either from the anterior or lateral direction or vertical shear, or combinations of rotational stress on the iliac wings. Initial evaluation of pelvic injuries includes an AP radiograph. Further imaging includes inlet and outlet views. Associated acetabular fractures and lumbar spine injuries require 45-degree oblique (Judet) views and AP and lateral radiographs of the lumbosacral spine. Most pelvic injuries will also need a CT scan with 3-mm cuts to evaluate a posterior injury to the pelvis. A CT scan is best used for evaluation of the sacrum and sacroiliac joints.

Continued, unexplained blood loss despite fracture stabilization and aggressive resuscitation is an indication for angiography. Early recognition of potential arterial bleeding should include early notification of the interventional radiology team. Angiography and embolization may be required in up to 20 percent of AP injuries, vertical shear injuries, and combined mechanical injuries.

Acetabular Fractures

Acetabular fractures are a subset of pelvic fractures that involve the acetabulum. These intraarticular fractures may result in posttraumatic arthritis of the hip and are sometimes associated with hip dislocations, which are discussed in the next section.

Thorough evaluation of acetabulum fractures requires 45-degree oblique views (Judet views) of the pelvis to assess the integrity of the anterior and posterior columns and the anterior and posterior walls. Additionally, CT scans are helpful in fully delineating fracture patterns and demonstrating the presence of intraarticular bony fragments. Nondisplaced or minimally displaced fractures are determined after complete evaluation of the radiographs and acetabular CT scans. Radiographs should be taken with traction removed and preferably with stress applied. Any degree of incongruence involving the weight-bearing surface of the acetabulum is unacceptable and is an indication for surgical treatment. Nondisplaced fractures may be treated with a period of traction followed by progressive weight bearing.

Hip Dislocation

Dislocation of the hip often is caused by a force applied to the femur and can be associated with fractures of the acetabulum or femoral head. The most common mechanism of injury is motor vehicles accidents. Force applied to an abducted hip can result in anterior dislocation, although striking the knee on a car dashboard with the hip flexed and adducted, results in posterior dislocations. Posterior dislocations often are associated with a fracture of the posterior wall of the acetabulum. Direct trauma to the greater trochanter from a lateral direction can result in medial wall fractures or central acetabular fractures/dislocations.

Thorough evaluation of hip dislocations often requires Judet radiographic views and additional CT scans. Similar to patients with pelvic fractures, these patients may have other major injuries and careful evaluation of the chest, abdomen, spine, and neurologic status is necessary. Prompt reduction of hip dislocations is essential in minimizing the incidence of osteonecrosis of the femoral head.

Femur Fractures

The mortality and morbidity of proximal femur fractures has significantly improved with modern methods of treatment. However, a proximal femur fracture still represents a major challenge to the health care system with the increasing age of our population. These fractures generally occur in the seventh and eighth decades of life. Femoral neck and intertrochanteric fractures occur with approximately equal frequency and similar epidemiology. Osteoporosis is a major contributing factor to hip fractures. An increasing awareness of this disease accompanied by new methods of treatment may facilitate the prevention of proximal femur fractures. This is extremely significant in light of the high mortality rate of hip fractures in older adults, which have been reported to be as high as 50 percent in the first year.

Femoral Neck Fractures

Femoral neck fractures most commonly are related to falls. The patient most often complains of pain in the groin or thigh and is unable to bear weight on the injured extremity. The lower extremity appears shortened and externally rotated. Most attempts at motion, especially rotational motion, cause severe pain. The diagnosis is confirmed by anteroposterior and lateral radiographs of the hip. The Garden classification is used to indicate the degree of displacement. A careful physical examination is necessary to rule out other injuries to the patient. Displaced femoral neck fractures can be treated with reduction and internal fixation. This method of treatment often is reserved for younger, active, individuals. The older adult patient is better treated with a hip replacement.

Intertrochanteric and Subtrochanteric Fractures

These fractures occur in older adults and are related to falls, and after significant trauma in younger individuals. Subtrochanteric femur fractures occur more distally below the level of the lesser trochanter. These fractures occur within 5 cm of the lesser trochanter. Below this level, the fracture is considered a femoral shaft fracture. The subtrochanteric region of the proximal femur is a high stress area. These fractures require strong implants to resist varus deformity and implant failure. Classically, the sliding hip screw with a side plate continues to be the preferred implant for most stable and unstable intertrochanteric hip fractures. More recently, fixed-angle sliding screws that incorporate an intramedullary nail to gain purchase to the shaft have been used to fix these fractures.

Fractures of the Femoral Shaft

Femoral shaft fractures may occur at any age from severe violence. However, these injuries may occur from less severe, direct torsional stress. Multiply injured trauma patients require evaluation of any associated injuries of the head, abdomen, and chest. These patients present with instability of the lower extremity, pain with motion, external rotational deformity, and shortening of the affected lower extremity. A complete neurovascular examination is essential because there may be injury to the sciatic or femoral nerve or femoral artery. Open femur fractures are associated with a 10 percent incidence of limb-threatening vascular injury. Associated femoral neck fractures or knee ligament injuries occur in approximately 5 percent of patients and must be intentionally looked for.

Femoral shaft fractures were historically treated in traction. This method had several disadvantages, such as shortening, rotational malunion, and knee stiffness. Traction is now mostly used as a temporizing measure until patients are stable enough to undergo definitive surgical stabilization. The gold standard of treatment of these fractures is reamed, locked, antegrade intramedullary nailing performed through a closed technique. Complications of treating femoral shaft fractures include infection (< 1 percent), delayed union, nonunion, malunion, compartment syndrome, neurologic injury, and heterotopic ossification. Nonunion is more common in patients with a history of smoking and diabetes.

Distal Femur Fractures

Distal femoral fractures occur in all age groups as a result of a variety of injuries. Older patients with osteoporotic bone may suffer this fracture from simple falls. Younger patients usually require higher-energy injuries, such as a motor vehicle accident, pedestrian injury, or falls from heights, to suffer supracondylar femur fractures. Patients usually present with pain, swelling, and deformity. Simple nondisplaced fractures may present only with a knee effusion. Supracondylar fractures are intraarticular fractures because of the large extension of the suprapatellar pouch of the knee. Even these fractures, which may be nonarticular, may result in scarring within the suprapatellar pouch and knee stiffness. Intracondylar fractures, by definition, involve the articular cartilage of the distal femur. Knee stiffness and posttraumatic arthritis is a major late complication of these fractures. Successful treatment of these fractures involves four major principles: (1) anatomic reduction of the fracture fragments, particularly intraarticular reduction; (2) preservation of the blood supply to the fracture fragments; (3) stable internal fixation; and (4) early, active, pain-free motion. Treatment is generally surgical for most of these fractures. Occasionally, a nondisplaced fracture is stable enough to be treated nonoperatively in a cast-brace. The majority of displaced fractures, including nondisplaced intraarticular fractures are treated with surgery.

In a patient with an open growth plate fractures that involve the growth plate may cause growth abnormalities. Absolute anatomic reductions are valuable in reducing this complication. Salter and Harris group fractures through the growth plate into five types. Type I is through the growth plate; type II is through the growth plate with extension into the metaphysis; type III is through the growth plate with extension into the epiphysis; type IV crosses the growth plate; and type V is a crush of the growth plate. The higher the type, the greater the risk of a growth abnormality. All growth plates can sustain fractures, but the most common site is the distal femur.

Patella Fractures

Patella fractures usually are caused by direct trauma to the patella but may also occur as a result of avulsion forces on the patella. This happens when the knee experiences sudden forced flexion while the quadriceps muscle is actively contracting. Fractures are classified by their geometry and location. The more common fractures are transverse secondary to avulsion forces; comminuted or stellate fractures may be caused by direct trauma. The patella functions as an integral part of the extensor mechanism and displacement of the patella usually is an indication that the extensor retinaculum has been interrupted. Disruption of the extensor retinaculum will make active extension of the knee impossible. Similar soft-tissue disruptions of either the quadriceps tendon or patellar tendon may result from a similar mechanism of injury and present with lack of active extension. These injuries usually present with tenderness and a palpable defect over the ruptured tendon. The treatment of the soft-tissue injuries is surgical repair. The treatment of patella fractures is to restore the extensor mechanism and reconstruct the articular surface of the patella.

Nondisplaced fractures of the patella require immobilization in extension. This can be accomplished with a plaster cylinder cast or knee immobilizer. Immobilization of 6–8 weeks should allow healing and prevent separation of the fragments. Displaced fractures require open reduction and internal fixation. The goal of treatment is to restore the articular surface and repair the fragments securely enough to start early ROM therapy.

Tibial Plateau Fractures

Tibial plateau fractures involve the articular surface of the proximal tibia. These fractures occur when the knee experiences a varus or valgus force, with or without a combined action or compression force. The force causes failure of the bone or ligaments, but rarely both within the same compartment. Lateral plateau fractures are the most common followed by bicondylar and finally medial fractures. Lateral plateau fractures usually occur from a force directed from the lateral side with a resultant valgus force. The amount of force and degree of osteopenia determines the magnitude of depression, displacement, and combination. Typically, younger patients have split-type fractures. Older adult patients with osteopenia usually have split-depression fractures.

The principles of treatment are to restore the articular surface, maintain alignment of the articular surface with the rest of the leg, and to resume early ROM exercise. These goals are best accomplished with internal fixation of the fracture. The challenge for the orthopaedic surgeon is to achieve these goals with avoidance of the severe complications that can occur with this fracture. An articular step-off of greater than 3 mm or a widening of greater than 5 mm are indicators for surgery. Instability of greater than 5 degree or angulation of greater than 5 degrees should also be treated surgically. Any bony avulsions of the cruciate ligaments should be repaired at the time of internal fixation. The menisci should be repaired and saved whenever possible.

Tibial Shaft Fractures

Tibia shaft fractures result from direct traumas such as motor vehicle accidents, sport injuries, and falls. All age groups are affected and approximately 30 percent of fractures are open injuries. The high incidence of open fractures is a result of the subcutaneous position of the bone. Nondisplaced fractures may present with localized pain and swelling, and an inability to bear weight, but lack obvious deformity. Displaced or angulated fractures are easily diagnosed on physical examination. The physician must perform a careful neurovascular examination of the extremity with a special concern to any signs or symptoms of compartment syndrome. There is no significant difference in the rate of healing of tibial fractures according to the location of the fracture, plane of the fracture, or treatment of the fracture. Rate of healing appears to be more a relationship with the severity of the trauma. Fractures caused by high-energy trauma with open wounds, such as those associated with automobile accidents, have the longest rate of healing.

Treatment options vary widely and should be discussed regarding open versus closed injuries. Closed tibia fractures, in general, can be treated successfully with closed reduction and cast immobilization. The indications for surgical treatment of closed tibia fractures remain relative and generally are at the discretion of the treating orthopaedic surgeon. Surgical treatment consists of reamed or nonreamed nailing of the fracture. Management of open tibia fractures remains a challenge to the orthopaedic surgeon. These fractures are usually the result of high-energy, direct trauma and there may be associated trauma elsewhere in the body. In some cases, the limb is so severely traumatized that salvage of the limb may be impossible.

Ankle Injury

Injuries to the ankle are common. The majority are ankle sprains that need temporary rest and completely heal with no residual consequences. There are more significant ligament injuries that occur to the ankle that can present like a simple ankle sprain. These more significant ligament injuries need to be treated with at least immobilization in a cast, and sometimes with surgery to allow maximum recovery. The patients with ankle fractures can be treated with a reduction and cast immobilization or open reduction and internal fixation. The patients also should have physical therapy after their injury has healed to regain their motion, strength, and ankle proprioception.

Depending on the degree of injury, the patient can sustain a strain, sprain, or complete disruption of the lateral ligaments. The degree of swelling and ecchymosis is directly correlated with the degree of ligamentous injury and is a simple means of determining the significance of the injury. If there is concern that the ligaments are completely torn and that the ankle is unstable, stress radiographs can be taken to evaluate the stability of the ankle. When the degree of the ligamentous injury is in question the initial management should be immobilization in a cast with a reassessment after the swelling and acute pain has subsided.

In general, ankle fractures that can be easily reduced and held with the foot in an anatomic position can be treated with a closed procedure. The patient is initially placed in a long-leg cast. This can be shortened to a well-molded short-leg cast after 3–4 weeks. Patients whose fracture cannot be reduced, or cannot be held reduced without placing the foot in an extreme position, should have open reduction and internal fixation.

The fibular is most often internally fixed with a plate, although the medial malleolus is held with one or two screws. If the deltoid ligament is torn but the talus reduces anatomically with reduction and fixation of the lateral malleolus, no surgery treatment of the deltoid is needed. If the reduction of the talus within the ankle mortis is not anatomic, the medial side of the ankle should be opened to remove any tissue that is preventing the reduction.

Talus

The most common fracture location is through the neck of the talus. The degree of displacement is both prognostically important and indicates the best treatment. Displaced fractures need reduction and internal fixation. Osteonecrosis of the proximal talus is a risk.

Calcaneus

Fractures of the calcaneus are common. They usually are caused by falls from heights. They may be associated with a lumbar fracture. The treatment depends on the amount of displacement and the expectations of the patient. Those with minimal displacement are treated closed. Involvement of the subtalar joint needs to be assessed and as close to an anatomic reduction of any intraarticular component is critical. Böhler angle is a radiographic measurement indicating the amount of displacement.

Midfoot Injury

Dislocations between the tarsal bones and proximal metatarsals are a more common injury than is realized. They often are seen after what seems to be a minor injury. The patient complains of pain in the midfoot and there is swelling. The plain radiographic findings are subtle and one has to suspect the injury to make the diagnosis. Often, it can be treated closed, but open reduction and internal fixation is indicated if the closed reduction is not anatomic or cannot be held reduced.

Metatarsal Fractures

Fractures of the metatarsals are usually a result of direct trauma (e.g., dropping a heavy object on the dorsum of the foot). These are easily treated by non–weight-bearing for 4–6 weeks, followed by gradual resumption of activities.

An exception is the base of the fifth metatarsal. There are two types of fractures at this site. Avulsion injuries occur when the peroneus brevis muscle pulls off the bone with a fragment of the bone. This can be treated closed and will be healed within 6 weeks. Bone union is not necessary for normal function. A Jones fracture is a fracture to the proximal fifth metatarsal through the metaphysic or proximal diaphysis. This injury has an increased risk of delayed union or nonunion. Often, internal fixation is recommended immediately and should be used if the bone is not united within 3 months.

Toes

Fractures of the phalanges of the toes are very common. Treatment is almost always only taping to the adjacent toe. If the great toe has a displaced fracture, pin fixation may be indicated.

Clavicle

More than 80 percent of fractures of the clavicle occur in the middle third of the clavicle, and almost all of the remainder occur in the distal third of the clavicle. The most common causes are a direct blow to the clavicle, a fall on the shoulder, or a fall on an outstretched arm. Clavicle fractures often are seen in patients with multiple injuries and should be specifically looked for in this situation because they can be easily missed. Swelling and tenderness are usually found at the fracture site and pain is associated with shoulder motion. Associated neurovascular injuries can occur, but are uncommon.

Fractures that occur in the middle third of the clavicle are treated by placing the injured arm in a sling. The patient should start to move the shoulder as soon as pain allows, usually within a few days to a week, to reduce the risk of developing restricted shoulder motion. Healing usually occurs in about 6–8 weeks with return to full function in about 3 months. Children will heal the fracture faster and start using their arm earlier than an adult. Nonunion is rare.

Distal-third clavicle fractures are less common and require more care. When there is minimal displacement nonoperative treatment is advised. When there is more than 100 percent displacement surgical treatment should be considered.

Acromioclavicular Separation

The mechanism of injury of the acromioclavicular (AC) joint is usually direct trauma to the acromion with a fall onto the shoulder. The patient presents with pain, swelling, and tenderness at the AC joint. Shoulder motion also causes pain. Direct pressure on the distal clavicle often demonstrates the instability of the joint. All AC joint separations can be treated nonoperatively. The more active the patient and the more displaced the more likely the patient will benefit from an open reduction and internal fixation. Those patients with persistent pain are operated on later.

Anterior Shoulder Dislocation

The glenohumeral joint is the most commonly dislocated large joint in the body. The humerus can dislocate anteriorly, posteriorly, or inferiorly relative to the glenoid. Anterior dislocations are by far the most common, accounting for more than 95 percent of cases. They generally occur after an indirect trauma with the arm abducted, externally rotated, and extended. Anterior dislocations often cause a tear in the glenoid labrum (Bankart lesion) and also can cause a compression fracture of the posterolateral aspect of the humeral head by the glenoid rim (Hill-Sachs lesion). When one of these occur, the patient usually develops recurrent dislocations of their shoulder.

Patients present with a painful shoulder held in slight external rotation and abduction. Physical examination may show squaring off of the shoulder with loss of the deltoid prominence, and fullness anteriorly, where the humeral head is situated. There is minimal active motion of the shoulder. A neurovascular exam should be performed. Sensation over the lateral deltoid region must be assessed, because the axillary nerve is the most common nerve injured. Anteroposterior, scapular Y, and axillary radiographs are obtained. Radiographs will demonstrate the anterior dislocation and any associated fractures of the proximal humerus or glenoid.

Reduction of the dislocated shoulder should be performed expeditiously. Narcotic analgesics and sedatives are usually necessary to facilitate reduction. Numerous reduction maneuvers have been described, but two of the more commonly used are the Stimson technique and the Hippocratic technique. The Stimson technique involves placing the patient prone with the involved arm hanging off the side of the table. Traction is applied by hanging weights from the patient's wrist. The patient must relax. Usually the shoulder reduces quickly, but it may take 15 min before the tensed shoulder muscles fatigue and allow the shoulder to reduce. In the Hippocratic technique, longitudinal traction is applied with the arm slightly abducted. Countertraction is applied in the axillary region, either with one's foot as originally described by Hippocrates or by an assistant holding onto a sheet wrapped around the patient's chest. Older patients are prone to develop shoulder stiffness so passive ROM, along with isometric exercises, is begun in 1–2 weeks. Rotator cuff tears are a common associated injury after shoulder dislocation in older adult patients. Slow progress with rehabilitation in this group should prompt one to evaluate for a cuff tear, because surgical cuff repair may be beneficial. Young patients are at risk for redislocation so they are kept immobilized from 3–4 weeks. Redislocation is the most common complication after shoulder dislocation. The age of the patient is the most important factor, with recurrence rates as high as 80–90 percent in patients younger than age 20 years, and as low as 10–15 percent in patients older than age 40 years.

If a shoulder joint has been dislocated for a few days, it becomes much harder to reduce by closed techniques. Open reduction is the only means to reduce the shoulder joint in this circumstance.

Posterior Shoulder Dislocation

Posterior shoulder dislocations most often are due to seizures or electric shock. Patients present with pain, the shoulder held in internal rotation, and adduction. The injury frequently is not recognized in the emergency room. Physical findings include a prominent coracoid process, fullness of the posterior shoulder, and limited external rotation and elevation of the shoulder. Anteroposterior, scapular Y, and axillary radiographs are obtained. The dislocation may be missed on the anteroposterior radiograph because the findings are subtle.

Proximal Humerus Fractures

Proximal humerus fractures are common in the older adult population and generally occur from a fall on an outstretched hand. They occur less commonly in young adults, but are often more serious with associated injuries such as shoulder dislocation because of the higher forces required to fracture nonosteoporotic bone. Patients present with pain, swelling, and tenderness about the shoulder and have difficulty with active motion. Three orthogonal radiographic views of the shoulder best demonstrate the displacement of the fracture. These consist of an anteroposterior view, a scapular Y view, and axillary view. The location(s) of the fracture can be categorized as anatomic neck, surgical neck, greater tuberosity, and lesser tuberosity. Displacement of the fracture fragments can be explained by the muscular forces that are applied to them. In surgical neck fractures, the shaft tends to displace anteromedially because of the pull of the pectoralis major. Greater tuberosity fractures are displaced superiorly and posteriorly by the attached supraspinatus, infraspinatus, and teres minor. Lesser tuberosity fragments are displaced medially by the subscapularis.

Minimally displaced fractures are treated with immobilization followed by early ROM. Closed reduction is attempted on displaced two-part surgical neck fractures, but if an adequate reduction cannot be obtained or maintained, surgical reduction and fixation is performed. Displaced greater tuberosity fractures usually require surgery as they may impinge on the undersurface of the acromion when the shoulder is elevated and block elevation and external rotation. Displaced three-part fractures usually are treated with closed reduction and percutaneous pin fixation, although four-part fractures often are treated with humeral head prostheses because of the high incidence of osteonecrosis of the humeral head. To minimize shoulder stiffness, early postoperative passive ROM exercise is begun if adequate stability was obtained with surgery.

Humeral Shaft Fractures

Fractures of the humeral shaft can be the result of either direct or indirect trauma. Patients present with pain, swelling, and difficulty moving the shoulder and elbow. Examination reveals swelling and tenderness of the arm with crepitus and motion at the fracture site. Radial nerve palsies are commonly associated injuries, particularly with fractures of the middle third of the humerus. Most of these are neurapraxias that resolve spontaneously within 3 to 4 months and therefore do not require operative nerve exploration.

A vast majority of humeral shaft fractures can be treated nonoperatively. A U-shaped plaster coaptation splint is commonly used initially. This is frequently converted to a humeral functional brace after 1–2 weeks, allowing better early ROM exercises of the shoulder and elbow. Operative stabilization of humeral shaft fractures is recommended in certain cases including inability to obtain an adequate alignment with a splint or brace, open fracture, floating elbow (fractures of humerus and radius/ulna), fracture with vascular injury, polytrauma, and pathologic fracture. Fracture fixation can be done with compression plate, intramedullary rod, or external fixation.

Elbow Fractures

Olecranon and distal humerus fractures are generally pure bone injuries with intact ligaments, barring iatrogenic injury. Open reduction and rigid internal fixation is recommended in the adult.

Supracondylar fractures are common in children and if minimally displaced, can be treated with a closed reduction and cast. A forearm compartment syndrome is not an uncommon complication. If displaced closed reduction and pin fixation most often is performed.

Forearm Fractures

The radius and ulna are the two bones of the forearm. Motor vehicle accidents, sports injuries, falls, or direct blows to the forearm may cause a fracture to one or both of these bones. The fracture may or may not have a significant associated soft-tissue or joint injury. Fractures of both bones of the forearm are described by their location (proximal, midshaft, or distal), by the amount of displacement (minimal, moderate, or complete), the degree of angulation, the extent of comminution, and whether the fracture is open (compound) or closed.

A fracture of the ulna with an associated dislocation of the radial head is known as a Monteggia fracture. A fracture in the distal third of the radius with an associated dislocation of the distal radioulnar joint is called a Galeazzi fracture. An isolated fracture of the ulna is called a "nightstick" fracture because being hit by a nightstick was a common mechanism of injury.

Recognizing a dislocation of the radial head from its normal articulation with the humeral capitellum can be difficult. A line perpendicular to the articular surface and through the central position of the radial head should bisect the capitellum. This relationship should be seen on all projections if the radial head is anatomically located. Generally, forearm fractures are treated with a closed manipulation and cast immobilization for children and open reduction and internal fixation in adults.

Distal Radius Fracture

Fractures of the distal radius are among the most common fractures encountered in children and in adults. There is a bimodal peak of incidence occurring in later childhood and after the sixth decade of life. Fractures in males contribute a greater number to the earlier peak, although fractures in females predominate in the later years. The most common mechanism of injury in both children and adults is a lower-energy fall from ground level onto an outstretched hand with the wrist extended. Fractures that do occur from higher-energy injuries have varying degrees of comminution, may occur in any age group, and have a higher incidence of associated injuries. Anteroposterior, lateral, and possibly oblique radiographs are usually all that are needed to assess distal radius fractures. In the presence of comminution and intraarticular involvement, a CT scan may be of use to assess the status of the radiocarpal, and especially the radioulnar, joints. Patients with distal radius fractures present with pain, swelling, and deformity. Examination must include a neurologic assessment prior to and after reduction of the fracture.

In children, the distal radius fractures are grouped into metaphyseal (more common) and physeal fractures. The metaphyseal fractures may be complete or incomplete (buckle or torus fracture). The physeal fractures are described according to the Salter-Harris classification. The majority of these fractures in children are treated by closed means. Buckle fractures are treated in plaster for 4 weeks. Angulated and/or displaced fractures are manipulated and kept in a cast for 6 weeks. If at least 2 years of growth remain, up to 20 degrees of angulation may be accepted because remodeling will occur. Physeal injuries are reduced by gentle distraction and manipulation avoiding repeated attempts and possible further physeal injury. The aim of treatment of distal radius fractures in adults is to restore the general alignment of the distal radius and ulna, avoiding radial shortening of greater than 3–5 mm, residual angulation greater than 10–15 degrees, and articular incongruity of greater than 2–3 mm. The degree of residual deformity accepted will depend on the age and functional needs of the individual patient. The majority of these fractures are extra-articular or have a minimally displaced, intraarticular component, and are treated successfully by closed reduction followed by 6 weeks of protection in a cast, splint, or brace. Closed reduction is obtained by finger-trap traction followed by manipulation and application of the splint of choice, usually under hematoma-block local anesthesia. Fractures with severe shortening, angulation, and comminution are usually unstable and require some form of fixation.

Spinal Injuries

Injuries to the spinal column are potentially the most devastating of orthopaedic injuries. They occur most often after high-energy trauma such as motor vehicle accidents and falls from significant heights. Initial stabilization of potential spinal injuries at the scene of the accident is done with rigid backboard to protect the thoracic and lumbar spine and with a rigid cervical collar to immobilize the cervical spine. All patients with high-energy injuries should be presumed to have spine injuries until proven otherwise.

Spine fractures, dislocations, and fracture/dislocations are caused by falls, major trauma, and diving accidents. The location of the fracture can be predicted by the mechanism of the injury. Diving accidents cause injuries to the cervical spine. This is one of the most common causes of paralysis. Often, patients present with a history of diving into water that was too shallow. Injuries to the thoracic spine, especially to the lower thoracic/upper lumbar spine, are usually a result of major trauma from an automobile accident or when a pedestrian is struck by a car. Lower lumbar injuries are more likely a result of a fall, with the patient landing on their feet or buttocks. Common combinations of injuries are calcaneal fractures with a lumbar burst fracture.

There are general categories of fractures. The most important initial differential is whether the patient has or does not have neurologic injury. The next differential is whether the spine is stable or unstable. Any neurologic injury indicates that the spine is unstable. All patients should be carefully log-rolled and the spinous processes along the entire spine palpated for tenderness. A rapid, but thorough neurologic examination should be performed. In patients with severe spinal cord injuries, it is important to determine whether the injury is complete (with total motor and sensory loss) or incomplete. The prognosis for complete spinal cord injuries is worse, with no return of functional strength below the level of injury. The presence of rectal tone, perianal sensation, or great toe flexor activity indicates that the injury is incomplete with sacral sparing and that the prognosis for recovery of nerve function is better. An absent bulbocavernosus reflex (anal sphincter contraction after pressure is applied to the glans penis or the clitoris or after gently tugging on the Foley catheter) indicates that spinal shock is present. Determination of whether a seemingly complete neurologic deficit is actually so cannot be made until spinal shock has resolved, which nearly always occurs within 24 h.

A lateral cervical spine radiograph is part of the initial "trauma series" that is obtained on all multitrauma patients. The radiograph must include the entire cervical spine from the occiput to the first thoracic vertebra. Inability to obtain a proper lateral radiograph necessitates additional views, such as swimmer's view, to visualize the lower cervical spine or a CT scan. Other views of the cervical spine that should be obtained after the patient is sufficiently resuscitated and stabilized are the AP and openmouth odontoid views. Anteroposterior, lateral thoracic spine, and lumbar spine radiographs are obtained in all unconscious or mentally impaired patients, and in conscious, alert patients with pain and/or tenderness in those regions.

Patients with neurologic injuries seen within 24 h of their injury are started on 30 mg/kg methylprednisolone, then 5.4 mg/kg per h for 24 h. Although there is some controversy regarding its efficacy, most believe the steroid improves the chance of recovery. Patients with spinal cord injuries may also have neurogenic shock with hypotension and bradycardia secondary to disruption of sympathetic outflow.

Cervical Spine

Stable injuries without nerve deficit can generally be treated with a cervical orthosis or a halo vest. The halo vest provides better immobilization than a cervical orthosis and is therefore preferred when there is a risk of instability. However, the halo vest does not completely restrict cervical motion and thus is not sufficient in patients with grossly unstable injuries. These types of patients require operative internal stabilization.

The presence of spinal cord compression with incomplete nerve injury generally necessitates operative decompression of the spine to facilitate recovery and prevent further damage to the cord. Most injuries are adequately seen on plain radiographs, but CT scans often are used to better appreciate the details of the bone fragments. For patients with neurologic injury an MRI is useful because the spinal cord and soft tissues within the canal can be visualized.

JOINT REPLACEMENT SURGERY

Total Hip Replacement

Pain and progressive disability in the face of failed conservative measures constitute the primary indication for total hip replacement. Total hip replacement is indicated in patients with deterioration of the hip joint, which may result from a number of causes, including degenerative arthritis, rheumatoid arthritis, osteonecrosis, ankylosing spondylitis, postinfectious arthritis, benign and malignant bone tumors of the hip joint, and hip fractures. Active infection, abductor muscle loss, progressive neurologic disease, and neurotrophic joints are specific contraindications to total hip replacement. Two types of fixation are employed: cement (polymethylmethacrylate, PMMA) and cementless. Cementless fixation is based on the use of a porous material that allows bone grow into the prosthesis. Roughened surfaces and biologically active coatings promote ingrowth of bone as a fixation method. For fixation of the acetabular component, cementless fixation is used in most healthy patients undergoing primary total hip replacement. Cemented fixation is used primarily in older adult patients (currently those older than 70 years of age), and in patients in which ingrowth is unlikely, such as those with significant prior irradiation to the pelvis. For fixation of the femoral component, both cemented and cementless stems are employed.

The major complications associated with total hip arthroplasty include infection, thromboembolism, heterotopic ossification, and dislocation. Infection is the most devastating consequence after total hip arthroplasty. The incidence of infection is 0.5–1 percent for primary total hip replacement. Thromboembolism is the most common complication following total hip arthroplasty and the leading cause of postoperative morbidity. The incidence of deep venous thrombosis, depending on how hard one looks, ranges from 8–70 percent with the occurrence of fatal pulmonary embolus, and from 1–2 percent in patients who are not given prophylaxis for thromboembolism. Multiple methods of postoperative prophylaxis (aspirin, warfarin, heparin, support hose, and sequential compression devices) are employed to lessen the incidence of deep vein thrombosis and pulmonary embolism. Despite the success of total hip arthroplasty, relatively short-term implant survival rates in active, young patients and in heavy laborers make its use in these groups problematic. As previously stated, the presence of an active infection is a contraindication to total hip arthroplasty. For patients in these situations, alternatives to hip arthroplasty include hip arthrodesis, hip osteotomies, and resection arthroplasty.

Total Knee Replacement

A total knee replacement resurfaces the distal femur with a metal prosthesis that articulates with a polyethylene surface that is attached to the tibia. Most commonly, the patella is also resurfaced with a dome-shaped implant made of high-density polyethylene. Fixation of the implants to the bone surfaces is either achieved with acrylic bone cement or by bone ingrowth into a roughened or coated prosthesis. Today, cemented knee replacements are the most commonly performed because of the excellent results achieved in long-term clinical studies.

As in other types of joint replacement, infection and deep venous thrombosis are significant systemic complications. Infection rates have been reported at 1–2 percent. Despite the indicated successes of total knee arthroplasty, younger patients continue to present a difficult challenge and often require alternate treatments. Osteotomy of the tibia or femur often is used to transfer weight-bearing load to an uninvolved tibiofemoral joint surface when there is unicompartmental disease. This procedure is most commonly done at the proximal tibia for medial compartmental disease but may also be performed at the distal femur in lateral compartment disease. Arthrodesis provides another surgical alternative for the management of young patients with unstable degenerative knees, the management of septic arthritis with extensive destruction of the joint, and in neuropathic joints. Arthrodesis and resection arthroplasty may be employed in patients with failed total knee replacement in which prosthetic implantation is not an option.

SHOULDER DISORDERS

Rotator Cuff and Biceps Tendon

The rotator cuff consists of four muscles: the supraspinatus, infraspinatus, teres minor, and subscapularis. All insert onto the tuberosities of the humeral head. The primary function of the rotator cuff is to provide dynamic stabilization of the glenohumeral joint by depressing the humeral head into the glenoid cavity. The rotator cuff separates the subacromial bursa from the glenohumeral joint. The acromion covers the bursa and can contribute to local problems. Tears of the rotator cuff, either partial or complete, are common in individuals older than age 40 years and increase with each subsequent decade. Patients with rotator cuff pathology present with pain (especially at night), weakness, and difficulties with the activities of daily living, particularly overhead motions. On physical examination, they have limited shoulder abduction because of pain. It is important to rule out referred pain from cervical spine pathology. Plain radiographs are indicated, but MRI is the most useful means of evaluating the rotator cuff.

The biceps muscle has two heads—a long and short. The long head tendon is intraarticular. It originates on the supraglenoid tubercle of the glenoid and lies between the lesser and greater tuberosities of the humeral head. The long head can be inflamed and can be a source of shoulder pain. Rupture of the long head of the biceps can lead to the characteristic "Popeye" deformity of the arm. This is caused by the muscle bunching in the upper arm. This is treated in young, active patients, but not in older patients.

Frozen Shoulder

Patients with adhesive capsulitis or "frozen section" present with shoulder pain and limited motion. Because the scapula moves on the chest wall, patients often do not appreciate how limited their motion is. Careful examination reveals complete loss of motion at the glenohumeral joint. Most often this occurs after a short period of immobilization of the shoulder. Other patients have no inciting event. Diabetics have a higher incidence of adhesive capsulitis than do nondiabetics. Physical therapy is the mainstay of treatment and it often takes up to 1 year to regain full motion. Rarely is surgical intervention necessary.

Glenohumeral Instability

Glenohumeral instability is a spectrum of disorders, which can vary in severity (subluxation to complete dislocation), direction (anterior, posterior, or multidirectional), and duration (acute, recurrent, or chronic). An acute, traumatic, anterior dislocation is the most common instability situation. The risk of developing recurrent subluxation or dislocations is inversely proportional to age, with those patients who have their first acute dislocation before they are 20 years of age having more than an 80 percent incidence of recurrence. Recurrent instability most often is caused by a tear of the anterior labrum off the anterior glenoid; the so-called Bankart lesion. Most patients who have repeated dislocations of their shoulder require surgical repair. Posterior dislocations more often are caused by a seizure or a fall in an older adult patient. This dislocation is often missed by the unsuspecting physician.

Glenohumeral Arthritis

Arthritis of the shoulder joint occurs less often than arthritis of the hip or knee. Idiopathic osteoarthritis is the most common cause of shoulder degeneration; however, other arthritic conditions can produce shoulder damage (e.g., rheumatoid, septic, posttraumatic, and rotator cuff deficiency arthropathy). Pain, weakness, limited motion in all planes of motion, and crepitus are common complaints. If conservative measures such as heat, activity modifications, and nonsteroidal antiinflammatory medications (NSAIDs) do not produce relief, total shoulder arthroplasty may be indicated.

ELBOW DISORDERS

Epicondylitis most often affects the lateral epicondyle; however, the incidence of medial epicondylitis has increased with the popularity of golf. Another common, nontraumatic elbow condition is ulnar nerve compression (cubital tunnel syndrome), which is caused by compression of the ulnar nerve in the cubital tunnel or proximal flexor carpi ulnaris muscle, and causes pain and dysesthesias in the little and ulnar border of the ring fingers. Compression of the radial nerve or posterior interosseous nerve beneath the supinator muscle is much less common than ulnar nerve compression. The vague forearm aching and pain associated with this syndrome may respond to neurolysis, but electrodiagnostic studies, unlike cubital tunnel syndrome, are not diagnostic.

Rupture of the distal biceps tendon attachment to the bicipital tuberosity of the proximal radius may occur as a consequence of a chronic, degenerative tendinopathy. Treatment may be conservative or surgical repair may be performed. If treated conservatively, the patient can expect good flexion strength, but notable weakness of supination and aching with heavy use.

SPINE DISORDERS

Low Back Pain

Pain in the lumbar area and buttock is one of the most common complaints heard in medicine. The majority of adults will have at least one episode of low back pain during their life, and many adults have recurrent episodes. Most instances of low back pain will not have a specific diagnosis and the cause is generally muscular strain and spasm. More significant abnormalities need to be excluded when a patient with low back pain is evaluated. The most important spinal diagnosis to exclude is a neoplasia; however, it is also the least likely cause. Patients with aortic aneurysms and pancreatic cancer can present with low back pain and these diagnoses must be considered. Degenerative arthritis is a more common cause of low back pain, but a delay in making this diagnosis is not significant. Herniated disc with nerve compression is a relatively common cause of back pain associated with leg pain and should be recognized from the patient's history and physical examination.

The initial evaluation includes the taking of a history to determine how the pain started, how long it has persisted, how severe it is, what makes it worse, and what makes it better. The abdomen should be examined. The patient's back is examined for tenderness, masses, muscular spasm, alignment, and motion. A neurologic examination should be done and a rectal examination is recommended. If no abnormalities are noted, except decreased motion and muscular spasm, the patient can be treated with a few days of rest and mild pain medication. If pain persists, a more complete evaluation is indicated.

Patients with a herniated disc without compression of a nerve root do not need specific treatment. They present with low back pain and virtually all will improve with nonoperative care. Those with compression of a nerve root will have pain that is distributed in the dermatome of the compressed nerve root. The patient usually has a positive straight-leg-raise test. Initially, nonoperative treatment is recommended, and most patients will have relief. Those with persistent pain or recurrent pain should undergo disc removal.

Discitis is an infection of the disc. This is not uncommon is children but is unusual in adults unless they are immunosuppressed or IV drug users. These patients will have unremitting back pain. On a radiograph there will be a loss of disc height; however, this may not be apparent until sometime after the patient has sought medical treatment.

Degenerative arthritis occurs in older adults, and typically can be managed with physical therapy and anti-inflammatory medication. Some patients will develop spinal stenosis as a result of compromise of the spinal canal. These patients may require decompression.

Another common cause of back pain, although usually seen more in the mid-back than in the lower back, is a compression fracture. Most compression fractures occur in osteoporotic bone and are caused by minimal trauma. Compression fractures can occur in patients with normal bone and are usually caused by significant trauma. However, the most common scenario is an older adult female who complains of acute onset back pain after a minor fall or automobile accident. There will be anterior wedging of a mid-thoracic vertebra. These patients are treated nonoperatively, usually with an extension brace.

Neck Pain

Like low back pain, neck pain is common. Usually it occurs after a minor injury and often is referred to as "whiplash." The usual patient has pain in the neck without a radicular component, loss of motion, and muscular spasm.

MUSCLE AND TENDON INJURIES

The most commonly injured muscles in the lower extremity are the hamstrings, quadriceps, and gastrocnemius. Injuries to these muscles either originate from a direct blow or, more typically, from a sudden eccentric contraction (acute lengthening of muscle as it is trying to shorten). This, in turn, ruptures muscle fibers. In severe cases, a defect in the muscle can be palpated; however, in most cases there is no gross defect. A well-defined sequence of events then occurs: bleeding, damage to muscle cells, and an inflammatory response that leads to a repair. Scar tissue then forms, ultimately leaving the muscle stiffer (less elastic) and more prone to re-injury. Treatment, therefore, involves controlling the pain and inflammation acutely and stretching as the muscle heals to try to keep it at its normal resting length. In severe cases in which there is a disruption in the muscle tissue, both remodeled muscle tissue and postinjury muscle strength are improved by suturing the torn muscle tissue together.

Another sequence of events that can be spawned from a quadriceps contusion is myositis ossificans (MO). Myositis ossificans also is called heterotopic bone formation. The majority of patients with MO will recover full function and can be successfully treated nonoperatively. Rarely, a patient will have persistent loss of motion and need the ectopic bone removed. This should not be done until 1 year or more after the injury. A careful history should be taken with someone who has ossification within a muscle, because MO histologically resembles osteosarcoma, and an incorrect diagnosis either way can be disastrous.

Tendinitis and bursitis are commonly caused by overuse, trauma, or through compensation for another injured area. The presence of a bursa is a normal. It is a thin fluid-filled sac with a lining of blood vessels and nerve endings. Bursa occur in any area that has soft tissue repetitively rubbing over a bony prominence. Once irritated, they swell and become painful. The most common sites to develop bursitis around the knee are overlying the patella and the patella tendon (prepatella bursitis), at the anteromedial aspect of the proximal tibia in which the pes anserine tendons (sartorius, gracilis, and semitendinosus) insert (pes anserine bursitis), and at the posteromedial corner of the tibia in which the semimembranosus inserts (semimembranosus bursitis). Other common sites of bursitis are the bursa inferior to the acromion (subacromial bursa), the bursa over the greater trochanter of the femur (greater trochanter bursa), and the bursa over the olecranon (olecranon bursa).

Initial treatment involves decreasing the inflammation through icing, antiinflammatory medication, and removing the offending insult. With the patella, in particular, it is important to avoid pressure through kneeling or bumping the knee. If this fails, the next step is to use a cortisone injection, aspirating the bursa first, if necessary. Finally, if conservative treatment fails, an excision of the bursa can be performed.

Tendinitis typically occurs from overuse. Endurance sports, such as running and cycling and power sports such as basketball, volleyball, and racquet sports are most frequently involved. The tendons are injured by cumulative microtrauma in which there is a failed adaptation of the cells and extracellular matrix to repetitive activities at submaximal load. Essentially the micro-injuries are unable to heal themselves quickly enough, leading to fatigue of the tendon and, finally, to symptomatic injury. At the knee, the hamstring tendons are most commonly involved and iliotibial band friction syndrome is the most common cause of lateral-based knee pain in runners. The iliotibial band repetitively rubs over the lateral femoral epicondyle, causing both a bursitis and a tendinitis. Other common sites for tendinitis are the biceps tendon (both proximal and distal), common wrist extenders (tennis elbow), the abductor pollicis longus (de Quervain disease), Achilles tendon, and posterior tibial tendon.

Treatment is focused on calming the inflammation and pain. Ice and rest are the initial modalities. Antiinflammatory medications are usually prescribed. As the pain subsides, stretching of all tight structures and the use of modalities such as ultrasound and electrical stimulation may be beneficial. Rarely is surgical intervention required. When needed, surgical procedures include tendon sheath débridement (for tenosynovitis), tendon-relaxing incisions or lengthening, or tendon advancement.

THE ATHLETIC KNEE

Meniscal Injuries

Each knee has a medial and lateral meniscus. These are C-shaped fibrocartilage rings, triangular in cross-section, that serve as shock absorbers and secondary restraints to the ligaments. The lateral meniscus is more circular than the medial meniscus, but less-well attached to the capsule, particularly posteriorly. Because the medial meniscus is more constrained, it is subjected to higher forces and tears more frequently than the lateral meniscus. The peripheral 25 percent of the meniscus is vascularized, thus making it amenable to repair. The inner 75 percent has no blood supply, will not repair a tear, and requires resection if torn and symptomatic. A twisting or hyperflexion event is the usual cause of tears in the athletic population; however, in older individuals, tears may occur without a defined moment, presumably via a cumulative microtraumatic degenerative mechanism.

People with symptomatic tears may recall hearing a pop or tear and then the development of swelling. They complain of pain at the involved joint line, a sense of catching or locking, and often have difficulty with deep flexion. Typically, they cannot squat. On exam there is tenderness over the joint line, particularly posteromedially or laterally, there is pain with hyperflexion. Further confirmation of a tear can be made with greater than 90 percent accuracy with an MRI. Occasionally, a meniscus will tear peripherally and the central torn segment will flip over and stick in the notch of the knee. This is called a bucket-handle tear. The bucket handle often "locks" the knee, preventing extension. This is considered a semi-urgent situation requiring surgery. An arthroscopic repair or trimming is the treatment of choice for symptomatic meniscal tears.

Ligament Injuries

The ACL and posterior cruciate ligament (PCL) are the central pivots to the knee. The ACL provides anterior translation restraint and anterolateral rotatory stability, although the PCL provides mostly posterior translation restraint. They also act as secondary restraints for the collateral ligaments (medial collateral ligament [MCL] and lateral collateral ligament [LCL]), which provide valgus and varus control.

A patient presenting with knee pain after a twisting injury or a varus or valgus torque to their knee with immediate swelling and who reports hearing a pop should be evaluated for a ligament tear. The knee should be examined for instability. The medical collateral ligament and anterior cruciate ligament are the most commonly injured ligaments.

The Dislocated Knee

This condition can be a limb-threatening injury. It usually occurs with high-speed vehicular trauma or with a fall from heights, but can also happen in sporting activities, typically a contact sport. Usually the ACL, PCL, and one of the collateral ligaments are disrupted. There is a high incidence of popliteal artery, tibial nerve, and peroneal nerve injury; therefore, close attention should be paid to the neurovascular status during evaluation of a dislocated knee.

Articular Cartilage Injuries

Articular cartilage does not repair itself. For this reason, it is always best to save as much articular cartilage possible. Whenever possible, any cartilaginous body that has been knocked loose should be replaced into the defect.

FOOT AND ANKLE DISORDERS

Complaints concerning the foot and ankle are common. Ankle injuries are common. Patients with these complaints are some of the most appreciative patients once their condition has been improved.

Tendon Disorders

Tendon disorders of the foot and ankle are common problems, with chronic tendinosis, tendinitis, and frank rupture of the Achilles tendon constituting the majority. The Achilles tendon is the most commonly affected and tendinosis, or a chronic partial tear of the Achilles tendon, presents with thickening of the tendon and pain with palpation. MRI shows degeneration within the tendon and thickening. Tendinitis of the Achilles tendon also presents with pain and inflammation around the tendon. MRI shows fluid around the tendon within the paratenon surrounding the tendon. Tendinosis and tendinitis are treated nonsurgically with NSAIDs, gentle stretching, bracing, and a heel lift. Steroid injections should be avoided in this area because of the risk of rupture of the tendon.

History and physical examination easily diagnose complete rupture of the tendon. Patients report a feeling of being struck in the back of the leg and an inability to ambulate following the injury. It is unusual for a patient with a ruptured Achilles tendon to have had tendinitis of the Achilles tendon. The Thompson test is useful in diagnosing a complete Achilles tendon rupture. This is performed with the patient prone and knees flexed to 90 degrees. The calf is then squeezed on both the affected and normal leg. The normal side will show plantar flexion of the foot with calf compression, although the affected side will not. Absence of plantar flexion is a positive indicator for a disrupted tendon. Nonsurgical treatment of a ruptured Achilles tendon consists of casting the ankle in slight plantar flexion or functional bracing. Surgery often is recommended to repair the ruptured tendon, however, wound complications are common.

Peroneal tendinitis is a common cause of lateral ankle pain following an inversion injury. Symptoms include lateral ankle swelling and pain with resisted eversion of the ankle. Tenderness to palpation is seen over the area just posterior to the distal fibula, and pain may be elicited with passive inversion. MRI often is helpful in imaging the peroneal tendons. Nonsurgical treatment includes rest, a stirrup ankle support, NSAIDs, and physical therapy. Surgery may include direct repair of the tendon and tenodesis to the adjacent peroneal tendon, and tendon transfer.

Posterior tibial tendon insufficiency, often referred to as the adult acquired flat foot, has three distinct stages and presents with pain along the medial side of the ankle and progressive flattening of the longitudinal arch. In stage I, there is swelling and pain along the medial side of the ankle; however, the foot alignment remains normal. In stage II, the posterior tibial tendon and the ligaments supporting the arch begin to stretch, allowing lowering of the longitudinal arch. The heel drifts into valgus and the forefoot abducts; however, the deformity is still flexible. In stage III of posterior tibial tendon insufficiency, arthritis of the hindfoot develops and the hindfoot remains fixed in valgus. At this stage, patients often report pain on the lateral aspect of the ankle, which is caused by impingement between the calcaneus and fibula. Stage IV occurs with long-standing deformity and consists of tilting of the talus within the mortise of the ankle. Radiographs are useful in assessing the position of the foot and ankle and determining the presence of arthritic changes. MRI is very helpful in assessment of the integrity of the posterior tibial tendon. Nonsurgical treatment consists of braces and orthoses, NSAIDs, and cast immobilization. Physical therapy does not usually help in this condition. Surgical treatment consists of tendon transfer with calcaneal osteotomy or lateral column lengthening. Often, an Achilles tendon lengthening is combined with these procedures. For patients with arthritic changes, selective arthrodesis of the hindfoot is necessary.

Heel Pain

Plantar heel pain, most often caused by plantar fascitis, is one of the most common problems seen in the foot. Patients report severe pain with the first step after arising from sleep or after prolonged periods of sitting. The pain usually subsides after a few min of walking and often recurs later in the day after prolonged standing or walking. Usually plantar fascitis is atraumatic in onset. Examination reveals point tenderness along the medial origin of the plantar fascia on the calcaneus. Heel cord contracture often is present. Approximately 40 percent of patients with plantar fasciitis also will have evidence of compression of the first branch of the lateral plantar nerve. Imaging studies should be used to eliminate other causes of heel pain such as a calcaneal stress fracture or insertional Achilles tendinitis. Treatment consists of plantar fascia and heel cord stretching, padding, custom-molded orthoses, NSAIDs, and a night splint to maintain passive stretch on the Achilles tendon and fascia. Cortisone injection can help relieve pain and inflammation. Surgery rarely is necessary and consists of releasing a portion of the plantar fascia along with decompression of the lateral plantar nerve.

Hallux Valgus

Hallux valgus is commonly known as a bunion. The great toe is deviated toward the second toe. The angle between the first metatarsal and proximal phalanges of the great toe is a valgus angle. The common causes of hallux valgus are genetic predisposition combined with improper shoes. Many patients will not have symptoms and do not need treatment. Others complain of pain over the medial eminence and difficulty fitting shoes. Lesser toe deformities often accompany hallux valgus as the migration of the great toe pushes the lateral toes out of proper alignment.

Stress Fractures

Stress fracture, or fatigue fracture of the metatarsals, is a common cause of forefoot pain. Most commonly affected are the second and third metatarsals. Athletes and dancers commonly suffer this problem, along with patients with underlying bone disorders. Symptoms consist of swelling and warmth in the foot, with point tenderness over the affected metatarsal. Radiographs are often negative initially; however, the healing fracture usually is evident by the third week of symptoms. Treatment consists of supportive shoes and temporary cessation of the activity that led to the fatigue fracture. Surgery rarely is necessary.

Ankle Instability

Fifteen percent of patients with an ankle sprain will develop chronic instability of the ankle requiring treatment. Usually an inversion injury causes damage to the lateral ligament complex, including the anterior talofibular and calcaneofibular ligaments. Patients report pain and swelling on the lateral aspect of the ankle, often associated with feelings of "giving way" or weakness of the ankle. Physical examination consists of the anterior drawer test and inversion stress test. Stress radiographs help confirm the diagnosis.

Diabetic Foot

Diabetes commonly affects the foot and can lead to devastating complications, including amputation. Diabetes is the most common cause of neuropathy leading to loss of protective sensation on the plantar aspect of the foot. Charcot arthropathy is a form of arthritis seen in the neuropathic foot and leads to severe deformity. The combination of deformity with a lack of protective sensation leads to pressure ulceration and infection. This can develop into osteomyelitis, and often requires bony resection or amputation. Patients with neuropathy as a consequence of diabetes should be treated with protective shoes consisting of a soft orthoses and accommodative shoes with a soft, leather upper. Pressure relief may be obtained with bracing and shoe modifications. In those patients with deformity not treatable with shoe modifications, surgery is necessary. The goals of surgery are resection of bony prominences, and restoration of normal foot architecture. Surgical débridement should remove all necrotic tissue while producing a stable, plantigrade foot. Correction of the deformity can be successful given the patient has adequate circulation. Preoperative vascular evaluation is often necessary. Adequate glucose control promotes healing of ulcerations, and surgical wounds.

Interdigital Neuroma

Interdigital neuroma often is called a Morton neuroma. The patient's symptoms are a burning or tingling in the plantar aspect of the forefoot radiating into the toes. It most often occurs in the third web space and may be seen between the second and third toes.

Tarsal Tunnel Syndrome

Tarsal tunnel syndrome occurs with compression of the tibial nerve as it passes beneath the flexor retinaculum of the ankle. Patients present with vague symptoms, usually consisting of numbness and tingling on the plantar aspect of the foot. A positive Tinel sign is present over the tibial nerve; however, sensation usually is preserved. Examination should also include the lower spine to rule out a radiculopathy as the source for the symptoms. MRI often is helpful to rule out a space-occupying lesion within the tarsal canal causing compression of the nerve.

PEDIATRIC DISORDERS

Developmental Dysplasia of the Hip

Developmental dysplasia of the hip (DDH) is a spectrum of disorders involving degrees of instability of the hip and underdevelopment of the acetabulum (socket). The term used in the past was congenital dislocation of the hip, but this is currently out of favor. The disorder is usually diagnosed shortly after birth because all newborns are screened for the condition by physical examination and, in some areas, by ultrasonography. DDH can present in the toddler, although controversy exists regarding whether these cases represent missed diagnoses.

The physical examination consists of two provocative maneuvers: the Ortolani test and the Barlow test. The Ortolani maneuver attempts to relocate a dislocated or subluxed hip. The Barlow maneuver attempts to dislocate or subluxate a reduced, but unstable hip.

Slipped Capital Femoral Epiphysis

A slipped capital femoral epiphysis (SCFE) is a developmental disorder in which there is dissociation between the epiphysis and metaphysis of the proximal femur. The term is a misnomer because the epiphysis is fixed in the acetabulum and it is the metaphysis, along with the rest of the femur, which slips. In the vast majority of slips, the epiphysis is posteromedial with respect to the metaphysis. A SCFE usually occurs during the adolescent growth spurt and is bilateral in about one third of cases. Sixty to 65 percent of patients are above the 90th percentile for weight. Patients usually present with pain and a limp. The extremity usually is rotated externally and the time spent on the leg is less than the unaffected leg.

Legg-Calvé-Perthes Disease

Legg-Calvé-Perthes disease (LCP) is defined as idiopathic osteonecrosis of the proximal femoral epiphysis. It occurs between the ages of 2 and 12 years with a peak incidence between 5 and 7 years of age. This corresponds to the period when the blood supply to the epiphysis is discreet. LCP is 3–5 times more common in males than in females, and is bilateral in 10–20 percent of cases. Patients with LCP present with pain in the groin, thigh, or knee. They may have an antalgic or a Trendelenburg gait. Plain radiographs and MRI help to classify the degree of head involvement, which has prognostic significance.

Talipes Equinovarus

Talipes equinovarus (TEV) is referred to as "clubfoot." TEV is an idiopathic congenital deformity of the foot in which there is equinus at the ankle joint, varus and medial rotation at the subtalar joint, and adduction of the midfoot and forefoot. It occurs in 1–2 individuals per 1000 live births and is bilateral in 50 percent of cases.

Metatarsus Adductus

Metatarsus adductus (MA) is differentiated from talipes equinovarus because these patients have a normal midfoot and hindfoot. Ordinarily, the lateral border of the foot is straight; in MA, the lateral border curves inward at the tarsal–metatarsal joints, producing a bean-shaped foot.

Tarsal Coalition

A tarsal coalition is an abnormal congenital connection between two or more tarsal bones. The calcaneonavicular and talocalcaneal joints most commonly are affected. Tarsal coalition is bilateral in 50–60 percent of patients. The cause is a failure of differentiation and segmentation during embryogenesis and is likely to be genetic. Tarsal coalition is estimated to occur in 1–3 percent of the population, and can be asymptomatic. When symptoms occur, they usually do so in early adolescence, when the coalition begins to ossify. Symptoms consist of activity-related foot and ankle pain associated with a fairly inflexible flat foot.

Plain radiographs may be sufficient to visualize the coalition, particularly when special oblique projections are used. When plain radiographs are not diagnostic, CT and MRI can be used. CT is best for bony coalitions and MRI is best for cartilaginous or fibrous coalitions.

Blount Disease

Infantile Blount disease is a disorder of toddlers in which the physiologic genu varum becomes progressive, damaging the anteromedial physis of the proximal tibia. As the bowing continues, increasing pressure on the anteromedial physis inhibits growth medially, which perpetuates the bowing.

Infantile Blount disease is diagnosed between the ages of 18 and 24 months. Affected children are generally early walkers who are above the 80th percentile for weight. Clinically, patients present with increasingly bowed legs and lateral instability of the knee evidenced by a thrust during single-leg stance of gait. Because the anterior portion of the medial physis is more affected than the posterior portion, these patients tend also to have increased internal tibial torsion.

Radiographs are used to measure the metaphyseal–diaphyseal angle (MDA) of Drennan. A measurement of greater than 11–16 degrees in the 18–24-month-old infant is predictive of progression. Classification systems of severity exist and depend on the extent of medial depression of the physis.

Patients with significant genu varum but a normal MDA are simply observed at 6–8-week intervals. Patients with an abnormal MDA and lateral instability are treated with bracing. The brace is designed to apply three-point pressure to the extremity to provide a valgus force, which unloads the medial physis. Controversy exists regarding whether the brace should be worn full-time, only during weight bearing, or while sleeping. Bracing is effective in reversing the progression in approximately 50 percent of cases, which reversal can be observed within 3 to 6 months.

Patients who either progress despite brace treatment or recur following treatment should have a proximal tibial osteotomy to restore the physiologic valgus alignment. An oblique osteotomy is made in the proximal metaphysis. Rotation at the osteotomy site corrects both the varus and torsion.

Adolescent Blount disease is a similar entity that occurs during the adolescent growth spurt. The MDA as an indicator of the significance of the genu valgum in adolescents has not been established. Adolescent Blount disease does not respond to bracing. The treatment is a proximal tibial osteotomy to realign the mechanical axis of the knee. These osteotomies are stabilized with an external fixator to accommodate the generally large size of the patient.

Osgood-Schlatter Disease

Growth cartilage that serves as the origin or insertion of a tendon is called an apophysis. If the muscle associated with the tendon becomes tight, the tendon pulls with excessive force on the apophysis, which becomes inflamed. This condition is known as traction apophysitis. Traction apophysitis can occur at virtually any apophysis and affects different apophyses at different ages. The most common location is the tibial tubercle in which the condition is known by the eponym Osgood-Schlatter disease (OSD).

OSD is caused by a tight quadriceps and typically is seen in patients 12–14 years old. Patients with OSD complain of activity related pain very specifically at the tibial tubercle. The pain can be severe and may also occur after prolonged sitting. On physical exam, the tubercle is prominent and tender and the quadriceps are tight. Stretching of the quadriceps generally reproduces the pain. In unilateral cases, radiographs should be obtained to rule out occult lesions. The treatment is activity modification as dictated by the symptoms and physical therapy to stretch the quadriceps.

Other areas of traction apophysitis include, but are not limited to, the calcaneus (Sever disease), inferior pole of the patella (Sinding-Larsen-Johansson disease), anterior inferior iliac spine, and base of the fifth metatarsal.

Acknowledgment

This chapter was cowritten by members of the Leni and Peter W. May Department of Orthopaedics at the Mount Sinai School of Medicine; Evan Flatow, MD and Professor; Michael Hausman, MD and Professor; Roger Levy, MD and Professor; Sheldon Lichtblau, MD; Randy Rosier, MD and Professor; Elton Strauss, MD and Associate Professor; Edward Yang, MD and Associate Professor; Richard Ghillani, MD and Assistant Professor; James Gladstone, MD and Assistant Professor; Judith Levine, MD and Assistant Professor; Michael Parks, MD and Assistant Professor; and Steven Weinfeld, MD and Assistant Professor.

Suggested Readings

Bucholz RW, Heckman JD, Kasser JR, et al: Rockwood, Green, Wilkins' Fractures, 5th ed. Philadelphia: Lippincott, Williams, and Wilkins, 2001.
Canale ST: Campbell's Operative Orthopaedics, 10th ed. St. Louis: Mosby, 2003.
Canale ST, Beaty JH: Operative Pediatric Orthopaedics, 2nd ed. St. Louis: Mosby, 1995.
Chapman MW, et al: Chapman's Orthopaedic Surgery, 3rd ed. Philadelphia: Lippincott, Williams, and Wilkins, 2000.
Fitzgerald RH, Kaufer H, Malkani AL: Orthopaedics. St. Louis: Mosby, 2002.
Herring JA: Tachdjian's Pediatric Orthopaedics, 3rd ed. St. Louis: Mosby, 2002.
Morrissy RT, Weinstein SL: Atlas of Pediatric Orthopaedic Surgery, 3rd ed. Philadelphia: Lippincott, Williams, and Wilkins, 2000.
Nordin M, Frankel VH: Basic Biomechanics of the Musculoskeletal System. Philadelphia: Lea and Febiger, 1989.
Reider B: The Orthopaedic Physical Examination. St. Louis: Mosby, 1999.
Simon SR: Orthopaedic Basic Science. Rosemont, IL: American Academy of Orthopaedic Surgeons, 1994.

43 | Plastic and Reconstructive Surgery

Saleh M. Shenaq, John Y. S. Kim, Alan Bienstock, Forrest S. Roth, and Eser Yuksel

HISTORY

Plastic surgery is derived from the Greek word, "plastikos," meaning to mold. The unifying objective of all plastic surgeons is the ability to improve or restore form and function through the possibilities inherent in the manipulation and remodeling of tissue. Historically, the premise for plastic surgery dates back several millennia to the Egyptian, "Edwin Smith papyrus," believed to be written in 1700 BC, which heralds modern fastidiousness with wound care, emphasizing the importance of débridement and meticulous surgical technique. During World Wars I and II, plastic surgery as a specialty evolved as surgeons were confronted with complex, massive, traumatic defects of the maxillofacial region and extremities. The reconstructive challenge crossed traditional boundaries of all other surgical specialties. In 1937, the American Board of Plastic Surgery was founded and plastic surgery was truly recognized as a distinct surgical specialty. As medical and technologic innovation resulted in the development of novel and advanced surgical techniques, subspecialization in plastic surgery developed, particularly in craniofacial, hand, aesthetic, and microsurgery. In 1962, Cronin and Gerow introduced the breast implant that sparked a heightened interest in aesthetic and reconstructive breast surgery and a general interest in applying alloplastic materials to plastic surgery.

WOUND HEALING

There are three general types of wound healing: primary, delayed primary and secondary. Primary wound healing is characterized by the physical opposition of wound edges. Delayed primary wound healing occurs when wound margins are intentionally left unopposed in face of presumed infection. If the signs of infection resolve, the wound may then be closed primarily at that time. Secondary wound healing occurs by granulation and wound contraction.

Paramount to wound healing are angiogenesis and the inflammatory reaction created by cells such as polymorphonuclear neutrophils, macrophages, lymphocytes, fibroblasts, and the cytokines they release. The fundamental limiting step to both wound healing and tissue reconstruction is adequate vascularity.

Impaired Wound Healing

Radiation is often an issue for reconstruction of ablative defects. Among other effects, radiation may result in ischemia via microangiopathic damage. Diabetic patients also experience impaired wound healing.

Dysfunctional healing may manifest as abnormal scars. Hypertrophic scars and keloids are manifestations of altered collagen deposition and breakdown. Hypertrophic scars are raised, collagen-rich lesions that do not extend beyond the initial boundaries of injury, whereas keloids are scars that have progressed beyond these margins.

1169

Treatment of scars includes pressure, silicone sheets and gels, intralesional corticosteroids, and topical vitamins A and E. For recalcitrant keloid formation, radiation therapy and surgical excision may be required.

Basic Technique of Skin Closure

The choice of suture material may vary from monofilament to polyfilament and absorbable to nonabsorbable. Minimizing skin tension is essential to maintaining wound closure and preventing excessive scar formation. Techniques to minimize tension include multilayered closures and placement of skin incisions along relaxed-skin tension lines.

Suture Technique

Cutaneous sutures generally are placed through the epidermis and into the deep dermis approximately 2 mm from the skin edge and 7–10 mm apart. Care is taken with any suture placement to ensure that the needle enters the skin as nearly perpendicular as possible. Slight eversion of the skin edges facilitates maximal dermal opposition and closure without contracting depression of the scar.

Vertical and horizontal mattress sutures may yield a more substantial eversion. However, there is a greater theoretical concern of local tissue ischemia and inhibition of tissue healing. Simple or mattress sutures are usually constructed with nonabsorbable material and should be removed as expeditiously as possible to prevent scarring. The buried dermal and fascial sutures should provide the majority of strength of deeper wounds.

Subcuticular sutures are running, superficial dermal sutures that avoid the external scar of cutaneous sutures. However, they should not be relied on to provide the strength of a closure. Simple running cutaneous sutures allow for rapid closure of tissue with some element of hemostasis, especially if performed in a "locking" fashion. Staples also may be used for cutaneous closure. In combination with deeper sutures they may augment the strength of the closure. In general, sutures should not be left in longer than 1 week to avoid unsightly scars. Biosynthetic tissue adhesives such as cyanoacrylate are advantageous when tensionless closure has been accomplished with deeper sutures. They also may obviate the need for local anesthetic. Steri-Strips and other tapes may similarly be used when simple apposition of the superficial skin is required.

Reconstruction of more complex defects may require the recruitment of local or distant tissue. The "reconstructive ladder" algorithm for reconstruction of a given defect are primary closure, skin grafts, skin flaps, tissue expansion, local muscle flaps and free flaps.

SOFT TISSUE RECONSTRUCTION

Skin Grafts

The term graft indicates that the vascular supply has been severed during the procurement of the tissue. Graft survival depends on three sequential events: (1) imbibition—the absorption of nutrients from recipient capillary beds during the first 24 h; (2) inosculation—the alignment of donor and recipient vessels during the 24–72-hour period; and (3) angiogenesis—ingrowth of vessels from the recipient bed into the graft after 72 h. Factors that may interrupt this process include fluid collection under the graft or mechanical shear forces. This is in contradistinction to a flap in which the blood supply to the tissue remains at least partially intact.

The type of skin graft is described according to its thickness. A split-thickness skin graft is comprised of epidermis and a portion of the dermis. Split-thickness skin grafts may be harvested from various donor sites depending on the thickness, color, and quality of skin needed. They may then be meshed to expand the potential coverage area. However, the cosmetic appearance of meshed grafts is inferior and they have a propensity to contract. In patients with significant skin requirements or when there may be a relative paucity of donor sites, skin grafts may be used in conjunction with skin substitutes.

A full-thickness skin graft includes the full complement of the epidermis and dermis (Table 43-1). Thicker grafts have more difficulty with adherence and survival because of their greater demand on vascular ingrowth. However, the greater the thickness of dermis, the greater the inhibition of myofibroblast activation and graft contraction. The full-thickness skin graft may also retain functional hair follicles and sweat glands. Full-thickness skin grafts are taken from areas in which primary closure can be accomplished.

Skin grafts may be immobilized for five days with compressive dressings to prevent graft loss because of fluid accumulation and shear forces. Donor sites for split-thickness grafts are allowed to re-epithelialize under occlusive dressings (OpSite, Tegaderm), petroleum (Scarlet Red) or antibiotic impregnated gauze (Xeroform). Re-epithelialization typically occurs in 7–14 days.

Skin Flaps

A flap is a volume of tissue that can be translocated and survive in a new location on its native blood supply. A flap may consist of skin and subcutaneous tissue, muscle, or a composite of all three. The vessels supplying a random flap are smaller and more diffuse than those of an axial pattern flap, in which the tissue has a consistent pedicle.

A Z-plasty is a method of constructing adjacent skin flaps at specific angles to lengthen or reorient a scar. A W-plasty is a camouflaging technique used to disperse the continuity of a linear scar. A V-Y advancement flap is a method of recruiting tissue from a region of relative excess to a soft tissue defect. Skin flaps may also be rotated on a dermal or subdermal pedicle. If the tension is too great, a back cut known as a "Burow triangle" may be created to increase the arc of rotation. A bilobed flap is transposed in sequence via two flaps with the most distal flap donor site being closed primarily. An

TABLE 43-1 Split-Thickness vs. Full-Thickness Skin Grafts

	Split-Thickness Graft	Full-Thickness Graft
Reliable take	+	
Available donor sites	+	
Primary contracture	+	
Secondary contracture		+
Mechanical durability		+
Ability to grow hair, secrete sweat and sebum		+
Pigmentary changes	+	

TABLE 43-2 Mathes and Nahai Muscle Flap Vascular Anatomy Classification

Type I	One vascular pedicle
Type II	Dominant and minor pedicle
Type III	Two dominant pedicles
Type IV	Segmental pedicles
Type V	One dominant pedicle and segmental pedicle

island flap is one in which the vessel is isolated from surrounding tissue, over an intervening segment. A free flap is one in which the vascular supply and flap are severed to be reattached via microvascular technique at a distant location.

Muscle-Based Flaps

The Mathes and Nahai Classification describes muscle flaps according to their pattern of dominant, minor, and/or segmental vascular supply (Table 43-2). Wounds that are prone to infection or irradiated benefit from muscle flaps because of their rich vascularity which ameliorates the delivery of antibiotics and immunological cells.

The vascular supply of a muscle flap may be enhanced by selective surgical ligation of one or several of the dominant feeding arteries. This delay phenomenon occurs as the vessels which connect adjacent angiosomes known as choke vessels dilate followed by neoangiogenesis. The ischemic tissue then acclimates to relying on the nonoccluded arterial supply. After a period of 10–14 days, the flap may be safely transferred with decreased risk of ischemic complications.

Tissue Expansion

The viscoelastic properties of skin allow a significant degree of stretch to be applied to the skin and subcutaneous tissue without undue ischemia. Tissue expanders inflated at staged intervals generate and recruit tissue via a process known as biologic creep. Histologic analysis of expanded skin shows increased mitotic activity and angiogenesis. The epidermis thickens in contrast to dermal attenuation.

Free Flaps and Microsurgery

Microsurgery is the technique which makes possible neurovascular repair in tissues transferred to distant locations. Microscopes or high-magnification loupes are required to visualize the nerves, vessels, instruments, and sutures. Interrupted or continuous sutures may be used to accomplish tensionless vascular anastomosis or neural coaptation. The configuration of the repair may be in an end-to-end or end-to-side fashion.

The vessels must be handled meticulously and minimally to prevent vasospasm and intimal injury. Papaverine, lidocaine, and heparinized saline may be applied intraoperatively to ameliorate vasospasm. Free flap thrombosis is a surgical emergency and vascular flow must be restored within a finite period of time. Factors contributing to thrombosis include anticoagulant deficiency, smoking, caffeine, hypovolemia, hypothermia, and cardiovascular disease. Venous congestion is more common than arterial complications and often resolves with leach therapy.

PERIPHERAL NERVE SURGERY

Compressive neuropathies are encountered in areas such as the carpal, cubital, and tarsal tunnels. Motor function may be assessed by various objective scales including the British Medical Research Council Muscle Grading Scale. Electrodiagnostic tests, such as nerve conduction studies, needle electrode examination, and somatosensory evoked potentials, are useful in determining the magnitude, location, and prognosis of the lesion.

Nerve injuries generally are graded according to the Sunderland Classification. A first-degree injury or neurapraxia results in focal axonal demyelination and transient conduction block. A second-degree injury or axonotmesis occurs as axonal injury results in Wallerian degeneration. Both first- and second-degree injuries are self-limited and complete recovery may be anticipated within 3 months. The third and fourth types of injury occur as significant force is applied to the nerve to result in a neuroma-in-continuity. The third-degree injury results in partial endoneural scarring and regenerating axons only are able to partially traverse the zone-of-injury. Recovery is generally incomplete. Fourth-degree injury results in complete obliteration of the nerve by scar tissue and axonal regeneration is not possible. Lastly, a fifth-degree injury or neurotmesis results from complete transection of a nerve. Microsurgical repair is required for fourth- and fifth-degree injuries within a finite period of time to prevent irreversible motor end-plate degeneration. Mackinnon described a sixth-degree injury in which variable degrees of injury occur at various segments of the injured nerve.

If signs and symptoms of nerve repair and regeneration are not present within three months, exploration and intraoperative nerve testing is warranted. Conduction distal to a partially conducting neuroma may be augmented by jump grafts in an side-to-side fashion, or excision of the neuroma followed by end-to-end cable grafts. If a proximal donor is not available as in the case of nerve root avulsions, adjacent nerve transfers may be performed to restore distal innervation.

CRANIOFACIAL SURGERY

Cleft Lip and Palate

In normal embryologic growth, five facial elements (the frontonasal, lateral maxillary, and mandibular segments) merge via mesenchymal migration. According to the classic theory of cleft lip embryogenesis, failure of fusion of the maxillary processes and frontonasal processes during this time interval yields a cleft of the primary palate. However, the mesodermal penetration theory describes palate closure as dependent on mesodermal penetration without which results in epithelial apoptosis and cleft formation.

The primary palate consists of the lip, alveolus, and hard palate anterior to the incisive foramen, although the secondary palate comprises the hard and soft palate structures posterior to the incisive foramen. Cleft lips are complete if the cleft extends in to the nostril floor and incomplete if a tissue bridge unites the lateral and central lip.

Incidence of cleft lip and palate is 46 percent versus 33 percent in patients with isolated cleft palates or 21 percent with isolated cleft lips. Unilateral left cleft lips occur more often than right-sided or bilateral cleft lips, 6:3:1 respectively. Furthermore, the ratio of incidence of cleft lip varies with ethnicity: 0.41:1000 in African Americans; 1:1000 in whites; and 2.1:1000 in Asians.

The etiology of cleft lip is multifactorial and potential risk factors include anticonvulsants, parental age, lower socioeconomic class, smoking, alcohol intake, prenatal nutrition, and family history. Families in which a parent or sibling has a cleft have a 4 percent risk of a subsequent child being born with cleft lip and/or palate.

Timing of surgical repair often is dictated by the rule of tens: 10 weeks of age, 10 lbs, and 10 mg of hemoglobin. A Latham appliance may be fitted intraorally prior to definitive surgical repair to facilitate alveolar segment alignment.

Cleft Palate

Palatal shelves develop as swellings of the medial maxillary prominences. After downward growth adjacent to the tongue, the shelves become horizontal and fuse at 12 weeks of gestation. Incomplete closure of these palatal shelves results in a cleft palate. A cleft palate is described as complete if there is extension into the nose or incomplete if a partition exists.

A submucous cleft palate is the most common type and is characterized by a bifid uvula, thin membranous central portion, and a posterior palpable notch. Cleft palates are associated with greater than 200 syndromes and malformations. Incidence is approximately 0.05 percent and associated risk factors include teratogens, alcohol, dietary deficiencies, and maternal epilepsy.

Approximately 5 percent of patients after cleft palate repair will have persistent velopharyngeal insufficiency. Consequently, incomplete oropharyngeal occlusion and abnormal intraoral pressures and ineffective sucking, feeding, facial growth disturbances, middle ear disease, and recurrent otitis media. Surgical management includes pharyngeal flap, pharyngoplasty, palatoplasty and intravelar veloplasty.

Hemangiomas and Vascular Malformations

Hemangiomas are common vascular tumors 30 percent of which are present at birth and 80 percent during the first month of life. Distinguished as a small red or deep bluish patch, they rapidly proliferate during the first 2 years. Following this proliferative phase, hemangiomas steadily involute and spontaneous resolution occurs in 50 percent of patients by 5 years of life and in 70 percent by 7 years of life. Females are more inclined to develop hemangiomas and the majority of such lesions preside in the head and neck.

Treatment is indicated in patients with visual or airway impairment, bleeding or ulceration, infection, Kasabach-Merritt syndrome, or congestive heart failure. Noninvasive modalities include systemic corticosteroids, intralesional corticosteroids, and subcutaneous interferon α-2a. More invasive techniques include surgical excision, laser or cryotherapy, and embolization.

Vascular malformations are structural abnormalities which arise as a consequence of embryogenic dysmorphogenesis. They are all present at birth and grow concurrently with the patient. They have no sexual predilection and do not display the typical rapid proliferation or regression phases of hemangiomas. They are classified as either slow-flow or fast-flow lesions. The former include capillary, lymphatic, or venous malformations, whereas the later comprise arterial aneurysms, arteriovenous fistulas, and arteriovenous malformations. Skeletal distortion or hypertrophy, increased skin temperature, bruit or thrill, high-output cardiac failure, bleeding or ulceration, pain, and tissue overgrowth may accompany vascular malformations. The more severe vascular malformations may have a propensity to bleed and have high morbidity and mortality rates. Arteriography and superselective embolization followed by surgical resection remains the standard of care. Other treatment modalities include sclerotherapy, compression garments, laser thermolysis, and surgical excision.

Craniosynostosis

Craniosynostosis is defined as the premature closure of one or more cranial sutures. Based on the law of Virchow, premature closure results in limited skeletal growth perpendicular to the suture line and overgrowth parallel to the suture. The incidence of craniosynostosis is 0.1 percent and its etiology is multifactorial.

Craniosynostosis may interfere with brain growth and result in increased intracranial pressures. Craniosynostosis may be an isolated manifestation or associated with a craniofacial syndrome. Classification is described according to the calvarial sutures involved and subsequent malformation: frontal plagiocephaly occurs with coronal synostosis; scaphocephaly with sagittal synostosis; trigonocephaly with metopic synostosis; and brachiocephaly with bicoronal synostosis.

Craniosynostosis Syndromes

Crouzon syndrome is characterized by brachycephaly, mid-face hypoplasia, strabismus, exophoria, antimongoloid palpebral fissures, and exophthalmos. Apert syndrome is similar to Crouzon syndrome with the addition of ocular muscle palsies, hypertelorism, and syndactyly. Saethre-Chotzen syndrome is distinguished by brachycephaly, low hairline, and syndactyly. Lastly, Pfeiffer syndrome is typified by brachycephaly and is distinguished by broad thumbs and toes. Craniofacial reconstructive surgery entails decompression by craniotomy followed by cranial vault remodeling and fixation with absorbable plates between 6 and 12 months of age.

Laterofacial Microsomias

Patients with hemifacial microsomia, the most common craniofacial anomaly, presents with unilateral or bilateral microtia, macrostomia, dysplastic mandible, zygoma, maxilla, temporal bone, facial muscles, muscles of mastication, palatal muscles, tongue, parotid gland, macrostomia, and cranial nerve involvement. Treacher-Collins syndrome includes maxillary and zygomatic dysplasia, eyelid colobomas, antimongoloid slant, hypoplastic mandible and maxilla, macrostomia, and microtia.

Orthognathic Surgery

The mandible and/or maxilla may be disproportionate because of traumatic or congenital anomalies. Dental occlusive relationships are characterized by Angle classification of malocclusion. In Angle class I, or normal occlusion, the mesiobuccal cusp of the maxillary first molar articulates with the buccal groove of the lower first molar. In class II occlusion, the maxillary first molar articulates anterior to the buccal groove of the lower first molar, although in class III occlusion, the maxillary first molar articulates posterior to the mandibular first molar.

Cephalometric analysis will determine vertical face, horizontal midface, horizontal lower face, and dental relationships. The mandible and maxilla may require advancement, division, or setback by LeFort osteotomies and genioplasty.

MAXILLOFACIAL TRAUMA

Most facial fractures occur during motor vehicle accidents or aggravated assault and 50–70 percent of patients with facial fractures/injuries will have concomitant injuries. Treatment may be emergent, early or delayed. Emergency treatment for life-threatening facial fractures includes respiratory obstruction, aspiration and hemorrhage. Facial fractures are suspected in patients with contusions, tenderness, lacerations, neurologic deficit, malocclusion, visual disturbances and facial asymmetry. Examination of the face should be carried out in an orderly, concise manner, proceeding from either superior to inferior or inferior to superior and should entail:

- Visual evaluation for asymmetry and deformity.
- Palpation of entire craniofacial skeleton for irregularities or crepitus.
- Trigeminal and facial nerve examination.
- Intranasal inspection for septal hematoma.
- Ophthalmologic examination for extraocular entrapment or optic nerve deficit.
- Intraoral examination for malocclusion, and fractured or missing teeth.

Mandibular Fractures

The mandible is the second most commonly injured facial bone and represents 10–25 percent of all facial fractures. The most common locations for fracture to occur are the body, the angle and condyle, and the ramus and symphysis, from most to least common, respectively. Mandibular fractures often are multiple and a thorough investigation for a second should always be undertaken.

The mandible has the potential for multiple vector displacements depending on the muscular attachments of the fracture fragments. Surgical management includes open versus closed reduction and intermaxillary fixation.

Frontal Sinus Fracture

Frontal sinus fractures should be suspect in patients with forehead trauma. They often are not associated with any acute signs or symptoms and may be evaluated by computed tomography.

Management includes palliative care, open reduction internal fixation of anterior wall fractures, and cranialization of posterior wall fractures. All patients should be evaluated over a period of time for sinus opacification indicative of nasofrontal duct obstruction.

Nasoethmoidal Orbital Fractures

Nasoethmoidal (NOE) fractures involve injuries to both the nose and frontal processes of the maxilla. These fractures may result in telecanthus if the medial canthal tendon is involved. NOE fractures should be suspected in patients with epistaxis, depressed or comminuted nasal fractures, maxillary frontal process tenderness and periorbital hematomas. Computerized tomography remains the standard for accurate diagnosis and treatment usually requires open reduction and interfragmentary fixation.

Orbital Fractures

The most frequent orbital fracture is the "blow-out fracture," which pertains to the medial and lower medial orbital walls. Orbital floor blow-out fractures may result from direct blunt trauma to the orbit or by an acute increase in intraorbital pressure. Signs and symptoms include periorbital hematoma, sub-conjunctival hemorrhage, diplopia, infraorbital nerve injury, enophthalmos, and visual acuity changes. Ophthalmologic and forced duction tests should be performed.

Indications for operative exploration include symptomatic diplopia greater than 2 weeks, positive forced duction test, muscle entrapment, orbital content herniation, orbital floor defect, and enophthalmos. Goals of treatment are reduction of herniated contents and restoration of normal architecture and orbital volume. Surgical treatment includes rigid fixation with either autologous or alloplastic materials.

Nasal Fractures

The nose is the most commonly fractured bone in the face. The nose may be laterally or posteriorly displaced, and the fracture may involve the cartilaginous septum and/or the nasal bones. Patients commonly present with edema, deformity, epistaxis, septal deviation, and/or crepitus. Intranasal inspection for septal hematoma should be performed and drained immediately if present. Diagnosis by computed tomography (CT) scan is useful to rule out concomitant injuries. Treatment consists of fracture reduction and midline positioning of the septum followed by splinting. Residual deformities may require formal rhinoplasty after inflammation and edema have resolved.

Zygoma Fractures

Signs and symptoms of zygomatic fractures include diplopia, trismus, depressed malar eminence, subconjunctival hemorrhage, infraorbital nerve injury and epistaxis. On examination, there may be a step-off deformity or tenderness. Fractures may be confirmed by plain films or CT scan. Surgical management includes open reduction and fixation with wires or plates.

Midface Fractures

The LeFort Classification is commonly used to describe the three classical midface fractures. Symptoms found with maxillary fractures are periorbital hematoma, epistaxis, and mobile maxillary segments. Surgical management includes open reduction and fixation.

MAXILLOFACIAL RECONSTRUCTION

Ear

Surgery may be performed in children with microtia once the rib cartilage has reached an appropriate size for ear reconstruction at 6–8 years of life. A radiograph tracing is made of the normal ear if present. In the first stage, the helix and antihelix are constructed from the patients costal cartilage. This framework is then implanted underneath a retroauricular skin envelope. In subsequent stages, the lobule and tragus are reconstructed.

Common causes of prominent ears include conchal overdevelopment, underdeveloped antihelical folds, or both. Surgical management includes imbrication of the conchal cartilage with mattress or Mustardé sutures, by excision of excess conchal cartilage, or by scoring of the anterior conchal cartilage. In infancy, prominent ears may be permanently corrected by taping and splinting.

Lip

The majority of lip defects are secondary to basal cell cancer of the upper lip and squamous cell carcinoma of the lower lip. Extirpation and/or radiotherapy are essential for possible cure. Goals of reconstruction are to maintain vermilion continuity, lip sensation and oral competence by reapproximation of the orbicularis oris. Upper and lower lip defects less than 30 percent may be repaired primarily. In defects greater than 30 percent, the Abbé flap or variations thereof may ameliorate reconstruction. Lower lip defects greater than 65 percent may be restored by Karapandzic or Webster-Bernard techniques. Larger lip/soft-tissue defects may require larger pedicle flaps or free tissue transfer.

Cheek

The cheek is divided into three esthetic units: zone I (suborbital), zone II (preauricular), and zone III (buccomandibular). If primary close or local flap coverage cannot be achieved, or if lower lid ectropion occurs, serial excision, full-thickness skin grafting, or tissue expansion may be considered. Otherwise, cervicofacial advancement, regional flaps, or even free tissue transfer may be required.

Nasal

The nose is divided into nine subunits based on surface, skin thickness, color, and texture. Reconstruction of each individual unit must achieve:

- Similar skin dimension and quality
- A cartilaginous framework to maintain shape and support
- Restoration of an adequate vascular supply

Reconstruction of nasal subunits may be achieved by secondary healing, skin grafting, or local flaps. Secondary healing is successful in a defect adjacent to a nonmobile unit where contraction will not cause distortion. Skin grafts are generally acceptable for the upper two thirds of the nose and local flaps for alar and tip defects.

The nasolabial flap based on the facial artery may be used to resurface the nasal ala. The paramedian forehead flap based on the supratrochlear–supraorbital vessels provides soft tissue coverage especially of the tip, dorsum, and areas of missing cartilage.

Eyelid

The goals of eyelid reconstruction are:

- Preservation and restoration of function
- Shape and symmetry
- Incisions within natural lid creases
- Aesthetic skin grafts and flaps

Primary closure may be achieved in defects that are less than one third the length of the lid margin. A lateral canthotomy with lateral advancement may be performed in defects greater than 25 percent. When there is skin loss of the lower lid, skin grafts from the upper lid, supraclavicular or preauricular region are excellent donor sites. When a full-thickness defect is greater than 25 percent, the cartilage and conjunctival lining will require septal or conchal cartilage with either conjunctiva from another lid, oral or nasal mucosa or a composite graft.

In general, local flaps provide the best color and texture match. For full-thickness lower-lid defects, local flap options include the nasolabial flap, V-Y advancement, and Mustardé cheek flap. In upper lid defects, a temporal skin flap may be designed to reconstruct defects greater than one half of the lid. Cross-lid flaps (e.g. Cutler-Beard or Hughes flaps) may be performed to restore either upper or lower lid defects involving the tarsus greater than 25 percent. Medial canthopexy may be performed when repairing the inner canthus to prevent telecanthus, or a tarsal strip and lateral canthopexy may be performed to prevent ectropion.

Ptosis may be congenital or acquired. Congenital ptosis may be caused by lid anomalies, ophthalmoplegia, and synkinesis, although acquired ptosis may be neurogenic, myogenic, or traumatic. Horner syndrome is a form of neurogenic ptosis in which sympathetic disruption results in ptosis, miosis, anhydrosis, and enophthalmos.

In patients with absent levator function, a frontalis sling procedure may be performed. In more mild forms of ptosis, Mueller resection, Fasanella-Servat advancement, or levator resections may suffice.

Scalp

The scalp is composed of five layers: skin, subcutaneous tissue, galea, loose areolar tissue, and pericranium. Scalp defects are classified as partial or full thickness. In partial-thickness defects, local flap elevation and advancement scalp flaps or multiple axial flaps may achieve closure with donor-site skin grafting. Larger defects may require a full scalp flap based on either the superficial temporal or posterior auricular arteries, pericranial flaps with skin grafting, or microvascular flap coverage. In patients with alopecia, tissue expansion with local tissue advancement performed to restore hair-bearing tissue or hair transplantation may be performed.

In full-thickness defects, skin grafts can be administered to the calvarium after the outer calvarial table is removed and burred. Calvarial defects may be reconstructed with autogenous bone (e.g., split rib grafts or calvarial bone grafts). Alloplastic materials also are available such as methylmethacrylate, LactoSorb, and hydroxyapatite. However, they generally have a higher rate of infection and extrusion.

Facial Paralysis

Lesions resulting in facial paralysis may be classified as intracranial, intratemporal, and extracranial. Idiopathic or Bell palsy is the most common etiology and 70 percent of such patients spontaneously recover without neurologic deficit.

The goals of facial reanimation surgery are:

- Restoration of resting facial symmetry
- Spontaneous, symmetrical facial animation

- Corneal protection
- Oral competence

Reconstruction depends on the duration of facial nerve injury. After eighteen months, the facial muscles atrophy and the motor end plate density is insufficient for reinnervation. If reinnervation is achieved within 18 months, primary repair, nerve grafting, or nerve transfers may be performed. If tensionless nerve repair is not feasible, then a nerve graft (e.g., sural nerve) will be interposed in between the proximal trunk and distal branches. When a proximal nerve is not available, cross-facial nerve grafting from the contralateral facial nerve and/or neurotization from the ipsilateral motor branch to the masseter may be performed.

Static or dynamic slings and free muscle transfers may be performed to restore facial and oral motor function. Static slings (e.g., Gore-Tex, fascia, temporalis, or masseter muscle) may be attached to the oral commissure to achieve both smile and oral competence. Gold weights are often placed in the upper eyelids to ensure corneal protection. Facial reanimation may be achieved by free muscle flaps.

HEAD AND NECK ONCOLOGIC RECONSTRUCTION

Small floor-of-mouth and tongue tumors may be treated with a skin graft. Larger defects will require more pliable tissue for an intraoral lining and allow for tongue mobility such as a radial forearm flap. In the setting of maxillectomy and/or orbitectomy, the palate and oral contents must be separated from the midface. If the palate is resected, a palatal obturator may be applied, but adequate soft-tissue coverage (i.e., rectus abdominis or scapular flap) is required. When the orbital floor is resected but the orbital contents are preserved, a bone graft is frequently used for reconstruction. Nevertheless, local flaps such as the temporalis muscle or temporoparietal flap offer adequate soft-tissue coverage in these defects.

More advanced lip and/or oral cancers may invade the maxilla and mandible. If the mandibular defect is smaller than 6 cm, a nonvascularized bone graft may fill the defect. However, if the defect is larger than 6 cm or the ablative field is to be irradiated, a free vascularized bone flap is required for durable reconstruction. Options for vascularized bone flaps include the fibula, iliac crest, and the scapula. These bone flaps may be accompanied with skin and soft tissue to obviate any dead space and provide an epithelialized lining.

In the neck, complete esophageal defects may be reconstructed with a jejunal flap. Hypopharyngeal defects, either circumferential or partially circumferential, may also be reconstructed with a jejunal flap if circumferential. Other tubed fasciocutaneous free flaps and the anterolateral thigh flap are reasonable alternatives that have the added benefit of not having the morbidity associated with entering the abdominal cavity.

BREAST SURGERY

Breast Reconstruction

Breast reconstruction following mastectomy may be performed with autogenous tissue or alloplastic implants. Autogenous tissue reconstruction may be considered in patients who require radiation postoperatively, or in patients who understand the morbidity of the procedure but desire the aesthetic benefits. Potential donor flaps include the transverse rectus abdominis myocutaneous (TRAM) flap, the latissimus dorsi flap, the superior inferior epigastric artery flap, gluteal flap, and the deep circumflex iliac artery flap (DIEP).

The pedicle TRAM flap is purported to have more fat necrosis and radiation-induced problems than the free TRAM. Additionally, smoking is a relative contraindication for a pedicle TRAM, but not for a free TRAM. The free TRAM has a slightly longer operative time and a failure rate of approximately 5 percent. Both of these types of breast reconstruction require sacrifice of the rectus muscle, and mesh reconstruction of the abdominal wall may be employed if the fascial defect is significant. Muscle-sparing techniques or intramuscular dissection of the perforating vessels (DIEP flap) may be preferable surgical techniques.

The choice of recipient vessels for microvascular anastomosis of these flaps includes the thoracodorsal and the internal mammary arteries and veins.

Tissue Expansion and Implant Reconstruction

The principal benefit of using tissue expansion and implants versus autologous tissue is lower complication and donor-site morbidity rates. However, the aesthetic result is often superior after autogenous reconstruction and the use of radiation may limit other techniques. Furthermore, most mastectomy defects result in a loss of skin and soft tissue, and expansion of the skin flaps over several months may be required prior to the definitive implant procedure.

Implants are available in a range of volumes and shapes and may be smooth or textured. The expander soft-tissue pocket generally is placed beneath the pectoralis and serratus muscle, which affords greater coverage of the implant and may soften the resultant contour.

Reduction Mammoplasty

Gigantomastia may result in significant morbidity including back and shoulder pain. Reconstruction is based on inferior, superior, or medial pedicle techniques. Occasionally, women with extremely large breasts may require a free nipple-areolar complex graft if the pedicle is too long to sustain adequate perfusion to the nipple.

A potential complication is the descent of the reduced breast volume below the nipple level or "bottoming out," hematoma, delayed wound healing, loss of nipple sensation, and impaired ability to breast-feed.

Mastopexy

The descent of breast tissue often occurring with age is known as ptosis. For mild ptosis, skin excision along a superior crescent or a periareolar "doughnut" mastopexy may be used. A subglandular augmentation may ameliorate lift of the breast in select patients. For more severe forms of ptosis, an inverted T-shaped incision may be necessary to achieve sufficient lift and projection to the breast.

Breast Augmentation

FDA-approved breast implants are saline filled with a silicone-based shell. The four most commonly used incisions for placement of the breast implants for augmentation are inframammary, periareolar, axillary, and transumbilical. The implants may then be placed in a subglandular or subpectoral position.

Capsular contracture occurs in 8–38 percent of patients who undergo augmentation mammoplasty. If significant contracture occurs resulting in surface deformity, asymmetry, or pain, then capsulotomy or capsulectomy with implant exchange may be required. Other potential complications include leak, rupture, hematoma, seroma, infection, and hypertrophic scarring occurs in less than 5 percent of patients. A study surveying augmented and nonaugmented patients found no statistical difference in survival or detection of carcinoma between the two cohorts.

Gynecomastia

Excessive breast tissue in males, or gynecomastia, may be associated with liver dysfunction, endocrine abnormalities, Klinefelter syndrome, and renal disease. Oncologic etiologies include testicular tumors, adrenal or pituitary adenomas, pulmonary carcinomas, and male breast cancer. Pharmacologic causes include marijuana use, digoxin, spironolactone, cimetidine, theophylline, diazepam, and reserpine. Occasionally, patients may respond to testosterone, tamoxifen, or danazol. Surgical treatment includes mastectomy and/or liposuction. Although most gynecomastia is not associated with male breast cancer, those patients with Klinefelter syndrome are at a higher risk.

Congenital Reconstruction

Congenital deformities of the breast include amastia, hypomastia, tuberous breast, and Poland syndrome. These are relatively rare conditions that may have psychosocial sequelae. Amastia and hypomastia may be addressed by augmentation with tissue expanders or adjustable implants. Tuberous breast deformities often have a degree of ptosis and herniation of breast tissue which may improve with subglandular implant placement. Poland syndrome is characterized by hypoplasia or aplasia of chest and limb structures including the breast. Reconstruction often is achieved in these patients with a latissimus dorsi flap and submuscular implant.

TRUNK, ABDOMEN, AND GENITOURINARY RECONSTRUCTION

Chest Reconstruction

If a significant bony defect exists (> 5 cm or four or more resected ribs), then the reconstruction may require a bone graft, mesh, or muscle flap. In patients with sternal wound infections, aggressive débridement and removal of infected hardware is essential. Serial débridements and quantitative culture data may be performed prior to definitive closure. Unilateral or bilateral pectoralis, rectus abdominus, and latissimus flaps or omentum may be used to provide soft tissue coverage. Complications such as re-infection, dehiscence, flap loss, or failure are relatively low with the integrated management of flap reconstruction and culture specific antibiotic therapy.

Posterior and lateral chest wall defects, occurring secondary to trauma or oncologic ablation, may require concomitant bony reconstruction. Marlex mesh, methylmethacrylate, and bone grafts are used to bridge rib gaps. The latissimus, trapezius, rectus, and pectoralis are all potential options for soft-tissue reconstruction.

Abdominal Wall Reconstruction

Component separation is a technique whereby differential release of the abdominal wall musculature allows for primary closure of moderately sized open defects. For larger fascial defects PTFE (Gore-Tex), polypropylene (Prolene), polyglactin (Vicryl), or polyester (Mersilene) may be used. PTFE may predispose to infection and seroma but provides strength with minimal adhesion formation. Polypropylene mesh provides strength but may also result in adhesion formation. Polyglactin mesh integrates readily with low infection rates but provides relatively less strength. Any type of alloplastic mesh should be covered with well perfused skin and soft tissue flaps. Occasionally, tissue expanders may be used to allow sufficient local tissue to be generated for primary closure.

The rectus abdominis, tensor fascia lata, rectus femoris, latissimus dorsi muscle, omentum, and anterolateral thigh flap are excellent potential local flaps. Vacuum-assisted coverage systems are particularly useful in patients with enterocutaneous fistulas.

Traumatic, oncological, or infected abdominal defect may not be able to be reconstructed immediately and a skin graft or dermal graft may be placed over viscera and allowed to heal. The fascial defect may then be repaired during a second stage procedure.

Genitourinary Reconstruction

The gracilis myocutaneous flap or the vertical rectus abdominis myocutaneous flap may provide durable soft-tissue in patients with vaginal cancer. For congenital defects of the vagina such as Mayer-Rokitansky-Küster syndrome (congenital absence of the vagina), variants of the McIndoe procedure can be applied. A judicious dissection of the potential vaginal vault space is followed by split-thickness grafting. A bolster expander is kept in place to maintain the space.

Hypospadias is an abnormality of male urethral development characterized by proximal urethral termination. Associated anomalies, such as inguinal hernias and undescended testes, occur in 9 percent of patients. The Mathieu procedure uses a ventral, meatal-based flap, whereas the meatal advancement and glanuloplasty techniques are ideal for distal hypospadias with a more compliant urethra. Proximal hypospadias may be repaired with preputial island flaps. Bladder exstrophy reconstruction is a multistage procedure in which the external genitalia is reconstructed with local flaps.

Traumatic or oncologic defects of the perineal region may be reconstructed with gracilis, rectus abdominis, tensor fascia lata or gluteal thigh flaps. Anal sphincter reconstruction may also be performed with local gracilis or gluteus maximus flaps. Avulsion injuries or Fournier's gangrene may result in full-thickness defects requiring skin grafting. Complete penile reconstruction is a complex problem that may be managed with tubed pedicle or free flaps, such as the radial forearm flap.

The cavernous nerves may be injured during radical prostatectomy. Grafting across the nerve defect with sural nerve grafts may be performed to restore erectile function.

PRESSURE ULCERS

Pressure ulcers occur when the external pressure, especially in the areas over bony prominences, exceeds capillary filling pressures (32 mmHg). Factors associated with pressure ulcers include tissue friction, moisture, nutritional status, and advanced age. Commonly affected areas include the sacrum, heel, ischium, and trochanters. A grading system for pressure ulcers has been developed.

Treatment of pressure ulcers must incorporate adequate débridement of infected and necrotic tissue, pressure relief, local wound care, and antibiotics.

A diagnostic evaluation for osteomyelitis may include plain film, bone scan, MRI, and bone biopsy. Leukocytosis and elevated erythrocyte sedimentation rates increase the predictive value of other digestive tests. Aggressive bony débridement, vascularized flap coverage, and treatment with intravenous antibiotics are essential to successful management.

Dressings for pressure ulcers include wet-to-dry saline dressings with or without antibiotics, and enzymatic débriding ointments. Povidone-iodine or hypochlorite combinations are often useful in infected ulcers. For stage I and II ulcers, hydrocolloid dressings promote reepithelialization by providing a moist environment. Calcium alginate dressings may help to absorb wound exudates. Growth factor and basic fibroblast growth factor may also ameliorate wound healing.

The principles of pressure ulcer management include prevention of fecal contamination with bowel preparations, postoperative pharmacologic constipation, and occasionally, colostomy. Sensate pedicle fasciocutaneous flaps may provide added protection for ulcer-prone areas. For the sacrum, fasciocutaneous advancement flaps or muscle-based flaps include one or both gluteus maximus flaps. Treatment of ischial ulcers often requires ostectomies and/or bursectomies and posterior thigh flaps. Alternatively, in nonambulatory patients, V-Y advancement quadriceps flaps provide durable coverage. Less commonly, the gracilis, gluteus maximus, or even rectus abdominis muscle-based flaps may be used. The treatment of trochanteric ulcers often includes concomitant ostectomy of the exposed femoral head. The tensor fascia lata flap, gluteus maximus, posterior thigh flap, and the vastus lateralis myocutaneous flap have all been used for coverage of this region.

Recurrence occurs in 50–80 percent of patients, with higher recurrence rates found in the paraplegic population. The use of air mattresses and positional changes are useful to relieve pressure on the flap reconstruction. A rare complication of pressure ulcers is the development of Marjolin carcinoma 15–20 years after ulcer formation.

LOWER-EXTREMITY RECONSTRUCTION

After a thorough primary and secondary survey, the multidisciplinary team must assess the trauma patient in regard to neurovascular status, soft-tissue defects, and fractures. The Gustillo classification is a useful method to grade patients with open fractures of the lower extremity. A Doppler exam or arteriogram may help identify any concomitant, vascular injury.

Split-thickness skin grafts are reasonable for coverage of exposed healthy muscle or soft tissue. Local flaps are used to cover small to moderate exposed bony defects of the lower or middle third of the leg. For larger, soft-tissue defects with bony exposure, particularly of the lower one third, free tissue transfer may be required. If no recipient vessels are available, the plastic surgeon may use a cross-leg flap as a last alternative.

Chronic osteomyelitis may complicate lower extremity reconstruction. The treatment for chronic osteomyelitis includes intravenous antibiotics, débridement of necrotic tissues, and replacement with well-vascularized soft tissue.

Diabetic Foot Ulcers

The pathophysiology of diabetic foot ulceration is divided into three components: peripheral neuropathy, peripheral vascular disease, and immunodeficiency. Because of profound sensory neuropathy, profound pressures may result in ischemia and subsequent ulcer formation. In the setting of microvascular disease, the oxygen-carrying capacity of the site is reduced, which predisposes to ulceration and diminished wound-healing capabilities. Finally, the diabetic patient's immune system is altered in terms of chemotaxis, phagocytosis, and bactericidal capacity predisposing the patient to polymicrobial bacterial and fungal infections.

Blood sugar levels must be controlled for expedient and successful wound healing. Furthermore, radiographs, bone scans, or MRI must be acquired to assess if there is osteomyelitis. Finally, a thorough vascular exam must be performed, either by duplex scanning or angiography. If significant vascular disease is present, the patient may require lower-extremity bypass.

All gross infection or foci of osteomyelitis must be débrided. Newer agents and modalities have emerged to enhance granulation and wound healing such as Regranex and the vacuum-assisted closure device. In certain circumstances, a skin graft may be appropriate, but are frequently unsuccessful because of the shear forces, particularly in weight-bearing areas. Local flaps, such as the reverse sural artery or lateral calcaneal artery flap, or free tissue transfer may provide durable tissue in weight-bearing areas.

Lymphedema

Lymphedema is classified by etiology. Primary or idiopathic lymphedema implies includes: (1) Milroy disease which is a congenital lymphedema that has an X-linked inheritance pattern; (2) lymphedema praecox which appears after puberty but before 35 years of age; and (3) lymphedema tarda which appears after the age of 35 years. Secondary lymphedema results from the mechanical obstruction of lymphatic channels.

The pathophysiology of lymphedema is based on abnormal pressure gradients in lymphatic channels. Normally, the pressure in the lower-extremity lymphatic system is subatmospheric and results in afferent lymphatic flow. However, in patients with lymphedema, the lymph spills into the dermis and subcutaneous tissue. Clinically, this is manifested as firm, nonpitting edema. CT or MRI may be helpful in differentiating lymphedema from venous insufficiency or lipodystrophic edema. Lymphoscintigraphy is useful to determine the lymphatic anatomy and quantitate the lymphatic flow.

Treatment of lymphedema is generally conservative and includes the use of external compressive garments and devices. Careful hygiene must also be instituted to avoid cutaneous fungal infection. Surgical treatments include excision of skin, subcutaneous tissue, and fascia as in the Charles procedure; suction lipectomy; lymphatic anastomosis or bridging procedures. Especially following oncologic ablation, the onset of lymphedema must be differentiated from neoplastic invasion of the lymphatics or lymphangiosarcoma.

AESTHETIC SURGERY

Body Contouring and Liposuction

The assessment of body contour deformities requires evaluation of skin excess, lipodystrophy, and musculoaponeurotic laxity. Suction assisted lipectomy (SAL) is a technique that allows subcutaneous fat to be aspirated. Lipodystrophy without significant skin excess or musculoaponeurotic laxity may be treated with liposuction alone. Tumescent fluid is first infiltrated subcutaneously with lidocaine and epinephrine for analgesia and vasoconstriction, respectively. Significant fluid shifts may occur when large amounts of fat is aspirated and careful monitoring of urine output, intravenous fluids, and hemodynamics are required to ensure patient safety.

When excess skin and subcutaneous tissue is present or when the skin tone is compromised by age or loss of intrinsic elasticity, then frank excision of the excess tissue and skin may be necessary. If this excess occurs in the abdominal region, then abdominoplasty is performed to excise excess skin and subcutaneous tissue and plication of the rectus fascia through a low transverse incision.

Lower-body lipodystrophy may be genetic or occur after significant weight loss. If the problem is recalcitrant lipodystrophy without significant skin excess, then liposuction alone may be sufficient. However, if redundancy occurs in both the skin and subcutaneous tissue, then a lower body lift may be necessary. The entire buttock and thigh region can be elevated and advanced over the fascia and then fixed into a more cephalad position. In the upper arm, brachioplasty entails excision of skin and subcutaneous tissue through an elliptical medial inner arm incision.

Blepharoplasty and Browlift

Excess skin in the upper eyelid or dermatochalasia may be approached through an elliptical incision. Careful markings of the degree of excess skin are required to prevent overresection of skin and resultant lagophthalmos. A strip of orbicularis muscle may be excised to accentuate the fold of the eyelid. Excess postseptal fat also is resected.

When there is ptosis of the brow, elevation of the forehead in a subperiosteal or subcutaneous plane may be performed. A coronal, mid-forehead, brow, anterior hairline, or endoscopic incision can be made followed by advancement and suspension with sutures or screws.

Rhytidectomy

Excess skin and musculoaponeurotic laxity of the face may be treated with elevation of skin flaps and skin excision. Preauricular incisions are extended superiorly into the temporal hairline and posteriorly to the retroauricular region. The superficial musculoaponeurotic system (SMAS) lies immediately deep to the skin and may be plicated or excised. Often, the cervical region also is included and treated concurrently.

Rhinoplasty

Nasal airway obstruction may occur from internal or external structural defects. A deviated septum may disrupt the airflow. Through the nasal canal, the internal nasal valve consists of the upper lateral cartilage and septum and is a common location for nasal airway obstruction. Improvement in airflow with lateral traction of the cheek (Cottle sign) is an indication that spreader graft placement may improve obstructive symptoms. Deformities of the internal valve or septum may be corrected by resection or manipulation of the nasal cartilages. Excessive dorsal hump and tip deformities may be corrected by open or closed techniques. Resection or rasping of cartilage often is combined with cartilage grafts placed in critical structural locations. Cartilage may be harvested from the septum, concha, or costal margin and placed in the columella, tip, dorsum, and ala. Internal sutures may also help alter the shape of cartilaginous structures. Osteotomies may improve the relation between the nasomaxillary bony structure and the reshaped nose. The interrelatedness of the nasal subunits must be observed during any manipulation of a single structure.

CONCLUSION

Plastic and reconstructive surgery continues to implement advances in technology and basic science into clinical practice. Permutations of older techniques have resulted in more precise and refined alternatives in reconstruction surgery. Ongoing research in tissue engineering, gene therapy, and alloplastic materials are evolving into novel treatments of defects and more durable reconstructions.

Suggested Readings

McGregor I: Fundamental Techniques in Plastic Surgery and Their Surgical Applications, 7th ed. Edinburgh: Churchill-Livingstone, 1995.

McCarthy J: Plastic Surgery. Philadelphia: WB Saunders, 1990.

Jackson IT: Local Flaps in Head and Neck Reconstruction. St. Louis: Mosby, 1985.

Mathes SJ, Najai F: Reconstructive Surgery: Principles, Anatomy, and Technique. New York: Churchill-Livingstone 1997.

Beasley R, Thorne C, Aston S: Grabbe and Smiths Plastic Surgery, 4th ed. Philadelphia: Lippincott-Raven, 1997.

Mackinnon SE, Dellon AL: Surgery of the Peripheral Nerve. New York: Thieme, 1988.

Spear SL, Little JW, Lippman ME, et al: Surgery of the Breast: Principles and Art. Philadelphia: Lippincott-Raven, 1998.

Rees TD, LaTrenta GS: Aesthetic Plastic Surgery, 2nd ed. Philadelphia: WB Saunders, 1994.

Cohen M: Mastery of Plastic and Reconstructive Surgery. Boston: Little, Brown, 1994.

Georgiade GS, Riefkohl R, Levin LS: Plastic, Maxillofacial and Reconstructive Surgery, 3rd ed. Baltimore: Williams & Wilkins, 1997.

Sheen JH: Aesthetic Rhinoplasty. St Louis: Mosby, 1987.

44 Surgical Considerations in Older Adults

Rosemarie E. Hardin and Michael E. Zenilman

GENERAL CONSIDERATIONS

It is estimated that by the year 2025, persons older than age 65 will constitute 25 percent of the United States population. This ever-growing older adult population will increasingly require surgical consultation and intervention. A 1996 review showed that more than 4 million patients older than 65 years of age underwent surgical procedures, with the most common interventions being coronary artery bypass grafting, orthopedic procedures, and cholecystectomy. Older adult surgical patients account for 50 percent of surgical emergencies and 75 percent of perioperative deaths.

Chronologic age is rarely an accurate predictor of morbidity and mortality from surgical interventions. It is, however, an accurate marker for declining physiologic reserve and the presence of multiple comorbid conditions. These, in turn, place older adult patients at higher risk because of depressed cardiac, pulmonary, renal, and neurologic reserves, thereby increasing the morbidity and mortality of surgical interventions.

PREOPERATIVE EVALUATION

Surgical risk increases with advancing age as a consequence of physiologic decline and the development of comorbid conditions leading to postoperative complications, which are poorly tolerated because of decreased reserve.

The higher prevalence of comorbid disease in older adult patients places them in a higher American Society of Anesthesiologists (ASA) class; with approximately 80 percent falling into ASA class 3 or higher (Table 44-1). This physiologic fact leads to higher complication and mortality rates in patients 65 years of age or older. Mortality rates of major surgical intervention in patients older than 65 years of age without comorbid disease is approximately 5 percent but rises to approximately 10 percent with the presence of three comorbid illnesses.

A particular problem encountered in the older adult population is potential delay in surgical intervention. This may be caused by misdiagnosis of urgent surgical disease because of atypical presentations leading to higher risk of complications. Elective procedures may be delayed because of provider misconception that older adult patients will suffer complications and poor outcomes. The two main predictors of postoperative morbidity and mortality are advancing age and its accompanying physiologic decline and comorbid disease and the emergent nature of surgical interventions.

An important variable in the proper perioperative evaluation of an older adult patient is nutritional status. Older adult patients may have poor nutritional status because of either poor intake or underlying illness and comorbidities. Protein calorie malnutrition can occur in nil per os (nothing by mouth [NPO]) patients with inadequate nutritional reserve. This may occur in a short period in the older adult, malnourished surgical patient in a hypermetabolic state

TABLE 44-1 American Society of Anesthesiologists' Physical Status Classification

ASA risk stratification for anesthetic/surgical risk	
Class 1	Healthy patient
Class 2	Mild systemic disease
Class 3	Severe (but not incapacitating) systemic disease
Class 4	Severe systemic disease posing a constant threat to life
Class 5	Moribund with life expectancy < 24 h, independent of operation
Class 6 (by definition)	Organ donor

Note: Suffix "e" is added to the class for emergency operations.
Source: Rudolph R, Ballantyne DL: Skin grafts, in McCarthy J (ed): *Plastic Surgery* Philadelphia: WB Saunders, 1990, p. 221.

induced by stress of illness and surgery. Older adult patients, therefore, need accurate assessment of nutritional status and, if clinically indicated, immediate appropriate nutritional support to meet caloric requirements.

Cardiac complications are the leading cause of perioperative complications and death in surgical patients of all age groups, but particularly among the older adult who may have underlying cardiac disease in addition to normal physiologic decline. Myocardial infarction or congestive heart failure comprises one quarter of all cardiac complications and perioperative deaths in older adult patients. Therefore, identifying correctable and uncorrectable cardiovascular disease is critical prior to elective surgical intervention.

Pulmonary complications are a major source of morbidity and mortality in surgical patients, with the older adult at an even greater risk because of the increased possibility of underlying pulmonary disease and decreased reserve. Pulmonary complications account for up to 50 percent of postoperative complications and 20 percent of preventable deaths. However, age alone is a minimal factor when adjusted for comorbidities, leading to a twofold risk of pulmonary complications.

Older adult surgical patients also are at increased risk of renal compromise in the perioperative period. The physiologic changes in renal function in these patients increase the susceptibility to renal ischemia perioperatively and to nephrotoxic agents. This functional decline with age is caused by glomerular damage and sclerosis leading to a decreased glomerular filtration rate (GFR). The GFR decreases by approximately 1 mL/min for every year over the age of 40. The GFR for a healthy 80-year-old patient is one half to two thirds of the value at age 30 years.

Acute renal failure is proven to dramatically increase morbidity and mortality in older adult patients. The mortality of perioperative acute renal failure is 50 percent, and may be even higher in older adult patients. Therefore, careful management of fluid and electrolytes status is prudent to avoid imbalances and limit exposure to nephrotoxic diagnostic studies and medications in the perioperative management of older adult patients. Prompt recognition of renal compromise, marked by an elevation of blood urea nitrogen (BUN) or creatinine levels, or oliguria requires aggressive correction of underlying causes.

SPECIFIC CONSIDERATIONS

Minimal Access Laparoscopic Surgery

The increasing experience with laparoscopic techniques, combined with minimized pain, decreased length of hospital stay, and low morbidity and mortality rates, has led to the increased use in minimal-access procedures among the older adult.

Laparoscopic surgery reduces common postoperative complications such as decreased atelectasis, ileus, and wound infections. In older adult surgical patients, these complications easily progress to pneumonia, deep vein thrombosis (DVT), moderate metabolic and electrolyte disturbances, and even sepsis. Decreased postoperative pain from smaller incisions leads to a faster return to a preoperative level of functioning including early ambulation, which decreases complications from prolonged bed rest such as DVT and pneumonia from poor pulmonary mechanics.

The cardiopulmonary effects induced by pneumoperitoneum are secondary to carbon dioxide insufflation and the increased intraabdominal pressure. CO_2 insufflation is associated with hypercarbia and acidosis, both of which are proven direct myocardial depressants. Hypercarbia becomes especially problematic in patients with preexisting pulmonary disease with chronic carbon dioxide retention such as chronic obstructive cardiopulmonary disease (COPD). However, in patients without preexisting disease, these alterations can be minimized with increased minute ventilation. The increase in intraabdominal pressure during insufflation can lead to increased afterload, increased peripheral vascular resistance and mean systemic pressure, and decreased preload because of decreased venous return.

Maintenance of adequate preload using appropriate preoperative and intraoperative volume control and careful mechanical ventilation to control hypercarbia and acidosis are basic concepts that allow safe application of minimally invasive techniques in the older adult.

A particularly valuable application of minimally invasive techniques in the older adult population is the evaluation of acute abdominal pain and to rule out a surgical abdomen. Vague, poorly localized pain with several confounding comorbid conditions that obscure the diagnosis, the risk of general anesthesia, and negative exploratory laparotomy would be life-threatening for an older adult, critically ill patient.

Endocrine Surgery

Breast Surgery

In the United States, breast cancer incidence continues to rise with advancing age; approximately two thirds of newly diagnosed breast cancer patients are age 55 years or older. Additionally, 77 percent of deaths caused by breast cancer occur in patients older than 55 years of age. There also is an increase in mortality rates for each successive 5-year age group, with patients 85 years and older having the highest mortality rate, estimated at approximately 200 deaths per 100,000 population. However, older adult patients have not been shown to present at later stages nor do they suffer increased morbidity and mortality after standard therapies.

The estimated mortality for a patient 70 years of age or older undergoing a mastectomy is less than 1 percent. Older adult women should be offered, and typically prefer, breast-conserving surgery. It has been suggested that older adult women have a low rate of recurrence after lumpectomy, axillary dissection, and radiotherapy, making this a viable option. Radiation therapy is well tolerated by older adult women, with a minimal increase in morbidity and mortality, when added to breast-conserving procedures.

Routine axillary lymph node dissection with breast-conserving surgery remains controversial in older adult patients. There has been a trend toward providing adjuvant therapy with tamoxifen to patients with node-positive and node-negative disease, making axillary lymph node dissection (ALND) unnecessary. Furthermore, because ALND is associated with some morbidity, older adult women are considered at greater risk of chronic lymph edema and decreased shoulder mobility. In patients with clinically node-negative status, the axillary field also can be added to the radiation port to provide local control rates equivalent to those achieved with axillary dissection. However, ALND remains necessary in patients with clinically palpable axillary lymph nodes for adequate local control.

Older adult women with multiple comorbid conditions that lack the physiologic reserve to undergo the stress of surgical intervention should be offered conservative management with tamoxifen as the sole treatment. Adequate response rates have been observed and range from 10–50 percent, with failure rates ranging between 33 and 58 percent.

Thyroid Surgery

The prevalence of thyroid disease increases with advancing age. The etiologies, risk factors, and presentations of thyroid disease are similar across all ages and, therefore, are not discussed in detail. Of note, however, is that older adult patients more often present with cardiac manifestations of hyperthyroidism such as atrial fibrillation than do their younger counterparts. A common finding requiring evaluation in older adult patients is the presence of a thyroid nodule, usually detected by physical examination. These nodules are usually single and are four times more common in women, making them a particular concern for postmenopausal older adult women. Indications for surgical intervention for thyroid nodules are dependent on the characteristics of the nodule (i.e., whether it is benign or malignant, or whether the patient is euthyroid or thyrotoxic). Additionally, surgical intervention becomes necessary if the nodule enlarges, producing compressive symptoms.

Papillary carcinoma in older adult patients tends to be sporadic with a bell-shape distribution of age at presentation, occurring primarily in patients age 30–59 years. The incidence of papillary carcinoma decreases in patients older than 60 years of age. However, patients older than 60 years of age have increased risk of local recurrence and for the development of distant metastases. Metastatic disease may be more common in this population secondary to delayed referral for surgical intervention because of the misconception that the surgeon will be unwilling to operate on an older adult patient with thyroid disease. Age is also a prognostic indicator for patients with follicular carcinoma. There is a 2.2 times increased risk of mortality from follicular carcinoma per 20 years of increasing age. Therefore, prognosis for older adult patients with differentiated thyroid carcinomas is worse when compared to younger counterparts. The higher prevalence of vascular invasion and extracapsular extension among older patients is in part responsible for the poorer prognosis in geriatric patients. Advancing age leads to increased mortality risk for patients with thyroid cancer and is demonstrated by the AMES (age, metastases, extent of primary tumor,

TABLE 44-2 AMES Classification of Thyroid Cancers

		Low Mortality Risk	High Mortality Risk
A:	Age	Men: < 41 y of age Women: < 51 y of age	Men: > 41 y of age Women: > 51 y of age
M:	Metastases	Absence of distant metastases	Presence of distant metastases
E:	Extent of primary tumor	Intrathyroidal papillary cancer (confined to thyroid)	Extrathyroidal papillary cancer
		Follicular cancer with minor capsular involvement	Follicular cancer with major capsular involvement
S:	Size of tumor	Primary tumor < 5 cm in diameter	Primary tumor ≥ 5 cm in diameter (regardless of extent of disease)

Note: Older patients (men > 41 years of age and women > 51 y of age) one included in the low-risk group if tumors are less than 5 cm, intrathyroidal, or follicular with minor capsular involvement.
Source: Adapted from Sanders LE, Cady B: Differentiated thyroid cancer. *Arch Surg* 133:419,1998.

and size of tumor) classification system developed by the Lahey Clinic (Table 44-2).

Anaplastic carcinoma is a highly aggressive form of thyroid carcinoma with a dismal prognosis. It accounts for approximately 1 percent of all thyroid malignancies; however, it occurs primarily in older adult patients. This poorly differentiated tumor rapidly invades local structures, leading to clinical deterioration and eventually tracheal obstruction. These patients may present with a painful, rapidly enlarging neck mass accompanied by dysphagia and cervical tenderness. This leads to respiratory compromise and impingement of the airway. Unfortunately, because of the aggressive nature of the disease and the dismal prognosis, surgical resection of the tumor is not attempted for cure. Furthermore, radiation therapy and chemotherapy offer little benefit. Airway blockage, however, may necessitate surgical palliation or permanent tracheostomy to alleviate symptoms of respiratory distress.

Parathyroid Surgery

Approximately 2 percent of the geriatric population, including 3 percent of women 75 years of age or older, will develop primary hyperparathyroidism. Geriatric patients are usually referred to surgery only when advanced disease is present because of concerns regarding the risks of surgery, but low morbidity and negligible mortality rates combined with high cure rates of approximately 95–98 percent make parathyroidectomy safe and effective.

Limited parathyroidectomies with minimal dissection in geriatric patients are an effective alternative. This is a viable option in patients with multiple comorbid conditions in whom the increased risk of surgical intervention or general anesthesia remains a concern. One study demonstrated that preoperative localization of the hyperfunctioning gland with the aid of 99mTc-sestamibi nuclear scanning, and intraoperative parathyroid hormone (PTH) assays to rapidly confirm that all hypersecreting glands have been removed, allows limited parathyroidectomy to be performed with accuracy in older adult patients.

This procedure is described as "limited" because bilateral neck dissection for identification and biopsy of the remaining glands in order to determine if they are hypersecreting becomes unnecessary.

Cardiothoracic Surgery

Coronary Artery Bypass Grafting

There has been a significant trend in providing definitive operative intervention to older adult patients requiring coronary artery bypass grafting (CABG). Although older patients have higher morbidity and mortality rates after cardiac surgery than do younger patients, these rates are decreasing significantly over time. This decline in morbidity and mortality rates among older adult patients undergoing cardiac surgery reflects better preoperative assessment and patient selection. Older adult patients are more likely to have significant triple-vessel disease accompanied by poor ejection fraction, left ventricular hypertrophy, significant valvular disease, and previous history of myocardial infarction than are younger patients. Older adult patients also are more likely to be classified at New York Heart Association (NYHA) functional class III or higher and are more likely to present on an emergent basis. Despite the increased risk of morbidity and mortality compared to younger patients, older adult patients, including those older than age 80 years, can undergo CABG with acceptable mortality risk. The overall mortality rate is approximately 7–12 percent for older adult patients, including cases performed under emergency conditions. This figure decreases to approximately 2.8 percent when CABG is performed electively with careful preoperative evaluation.

Valve Replacement

There also is an increasing percentage of the geriatric population presenting with symptomatic valvular disease requiring intervention. The most common valvular abnormality present in older adult patients is calcific aortic stenosis, which can lead to angina and syncope. The operative mortality from aortic valve replacement is estimated to be between 3 and 10 percent, with an average of approximately 7.7 percent. If aortic stenosis is allowed to progress without operative intervention, congestive heart failure will ensue. The average survival of these patients is approximately 1.5–2 years. Older adult patients require surgery for mitral valve disease when ischemic regurgitation is present. Surgery for mitral valve disease carries a higher morbidity and mortality than for aortic intervention, with an estimated mortality rate as high as 20 percent. Left ventricular function is usually compromised in patients requiring intervention, leading to a poorer outcome in these patients. The surgical outcome for mitral valve procedures depends on the extent of the disease, age of the patient, presence of pulmonary hypertension, and extent of coronary artery disease.

Another concern regarding older adult patients who require surgery for valve disease is the additional requirement for coronary revascularization. This increases the morbidity and mortality from surgical intervention. An older adult patient with many comorbid conditions in need of a combined procedure should only have critically stenosed vessels bypassed.

An important consideration in valve replacement procedures in older adult patients is the type of prosthesis to be used. Older adult patients are at increased risk from bleeding-associated anticoagulation complications. This is especially significant in patients who have experienced falls and minor trauma that have resulted in significant intracranial hemorrhage. To avoid the life-long requirement for anticoagulants, bioprosthetic valves should be used in place of mechanical valves whenever possible.

Trauma

Geriatric patients older than 65 years of age currently account for approximately 23 percent of total hospital trauma admissions—many of which are multisystem and life-threatening. This percentage is expected to rise to as high as 40 percent, making this a growing concern for potential long-term morbidity, mortality, rehabilitation, and cost. Trauma is the sixth most common cause of death in patients 65–74 years of age. Older adult patients are particularly susceptible to trauma because of changes that occur with aging, such as gait instability, decreased hearing and visual acuity, presence of confusion and dementia, or underlying disease. The presence of preexisting comorbid conditions increases the odds of an older adult patient experiencing a complication by a factor of three.

It is crucial to determine the medication regimen of older adult trauma patients. Medication such as beta blockers, calcium channel blockers, diuretics, and afterload reducers may impair augmentation of myocardial function in trauma patients, especially if they are hypovolemic.

Not only are older patients at increased risk of death from trauma, there is also an increased occurrence of delayed death when compared to younger patients. Preexisting cardiovascular or liver disease and the development of cardiac, renal, or infectious complications are independent predictors of delayed mortality.

The most common mechanism for injuries in the older adult is from falls, which account for approximately 20 percent of severe injuries. Many underlying chronic and acute diseases common to older patients place them at increased risk for falls. These diseases include postural hypotension leading to syncopal "drop attacks," dysrhythmia from sick sinus syndrome, autonomic dysfunction from polypharmacy with improper dosage of antihypertensive or oral hypoglycemic agents resulting in hypotension, and hypoglycemia.

Blunt thoracic trauma accounts for approximately 25 percent of all trauma deaths in North America. Rib fractures occur in up to two thirds of all cases of chest trauma and are associated with pulmonary complications in approximately 35 percent of cases. More than 50 percent of patients older than age 65 years sustain rib fractures from falls from less than 6 feet, which includes falls from the standing position. This injury in particular leads to morbidity and mortality for older adult patients as a consequence of the increased risk of development of pulmonary contusions and subsequent pneumonia, the latter of which occurs in 27 percent of older patients, as compared to 13 percent of younger patients.

In addition to higher mortality, older adult patients suffer from poorer functional recovery from trauma despite survival of injury, with approximately 20–25 percent of patients requiring discharge to a skilled nursing facility for long-term care and rehabilitation.

Kidney Transplantation

A new trend provides older adult patients with an increasing opportunity for organ donation and receipt, which increases the pool of potential organ donors. According to the United Network for Organ Sharing (UNOS) data, the percentage of older adult organ donors increased from 2–24 percent between 1982 and 1995. In 1997, 44 percent of cadaveric renal transplant donors were older than 50 years of age. This trend is expected to increase given the expanding older adult population in the United States.

In the 1970s, experience with kidney transplantation in older patients was associated with poor prognosis. It was estimated that the 1-year patient and graft survival rates for patients older than age 45 years was 40 and 20 percent, respectively. This was thought to be a result of the decline in renal function and changes within the kidney as a result of damage from the aging process. It was therefore adopted that cadaveric transplants were not to be given to patients older than 45 years of age. However, advancements in immunosuppression have significantly improved quality of life off dialysis and have improved survival in this population. The significance of better survival outcomes in older patients receiving transplantation today is that older adult patients have the potential for prolonged life expectancy. The importance of this advancement is evident in the fact that in 2000, approximately 60 percent of end-stage renal disease (ESRD) patients were older than 65 years of age, and approximately 50 percent of newly diagnosed patients with ESRD belong to older age cohorts.

Older adult patients have better graft function, with decreased incidence of delayed graft function and fewer episodes of acute rejection, than do younger patients. This may be the result of decreased immune competence with aging. With the lower occurrence of both acute and chronic rejection in older adult patients, it has been suggested that older adult patients would benefit from lower doses of immunosuppressive agents. However, this decreased competence is balanced by the increased incidence of infections from viruses such as herpes, cytomegalovirus (CMV), and Epstein-Barr, and posttransplant neoplasia, including lymphoproliferative disorders.

The adoption of dual-kidney donation from older adult patients with depressed innate kidney function expanded the donor population to more than 75 years of age; greater than 15 percent of whom were glomerulosclerotic. The increased nephron mass achieved with dual-kidney transplantation compensated for the possible declining renal function with advanced age.

PALLIATIVE SURGERY

Palliative surgery is defined as surgical intervention targeted to alleviate a patient's symptoms, thus improving the patient's quality of life despite minimal impact on the patient's survival.

With an increasing number of aging surgical patients who often present with advanced disease, surgeons must be familiar with the concept of palliation to control disease. This concept focuses on providing the maximal benefit to the patient using the least-invasive intervention. Ultimately, this leads to symptom relief and preservation of the quality of life in terminal disease states.

There currently is no evidence to support that palliative surgery is less effective for older adult patients with surgically unresectable disease. Younger patients undergoing palliative interventions do not have a demonstrated improved outcome when compared to disease-matched older patients. Therefore, it is important to recognize that age is not a limitation to surgical intervention and that all interventions should be individualized based on the severity of symptoms and the predicted benefit.

Surgical palliative care can range from nonoperative management of malignant obstructions by percutaneous methods to laparoscopic surgery for the treatment of life-threatening illness by minimally invasive technique. An interesting challenge in palliative care is the determination of the actual cause of a patient's symptoms in order to offer the most beneficial, but least invasive, intervention.

Palliative intervention for symptom relief and prevention of complications can be demonstrated in the management of terminal pancreatic cancer and metastatic colorectal cancer. Two-thirds of patients with pancreatic cancer present with advanced disease, which is often diagnosed after evaluation of obstructive jaundice. Despite advanced disease, surgical intervention improves quality of life through relief of biliary obstruction. Percutaneous transhepatic stenting has emerged as a viable alternative to surgical bypass, achieving similar results and lowering mortality rates with the occurrence of fewer early complications. Endoscopic stenting is yet another option. If a patient does not have multiple comorbidities with good functional status, surgical intervention then can provide a definitive diagnosis and permanent biliary decompression and gastric drainage. Additionally, an important palliative intervention that can be provided to patients with the open procedure is chemical splanchnicectomy, which is infiltration of the celiac plexus with an agent such as alcohol for effective relief of intractable pain from tumor invasion of the celiac plexus. A gastroenterostomy drainage procedure is effective protection against gastric outlet obstruction, which inevitably develops in 30 percent of patients.

Palliative surgery for disseminated colorectal cancer should be aimed at the reduction of symptoms such as pain, obstruction, or hemorrhage. Bowel obstruction can be relieved with intestinal bypass or a diverting colostomy. The most common site of disseminated disease is the liver, and uncontrolled liver metastasis is responsible for pain, abdominal distention, jaundice, and inferior vena caval obstruction. Many patients with liver metastasis are not candidates for resection and therefore may be considered for ablation of the lesions by local destruction, cryotherapy, or radiofrequency ablation. More traditional means, such as chemotherapy, which can be administered via the hepatic artery, or radiation, also may be employed. Systemic corticosteroid therapy can be used in patients with advanced metastatic disease to reduce pain caused by swelling of the liver capsule. If bone metastases are present, pain may be controlled by irradiation, and prophylactic fixation of long bones may be considered to decrease pain and morbidity from pathologic fractures.

Specific Symptom Management

Gastrointestinal Disturbances

The distressing symptoms often faced by terminally ill patients either result from the disease process or as a side effect of treatment. The causes of nausea and vomiting in terminally ill patients are multifactorial and can be attributed to various medications or chemotherapy treatments, gastric stasis, obstruction of the gastrointestinal tract, mesenteric metastases, irritation of the gastrointestinal (GI) tract, raised intracranial pressure from cerebral metastasis, or anxiety-induced emesis. Treatment should be focused on prevention of dehydration and malnutrition from poor oral intake. Antiemetics may be administered for control of nausea and vomiting. The oral route of administration is the best option for prophylaxis prior to chemotherapy treatments. However, other preparations, such as suppositories or injections, can be appropriate for patients who are unable to tolerate oral medications.

Diarrhea and constipation also are common GI disturbances in terminal patients. Constipation is particularly common in patients receiving chronic narcotic medications. Constipation also can be caused by such events as tumor invasion leading to intestinal obstruction, metabolic abnormalities such as hypercalcemia from metastatic disease, and dehydration. Because constipation may be worsened by dehydration, adequate fluid intake often helps to alleviate symptoms. Constipation can lead to fecal impaction, nausea, and colicky abdominal pain. If there is difficulty distinguishing between constipation and early bowel obstruction, diagnostic tests are useful, but should be kept to a minimum in terminal patients. Patients can be treated with stool softeners and stimulant agents. Laxatives with peristalsis-stimulating action such as senna or bisacodyl should be used with caution because of the potential for causing intestinal colic.

The occurrence of diarrhea also is multifactorial and can be caused by medications, overload incontinence with fecal impaction, from the disease process itself, malignant bowel obstruction, or improper laxative therapy. Radiation therapy can cause diarrhea by damage of the intestinal mucosa, which results in the release of prostaglandins and the malabsorption of bile salts that increases peristalsis. Once the underlying causes are identified and appropriately managed, patients can be given bulk-forming agents and opiate derivatives to aid in symptomatic improvement.

Cachexia and Anorexia

Cachexia refers to catabolic changes associated with progressive wasting that is present in patients with advanced illness; prominent symptoms include anorexia, weight loss, and asthenia. A subsequent loss of muscle and fat leading to anemia, hypoalbuminemia, and hypoproteinemia also is common. This is a chronic form of malnutrition and is not reversible with short-term nutritional support and hyperalimentation. Malnourished cancer patients with cachexia have reduced response to antineoplastic medications, radiation, and chemotherapy, and decreased survival rates. The mechanism of cachexia is poorly understood, but hypotheses include actions of interleukin-6, tumor necrosis factor, and interferon-mediating metabolic changes in chronic illness.

Management of cachexia begins with the identification of correctable causes. Patients may have underlying metabolic derangements, and dehydration, that must be appropriately treated. Poorly controlled pain, anemia, and sleep disturbances also may exacerbate symptoms of cachexia, leading to malnutrition and wasting. Patients with terminal disease additionally often suffer from gastrointestinal disturbances, such as constipation and nausea, which may lead to anorexia. Malabsorption is common in patients with pancreatic cancer, and supplementation of pancreatic enzymes may improve absorption and help to improve nutritional status. Nausea and vomiting should be appropriately managed. It is important to rule out mechanical causes of malnutrition that can effectively be treated with nonoperative management such as bowel rest and nasogastric tube compression or operative intervention.

If no underlying correctable abnormalities are identified, patients may benefit from pharmacologic intervention with dexamethasone and prednisone, which increase appetites in patients with advanced cancer, leading to improved quality of life. Other agents, such as progestational drugs, namely megestrol acetate (Megace), also stimulate appetite and cause weight gain in cachexia patients.

Malignant Bowel Obstruction

Patients with malignant bowel obstruction typically present with cramping abdominal pain, nausea, and vomiting, which may be a common complication of advanced terminal disease secondary to gastrointestinal malignancy or from extrinsic compression of bowel loops from progressive tumor burden. Conservative management can be effective and includes NPO, intravenous hydration, and nasogastric decompression. Medical management with pharmacologic agents such as somatostatin analogues to decrease gastrointestinal output may also be considered for symptom alleviation along with analgesics and antiemetics. However, surgical palliation via bypass procedures, decompressing, or diverting ostomies may be required.

Surgical intervention may provide permanent alleviation of obstruction and eliminate the need for repeated nasogastric decompressions that can limit patient comfort. This must be balanced against the risk of perioperative mortality from surgical intervention, which ranges from approximately 12–20 percent, and the potential for mortality from wound infection, poor wound healing, and fistula formation. Patients in whom the risk of surgical intervention outweighs the benefit of palliation include patients who have ascites or multiple sites of obstruction accompanied by poor functional status and poor nutrition with serum albumin levels less than 3 g/dL. Should conservative management fail in a patient who is unfit to undergo surgical intervention, alternatives include a venting gastrostomy or jejunostomy, which can be inserted percutaneously.

ETHICAL CONSIDERATIONS

Ethical considerations and end-of-life care dilemmas have gained prominent focus in the care of older adult patients, especially in the terminal stages of illness. This is a particularly important issue given the increasing effectiveness of modern therapies and sophisticated intensive care available to patients with the technical ability to sustain life indefinitely. It is therefore critical to begin to address these issues early in the course of disease to properly interact with patients and family members regarding prognosis, treatment options, alternatives, and plan of care in terminal stages. Development of a clear plan of care for a terminally ill patient eases the transition from curative therapy to palliation. Open discussions regarding end-of-life care, withholding or withdrawal of life support, and medical futility are critical issues for patients, family, and caregivers and should be held as soon as is appropriate.

Defining medical futility remains controversial in practical definitions and in clinical determinations. The American Thoracic Society has stated that "a life-sustaining intervention is futile if reasoning and experience indicate that the intervention would be highly unlikely to result in meaningful survival for the patient," with attention paid to both the duration of survival and existing quality of life. In actual clinical practice, it is difficult to predict that a particular therapy will in fact be futile in a given patient. It is helpful to clarify a patient's wishes regarding life-sustaining treatment via advance directives, living wills, and do not resuscitate (DNR) orders to avoid unnecessary prolongation of futile treatment.

The governing principle in end-of-life decision making is patient autonomy, which takes precedence over physicians' judgment of what is most appropriate care. Patients have a right to refuse treatment, even if it delays appropriate treatment or results in the patient's death. However, these preferences need to be documented during a time of mental competency. Surrogate decision making is tantamount to patient's wishes, giving surrogates complete decision-making responsibilities.

Physicians are not required to provide futile care. The Patient Self-Determination Act allows a patient to document preferences for life-sustaining interventions and resuscitation before undergoing treatments in the form of advance directives and living wills. These documents define the patient's wishes regarding life support measures. Additionally, a surrogate for decision making can be appointed by the patient to make decisions regarding plan of care in the event the patient becomes mentally incapacitated. Unfortunately, most DNR orders are written only within days of a patient's death. This issue should always be addressed with patients prior to operative intervention.

Another important principle is open communication. Patients must be informed honestly of their diagnosis and prognosis, and of the risks and benefits of all treatment options. It can be difficult to accurately portray a patient's prognosis to either the patient or family members because it often is unclear. Although this may be impossible to predict with certainty, patients and their families can be given honest information based on a physician's prior clinical experience with similar patients.

One of the most difficult issues faced in palliative care is resolution of conflicts that arise between the physician and the patient's family. Withdrawal and withholding of life-sustaining therapies is often a source of conflict between the physician, patient, and family members. It has been demonstrated that the most frequently identified cause of conflict, accounting for approximately 63 percent of disputes, was in regard to decisions for withdrawal or withholding of treatment. Strategies to avoid conflict regarding termination of care or withholding further measures that are deemed futile is to identify a single decision maker early in the course of illness and to establish a clear line of communication between the physician and family members regarding diagnosis, treatment plans, and transition to palliative care. The easiest way of avoiding conflict is by maintaining a relationship with the patient and the patient's family throughout the course of hospitalization.

End-of-life decisions are considerably easier when a patient elects a surrogate decision maker to make all necessary decisions in event of incapacitation via written documentation prior to admission to the hospital. Additionally, continuity of care must be established with flexibility in treatment plans. One method is to establish limits to therapy prior to, and during, therapy. This is helpful in demonstrating whether a patient is likely to respond to therapy and helps to alleviate family doubt regarding the likelihood of the patient's recovery and can confirm the physician's assessment that further care would be futile. If conflicts continue, involvement of an ethical committee is the next appropriate step. It is important for a physician to alleviate the fear of legal liability for the family member or proxy responsible for making the decision to withdraw or withhold life-sustaining therapies.

Suggested Readings

Keating HJ, Luben MF: Perioperative considerations of the physician/geriatrician. Clin Geriatr Med 6:459, 1990.

Ballista-Lopez C, Cid JA, Poves I, et al: Laparoscopic surgery in the elderly patient: Experience of a single laparoscopic unit. Surg Endosc 17:333, 2003.

Yanik R, Wesley MN, Ries LA, et al: Effect of age and comorbidity in post-menopausal breast cancer patients aged 55 years and older. JAMA 285:885, 2001.

Berger DH, Roslyn JJ: Cancer surgery in the elderly. Clin Geriatr Med 13:119, 1997.

Irvin GL, Carneiro DM: "Limited" parathyroidectomy in geriatric patients. Ann Surg 233:612, 2001.

Aziz S, Grover FL: Cardiovascular surgery in the elderly. Cardiol Clin 17:213, 1999.

Richmond TS, Kaunder D, Strumpf N, et al: Characteristics and outcomes of serious traumatic injury in older adults. J Am Geriatr Soc 50:215, 2002.

Lee CM, Carter JT, Weinstein RJ, et al: Dual kidney transplantation: Older donors for older recipients. J Am Coll Surg 189:82, 1999.

McCahill LE, Krouse RS, Chu DZ, et al: Decision making in palliative surgery. J Am Coll Surg 195:411, 2002.

Dunn GP, Milch RA, Mosenthal AC, et al: Palliative care by the surgeon. J Am Coll Surg 194:509, 2002.

45 | Anesthesia of the Surgical Patient

Robert S. Dorian

The discipline of anesthesia embodies control of three great concerns of humankind: consciousness, pain, and movement. The field of anesthesiology combines the administration of anesthesia with the perioperative management of the patient's concerns, pain management, and critical illness. The fields of surgery and anesthesiology are truly collaborative and continue to evolve together, enabling the care of sicker patients and rapid recovery from outpatient and minimally invasive procedures.

BASIC PHARMACOLOGY

Pharmacokinetics "What the Body Does to the Drug"

Pharmacokinetics describes the relationship between the dose of a drug and its plasma or tissue concentration. It depends on absorption (into the bloodstream), distribution, and elimination. Route of administration, metabolism, protein binding, and tissue distribution all affect the pharmacokinetics of a particular drug.

Administration, Distribution, and Elimination

The route of administration of a drug affects its pharmacokinetics, as there will be different rates of drug entry into the circulation. For example, the oral and intravenous routes are subject to first-pass effect of the portal circulation; this can be bypassed with the nasal or sublingual route. Other routes of drug administration include transdermal, intramuscular, subcutaneous, or inhalation.

Distribution is the delivery of a drug from the systemic circulation to the tissues. Once a drug has entered the systemic circulation, the rate at which it will enter the tissues depends on several factors:

1. Molecular size of the drug, capillary permeability, polarity, and lipid solubility. Small molecules will pass more freely and quickly across cell membranes than large ones, but capillary permeability is variable and results in different diffusion rates. Renal glomerular capillaries are permeable to almost all non–protein-bound drugs; capillaries in the brain are fused (i.e., they have tight junctions) and are relatively impermeable to all but the tiniest molecules (the blood-brain barrier). Unionized molecules pass more easily across cell membranes than charged molecules; diffusibility also increases with increasing lipid solubility.
2. Plasma protein and tissue binding. Many drugs bind to circulating proteins like albumin, glycoproteins, and globulins. Disease, age, and the presence of other drugs will affect the amount of protein binding; drug distribution is affected because only the unbound free portion of the drug can pass across the cell membrane. Drugs also bind reversibly to body tissues; if they bind with high affinity they are said to be sequestered in that tissue (e.g., heavy metals are sequestered in bone).

The fluid volume in which a drug distributes is termed the volume of distribution (Vd). This mathematically derived value gives a rough estimation of the overall physical distribution of a drug in the body. A general rule for volume distribution is that the greater the Vd, the greater the diffusibility of the drug. Because drugs have variable ionization rates and bind differently to plasma proteins and tissues, the Vd is not a good predictor of the actual concentration of the drug after administration. Determining the apparent volume of distribution (dose/concentration) is an attempt to more accurately ascertain the drug dose administered and its final concentration. This in turn is complicated by the immediate elimination of a drug after administration.

Drug elimination varies widely; some drugs are excreted unchanged by the body, some decompose via plasma enzymes, and some are degraded by organ-based enzymes in the liver. Many drugs rely on multiple pathways for elimination (i.e., metabolized by liver enzymes then excreted by the kidney). When a drug is given orally, it reaches the liver via the portal circulation and is partially metabolized before reaching the systemic circulation. This is why an oral dose of a drug often must be much higher than an equally effective intravenous dose. Some drugs (e.g., nitroglycerin) are hydrolyzed presystemically in the gut wall and must be administered sublingually to achieve an effective concentration.

It is important to remember that the response to drugs varies widely. The disposition of drugs is affected by age; weight; sex; pregnancy; disease states; the concomitant use of alcohol, tobacco, and other licit and illicit drugs; and genetic factors. The most important monitor in the operating room is the anesthesiologist, who continuously assesses the patient's response and adjusts the doses of anesthetic agents to match the surgical stimulus.

Pharmacodynamics "What the Drug Does to the Body"

Pharmacodynamics, or how the plasma concentration of a drug translates into its effect on the body, depends on biologic variability, receptor physiology, and clinical evaluations of the actual drug. An agonist is a drug that causes a response. A full agonist produces the full tissue response, and a partial agonist provokes less than the maximum response induced by a full agonist. An antagonist is a drug that does not provoke a response itself, but blocks agonist-mediated responses. An additive effect means that a second drug acts with the first drug and will produce an effect that is equal to the algebraic summation of both drugs. A synergistic effect means that two drugs interact to produce an effect that is greater than expected from the two drugs' algebraic summation.

Hyporeactivity means a larger than expected dose is required to produce a response, and this effect is termed tolerance, desensitization, or tachyphylaxis. Tolerance usually results from chronic drug exposure, either through enzyme induction (e.g., alcohol) or depletion of neurotransmitters (e.g., cocaine).

Potency, Efficacy, Lethal Dose, and Therapeutic Index

The potency of a drug is the dose required to produce a given effect, such as pain relief or a change in heart rate. The average sensitivity to a particular drug can be expressed through the calculation of the effective dose; ED50 would have the desired effect in 50 percent of the general population. The efficacy of any therapeutic agent is its power to produce a desired effect. Two drugs may have the same efficacy but different potencies. The difference in potency of the two drugs is described by the ratio EDb50/EDa50 in which a is the less potent drug. If the EDb50 equals 4 and the EDa50 equals 0.4, then drug a is 10 times as potent as drug b. For example, 10 mg of morphine produces analgesia equal to that of 1 mg of hydromorphone. They are equally effective, but hydromorphone is 10 times as potent as morphine.

The lethal dose (LD50) of a drug produces death in 50 percent of animals to which it is given. The ratio of the lethal dose and effective dose, LD50/ED50, is the therapeutic index. A drug with a high therapeutic index is safer than a drug with a low or narrow therapeutic index.

ANESTHETIC AGENTS

Anesthesia can be local, regional, or general (Table 45-1).

Local anesthesia is accomplished using a local anesthetic drug that can be injected intradermally, and is used for the removal of small lesions or to repair traumatic injuries. Local anesthesia is the most frequent anesthetic administered by surgeons, and may be accompanied by intravenous sedation to improve patient comfort.

Local Anesthetics

Local anesthetics are divided into two groups based on their chemical structure: the amides and the esters. In general, the amides are metabolized in the liver and the esters are metabolized by plasma cholinesterases, which yield metabolites with slightly higher allergic potential than the amides.

Amides

The amide local anesthetics include lidocaine, bupivacaine, mepivacaine, prilocaine, and ropivacaine. Lidocaine has a more rapid onset and is shorter acting than bupivacaine; however, both are widely used for tissue infiltration, regional nerve blocks, and spinal and epidural anesthesia. Ropivacaine is the most recently introduced local anesthetic, clinically similar to bupivacaine with a slow onset and a long duration, but less cardiotoxic. All amides are 95 percent metabolized in the liver, with 5 percent excreted unchanged by the kidneys.

Esters

The ester local anesthetics include cocaine, procaine, chloroprocaine, tetracaine, and benzocaine. Unique among local anesthetics, cocaine occurs in nature, was the first used clinically, produces vasoconstriction (making it useful for topical application; e.g., for intranasal surgery), releases norepinephrine from nerve terminals resulting in hypertension, and is highly addictive. Cocaine is a Schedule II drug. Procaine, synthesized in 1905 as a nontoxic substitute for cocaine, has a short duration and is used for infiltration. Tetracaine has a long duration and is useful as a spinal anesthetic for lengthy operations. Benzocaine is for topical use only. The esters are hydrolyzed in the blood by pseudocholinesterase. Some of the metabolites have a greater allergic potential than the metabolites of the amide anesthetics, but true allergies to local anesthetics are rare.

The common characteristic of all local anesthetics is a reversible block of the transmission of neural impulses when placed on or near a nerve membrane. Local anesthetics block nerve conduction by stabilizing sodium channels in their closed state, preventing action potentials from propagating along the nerve. The individual local anesthetic agents have different recovery times

TABLE 45-1 Anesthetic Agents, Their Actions, and Their Clinical Uses

Effect	Monitor	Intravenous drugs	Potent gases	Weak gases	Local anesthetics
Unconsciousness, amnesia, anxiolysis	*Eeg;* clinical signs	*Benzodiazepines* Midazolam Diazepam Lorazepam *Barbiturates* Propofol Etomidate Ketamine[a]	Sevoflurane Desflurane Isoflurane Enflurane Halothane	Nitrous oxide	
Analgesia	Heart rate, blood pressure, respiratory rate, clinical signs	*Opioids* Morphine Meperidine Hydromorphone Fentanyl *NSAID* Ketorolac Parecoxib	Sevoflurane Desflurane Isoflurane Enflurane Halothane	Nitrous oxide	*Esters* Cocaine Procaine Chloroprocaine Tetracaine Benzocaine *Amides* Lidocaine Bupivacaine Mepivacaine Prilocaine Ropivacaine *Regional peripheral* Brachial plexus Lower extremity Cervical plexus *Regional central* Spinal Epidural
Muscle relaxation, paralysis	Nerve stimulator; clinical signs; tidal volume, hand grip; 5-second head lift	*Depolarizing agent* Succinylcholine *Nondepolarizing agents* Pancuronium Vecuronium Rocuronium Atracurium Cis-atracurium Mivacurium	Sevoflurane Desflurane Isoflurane Enflurane Halothane	—	

[a]Note that the intravenous agents are quite specific in their effects, except for ketamine, which has both amnestic and analgesic qualities.
The potent inhalational anesthetics contribute to all three components of anesthesia, but nitrous oxide has weak amnestic and analgesic properties, and provides no muscle relaxation at all.
The local anesthetics produce excellent analgesia and muscle relaxation, but contribute nothing to amnesia or anxiolysis, these anesthetics must be supplemented with an intravenous sedative.
General anesthesia entails all three elements of anesthesia (amnesia, analgesic, and muscle relaxation).

based on lipid solubility and tissue binding, but return of neural function is spontaneous as the drug is metabolized or removed from the nerve by the vascular system.

Toxicity of local anesthetics results from absorption into the bloodstream or from inadvertent direct intravascular injection. Toxicity manifests first in the more sensitive central nervous system, and then the cardiovascular system.

Central nervous system. As plasma concentration of local anesthetic rises, symptoms progress from restlessness to complaints of tinnitus. Slurred speech, seizures, and unconsciousness follow. Cessation of the seizure via administration of a benzodiazepine or thiopental and maintenance of the airway is the immediate treatment. If the seizure persists, the trachea must be intubated with a cuffed endotracheal tube to guard against pulmonary aspiration of stomach contents.

Cardiovascular system. With increasingly elevated plasma levels of local anesthetics, progression to hypotension, increased P-R intervals, bradycardia, and cardiac arrest may occur. Bupivacaine is more cardiotoxic than other local anesthetics. It has a direct effect on ventricular muscle, and because it is more lipid soluble than lidocaine, it binds tightly to sodium channels (it is called the fast-in, slow-out local anesthetic). Patients who have received an inadvertent intravascular injection of bupivacaine have experienced profound hypotension, ventricular tachycardia and fibrillation, and complete atrioventricular heart block that is extremely refractory to treatment. The toxic dose of lidocaine is approximately 5 mg/kg; that of bupivacaine is approximately 3 mg/kg.

Calculation of the toxic dose before injection is imperative. It is helpful to remember that for any drug or solution, 1 percent = 10 mg/mL. For a 50-kg person, the toxic dose of bupivacaine is approximately 3 mg/kg, or 3 × 50 = 150 mg. A 0.5 percent solution of bupivacaine is 5 mg/mL, so 150 mg/5 mg/mL = 30 mL as the upper limit for infiltration. For lidocaine in the same patient, the calculation is 50 kg × 5 mg/mL = 250 mg toxic dose. If a 1 percent solution is used, the allowed amount would be 250 mg/10 mg/mL = 25 mL.

Additives. Epinephrine has one physiologic and several clinical effects when added to local anesthetics. Epinephrine is a vasoconstrictor, and by reducing local bleeding, molecules of the local anesthetic remain in proximity to the nerve for a longer time period. Onset of the nerve block is faster, the quality of the block is improved, the duration is longer, and less local anesthetic will be absorbed into the blood stream, thereby reducing toxicity. Although epinephrine 1:200,000 (5 μg/mL) added to a local anesthetic for infiltration will greatly lengthen the time of analgesia, epinephrine-containing solutions should not be injected into body parts with end-arteries such as toes or fingers, as vasoconstriction may lead to ischemia or loss of a digit.

Regional Anesthesia

Peripheral

Local anesthetic can be injected peripherally, near a large nerve or plexus to provide anesthesia to a larger region of the body. Examples include the brachial plexus for surgery of the arm or hand, blockade of the femoral and sciatic nerves for surgery of the lower extremity, ankle block for surgery of the foot or toes, intercostal block for analgesia of the thorax postoperatively, or blockade of the cervical plexus, which is ideal for carotid endarterectomy. Risks of peripheral regional nerve blocks are dependent on their location. For example, nerve blocks injected into the neck risk puncture of the carotid or vertebral arteries, intercostal nerves are in close proximity to the vascular bundle and have a high rate of absorption of local anesthetic, and nerve blocks of the thorax run the risk of causing pneumothorax. All peripheral nerve blocks may be supplemented intraoperatively with intravenous sedation and/or analgesics.

Central

Local anesthetic injected centrally near the spinal cord—spinal or epidural anesthesia—provides anesthesia for the lower half of the body. This is especially useful for genitourinary, gynecologic, inguinal hernia, or lower-extremity procedures. Spinal and epidural anesthesia block the spinal nerves as they exit the spinal cord. Spinal nerves are mixed nerves; they contain motor, sensory, and sympathetic components. The subsequent block will cause sensory anesthesia, loss of motor function, and blockade of the sympathetic nerves from the level of the anesthetic distally to the lower extremities. Subsequent vasodilation of the vasculature from sympathetic block may result in hypotension, which is treatable with intravenous fluids and/or pressors.

Spinal anesthesia. Local anesthetic is injected directly into the dural sac surrounding the spinal cord. The level of injection is usually below L1–L2, where the spinal cord ends in most adults. Because the local anesthetic is injected directly into the cerebrospinal fluid (CSF) surrounding the spinal cord, only a small dose is needed, the onset of anesthesia is rapid, and the blockade thorough. Lidocaine, bupivacaine, and tetracaine are commonly used agents of differing durations; the block wears off naturally via drug uptake by the CSF, blood stream, or diffusion into fat. Epinephrine as an additive to the local anesthetic will significantly prolong the blockade.

Possible complications include hypotension, especially if the patient is not adequately prehydrated; high spinal block requires immediate airway management; and postdural puncture headache sometimes occurs. Spinal headache is related to the diameter and configuration of the spinal needle, and can be reduced to approximately 1 percent with the use of a small, 25- or 27-gauge needle.

Cauda equina syndrome is injury to the nerves emanating distal to the spinal cord resulting in bowel and bladder dysfunction, and lower-extremity sensory and motor loss. It has mainly been seen in cases in which indwelling spinal microcatheters and high (5 percent) concentrations of lidocaine were used. Indwelling spinal catheters are no longer used.

Epidural anesthesia. Epidural anesthesia also could be called extradural anesthesia, because local anesthetics are injected into the epidural space surrounding the dural sac of the spinal cord. Much greater volumes of anesthetic are required than with spinal anesthesia, and the onset of the block is longer—10–15 min. As in spinal anesthesia, local anesthetic bathes the spinal nerves as they exit the dura; the patient achieves analgesia from the sensory block, muscle relaxation from blockade of the motor nerves, and hypotension from blockade of the sympathetic nerves as they exit the spinal cord. Note that regional anesthesia, whether peripheral or central, provides only two of the three major components of anesthesia—analgesia and muscle relaxation. Anxiolysis, amnesia, or sedation must be attained by supplemental intravenous administration of other drugs (e.g., the benzodiazepines or propofol infusion).

Complications are similar to those of spinal anesthesia. Inadvertent injection of local anesthetic into a dural tear will result in a high block, manifesting as unconsciousness, severe hypotension, and respiratory paralysis requiring immediate aggressive hemodynamic management and control of the airway. Indwelling catheters often are placed through introducers into the epidural space, allowing an intermittent or continuous technique, as opposed to the single-shot method of spinal anesthesia. By necessity, the epidural-introducing needles are of a much larger diameter (17- or 18-gauge) than spinal needles, and accidental dural puncture more often results in a severe headache that may last up to 10 days if left untreated.

General Anesthesia

General anesthesia incorporates a triad of three major and separate effects: unconsciousness (and amnesia), analgesia, and muscle relaxation (see Table 45-1). Intravenous drugs usually produce a single, discrete effect, although most inhaled anesthetics produce elements of all three. General anesthesia is achieved with a combination of intravenous and inhaled drugs, each used to its maximum benefit. The science and art of anesthesia is a dynamic process: as stimuli to the patient change during surgery, the patient's vital signs are used as a guide and the quantity of drugs is adjusted, maintaining an equilibrium between stimulus and dose. General anesthesia is what patients commonly think of when they are to be "put under," and can be a cause of considerable preoperative anxiety.

Intravenous Agents

Unconsciousness and amnesia. The intravenous agents that produce unconsciousness and amnesia are frequently used for the induction of general anesthesia. They include barbiturates, benzodiazepines, propofol, etomidate, and ketamine. Except for ketamine, the following agents have no analgesic properties, nor do they cause paralysis or muscle relaxation.

Barbiturates. The most common barbiturates are thiopental, thiamylal, and methohexital. The mechanism of action is at the gamma-aminobutyric acid (GABA) receptor, where they inhibit excitatory synaptic transmission. They produce a rapid, smooth induction within 60s, and wear off in about 5 min.

Propofol. Propofol is an alkylated phenol that inhibits synaptic transmission through its effects at the GABA receptor. With a short duration, rapid recovery, and low incidence of nausea and vomiting, it has emerged as the agent of choice for ambulatory and minor general surgery. Additionally, propofol has bronchodilatory properties which make its use attractive in asthmatic patients and smokers. Propofol may cause hypotension, and should be used cautiously in patients with suspected hypovolemia and/or coronary artery disease (CAD), the latter of which may not tolerate a sudden drop in blood pressure. It can be used as a continuous infusion for sedation in the intensive care unit setting. Propofol is an irritant and frequently causes pain on injection.

Benzodiazepines. The most important uses of the benzodiazepines are for reduction of anxiety and to produce amnesia. Frequently used intravenous benzodiazepines are diazepam, lorazepam, and midazolam. They all inhibit synaptic transmission at the GABA receptor, but have differing durations of action. The benzodiazepines can produce peripheral vasodilatation and hypotension, and have minimal effects on respiration when used alone. They must be used with caution when given with opioids; a synergistic reaction causing respiratory depression is common. The benzodiazepines are excellent anticonvulsants, and only rarely cause allergic reactions.

Etomidate. Etomidate is an imidazole derivative used for intravenous induction. Its rapid and almost complete hydrolysis to inactive metabolites results in rapid awakening. Like the above intravenous agents, etomidate acts on the GABA receptor. It has little effect on cardiac output and heart rate, and induction doses usually produce less reduction in blood pressure than that seen with thiopental or propofol. Etomidate is associated with pain on injection and more nausea and vomiting than thiopental or propofol.

Ketamine. Ketamine differs from the above intravenous agents in that it produces analgesia and amnesia. Its principal action is on the N-methyl-d-aspartate (NMDA) receptor; it has no action on the GABA receptor. A dissociative anesthetic, it produces a cataleptic gaze and nystagmus. Patients may associate this with delirium and hallucinations while regaining consciousness; the addition of benzodiazepines has been shown to prevent these side effects. Ketamine can increase heart rate and blood pressure which may cause myocardial ischemia in patients with CAD. Ketamine is useful in acutely hypovolemic patients to maintain blood pressure via sympathetic stimulation, but is a direct myocardial depressant in patients who are catecholamine depleted. Ketamine is a bronchodilator, making it useful for asthmatic patients, and rarely is associated with allergic reactions.

Analgesia. The intravenous analgesics most frequently used in anesthesia today have little effect on consciousness, amnesia, or muscle relaxation. The most important class is the opioids, so called because they were first isolated from opium, with morphine, codeine, meperidine, hydromorphone, and the fentanyl family being the most common. The most important nonopioid analgesics are ketamine (discussed above) and ketorolac, an intravenous nonsteroidal antiinflammatory drug (NSAID).

Opioid analgesics. The commonly used opioids—morphine, codeine, oxymorphone, meperidine, and the fentanyl-based compounds—act centrally on μ-receptors in the brain and spinal cord. The main side effects of opioids are euphoria, sedation, constipation, and respiratory depression, which also are mediated by the same μ-receptors in a dose-dependent fashion. Although opioids have differing potencies required for effective analgesia, equianalgesic doses of opioids result in equal degrees of respiratory depression. Thus there is no completely safe opioid analgesic. The synthetic opioids fentanyl, and its analogs sufentanil, alfentanil, and remifentanil, are commonly used in the operating room. They differ pharmacokinetically in their lipid solubility, tissue binding, and elimination profiles, and therefore have differing potencies and durations of action. Remifentanil is remarkable in that it undergoes rapid hydrolysis that is unaffected by sex, age, weight, or renal or hepatic function, even after prolonged infusion. Recovery is within min, but there is little residual postoperative analgesia.

Naloxone and the longer-acting naltrexone are pure opioid antagonists. They can be used to reverse the side effects of opioid overdose (e.g., respiratory depression), but the analgesic effects of the opioid also will be reversed.

Nonopioid analgesics. Ketamine, an NMDA receptor antagonist, is a potent analgesic, but is one of the few intravenous agents that also causes significant sedation and amnesia. Unlike the μ-receptor agonists, ketamine stimulates respiration. It can be used in combination with opioids, but the dysphoric effects must be masked with the simultaneous use of sedatives, usually a benzodiazepine like midazolam.

Ketorolac is a parenteral NSAID that produces analgesia by reducing prostaglandin formation via inhibition of the enzyme cyclooxygenase (COX). Intraoperative use of ketorolac reduces postoperative need for opioids. Two forms of cyclooxygenase have been identified: COX-1 is responsible for the synthesis of several prostaglandins and prostacyclin (which protects gastric mucosa), and thromboxane, which supports platelet function. COX-2 is induced by inflammatory reactions to produce more prostaglandins. Ketorolac (and many oral NSAIDs, aspirin, and indomethacin) inhibits both COX-1 and COX-2, which causes the major side effects of gastric bleeding, platelet dysfunction, and hepatic and renal damage. Parecoxib is a parenteral COX-2 NSAID now being tested which would presumably produce analgesia and reduce inflammation with less gastrointestinal bleeding and platelet dysfunction.

Neuromuscular blocking agents. Neuromuscular blocking agents have no amnestic, hypnotic, or analgesic properties; patients must be properly anesthetized prior to and in addition to the administration of these agents. A paralyzed but unsedated patient will be aware, conscious, and in pain, yet be unable to communicate their predicament. Inappropriate administration of a neuromuscular blocking agent to an awake patient is one of the most traumatic experiences imaginable. Neuromuscular blockade is not a substitute for adequate anesthesia, but is rather an adjunct to the anesthetic. Depth of neuromuscular blockade is best monitored with a nerve stimulator to ensure patient immobility intraoperatively, and to confirm a lack of residual paralysis postoperatively.

Unlike the local anesthetics, which affect the ability of nerves to conduct impulses, the neuromuscular blockers have no effect on either nerves or muscles, but act primarily on the neuromuscular junction.

There is one commonly used depolarizing neuromuscular blocker—succinylcholine. This agent binds to acetylcholine receptors on the postjunctional membrane in the neuromuscular junction and causes depolarization of muscle fibers.

Although the rapid onset (< 60 s) and rapid offset (5–8 min) make succinylcholine ideal for management of the airway in certain situations, total body muscle fasciculations can cause postoperative aches and pains, an elevation in serum potassium levels, and an increase in intraocular and intragastric pressure. Its use in patients with burns or traumatic tissue injuries may result in a high enough rise in serum potassium levels to produce arrhythmias and cardiac arrest. Unlike other neuromuscular blocking agents, the effects of succinylcholine cannot be reversed. Succinylcholine is rapidly hydrolyzed by plasma cholinesterase, also referred to as pseudocholinesterase. Some patients have a genetic disorder manifesting as atypical plasma cholinesterase; the atypical enzyme has less-than-normal activity, and/or the patient has extremely low levels of the enzyme. The incidence of the homozygous form is approximately one in 3000; the effects of a single dose of succinylcholine may last several h instead of several min. Treatment is to keep the patient sedated and unaware he or she is paralyzed, continue mechanical ventilation, test the return of motor function with a peripheral nerve stimulator, and extubate the patient only after he or she has fully regained motor strength.

Two separate blood tests must be drawn: pseudocholinesterase level to determine the amount of enzyme present, and dibucaine number, which indicates the quality of the enzyme. Patients with laboratory-confirmed abnormal pseudocholinesterase levels and/or dibucaine numbers should be counseled to avoid succinylcholine (and mivacurium, which also is hydrolyzed by pseudocholinesterase). First-degree family members should also be tested. Succinylcholine is the only intravenous triggering agent of malignant hyperthermia (discussed below).

There are several competitive nondepolarizing agents available for clinical use. The longest-acting is pancuronium, which is excreted almost completely unchanged by the kidney. Intermediate-duration neuromuscular blockers include vecuronium and rocuronium, which are metabolized by both the kidneys and liver, and atracurium and cis-atracurium, which undergo breakdown in plasma known as Hofmann elimination. The agent with shortest duration is mivacurium, the only nondepolarizer that is metabolized by plasma cholinesterase, and like succinylcholine, is subject to the same prolonged blockade in patients with plasma cholinesterase deficiency. All nondepolarizers reversibly bind to the postsynaptic terminal in the neuromuscular junction and prevent acetylcholine from depolarizing the muscle. Muscle blockade occurs without fasciculation and without the subsequent side effects seen with succinylcholine. Table 45-2 lists the most commonly used agents of this type and their advantages and disadvantages.

The reversal of neuromuscular blockade is not a true reversal of the drug, as with protamine reversal of heparinized patients. Neuromuscular blocking reversal agents, usually neostigmine, edrophonium, or pyridostigmine, increase acetylcholine levels by inhibiting acetylcholinesterase, the enzyme that breaks down acetylcholine. The subsequently increased circulating levels of acetylcholine prevail in the competition for the postsynaptic receptor, and motor function returns. Use of the peripheral nerve stimulator is required to follow depth and reversal of motor blockade, but it is essential to correlate data from the nerve stimulator with clinical signs that indicate return of motor function, including tidal volume, vital capacity, hand grip, and 5-s sustained head lift.

TABLE 45-2 Advantages and Disadvantages to Common Nondepolarizing Neuromuscular Blocking Agents

Agent	Duration	Advantages	Disadvantages
Pancuronium	>1 h	No histamine release	Tachycardia; slow onset; long duration
Vecuronium	<1 h	No cardiovascular effects	Intermediate onset
Rocuronium	<1 h	Fast onset; no cardiovascular effects	
Mivacurium	<1 h	Fast onset; short duration	Histamine release

Source: Adapted with permission from Rutter TW, Tremper KK: Anesthesiology and pain management, in Petroni KC, Green R (eds). *Surgery: Scientific Principles and Practice,* 5th ed. Philadelphia: Lippincott & Williams, 1995, p 452.

Inhalational Agents

Unlike the intravenous agents, the inhalational agents provide all three characteristics of general anesthesia: unconsciousness, analgesia, and muscle relaxation. It would be impractical to use an inhalation-only technique in larger surgical procedures, because the dose required would cause unacceptable side effects, so intravenous adjuncts such as opioid analgesics and neuromuscular blockers are added to optimize the anesthetic. All inhaled anesthetics display a dose-dependent reduction in mean arterial blood pressure except for nitrous oxide, which maintains or slightly raises the blood pressure. Nitrous oxide, although not potent enough to use alone, provides partial anesthesia and allows a second potent agent to be used in smaller doses.

Minimum alveolar concentration (MAC) is a measure of anesthetic potency. It is the ED50 of an inhaled patient (i.e., the dose required to block a response to a painful stimulus in 50 percent of subjects). The higher the MAC, the less potent an agent is. The potency and speed of induction of inhaled agents correlates with their lipid solubility and is known as the Meyer-Overton rule. Nitrous oxide has a low solubility and is a weak anesthetic agent, but has the most rapid onset and offset. The "potent" gases (e.g., desflurane, sevoflurane, isoflurane, enflurane and halothane) are more soluble in blood then nitrous oxide and can be given in lower concentrations, but have longer induction and emergence characteristics.

Sevoflurane and desflurane are the two most recently introduced inhalational agents in common use. Because of their relatively lower tissue and blood solubility, induction and recovery are more rapid than with isoflurane or enflurane.

All of the potent inhalational agents (e.g., halothane, isoflurane, enflurane, sevoflurane, and desflurane), and the depolarizing agent succinylcholine, are triggering agents for malignant hyperthermia.

ANESTHETIC MANAGEMENT

Preoperative Evaluation and Preparation

The preoperative visit results in a summary of all pertinent medical findings, including a detailed history, current drug therapy, complete physical examination, and laboratory and specific testing results. Based on these findings, the anesthesiologist may find that the patient is not in optimal medical condition to undergo elective surgery. These findings and opinions are then discussed with the patient's primary physician and the surgery may be delayed or canceled until the patient's medical condition is further tested and optimized.

The detailed medical history obtained at the preoperative visit should include the patient's previous exposure and experience with anesthesia, and any family history of problems with anesthesia. History of atopy (medication, foods, or environmental) is an important aspect of this evaluation in that it may predispose patients to form antibodies against antigens that may be represented by agents administered during the perioperative period. A careful review of major organ systems and their function also should be performed.

The physical examination is targeted primarily at the central nervous system, cardiovascular system, lungs, and upper airway.

Concurrent medications that produce desired effects (i.e., β blockade, antihypertensive, and asthma medications) should be continued throughout the perioperative period; patients should be counseled to continue these medications up to and including the morning of surgery.

Preoperative laboratory data and specific testing for elective surgery should be patient- and situation-specific. For example, serum potassium if the patient is on diuretics, glucose in a diabetic patient, or hemoglobin concentration if the planned surgery has a high risk of blood loss. Coagulation tests are not necessary if the patient is not receiving anticoagulants or has no history, signs or symptoms of abnormal clotting. Otherwise healthy patients usually do not need preoperative laboratory testing, and tests performed within the previous 6 months usually are sufficient. Other tests that should be generated by history and physical exam include chest radiograph if there is evidence of chest disease, and pulmonary function tests in patients who are morbidly obese, severe asthmatics, or patients undergoing pulmonary resection surgery. An electrocardiogram (ECG) should be performed in all symptomatic patients, and in asymptomatic men age 45 years or older and asymptomatic women age 50 years or older. Urine pregnancy testing is recommended on the day of surgery in all menstruating females.

Risk Assessment

An integral part of the preoperative visit is for the anesthesiologist to assess patient risk. Risk assessment encompasses two major questions: (1) Is the patient in optimal medical condition for surgery? and (2) Are the anticipated benefits of surgery greater than the surgical and anesthetic risks associated with the procedure?

Originally designed as a simple classification of a patient's physical status immediately prior to surgery, the ASA physical status scale is one of the few prospective scales that correlate with the risk of anesthesia and surgery (Table 45-3).

Criticism of the ASA scale is primarily because of its exclusion of age and difficulty of intubation (discussed later in this chapter); the ASA scale remains useful and should be applied to all patients during the preoperative visit.

Evaluation of the Airway

The airway examination is employed to identify those patients in whom management of the airway and conventional endotracheal intubation may be difficult. It is vitally important to recognize such patients before administering medications that induce apnea.

Mallampati Classification

The amount of the posterior pharynx one can visualize preoperatively is important and correlates with the difficulty of intubation. A large tongue (relative to the size of the mouth) that also interferes with visualization of the larynx on laryngoscopy will obscure visualization of the pharynx. The Mallampati

TABLE 45-3 ASA Physical Status Classification System

P1	A normal healthy patient
P2	A patient with mild systemic disease
P3	A patient with severe systemic disease
P4	A patient with severe systemic disease that is a constant threat to life
P5	A moribund patient who is not expected to survive without the operation
P6	A declared brain-dead patient whose organs are being removed for donor purposes

classification is based on the structures visualized with maximal mouth opening and tongue protrusion in the sitting position.

Other predictors of difficult intubation include obesity, immobility of the neck, interincisor distance less than 4 cm in an adult, a large overbite, or the inability to shift the lower incisors in front of the upper incisors. The thyromental distance (i.e., the distance from the thyroid cartilage to the mentum [tip of the chin]) should be greater than 6.5–7 cm.

Consideration of Patients with Comorbidities

A thorough knowledge of the pathophysiology of concurrent medical conditions regardless of the reason for surgery is essential for optimal perioperative care. Optimal anesthesia extends beyond pharmacology and technical procedures. Specifically, ischemic heart disease, renal dysfunction, pulmonary disease, metabolic and endocrine disorders, central nervous system diseases, and diseases of the liver and biliary tract can have major impact on the management of anesthesia.

Ischemic Heart Disease

Ischemic heart disease is the result of the heart demanding more oxygen than its supply can provide. In the vast majority of cases, this is because of a reduction in the luminal area of coronary arteries secondary to atherosclerosis.

An estimated 14 million people in the United States have ischemic heart disease. Of these, as many as 4 million have few or no symptoms and are unaware that they are at risk for angina pectoris, myocardial infarction, or sudden death.

An important goal of the preoperative visit is for the anesthesiologist to ascertain the severity, functional limitations and possibility of previously undiagnosed ischemic heart disease. The risk of perioperative death because of myocardial infarction in patients without ischemic heart disease is approximately 1 percent. In contrast, the risk in patients with known or suspected ischemic heart disease is approximately 3 percent, and in patients undergoing surgery for peripheral vascular disease, the combined risk of death because of cardiac causes is 29 percent.

Major Risk Factors for Coronary Artery Disease

The risk of hypercholesterolemia is proportional to the increased serum level of low-density lipoprotein (LDL) cholesterol. Reduction achieved via decreased dietary fat or pharmacotherapy reduces risk.

Hyperlipidemia may be familial, and thus may account for the fact that a strong family history of premature CAD is a significant risk factor. High-density lipoprotein (HDL) cholesterol is protective.

Although definitely a risk factor, hypertension alone probably does not cause plaques. Rather, it may act synergistically with hypercholesterolemia by first causing mechanical wall stress and damage.

Smoking causes endothelial damage and therefore promotes plaque thrombosis. Cessation greatly reduces the risk of CAD.

Diabetes mellitus is a strong independent risk factor. A hypothesis is that glycosylation products cause release of growth factors that stimulate smooth muscle proliferation and blockage of coronary arteries.

Other risk factors. Hyperhomocysteinemia is becoming an established independent risk factor, but is still under evaluation. Reduction of levels by folate therapy may be beneficial.

Advanced age, male sex, obesity, and a sedentary lifestyle also can put a person at risk for developing ischemic heart disease.

Drugs used for the medical management of patients with ischemic heart disease and hypertension should be continued throughout the perioperative period.

Intraoperative anesthetic technique allows for the prompt control of hemodynamic variables; the maintenance of the balance between myocardial oxygen delivery and myocardial oxygen demand is probably the single most important factor in managing patients with ischemic heart disease. In patients with impaired left ventricular function, continued myocardial depression with volatile anesthetics may not be tolerated; the addition of short-acting opioids (e.g., fentanyl) is beneficial. In cardiac surgical patients, it is not uncommon for high-dose opioids to be used as the predominant anesthetic.

Pulmonary Disease

Chronic pulmonary disease has developed into a worldwide public health problem. Chronic obstructive pulmonary disease (COPD) is distinguished from asthma in that it is not reversible; it is a progressive disease that leads to the destruction of the lung parenchyma.

Infection, noxious particles, and gases can exacerbate COPD, but no specific parameters of lung function are predictive of postoperative lung complications. The highest predictive parameter found was upper abdominal surgery and thoracic surgery.

General anesthesia can be performed safely in patients with pulmonary disease; inhaled anesthetics often are used because of their bronchodilating properties.

Regional and local anesthesia has the benefit of avoiding tracheal irritation and stimulating bronchospasm. However, patients with COPD may become hypoxic while lying strictly supine, and sensory levels of anesthetic above T10 are associated with the impairment of respiratory muscle activity necessary for patients with COPD to maintain adequate ventilation.

Intraoperatively, mechanical ventilation using a slow breathing rate (8 breaths per min) should be used to allow for passive exhalation in the presence of increased airway resistance. This slow breathing, facilitated by high inspiratory flow rate, may allow for improved maintenance of normal Pao_2 and $Paco_2$ levels. Patients should also be well hydrated during the procedure with adequate crystalloid/colloid volume therapy, which may allow for less viscous pulmonary secretions following surgery.

Renal Disease

Five percent of the adult population may have preexisting renal disease that could contribute to perioperative morbidity. Additionally, the risk of acute renal failure is increased by certain events or patient characteristics independent of preexisting renal disease, such as hypovolemia and obstructive vascular disease. Ischemic tubular damage (i.e., acute tubular necrosis) is the most likely cause of acute renal failure in the perioperative period, reflecting events that cause an imbalance of oxygen supply to oxygen demand in the medullary ascending tubular cells.

Virtually all anesthetic drugs and techniques are associated with decreases in renal blood flow, the glomerular filtration rate, and urine output, reflecting multiple mechanisms such as decreased cardiac output, altered autonomic nervous system activity, neuroendocrine changes, and positive pressure ventilation. Renal blood flow (15–25 percent of the cardiac output) far exceeds renal oxygen needs, but ensures optimal clearance of wastes and drugs. Prehydration and the depth of anesthesia may influence the renal response to anesthesia.

Management of anesthesia in patients with chronic renal disease requires attention to intraoperative fluid management and tight control of ventilation, as respiratory alkalosis will shift the oxyhemoglobin dissociation curve, and respiratory acidosis could raise serum potassium to dangerous levels. Because of decreased excretion by the kidney, doses of opioids and neuromuscular blocking agents must be attenuated.

Hepatobiliary Disease

Data from the 1970s suggested that approximately 1 in every 700 adult patients who are scheduled for elective surgical procedures has unknown liver disease or is in the prodromal phase of viral hepatitis. Severe hepatic necrosis following surgery and anesthesia most often is because of decreased hepatic oxygen delivery rather than the anesthetic.

Regional anesthesia may be useful in patients with advanced liver disease, assuming coagulation status is acceptable. When general anesthesia is selected, administration of modest doses of volatile anesthetics with or without nitrous oxide or fentanyl often is recommended. Selection of nondepolarizing muscle relaxants should consider clearance mechanisms for these drugs. For example, patients with hepatic cirrhosis may be hypersensitive to mivacurium because of the lowered plasma cholinesterase activity. Perfusion to the liver is maintained by administering fluids (guided by filling pressures) and maintaining adequate systemic pressure and cardiac output.

The coexisting presence of liver disease may influence the selection of volatile anesthetics. Halothane is the anesthetic most studied regarding possible hepatotoxicity. Halothane hepatitis occurs rarely (approximately 1:25,000 patients) and may have an immune-mediated mechanism stimulated by repeated exposures to halothane. Halothane, enflurane, isoflurane, and desflurane all yield a reactive oxidative trifluoroacetyl halide and may be cross-reactive, but the magnitude of metabolism of the volatile anesthetics is a probable factor in the ability to cause hepatitis. Halothane is metabolized 20 percent, enflurane 2 percent, isoflurane 0.2 percent, and desflurane 0.02 percent; desflurane probably has the least potential for liver injury. Sevoflurane does not yield any trifluoroacetylated metabolites and is unlikely to cause hepatitis.

An estimated 15–20 million adults in the United States have biliary tract disease. Treatment of gallbladder disease by open or laparoscopic cholecystectomy most often is performed with general anesthesia supplemented with muscle relaxants. Complete biliary tract obstruction could interfere with the clearance of some muscle relaxants dependent on liver metabolism, such as vecuronium and pancuronium. Anesthetic considerations for laparoscopic cholecystectomy are similar to those for other laparoscopic procedures. Insufflation of the abdominal cavity with carbon dioxide results in increased intraabdominal pressure that may interfere with the ease of ventilation and venous return. During laparoscopic cholecystectomy, placement of the patient in the reverse

Trendelenburg position favors movement of abdominal contents away from the operative site and may improve ventilation. However, this position may further interfere with venous return and reduce cardiac output, emphasizing the need to maintain intravascular fluid volume. Mechanical ventilation of the lungs is recommended to ensure adequate ventilation in the presence of increased intraabdominal pressure and to offset the effects of systemic absorption of carbon dioxide used during insufflation of the abdominal cavity. High intraabdominal pressure may increase the risk of passive reflux of gastric contents. Tracheal intubation with a cuffed tube is advised to minimize the risk of pulmonary aspiration.

Metabolic and Endocrine Disease

Metabolic and endocrine disorders encompass a wide range of diseases. These diseases may be the primary reason for surgery or can exist in patients requiring surgery for other unrelated disorders. Preoperative evaluation of endocrine function consists of relevant medical history, glucose or protein in the urine, vital signs, history of fluctuations in body weight, survey of sexual function, and concomitant medications. The three metabolic and endocrine conditions that are most prevalent in patients undergoing surgery are diabetes mellitus, hypothyroidism, and obesity. The prevalence of all three conditions, either alone or in combination, in the general population has been steadily rising throughout the world for the past 20–30 years.

Patients with diabetes are at an increased risk for perioperative myocardial ischemia, stroke, renal dysfunction or failure, and increased mortality. Increased wound infections and impairment of wound healing also is associated with the preexistence of diabetes in patients undergoing surgery.

The stress response to surgery is associated with hyperglycemia in nondiabetic patients because of increased secretion of catabolic hormones, and a combination of reduced insulin secretion and increased insulin resistance. Improved glycemic control in diabetic patients undergoing major surgery has been shown to improve perioperative morbidity and mortality; avoidance of hypoglycemia and hyperglycemic events is the standard of care in these patients.

Anesthetic techniques in the diabetic patient can modulate the secretion of catabolic hormones. There is no evidence that regional anesthesia or general anesthesia, either alone or in combination, offers any benefit to the diabetic surgical patient in terms of morbidity or mortality.

Hypothyroidism is a deficiency in the secretion of the thyroid hormones, thyroxine (T4) and triiodothyronine (T3), by the thyroid gland. Over 5 million Americans have this common medical condition, and as many as 10 percent of women may have some degree of thyroid hormone deficiency. Controlled clinical trials have not shown an increase in risk when patients with mild to moderate hypothyroidism undergo surgery. Nevertheless, close monitoring of these patients for adverse effects of anesthesia including delayed gastric emptying, adrenal insufficiency, and hypovolemia, is warranted.

The prevalence of significant obesity continues to rise both in developed and developing countries, and is associated with an increased incidence of a wide spectrum of medical and surgical pathologies. In the United States, one third of people have a body weight more than 20 percent above their ideal weight. Body mass index (BMI) is calculated by dividing the weight in kilograms by the square of the height in meters. In the United States, the prevalence of a

BMI greater than 25 kg/m^2 is 59.4 percent for men, 50.7 percent for women, and 54.9 percent for adults overall. Patients with a BMI greater than 28 have increased perioperative morbidity over the general population.

Anesthetic management of the obese patient is problematic, and tasks such as establishing intravenous access, applying monitoring equipment, managing the airway, and transporting the patient are more difficult. Ventilation may be a particular problem because of obstructive sleep apnea or because obesity itself imposes a restrictive ventilatory state with decreased expiratory reserve and vital capacity. Induction of anesthesia is particularly challenging in the obese patient, as there is increased risk of pulmonary aspiration, and the increased mass of soft tissue about the head and neck make establishing and maintaining a patent airway difficult.

The impact of obesity on the pharmacokinetics of anesthetic drugs is variable. For example, blood volume often is increased in obese patients, which can decrease predicted concentrations of drugs, but adipose tissue has low blood flow, which could elevate blood concentrations of these agents. It is prudent to calculate the first dose of anesthetic based on ideal body weight, and base subsequent dosages on the patient's responsiveness.

Central Nervous System Disease

Diseases of the central nervous system (CNS) present unique situations for the anesthesiologist, and require an understanding of the relationship between intracranial pressure (ICP), cerebral blood flow (CBF), and cerebral metabolic rate of oxygen consumption (CMRO$_2$). Preoperative assessment of ICP is difficult, as symptoms of headache, nausea, and vomiting are nonspecific, and signs of retinal changes do not occur acutely. A midline shift on computed tomography (CT) scanning or magnetic resonance imaging (MRI) may indicate an expanding lesion in the brain.

Provision of anesthesia for intracranial procedures must balance hemodynamic factors such as fluid volume, mean arterial pressure (MAP), ICP, and CBF. For intracranial tumors, the mass effect of the tumor makes control of ICP and CBF critical. In intracranial aneurysm surgery, the goal of the anesthetic is to prevent sudden increases in systemic blood pressure that could rupture the aneurysm, especially during the stress of laryngoscopy and endotracheal intubation.

The relationship between MAP, ICP, and CBF is affected by pharmacologic agents. Inhalational agents in high concentrations (>0.6 MAC) cause dilation of the cerebral vasculature, decreasing cerebral vascular resistance. Cerebral blood flow is therefore increased in a dose-dependent fashion, despite decreases in CMRO$_2$.

Propofol decreases CBF, ICP, and CMRO$_2$. Propofol may also decrease systemic blood pressure, resulting in a decrease in cerebral perfusion pressure; however, propofol does not alter the autoregulation of CBF. Etomidate is a potent cerebral vasoconstrictor that reduces CBF and ICP, and should be used with caution in patients with epilepsy because of its excitatory effects seen on electroencephalograms.

Opioids decrease cerebral blood flow and may also decrease ICP under certain conditions. However, Sperry and associates have reported increases in ICP with the administration of fentanyl in head trauma patients. Additionally, opioids have a depressant effect on consciousness and ventilation that may increase ICP if accompanied by an increase in $Paco_2$; opioids should be used with caution in head trauma patients.

Regardless of the drugs or technique selected, maintenance of stable hemo-dynamics is optimal. Recovery from anesthesia should be smooth, avoiding pain, coughing, and straining, all of which can increase blood pressure and ICP, and cause bleeding at the surgical site.

Fluid therapy can increase cerebral edema and ICP when administered in large quantities, resulting in hypervolemia. Euvolemia should be the goal in head trauma patients, although hypervolemia may be beneficial for patients with intracranial aneurysms, to reduce vasospasm.

INTRAOPERATIVE MANAGEMENT

Induction of General Anesthesia

During induction of anesthesia, the patient becomes unconscious and rapidly apneic, myocardial function usually is depressed, and vascular tone abruptly changes. The induction of general anesthesia is the most critical component of practicing anesthesia, as the majority of catastrophic anesthetic complica-tions occur during this phase. There are several different techniques used for the induction of general anesthesia, each with significant advantages and dis-advantages. Each patient must be carefully evaluated during the preoperative period to ensure that the most efficacious and safe technique is used.

Intravenous induction, used primarily in adults, is smooth and is associ-ated with a high level of patient satisfaction. The addition of opioids will blunt the response of laryngoscopy and intubation to avoid hypertension and tachycardia.

In a patient with a full stomach, the standard induction technique may result in vomiting and pulmonary aspiration of stomach contents. The goal of rapid sequence induction is to achieve secure protection of the airway with a cuffed endotracheal tube while preventing vomiting and aspiration.

Rapid sequence induction is performed as follows:

1. Proceed only after evaluation of the airway predicts an uncomplicated intubation,
2. Preoxygenate the patient,
3. Rapidly introduce an intravenous induction agent, (e.g., propofol),
4. An assistant to the anesthesiologist presses firmly down on the cricoid cartilage to block any gastric contents from being regurgitated into the trachea, and
5. A muscle relaxant is injected and the trachea is quickly intubated. The assistant is instructed not to release pressure on the cricoid cartilage until the cuff of the endotracheal tube is inflated and the position of the tube is confirmed.

Patients undergoing inhalation induction progress through three stages: (1) awake, (2) excitement, and (3) surgical level of anesthesia. Adult patients are not good candidates for this type of induction, as the smell of the inhalation agent is unpleasant and the excitement stage can last for several min, which may cause hypertension, tachycardia, laryngospasm, vomiting, and aspiration. Children, however, progress through stage 2 quickly, and are highly motivated for inhalation induction as an alternative to the intravenous route. The benefit of postinduction intravenous cannulation is the avoidance of many presurgical anxieties, and inhalation induction is the most common technique for pediatric surgery.

Management of the Airway

After induction of anesthesia, the airway may be managed in several ways, including by face mask, with a laryngeal mask airway (LMA), or most definitively by endotracheal intubation with a cuffed endotracheal tube. Nasal and oral airways can help establish a patent airway in a patient being ventilated with a mask by creating an air passage behind the tongue.

The LMA is a cuffed oral airway that sits in the oropharynx. It is passed blindly and the cuff is inflated to push the soft tissues away from the laryngeal inlet. Because it does not pass through the vocal cords, it does not fully protect against aspiration. It should not be used in patients with a full stomach.

The accurate placement of an endotracheal tube requires skill, the proper equipment, and the proper conditions. Usually the patient is unconscious and immobile (including paralysis of the muscles of respiration). Intubation is typically performed under direct visualization by looking through the mouth with a laryngoscope directly at the vocal cords (direct laryngoscopy), and watching the endotracheal tube pass through the cords into the trachea. To obtain a direct line of sight, the patient is placed in the sniffing position. The neck is flexed at the lower cervical spine and extended at the atlanto-occipital joint. This flexion and extension is amplified during laryngoscopy. Laryngoscope handles contain batteries and can be fitted with curved (Macintosh) or straight (Miller) blades.

Some patients have physical characteristics or a history suggesting difficulty in placing an endotracheal tube. A short neck, limited neck mobility, small interincisor distance, short thyromental distance, and Mallampati class IV, may all represent a challenge to endotracheal intubation. Several devices have been developed to assist in management of the difficult airway. The Bullard rigid fiberoptic laryngoscope is a self-contained device that can be passed through a mouth with a narrow opening. The head and neck also can be kept in a neutral position, as a direct line of sight needed with a standard laryngoscope is not necessary.

The intubating laryngeal mask airway (ILMA) is an advanced form of laryngeal mask airway designed to maintain a patent airway and facilitate tracheal intubation with an endotracheal tube. The ILMA can be placed in anticipated or unexpectedly difficult airways as an airway rescue device and as a guide for intubating the trachea. An endotracheal tube can be passed blindly through the ILMA into the larynx, or the ILMA can be used as a conduit for a flexible fiberoptic scope.

The flexible fiberoptic intubation scope is the gold standard for difficult intubation. It is indicated in difficult or compromised airways in which neck extension is not desirable, or in cases with risk of dental damage. The scope is constructed of fiberoptic bundles and cables encased in a sheath. The cables permit manipulation of the tip of the scope by adjustments made at the operating end of the device. There is a port for suction and/or insufflation of oxygen. The scope gives excellent visualization of the airway with minimal hemodynamic stress when used properly. It can be used nasally or orally in an awake, spontaneously ventilating patient, whose airway has been treated with topical anesthetic. It requires skill for proper use, is expensive, and requires careful maintenance.

The ASA has developed algorithms for management of the difficult airway.

Fluid Therapy (See Chapter 2)

Transfusion of Red Blood Cells (See Chapter 3)

RECOVERY FROM ANESTHESIA

Reversal of Neuromuscular Blockade

The elimination of neuromuscular blocking agents from the body and subsequent resumption of neuromuscular transmission takes a considerable amount of time, therefore it has become routine to antagonize the neuromuscular block pharmacologically with the use of reversal agents. Reversal agents raise the concentration of the neurotransmitter acetylcholine to a higher level than that of the neuromuscular blocking agent. This is accomplished by the use of anticholinesterase agents, which reduce the breakdown of acetylcholine. The most commonly used agents are neostigmine, pyridostigmine, and edrophonium.

The common side effects of these three anticholinesterase agents are bradycardia, bronchial and intestinal smooth muscle contractions, and excessive secretions from salivary and bronchial glands. These effects are primarily mediated by effects on muscarinic receptors, which are effectively blocked by the concomitant use of antimuscarinic drugs such as atropine or glycopyrrolate. To ensure adequate ventilation postoperatively, it is important that the neuromuscular blocking agents are fully reversed, as assessed by monitoring twitch strength with a nerve stimulator and clinically correlating this with signs such as grip strength or 5-s head lift.

The Postanesthesia Care Unit

It is of primary importance that all patients awakening from anesthesia are followed in a recovery room, as approximately 10 percent of all anesthetic accidents occur in the recovery period. As more serious surgeries are performed on older and sicker patients, the number of patients requiring postoperative ventilation and medications to support their circulation increases with age. The new trend for postoperative pain control with continuous epidural administration of local anesthetics and narcotics demands close observation, because respiratory depression can occur. In most hospitals, the number of intensive care beds is too small to accommodate the increasing number of these patients. What originally began as the recovery room now must function as an intensive care unit setting for short stays. The name "recovery room" has been changed to "postanesthetic care unit" (PACU).

A variety of physiologic disorders that can affect different organ systems need to be diagnosed and treated in the PACU during emergence from anesthesia and surgery. Postoperative nausea and vomiting (PONV), airway support, and hypotension requiring pharmacologic support have been observed to be the most frequent complications in the PACU. However, abnormal bleeding, hypertension, dysrhythmia, myocardial infarction, and altered mental status are not uncommon.

Postoperative Nausea and Vomiting

Postoperative nausea and vomiting (PONV) typically occurs in 20–30 percent of surgical cases and generally is considered a transient, unpleasant event carrying little long-term morbidity; however, aspiration of emesis, gastric bleeding, and wound hematomas may occur with protracted or vigorous retching or vomiting. Troublesome PONV can prolong recovery room stay and hospitalization, and is one of the most common causes of hospital admission following ambulatory surgery. Prophylactic administration of antiemetics is not cost-effective in the surgical setting. Recent consensus guidelines using data from systematic reviews, randomized trials and studies, and data from logistic regression models recently have been published.

Agents usually administered for PONV are the serotonin receptor antagonists ondansetron, dolasetron, granisetron, and tropisetron. The safety and efficacy of the compounds when given at the end of surgery are virtually identical. Metoclopramide, when used in the standard dose of 10 mg, is ineffective for PONV. Although some studies have shown higher doses (20 mg) to have some effect on PONV, most evidence suggests that the serotonin receptor antagonists are the most efficacious choice.

Pain: The Fifth Vital Sign

Analgesic research methodology has been enhanced since the 1960s through the use of graduated and visual analog scales, tools that permit the standardization of pain scores. One frequently used graduated scale is a four-point measure of pain intensity (0 = no pain, 1 = mild pain, 2 = moderate pain, and 3 = severe pain) and a five-point measure of relief (0 = no relief, 1 = a little relief, 2 = some relief, 3 = a lot of relief, and 4 = complete relief).

Acute postoperative pain and its treatment (or prophylaxis) is a significant challenge for the health care professional. Despite the recent development of new nonnarcotic analgesics, and a better understanding of the side effects associated with pain medication of all types, acute postoperative pain remains a significant concern for patients, and represents an extremely negative experience for patients undergoing surgery. Many patients experience pain in the postoperative period despite the use of potent techniques such as patient-controlled analgesia, epidural analgesia, and regional anesthesia. The culture of acceptance of postoperative pain is changing. The American Pain Society has advocated the assessment of pain as the fifth vital sign, along with temperature, pulse, blood pressure, and respiratory rate. The four vital signs provide a quick snapshot of a patient's general condition, but pain management advocates claim the picture is not complete without including pain as the fifth vital sign. This approach may improve the efficacy of pain treatment.

MALIGNANT HYPERTHERMIA

Malignant hyperthermia (MH) is a life-threatening, acute disorder, developing during or after general anesthesia. The clinical incidence of malignant hyperthermia is about 1:12,000 in children and 1:40,000 in adults. A genetic predisposition and one or more triggering agents are necessary to evoke MH. Triggering agents include all volatile anesthetics (e.g., halothane, enflurane, isoflurane, sevoflurane, and desflurane), and the depolarizing muscle relaxant succinylcholine. Volatile anesthetics and/or succinylcholine cause a rise in the myoplasmic calcium concentration in susceptible patients, resulting in persistent muscle contraction. The classic MH crisis entails a hypermetabolic state, tachycardia, and the elevation of end-tidal CO_2 in the face of constant minute ventilation. Respiratory and metabolic acidosis and muscle rigidity follow, and rhabdomyolysis, arrhythmias, hyperkalemia, and sudden cardiac arrest. A rise in temperature is often a late sign of MH.

Treatment must be aggressive and begin as soon as a case of MH is suspected:

1. Call for help.
2. Stop all volatile anesthetics and give 100 percent oxygen.
3. Hyperventilate the patient up to three times the calculated minute volume.
4. Begin infusion of dantrolene sodium, 2.5 mg/kg IV. Repeat as necessary, titrating to clinical signs of MH. Continue dantrolene for at least 24 h after the episode begins.
5. Give bicarbonate to treat acidosis if dantrolene is ineffective.
6. Treat hyperkalemia with insulin, glucose, and calcium.
7. Avoid calcium channel blockers.
8. Continue to monitor core temperature.
9. Call the malignant hyperthermia hotline to report the case and get advice: 1-888-274-7899.

Suggested Readings

Stoelting RK, Miller RD: Basics of Anesthesia. Philadelphia: Churchill-Livingstone, 2000, p 436.

Stoelting RD, Dierdorf SF: Anesthesia and Co-Existing Disease, 4th ed. Philadelphia: Churchill Livingstone, 2003.

Butterworth JF IV: Local anesthetics and regional anesthesia, in Hemmings H, Hopkins PM (eds): Foundations of Anesthesia. London: Mosby, 2000, p 298.

Cullen DJ, Apolone G, Greenfield S, et al: ASA physical status and age predict morbidity after three surgical procedures. Ann Surg 220:3, 1994.

Zollinger AH, C Pasch T: Preoperative pulmonary evaluation: Facts and myths. Curr Opinion Anesthesiol 14:59, 2002.

Das UN: Insulin and the critically ill. Crit Care 6:262, 2002.

Adams JP, Murphy PG: Obesity in anaesthesia and intensive care. Br J Anaesth 85:91, 2000.

Practice guidelines for management of the difficult airway: An updated report by the American Society of Anesthesiologists Task Force on Management of the Difficult Airway. Anesthesiology 98:1269, 2003.

Gan TJ, Soppitt A, Maroof M, et al: Goal-directed intraoperative fluid administration reduces length of hospital stay after major surgery. Anesthesiology 97:820, 2002.

Gan TJ, Meyer T, Apfel CC, et al: Consensus guidelines for managing postoperative nausea and vomiting. Anesth Analg 97:62, 2003.

46 | ACGME Core Competencies

*Liz Nguyen, Mary L. Brandt, Samir S. Awad,
Ruth Bush, David H. Berger, and F. Charles Brunicardi*

Medicine has undergone several important changes over the last decade. Technologic and molecular advances have fundamentally changed the way diseases are treated. Access to the internet has changed the way both physicians and patients learn about diseases. Political and economic pressures have changed the way society views and reimburses medical care. The end result is that access to medical care, access to information about medical care and the very nature of the doctor-patient relationship have changed. These changes in medicine have resulted in a need for new approaches to medical education as well. The Accreditation Council for Graduate Medical Education (AGME) developed the core competencies as a way to articulate, and measure, the specific goals of medical education in the United States.

The core competencies offer an effective conceptual framework to train surgeons and are designed to ensure that surgical residents will learn the skills necessary to competently and compassionately treat patients as they enter practice. The six core competencies, as designated by the ACGME are: patient care, medical knowledge, practice-based learning and improvement, interpersonal and communication skills, professionalism, and systems-based practice. These are principles that should make up the basis of competent surgical practice in the 21st century. Articulating these competencies, and mandating documentation that they have been learned, should lead to greater and more universal compliance with these principles. Even though the ACGME has mandated that all residency programs must train their residents in the six core competencies there is enormous flexibility in how this is to be accomplished. Training surgical residents in the modern health care system is an especially challenging endeavor. Not only must educators impart the medical knowledge of caring for patients and new advances in patient care but they must also impart the technical skills necessary to perform complex surgical procedures. Furthermore, with the burgeoning field of genomics and molecular biology, the surgical trainee must become adept at understanding and applying the latest in molecular medicine. The challenge of the surgical educator is to develop innovative and focused learning techniques to accomplish all six core competency mandates within an 80-h work week.

CORE COMPETENCIES

The six core competencies include six specific areas that have been designated as critical for resident training. Each surgical training program should provide an environment that is conducive for training of these six core competencies and proper assessment of that training (Table 46-1). The areas of training include:

1. Patient care. Residents must be able to provide patient care that is compassionate, appropriate, and effective for the treatment of health problems and the promotion of health.

TABLE 46-1 Accreditation Council for Graduate Medical Education Core Competencies [ACGME].

Core competency	Description
Patient Care	To be able to provide compassionate and effective health care in the modern day health care environment.
Medical Knowledge	To effectively apply current medical knowledge in patient care and to be able to use medical tools (e.g., PubMed) to stay current in medical education.
Practice-Based Learning and Improvement	To critically assimilate and evaluate information in a systematic manner to improve patient care practices.
Interpersonnel/Communication Skills	To demonstrate sufficient communication skills that allow for efficient information exchange in physician-patient interactions and as a member of a health care team.
Professionalism	To demonstrate the principles of ethical behavior (e.g., informed consent, patient confidentiality) and integrity that promotes the highest level of medical care.
Systems-Based Practice	To acknowledge and understand that each individual practice is part of a larger health care delivery and to be able to use the system to support patient care.

   a. Communicate effectively and compassionately with patients and patient family members.

   b. Use the latest medical information to effectively formulate and implement a patient management plan.

   c. Competently interpret diagnostic information and perform all diagnostic or therapeutic procedures essential for patient care.

   d. Collaborate with other health care professionals to deliver excellent patient care.

2. Medical Knowledge. Residents must demonstrate knowledge about established and evolving biomedical, clinical, and cognate (e.g., epidemiological and social-behavioral) sciences and the application of this knowledge to patient care.

   a. Understand and apply the basic and clinical sciences that are necessary for practice in the appropriate discipline.

3. Practice-Based Learning and Improvement. Residents must be able to investigate and evaluate their patient care practices, appraise and assimilate scientific evidence, and improve their patient care practices.

   a. Systematically appraise and analyze one's clinical practice and practice-based outcomes. Apply this information for improvement in patient care.

   b. Understand the basics of statistical methodology and its application for the appraisal of clinical studies.

   c. Apply information technology tools for efficient management of patient information, support of clinical care, and patient education.

4. Interprofessional and Communication Skills. Residents must be able to demonstrate interpersonal and communication skills that result in effective

information exchange and teaming with patients, patient families, and professional associates.

  a. Develop the skills necessary to lead a medical team that may consist of consultants and allied health care professionals.
  b. Effectively elicit patient interaction and participation in their care through nonverbal communication skills.
  c. Create a skill set that will allow trainees to sustain a healthy patient-physician relationship based on trust and integrity.

5. Professionalism. Residents must demonstrate a commitment to carrying out professional responsibilities, adherence to ethical principles, and sensitivity to a diverse patient population.

  a. Demonstrate the principles that are inherent for practice as a physician such as integrity, respect, and a responsiveness to patient care and society that may supersede self-interest.
  b. Act responsibly with a commitment to excellent patient care.
  c. Understand and practice the ethical obligations for patient confidentiality, informed consent, and business practice.
  d. Awareness of a possible patient cultural difference and to be sensitive and respectful of these differences.

6. Systems-Based Practice. Residents must demonstrate an awareness of and responsiveness to the larger context and system of health care and the ability to effectively call on system resources to provide care that is of optimal value.

  a. Acknowledge the importance of understanding that each individual medical practice is a component of the entire health care system and that each individual practice impacts the overall delivery and access of health care.
  b. Practice cost-efficient health care so that resources may be properly allocated and health-care costs controlled.
  c. Advocate for the improvement in health care delivery, quality health care, and improvement of patient access.
  d. Develop a knowledge base of how to partner with health care organizations and health care providers to improve health care access, delivery, and cost-control.

Patient Care

Patient care is the foundation for the practice of clinical medicine and must be addressed early and continuously during residency. In the past, patient care was taught by an apprenticeship model, in other words, spending time with attending physicians on the wards or in the operating room. This model, which started with true "house officers" (i.e., residents that lived full-time in the hospital), is inherently inefficient. The unnecessary h spent between times of real learning are an experience the former generation will not forget and the current generation cannot afford. Training surgeons involves not only imparting sufficient knowledge, but, much like training pilots, also requires "hours" of practice, to ensure mastery of the technical skills needed to competently practice the art of surgery. With the 80-h work week, residents and educators must become more focused and efficient to provide adequate time to learn complex procedures and complex issues of patient care. The application of resident time motion studies may aid in properly allocating time to high-yield patient care. For example, optimal teaching occurs when residents participate in educationally appropriate operations with attending physicians that have a dedication to teaching. This ideal cannot always be met, but programs have to struggle with how to limit the time residents spend doing inherently simple problems and procedures to allow them to concentrate on more complex issues. Other methods of maximizing the resident educational experience include adding ancillary professionals (e.g., physician assistants or nurse practitioners) to help with the day-to-day simple necessities of patient care so that the surgical residents can spend more time on high-yield tasks. Other innovative educational philosophies and techniques also can be applied to surgical education to optimize resident training. For example, lessons learned in the training of pilots have direct applicability to the training of surgeons. The use of simulators, whether mechanical or "table simulators" (e.g., discussing the case before scrubbing) is one example of how these techniques can be applied to surgical training.

Medical Knowledge

The rapidly changing medical research environment also has created a responsibility among medical trainees to understand evolving research and its application to patient care. With this in mind, the ACGME has stated that "residents must demonstrate knowledge about established and evolving biomedical, clinical, and cognate (e.g., epidemiological and social-behavioral) sciences and the application of this knowledge to patient care." Surgery has undergone an exponential growth in new procedures and technologies. With this explosion in medical innovation, surgical training programs are posed with the daunting task of teaching new and complex skills to surgical trainees. From laparoscopic procedures to endovascular stenting, the evolving indications and techniques for each new surgical procedure must be continuously taught to the residents. Furthermore, the field of molecular biology and its application to surgical diseases has mandated that surgeons understand the basic molecular mechanisms of each disease. "Molecular surgery" has become a term that can describe the training of future surgeons and the knowledge base that surgeons will need to function in the 21st century medical field. The new era of molecular biology requires understanding the complex science that will lead to such innovations as molecular fingerprinting techniques to tailor treatments that are specific for each individual patient. Other, more cognitive tools such as the ability to critically review literature and logically apply the relevance of a study must also be imparted to residents so that they can correctly apply the latest medical studies to each individual patient.

The ability of a surgical program to adequately meet this educational challenge can be improved by using innovative learning techniques. Educational systems such as the SQR system of studying, the Pimsleur model and Rosetta Stone learning techniques are all tools that can aid in the understanding and application of a rapidly advancing surgical field. Finally, it must be conveyed to surgical trainees that surgery is a life-long learning process and the ability to continue building on one's medical knowledge is critical for a successful surgical career.

Practice-Based Learning and Improvement

The third ACGME mandate concerns the ability of the trainee to learn from real-life scenarios to improve their own performance and patient outcomes. The mandate states "residents must be able to investigate and evaluate their patient care practices, appraise and assimilate scientific evidence, and improve their patient care practices." The goal of this mandate is to teach the surgical trainee the ability to critically evaluate their practice patterns and outcomes in a systematic fashion. Currently, the simplest example of this mandate is the surgical morbidity and mortality conference. This conference allows for in-depth discussions on how to improve patient care and patient outcomes through review of weekly surgical cases. To further improve practice patterns the ACGME also has suggested that trainees should be trained on the use of information technology systems to manage patient information and support clinical care. As hospitals increasingly move toward computer-based patient information systems, surgical trainees must receive formal training on the use and application of these systems. One of the best examples of the use of information technology and computerized patient database systems is the Computerized Patient Record System (CPRS) that is employed by the Veterans Affairs (VA) Hospital System. This fully computerized patient database allows easy access to all patient clinical data, including lab tests, radiologic studies, physician notes, and appointment times. This central core information system has allowed the VA health system to develop the National Surgical Quality Improvement Program (NSQIP). Using information from CPRS, nurse reviewers are able to gather and input information into the NSQIP system. NSQIP has been the first prospective risk-adjusted outcome based program for comparing and improving surgical outcomes across multiple institutions. This program has revolutionized the reporting and quality control of surgical services within the VA system. With the VA system as an example of improvement in not only information technology management but also surgical outcomes monitoring, the surgical trainee will need to stay abreast of the changes in new information technology systems and its application to patient care.

Interprofessional and Communication Skills

Communication is essential to the successful and competent practice of medicine. Developing advanced communication skills not only improves patient-physician interaction but also improves interactions with physicians and other health-care professionals. To be an effective leader, which is necessary to achieve optimal patient care, surgical trainees must be taught to effectively communicate with patients, families, consultants and ancillary health care personnel. Formal leadership training has been shown to improve communication skills in surgical residents. After institution of a formal collaborative leadership training program, Awad and associates described a 12 percent increase in resident perceived communication skills. Other studies also have shown that formal physician leadership training improves communication and conflict resolution skills. The use of leadership training provides the tools necessary for successful team building. All of these components will allow the trainee to work effectively as a member or leader of a health care team.

Professionalism

The core competency of professionalism is expressed as follows: "residents must demonstrate a commitment to carrying out professional responsibilities, adherence to ethical principles, and sensitivity to a diverse patient population." The trainee should demonstrate respect, compassion, and integrity while involved in patient care. The adherence to the principles of patient confidentiality and informed consent also are involved in professionalism. Of all the core competencies, this one may be the most difficult to teach, and the one that relies the most on successful role models and mentors. However, with less time spent in the hospital, the ability to learn from real-life situations is decreased.

Therefore, these principles need to be creatively taught to the residents, either through didactic lectures or problem-based learning. As with communication, formal leadership training may be an effective method of teaching the basic principles of professionalism. In one study, residents increased their scores on the integrity section of an Internal Strength Scorecard Survey by 12 percent (p-value < 0.04) after completion of a formal leadership training program. Professionalism also can be taught with training in negotiating and problem-solving skills. Teaching residents how to navigate difficult situations can further promote an environment of integrity and mutual respect. Fisher and Ury have described five principles to successful conflict resolution: (1) maintain objectivity by not focusing on the participants but by focusing on the problem, (2) relinquish the position of power and inflexibility to focus more on individual interests, (3) create outcomes in which both parties will have gains, (4) make sure there are objective criteria for the negotiating process, and (5) maintain an open mind and dialogue, yielding to principles not pressure. These five principles can best be taught with role-playing and small group discussions and are essential skills for the surgical trainee. The role of the individual surgical educator in teaching professionalism cannot be overstated. The daily interaction of residents with their attending physicians is the single most important component of teaching professionalism. Therefore, it is the responsibility of each surgical educator to maintain the highest standards of integrity, for they are serving as role models for the next generation of surgeons.

Systems-Based Practice

With increasing health care costs and an aging population, surgical trainees need to recognize that they are part of a larger health care system which struggles to balance resources and principles. The ACGME has concluded it is important that "residents demonstrate an awareness of and responsiveness to the larger context and system of health care and the ability to effectively call on system resources to provide care that is of optimal value." In today's medical world, resources and finances are limited and each health care provider must understand that what they do impacts the greater health care system. Dimick and associates described a 1-year analysis of a private sector hospital participating in the private sector NSQIP program and showed that surgical complications significantly increased hospital costs. Major complications increased costs by almost $12,000 per admission. Their conclusion was that to successfully manage health care costs, private sector hospitals should model their outcomes analysis and surgical improvement programs after the VA NSQIP system. This initial feasibility analysis of using the VA NSQIP system in the private sector has already been performed and demonstrated that use of the NSQIP system can generate reasonable predictive models in non-VA hospital.

Further integration of the NSQIP program into mainstream private health care is continuing and is a major focus of the American College of Surgeons.

As health care costs have grown, so have health care management organizations. Learning how to interact with these organizations is crucial for the improvement of health care delivery and allocation of resources. Recent reports have demonstrated that surgeons feel deficient in the understanding of the public health and business aspect of surgery. These principles can be taught by individuals who have an expertise in health care delivery systems and overall health care management. If necessary, surgical departments could enlist these experts to concisely review the important components of the health care delivery system to surgical trainees. In the daily care of patients, costs and appropriate utilization of resources should be discussed as another way to teach this important principle.

Assessment of the Core Competencies

The ACGME has not only mandated the teaching of these six core competencies, but also has stated that residents must be evaluated to ensure they have acquired these skills. In the future, there is little doubt that these, or similar, core competencies will be used to assess practicing surgeons as well. Hence, the need to document the acquisition and maintenance of these competencies is important to all surgeons, not just those in training. Historically written medical examinations, such as the American Board of Surgery in Service Training Exam, have previously been the only measure of the educational success of a training program. However, this exam evaluates only two of the core competencies (i.e., medical knowledge and patient care). To accurately assess the other core competencies, different assessment tools need to be developed, and will vary from program to program. Small group and problem-based learning sessions are effective environments for faculty to assess the success of residents in learning the core competencies such as professionalism and communication. Sidhu and associates suggested that regular meetings with residents should be scheduled to allow frequent feedback of resident performance. Furthermore, clinical evaluations should incorporate rating systems for professionalism and interpersonal skills. If a resident is consistently rated as deficient in these categories, further counseling and training can be used to address the deficiencies.

CONCLUSION

The goal of the ACGME core competency mandate has been to ensure that patient care continues to improve into the 21st century. The goal of the modern surgical educator is to develop better means to ensure that the material is properly taught and, even more importantly, truly learned. This provides an exciting venue for introduction of new educational initiatives and development of innovative educational programs. These innovations should serve to move surgical education forward, allowing better training of the surgeons of the future.

Suggested Readings

ACGME. Accessed March 1, 2005, from http://www.acgme.org/outcome/comp/comp Full.asp. Accreditation Council for Graduate Medical Education.

Brunicardi FC, Chen C: Second molecular surgeon symposium on pancreatic cancer and other cancers: An introduction. World J Surg 30(10), 2005.

Brunicardi FC, Hobson FL. Time management: A review for physicians. J Natl Med Assoc 88(9):581–587, 1996.

Accessed December 20, 2004, from http://www.studygs.net. Study Guides and Strategies.

Accessed November 10, 2004, from http://en.wikipedia.org/wiki/Pimsleur_language_learning_system. Wikipedia, The Free Encyclopedia.

Accessed December 20, 2004, from http://www.rosettastone.com. Rosetta Stone© Language, Learning, Success.

Nguyen L, Brandt ML, Bush RC, Awad SS, et al: The role of learning theory and learning techniques for education of the modern day surgical resident. In Press.

Khuri SF, Daley J, Henderson W, et al: The Department of Veterans Affairs' NSQIP: The first national, validated, outcome-based, risk-adjusted, and peer-controlled program for the measurement and enhancement of the quality of surgical care. National VA Surgical Quality Improvement Program. Ann Surg 228(4):491-507, 1998.

Itani KM, Liscum K, Brunicardi FC: Physician leadership is a new mandate in surgical training. Am J Surg 187(3):328–31, 2004.

Schwartz RW: Physician leadership: a new imperative for surgical educators. Am J Surg 176:38–40, 1998.

Awad SS, Hayley B, Fagan SP, Berger DH, et al: The impact of a novel resident leadership training curriculum. Am J Surg 2004 188(5):481–484, 2004.

Schwartz RW, Pogge C: Physician leadership: essential skills in a changing environment. Am J Surg 180(3):187–192, 2000.

Fisher R, Ury W: Getting to Yes. New York: Publisher, pp 1–14, 1991.

Dimick JB, Chen SL, Taheri PA, Henderson WG, et al: Hospital costs associated with surgical complications: A report from the private-sector National Surgical Quality Improvement Program. J Am Coll Surg 199(4):531–537, 2004.

Fink AS, Campbell DA Jr, Mentzer RM Jr, Henderson WG, et al: The National Surgical Quality Improvement Program in non-veterans administration hospitals: initial demonstration of feasibility. Ann Surg 236(3):344–353, 2002.

Satiani B: Business knowledge in surgeons. Am J Surg 188(1):13–16, 2004.

Sidhu RS, Grober ED, Musselman LJ, Reznick RK: Assessing competency in surgery: where to begin? Surgery 135(1):6–20, 2004.

Index

Note: Numbers followed by *f* indicate figures; those followed by *t* indicate tables.